UNDERSTANDING ANESTHETIC EQUIPMENT AND PROCEDURES

A Practical Approach

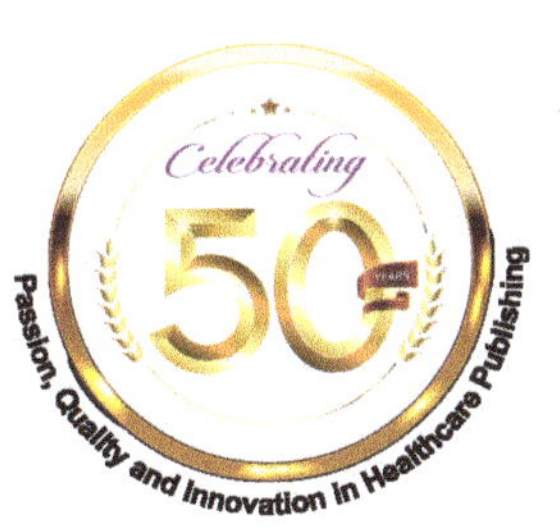

VIDEO CONTENTS*

**The videos are available on www.emedicine360.com.*

UNDERSTANDING ANESTHETIC EQUIPMENT AND PROCEDURES

A Practical Approach

(Revised and Updated with Section on Anesthetic Scenario in COVID-19 Pandemic)

Third Edition

Editors

Dwarkadas K Baheti MD
Consultant Pain Physician
Lilavati, Shushrusha, and Raheja Hospitals, Mumbai
Head of Pain Division
Department of Anesthesiology
Lilavati Hospital and Research Centre, Mumbai
Former Professor and Head
Department of Anesthesia and Pain Management
Bombay Hospital Institute of Medical Sciences
Mumbai, Maharashtra, India

Vandana V Laheri DA MD
Former Professor and Head
Department of Anesthesia
ESI PGIMSR and
Mahatma Gandhi Memorial Hospital
Mumbai
Former Professor
Department of Anesthesia
Lokmanya Tilak Municipal Medical College and
General Hospital
Mumbai, Maharashtra, India

Foreword

Dipankar Das Gupta

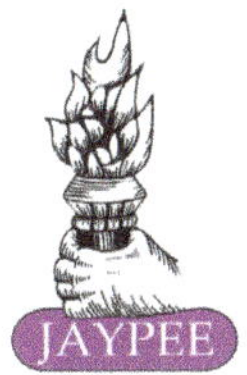

JAYPEE BROTHERS MEDICAL PUBLISHERS
The Health Sciences Publisher
New Delhi | London

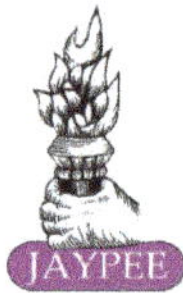

Jaypee Brothers Medical Publishers (P) Ltd.

Headquarters
Jaypee Brothers Medical Publishers (P) Ltd
EMCA House, 23/23-B
Ansari Road, Daryaganj
New Delhi 110 002, India
Landline: +91-11-23272143, +91-11-23272703
+91-11-23282021, +91-11-23245672
Email: jaypee@jaypeebrothers.com

Corporate Office
Jaypee Brothers Medical Publishers (P) Ltd
4838/24, Ansari Road, Daryaganj
New Delhi 110 002, India
Phone: +91-11-43574357
Fax: +91-11-43574314
Email: jaypee@jaypeebrothers.com

Overseas Office
JP Medical Ltd.
83, Victoria Street, London
SW1H 0HW (UK)
Phone: +44 20 3170 8910
Fax: +44 (0)20 3008 6180
E-mail: info@jpmedpub.com

Website: www.jaypeebrothers.com
Website: www.jaypeedigital.com

Understanding Anesthetic Equipment and Procedures: A Practical Approach

First Edition: 2015
Second Edition: 2018
Third Edition: 2022

ISBN: 978-93-5465-006-2

Dedicated to

All Doctors, Scientists, Engineers and Technicians who have made Anesthesiology what it is today as also to all the VALIANT COVID Warriors who are currently engaged in the control of this COVID-19 pandemic

CONTRIBUTORS

Anil Agarwal MD MNAMS
Professor
Department of Anesthesia
Sanjay Gandhi Postgraduate Institute of Medical Sciences
Lucknow, Uttar Pradesh, India

Masood Ahmed
MBBS MD (Anesthesia) DNB-SS (Critical Care Medicine)
Resident
Department of Critical Care Medicine
Apollo Hospital
Navi Mumbai, Maharashtra, India

Amruta A Ajgaonkar
MBBS DNB Post-doctoral Fellowship (ISNACC) in Neuroanesthesia
Consultant Anesthesiologist
Department of Anesthesiology
Fortis Hospital, Mulund
Mumbai, Maharashtra, India

Vasundhra R Atre
MD (Anesthesiology) MPhil HHSM (BITS, Pilani) DHA PGDMLS
Director Medical Operations
Medical Services and Operations Group
Fortis Healthcare
Bengaluru, Karnataka, India

Dwarkadas K Baheti MD
Consultant Pain Physician
Lilavati, Shushrusha, and Raheja Hospitals
Mumbai
Head of Pain Division
Department of Anesthesiology
Lilavati Hospital and Research Centre
Mumbai
Former Professor and Head
Department of Anesthesia and Pain Management
Bombay Hospital Institute of Medical Sciences
Mumbai, Maharashtra, India

Lipika A Baliarsing MD
Professor
Department of Anesthesia
Topiwala National Medical College and BYL Nair Hospital
Mumbai, Maharashtra, India

Vaibhavi Baxi DA FCPS DNB
Consultant Anesthetist
Department of Anesthesia
Lilavati Hospital and Research Centre
Mumbai, Maharashtra, India

Chinmaya P Bhave
MBBS DNB Post Doctoral Fellowship in Neuroanesthesia (NIMHANS)
Consultant Anesthesiologist
Department of Neuroanesthesia
Kokilaben Dhirubhai Ambani Hospital and Medical Research Institute
Mumbai, Maharashtra, India

Shashank A Budhakar MD FRCA
Consultant
Department of Anesthesia
Lilavati Hospital and Research Centre
Mumbai, Maharashtra, India

Aparna S Budhakar MD FRCA
Consultant
Department of Anesthesia
Jaslok Hospital
Mumbai, Maharashtra, India

Indrani Hemantkumar Chincholi
MBBS DA MD DNB
Professor and Head
Department of Anesthesiology, Pain Medicine and Critical Care
Seth GS Medical College and KEM Hospital
Mumbai, Maharashtra, India

Naina P Dalvi MD DNB MNAMS FCPS DA
Additional Professor
Department of Anesthesia
HBT Medical College and
Dr RN Cooper Municipal General Hospital
Mumbai, Maharashtra, India

Nandini M Dave
MD DNB MNAMS PGDHHM PGDMLS
Senior Consultant
Department of Anesthesia
NH SRCC Children's Hospital
Mumbai, Maharashtra, India

Madhavi D Desai DA DNB
Associate Professor
Department of Anesthesia, Critical Care, and Pain
Tata Memorial Centre
Mumbai, Maharashtra, India

Charulata M Deshpande MD DA
Professor
Department of Anesthesia
Topiwala National Medical College and BYL Nair Hospital
Mumbai, Maharashtra, India

Vasumathi M Divekar BSc DA MD MNAMS
Emeritus Professor
Department of Anesthesia
PDY Patil Medical College
Mumbai, Maharashtra, India

Jeson R Doctor MD DNB
Assistant Professor
Department of Anesthesia, Critical Care, and Pain
Tata Memorial Hospital
Mumbai, Maharashtra, India

Sarita Fernandes MD
Additional Professor
Department of Anesthesia
Topiwala National Medical College and BYL Nair Hospital
Mumbai, Maharashtra, India

Rajashree U Gandhe MD
Consultant Neuroanesthesiologist
Department of Neuroanesthesia
Kokilaben Dhirubhai Ambani Hospital and Medical Research Institute
Mumbai, Maharashtra, India

Sujeet KS Gautam MD FIPP
Assistant Professor
Department of Anesthesia
Sanjay Gandhi Postgraduate Institute of Medical Sciences
Lucknow, Uttar Pradesh, India

Raghbirsingh P Gehdoo
DA MD (Anesthesia) FICA FIAPM
Professor and Head
Department of Anesthesiology
Dr DY Patil Medical College, Nerul
Navi Mumbai, Maharashtra, India

Sunil Gvalani MBBS DA DNB
Professor and Head
Department of Anesthesia
HBT Medical College and
Dr RN Cooper Municipal General Hospital
Mumbai, Maharashtra, India

Sarika Ingle MD
Associate Professor
Department of Anesthesia
Topiwala National Medical College and
BYL Nair Hospital
Mumbai, Maharashtra, India

Dinesh K Jagannathan
MBBS DA DABA Fellowship in Obstetric Anesthesiology
Consultant Anesthesiologist
Department of Anesthesiology
Fortis Malar Hospital
Chennai, Tamil Nadu, India

Azra Z Kakroo MBBS
Resident in Anesthesiology
Department of Anesthesiology
Dr DY Patil Medical College, Nerul
Navi Mumbai, Maharashtra, India

Neeta V Karmarkar
MBBS DA DNB Post-doctoral Fellowship (ISNACC) in Neuroanesthesiology
Head Neuroanesthesia
Kokilaben Dhirubhai Ambani Hospital
and Medical Research Institute
Mumbai, Maharashtra, India

Pallavi Kharat
DA DNB (Anesthesia) IDCCM
Assistant Professor
Department of Anesthesia
HBT Medical College and
Dr RN Cooper Municipal General Hospital
Mumbai, Maharashtra, India

Bhavani S Kodali MD
Vice Chairman (Clinical Affairs)
Department of Anesthesiology
Brigham and Women's Hospital
Boston, MA, USA
Associate Professor
Department of Anesthesiology
Harvard Medical School
Westwood, MA, USA

Pradnya C Kulkarni
MD DA DAFRCA
Professor and Head
Department of Anesthesia
Bombay Hospital and Medical Research Centre
Mumbai, Maharashtra, India

Satish K Kulkarni MD FRCA
Consultant
Department of Anesthesia
Lilavati Hospital and Research Centre
Mumbai, Maharashtra, India

Samhita Kulkarni DNB
Consultant Cardiologist
Department of Cardiology
Dr DY Patil Hospital
Navi Mumbai, Maharashtra, India

Vandana V Laheri DA MD
Former Professor and Head
Department of Anesthesia
ESI PGIMSR and Mahatma Gandhi
Memorial Hospital, Mumbai
Former Professor
Department of Anesthesia
Lokmanya Tilak Municipal Medical
College and General Hospital
Mumbai, Maharashtra, India

Harprit Kaur Madan
MBBS DA DNB FCCM PGDHHM
Associate Professor
Department of Anesthesia
HBT Medical College and
Dr RN Cooper Municipal General Hospital
Mumbai, Maharashtra, India

Anila D Malde MD DA
Professor and Head
Department of Anesthesiology
Lokmanya Tilak Municipal Medical
College and General Hospital, Sion
Mumbai, Maharashtra, India

Aaliya Mehmood MBBS DA
Senior Resident
Department of Anesthesiology and
Pain Management
Lilavati Hospital and Research Centre
Mumbai, Maharashtra, India

Preeti G More MD FPCI
Professor
Department of Anesthesiology
KJ Somaiya Medical College and Hospital
Mumbai, Maharashtra, India

Manjari S Muzoomdar MD DA
Consultant Anesthesiologist
Department of Anesthesia
Breach Candy, Saifee, and Dalvi Hospitals
Mumbai, Maharashtra, India

Sheila N Myatra MD FICCM
Professor
Department of Anesthesia, Critical Care,
and Pain
Tata Memorial Hospital
Mumbai, Maharashtra, India

Prashant S Naphade MD DNB
Radiologist
Department of Radiology, ESIS Hospital
Mumbai, Maharashtra, India

Aparna A Nerurkar MD DNB
Additional Professor
Department of Anesthesia
Lokmanya Tilak Municipal Medical
College and General Hospital
Mumbai, Maharashtra, India

Balkrishna D Nimavat
MBBS MD DNB (Anesthesia) IDCCM FNB (Critical Care) EDIC EDAIC
Consultant Critical Care
Department of Critical Care
Sir HN Reliance Hospital
Mumbai, Maharashtra, India

Gunadhar Padhi
MBBS MD DICM FCCCPM IDIE (Paris)
FIMSA (Critical Care Medicine)
Consultant Intensivist
Department of Critical Care Medicine
Apollo Hospital
Navi Mumbai, Maharashtra, India

Amit Padvi
MD Fellowship in Pediatric Anesthesia (MUHS)
Assistant Professor
Department of Anesthesia
Seth GS Medical College and KEM Hospital
Mumbai, Maharashtra, India

Preeti A Padwal
DNB Anesthesia and Critical Care
Fellowship Paediatric Anesthesia
Freelance Practitioner Anesthesiologist
Mumbai, Pune, Maharashtra, India

Ameya Panchwagh MD
Consultant Anesthetist
Department of Anesthesia
Global Hospital
Mumbai, Maharashtra, India

Anil Parakh MD
Consultant Anesthesiologist
Department of Anesthesia
Global Hospital
Mumbai, Maharashtra, India

Devangi A Parikh MD DNB
Associate Professor
Department of Anesthesia
Lokmanya Tilak Municipal Medical
College and General Hospital
Mumbai, Maharashtra, India

Vijaya P Patil
MD Diploma in Hospital Administration
Professor
Department of Anesthesia, Critical Care,
and Pain
Tata Memorial Hospital
Mumbai, Maharashtra, India

Ajit C Pillai MD
Consultant Anesthesiologist
Department of Anesthesia
Wockhardt Hospital
Mumbai, Maharashtra, India

Anjali A Pingle
MBBS DA DNB FRCA
Consultant Anesthesiologist
Department of Anesthesia
PD Hinduja Hospital and Research Centre
Mumbai, Maharashtra, India

Abhijit A Raut MD
Consultant
Department of Radiology
Kokilaben Dhirubhai Ambani Hospital
Mumbai, Maharashtra, India

M Ravishankar MD DA FRCP
Professor and Head
Department of Anesthesia and
Critical Care
Mahatma Gandhi Medical College and
Research Institute
Puducherry, India

Anjana D Sahu MD
Assistant Professor
Department of Anesthesia
Topiwala National Medical College and
BYL Nair Hospital
Mumbai, Maharashtra, India

Amit K Sarkar BE PGDIM
Deputy General Manager–MES Sales
Department of Health Care
Linde India Limited
Kolkata, West Bengal, India

Nazmeen I Sayed
MBBS DNB PDCC
Assistant Professor
Department of Anesthesia
Lokmanya Tilak Municipal Medical
College and General Hospital
Mumbai, Maharashtra, India

Prerana N Shah MD
Additional Professor
Department of Anesthesia
Seth GS Medical College and
KEM Hospital
Mumbai, Maharashtra, India

Falguni R Shah
MD (Anesthesiology) DNB FCPS MNAMS
PGDHHM PGDMLS
Senior Consultant Anesthesiologist
Department of Anesthesiology
Lilavati Hospital and Research Centre
Mumbai, Maharashtra, India

Manoj R Shahane MD
Chair of Anesthesia
Summit Anesthesia Associates
Overlook Medical Center
Summit, NJ, USA

Smita D Sharma DNB
Consultant Anesthetist
Department of Anesthesia
Bombay Hospital and Medical
Research Centre
Mumbai, Maharashtra, India

Sohan L Solanki MD PDCC MAMS
Professor
Department of Anesthesia, Critical Care
and Pain
Tata Memorial Hospital
Tata Memorial Centre
Mumbai, Maharashtra, India

R Sripriya DNB (Anesthesia) FUGRA
Professor
Department of Anesthesiology
Mahatma Gandhi Medical College and
Research Institute
Puducherry, India

Maithili Thakur MD DNB PGDHHM
Assistant Professor
Department of Anesthesiology
HBT Medical College and
Dr RN Cooper Municipal General Hospital
Mumbai, Maharashtra, India

Bhakti D Trivedi MD
Assistant Professor
Department of Anesthesia, Critical Care,
and Pain
Tata Memorial Centre
Mumbai, Maharashtra, India

FOREWORD

When the world is reeling under disastrous COVID—an unseen infectious disease never thought or imagined in the history of mankind, Dwarkadas K Baheti kept himself completely occupied. He complied the third edition of *Understanding Anesthetic Equipment and Procedures: A Practical Approach*. With his success of two earlier editions, he with his team dreamt the much deserving third edition. He respected the dictum that one who remains stationary and does not move forward automatically falls behind.

In the third edition he has updated a number of chapters, to give a contemporary look, where he has proved to be outstanding is creating a section on "COVID and Anesthesiology".

During 2020-21 exceptional efforts to understand and treat COVID, developed laboratory, treatment, and research. Anesthesiologists shared a vital role to treat and develop monitors, emergency care, laboratory facility, resuscitation and life support. There are revolutionary developments of equipment. Dr Baheti has very wisely thought of benefiting medical fraternity with the knowledge and created a much-desired chapter on COVID and Anesthesiology.

With my best efforts, I had written the forward note of the second edition of his book and today I am equally honored to add my justified word of praise for the authors and congratulate them.

I wish Dwarkadas K Baheti, Vandana V Laheri and their team members for the third edition and this is precisely the hallmark. This should be the standard textbook for the students as well as the teachers.

Yours sincerely,

Dipankar Das Gupta
Director
Department of Anesthesiology
Jaslok Hospital and Research Centre
Mumbai, Maharashtra, India

PREFACE TO THE THIRD EDITION

We are grateful to the readers who did mouth to mouth publicity which led to heavy demand for the second edition of book *Understanding Anesthetic Equipment and Procedures—A Practical Approach.*

It happened so that we had to bring the revised third edition in record two and half months' time.

The COVID pandemic came as great challenge to COVID warriors all over the world.

The anesthetic management of these patients posed new challenge to anesthesiologist too. Hence, we have added new section on *Corona/COVID-19—Anesthetic Scenario in Corona Pandemic.*

We express our heartfelt gratitude to the readers for stupendous response to the first and second editions which further boosted our confidence to bring out the third edition.

The medical world is witnessing medical, technological, and medical engineering advances. Anesthesiology as specialty and anesthesiologist are also adapting themselves to the technological and monitoring devices. These advances are at times challenging for practicing anesthesiologists which they are happily accepting.

The feedback and response from undergraduates and postgraduates have prompted us to re-edit many chapters and add COVID section.

We are confident the revised third edition will find readers extremely helpful in their day-to-day practice and science of anesthesia.

We express our heartfelt gratitude to all the contributors; without their help, this herculean task would be impossible.

We have taken utmost care to bring out the book of an international quality at an affordable price. The credit goes to the team at M/s Jaypee Brothers Medical Publishers (P) Ltd, New Delhi, India.

We sincerely hope that our efforts to bring out with the third revised edition will further benefit the undergraduates, postgraduates, and practicing anesthesiologists.

This will ultimately provide better patient care, improve surgical outcome, and more cost effective.

Dwarkadas K Baheti
Vandana V Laheri

CONTENTS

Historical Perspective

SECTION 1

Evolution of Anesthesia Practice

Vandana V Laheri, Preeti G More

ABSTRACT

It is the evolution in anesthetic techniques, anesthetic agents, anesthetic equipment's and the development of the specialty that made performance of complex surgical procedures possible without complications. It is therefore important for any anesthesiologist to know how the branch that he or she practises evolved. This chapter gives an idea of the evolution of this specialty. However, more stress is given on the development of equipment and procedures rather than drugs, since the book is all about equipment and procedures.

INTRODUCTION

In the first century, the Greek philosopher Dioscorides (40–90 AD) described the use of wine made from *Mandragora* spp. (a plant known as mandrake) to produce a deep sleep in patients undergoing surgery. Dioscorides used the Greek word "anesthesia" to describe this sleep. The Greek poet Homer (author of the *Illiad* and the *Odyssey*) referred to the pain-killing effects of the potion nepenthe. The present use of the term "anesthesia" to denote the sleep like state that makes painless surgery possible is credited in 1846 to Oliver Wendell Holmes, professor of anatomy and physiology at Harvard Medical School.[1-3]

In the United States, use of the term "anesthesiology" to denote the practice or study of anesthesia was first proposed in the second decade of the twentieth century to emphasize the growing scientific basis of the specialty.[1]

However, surgical procedures were taking place by the times of the Greeks and Romans. In the era 1000 BC, Indians were using wine to produce insensibility. Early Chinese practitioners used acupuncture and the smoke of Indian hemp to dull a person's awareness of pain. Ancient Hindu (East Indian) civilizations used henbane (a plant), wine, and hemp.[2]

Ancient civilizations have used various agents like alcohol, opium (poppy), mandrake root, hyoscine, *Cannabis* (hemp), coca leaves, and even phlebotomy (to the point of unconsciousness) to relieve pain and allow surgeons to operate **(Table 1)**.[2]

From the ninth to the thirteenth centuries, the "soporific sponge" was a dominant mode of providing pain relief during surgery. Mandrake leaves, along with black nightshade, poppies, and other herbs were boiled together and cooked onto a sponge. The sponge was then reconstituted in hot water and placed under the patient's nose before surgery.[4]

Literature quotes first reliable documentation of general anesthesia for surgery on October 13, 1804 from Japan[5] where Seishi Hanaoka removed a breast tumor from Kan Aiya, a woman who had lost all her sisters due to the same disease. The anesthetic was called "tsüsensan" and consisted of an oral herbal concoction, which included scopolamine, hyoscyamine, atropine, aconitine, and angelic toxin, that had been developed by the surgeon himself. When consumed in sufficient quantity, tsüsensan produced a state of general anesthesia and skeletal muscle paralysis.[5,6] This was the way general anesthesia was given. Hanaoka performed many operations using tsüsensan, including resection of malignant tumors, extraction of bladder stones, and extremity amputations. Before his death in 1835, Hanaoka performed more than 150 operations for breast cancer.[5,6]

Throughout history pain prohibited surgical advances, and therefore, development of surgical anesthesia is considered one of the most important discoveries in the history of medicine. The history of anesthesia enables us to appreciate the way this specialty grew.

The development of the specialty can be appreciated well if we look at it under the following heads:

- Anesthetic techniques and anesthetic equipment's
- Anesthetic agents
- Anesthesiology as a medical specialty.

TABLE 1: Relief of pain in ancient times.[2,3]

Drugs available for relief of pain	*Nondrug methods*	*Regional anesthesia method*
• Alcohol • Cannabis (hemp) • Cocaine • Hyoscine (mandrake + others) • Opium (poppy)	• Cold • Concussion • Carotid compression • Nerve compression • Hypnosis • Bloodletting	Compression of nerve trunks (nerve ischemia) or the application of cold (cryo analgesia)

ANESTHETIC TECHNIQUES AND ANESTHETIC EQUIPMENT

The anesthetic techniques evolved first with inhalation (general) anesthesia, followed by local and regional anesthesia, and finally, intravenous (IV) anesthesia.[1] Simultaneously, there was evolution in anesthesia equipment's and monitoring equipment.

General Anesthesia

The first general anesthetics were inhalational agents, because the invention of the hypodermic needle and syringe did not occur.[1] Inhalational anesthesia has been described in literature using a "soporific sponge" soaked in hashish, opium and other herbal aromatics and placed under the nose of the patients.[1,2] Intravenous anesthesia followed the invention of the hypodermic syringe and needle in 1855. Early attempts at IV anesthesia included the use of chloral hydrate with inhalational agents chloroform or ether and the combination of morphine and scopolamine **(Table 2)**.[1]

The demonstration of anesthesia with diethyl ether in 1846 at the Massachusetts General Hospital started a new era of pain-free operations. In nineteenth century, the discovery of nitrous oxide (NO_2), chloroform, oxygen (O_2), and ether made the possibility of operations being done under the state of unconsciousness.

Scientific discoveries in the late eighteenth and early nineteenth centuries laid down the foundation for the development of modern anesthetic techniques **(Table 2)**.

TABLE 2: Important events during the evolution of inhalational anesthesia.[1-10]

Year	Events
1020	Inhaled anesthesia described using a "soporific sponge" soaked in hashish, opium and other herbal aromatics and placed under the nose of the patient
1772	Nitrous oxide (N_2O) discovered by Joseph Priestly
1799	N_2O suggested for pain relief and called "laughing gas" by Sir Humphry Davy, a British chemist
1800	Humphry Davy published his experiments with nitrous oxide
1824	CO_2 used to produce unconsciousness in mice and dogs by Henry Hill Hickman in Shropshire and Paris
1842	Crawford Long administered diethyl ether by inhalational route
1844	Horace Wells administered NO_2 for dental analgesia in US
1846	William Morton gave public demonstration of diethyl ether at the Massachusetts General Hospital
1847	James Young Simpson administered chloroform for general anesthesia in England
1848	Heyfelder discovered anesthetic properties of ethyl chloride
1853	John Snow, an English physician, administered chloroform to Queen Victoria for the birth of Prince Leopold
1856	John Snow designed ether and chloroform inhalers so as to deliver the anesthetic agent at optimum levels. He used scientific principles and devised inhalers in which the concentration could be controlled. He also described some of the planes (stages) of anesthesia
1862	Thomas Skinner, a general practitioner and obstetrician from Liverpool designed the first wire frame for administration of anesthetic agents by open drop
1864	Report of the Chloroform Commission appeared
1868	Method of converting N_2O gas to liquid for storage in cylinder developed by George Barth and J Coxeter of Coxeter and Sons, England
1868	Edmund Andrews introduced the use of O_2 with N_2O in anesthetic practice in US
1870	Investigations for the use of chloroform and development of inhalational equipment for its administration by Joseph T Clover, an English surgeon, improved the techniques of gas delivery and he cautioned the physicians to monitor the vital signs
1876	JT Clover introduced gas–ether sequence in anesthesia in England
1882	SJ Hayes from US patented an apparatus for generating and applying anesthetic agents. Ether and chloroform mixtures were heated by water bath and air was pumped through this mixture
1883	Oxygen first liquefied by Zygmunt Wroblewski and Karol Olszewski in Krakow, Poland
1889	First reliable pressure-reducing valve introduced by Johann Heinrich and his son Bernhard, the founders of Dräger in Lubeck, Germany for the controlled release of gases from high pressure containers—called the "Lubeca valve"
1890	Curt Theodor Schimmelbusch, a German physician and pathologist in Berlin produced Schimmelbusch mask
1892	F Hewitt from England introduced the first practical gas and oxygen apparatus
1899	SS White from Germany introduced "gas machine" with proportioned gages
1902	Charles Teter from US introduced machine for administration of N_2O and O_2
1903	Ethyl chloride popularized in UK as general anesthetic by Dr WJ McCardie after reporting using it for dental anesthesia since 1901 at Birmingham Dental Hospital
1905	First soda lime CO_2 absorption cartridge was introduced in an elementary closed system by Drägerwerk, Germany with Professor Franz Kuhn, a surgeon—but proved to be inadequate
1906	Clark from US developed gas machine where a central valve with a slot for each gas was used to proportion the gas

Contd...

Contd...

Year	Events
1907	Frederick J Cotton and Walter M Boothby invented an apparatus for the delivery of NO_2, ether, and O_2
1907	First intermittent positive pressure ventilation (IPPV) device "pulmotor" was introduced by Dräger in Germany. This was used mainly by fire fighters
1908	AD Waller designed the chloroform balance which determined the concentration of the vapor received by the patient
1909	Introduction of self-administration of N_2O in obstetrics and office surgery by AE Guedel from US
1910	El Mckesson from US perfected their first "intermittent flow" N_2O and O_2 apparatus with an accurate percentage control for two gases and also introduced fractional rebreathing
1912	Heidbrink pressure relief valve was introduced by Jay A Heidbrink (dentist) of the Heidbrink Company of Minneapolis
1912	Ohio monovalve anesthesia machine was patented and put in US market
1914	Foregoer Company from New York produced Gwathmey O_2/N_2O/ether anesthetic apparatus and became heavily involved in producing different items for anesthesia
1915	CO_2 absorber was developed for use with closed circuit by Dennis E Jackson (pharmacologist), St Louis, USA
1917	Henry Edmund Gaskin Boyle, St Bartholomew's Hospital, London, developed the first English-designed anesthetic machine. This included cylinders for O_2 and N_2O, and a Boyle's bottle to vaporize diethyl ether. The machine was named in his honour (Boyle's machine) by the makers, Coxeters and British Oxygen Company
1921	CO_2 absorber concepts refined with development of Waters' "to-and-fro" canister, which used soda lime by Ralph M Waters, Iowa, USA, the first professor of anesthesiology in the world
1924	Circle breathing CO_2 absorption system first developed for acetylene anesthesia by Carl Gauss in Germany. Apparatus was manufactured by Drägerwerk of Lübeck. Same company produced systems for use with N_2O/O_2/ether, which were introduced into practise by Paul Sudeck and Helmut Schmidt
1927	Circle anesthetic system was developed into the United States by Foregger and Waters. This version was tested and modified by suggestions from several practitioners, including Brian Sword who reported 1,200 cases he had done by 1929
1928	Magill's circuit developed
1930	The circle absorption system was introduced in clinical practice by Brian Sword
1933	Minnitt's "gas and air" apparatus was produced for analgesia during labor by Robert James Minnitt, Liverpool, England
1934	First activated carbon filters to scavenge ether vapor in expiratory limb of anesthetic circuit introduced by Max Tiegel of Trier in the Tiegel-Dräger anesthetic apparatus
1937	Definitive "stages" of anesthesia described for ether with spontaneous breathing by Arthur E Guedel, an American anesthetist
1937	Ayre's T-piece developed—first designed for use with neurosurgical patients by Philip Ayre in England
1950	Jackson Rees added an open-ended bag to the expiratory limb of Ayre's T-piece that facilitated manual controlled ventilation
1952	Pin-index system for gas cylinder mounting on yokes introduced
1952	Manley ventilator introduced by Roger Manley of Westminster Hospital, London. This was the first ventilator powered entirely by gas from the fresh gas supply of the anesthetic machine
1954	William Wellesley Mapleson, a physicist working in the Department of Anaesthetics at the Welsh National School of Medicine published analysis of five semi closed breathing systems in use at that time the origin of which was not known. He classified them as Mapleson A, B, C, D and E
1972	JA Bain and WE Spoerel introduced Bain's breathing system

Evolution of Anesthesia Machines[1-8,10,11]

Intermittent flow devices (anesthesia machines with gases drawn as a result of the inspiratory efforts of patient) were commonly used in dentistry and obstetrics. Before 1900s, the SS White Company modified Frederick Hewitt's apparatus and marketed its continuous-flow machine. Anesthetists often carried all their equipment with them, but it was not practical for most circumstances to carry heavy, bulky cylinders.

In the late nineteenth century, demands in dentistry instigated development of the first freestanding anesthesia machines. Three American dentist-entrepreneurs, Samuel S White, Charles Teter, and Jay Heid brink, developed the original series of US instruments that used compressed cylinders of N_2O and O_2, and Frederick Hewitt's continuous-flow machine was refined by Teter in 1903.

- Anesthesia machine produced by Charles K Teter, Jay Heid brink, and Samuel S White in USA, known as Teter Anesthesia Machine (1903) incorporated compressed gas cylinders. Heid brink added reducing valves in 1912. Walter Boothby and Fred Cotton (Harvard) adapted it with water-bubble flowmeters. James Gwathmey (USA) produced O_2/N_2O/ether anesthesia apparatus and made it portable (1914)
- Henry Edmund Gaskin "Cockie" Boyle, St. Bartholomew's Hospital, London used the concepts of Gwathmey machine and developed the first English-designed "anesthesia machine" (1917). This included cylinders for O_2 and N_2O, and a "Boyle's bottle" to vaporize diethyl ether. The machine was named in his honor (Boyle's machine) by the makers, Coxeters and British Oxygen Company
  - Originally Boyle introduced N_2O–O_2 anesthesia through this machine, and it was a two-gas system with water sight-feed type of flowmeter

- In 1920s, modification was made by incorporating a vaporizing bottle to flowmeters
- In 1926, a second vaporizing bottle and bypass controls were added
- In 1927, addition of carbon dioxide cylinder
- In 1930s, addition of plunger to vaporizing bottles
- In 1933, dry bobbin type of flowmeter was introduced in place of water sight-feed type
- In 1937, rotameters displaced dry-bobbin type of flowmeters
- Later pin-index system, pressure regulators, trilene interlock, circle system, Tec vaporizers, compressed air, pressure relief valve/pop off valve, oxygen fail-safe mechanism, etc., got added

- During the same period in Lubeck, Germany, Heinrich Dräger and his son, Bernhaard, adapted compressed-gas technology, which they had originally developed for mine rescue equipment, to manufacture ether and chloroform-oxygen machines.

Dräger Anesthesia Machines[11]

In 1901 from Germany Heinrich, Bernhard Dräger and Otto Roth were the first made an anesthetic apparatus for oxygen and chloroform, was like bubbler devices in England. The same team developed a totally new, unique drip-feed device for liquid anesthetic agents with injector developed by them. To generate suction, the oxygen was passed through injector, not routed through the anesthetic agent.

The added components were the pressure-reducing device to control the gas flow from the cylinder and controlled and precise flow of anesthetic agent via the drip-feed device. To administer anesthetic agents Dräger developed three models with similar in design such as (i) oxygen/chloroform, (ii) oxygen/ether and (iii) oxygen/chloroform/ether. In 1911, Roth-Dräger-Krönig devised apparatus for anesthetist to ventilate oxygen enriched air with positive pressure.

The "to-and-fro system was introduced by Ralph M Waters and Circle system was by Brian C Sword and RV Foregger. The "Model A" first anesthetic machine with circle system was developed. To take advantages of O_2/N_2O and with features of new circle system "Model D" and "Model F" with O_2, N_20 and Ether was developed in 1946.

Dräger was first machine in which the gas flow was controlled by flowmeters/rotameters, with the option of connecting cyclopropane and carbon dioxide.

The "Model G" had the option of connecting 2–5 gases: two cylinders each of O_2 and N_2O, with cyclopropane, helium, and CO_2 as additional option.

Addition of Newer Advances and Safety Devices in the Development of Machines[1,3]

- Important safety features
  - The pin-index system for cylinders
  - Color coding of cylinders and pipelines
  - Pressure gages for cylinders
  - Preset pressure reducing valves
  - Nonreturn valves at the hanger yoke
  - Flow meter-color and touch coding, placement coding
  - Noninterchangeable system [(noninterchangeable quick couplers (NIQC), diameter index safety system (DISS), and noninterchangeable screw threads (NIST)] for gas delivery to the machine
  - Patient safety valves in the circuit and machine
- Antistatic wheels
- Entry of oxygen as the last gas admitted to the back bar so that a leak in the other rotameters cannot dilute the oxygen delivered
- The international oxygen knob with the oxygen knob set forward of all other knobs
- An antihypoxic device for use whenever N_2O is administered became a requirement
- Vaporizers developed from simple bubble through or flow over devices to devices that could guarantee a constant output over a given range of flow (Tec vaporizers)
- An oxygen failure warning device
  - The Ritchie whistle developed in the late 60s operated on residual oxygen in the system and did not rely on a second gas to provide the alarm
  - The Howison alarm, a refinement of the Ritchie whistle, cut off the N_2O as the whistle sounded and supplied oxygen at a reduced rate from a reserve cylinder.

American National Standards Institute (ANSI) way back in 1979 provided guidelines for manufacturers of anesthesia machines regarding minimum performance, design characteristics and safety requirements. These standards for anesthesia machines were designated as "ANSI Z79.8-1979". In 1988, American Society for Testing and Materials (ASTM) added their standards—ASTM F1161-88 which was modified in 1994 as ASTM F1161-94. These were discontinued in the year 2000 and were replaced by ASTM F1850-00.

The basic design of all the machines has been upgraded to perform more complicated functions since 1990s, with the advent of computer-controlled monitors into the operating room, especially pulse oximetry, capnography, gas analysis, anesthesia ventilators, airway pressure monitoring and various "fail safe" alarm systems leading to development of "anesthesia work stations", to name a few: Fabius GS®, Primus, Narkomed AV2+, Ohmeda 7800, Ohmeda 6400, Julian, BleaseSirius, anesthesia delivery unit (ADU) and many others.

All of these machines have following common features:

- Oxygen supply pressure failure alarms along with safety devices
- Flowmeters having proportioning systems, oxygen ratio monitor controller or sensitive oxygen ratio controller system

- Vaporizers being agent-specific, having keyed filling devices, interlock systems and being protected from overfilling
- Anesthesia ventilators with facility for compliance and leak testing, fresh gas decoupling or compensation and suitability for low flows
- Workstation self-tests.

There is development going on at all the time in the design and features of anesthesia workstations, e.g., vaporizers for the newer volatile anesthetic agents, after market add-on devices, ventilators with different features, latest monitoring gadgets, scavenging systems and so on. These newer features are added to provide safe anesthesia to patients.

Equipment for Endotracheal Anesthesia

Elective tracheal intubations during anesthesia were performed in the late nineteenth century by surgeons, Sir William MacEwen in Scotland, Joseph O'Dwyer in the US, and Franz Kuhn in Germany. Tracheal intubation during anesthesia was popularized in England by Sir Ivan Magill and Stanley Rowbotham in the 1920s **(Table 3)**.[1]

TABLE 3: Timeline of important events in evolution of endotracheal anesthesia.[1-10]

Year	Events
1743	First record of a laryngoscope by a French accoucher named Leveret who used a bent reflective spatula and even developed a snare for laryngeal polyps
1807	Early record of laryngoscopy by Philipp Bozzini in Germany. He developed an instrument called a "lichtleiter" (light conductor) for endoscopy of numerous body cavities, which was illuminated by reflected candlelight
1829	Indirect laryngoscopy first described by Benjamin Guy Babington
1829	Development of a laryngoscope that had both an epiglottic retractor and a laryngeal mirror by Benjamin Babington in a paper presented to the Hunterian Society in London
1844	Development of enhanced lighting for a laryngoscope by John Avery, a surgeon at Charing Cross Hospital, London. He modified a Miner's lamp to concentrate and focus candlelight down an aural speculum
1852	First direct laryngoscopy operation by Horace Green, the first specialist airway physician in the US. Using a bent spatula to displace the tongue and sunlight to see, he removed a laryngeal tumor in a child, which had been causing intermittent obstruction
1854	Description of mirrors used to view larynx by Manuel Patricio Rodriguez Garcia. He described the use of mirrors to view the larynx in a paper to the Royal Society of London
1869	First description of human endotracheal intubation via tracheotomy by Dr Friedrich Trendelenburg (German surgeon) for the purpose of administering general anesthesia
1878	First oral endotracheal tube introduced by Macewan which was made of flexible brass with 3/8 inches diameter
1880	The first recorded case of endotracheal insufflation anesthesia for an osteosarcoma of the hard palate with a catheter in the trachea by MacReddie for MacEwan's procedure
1889	Invention of cuffed tubes (these being endobronchial tubes) and double-lumen endobronchial tube by Henry, Head (physiologist and neurologist) at the University College Hospital, London. These were designed for physiological lung studies (to study differential lung function) in animals at The (now Royal) London Hospital. They were made of Indian rubber and were inflated using syringes filled with glycerine
1895	First direct laryngoscope by Alfred Kirstein (Germany) with transmitted light (auto scope)
1897	First rigid bronchoscopy performed to remove a pork bone under topical cocaine by Gustav Killian, Professor of Laryngology at University of Berlin
1903	Chevalier Jackson laryngoscope designed by Chevalier Jackson
1907	Intratracheal insufflation of chloroform was done
1909	Modern technique of surgical tracheostomy described by Chevalier Jackson (laryngologist), professor at six universities in the US and founder of the American Bronchoesophagological Association (ABEA)
1913	In 1913, Chevalier Jackson (1865–1958) introduced a new laryngoscope blade that had a light source at the distal tip, rather than the proximal light source used by Kirstein. This new blade incorporated a component that the operator could slide out to allow room for passage of an endotracheal tube or bronchoscope
1913	Tungsten bulb added as a light source to laryngoscope introduced by Professor Chevalier Jackson
1913	Henry H Janeway, an American, practising at Bellevue Hospital in New York City, developed a laryngoscope designed for the sole purpose of tracheal intubation. Similar to Jackson's device, Janeway's instrument incorporated a distal light source. Unique however was the inclusion of batteries within the handle, a central notch in the blade for maintaining the tracheal tube in the midline of the oropharynx during intubation and a slight curve to the distal tip of the blade to help guide the tube through the glottis. Janeway was instrumental in popularizing the widespread use of direct laryngoscopy and tracheal intubation in the practise of anesthesiology
1919	Red rubber endotracheal tubes developed by Sir Ivan Whiteside Magill at Queen Mary Hospital, Sidcup to help anesthetize for World War I facial injuries. Connections to anesthetic machine included a piece of car brake hose from a Morris MG car engine
1920	Magill and Rowbotham developed endotracheal anesthesia
1921	Magill's forceps developed by Sir Evan Magill

Contd...

Contd...

Year	Events
1926	Magill laryngoscope blade produced by Sir Ivan Magill and manufactured by Hamblin, London
1931	"Cuffed" endotracheal tubes produced
1933	Arthur Guedel designed a new "nontraumatic pharyngeal airway". The Guedel airway remains in use worldwide today
1941	Miller laryngoscope blade produced by Robert Miller
1943	Sir Robert Reynolds Macintosh introduced his new curved laryngoscope blade
1949	Macintosh published a case report describing the novel use of a gum elastic urinary catheter as an endotracheal tube introducer to facilitate difficult tracheal intubation
1949	Double-lumen endobronchial tube designed for humans by Eric Carlens, Sweden, for use in Broncho spirometry under local anesthesia
1950	Double-lumen endobronchial tube first used in humans for one-lung anesthesia by Dr Eric Carlens and Viking Björk, a thoracic surgeon
1953	First range of double-lumen endotracheal tubes produced for anesthesia by Frank Robertshaw, Manchester
1955	Percutaneous tracheostomy developed by C Hunter Shelden (neurosurgeon) et al. (USA)
1960s	First patient mannikin produced—"Resusci Anne" by Asmund S Laerdal in Norway
1961	Brian Arthur Sellick published a paper describing "cricoid pressure" to control regurgitation of stomach contents during induction of anesthesia in the Lancet
1966	Flexible bronchoscope invented by Shigeto Ikeda, Japanese physician working in concert with Machida Endoscope Company (later Pentax®) and Olympus Optical Company
1967	The concept of using a fibre optic endoscope for tracheal intubation was introduced by Peter Murphy, an English anesthetist
1967	Jet ventilation via injector developed by RD Sanders of Delaware, initially used for rigid bronchoscopy
1970s	Flexible fibre optic intubation technique developed by Andranik Ovassapian who later became Professor of Anesthesia and Critical Care at the University of Chicago
1971	High volume-low pressure cuffs for endotracheal tubes designed (initially for tracheostomy tubes) by Joel D Cooper et al., Pennsylvania
1973	P Hex Venn developed Eschmann endotracheal tube introducer. The material of Venn's design was different from that of a gum elastic bougie in that it had two layers: (i) a core of tube woven from polyester threads and (ii) an outer resin layer. This provided more stiffness but maintained the flexibility and the slippery surface. Other differences were the length: the new introducer was 60 cm (24 inches), which is much longer than the gum elastic bougie and the presence of a 35 curved tip, permitting it to be steered around obstacles
1975	Ring-Adair-Elwyn (RAE) endotracheal tubes developed and used by Wallace Ring, John Adair and Richard Elwyn, University of Utah, Primary Paediatric Hospital, Salt Lake City
1978	First disposable Robertshaw double-lumen tube produced by Mallinckrodt Medical, Althone, Ireland
1983	LMA Classic introduced by AIJ "Archie" Brain at the Royal London Hospital
1984	Ronald Sidney Cormack and John Robert Lehane published their landmark paper describing typical views during direct laryngoscopy
1985	Seshagiri Rao Mallampati and colleagues in Boston, Massachusetts published their airway classification—dividing patients into three groups according to which pharyngeal structures were visible
1987	Samsoon and Young in Portsmouth, UK, added a fourth class to Mallampati class
1987	Esophageal tracheal combi tube was introduced
1993	EP McCoy and RK Mirakhur introduced the McCoy laryngoscope blade
1997	Intubating LMA introduced
2000	Proseal LMA introduced
2001	The Glide scope, the first commercially available video laryngoscope, designed by vascular and general surgeon John Allen Pacey, Honorary Professor of Anesthesiology, Pharmacology and Therapeutics Department, University of British Columbia, Canada

(MG: Morris Garage; LMA: laryngeal mask airway)

Late twentieth century saw the evolution of different laryngoscopes, video laryngoscopes, airways, endotracheal tubes, endobronchial tubes and equipment's for management of difficult airway. The list is never ending as the devices still keep on evolving and getting improved.

Contributions of Sir Ivan Whiteside Magill (1888–1986):[12]

- *Magill endotracheal tubes:* Oral and nasal designs
- *An anesthetic breathing system:* Magill circuit and expiratory valve
- Magill's forceps
- Straight bladed laryngoscope
- *Catheter mount:* Endotracheal tube-to-circuit connector
- *Endotracheal tube connectors:* Oral and nasal versions
- Magill's spray
- Single-lung anesthesia
- Endobronchial tubes and bronchial blockers
- Bobbin flowmeters
- Helped establish the Diploma in Anesthesia
  Helped found the Association of Anesthetists in 1932.

Evolution in Operating Room Monitoring

Way back in 1870s, Joseph T Clover, an English surgeon, improved the techniques of gas delivery during anesthesia and cautioned the physicians to monitor the vital signs. In 1894, Cushing and a fellow student, Charles Codman, at Harvard Medical School initiated a system of recording patients' pulses to assess the course of the anesthetics.[4]

In 1881, sphygmomanometer developed by Samuel Siegfried Karl Ritter von Basch (Austrian physician) and in 1896 "Riva-Rocci blood pressure cuff" developed. George W Crile and Harvey Cushing developed a strong interest in measuring blood pressure during anesthesia. Cushing was the first American to apply the Riva Rocci cuff, which he saw while visiting Italy. Cushing introduced the concept in 1902 and had blood pressure measurements recorded on anesthesia records.[4]

Cushing continued the practice of monitoring and recording patient's blood pressure and pulse. The transition from manual to automated blood pressure devices, which first appeared in 1936 has been gradual. The development of inexpensive microprocessors has enabled routine use of automatic blood pressure cuffs in clinical settings.[4]

As the specialty grew further, in addition to monitoring of pulse and blood pressure, monitoring of ECG, airway pressure, breathing system disconnect alarms, monitoring of neuromuscular blockade, inspired oxygen, pulse oximetry, expired CO_2 ($EtCO_2$), respiratory gas monitoring of the five-potent inhaled anesthetic agents, N_2O, CO_2 and O_2 (RGM), anesthetic depth [bispectral index (BIS), entropy], transesophageal echocardiography and so on came in practice **(Table 4)**.

TABLE 4: Timeline of evolution of other important aspects.[1-10]

Year	*Evolution of other important aspects*
1767	The use of bellows for respiratory resuscitation officially recommended by Society of Resuscitation of Drowned Persons of Amsterdam
1771	The use of bellows for respiratory resuscitation officially recommended by Royal Humane Society of London
1774	The application of cricoid pressure first described by Alexander Monro Secundus, Professor of Medicine, Anatomy, and Surgery at Edinburgh University. He described the technique in order to "reduce water in the lungs and prevent gastric distension" (with air) while attempting to resuscitate victims of drowning using mouth-to-mouth or bellows for lung inflation
1825	Classic description of experiments with curare by Charles Waterton who proved that if ventilated, the animal survives after curare injection.
1828	First measurement of blood pressure using mercury-filled manometer by Jean-Louis-Marie Poiseuille, French physician and physiologist in Paris
1850	Curare's site of action described by a French physiologist, Claude Bernard
1853	Charles Gabriel Pravaz first to develop syringe made of silver with screw-down plunger to estimate dose
1853	Danial Ferguson developed glass syringe with a hollow needle
1853	Charles Hunter coined term "hypodermic" syringe and attached hollow needle designed by Alexander Wood. He injected local morphine to treat a woman with neuralgia using the Ferguson-produced syringe
1854	Henning Ruben invented a "Ambu Bag" with sprung bicycle spokes to aid automatic re-expansion and a refined one was marketed with help of Holger Hesse
1855	Claud Bernard described physiological effects of curare
1864	John Tyndall developed infrared absorption measurement of CO_2 in human breath
1868	George Barth and J. Coxeter developed method of converting N_2O gas to liquid for storage in cylinder
1869	Hermann Wülfing Luer made first all-glass syringe (Wülfing Luer Company)
1877	Joseph Clover designed emergency metal surgical airway promoted the anterior jaw thrust maneuver to pull the tongue forward off the posterior pharynx
1881	Samuel Siegfried Karl Ritter von Basch developed sphygmomanometer
1896	Scipione Riva-Rocci Riva developed Rocci blood pressure cuff
1902	Harvey Williams Cushing wrote first anesthetic record
1903	Professor Willem Einthoven developed Electrocardiogram (ECG or EKG) and awarded Nobel Prize in 1924
1905	Nikolai Korotkoff described auscultatory method of determining blood pressure using a Riva-Rocci cuff
1938	Clarence Crafoord used a mechanical ventilator—the Frecken "spiropulsator" for surgery
1940	Thore Olovson described long-term intravenous cannula for repeated injections and more permanent access from treatment of cases of deep vein thrombosis (DVT) with repeated injections of heparin. It became known as the "heparin needle"
1941	Professor Emery Andrew Rovenstine introduced American Society of Anesthesiologists (ASA) classification of patient health status
1942	Millikan created a lightweight ear-oximeter for aviation research and was first to coin the term "oximetry"
1943	Luft introduced the first infrared CO_2 measuring and recording apparatus
1945	Torsten Gordh described his modification of needle developed by Olovson, and it then became known as the "Gordh needle" for anesthesia and infusions.

Contd...

Contd...

Year	Evolution of other important aspects
1946	Mendelson's syndrome (aspiration pneumonitis) described
1949	John Haven Emerson designed first American mechanical ventilator
1954	Henning Ruben invented a "Ambu Bag" with sprung bicycle spokes to aid automatic re-expansion and a refined one was marketed with help of Holger Hesse
1955	Collier et al. established the accuracy of rapid infrared CO_2 analysis in determining alveolar CO_2 concentration
1959	Ranwell established the value of the end tidal sample
1960	Cardio scopes were introduced for cardiac surgery
1965	Guenter Corssen Edward Felix Domino and P Chodoff (USA) describe the term "dissociative anesthesia" for effects of Ketamine
1966	American Heart Association developed cardiopulmonary resuscitation (CPR) techniques
1967	Al Vaisman first to proposed the need for scavenging anesthetic gases in operating theaters
1968	Wellcome laboratories introduced monitoring of neuromuscular agents
1969	Abrahamson, JS Denson and RM Wolf developed first anesthesia simulator developed called "SIM 1" or "SIM ONE", and intubated and did IV cannulation on a mannequin. Which was computer controlled, with a heart-beat, temporal and carotid pulse and recordable blood pressure. It could open and close its mouth and blink its eyes. It can respond to intravenous drugs, gases. It was used for teaching intubation and induction of anesthesia
1970	Hewlett-Packard developed an eight-wavelength self-calibrating ear oximeter. However, it was too bulky to be used clinically
1971	Leonard Bachman redefined the concept of minimum alveolar concentration (MAC) in relation to ED50. It was defined by Merkel and E Eger in 1963 during animal studies and by E (Ted) Eger, L Saidman and B Brandstater in studies on human
1972	Takuo Aoyagi at Nihon Kohden developed clinical pulse oximeter
1976	First automated oscillometric noninvasive blood pressure machine—DINAMAP® by GE Medical Systems
1976	Transesophageal echocardiography reported (nonoperative) by MA Shirley and RB Roberts
1978	Zden Kalenda first adopted capnography for use in anesthesia
1979	Intraoperative transesophageal echocardiography study reported by Oka and Matsumoto in New York
1980	Biox Technology in USA commercialized the first clinically useful pulse oximeter
1980	TIVA developed
1980s	Screen-only computerized anesthesia simulators produced—versions called "SLEEPER", "BODY" and anesthesia simulator consultant (ASC)
1981	Smalhout and Kalenda pioneered the introduction of capnography into routine clinical practice in Netherlands
1984	Infrared-based gas analysis products such the Puritan-Bennett/Datex 222 Anesthetic Agent Monitor, came in the market. The Datex 222 was soon followed by the Datex Normac, Dräger's IRINA, Andros 4600 (analyser bench)/4700 (agent ID bench), Datex Capnomac, Nellcor 2500, Ohmeda RGM, and Criticare's POET II
1986	The American Society of Anesthesiologists first approved Standards for Basic Intraoperative Monitoring. It was last updated in 2010
1994	Bispectral index (BIS) monitoring as a guide to depth of anesthesia developed by (Organon, now Schering-Plough) Aspect Medical Industries, USA
1999	Ultrasound recommended for use in anesthesia and intensive care for nerve blocks and intravascular line placement by Hatfield and Bodenham at Leeds General Infirmary
2003	Datex-Ohmeda developed Spectral Entropy Monitoring as a guide to depth of anesthesia

Newly manufactured anesthesia workstations have monitors (as per ASTM F1850-00 standards) that measure:

- Continuous breathing system pressure
- Exhaled tidal volume
- Ventilatory CO_2 concentration
- Anesthetic vapor concentration
- Inspired oxygen concentration
- Oxygen supply pressure
- Arterial oxygen saturation of hemoglobin
- Arterial blood pressure
- Continuous ECG.

In the twentieth century, the safety and efficacy of general anesthesia was improved not only by the routine use of tracheal intubation, but also due to advanced airway management, ventilatory management techniques, advances in monitoring, addition of newer inhalational and intravenous anesthetic agents and newer muscle relaxants with improved pharmacodynamic characteristics.[3,5]

Regional Anesthesia[9]

The most potent alkaloid of the coca plant, cocaine, was isolated in 1855 by Friedrich Gaedcke. In 1884, Austrian ophthalmologist Karl Koller instilled a 2% solution of cocaine into his own eye and tested its effectiveness as a local anesthetic by pricking the eye with needles. He presented his findings at annual conference of the Heidelberg Ophthalmological Society. In 1885, William Halsted performed the first brachial plexus block and in the same year James Leonard Corning injected cocaine between the spinous processes of the lower lumbar vertebrae, first in a dog and then in a healthy man. His experiments are the first published descriptions of the principle of neuraxial blockade. On August 16, 1898, German surgeon August Bier performed surgery under spinal anesthesia in Kiel. A Swiss obstetrician, Oscar Kreis, recognized the advantages of regional anesthesia in obstetrics and administered the first spinal anesthesia for control of labor pain at the start of the twentieth century **(Tables 5 and 6)**.[9]

TABLE 5: Timeline of evolution in regional anesthesia.[1-10]

Year	Events
1855	Cocaine isolated from the coca plant by chemist Friedrich Gaedcke in Germany
1860	Cocaine purified by Albert Neimann, PhD student at University of Göttingen in Germany
1884	Demonstration of the local anesthetic properties of cocaine on the cornea by Austrian ophthalmologist Karl Koller
1884	The surgeon William Halsted demonstrated the use of cocaine for intradermal infiltration and nerve blocks including the facial nerve, the brachial plexus, the pudendal nerve, and the posterior tibial nerve
1885	James Leonard Corning, neurologist in New York, introduced spinal anesthesia for pain relief and he coined the term "spinal anesthesia" and was the first to describe post dural puncture headache in patients
1892	Schleich used infiltration LA
1987	The term "block" introduced to describe the use of local anesthetics by George Washington Crile, an American surgeon
1898	August Bier is credited for administering the first spinal anesthetic; he used 3 mL of 0.5% cocaine intrathecally
1898	Post dural puncture headache linked to CSF loss by Jean-Anthanase Sicard
1901	The term "regional anesthesia" introduced to describe the use of local anesthetics by Harvey Williams Cushing
1901	Ferdinand Cathelin and Jean Sicard introduced caudal epidural anesthesia
1901	Romanian surgeon Nicolae Racoviceanu-Piteşti was the first to use opioids for intrathecal analgesia; he presented his experience in Paris
1902	Adrenaline first added to local anesthetic agents by Heinrich Braun, a German surgeon with an interest in anesthesia. He initially added it to cocaine
1903	Amylocaine (Stovaine), the first synthetic local anesthetic developed
1904	Procaine was synthesized by Alfred Einhorn and within a year was used clinically as a local anesthetic by Heinrich Braun
1905	Procaine introduced as a local anesthetic
1908	August Bier was the first to describe intravenous regional anesthesia (Bier block)
1909	First caudal anesthesia given for labor pains by Professor Walter Stoeckel in Germany
1921	Spanish military surgeon Fidel Pagés developed the technique of "single-shot" lumbar epidural anesthesia, which was later popularized by Italian surgeon Achille Mario Dogliotti
1922	Use of fine needle (for dural puncture) inserted through larger needle (for skin puncture) suggested as means of reducing incidence of post dural puncture headache by Dr Hoyt
1931	Dogliotti described a "loss-of-resistance" technique, involving constant application of pressure to the plunger of a syringe to identify the epidural space whilst advancing the needle—a technique sometimes referred to as Dogliotti's principle
1931	Eugène Aburel Bogdan, a Romanian surgeon and obstetrician, described lumbar plexus block during early labor, followed by a caudal epidural injection for the expulsion phase
1940	William Lemmon introduced concept of continuous spinal anesthesia
1941	Robert Andrew Hingson, Waldo B Edwards and James L Southworth, working at the US Marine Hospital at Stapleton, on Staten Island in New York, developed the technique of continuous caudal anesthesia. They first used this technique in an operation to remove the varicose veins of a Scottish merchant
1942	The first use of continuous caudal anesthesia in a laboring woman in US for an emergency Cesarean section by Robert Andrew Hingson, Waldo B Edwards and James L Southworth. Because the woman suffered from rheumatic heart disease, her doctors believed that she would not survive the stress of labor but they also felt that she would not tolerate general anesthesia due to her heart failure. With the use of continuous caudal anesthesia, the woman and her baby survived
1943	Lidocaine synthesised by Nils Lofgren and Bengt Lundqvist—chemists at Institute of Chemistry at Stockholm University, Sweden.
1944	Edward Tuohy introduced the Touhy needle designed by Ralph L Huber, a Seattle dentist and inventor
1947	Pío Manuel María Martínez Curbelo performed placement of a lumbar epidural catheter with 16 gauge Tuohy needle. He introduced a 3.5 French ureteral catheter into the lumbar epidural space and repeatedly injected 0.5% percaine (cinchocaine, also known as dibucaine) for anesthesia.
1948	Lignocaine introduced into clinical practise by Torsten Gordh (first specialist anesthetist in Sweden having trained with Ralph Waters in the US) at Karolinska University Hospital
1960	Epidural blood patch introduced by JB Gormley
1965	Philip Raikes Bromage publishes his scoring system to assess the intensity of lower limb motor blockade after extradural analgesia or anesthesia
1979	First extradural morphine by Behar et al.

Contd...

Contd...

Year	Events
1979	Combined spinal and epidural (CSE) anesthesia introduced as a "double segment" technique by Professor Ioan Curelaru at Department of Anaesthesiology at Gothenburg University, Sweden
1981	Combined spinal and epidural introduced in England for Cesarean section by Dr Peter Brownridge
1982	CSE "single segment" technique first used
1988	Patient-controlled epidural anesthesia (PCEA) introduced by David R Gambling et al. in Canada
1999	First reviews got published recommending the routine use of ultrasound for regional nerve blocks and placement of central venous lines

(LA: local anesthesia; CSF: cerebrospinal fluid)

TABLE 6: Timeline of evolution of local anesthetics.

Local anesthetic	Year in which introduced clinically
Cocaine	1884
Procaine	1905
Dibucaine	1930
Tetracaine	1932
Lidocaine	1948
Chloroprocaine	1955
Mepivacaine	1957
Prilocaine	1960
Bupivacaine	1963
Etidocaine	1972
Ropivacaine	1996

Ropivacaine and levobupivacaine, an isomer of bupivacaine, are newer agents with the same duration of action as bupivacaine but with less cardiac toxicity.

The development of plexus blocks and other regional anesthesia techniques progressed to incorporate the use of nerve stimulators and ultrasound to facilitate locating nerves, thus enhancing the quality of the block.

ANESTHETIC AGENTS

Inhalational Anesthetics (Table 7)

Anesthesia Prior to Ether Era

Because the invention of the hypodermic needle did not occur until 1855, the first general anesthetics were destined to be inhalation agents.[1] Agents such as ethyl alcohol, *Cannabis* spp. and opium were inhaled by the ancients for their stupefying effects before surgery. Alchemist and physician Arnold of Villanova used a mixture of opium, mandragora, and henbane to make his patients insensible to pain. In the 1020s inhaled anesthesia was described using a "soporific sponge" soaked in hashish, opium and other herbal aromatics and placed under the nose of the patient. Around 1825 Henry Hickman carried out operations on animals using CO_2 with freedom from pain.[3]

Ether, Chloroform, and Nitrous Oxide Era

Valerius Cordus prepared Ether in 1540s and Crawford W Long and William E Clark used it independently on patients but not published.

TABLE 7: Timeline of inhalational anesthetic agents.[1,6]

Inhalational agent	Event
Nitrous oxide	First prepared in 1772 by Joseph B Priestley, suggested for pain relief and called "laughing gas" by Sir Humphry Davy in 1799, used by Horace Wells in 1844
Ether	First synthesized in 1540s by Valrius Cordus, administered by William Edward Clarke (a chemist and medical student at Berkshire Medical College) for the removal of a tooth, used by Crawford Williamson Long for surgical case in 1842, first successful public demonstration by William Morton in 1846
Chloroform	First prepared in 1831, first used clinically by Professor James Young Simpson of the University of Edinburgh in 1847, administered by John Snow to Queen Victoria for birth of eight child, Prince Leopold in 1853 and in 1857 for the birth of Princess Beatrice
Ethyl chloride	Anesthetic properties first described by Marie Jean Pierre Flourens in France in 1847, popularized in UK as general anesthetic by WJ McCardie after using it for dental anesthesia since 1901 at Birmingham Dental Hospital
Cyclopropane	Discovered by August Freund in 1881. Anesthetic properties discovered in 1929 by Velyien E Henderson at the University of Toronto on animals. Human trials were done by Ralph M Waters and Erwin R Schmidt at University of Wisconsin with results published in JAMA in 1934, introduced commercially in 1936
Trichloro-ethylene (Trilene)	First produced in 1920s when it was used as a solvent for variety of organic materials. Its major use was to extract vegetable oils from plant materials, such as soy, coconut, and palm. From 1935 it was used as an anesthetic. It was also used as an analgesic in dentistry and during labor
Halothane	Developed in 1951; released in 1956
Methoxy-flurane	Developed in 1948; released in 1960
Enflurane	Developed in 1963; released in 1973
Isoflurane	Developed in 1965; released in 1981
Sevoflurane	Developed in 1960; released in 1990
Desflurane	Developed in 1987; released in 1992

(JAMA: Journal of the American Medical Association)

William TG Morton gave public demonstration of general anesthesia by inhalation anesthesia using ether on 16th October 1846.[1]

Chloroform was independently prepared by von Leibig, Guthrie, and Soubeiran in 1831 and first used by Holmes Coote in 1847, and Sir James Simpson administered chloroform for pain relief of labor.

Joseph Priestley produced nitrous oxide in 1772, but Humphry Davy first noted its analgesic properties in 1800. Gardner Colton and Horace Wells first used nitrous oxide as an anesthetic in humans in 1844.

Chloroform initially superseded ether but reports of chloroform-related cardiac arrhythmias, respiratory depression, and hepatotoxicity eventually decreased its use and its discard.

However, in India till 1928, chloroform was the only anesthetic used. In fact, it became synonymous with anesthesia.[3,13]

Post-ether or Post-chloroform Era

The Ethyl chloride and ethylene were first formulated in the eighteenth century. Ethyl chloride was used as a topical anesthetic and counterirritant; it was so volatile that the skin transiently "froze" after ethyl chloride was sprayed on it. Its rediscovery as an anesthetic came in 1894, when a Swedish dentist named Carlson sprayed ethyl chloride into a patient's mouth to "freeze" a dental abscess. Carlson was surprised to discover that his patient suddenly lost consciousness.[4]

The Ethylene gas was the first alternative to ether and chloroform. Arno Luckhardt was the first to publish a clinical study on ethylene gas in February 1923. Within a month, Isabella herb in Chicago and W Easson Brown in Toronto presented two other independent studies. Ethylene was not a successful anesthetic because high concentrations were required and it was explosive. An additional significant shortcoming was a particularly unpleasant smell, which could only be partially disguised by the use of oil of orange or a cheap perfume. When cyclopropane was introduced, ethylene was abandoned.[4]

Cyclopropane's anesthetic action was inadvertently discovered in 1929. The Wisconsin group investigated the drug thoroughly and reported their clinical success in 1934.[4]

To reduce the danger of explosion during the incendiary days of World War II, British anesthetists turned to trichloroethylene.[4]

Modern Inhaled Anesthetics[1]

In twentieth century, the search for an ideal inhaled anesthetic led to the introduction ethyl chloride, ethylene, cyclopropane, trichloroethylene, and other volatile agents. Their disadvantages, such as strong pungency, weak potency, and flammability led to its discard.

The introduction of Fluorinated hydrocarbons made inhaled anesthetics more stable, less combustible, and less toxic.

Halothane was a superior anesthetic over its predecessors. The Methoxyflurane was withdrawn for its dose-related nephrotoxicity. Enflurane had limited use due to cardiovascular depression and seizures. Isoflurane was more difficult to synthesize and purify than enflurane.

Isoflurane, Sevoflurane and Desflurane and addition to nitrous oxide, constitute the mainstay of inhalation anesthetics.[1]

Evolution of Vaporizers

The open drop technique involved using a folded handkerchief with inhalational agent over the patient's face. Handkerchiefs were replaced by masks. These masks were generally open mesh frames that were covered with cloth; ether or chloroform was dropped on to the cloth. Further development of these masks involved a lip to prevent spillage of liquid onto the patient, e.g., a Schimmel Busch mask.

Masks for Inhalation Agents

- Skinner, a general practitioner and obstetrician from Liverpool designed the first wire frame for administration of open drop in 1862, called Skinner mask
- Johannes Esmarch from Germany developed Esmarch ether mask in 1879
- Curt Theodor Schimmel Busch introduced Schimmel Busch mask in 1890s
- Ferguson mask came in 1905
- Yankauer mask with drop bottle was introduced in 1910
- Ochsner mask
- Bellamy Gardner mask.

Vaporizers

The first anesthetics were given from inhalers. Morton gave his ether through a simple inhaler which was nothing more than a glass bottle with attached mouth-piece. A breathing tube was placed in the patient's mouth and valves separated the inspired and expired gases.

Joseph Clover, a British physician, was the first anesthetist to administer chloroform in known concentrations through the "Clover bag." He obtained a 4.5% concentration of chloroform in air by pumping a measured volume of air with a bellows through a warmed evaporating vessel containing a known volume of liquid chloroform.

Inhalers were nothing but primitive models of draw over vaporizers. Continuous flow (plenum) vaporizers were developed in parallel ever since the draw over vaporizers began to replace open-drop methods at the turn of the twentieth century.

Inhalers[7]

- *1847:* Snow ether inhaler invented by John Snow, within 2 weeks of first seeing ether administered in London in December 1846. Snow designed this forerunner of modern vaporizers
- *1856:* John Snow designed a chloroform inhaler

- *1862:* Clovers chloroform inhaler
- *1877:* Clover portable regulating ether inhaler
- *1903:* Vernon Harcourt chloroform inhaler
- *1908:* Ombredanne ether inhaler
- *1908:* Somnoform inhaler
- *1933:* Goldman Vinethene inhaler
- *1940:* Oxford Vinethene inhaler
- *1941:* Epstein, Macintosh, Oxford (EMO) inhaler
- *1947:* Cyprane trilene inhaler
- *1950:* Oxy-Columbus trilene inhaler
- *1952:* Duke trilene inhaler
- *1955:* Drager bar trilene inhaler
- *1968:* Penthrane analgizer.

Draw over Vaporizers

- Rowbotham vaporizer
- Bryce-Smith induction unit
- Triservice anesthesia kit
- Oxford vaporizer, a portable ether inhaler with a temperature regulating device was introduced in 1941 by Epstein, Macintosh and Mendelssohn
- *EMO:* The Epstein, Macintosh, Oxford vaporizer was designed in 1952 by HG Epstein and Sir Robert Macintosh of the Nuffield Department of Anesthetics at the University of Oxford, with the aid of their technician, Richard Salt. It was meant to be used for ether. Upgraded versions were Mark II, Mark III and Mark IV. EMO for trilene was available as "emotril"
- Goldman vaporizer mark I—1952, adapted from Leyland fuel pump by BOC (using technology of other industries, a carburettor used on a petrol engine) to be used for halothane. Upgraded to Mark II and Mark III
- Tecota Mark 6 was manufactured by Cyprane in 1952 and was meant for trilene
- Oxford miniature vaporizer—was introduced by Epstein and Macintosh in 1966. It had dials that could swivel. Depending on the agent that you use, you can select the dial for chloroform, trilene, halothane or methoxyflurane.

Plenum Vaporizers

They developed from simple bubble through or flow over devices often using technology of other industries to devices that could guarantee a constant output over a given range of flow, e.g., the Modern Days' Tec vaporizers which are temperature and flow compensated.

- A Boyle's vaporizing bottle for ether was added in 1920s and that for chloroform (which was later used for trilene) was added in 1926
- The Copper Kettle was the first temperature-compensated, accurate vaporizer. It had been developed by Lucien Morris at the University of Wisconsin in response to Ralph Waters' plan to test chloroform by giving it in controlled concentrations
- *Tec vaporizers:* Fluotec Mark I for halothane came in 1957, later upgraded to Mark 2, Mark 3 and Mark 4. That for isoflurane was known as Isotec and the one for methoxyflurane was known as Pentec. Datex Ohmeda Tec 4, Tec 5 and Tec 7, American Drager Vapor 19n and 20n are agent specific for a given agent. Tec 6 by Ohmeda is meant for desflurane only
- Aladdin cassettes vaporizer by Ohmeda are color coded, agent specific, electronically operated vaporizers in the form of cassettes.

Additional Safety Measures in Modern Day Vaporizers

Agent specific vaporizers with keyed filling system for preventing filling of vaporizer with wrong agent and "select-a-tec" or interlocking mechanism for vaporizer mounting to prevent inadvertent delivery of more than one vaporizing agent at any given time have been introduced as safety mechanisms in the modern-day vaporizers. Also tipping and overfilling has been prevented using modern technologies.

Intravenous Anesthetics (Table 8)

The invention of the hypodermic syringe by Charles Gabriel Pravaz [6] and invention of the hypodermic syringe and needle by Alexander Wood in 1855[1,6] made intravenous anesthesia popular.

The use of barbiturates for induction made a popular technique.[1]

John Lundy and Ralph Waters first used Thiopental, clinically. VK Stoelting used Methohexital for induction of anesthesia. The use of benzodiazepines diazepam (1959), lorazepam (1971) and midazolam (1976) for premedication, induction, supplementation of anesthesia, and IV sedation[1] increased since then.

Stevens synthesized Ketamine and clinically used by Corssen and Domino. Ketamine was the first IV agent associated with minimal respiratory depression.

The Etomidate had to be withdrawn due to reports of adrenal suppression after even a single dose.

The Propofol, was a major advance in outpatient anesthesia because of its short duration of action.[1]

It was the introduction of IV anesthesia with thiopental and later muscle relaxants along with progress in equipment's for airway maintenance, laryngoscopy, endotracheal intubation, ventilation and monitoring that brought about a major revolution in anesthesia practice.

Neuromuscular Blocking Agents

In 1804, animals paralyzed by curare were observed to be capable of surviving if artificially ventilated for a sufficient length of time. Classic description of experiments with curare appeared in 1825. In 1857, Claude Bernard discovered the effects of curare located at the myoneural junction. On January 23, 1942, the drug form of curare, Intocostrin, was

TABLE 8: Evolution of intravenous anesthetic agents and adjuvants.[1-10]

Year	Intravenous agent
1903	Barbiturates were synthesized, diethyl barbituric acid (barbital) was the first barbiturate used for IV induction
1927	Introduction of hexobarbital, first used in 1933
1932	Thiopental, synthesized in 1932 by Ernest H Volwiler, used clinically in 1934 by Ralph M Waters
1957	Methohexital first used clinically for induction
1957	Chlordiazepoxide synthesized
1959	Diazepam synthesized
1960	Diazepam approved for use; used for premedication, induction, supplementation of anesthesia, and intravenous sedation
1960	Fentanyl synthesized
1961	Droperidol discovered
1962	Ketamine synthesized
1964	Propanidid first used
1964	Etomidate synthesized
1970	Ketamine released, fentanyl anesthesia first reported
1971	*Lorazepam:* Used for premedication, induction, supplementation of anesthesia and intravenous sedation
1972	Althesin used for the first time
1972	Etomidate released
1974	Sufentanil synthesized
1975	Etomidate used clinically
1976	*Midazolam:* Used for premedication, induction, supplementation of anesthesia and intravenous sedation
1976	Alfentanil synthesized
1977	Propofol synthesized by JW Dundee et al.
1980	TIVA developed
1989	Propofol released
1996	Remifentanil approved

(TIVA: total intravenous anesthesia; IV: intravenous)

introduced into anesthesia practice by anesthesiologist, Harold R Griffith, and his resident, Enid Johnson, at Montreal Homeopathic Hospital.[1,6]

The facilitation of tracheal intubation and abdominal muscle relaxation produced by intocostrin during cyclopropane anesthesia heralded a new era for development of neuromuscular blocking agents. For the first time, operations could be performed on patients without having to administer relatively large doses of anesthetic to produce muscle relaxation. These large doses of anesthetic often resulted in excessive circulatory and respiratory depression as well as prolonged emergence and they were often not tolerated by frail patients.[1]

Succinylcholine was synthesized by Bovet in 1949 and released in 1951. Other neuromuscular blocking agents gallamine, decamethonium, metocurine, alcuronium, and pancuronium were soon introduced clinically. Because the use of these agents was often associated with significant side effects, the search for the ideal neuromuscular blocking agents (NMBA) continued. Recently introduced agents that come close to this goal include vecuronium, atracurium, pipecuronium, doxacurium, rocuronium, and *cis*-atracurium.[1]

Opioids

Friedrich Sertürner first isolated morphine from opium in 1804. He named it morphine after Morpheus, the Greek God of dreams and subsequently tried as an IV anesthetic. The morbidity and mortality associated with high doses of opioids caused many anesthetists to avoid opioids and use pure inhalation anesthesia.

Interest in opioids in anesthesia returned following the synthesis of meperidine in 1939. The concept of "balanced anesthesia" was introduced in 1926 by Lundy et al. and evolved to consist of thiopental for induction, NO_2 for amnesia, meperidine (or any opioid) for analgesia, and curare for muscle relaxation.

In 1960s, Jannsen Pharmaceutica synthesized fentanyl. Fentanyl was followed by sufentanil (1974), alfentanil (1976), carefentanil (1976), lofentanil (1980) and remifentanil (1996).[5,6]

In 1969, Lowenstein introduced the concept of high doses of opioids as complete anesthetics. Morphine was initially employed, but fentanyl, sufentanil, and alfentanil were all subsequently used as sole agents. As experience grew with this technique, its limitations in reliably preventing patient awareness and suppressing autonomic responses during surgery were realized.

It can be appreciated from the facts mentioned above that in the twentieth century the progress of general anesthesia occurred due to the development of various equipment's and anesthetic drugs. The equipment's allowed the anesthesiologists to deliver combination of inhalational agent with N_2O and O_2 in a controlled manner initially and later with a precise known concentration. Also the anesthesiologists could ventilate the patients whenever the need arose.

ANESTHESIOLOGY AS A MEDICAL SPECIALTY[1-10]

The field of anesthesiology as a recognized medical specialty. Initially lack of formal training in anesthesia and trained anesthetists, the nurses administered anesthesia Ralph Waters, Thomas D Buchanan and John Lundy established anesthesia departments and training programs.

Thomas D Buchanan was appointed the first Professor of Anesthesiology at the New York Medical College in 1904. The American Board of Anesthesiology was established in 1938 with Buchanan as its first president. In England, the first examination for the Diploma in Anesthetics took place in 1935, and the first Chair in Anesthetics was awarded to Sir Robert Macintosh in 1937 at Oxford University **(Table 9)**.

TABLE 9: Timeline of evolution of anesthesiology as a medical specialty.[1,3,6,10]

Year	Event
1893	The Society of Anaesthetists founded in London—the first such body in the world. Initiated by John F Silk of Kings College Hospital. It was not limited to the UK but also included representatives from the US, Canada, Australia, South Africa and Switzerland
1905	Long Island Society of Anaesthetists founded
1911	Long Island Society of Anaesthetists became the New York Society of Anesthetists
1922	The first edition of "Anesthesia and Analgesia" was published under the auspices of the International Anesthesia Research Society. Edited by Francis McMechan, this became the first dedicated journal of anesthesia
1923	The British Journal of Anaesthesia (BJA) founded
1927	Ralph Waters established first anesthesiology postgraduate training program at the University of Wisconsin-Madison
1932	Association of Anaesthetists of Great Britain and Ireland (AAGBI) founded
1934	Australian Society of Anesthetists founded
1935	Diploma in Anaesthetics (DA) examinations introduced in Great Britain
1936	New York Society of Anesthetists became the American Society of Anesthetists
1937	Macintosh first European chair of anaesthesia
1938	The American Board of Anesthesiology (ABA) founded
1943	The Canadian Anesthesiologists' Society founded (originally called Canadian Anesthetists' Society, founded in 1920s and subsumed into the section on Anesthesia of the Canadian Medical Association in 1928)
1945	American Society of Anesthetists became the American Society of Anesthesiologists (ASA)
1946	"Anaesthesia", the journal of the AAGBI first published
1947	Faculty of Anaesthetists of the Royal College of Surgeons of England is founded
1948	National Health Service is established in Great Britain. Negotiation by the AAGBI ensured that anaesthetists received consultant status
1952	The Faculty of Anesthetists of the Royal Australasian College of Surgeons founded
1953	Fellowship of the Faculty of Anaesthetists of the Royal College of Surgeons (FFARCS) examinations introduced. These became the Fellow of the College of Anaesthetists (FCAnaes) examinations in 1989 and Fellow of the Royal College of Anaesthetists (FRCA) examinations in 1992
1954	The Society of Anaesthetists of Hong Kong founded
1955	World Federation of Societies of Anesthesiologists (WFSA) founded
1955	The BJA, the second oldest journal of anaesthesia, was the first to be published monthly
1972	The Australian Society of Anaesthetists commenced publishing its "Anaesthesia and Intensive Care" journal
1982	United Kingdom Resuscitation Council formed
1985	Anesthesia Patient Safety Foundation (APSF) established
1986	Standards for basic anesthesia monitoring approved by the ASA House of Delegates
1988	College of Anaesthetists founded replacing the Faculty of Anaesthetists of the Royal College of Surgeons of England
1989	Hong Kong College of Anaesthesiologists founded
1990	BJA became the journal of the College of Anaesthetists
1993	Faculty of Intensive Care (FIC) of the Australian and New Zealand College of Anaesthetists (ANZCA) founded
1993	ANZCA's Faculty of Intensive Care founded

CONCLUSION

Development in anesthesia took place simultaneously as well as independently in different parts of the world. It is difficult to compile everything. But it can be said that scientific discoveries in the late eighteenth and early nineteenth centuries lead to the development of modern anesthetic techniques. An attempt is made in this review to include most of the important developments with their timeline that helped the anesthesiologists to practice anesthesia today with great safety for the patients' lives and the ease of administration for the anesthesiologists.

REFERENCES

1. Morgan E, Mikhail MS, Murray MJ. The practice of anesthesiology. In: Morgan E, Mikhail MS, Murray MJ (Eds). Clinical Anesthesiology, 5th edition. New York: The McGraw-Hill Medical Companies Inc.; 2013
2. Medical Discoveries. Anesthetics. [online] Available from http://www.discoveriesinmedicine.com/A-An/Anesthetics.html#ixzz2o5aVnXqD. [Last accessed March, 2014].
3. New Zealand Society of Anaesthetists. (2006). The History of Anaesthesia, extract from material prepared by Society member Dr Andrew Warmington, 2006, for the paper Anaesthesia I in Diploma in Applied Science (Anaesthesia Technology) for AUT University, Auckland. [online] Available from http://www.anaesthesia.org.nz/public/history-anaesthesia. [Last accessed March, 2014].
4. Barash PG, Cullen BF, Stoelting RK, et al. Chapter 1: The history of anaesthesia. In: Clinical Anesthesia, 7th edition. Philadelphia: Lippincott Williams & Wilkins; 2013.
5. Wikipedia. (2012). History of general anesthesia. [online] Available from http://en.wikipedia.org/wiki/History_of_general_anesthesia#cite_note-Corrsen1966-117. [Last accessed March, 2014].
6. Cammack R. Timeline of some significant events in the evolution/history of anaesthesia, an ongoing project; 2012.
7. Shephard DAE, Chalklin J, Pope F. An exhibit of inhalers and vaporizers (1847–1968): illustrating aspects of the evolution of inhalation anesthesia and analgesia from ether to methoxyflurane. Artifacts from the Canadian Anesthesiologists' Society Archives, Ottawa; 2003.
8. Florida International University. (2012). History of Anesthesia: a timeline through the ages 4004 BC–2000 AD. [online] Available from http://chua2.fiu.edu/Nursing/anesthesiology/courses/Semester%203/ngr%206760%20ane%20prof%20aspects/prof%20study%20guide/anesthesia%20history%20timeline.pdf. [Last accessed March, 2014].
9. Wikipedia. History of neuraxial anesthesia. [online] Available from http://en.wikipedia.org/wiki/History_of_neuraxial_anesthesia. [Last accessed March, 2014].
10. History of Anaesthesia Society (2011). Timeline of important dates and events in the development of anaesthesia. [online] Available from www.histansoc.org.uk. [Last accessed March, 2014].
11. Dräger: Technology for Life. (1970). The history of anaesthesia at Dräger. [online] Available from www.draeger India, www.draeger.net/media. [Last accessed March, 2014].
12. Wikipedia. Ivan Magill. [online] Available from http://en.wikipedia.org/wiki/Ivan_Magill. [Last accessed March, 2014].
13. Divekar VM, Naik LD. Evolution of anaesthesia in India. J Postgrad. 2001;47:149-52.

Anesthesia Equipment in India: A Historical Perspective

Vasumathi M Divekar

"The farther we look back, the further we can see."
—Winston Churchill

ABSTRACT

Pain relief for surgery is more than 2-millennia-old in India, from Sushruta and Ayurvedic practices to date. The modern era started with the introduction of ether in United States. An attempt has been made to mention all the equipment, apparatus, vaporizers, and ventilators as they were introduced in India.

INTRODUCTION

The advent of modern anesthesia was a medical revolution which made possible painless surgery. Besides, it is one of the factors for the development of stupendous advances in surgery, intensive care, acute and chronic pain relief. The basic factors responsible for these advances are the introduction of various new drugs and equipment. In India, we have both the latest equipment as well as some of the old ones still in use in different centers.

ANCIENT INDIA

Surgery and pain medications were prevalent in India since 2,500 years. Primitive means of making patient unconscious was by a knock on the head **(Fig. 1)**. The first event in the "chronology of events in anesthesia" in the world is of Sushruta of ancient India in Takshashila now near Islamabad in Pakistan **(Fig. 2)**. He performed eye surgery and is still remembered for median forehead flap for cut nose. Patients were sedated with concoction of opium and vapors of hemp from metal and earthen containers. There is a reference by Raja Bhoj (527 AD) of surgery on himself where he was given concoctions of herbs for pain relief called Sammohini for induction and Sanjivani for recovery. During the Muslim reign alcohol was widely used **(Fig. 3)** for pain relief.

NINETEENTH CENTURY

Modern anesthesia first started in India on March 22, 1847 (5 months after Morton's first administration of ether on October 16, 1846 in Boston, USA). It was administered on a handkerchief in Calcutta Medical College and Hospital **(Fig. 4)**. The first chloroform anesthesia was administered on January 12, 1848 in Calcutta (first administered on November 15, 1847 in Edinburgh by Dr Simpson, an obstetrician). Hyderabad is credited with the great anesthesia research of 19th century by Edward Lawrie to prove the safety of chloroform **(Fig. 5)**. The British Medical Association proposed the research program and it was funded by the Nizam of Hyderabad. Experiments were carried out on 430 animals (dogs, monkeys, horses, goats, rats, rabbits, cats, and humans). The device used was "the Hyderabad cone" used in Britain also at that time **(Fig. 6)**.

The first endotracheal anesthesia was in 1880 by McReddie for osteosarcoma of hard palate in Calcutta. Hypodermic morphine by syringe was first used in Calcutta by Alexander Crombie for premedication (the first report in the world confirmed by Gwathmey and Miller, Ind Med Gaz. 1888. 23, 34). In the early 1900s, Flagg's metal can was used. This was modified into a bottle in 1929—the KEM bottle with a cap and two holes **(Fig. 7)**.

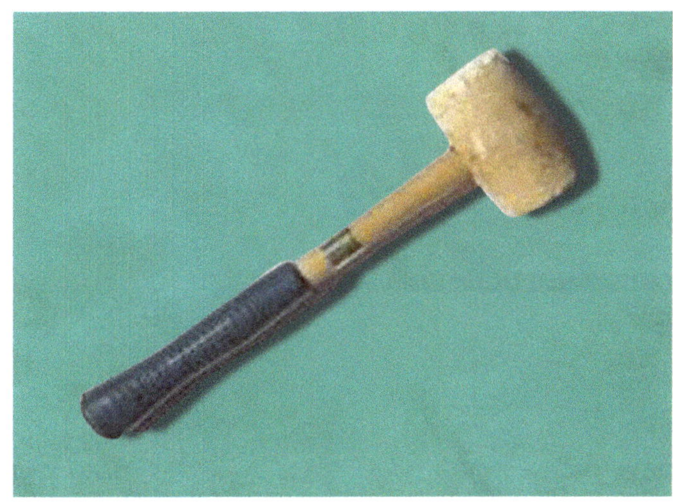

Fig. 1: The hammer used to knock the patient unconscious.

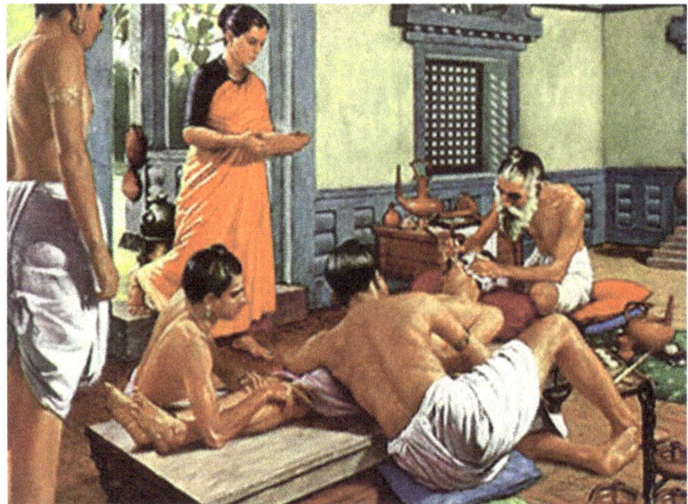

Fig. 2: Sage Sushruta performing surgery around 2000 BC.

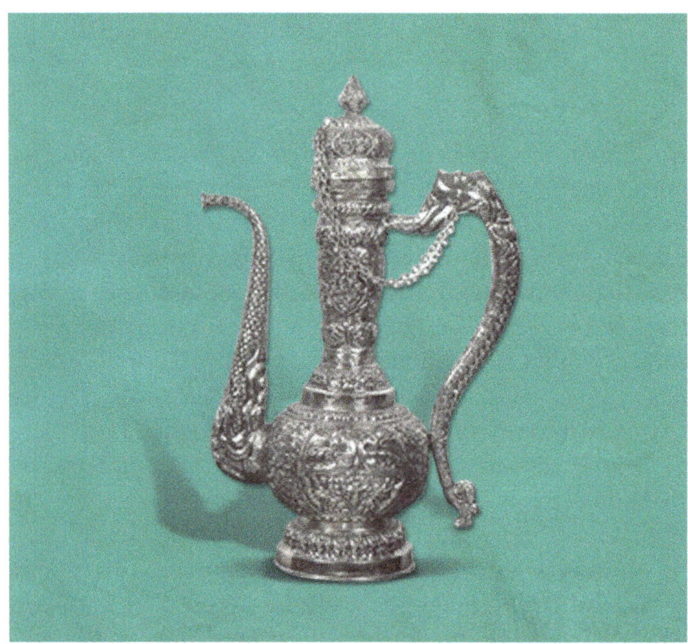

Fig. 3: The pitcher used for dispensing alcohol in the 15th century.

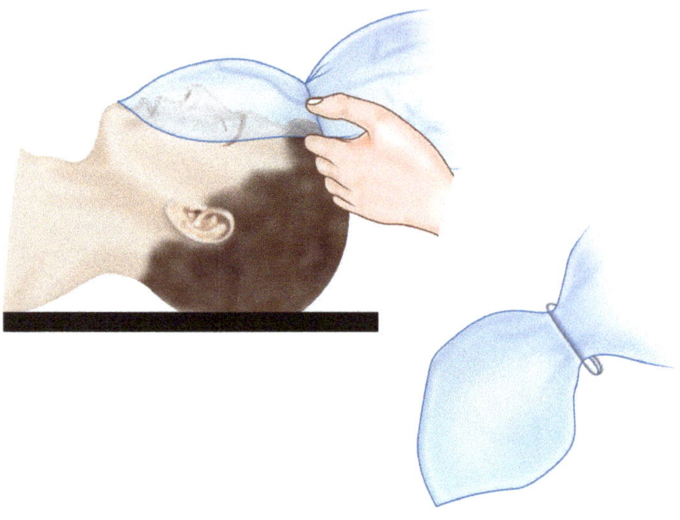

Fig. 4: A handkerchief corner used as a mask for ether administration in Calcutta.

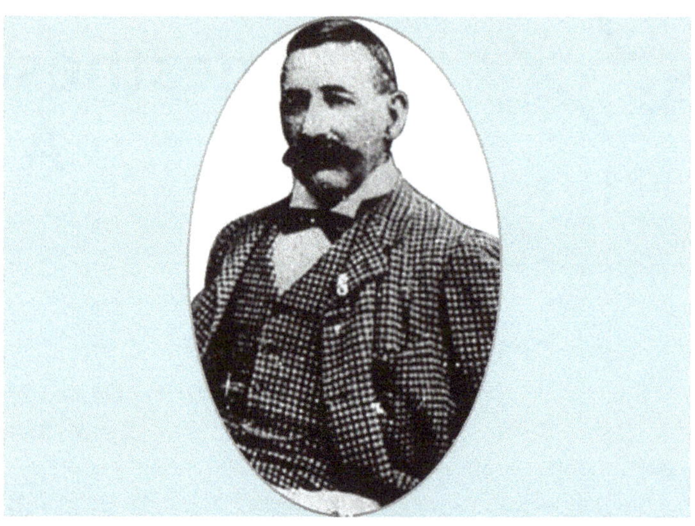

Fig. 5: Edward Lawrie of Hyderabad Chloroform Commission.

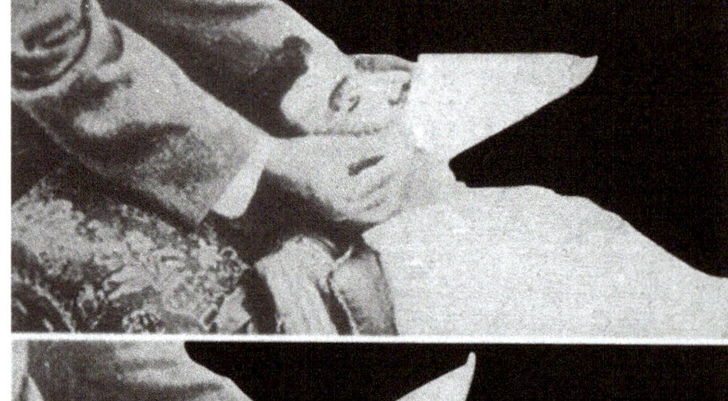

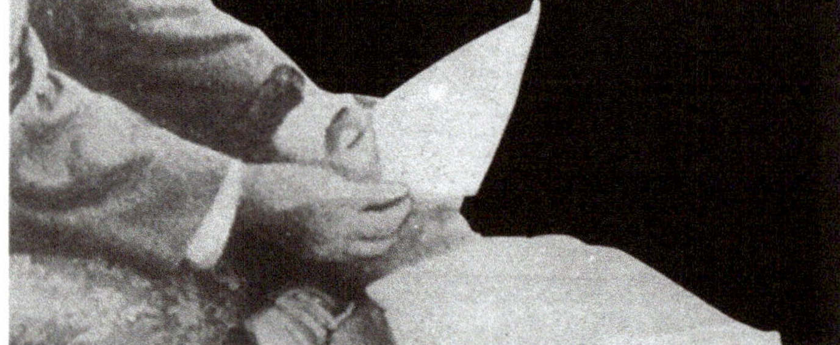

Fig. 6: The Hyderabad cone for administering chloroform.

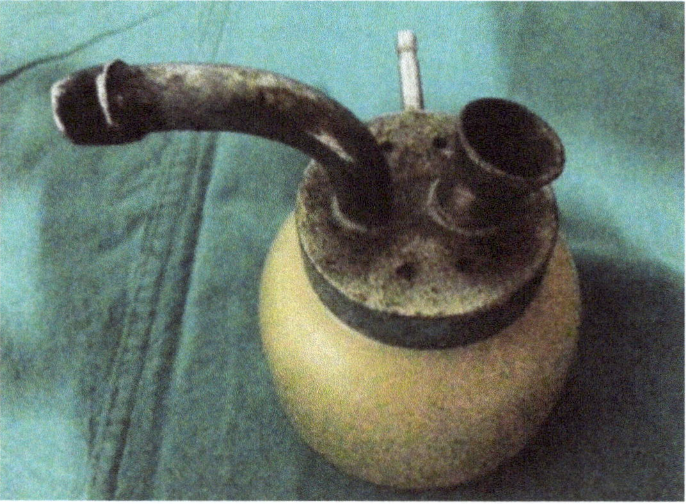

Fig. 7: The KEM bottle—an indigenous adaptation of the Flagg's can.

MACHINES AND GASES

On January 22, 1935, the first Boyle's apparatus arrived in Calcutta from England, it did not have pressure reducing valve, only adjustment valves and water sight feed bottle meter for ether vaporization and a two-way stopcock for rebreathing and nonrebreathing. It also included the Shipway's carbon dioxide (CO_2) absorption apparatus with four cylinders of oxygen (O_2) and nitrous oxide (N_2O) **(Fig. 8)**. The cost of apparatus, including delivery charges was ₹645. The gases were imported from England which took 3 months to replace.

The first O_2 producing plant was installed by BOC India Ltd. in Calcutta in 1935. Nitrous oxide was imported from England by ship till 1962. The first O_2 pipeline was installed in Vellore in 1954 and by 1979 over 150 centers had the piped O_2. Liquid O_2 was introduced in 1980 in Metro cities.

The first indigenous Boyle "F" wheeled out of Indian Oxygen Co. of Calcutta in 1950 with imported parts **(Fig. 9)**. By 1956, it was entirely manufactured in India except the cylinders. The Epstein Macintosh and Oxford (EMO) draw-over vaporizer **(Figs. 10A and B)** was used after the 2nd world war. Subsequently, the Oxford Miniature Vaporizer was devised with interchangeable agent specific percentages by Penlon, widely marketed in India **(Fig. 11)**.

During the first Indo-Pak war in 1965 the Porta Boyle **(Fig. 12)** was developed, as well as an indigenous draw-over vaporizer.

For use on the war front an "Air-Trilene apparatus" **(Fig. 13)** was devised with feedback from Dr Nawathe of Mumbai.

Ventilators

In 1945, Lord Nuffield of Oxford, a car magnate who had his tooth extracted under anesthesia by Professor Mackintosh was hailed as a benefactor to the anesthesia fraternity for two reasons. One was for instituting a chair in anesthesia

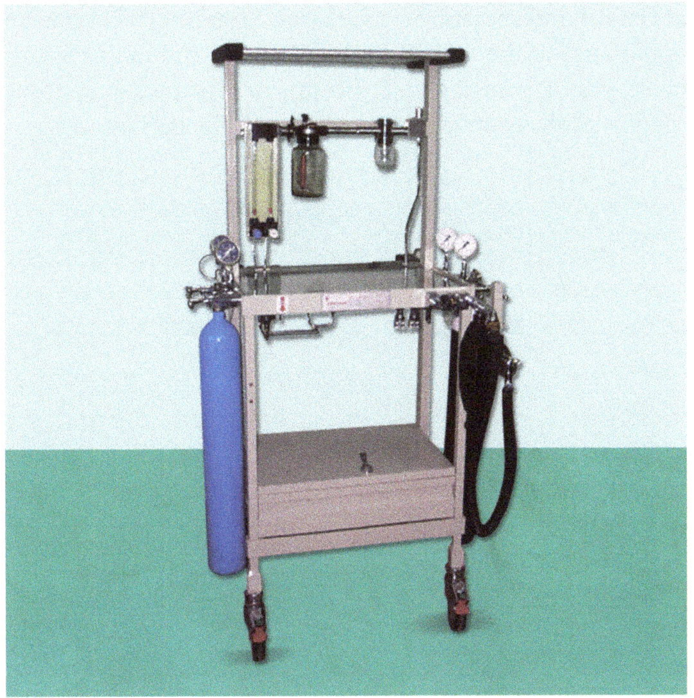

Fig. 9: Prototype of the first anesthesia apparatus manufactured in Calcutta in 1935.

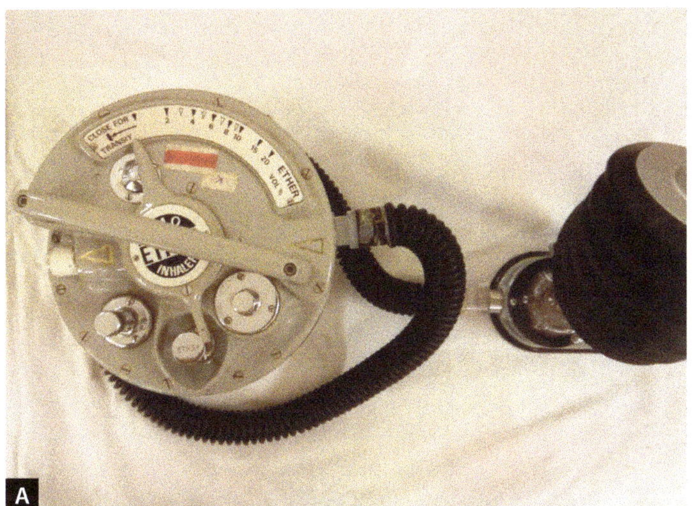

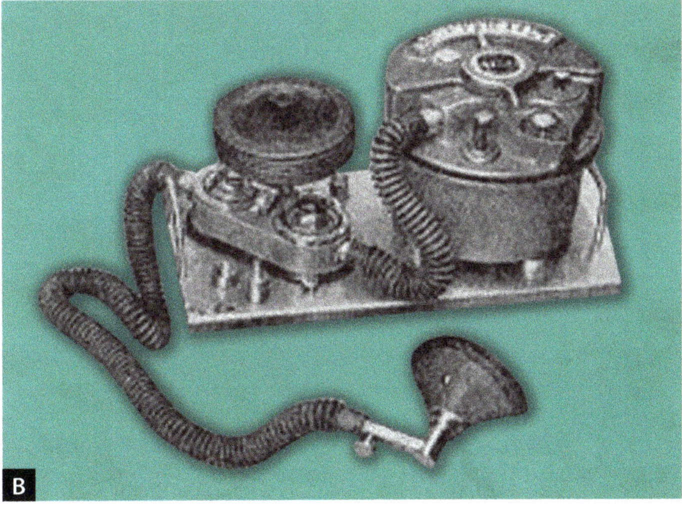

Figs. 10A and B: The Epstein Macintosh Oxford vaporizer and circuit.

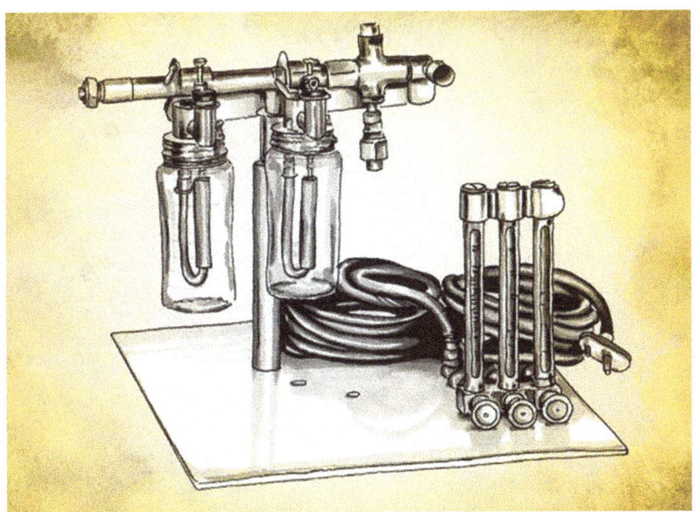

Fig. 8: One of the first Boyle apparatus imported into India.

at Oxford and secondly for donating "iron lungs" (Drinker's apparatus) to the Armed Forces Hospital and major Metro cities—KEM Hospital, JJ Group of Hospitals, Madras Medical College and Calcutta Medical College **(Fig. 14)**.

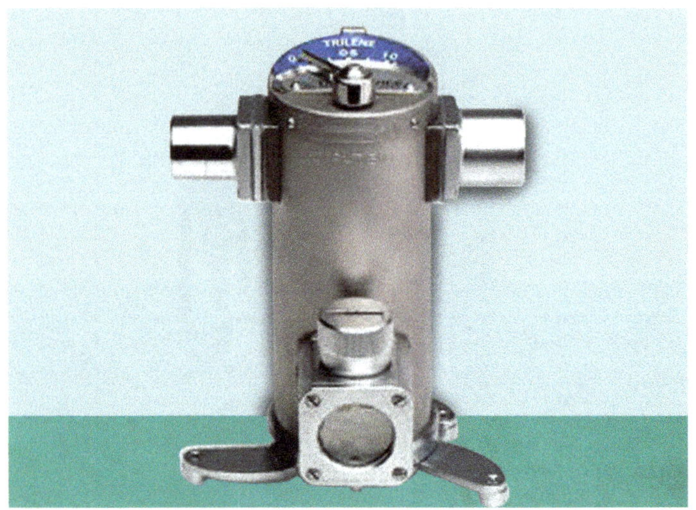

Fig. 11: The Oxford Miniature Vaporizer.

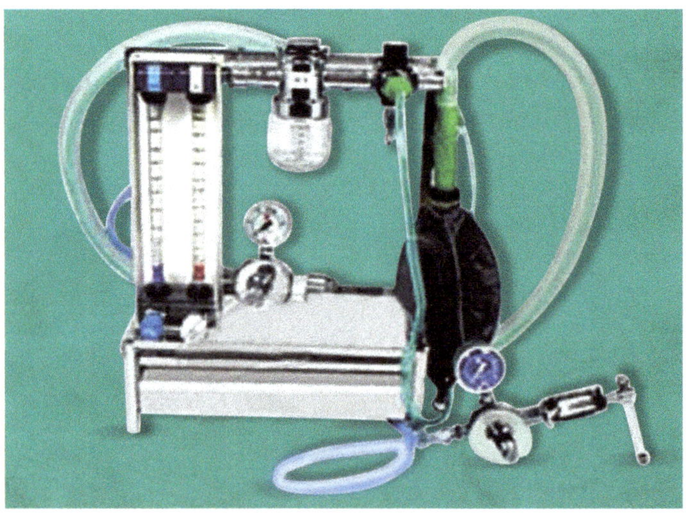

Fig. 12: The Porta Boyle.

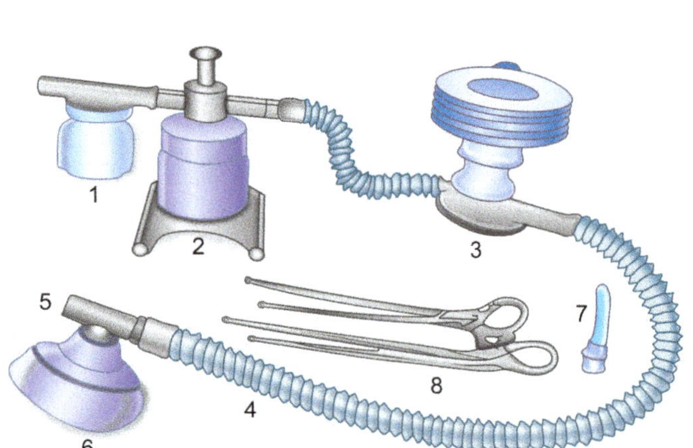

Fig. 13: Air trilene draw-over vaporizer and circuit (Rao's apparatus).

Occasionally, "Dog-pumps" were used in experimental surgery at KEM and Nair Hospitals **(Fig. 15)**. The "Beaver" and "Bird Mark 7" **(Figs. 16 and 17)** ventilators were introduced in 1960. Attempts were made to manufacture

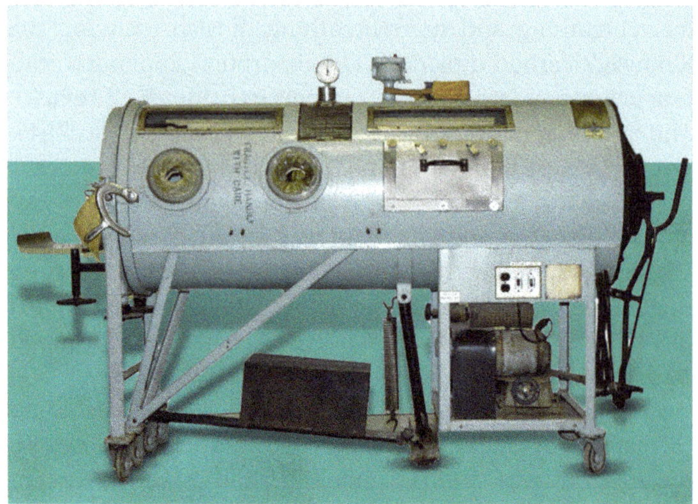

Fig. 14: The iron-lung—Drinker's apparatus.

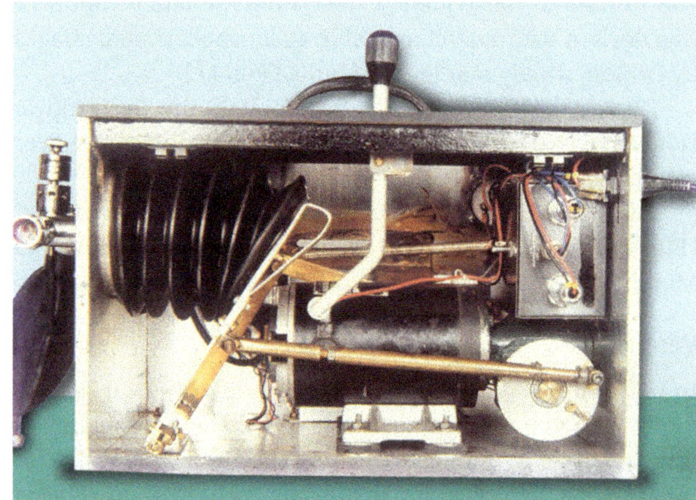

Fig. 15: The dog pump.

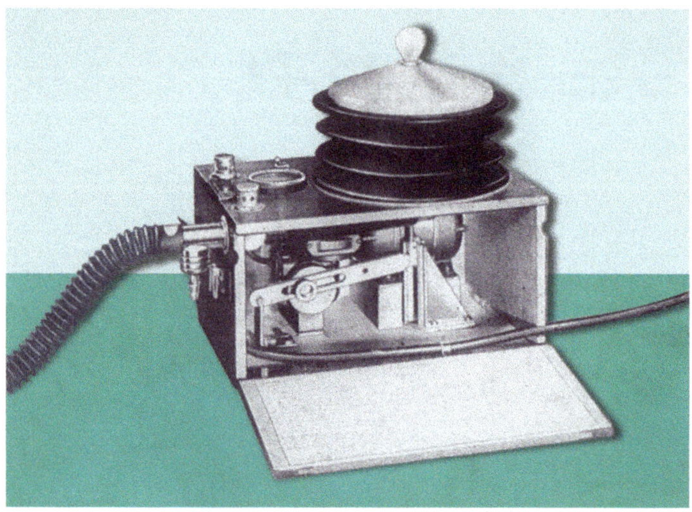

Fig. 16: The Beaver respirator.

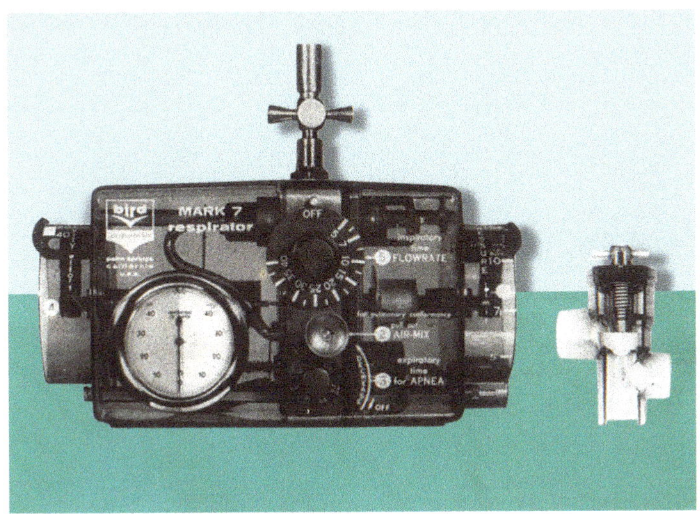

Fig. 17: The bird mark 7 ventilator and expiratory-valve assembly.

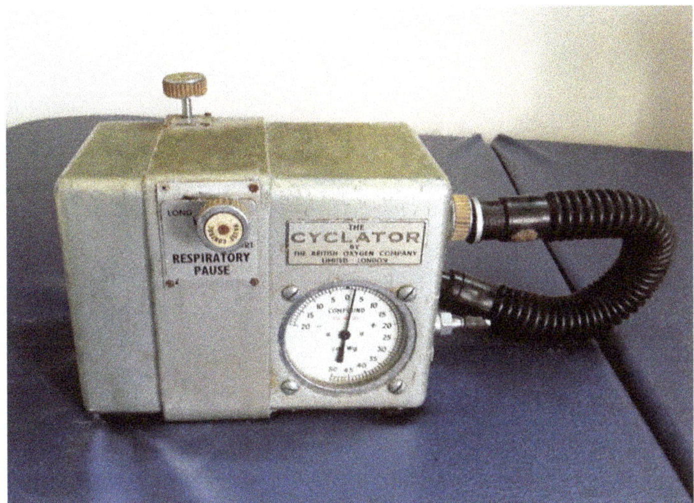

Fig. 18: The cyclator ventilator—the first with a trigger in India.

triggered ventilators in 1970 without success. The "Cyclator" was the first triggered ventilator to be used in anesthesia and postoperative ventilation **(Fig. 18)**.

The first single channel "Cardioscope" was introduced in 1960 for use in cardiac surgery. Pulse oximeters and end-tidal CO_2 were first introduced in mid-1980s in India.

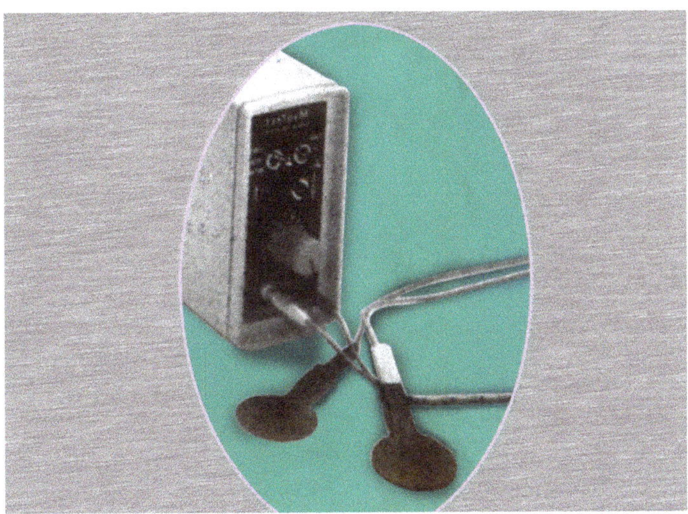

Fig. 19: The Wellcome nerve stimulator.

Neuromuscular monitoring was first introduced in 1968 in India by Wellcome Laboratories in Mumbai **(Fig. 19)** and other Metros with only single and tetanic stimulation.

CONCLUSION

In India, about a century and a half of anesthesiology, the youngest specialty in medicine from the days of Sushruta to the modern era shows that India had a major and important role in this field of medicine.

BIBLIOGRAPHY

1. Anesthesia and Intensive Care. 1999;27:110.
2. Divekar VM. A Historical Perspective, Souvenir, The Golden Jubilee Year - Indian Society of Anaesthetists; 1997.
3. Eckenhoff JE. Anesthesia from Colonial Times: A History of Anesthesia at the University of Pennsylvania, 1st edition. Philadelphia: JB Lippincott Co.; 1966.
4. Keys TE. The History of Surgical Anesthesia, New York, Schuman: Dover Publications; 1945. Chronicle of events 4004 BC to 1944. pp. 111, 113.
5. Sally Graham. Personal Communication. Park Ridge, Illinois: Wood Library-Museum of Anesthesiology.
6. Souvenir—Centenary of the Afzalganj Hospital and Diamond Jubilee Osmania Hospital, Hyderabad, March 1988.
7. Souvenir—III Joint Indo-US Anesthesiology—update cum workshop; 1994. p. 15.
8. Sushruta Samhita—Ayurveda 500 BC.

Role of Physical Principles

SECTION 2

Utility of Physical Principles in Anesthetic Practice

Aparna S Budhakar, Shashank A Budhakar

ABSTRACT

Concept of pressure needs to be understood by the anesthetist. It is measured by various devices depending upon the range of pressure measured. The gas laws help us predict behavior of gases whenever there is a change in temperature and pressure. Flow can be laminar or turbulent. Laminar flow becomes turbulent when it is flowing at a high velocity, in large diameter tubes and when the fluids are relatively dense. Solubility is the ability of a substance to dissolve. The amount of a gas, which dissolves in a liquid, is directly proportional to the partial pressure of the gas in equilibrium with the liquid. Understanding of blood/gas partition coefficient and oil/gas partition coefficient are important. Diffusion of a fluid depends on various factors.

INTRODUCTION

Understanding of physical principles is very important, since it gives us in-depth understanding of not only anesthetic machine and equipment but also physics applicable to behavior of gases and liquids. Simple anesthesia machines have now been replaced with anesthesia workstations. It is necessary to understand their working principles. This understanding helps us to be a better and safer anesthetist.

This chapter will be covering common physical principles applicable to anesthesia practice. Since this book deals with equipment and has individual chapters on different equipment and monitors, duplication of their physics is avoided. We have tried to simplify this topic and explained with examples wherever possible. Readers are requested to go through dedicated books on physics for anesthetist for further understanding.

PRESSURE

Knowledge of pressure is very important to anesthetist. Understanding the various concepts of pressure is a necessity. Vacuum is a space where there is zero pressure. We do not find vacuum routinely. At sea level, the pressure of air surrounding us is 1 atm. Pressure is defined as force acting per unit area (P = f/a). Pressure is measured in various units. In SI system, pressure is measured in Pascal (Pa) where 1 Pa is a pressure of 1 N acting over an area of 1 m^2. Since 1 Pa represents a tiny pressure, it is more commonly represented as kilopascal (kPa). There are several units used to measure pressure as shown in **Table 1**.

RELATION BETWEEN PRESSURE AND FORCE

In clinical practice, we often use different capacity of syringes to inject medicine intravenously. The knowledge of interrelationship of pressure and force helps us prevent generation of excessive pressures, which may cause extravasation of medicines. Consider injecting medicine with a 2 mL and 20 mL syringe.[1] If the force of injection is the same, since the area and pressure are inversely proportional to each other (P = f/a), the pressure generated is high in a 2 mL syringe **(Fig. 1)**. Hence, care should be taken when injecting through small volume syringes. Even while injecting medicine during an intravenous

TABLE 1: Pressure conversion table.

	atm	*kg/cm²*	*bar*	*psi*	*kPa*	*cmH₂O*	*mm Hg*
atm	1	1.033	1.013	14.7	101.325	1,034	760
kg/cm²	0.968	1	0.980	14.22	98.067	1,001	735.6
bar	0.987	1.02	1	14.504	100	1,021	750.1
psi	0.068	0.070	0.068	1	6.895	70.38	51.715
kPa	0.009	0.010	0.01	0.145	1	10.207	7.5
cmH₂O	0.0009	0.001	0.0009	0.014	0.098	1	0.735
mm Hg	0.001	0.001	0.001	0.019	0.133	1.36	1

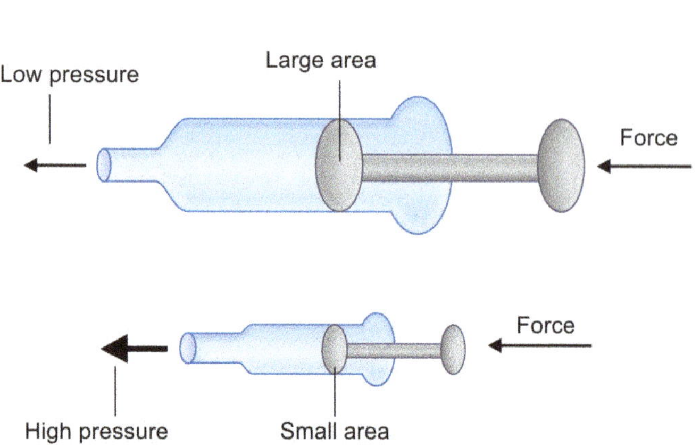

Fig. 1: Relationship between pressure and force.

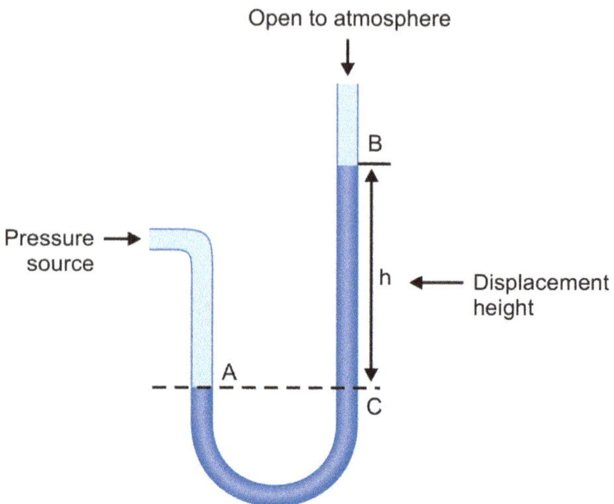

Fig. 2: Manometer.

regional anesthesia with a 20 mL syringe, the pressure generated can be as high as 120 mm Hg.

Pressure Measuring Devices

At sea level, all objects are subjected to 1 atm. All pressure measurements are done keeping this (1 atm) as a zero point, and hence they are called relative pressures (also known as gauge pressure).

Manometer

This is a simplest way of measuring pressure. The pressure is simply measured by vertical displacement of the liquid in the manometer tube. The measuring pressure source is applied at one end and the other end is kept open to atmosphere. The displacement is also dependent on the density of the liquid. Such manometer is routinely used to measure blood pressure (where mercury is used as a liquid) and also while measuring central venous pressure (where saline is used as a liquid) **(Fig. 2)**.

Bourdon Tube Gauge

When higher pressures are required to be measured like pressures in gas cylinder, simple manometer cannot be used. These higher pressures can be measured using a Bourdon tube gauge. This was devised by French industrialist Eugene Bourdon. It consists of semicircular hollow tube. One end of it is sealed while at the other end, a pressure source is applied. Depending on the pressure of the source, the hollow tube extends outward at the sealed end moving the pointer attached to it over a calibrated dial **(Fig. 3)**.

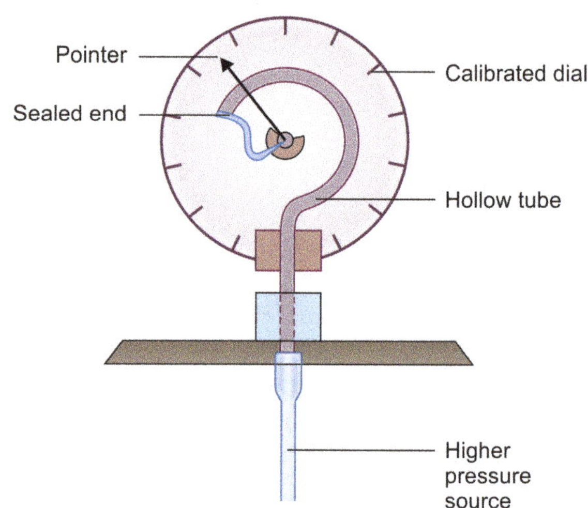

Fig. 3: Bourdon tube gauge.

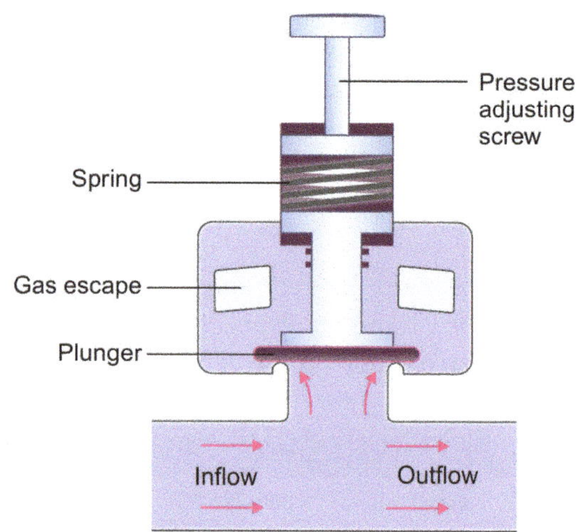

Fig. 4: Pressure relief valve.

Pressure Relief Valve

As the name suggests, these valve relieves the excess pressure beyond a specific limit to which it is set. They are available in the anesthesia circuits as well as on workstations. Since they prevent excess pressure build up, they are also known as safety valves. **Figure 4** shows typical layout of pressure relief valve. Spring is attached to a plunger, which prevents escape of air in a closed position. The spring tension can be varied to maintain a set amount of pressure in the system. When that pressure is exceeded in the system the plunger is lifted up and it allows escape of the gas thus maintaining the pressure to prevent damage. This type of valve is also called a nonreturn valve, since the gas is expelled in the surrounding.

Pressure Regulator Valves

These types of valves do the work of reducing a high pressure to a low pressure, and hence, they are also called pressure-reducing valves.

Figure 5 illustrates the component of a typical pressure-reducing valve. In this, the spring is also attached to a piston with a bulbous end, which passes through a valve that controls gas supply. The required pressure can be set by the adjusting screw to maintain spring tension over the piston. This allows the gas to pass through the valve, so that the outflow is maintained. Depending on the requirement of the outflow gas, the pressure in the chamber can be maintained at a narrow range. Thus, the high pressure in the cylinder does not reach the outflow end preventing damage (barotrauma).

Two-stage Pressure Regulator

The good example of this type of regulator is the Entonox® valve. The first stage of pressure reduction is same as the one-stage pressure regulator; the outflow of this is passed into the second regulator valve.

THE GAS LAWS

The gas laws help us predict behavior of gases whenever there is a change in temperature and pressure.

So lets define gas first. A gas is a substance that is in gaseous phase above its critical temperature. Critical temperature is the temperature above which a gas cannot be liquefied no matter how high the pressure. A vapor in contrast is a substance in the gaseous phase, but is below its critical temperature.

"Boyle's law" states that at constant temperature, the volume of a given mass of gas varies inversely with the absolute pressure (at constant T, $V \propto 1/P$ or $PV = k_1$), e.g., if a gas is forced in smaller cylinder from larger cylinder, pressure inside the smaller cylinder will be much higher than larger cylinder.

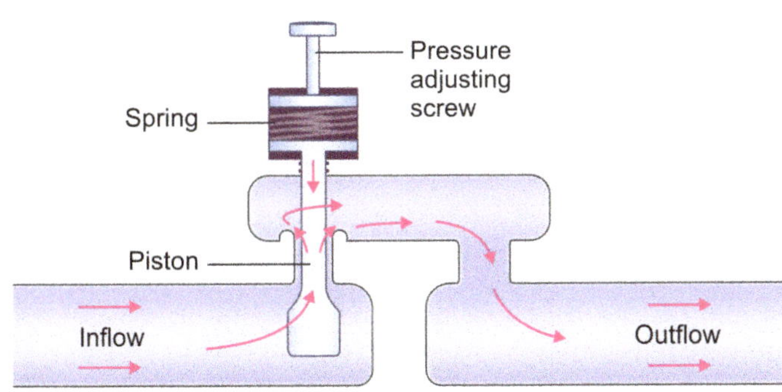

Fig. 5: Pressure regulator valve.

"Charles' law" states that at constant pressure, the volume of a given mass of gas varies directly with the absolute temperature (at constant P, $V \propto T$ or $V/T = k_2$), e.g., gases expand when they are heated and become less dense, thus hot air rises.

"The third perfect gas law (Gay-Lussac's law)" states that at constant volume, the absolute pressure of a given mass of gas varies directly with the absolute temperature (at constant V, $P \propto T$ or $P/T = k_3$). For this reason, gas cylinders should be filled keeping in mind ambient temperature of storage. If temperature in storage place is high, the pressure inside the cylinder will increase leading to explosion.

The Combined Gas Law

It is the combination of all the gas laws:

$$PV = k_1 \quad V/T = k_2 \quad P/T = k_3$$

Therefore,

$$PV/T = \text{Constant}$$

The combined gas law states that product of pressure and volume is proportional to the absolute temperature ($PV \propto T$).

"Avogadro's law" states that equal volume of gases, at the same temperature and pressure, contain the same number of molecules.

If Avogadro's law is applied to combined gas law, it gives "universal" gas law.

$$PV = nRT$$

Where, n = the number of moles of the gas

R = the universal gas constant (8.31 JK^{-1}).

The practical application of this law is the use of pressure gauges to assess the contents of a cylinder. If the volume, temperature and gas constant remain the same then pressure is proportional to n, the number of moles.

"Dalton's law of partial pressures" states that in a mixture of gases, the pressure exerted by each gas is the same as that which it would exert if it alone occupied the container. That means the total pressure in a gas mixture is the sum of the partial pressure of each individual gas **(Fig. 6)**.

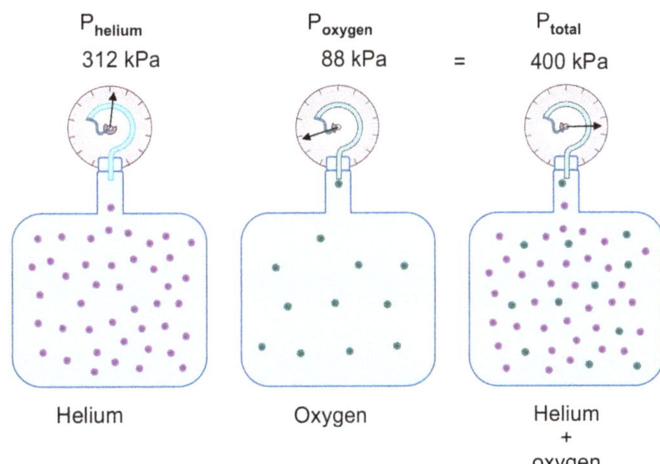

Fig. 6: Dalton's law of partial pressure.

So if a cylinder of gas mixture at 400 kPa contains 21% oxygen and 79% helium, then if the oxygen existed on its own it would exert a partial pressure of 21% of 400 kPa = 88 kPa. The helium, therefore, exerts a partial pressure of 400 - 88 = 312 kPa.

FLOW

Flow is defined as the quantity of a fluid passing a point in unit time.

Flow Types

Flow can be described as laminar or turbulent.

Laminar Flow

In a laminar flow, the molecules of the fluid move in numerous "layers" or laminae. There are no eddies or turbulence. Laminar flow is generally seen in smooth tubes and at low flow rates. The velocity of flow is highest at center compared to periphery **(Fig. 7)**. Generally, flow through cannula and endotracheal tube (ETT) is laminar.

For flow to occur, there must be pressure difference between ends of tube. Flow across the tube also depends on diameter of tube, length of tube and viscosity of fluid.

Tube diameter: If the diameter of the tube is halved, the flow through it reduces to 1/16. This means that flow is directly proportional to d.[2] That is why fluid flows rapidly through 16 G cannula compared to 22 G. Also small size ETT may cause a tremendous decrease in the flow of gases.[3]

Length: If the length is doubled the flow is halved; therefore, flow is inversely proportional to the length of the tube. Therefore, fluid flows slowly through central line compared to peripheral cannula.

Viscosity: This is a measure of the frictional forces acting between the layers of the fluid as it flows along the tube. As the viscosity increases the flow decreases proportionally, thus flow and viscosity are inversely proportional. Therefore, it is often seen that increased viscosity increases risk of vascular occlusion.[4] This relationship between flow and factors affecting flow is represented by the "Hagen-Poiseuille" equation:

$$Q = \pi P d^4 / 128\, \eta l$$

where, Q = flow, P = pressure across the tube, d = diameter of the tube, η = viscosity, l = length of the tube, π/128 = constant.

Turbulent Flow

In a turbulent flow, fluid no longer flows in steady manner. There is formation of eddy currents. This happens when fluid is flowing at a high velocity, in large diameter tubes and when the fluids are relatively dense. In turbulent flow, the flow rate is proportional to the square root of the pressure gradient. This means that to double the flow, the pressure across the tube must be quadrupled **(Fig. 8)**.

Reynolds Number

Reynolds number tells us about the point at which flow changes from laminar to turbulent.

$$\text{Reynolds number} = v\, \rho\, d / \eta$$

Where, v = velocity, ρ = density, d = diameter, η = viscosity

If Reynolds number is less than 2,000, flow is laminar. If Reynolds number is more than 2,000, flow is turbulent. Whenever there is narrowing or sharp bend in tubing, velocity of fluid increases leading to turbulent flow. That is why it is important that breathing system should have gradual bends and no narrowing. Since density plays important role in turbulent flow, helium in oxygen can be used in patient with airway obstruction to reduce extent of turbulent flow (oxygen density—1.3, helium density—0.16). In rotameter at low flow rate gas flow is laminar, and hence, the viscosity of the gas is important. But at high flows, the diameter of the rotameter becomes greater where the space between bobbin and rotameter wall acts like orifice. So at this point, the density of the gas is important.[3] This property of gas is kept in mind while calibrating individual rotameter.

Bernoulli's Principle

Bernoulli's principle shows that as fluid passes through constriction, there is an increase in velocity of the fluid, as the total energy must remain constant, the potential energy falls.

Venturi Effect

This is the consequence of the Bernoulli's principle described previously. The pressure drop induced by the increase in velocity of a fluid passing through a narrow orifice can be used to entrain air, e.g., Venturi masks, nebulizers, and suction apparatus **(Fig. 9)**.

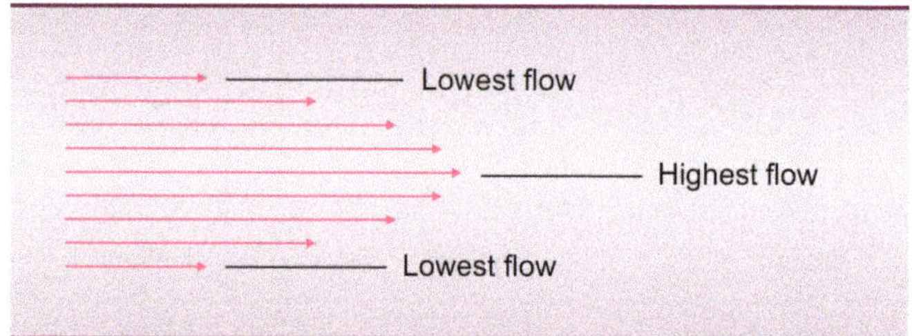

Fig. 7: Laminar flow.

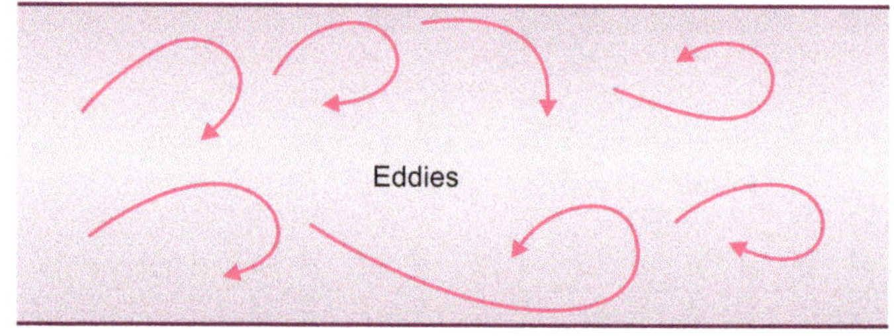

Fig. 8: Turbulent flow.

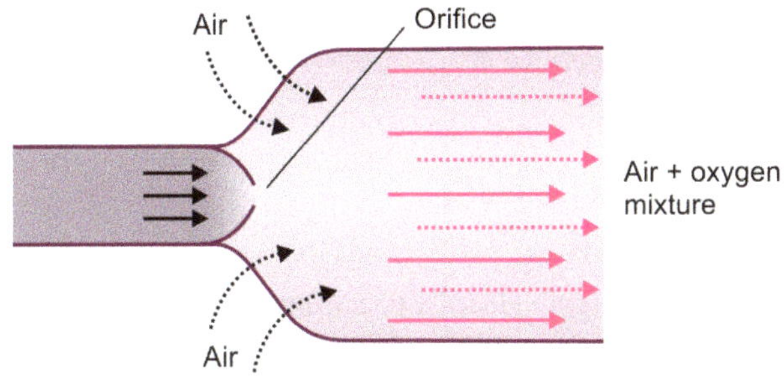

Fig. 9: Venturi effect.

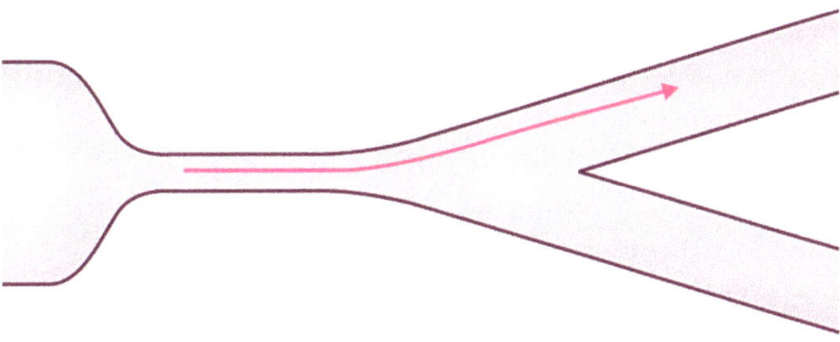
Fig. 10: Coandă effect.

Venturi Masks

These masks are designed in such a way that with appropriate flow of oxygen, there is large degree of entrainment of air through side hole on the mask. This leads to very high total gas flow rate which exceeds patients peak expiratory flow rate. This helps maintain designed inspired oxygen concentration. For example, if a mask is designed to supply 28% oxygen, recommended oxygen flow rate is 4 L/min. At this flow rate, approximately 41 L/min of air is entrained and total flow of 45 L/min is provided to patient.

Coandă Effect

Whenever gas flows through a tube and enters Y junction, gas tends to cling either to one side of the tube or to the other. This is often seen in a constricted portion of bronchiole, gas flow will stream along one fork of the division leading to unequal distribution of gas flow **(Fig. 10)**.

SOLUBILITY

Solubility is the ability of a substance to dissolve. It is defined as the amount of a solute that can be dissolved in unit volume of solvent under specified conditions.

"Henry's law" states that at a given temperature, the amount of a gas which dissolves in a liquid, is directly proportional to the partial pressure of the gas in equilibrium with the liquid.

But, above law does not hold true if temperature changes. As temperature increases, solubility decreases. We see frequently that bubbles of air are formed when intravenous infusion passes through fluid warmers. Solubility of gas also depends on the gas and liquid concerned.

Solubility Coefficients

The "Bunsen solubility coefficient" is the volume of gas, which dissolves in unit volume of the liquid at the temperature concerned, where the partial pressure of the gas above the liquid is 1 standard atmosphere pressure. This solubility coefficient is generally used in scientific books. For anesthesia practice, "Ostwald solubility coefficient" is preferred. The Ostwald solubility coefficient is the volume of gas, which dissolves in unit volume of the liquid at the temperature concerned. The advantage of Ostwald solubility coefficient is that it does not depend on pressure.

The "partition coefficient" is defined as the ratio of the amount of substance present in one phase compared with another, the two phases being of equal volume and in equilibrium. Unlike Ostwald coefficient, the partition coefficient may be applied to two liquids.

Solubility of an anesthetic agent in blood is quantified as the "blood/gas partition coefficient," which is the ratio of the concentration of an anesthetic in the blood phase to the concentration of the anesthetic in the gas phase when the anesthetic is in equilibrium between the two phases. Anesthetic agents with high blood/gas partition coefficient (blood solubility) are carried away from lungs more rapidly compared to agents with low blood/gas partition coefficient. Therefore, their concentration in the alveolar air builds up more slowly compared to agents with low blood/gas partition coefficient. Since the concentration of anesthetic agent in brain is close to the alveolar concentration, there is rapid onset of anesthesia with agent with low blood/gas partition coefficient, e.g., sevoflurane and desflurane.

Oil/gas partition coefficient is the ratio of the concentration of an anesthetic in the oil phase (i.e. adipose tissue) to the concentration of the anesthetic in the gas phase, when the anesthetic is in equilibrium between the two phases.

An anesthetic agent with high oil/gas partition coefficient (one with high oil solubility) is effective at a lower alveolar concentration and has a high potency. Differences in the solubility of inhaled anesthetic agents in blood and tissue have important implications for patient recovery from anesthesia.

Recovery from anesthesia with desflurane is more rapid than recovery after sevoflurane anesthesia, and recovery after sevoflurane anesthesia is more rapid than recovery after anesthesia with isoflurane. The highly soluble anesthetic agent in fat has higher uptake in fat tissue. So, if the anesthetic procedure is long, the recovery will be prolonged.

DIFFUSION

Diffusion is defined, as the process by which there is movement of a substance from an area of high concentration of that substance to an area of lower concentration.

Factors Affecting the Rate of Diffusion

- *Concentration gradient across the membrane:* "Fick's law" states that the rate of diffusion of a substance across unit area is proportional to the concentration gradient. As per modified Fick's law, rate of diffusion of a substance across a membrane is proportional to the tension gradient/partial pressure, e.g., diffusion of nitrous oxide into cuff of endotracheal tube or air filled cavities like middle ear and pneumothorax.
- *Molecular size:* Graham's law states that the rate of diffusion of a gas is inversely proportional to the square root of its molecular weight/density. That means heavier gases takes longer time to diffuse.
- *State of matter:* Molecules move easily in gaseous state compared to liquid state. Therefore, local anesthetic solution should be deposited as close to nerve fiber as possible for it to be effective.[4]
- *Solubility coefficient:* Gases with higher solubility coefficient diffuses easily compared to those with lower solubility coefficient, e.g., carbon dioxide diffuses more rapidly across the alveolar membrane compared to oxygen.[4] Therefore, diseases where gas exchange is affected hypoxia is more common compared to hypercarbia.
- *Membrane area and thickness:* Diffusion is directly proportional to the surface area of the membrane and inversely proportional to thickness of membrane, e.g., impaired diffusion due to decrease in surface area after lobectomy and due to increase thickness of alveolar membrane in fibrosing alveolitis.

HUMIDITY

Water vapor present in the air constitutes humidity. The amount of water vapor present in air is directly proportional to the temperature. At a particular temperature, the maximum water vapor pressure present is called the saturated vapor pressure.

Humidity is measured in two ways:

1. *Absolute humidity:* This is the mass of water vapor present in a given volume of air expressed as grams per cubic meter (g^{-3}). This will depend on the temperature at which the measurement is done. At 20°C when air is fully saturated it contains 17 g^{-3} whereas at 37°C, it contains 44 g^{-3}.
2. *Relative humidity:* It is the percentage of moisture that air holds relative to the amount it can hold when fully saturated at the given temperature. Thus, it is expressed as percentage as follows:

$$\text{Relative humidity} = \frac{\text{Actual vapor density}}{\text{Saturated vapor density}} \times 100\%$$

Or

$$\text{Relative humidity} = \frac{\text{Actual vapor pressure}}{\text{Saturated vapor pressure}} \times 100\%$$

Relative humidity is the most common term used and routinely measured as it is easier to measure then absolute humidity.

Measurement of Humidity

Relative Humidity

- *Hair hygrometer:* Humidity causes changes in physical, chemical, and electrical properties of several materials. This property can be used to measure relative humidity. Absorption of moisture causes the hair to increase its length. This increase in length is proportional to the increase in relative humidity **(Fig. 11)**. This simple arrangement works accurately for relative humidity between 30 and 90%.
- *Wet and dry bulb hygrometer:*
  - It is also called as whirling hygrometer or sling psychrometer.
  - This consists of two thermometers, one is exposed to ambient air to measure ambient temperature and the other is covered by a wick which takes water from a reservoir. Both thermometers are enclosed in a casing which is attached to a handle which swings the thermometers together **(Fig. 12)**.
  - The instrument is swung for 30 seconds, holding it away from the body after which the temperature in both thermometers is noted. Three such successive readings are taken to check that they are similar. The relative humidity is then determined from a table which requires the difference in the readings of dry and thermometer.

Absolute Humidity

- *Regnault's dew point hygrometer:*
  - *Dew point:* It is the temperature at which air is saturated with water vapor and condensation begins.
  - In this instrument, silver tube containing ether is used. Air is blown through ether, this causes cooling of ether. This initiates condensation at the

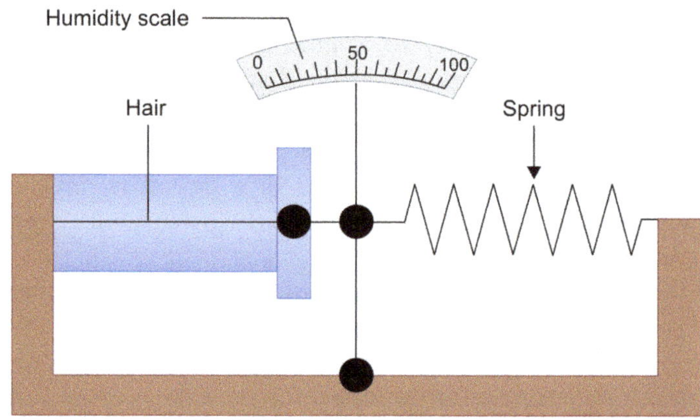

Fig. 11: Hair hygrometer.

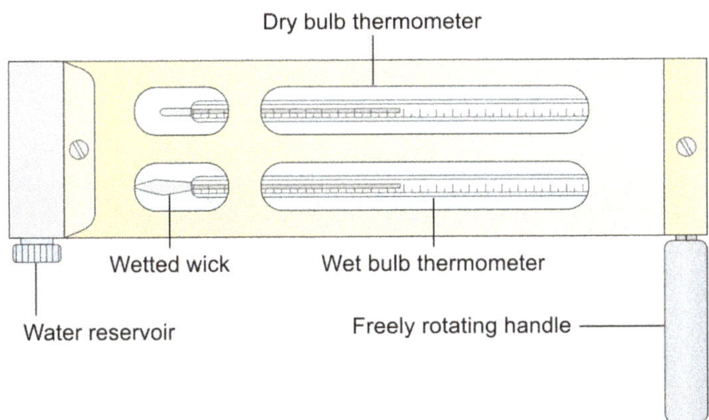

Fig. 12: Sling psychrometer.

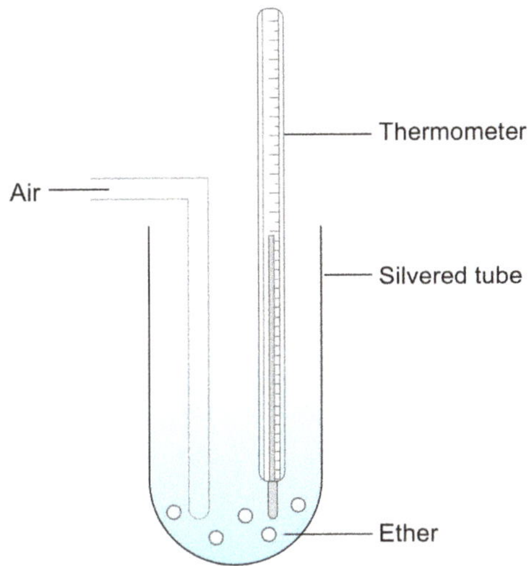

Fig. 13: Regnault's hygrometer.

outer surface of the tube. The temperature at which it occurs is noted from which both absolute and relative humidity can be calculated **(Fig. 13)**.

- *Chilled mirror hygrometer:* It contains a metallic mirror (silver or copper) plated with inert material such as iridium. The metallic mirror is chilled using thermoelectric cooler until the water vapor in the gas sample which is passed over the surface starts condensing (dew point). This dew point is detected by a LED beam reflected from the surface **(Fig. 14)**. This temperature is noted and the humidity (absolute and relative) can be calculated from it using the NIST (National Institute of Standards and Technology) tables.

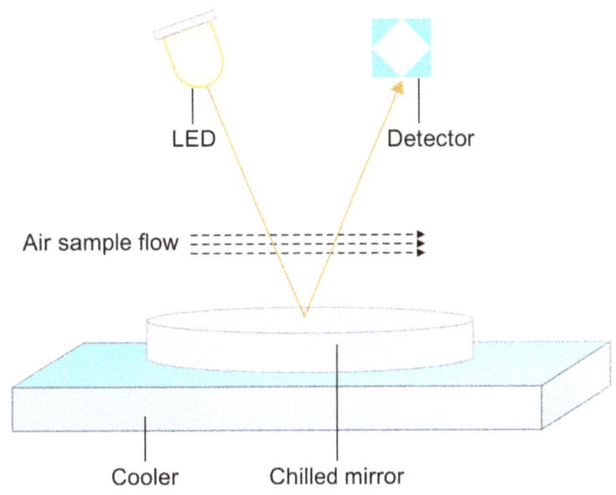

Fig.14: Chilled mirror hygrometer.

- *Mass spectroscopy:* This measures breath to breath humidity in the gas sample.
- *Humidity transducers:* This works on the principle that electrical resistance or capacitance changes with increasing humidity.

CONCLUSION

Physics is an integral part of learning for anesthesiologist. It is not limited to understanding of only equipment but to knowing the behavior of matter in its various states.

REFERENCES

1. Middleton B, Phillips J, Thomas R, et al. Physics in Anaesthesia. Oxford: Scion Publishing Ltd; 2012.
2. Davis PD, Kenny GN. Basic Physics and Measurement in Anaesthesia, 5th edition. Butterworth-Heinemann; 2003.
3. Aitkenhead AR, Rowbotham DJ, Smith G. Textbook of Anaesthesia, 5th edition. Philadelphia: Churchill Livingstone Elsevier; 2007.
4. Paul Clements, Carls Gwinnutt. (2008). The physics of flow, Update in Anaesthesia. [online] Available from http://update.anaesthesiologists.org/wp-content/uploads/2008/12/Flow.pdf. [Last accessed April, 2021].

Medical Gases and Distribution System

SECTION 3

Medical Gas Supply, Storage, and Safety

Vandana V Laheri, Amit K Sarkar

ABSTRACT

Gases used in anesthesia as well as medical practice are either provided in the form of cylinders or medical gas piping system. It is very important for anesthesiologists to understand the intricacies of these systems, safety measures to be undertaken so as to be able to rectify and prevent the mishaps like crossover of gas connections, system running out of supply and so on that can lead to disasters. This chapter, therefore, covers in detail the most important aspects of methods of delivery of gases used in anesthesia as well as medical practice, their storage, and safe use.

INTRODUCTION

The practice of anesthesia involves the use of compressed gases day in and out. A well-planned gas delivery system is an efficient, economic, and highly dependable medical life support network that carries medical gases, vacuum and compressed air towards, operation theaters, intensive care units (ICUs), remote areas for anesthesia and allows better patient care in all the areas of the healthcare institutes.

The medical gases used in "anesthesia practice" are supplied under high pressure either in the form of cylinders or as a piped gas supply. Smaller cylinders up to a certain specific sizes can be fitted to anesthesia machine or anesthesia work stations, medium sizes are used in ICU, wards and remote areas where central supply is not available and bigger cylinders are used in a central manifold room (bank of large cylinders) and from there the gases are supplied via pipelines to operating rooms, wards ICUs, and remote areas where gases are needed. The central area can have large cylinders, or it can receive gas from a large insulated tank of liquid gas (e.g., liquid O_2) caged in an open area and protected from having thoroughfare. Each gas in the cylinder is supplied at specific pressure. Some gases at that specific pressure are in liquid form, e.g., N_2O, CO_2 and cyclopropane whereas O_2, air, N_2, and He are in gaseous form.

COMPRESSED GAS CYLINDERS

The cylinders are mounted on hanger yokes of anesthesia machines as a primary source of gases or as backup for anesthesia machine **(Figs. 1A and B)**, should the central piping gas supply fail. However, they are the primary "source supply" for the central piping system. The cylinders used in medical practice are either solid drawn or made from seamless steel tube and never welded at ends. After manufacturing, the cylinders are kept in a furnace at a

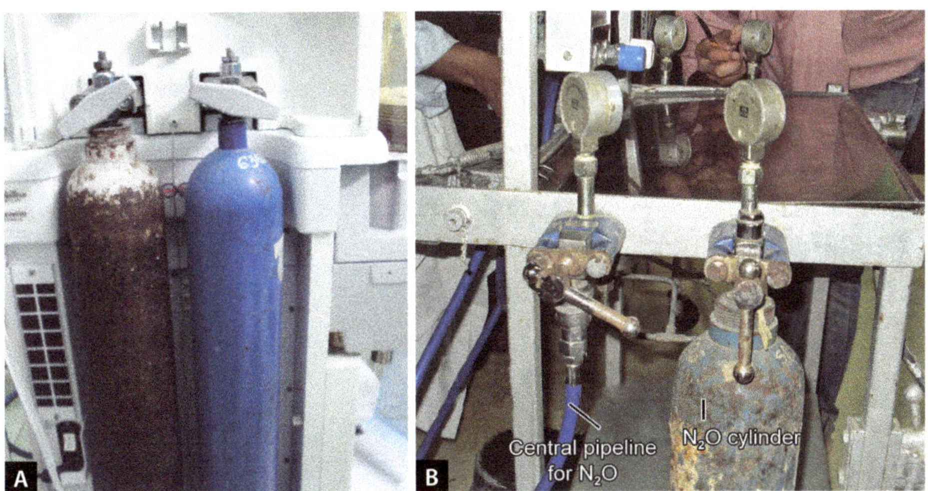

Figs. 1A and B: Cylinders on anesthesia machine as reserve stock.

temperature of 860–890°C and then carefully removed and cooled at atmospheric pressure.[1]

As the cylinders have to withstand a high gas pressure and rough handling during transport, they are subjected to mechanical testing before marketing for use. The tensile test, flattening test, impact test, and bend test are performed on one cylinder from a batch of every 100 finished cylinders.[1] Hydraulic test or pressure test is performed on every finished cylinder from the batch before filling and marketing. This test confirms that the cylinder is leak proof. The manufacturer should regularly check cylinders for faults during the process of refilling of the cylinders. Cylinders must be tested at least every 5 years.

The size and capacity of the cylinder may vary from country to country and with the manufacturer. In USA, the sizes of cylinders are labeled alphabetically from A (smallest) to J (largest). Cylinders used on anesthesia machine are C, D, and E size. In other countries, the sizes are labeled as cubic feet (free gas capacity/volume at normal temperature and pressure), gas capacity in liters, water capacity that the cylinder would hold in liters and so on.

Though the sizes may vary from smallest (size A) to the largest (size J), each cylinder contains a gas under specified pressure, which is known as service pressure. Service pressure is the maximum pressure at 70°F to which the cylinder is ordinarily filled.[2,3] Pressure in a filled cylinder at 70°F may not exceed the service pressure marked on the cylinder. O_2, He, He-O_2, CO_2-O_2 are allowed additional 10%[2,3] (**Table 1**).

Units of Pressure Used

- psi = pounds per square inch
- psig = pounds per square inch gauge (difference between measured pressure and surrounding atmospheric pressure)
- psia = pounds per square inch absolute [based on a reference point of "0" pressure (vacuum)], i.e., psia = (psig + local atmospheric pressure)

One atmospheric pressure = 760 mm Hg = 14.7 psi = 1,030 cmH_2O = 100 kPa = 1,000 mbar.

Oxygen, N_2, air, and He are in the form of compressed gases in the cylinder at service pressure, but N_2O, CO_2, and cyclopropane are in the liquid form in the cylinders. The cylinders are not fully filled with liquids otherwise a rise of temperature may cause a rise of pressure leading to bursting. They are filled up to the specified filling ratio which is different for each gas. The filling ratio is the weight of gas with which the cylinder is filled, divided by the weight of the water the cylinder could hold. Filling ratio for N_2O and CO_2 is 0.66 (IS 8866),[5,6] and that for cyclopropane

TABLE 1: Cylinders sizes, color, capacity and service pressure.[4]

A. Used on anesthesia machine with pin index valves

Gas	Color	Pin index	Size	Free gas capacity at 15°C and 1 atmospheric pressure	Water capacity	Full Wt. In kg	Service pressure
Oxygen	Black body, White shoulder	2:5	C	170 L/6 ft³	1.2 L	2.5	1987 psi/137 bar
			D	340 L/12 ft³	2.32 L	3.9	
			E	680 L/24 ft³	4.68 L	6.5	
Nitrous oxide	Blue body, Blue shoulder	3:5	C	450 L/16 ft³/ 100 gallons	1.2 L	3.0	750 psi/51 bar
			D	900 L/32 ft³/200 gallons	2.32 L	5.0	
			E	1800 L/64 ft³/400 gallons	4.68 L	9.0	
Carbon dioxide	Gray body, Gray shoulder	1:6	C	450 L/16 ft³/ 100 gallons	1.2 L	3.0	725 psi/50 bar
			D	900 L/32 ft³/200 gallons	2.32 L	5.0	
			E	1800 L/64 ft³/400 gallons	4.68 L	8.5	

B. Attached to anesthesia machine with flexible hoses/used in wards with flow meters Or attached to central manifold

Gas	Color	Valve type	Size	Free gas capacity at 15°C and 1 atmospheric pressure	Water capacity	Full Wt. In kg	Service pressure
Oxygen	Black body, White shoulder	Bull-nosed valves Or Hand wheel	F	1360 L/48 ft³	9.4 L	17.0	1,987 psi/137 bar
			G	3400 L/120 ft³	23.6 L	39.0	
			J	6800 L/240 ft³	47.2 L	78.0	
Nitrous oxide	Blue body, Blue shoulder		F	3600 L/128 ft³/ 800 gallons	9.4 L	22.0	750 psi/51 bar
			G	9000 L /320 ft³/2000 gallons	23.6 L	52.0	
			J	18000 L/640 ft³/4000 gallons	47.2 L	105.0	

ft³, cubic feet.

Units of pressure used:

psi = pounds per square inch

psig = pounds per square inch gauge (difference between measured pressure and surrounding atmospheric pressure)

psia = pounds per square inch absolute, (based on a reference point of '0' pressure (vacuum), i.e., psia = (psig + local atmospheric pressure).

is 0.48 (IS 3710).[5,6] Until recently, cylinders of cyclopropane and CO_2 were commonly found on anesthetic machines. Cyclopropane is now rarely used and CO_2 should only be attached if the anesthetist wants to use it for a specific reason.

PARTS OF CYLINDER

- Body
- Valve
- Port
- Stem
- Pressure relief devices

Body

Cylinders are made of molybdenum steel. Alloy containing molybdenum (0.15–0.25%) and/or chromium (0.8–1.1%)[1] is used to increase strength and to minimize weight and wall thickness. Walls of the cylinders are on an average 5/64 to 1/4 inch thick.[1] Magnetic resonance imaging (MRI) compatible cylinders are made of aluminum. Cylinders that have marked "3AA" are manufactured by using steel. The marking "3AL" or "3ALM" indicates that the cylinders made from aluminum. Bodies of the cylinders have flat or concave bases. The other end taper into a neck with screw threads to which is fitted the cylinder valve. The body of the cylinders have a label[3] **(Fig. 2A)** and certain markings[3] **(Fig. 2B)** engraved on the body.

Valve

The cylinder outlet valves **(Figs. 3A to D)** are made of bronze or brass, which is heavily plated with nickel and chromium (IS 3745) so as to allow a rapid dissipation of heat of compression.[1] The end, which enters the neck of the cylinder, is threaded to fit a corresponding screw thread inside the neck itself. A sleeve or washer of soft alloy (containing a high proportion of lead) completes the gas-tight seal as the valve is screwed into the neck of a cylinder. The spindle or screw-pin (stem) of the valve is made of very hard steel. The inner end is cone-shaped and beds into a cone shaped hollow within the valve through which gas is admitted. Longitudinal spindle is set within a gland, which is screwed into the valve block. Turning the longitudinal spindle opens the valve.

Cylinders are filled and discharged through the cylinder valve. The valve is marked with the chemical symbol of gas that it contains, tare weight of the cylinder, pressure at the last hydraulic test, and a serial number **(Fig. 3D)**. Leaks are prevented by the compression of a nylon ring around the spindle. A safety outlet is fitted between the cylinder neck and the valve block. This melts at relatively low temperatures to allow gas to escape in case of fire and minimize the risk of explosion.

Cylinder valves are of various types. Those to be used on anesthesia machines are "flush" type which fits with the pin index system on the machine **(Figs. 3A, B, D and 4A)** and for the medium and large capacity cylinders the valves are "bullnose" type **(Figs. 3C and D)**. Valves have certain markings engraved on it **(Fig. 3D)**.

Cylinder valve designs are of two types, packed type and diaphragm type.

Packed Type[7]

This type of valve is capable of withstanding high pressures. This type of valve is also called direct acting valve. This is because turning the stem makes the seat also to turn. Here, stem is sealed by a resilient packing, such as Teflon®. This prevents leaks around the threads. It withstands high pressure. It is opened by two to three full turns. In a large cylinder valve, the force is transmitted by means of a driver square.

Diaphragm Type[7]

Here, the stem is separated from the seat. A disk or diaphragm separates upper and lower stems. The stem may be permanently attached to the diaphragms. The upper stem is actuated by a manual or automatic means whereas the lower stem shuts or permits flow through the valve.

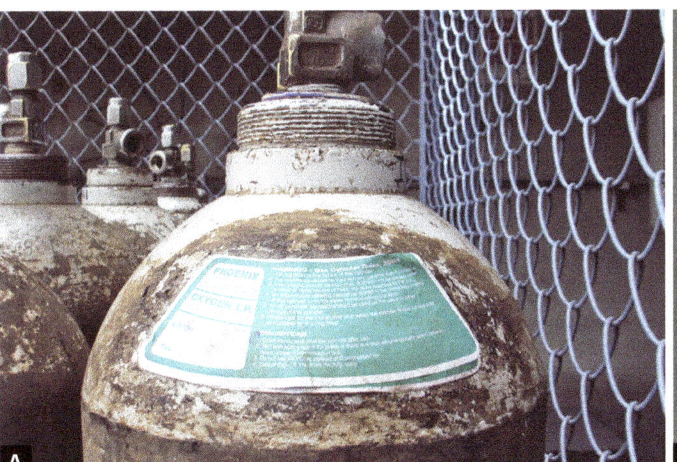

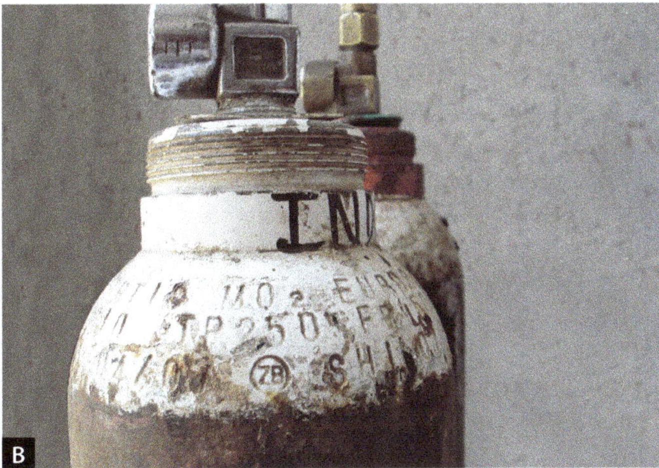

Figs. 2A and B: Labels and markings on the cylinder body.

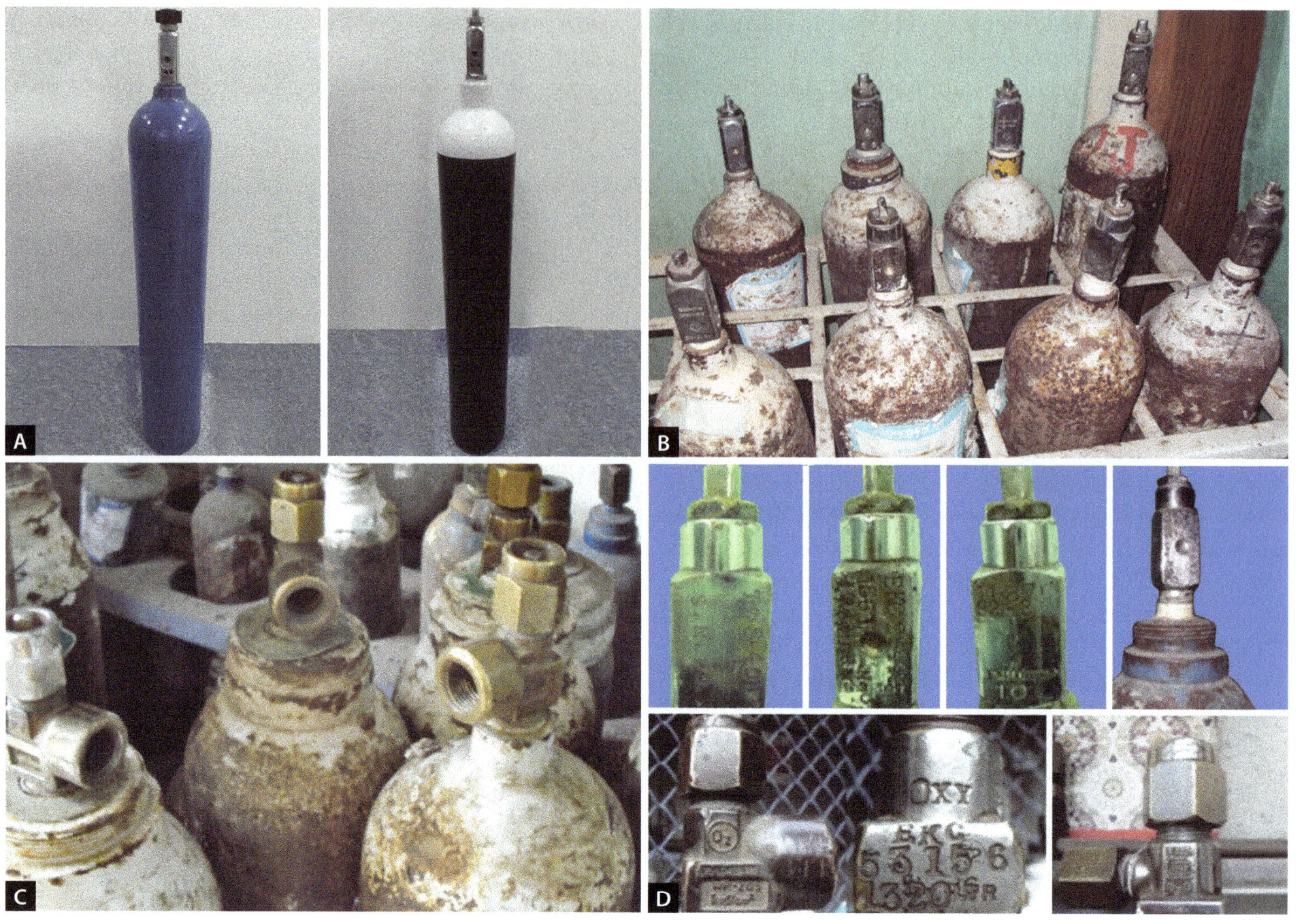

Figs. 3A to D: Types of cylinder valves and markings on cylinder valves. (A) N_2O and O_2 cylinders; (B) Flush type valves; (C) Bull-nose valves; (D) Markings on body of valves.

The advantages of this type of valve is that it can be opened fully using a one-half to three quarters turn, the seat does not turn and therefore it is less likely to leak.

In UK and some countries, compressed medical O_2 cylinders are supplied with two main types of cylinder valves,[4] depending upon the cylinder filling pressure and the type of application. Conventional cylinder valves are fitted to cylinders, which are filled to 137 bar pressure and are designed to be used with a pressure regulator. All such cylinders are fitted with valves with outlet connections that conform to either ISO 407 (pin index) or BS 341 (5/8" BSP F).[4] The cylinders with an outlet pressure of 3–4 bar is fitted with valves that have an integral pressure regulator. These regulated valves are fitted with an ISO 5145 product specific filling connection and either a product specific BS 5682 Schrader outlet connection or a standard 6 mm fir tree outlet.

Port

The port **(Fig. 4A)** is the point of exit for the gas. It fits into the nipple **(Fig. 4B)** on the hanger yoke of the anesthesia machine. It should be protected in transit by a covering. When installing a cylinder on anesthesia machine, it is important for the user not to mistake the port for the conical depression. Conical depression **(Fig. 4A)** is situated on the opposite side of the port on the cylinder valve and is situated above the safety relief device. It is present on those cylinders which are designed to fit on anesthesia machines. The conical depression is designed to receive the retaining screw **(Fig. 4B)** on the yoke of the anesthesia machine. Screwing the retaining screw into the port may damage the port and/or index pins.

Stem

Each valve contains a stem (spindle/screw-pin) **(Fig. 4A)** or shaft that is rotated to open or close the cylinder valve. It is made up of very hard steel. Stem closes the valve by sealing against the seat. To close the valve, the stem seals against the seat that is part of the valve body. When the valve is opened, the stem moves upward and allows the gas to flow to the port.

Pressure Relief Devices

Every cylinder is fitted with pressure relief (safety relief/ safety) device **(Fig. 4A)**. The whole purpose of this device is to vent the cylinder's content to atmosphere rather than the cylinder bursting if the pressure of enclosed gas increases to dangerous level.

Types[7]

- Rupture disk
- Fusible plug
- Combination of both
- Pressure relief valve (spring loaded)

Rupture disk:[7] When predetermined pressure is reached, the disk ruptures and allows the cylinder content to be discharged. It is a nonreclosing device held against an orifice. It protects against excess pressure as a result of high temperature or overfilling.

Fusible plug:[7] The fusible plug is thermally operated. It is a nonreclosing pressure relief device where the plug held against the discharge channel. It does offer protection from excessive pressure caused by a high temperature (yield temperature), but it does not protect against excessive pressure from overfilling. The yield temperature is the temperature at which the fusible material becomes sufficiently soft to extrude from its holder so that cylinder contents are discharged.

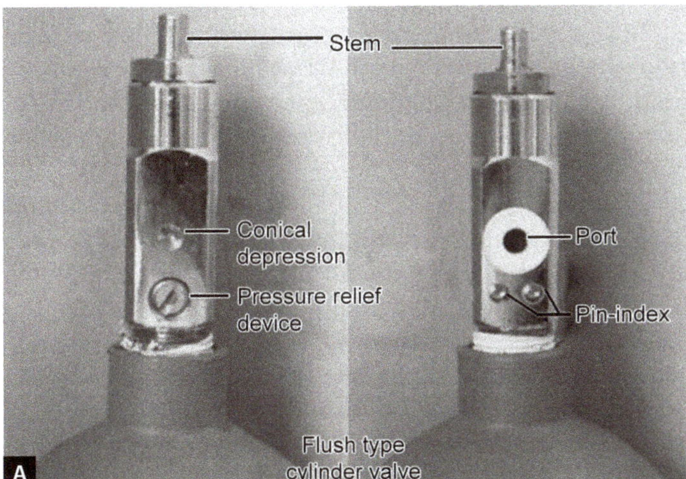

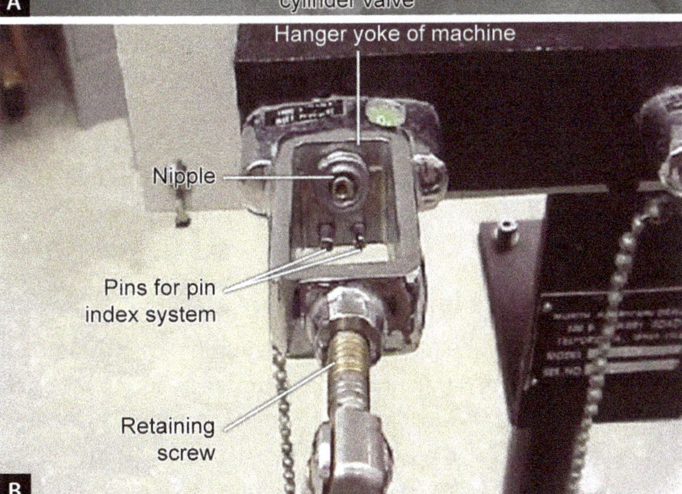

Figs. 4A and B: Flush type cylinder valve and hanger yoke of anesthesia machine.

Spring-loaded pressure relief valve:[7] It is a reclosing device. When the set pressure is exceeded, the pressure in the cylinder forces the spring to open the channel for letting out gases and gas flows around the safety valve seat to the discharge channel till the excess pressure is relieved.

SAFETY FEATURES OF CYLINDERS

- Molybdenum steel alloy construction. This is stronger and lighter than its carbon steel predecessor
- Color-coding for each gas or vapor
- *Pin-index system:* This prevents the accidental connection of a cylinder/yoke block of one gas to the hanger yoke of another gas on the anesthesia machine or work station
- *Bodok seals (bonded disk):* These are noncombustible small metal and neoprene seal (neoprene washers with aluminum edges) to ensure a gas-tight fit between the cylinder and anesthetic machine yoke
- *Cylinder pressure indicator (gauge):* Bourdon pressure gauges are fitted adjacent to each yoke and pipeline connection on the machine. These are calibrated, labeled, and color-coded for each gas.

Color-coding (Table 2, Figs. 1A and 3A)

There is no unique international color-coding system for the contents of anesthetic gas cylinders (or pipelines). In USA, O_2 is supplied in green cylinders; in UK and India (IS 3933), O_2 cylinders have black body with white shoulders, and in Germany, they are blue.

As per the data by BOC,[4] for a limited period, O_2 cylinders may have black bodies. These cylinders do not have the name "oxygen" on the body of the cylinder. The program to convert all compressed medical oxygen cylinders to white bodies and carrying the name "oxygen" on the body of the cylinder will be completed by 2025.

Pin-index Safety System (Fig. 5 and Table 3)

The use of pin-index system began in 1952. In order to ensure that the correct cylinder or central pipeline supply is attached to the appropriate hanger yoke of the anesthesia machine/work station, a series of pins on the hanger yoke is made to fit into corresponding indentations (pits/holes) drilled into the cylinder valve or yoke block **(Figs. 4 and 5)**.

TABLE 2: Color-coding of cylinders in India (IS 3933).[5,6]

Gas	Body	Shoulder
O_2	Black	White
N_2O	Blue	Blue
Cyclopropane	Orange	Orange
CO_2	Gray	Gray
Air	Gray	White/Black quarters
Nitrogen	Black	Black
$N_2O + O_2$, 50:50	Blue	White/Blue quarters

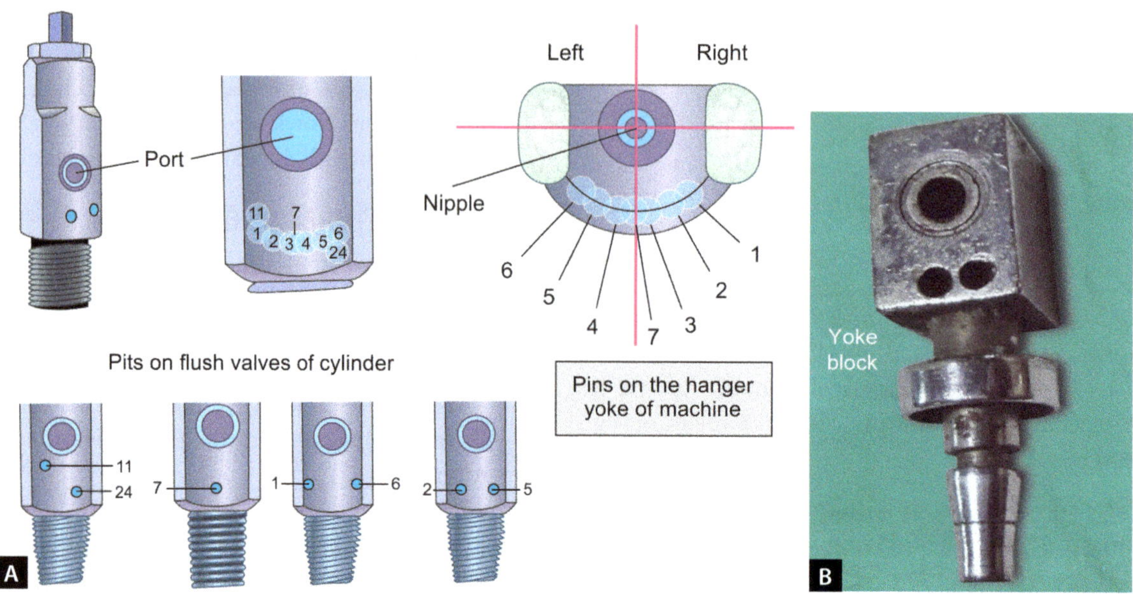

Figs. 5A and B: Pin-index system.

TABLE 3: Pin-index for various gases (IS 3745).[5,6]

Gas	*Index pins*	*Gas*	*Index pins*
O_2	2, 5	O_2–CO_2 (CO_2 <7.5%)	2, 6
N_2O	3, 5	O_2–CO_2 (CO_2 >7.5%)	1, 6
Cyclopropane	3, 6	O_2–He (He >80.5%)	4, 6
Air	1, 5	O_2–He (He <80.5%)	2, 4
N_2	1, 4	N_2O–O_2 (N_2O 47.5–52.5%)	7

This pin-index system is used on small cylinder (sizes A to E) valves and yoke blocks.

The indentations (pits/holes) on the cylinder valve/yoke block are counted 1–6 from left to right whereas pins on hanger yoke of the machine are counted 1–6 from right to left **(Fig. 5)**, in reverse direction than pits on cylinder valves/yoke blocks. There are seven positions for pins and holes (IS 3745). The pins are 4.75 mm in diameter and 6 mm long, except for pin number 7. Pin number 7 is slightly thicker and it is placed in the center, between pin number 3 and 4. Positions of seven holes (indentations) on the cylinder valve are on the circumference of a circle of 9/16 inch (14.3 mm) radius cantered on the port. The port has a diameter of 7.00 mm. The distance between the center and the lower part of yoke should be 20.6 mm. In a similar fashion, the index pins are mounted in an arc below the nipple. The distance between the center of first pin and the sixth pin should be 16 mm.

If both, the pins and the indentations are not aligned, port of the cylinder would not seat against the nipple on the yoke. Pin-index system is not foolproof as the pins may be deliberately removed allowing the wrong cylinder to be fitted to the machine.

Index pins numbers 11 and 24 have been added by Compressed Gas Association (CGA) for various non-inflammable, noncorrosive medical gases.

Bodok Seal

A small disk of neoprene with metal periphery ensures a gas-tight fit between the cylinder and anesthetic machine yoke in the form of seal **(Figs. 6A and B)**. Under no circumstances, may oil or grease be used as a seal; the pressurized gases give off heat as they are released from the cylinder and may cause explosions if oil is used. Before attaching a full cylinder to the machine briefly open and close the cylinder valve to clear any dirt from the port. This is called cracking the cylinder.

Additional safety features are on the anesthesia machine. Each gas entering the machine from a cylinder flows through a filter, one-way check valve and pressure regulator. Nonreturn valves prevent empty cylinders still attached to the machine from refilling from fresh cylinders. The pressure in anesthetic gas pipelines is 4 bar (the same as the working pressure of the anesthetic machine). All anesthetic machines, including those having pipeline gases, have provision to attach reserve gas cylinders. These cylinders should be turned off when pipeline pressure is sufficient.

Anesthetic machines operate at 4 bar pressure and therefore the compressed medical gases in cylinders pass through reducing valves to bring the gas pressure to a constant 4 bar. Nonreturn valves prevent empty cylinders still attached to the machine from refilling from fresh cylinders.

Cylinder Pressure Indicator (Gauge)

The anesthesia workstation standard requires that there be a pressure indicator to displays the cylinder pressure for each gas supplied by cylinders. The indicator may be located near the cylinders **(Fig. 7A)** or on a panel on the front of the machine **(Fig. 7C)**. The scale is 33% greater than the maximum filling pressure of the cylinder or the "full indication" position.

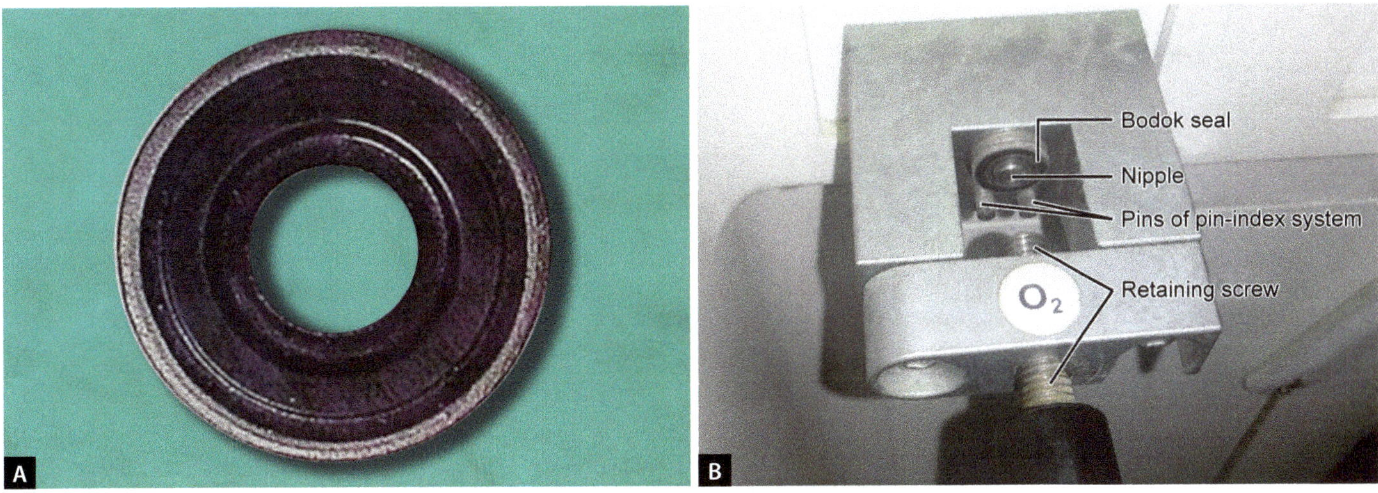

Figs. 6A and B: (A) Bodok seal; (B) Bodok seal *in situ*.

Many indicators are of the Bourdon tube (Bourdon spring, elastic element) type **(Figs. 7B and D)**. A hollow metal tube is bent into a curve. One end is sealed and linked to a clocklike mechanism. The other end which is open is connected to the gas source. An increase in gas pressure inside the tube makes the curved tube to straighten out depending on the change in pressure. As the pressure falls, the tube resumes its curved shape. The open end is fixed and the sealed end moves. Movement of the sealed end is transmitted to the indicator, which moves over a calibrated scale. Cylinder pressure gauges are calibrated in kg/cm^2, pounds/inch^2 or kilo Pascals (kPa).[7]

Some electronic machines have light-emitting diodes (LEDs) to indicate cylinder pressure. LED is green if the pressure is adequate when the cylinder valve is opened. But, if the pressure is inadequate when the cylinder valve is opened, LED will flash red. It will be dark if the cylinder valve is not open. These machines may also display the actual pressure for pipelines and cylinders on a screen during the checkout. The readings can be available on a continuous basis or on demand.[7]

As the cylinder content gets empty, the pressure in the cylinder falls proportionately if the cylinder contents are in gaseous form. If half of the content is over, the pressure drops to half of the original and so on. The same is not true for the gases in the liquid form. The pressure in the cylinder containing gases in liquid form remains as "full cylinder pressure" until the last drop of liquid form of gas vaporizes. This is because the pressure gauge reads the saturated vapor pressure of the liquid gas. Once all the liquid has evaporated, the pressure drops much faster till all the gaseous contents are over. However, during use the cylinder pressure does drop because the latent heat of vaporization is provided by the liquid gas for vaporization into gaseous form leading to drop in temperature of the liquid and hence fall in saturated vapor pressure of the liquid. If the entire cylinder is used at single sitting then the pressure drop is gradual and becomes zero when contents are over. But, after using part of the cylinder contents, if the gas flow is discontinued, the pressure rises to "full cylinder pressure" as the gases gain the heat from atmosphere to come back to room temperature.

Cylinder Key (Handle) or Handwheel

A cylinder key (handle) or handwheel is used to open or close a cylinder valve. It is turned counterclockwise to open the valve and clockwise to close it. This causes the stem to turn. A cylinder key (handle) is used to open a small cylinder valve. They come in a variety of shapes **(Fig. 8A)**.

Rules for Safe Use of Cylinders

- To be handled only by trained staff
- Store cylinders in a cool, clean room with adequate ventilation
- Do not drape cylinders with any material during storage
- Cylinders are best stored upright in a cylinder stand **(Figs. 8B and C)**
- Should be grouped by contents or sizes **(Figs. 8B and C)**
- Good segregation between empty and full cylinders
- To be kept away from oils, rubber, and other combustible substances
- Never to expose cylinders to heat or higher temperatures
- Never interchange parts of cylinder used for one gas with other
- Take care to avoid obstructions to discharge ports
- Keep the valve closed when not in use
- Identify contents by label
- Remove wrappings (protective cover) before using
- Remove dust and foreign bodies before connecting
- "Cracking" to be done to reduce possibility of flash fire
- A sealing washer in good condition should be used
- Flow control valve should be closed before the cylinder valve is opened

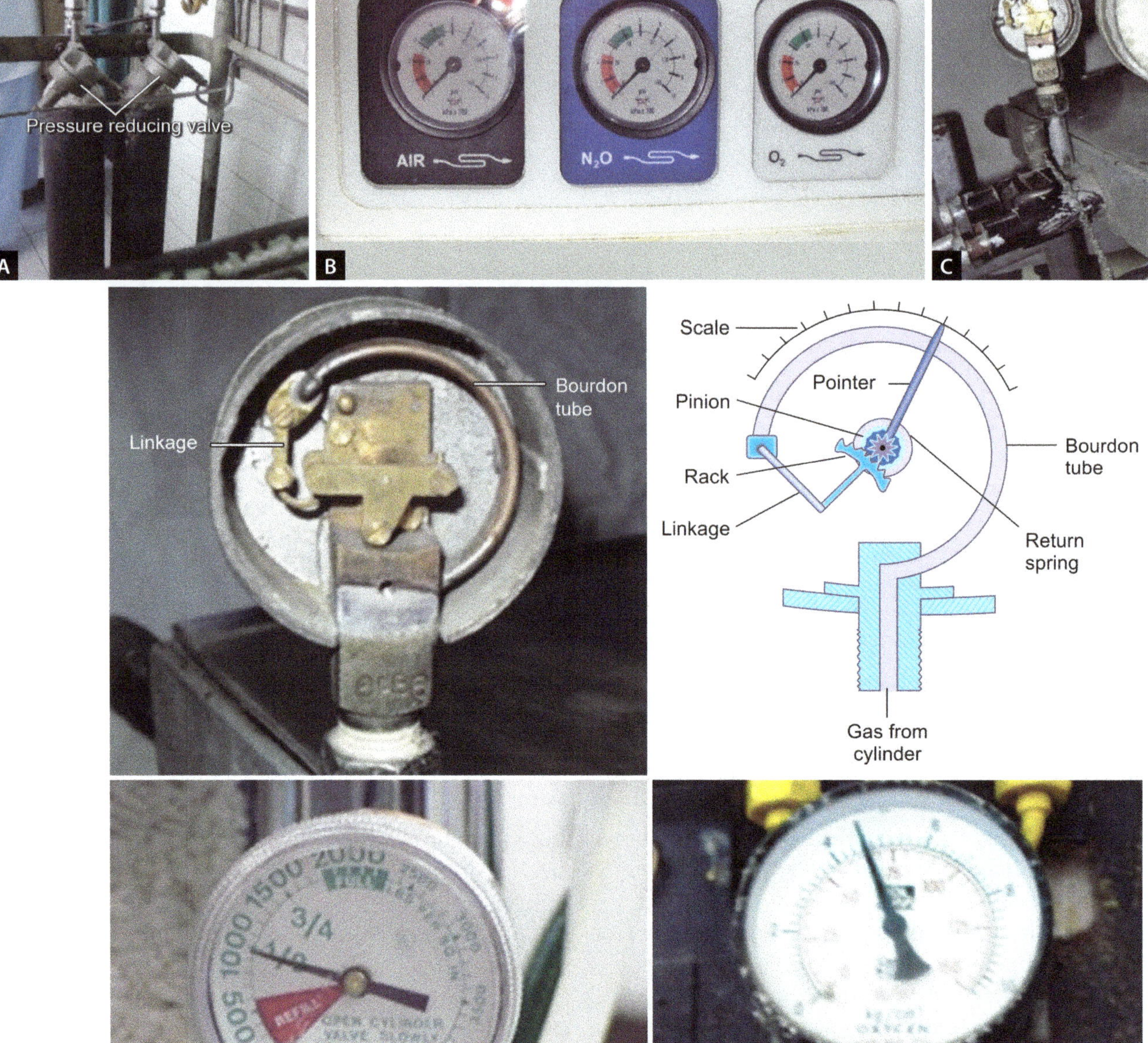

Figs. 7A to D: Cylinder pressure gauges.

- While opening, stand to the side; not in front or back
- Quick opening to be avoided as it can generate heat leading to flame
- Valve should be fully opened when in use
- Valve should be closed before removing from a regulator or yoke
- Lower part of the tag should be removed when cylinder is empty.

Hazards

- Incorrect cylinder contents
- Incorrect valve
- Incorrect color, labeling
- Inoperable valve, damaged valve
- Suffocation, fires, explosion, and thermal injury
- Contamination of contents
- Overfilling

STANDARDS FOR CYLINDERS IN INDIA

The rules governing handling of compressed gases in India are the Gas Cylinders Rules, the SMPVs (U) Rules and the Indian Standards (IS).

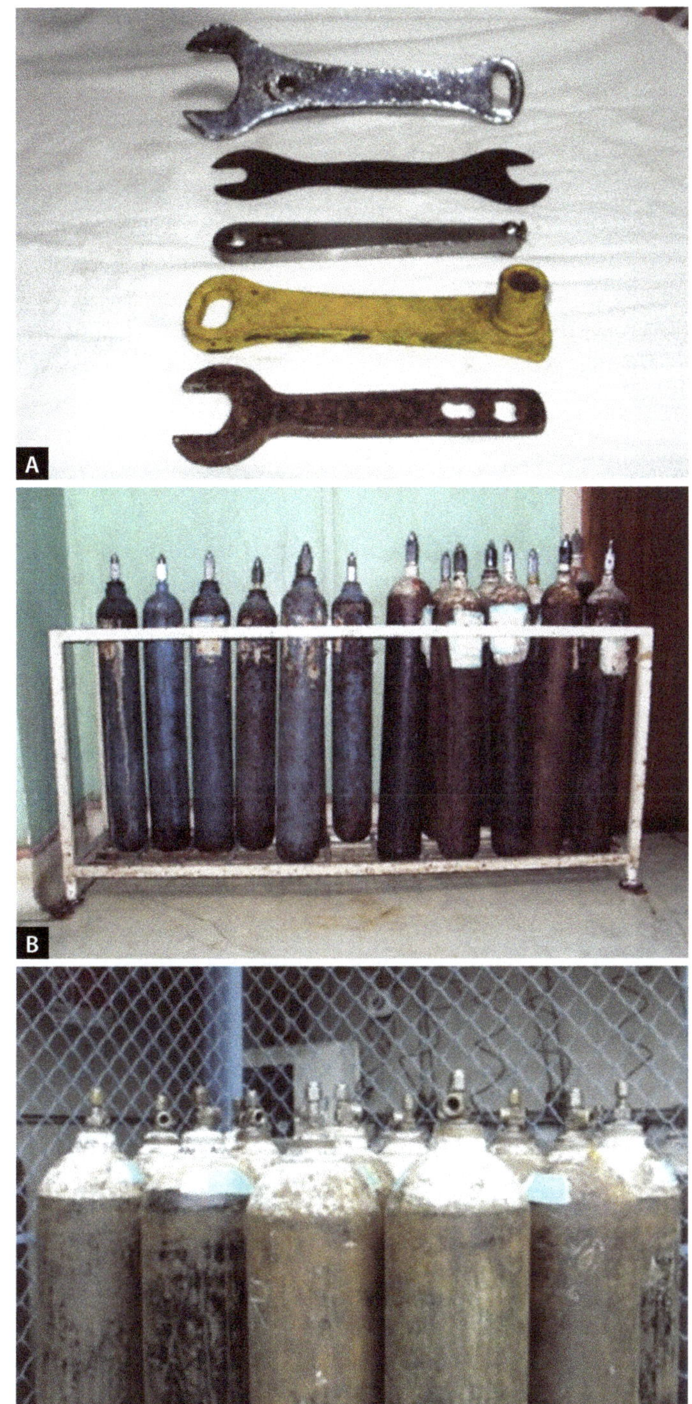
Figs. 8A to C: Cylinder keys and cylinder stand/storage.

Gas Cylinders Rules, 1981[2]

These rules were published by the Government of India to maintain the standards for the manufacturing, transport, storage, and safe use of gas cylinders. In supersession of the Gas Cylinders Rules, 1981, the Central Government published Gas Cylinders Rules, 2004[3] in the Gazette of India dated September 21, 2004. It contains 73 rules distributed topic wise in nine chapters, and it contains five schedules. Gas Cylinders Rules, 2004 are primarily aimed at prevention of accidents by ensuring safe design, manufacture, inspection and quality control of cylinders, valves, and regulators.[3] Rules also cover safety aspects concerning filling, possession, transport, and import of compressed gases in cylinders.[3] In 2010, amendments were made via Gas Cylinders (Amendment) Rules, 2010.[3]

Static and Mobile Pressure Vessels (Unfired) Rules 1981[8]

These rules prescribe separate licenses for storage and transportation of compressed gases and list safety in the design, manufacture and location of pressure vessels, safety during filling and during transportation, safety status of the vehicles transporting the vessels and certificate of safety.

As per the policy of Government of India, the rules are revised from time to time to meet the changing requirements of industry due to technological developments, globalization, opening up of economy including environmental concerns. Gas Cylinders Rules 1981 were superseded by Gas Cylinders Rules 2004, and Static and Mobile Pressure Vessels (Unfired) [SMPV(U)] Rules 1981[8] were amended from time to time for introduction of liquefied petroleum gas (LPG), compressed natural gas (CNG), hythane, tube cylinders, cryogenic liquids, composite cylinders, mounded/underground tanks, cavern storages, LOT, ATD, etc. SMPV (U) Rules 1981 and the Gas Cylinders Rules 2004 were reviewed by Petroleum and Explosive Safety Organization (PESO) at Nagpur on March 16, 2012.

Indian Standards[5,6]

Bureau of Indian Standards (BIS) has issued a number of standards pertaining to the design, transportation, and handling of compressed gases, e.g., specifications of color-codes for medical gas cylinders (IS 3933), the methods for hydrostatic stress testing (IS 5844), periodical inspection interval for gas cylinders in use (IS 8868), etc.

Bureau of Indian Standards is a statutory institution established under the BIS Act, 1986[5,6] to promote harmonious development of the activities of standardization, marking, and quality certification of goods and attending to connected matters in the country. Amendments are issued to IS are reviewed periodically; a standard along with amendments is reaffirmed when such review indicates that no changes are needed; if the review indicates that changes are needed, it is taken up for revision. Users of IS should ascertain that they are in possession of the latest amendments or edition by referring to the latest issue of "BIS catalogue" and "standards: Monthly additions".

CONTENTS OF "GAS CYLINDER RULES, 2004" OF INTEREST TO ANESTHESIOLOGISTS

Definitions from Chapter I[3]

- "Gas cylinder" or "cylinder" means any closed metal container having a volume exceeding 500 mL but not exceeding 1,000 L intended for the storage and transport of compressed gas **(Fig. 9)**

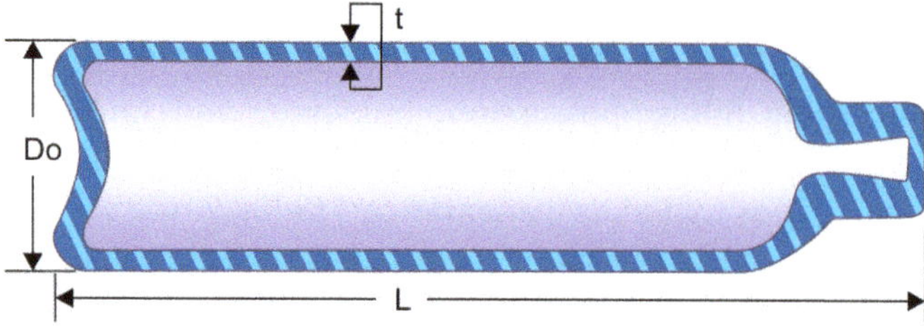

Fig. 9: Internal anatomy of gas cylinder.[3]

- "Compressed gas" means any permanent gas, liquefiable gas or gas dissolved in liquid under pressure or gas mixture which in a closed gas cylinder exercises a pressure either exceeding 2.5 kgf/cm^2 absolute (1.5 kgf/cm^2 gauge) at +15°C or a pressure exceeding 3 kgf/cm^2 absolute (2 kgf/cm^2 gauge) at +50°C or both
- "Flammable gas" means any gas which, if either a mixture of 13% or less (by volume) with air forms a flammable mixture or the flammability range with air is greater than 12% regardless of the lower limit and these limits shall be determined at atmospheric temperature and pressure. "Flammability range" means the difference between the minimum and maximum percentages by volume of the gas in mixture with air that forms a flammable mixture
- "Inert gas" means a gas which is resistant to chemical action under normally encountered conditions
- "Permanent gas" means a gas whose critical temperature is below –10°C that is to say a gas which cannot be liquefied under any pressure at a temperature above –10°C
- "Filling pressure" means the maximum permissible gauge pressure, converted to +15°C, at which a gas cylinder for permanent gas or gas dissolved under pressure can be filled
- "Filling ratio" means the ratio of the weight of a liquefiable gas introduced in the cylinder to the weight of the water the cylinders will hold at 15°C
- "Liquefiable gas" means a gas that may be liquefied by pressure at -10°C, but will be completely vaporized when in equilibrium with normal atmospheric pressure (760 mm Hg) at 17.5°C which value shall be increased to 30°C for toxic gases
- "High-pressure liquefiable gas" means a liquefiable gas having a critical temperature between -10 and +70°C
- "Low-pressure liquefiable gas" means a liquefiable gas having critical temperature higher than +70°C
- "Critical temperature" means the temperature above which gas cannot be liquefied by the application of pressure alone
- "Tare weight" for liquefiable gas cylinder means the weight of the cylinder together with any fittings permanently attached thereto and includes the weight of valve; and that for permanent gas cylinder means the weight of the cylinder together with any fittings permanently attached thereto and excludes the weight of valve
- "Hydrostatic test" means the test to which a cylinder is subjected to a hydrostatic pressure equal to the test pressure of the cylinder
- "Hydrostatic stretch test" means subjecting the cylinder to a hydrostatic pressure equal to the test pressure of the cylinder and recording the permanent stretch undergone by the cylinder
- "Test pressure" means the internal pressure required for the hydrostatic test or hydrostatic stretch test of the cylinder
  - For permanent and high pressure liquefiable gases, it should be calculated from the following:

$$Ph = 200 \times t \times Re/1.25\,(Do - t)$$

where Ph is test pressure in kgf/cm,^{2} Do is outside diameter of the cylinder in mm, t is minimum calculated wall thickness of the cylinder shell in mm, and Re is minimum specified yield strength of the material of cylinder in kgf/mm.^{2} It is limited to 75% of the minimum value of the tensile strength in the case of normalized cylinder and 85% of the minimum value of the tensile strength for quenched and tempered cylinder, provided that the value of test pressure shall not exceed 80% of the yield strength
  - For low pressure liquefiable gas—one and a half times the saturated vapor pressure of the gas at 65°C or as specified in IS 8867, whichever is higher
- "Yield strength" means the stress corresponding to a permanent strain of 0.2% of the original gauge length in a tensile test. For practical purpose it may be taken as a stress at which elongation first occurs in the test piece without the increase of load in a tensile test
- "Water capacity" means the volume of water in liters, a cylinder will hold at 15°C
- "Working pressure for low-pressure liquefiable gas" means the saturated vapor pressure at 65°C; the values of saturated vapor pressure of different gases are specified in IS 3710
- "Working pressure for permanent gas" means the internal pressure of the gas in the cylinder at a temperature of 15°C.

General Provisions from Chapter II[3]

For Filling, Possession, Import, and Transport of Cylinders

- Cylinder and its valve to be constructed to a type and standard specified in schedule I as amended from time to time by an order issued by the chief controller
- The test and inspection certificates issued by the inspecting authority in respect of cylinder and its valve to be made available to the chief controller and prior approval of the said authority to be obtained
- The test and inspection certificates required to be obtained from the inspecting authority in respect of

cylinders and valves inspected and certified by it in accordance with the approved design and specification or code shall give the information included in schedule II.

Valves

- Valves fitted to gas cylinders shall comply in all respects with the following specifications:
  - IS 3224 in respect of industrial gas cylinders
  - IS 3745 in respect of medical gas cylinders
  - IS 7302 as amended from time to time in respect of cylinders used with breathing apparatus
- The valves fitted to CO_2 cylinders must provide with a safety release consisting of softened copper disk so arranged as to burst at a pressure between 200 kg/cm^2 and 220 kg/cm^2
- The valves containing flammable gases not listed in IS 3224 should have outlets provided with left-handed screw threads for the pipes or other connections. And all other valves shall have outlets with right-handed screw threads
- The valves shall be attached to the cylinder neck by screwing and not by any permanent attachment or inserting adapter in between
- The design of spindle-operated valves shall be such that when fitted to the cylinders it shall not be possible to withdraw the spindle under normal operating conditions.

Safety Relief Devices

- The safety relief devices for cylinders manufactured in India must be manufactured and maintained in accordance with IS 5903
- No safety devices should be provided to the cylinders containing obnoxious or poisonous gases
- The cylinders manufactured in foreign countries and approved for use the fitted safety relief devices must be maintained in accordance with specification to which they were made originally.

Marking on Cylinders

- Each gas cylinder shall be clearly and permanently marked in accordance with following conditions by stamping, engraving, or similar processes:
  - On the shoulder of the cylinder which shall be reinforced by forging or other means, or
  - On such a part which is inseparably bound with the cylinder and which is not or only negligibly affected by the stresses due to the gas pressure within it
- The nameplate shall not be affixed to the cylinder by soldering if there is a risk of corrosion or embrittlement
- In conjunction with the original marking, space shall be provided for stamping the test date obtained at the periodic inspection
- Markings shall be so carried out and the letters and numerals used shall be of such shape and size that the marking is clear and easily readable and does not give place for misreading.

Marking on permanent and liquefiable gas cylinders:

- Every cylinder shall be marked with the following markings, namely:
  - Manufacturer's, owner's, and inspector's marking and rotation number (these markings shall be registered with the chief controller)
  - Specification to which the cylinder has been made
  - A symbol to indicate the nature of heat treatment given to the cylinder during manufacture or after repairs
  - The date of the last hydrostatic test or hydrostatic stretch test, as the case may be, with the code mark of recognized testing station where the test was carried out and the code mark shall be registered with the chief controller
  - Working pressure and test pressure
  - Tare weight
  - Water capacity
- All the markings, except the manufacture's markings, which may be on the base, shall be stamped on the neck end of the cylinder. However, seamless cylinders having no foot ring or skirt shall be stamped with the manufacturer's marking on the neck end of the cylinder.

Markings on Valves

The valves fitted to the cylinder shall be clearly and durably marked in accordance with the following provisions by stamping, engraving, or similar processes:

- The specification of the valves
- Year and month or quarter of manufacture
- Symbol of manufacturer
- Working pressure
- The name or chemical symbol of the gas for which the valve is to be used
- The type of screw threads on the outlet, in case of left handed as (l.h.), i.e., l for left and h for hand
- Inspector's stamp.

Identification Colors

All cylinders with compressed gas to be painted with appropriate identification colors specified in IS 4379 for industrial cylinders and IS 3933 for medical cylinders to be stored.

Labeling of Cylinders

- All cylinders shall be labeled with the name of the gas and the name and address of the person by whom the cylinder was filled with
- A warning in the following terms shall be attached to every cylinder containing permanent or liquefiable gas, namely:

"WARNING"

Gas Cylinders Rules, 2004

- Do not change the color of this cylinder
- This cylinder should not be filled with any gas other than the one it now contains
- No flammable material should be stored in the close vicinity of this cylinder or in the same room in which it is kept
- No oil or similar lubricant should be used on the valves or other fittings of this cylinder
- Please look for the next date of test, which is marked on a metal ring inserted between the valve and the neck of the cylinder, and if this date is over, do not accept the cylinder for filling.

General Precautions

- All cylinders with their valves and other fittings and the identification colors must be maintained in good condition
- No oil or similar lubricant shall be used on any valves or other fittings of any cylinder
- No cylinder shall be subjected to any heat treatment or exposed to a high temperature or to the Sun or stored with any other flammable or explosive material
- Every cylinder containing compressed gas shall have its valve securely closed so as to prevent leakage
- If a leak in the valve cannot be rectified by tightening the gland nut or the spindle, the cylinder shall be removed to an open space where it is least dangerous to life and property and the filler shall be informed.

Handling and Use

- During handling cylinders should be adequately supported
- The shifting of cylinder should be done with the help of conveyors, trolleys, and cradles
- The cylinders shall be handled carefully and not be allowed to fall upon one another or otherwise subjected to any undue shock
- Avoid sliding, dropping, or playing with cylinders
- Cylinders containing liquefiable gases shall always be kept in an upright position and shall be so placed that they cannot be knocked over
- Cylinders used in horizontal position shall be secured to avoid roll
- These cylinders contain flammable gases so open flames, lights, use of mobile phones, lighting of fires, welding, and smoking shall be prohibited near it
- Working places shall not be classified as storage places for licensing.

Storage of Cylinders

- All cylinders shall be stored in a cool, dry, well-ventilated place under cover and kept away from boilers, open flames, steam pipes, or any potential sources of heat
- The storage room or shed shall be of fire-resistant construction
- Thin wall cylinders such as LPG cylinders and dissolved gas cylinders shall not be stacked in a horizontal position
- The cylinders containing flammable gases and toxic gases shall be kept separated from each other and from cylinders containing other types of gases by an adequate distance or by a suitable partition wall
- The cylinders shall not be stored under conditions, to avoid corrosion
- Cylinders shall not be stored along with any combustible material
- Empty cylinders shall be segregated from the filled ones and care shall be taken that all the valves are tightly shut.

Purity of Gas

- Compressed gases shall be free from impurities, which are likely to corrode the metal of the cylinder or form an explosive substance with it or cause the gases to decompose or explode
- The gases shall be as dry as possible and in no instance shall the aqueous phase separate when a liquefied gas is cooled to 0°C.

Retesting of Cylinder

A cylinder for which prescribed periodical retest has become due shall not be charged and transported until such retest has been properly made.

Examination and Testing of Cylinders from Chapter IV[3]

Periodicity of Examination and Testing of Cylinders

- No person shall fill any cylinder with any compressed gas unless the cylinder has been examined and subjected to hydrostatic test or hydrostatic stretch test, as the case may be, and other tests set forth in Schedule IV within such period as is specified in IS 8868 issued by BIS or as approved in writing by the chief controller
- Any testing station desiring to obtain recognition for periodical testing and examination of cylinders shall provide the facilities set forth in Schedule IV and shall submit to chief controller the particulars of the facilities provided and scrutiny fee specified in Schedule "V".

Condemning of Cylinders

Any cylinder which fails to pass periodic examination or test or which loses in its tare weight by over 5% or which for any other defect is found to be unsafe for use or after expiry of the service life of the cylinder shall not be filled with any compressed gas and shall be destroyed by flattening it as a whole or after being cut into pieces in such a manner that the pieces cannot again be joined together by welding or otherwise to form a cylinder, under intimation to the owner of the cylinder, as specified in IS 8198.

Filling and Possession from Chapter VI

Working Pressure and Filling Ratios

- The working or internal pressure in any cylinder charged with a permanent gas shall not exceed two-thirds of the test pressure
- Cylinders charged with liquefiable gases shall not be filled in excess of the filling ratios specified in IS 3710 for low-pressure liquefiable gases and IS 8866 for high-pressure liquefiable gases.

CONTENTS OF VARIOUS SCHEDULES OF THE "GAS CYLINDER RULES" OF INTEREST TO ANESTHESIOLOGISTS[3]

Schedule I[3]: Types and Standards of Cylinders and Valves

Cylinders and Containers

- *Indian origin:* Seamless steel cylinders manufactured to IS 7285
- *UK origin:* Seamless steel cylinders for permanent and liquefiable gases conforming to BS:5045:Part I (BS = British Standards)
- *USA origin:* Steel cylinders—inspected and certified by appropriate authority, conforming to specifications of Department of Transportation (DOT):3A/3AA for permanent and liquefiable gases, aluminum alloy cylinders conforming to DOT:3AL specification.

Valves

Indian origin: Valves and regulators in respect of medical gas cylinder manufactured to IS 3745 and valves in respect of cylinders used with breathing apparatus to IS 7302, certified by BIS and approved by the chief controller.

Schedule II[3]

Information regarding the test and inspection certificates to be obtained from the inspecting authority in respect of cylinders and valves manufactured in accordance with the approved design and specification or code.

Schedule III[3]

Information regarding particulars to be submitted by person who is desiring to fabricate cylinder, valves, and other fittings.

Schedule IV[3]

Facilities required for cylinder testing stations.

Schedule V[3]

Information regarding license fees, fees other than license fees, and various forms.

CENTRAL PIPELINE SYSTEMS

Nonflammable gases, such as O_2, N_2O, air, CO_2, and N_2 can be delivered to operating rooms and other patient care areas via central piping system. Central piping systems are installed by contractors or suppliers dealing with medical gas pipelines and are maintained by the bioengineering or the maintenance department of the healthcare institute. To begin with system design is the most important aspect of centralized medical gas pipeline systems for any hospital which will determine the perfect capacity of source equipment and size of piping layout to ensure supply of medical gases/vacuum at each outlet point at desired pressure and flow.

Gases from the central manifold are fed into labeled and color-coded pipeline distribution network, which terminates in self-sealing noninterchangeable sockets either as diameter-index safety system (DISS), noninterchangeable screw threads (NIST) or as noninterchangeable quick couplers (NIQC) at the user point as wall outlets, ceiling pendants, ceiling columns, or bed head panels.

Piped O_2 is provided from a central O_2 source, which may be in the gaseous form, i.e., a cylinder manifold, gas in manifold cylinders on a trailer or pallet; or in the liquid form, i.e., a vacuum insulated evaporator or an O_2 concentrator. Piped medical air may be supplied from either a cylinder manifold or a compressor with an outlet filter. Nitrous oxide is generally supplied from a cylinder manifold.

Standards and Sources of Information[7]

The Canadian Standards Association (CSA), the CGA, the International Standards Organization (ISO) and the National Fire Protection Association (NFPA) have published numerous documents related to piping systems. Many of their provisions are incorporated into law. There are also many state and local codes that supersede these standards. Compliance with the appropriate standard is the responsibility of the individual contractor or supplier of medical gas piping system and the healthcare institute.

Standard in our country regarding designing of medical gas pipeline system, selection of its equipment, installation and commissioning is IS.[9]

- *IS 12827/ISO 7396:* Nonflammable medical gas pipeline systems
- *IS/ISO 7396-1:* Pipeline systems for compressed medical gases and vacuum
- *IS/ISO 9170-2:* Terminal units for use with compressed medical gases and vacuum
- *IS 2379:1990:* Pipelines identification color-code.

Components of Central Piping System

- *Source equipment:* Central manifold containing cylinders, liquid tank, or central plant containing generators for piped compressed air and vacuum
- *Pipeline distribution system:* Piping emerging out from source equipment and extending to locations where the gas may be required

- *Terminal units:* Wall outlets, ceiling pendants, and bed head panels at the user points
- Suction and O_2 therapy products.

Source Equipment (Central Manifold or Plant Room)

It comprises of O_2 and N_2O manifold or plant room for central compressed air and vacuum system.

The source of supply may consist of one or more of the following (IS 12827/ISO 7396):[9]

- Gas in manifolded portable cylinders
- Gas in manifolded cylinders on a trailer or pallet
- Cryogenic liquid in portable cylinders (sometimes manifolded)
- Cryogenic liquid in manifolded cylinders on a trailer
- Cryogenic liquid in a stationary vessel(s)
- Liquefied gas in a vessel
- Medical air-compressing system
- Medical vacuum-pumping system
- Proportioning system
- Medical O_2 concentrator.

These manifolds/plants are located outdoors (with the control panel protected from the weather) in an enclosure used only for this purpose or in a room or enclosure within a building. Access to the central supply area is restricted to individuals familiar with and responsible for the system, namely biomedical and the maintenance department people, company personnel responsible for filling or replacing the manifold cylinders or liquid tank.

General Criteria for Manifold Room Selection

- Oxygen, N_2O manifold room must be at ground level so as to have easy access for cylinder delivery vehicles
- Access should be from the open air, not from corridors or other rooms
- Floor level of the manifold room should be approximately 1 m higher than the ground floor level for ease of handling of cylinders from the truck.

General Criteria for Plant Room Selection

- Should not be located in the medical gases manifold room
- Should not be used for storing full or empty medical gas cylinders
- Should be in close proximity to the manifold room
- Should avoid contamination of other systems by oil or oil mist and to fire or explosion hazards.

Medical Oxygen and Nitrous Oxide Manifolds

Manifolds comprise of O_2 and N_2O cylinders with control panels. The size of the manifold varies from a "double two", i.e., two banks (one right-sided bank and one left-sided bank) of two cylinders each (usually G and H size cylinders) to a "double 20" (two banks of 20 cylinders each). The manifold system controls duplex banks of high pressure cylinders, constantly monitors the condition of the supply and transmit appropriate information to ensure continuity of supply. Operation of control panel for O_2 and N_2O is exactly the same in each case whether older **(Figs. 10A to D)** or newer control panels. However, the parts and the designs of the newer control panels **(Figs. 11A to D)** differ from those of old control panels.

The cylinders are connected to a common manifold (header). A check (nonreturn) valve is placed between each cylinder lead and the header to prevent loss of gas from the cylinders if there is a leak in an individual cylinder or lead. The primary (running) supply is the bank of cylinders from which the gases are being used at that given point of time, while the other bank of cylinders is the secondary (standby/reserve) supply. When the pressure of primary (running) supply drops to a predetermined level due to emptying of cylinders, the secondary supply automatically starts and becomes the primary (running) supply. The system indicates the change of "running supply" in the alarm panel designed for the system so that the concerned authority can change the cylinders in the empty bank.

The pressures at which gases are piped vary, depending on the country. In the US, gases other than N_2 and instrument air are normally piped at 345–380 kPa (50–55 psi). In India, medical gases are piped at 4–4.2 bar (55–60 psi). Nitrogen and instrument air are usually delivered at 700 kPa (100 psi). The NFPA now permits pressures up to 2,068 kPa (300 psi).

Liquid Oxygen Supply[7]

Liquid O_2 containers are installed when large amounts of O_2 are required. They are situated at ground level **(Figs. 12A to D)** so that they can be readily accessible to supply trucks. The containers should be located where exposure to potential ignition sources is minimal. Standards for installation of liquid gas container specify how far the container must be from sidewalks, parked vehicles, and other objects. Liquid O_2 containers are refilled from supply trucks without interrupting service. Alternatively, filled liquid containers may be transported between the supplier and the institute.

To prevent the liquid from evaporating, it is kept at or below its boiling point (-184°C) by keeping it in special insulated vessels. They are constructed like thermos bottles with outer and inner metal jackets separated by insulation and a layer that is near vacuum to retard heat transfer from the exterior. These containers vary in size and shape. Each container has a contents indicator and low liquid level alarm. Gaseous O_2 is drawn off as required and passed through an atmospheric vaporizing coil **(Figs. 12A and B)** to bring it up to ambient temperature and raise its pressure.

Although the tank is well-insulated, a small amount of heat will be continuously absorbed from the surroundings, causing the liquefied gas to evaporate. This will slowly increase the pressure in the container which will open the safety relief valve venting O_2 to atmosphere. Therefore, if a liquid system is left standing unused for a long period of time, a significant amount of O_2 will be lost. Using liquid containers is economical only when there is a fairly constant demand. Having the proper size container will minimize O_2 loss from venting.[7]

Most of the time, the O_2 is kept cold by the latent heat of vaporization as gaseous O_2 is removed and the temperature falls. As the temperature falls, the pressure within the tank also falls. To maintain pressure, a portion of liquid O_2 must be removed from the tank and passed through a vaporizer (evaporator, vaporizing column, gasifier to form gaseous O_2 and recycled to increase the pressure inside the tank).

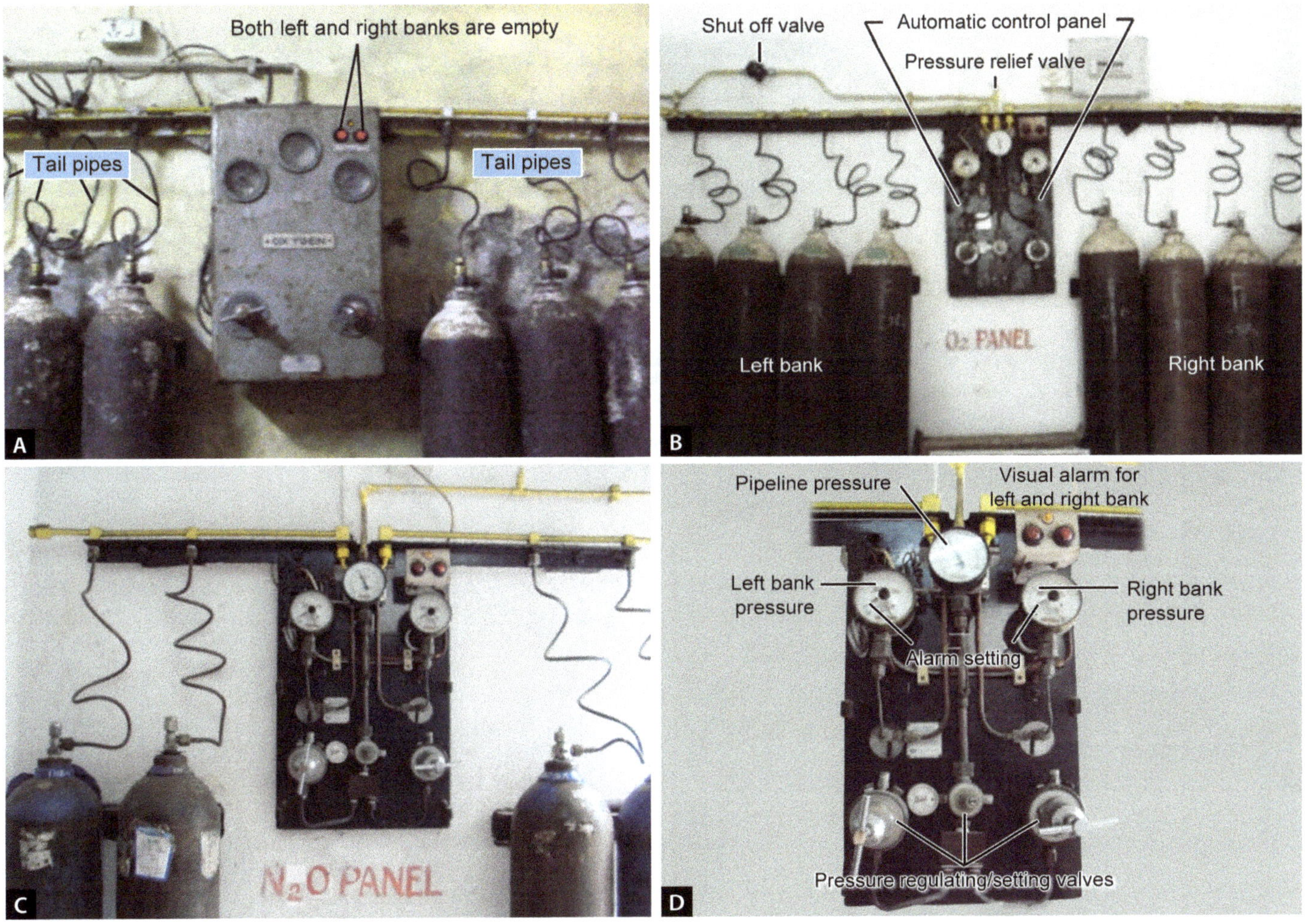

Figs. 10A to D: Central pipeline manifolds—old design. (A) O_2 manifold with control panel cover; (B) O_2 manifold with control panel cover open; (C) N_2O manifold with control panel cover open; (D) Parts of old manifold and control panel.

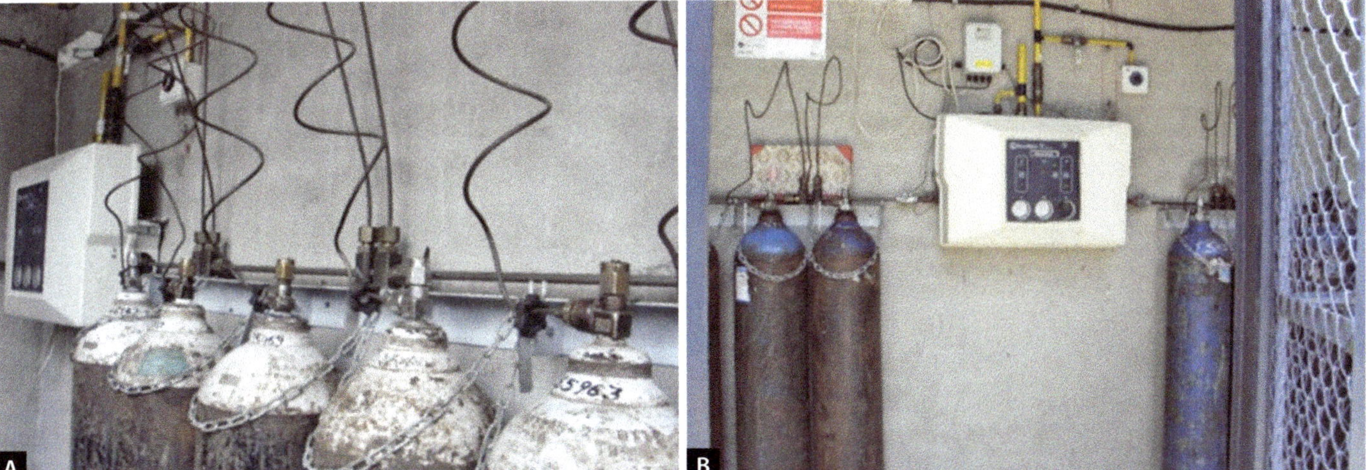

Figs. 11A and B

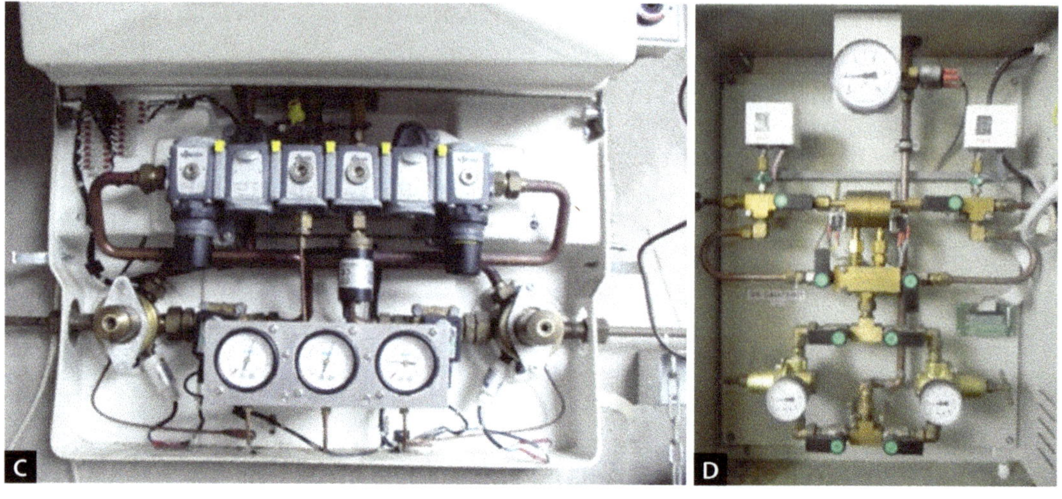

Figs. 11C and D

Figs. 11A to D: Central pipeline manifolds—newer designs. (A) O_2 manifold with control panel cover; (B) N_2O manifold with control panel cover; (C and D) Modern control panel.

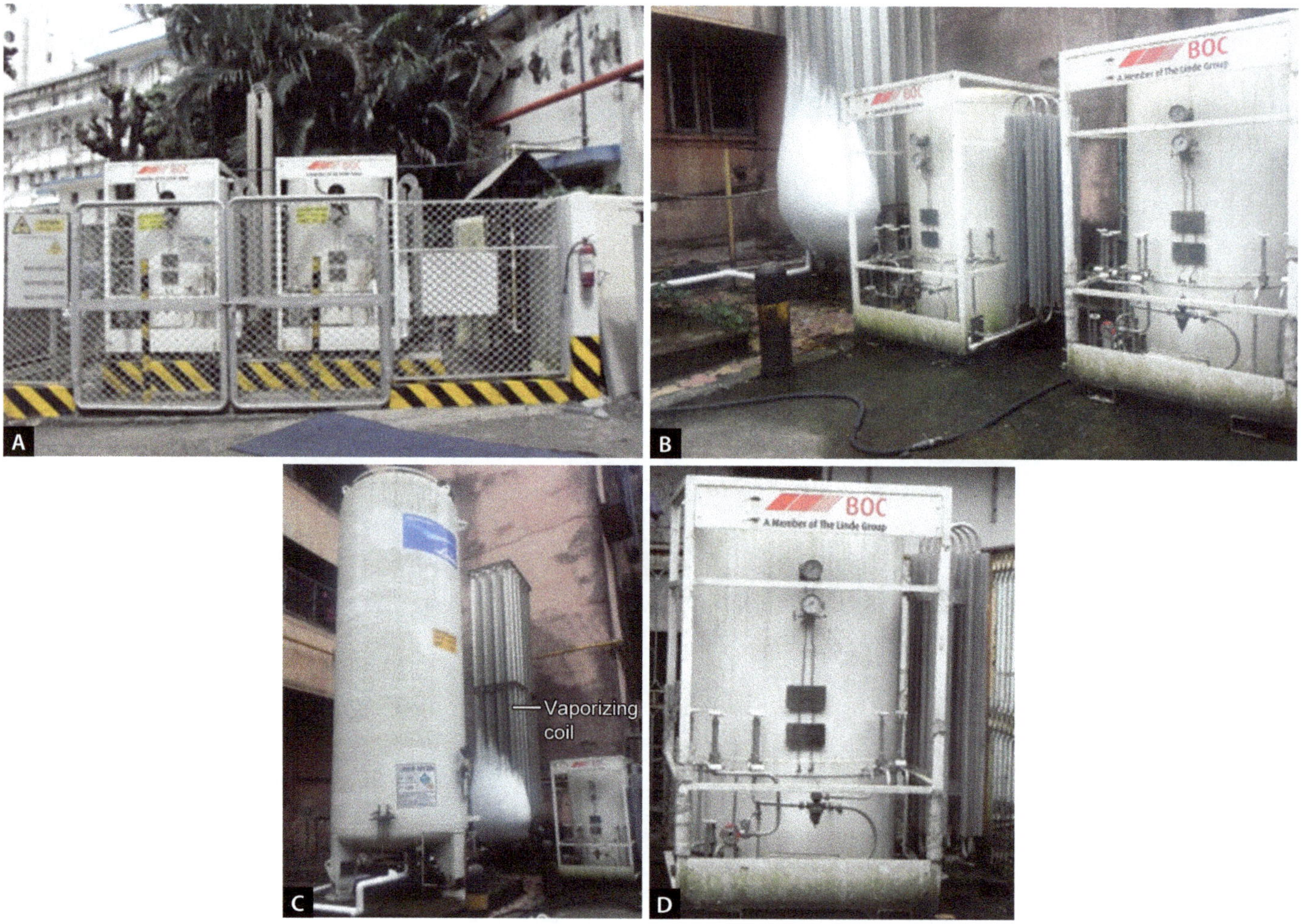

Figs. 12A to D: Various liquid O_2 tanks/vessels.

Oxygen Concentrator[10]

For remote locations where liquid/cylinder O_2 is not available, O_2 pipeline is fed with O_2 concentrators though purity of O_2 is not up to the desired level. Oxygen concentrators extract O_2 from air by differential absorption. Molecular sieve of hydrated aluminum silicates of the alkaline earth metals in a powder or granular form (zeolites) is used. Ambient air is filtered and pressurized by a compressor. Air is exposed to a zeolite molecular sieve column at a certain pressure. The sieve selectively retains N_2 and

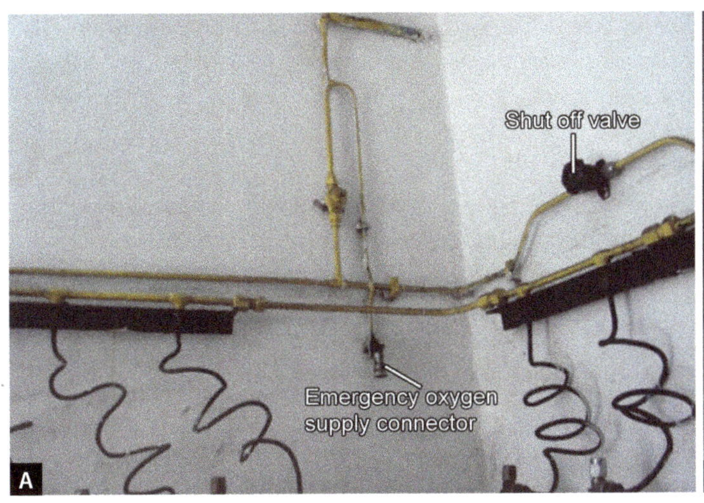

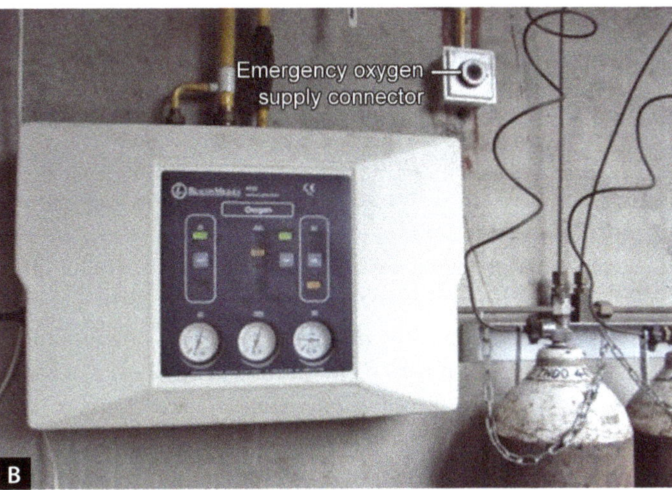

Figs. 13A and B: Emergency O_2 supply connector to central manifold. (A) Old design; (B) Newer design.

other unwanted components of air which are released into the atmosphere after heating the column and applying a vacuum. The maximum O_2 concentration achieved is 95% by volume.[10] Argon is the main remaining constituent.

Emergency Oxygen Supply Connector

A fitting for connecting a temporary auxiliary supply source for emergency or maintenance situations is required. The pipe from this fitting attaches to the main supply line immediately downstream of the main line shut-off valve **(Figs. 13A and B)**. The inlet should be located where a supply vehicle will have year-round access.

Medical (Compressed) Air[7]

Air may be supplied from manifolded cylinders, a proportioning device that mixes gas from O_2 and N_2 cylinders, or motor-driven compressors. For clinical purposes it is supplied at a pressure of 400 kPa and for driving power tools it is supplied at 700 kPa.

The vast majority of piped air systems employ two or more compressors that operate alternately or simultaneously, depending on demand, but always there should be a standby compressor. A typical system consists of compressor with electric motor, after cooler, air receiver, air dryer, filtration, pressure reducing station with suitable mountings for installation. Each compressor takes in ambient air, compresses it to above the working pressure, and supplies it to one or more receivers (accumulators, reservoir tanks, storage receivers, reservoirs, holding tanks, receiver tanks) from which air can be withdrawn as needed **(Fig. 14)**. The receiver is equipped with a pressure relief valve, automatic drain, sight glass to permit visual checking that the drains are operating properly, and a pressure gauge.

The intake location is important to ensure that the air is free of contaminants as far as possible, i.e., free of dirt, fumes, and odors. The air at the intake is checked periodically as the air quality varies with time and may exceed the contaminant limits. To render the air suitable for medical use, its water content must be reduced. An after-cooler in which the air is cooled and the condensed moisture is removed is usually installed downstream of each compressor. More water may condense in the receiver. Additional water may be removed by running the air through a dryer. Air downstream of the dryers and upstream of the piping system must be monitored for CO and dew point and with certain types of compressors, for gaseous and liquid hydrocarbons. Valves, pressure regulators, and alarms analogous to those in O_2 supply systems are needed. The reserve supply may be manifolded cylinders or a separate compressor system.

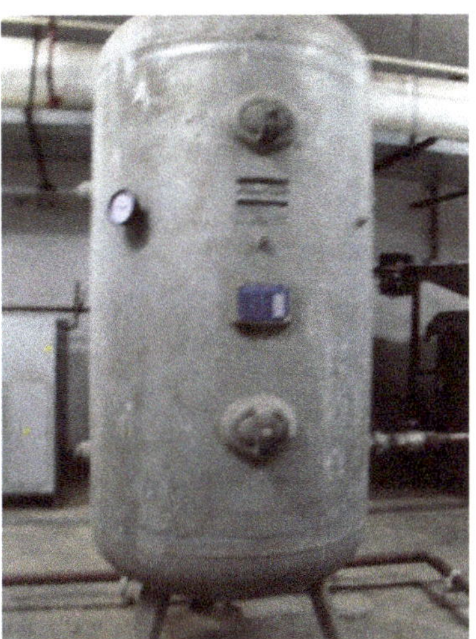

Fig. 14: Central compressed air reservoir.

Central Vacuum System

The unit consists of vacuum pump complete with electric motor with suitable mountings for installation. A cylindrical reservoir tank which stabilizes the present pressure of the pipeline system between 305 and 635 mm of mercury at all outlet points is connected to the pump. Automatic start and stop of the motor is controlled by a negative pressure switch. The vacuum pumps are at least duplexed where one vacuum pump will be in running condition whereas the other will remain as standby.

Pipeline Distribution System

Clean and degreased nonarsenical copper pipes of the appropriate grade and standard are utilized to convey gases from source equipment to outlet points. The pipeline is installed at various wings and floors of the healthcare facility as per the requirement of distribution of medical gases/ vacuum. All pipes are normally joined by flux less brazing to ensure maximum internal cleanliness. Branched outlines are normally fitted with stop valves to enable them to be isolated should the necessity arise.

For all other systems except vacuum, an alternative emergency inlet point (T fitting for connecting auxiliary source of the gas) is generally provided, to which only gas-specific connector can be attached **(Figs. 11 and 13)**. Branched outlines are normally fitted with stop (shut-off) valves to enable them to be isolated should the necessities arise.

There are three general classes of piping:

1. *Main lines:* Pipes connecting the source to risers or branch lines or both
2. *Risers:* Vertical pipes connecting the main line with branch lines on various levels of the healthcare facility
3. *Branch (lateral) lines:* Sections of the piping system that service a room or group of rooms on the same level of the facility.

Medical Gas Pipeline Installation and Testing Procedure

Generally, vacuum is installed in 15 mm outer diameter (OD) and other gases in 12 mm OD pipes. Pipes are marked at least every 20 feet and at least once in every room so as to identify the gases that they contain. The name and pressure of the gas inside the pipe and its flow direction is displayed.

It is advisable to keep medical gas pipelines away from following:

- From mechanical damage
- From chemical damage
- Excessive heat
- Avoid contact with oil, grease, or bituminous compounds and from splashing and dripping
- Avoid electrical sparks in and around pipeline areas.

The area of service ducts or void should have adequate ventilation, so in event of leakage higher gas concentrations can be prevented. The pipeline should be installed any areas to house combustible materials such as kitchen, boiler houses, electric cables.

The pipelines for distribution of medical gases in hospitals and visible connecting tubing of anesthetic apparatus are marked with bands at least at each end and at every joint by the color appropriate for the gases **(Table 4, Figs. 15 and 16A)**. Flexible hoses are restricted to exposed areas where they can be inspected and maintained. They cannot penetrate or be concealed in walls, floors, ceilings, or partitions.

Shut-off Valves

Shut-off (stop) valves permit specific areas of the piping system to be isolated in the event of a problem as well as

TABLE 4: Color-code for medical gases pipelines IS 2379 (1990).*

Gas	*Ground color band*	*First color band*	*Second color band*
O_2	Canary yellow	White	–
N_2O	Canary yellow	French blue	Signal red
Vacuum	Sky blue	Black	–
Air	Sky blue	White	Black
N_2	Canary yellow	Black	–
CO_2	Canary yellow	Light gray	–
O_2 and CO_2 mixture	Canary yellow	White	Light gray
He	Canary yellow	Light brown	–
O_2 and He mixture	Canary yellow	White	Light brown

*The direction of flow is indicated.

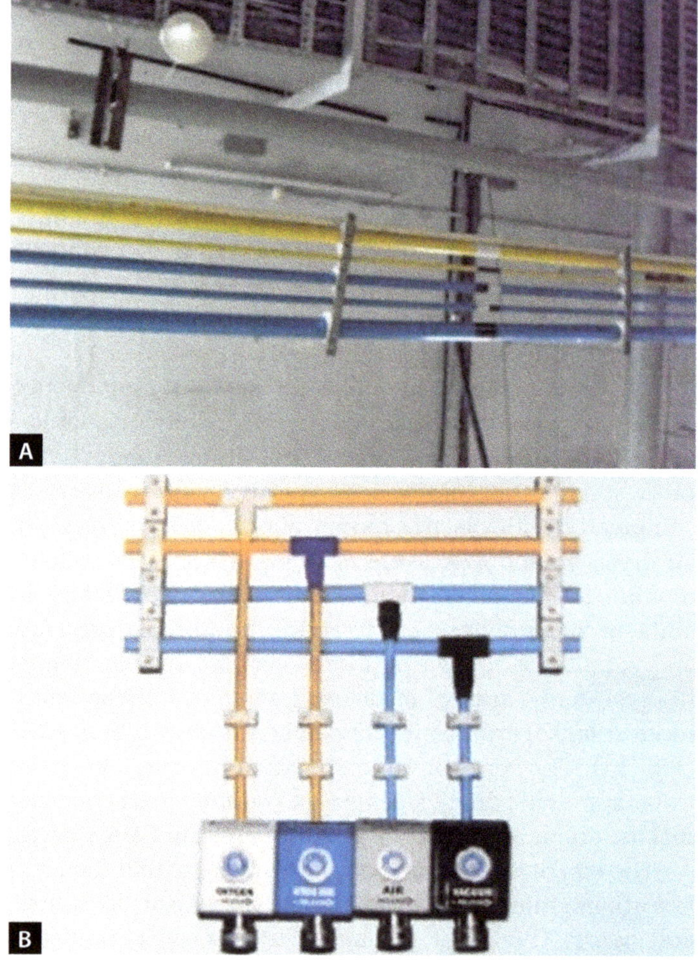

Figs. 15A and B: Color-coding of central pipelines. (A) Main lines; (B) Branch lines.

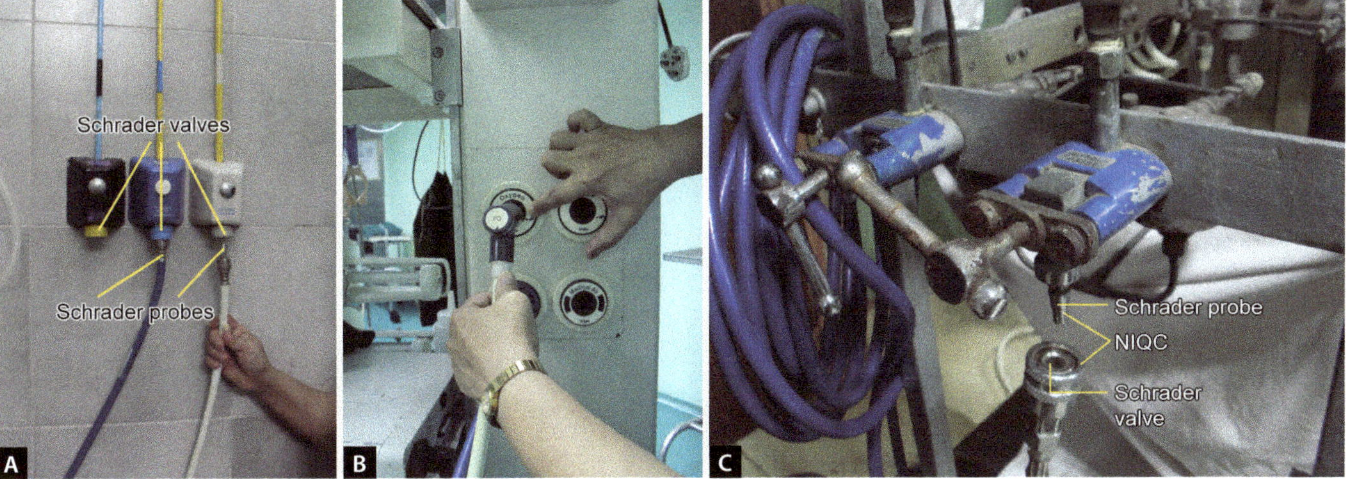

Figs. 16A to C: Noninterchangeable quick connectors (NIQC). (A) Wall outlets; (B) Ceiling column; (C) Anesthesia machine.

for maintenance, repair, testing or expansion without the whole system being turned "off". There are two types of shut-off valves: (1) manual and (2) service. Manual shut-off valves are installed where they are visible and accessible at all times for authorized persons. Service shut-off valves are designed to be used only by authorized personnel. They are in locked cases or have their handles secured and tagged to prevent accidental closing.

Shut-off valves are classified as follows (IS 12827):[9]

1. Service shut-off valves:
   - Main service shut-off valve **(Figs. 13A and 17)**
   - Riser service shut-off valve
   - Lateral service shut-off valve
   - Equipment service shut-off valve.
2. Manual/Zone shut-off valves **(Figs. 18A to C)** in boxes with fixed covers or doors.

   Boxes enclosing zone shut-off valves have fixed covers or doors which can be locked in the closed position. The covers or doors have a means of quick access in case of emergency.

Pressure Relief Valves (Fig. 17A)

Each central supply system must have a pressure relief valve set at 33% above normal line pressure downstream of the line regulator(s) and upstream of any shut-off valve. This relief valve prevents pressure build-up if a shut-off valve is closed. The valve should close automatically when the excess pressure has been relieved.

TESTS AND CHECKS ON THE PIPELINE CARCASS[11]

The following tests must be carried out after installation of the pipeline carcass but before concealment:

- Visual check of pipeline labeling, marking, sleeving, and support
- Leakage test
- Documented tests for cross-connection
- Valve tests for closure, zoning, and leakage.

Gas Pipeline Pressure Drop or Leakage Test

One and half times the working pressure or 10.5 bar, whichever is higher, for 24 hours. Appreciable pressure drop should be less than 0.025% per hour.

This test should be carried out on the pipeline carcass with the area service units or other valves open.

During pressure testing, any safety valves and pressure-sensing devices installed may be removed and the connections blanked off.

It is not desirable to cross-link the carcasses to form a single system for the purpose of the carcass leakage test.

Valve Tightness Test

This test is to check pressure test on pipeline of all isolating valves for 15 minutes at 6.9, gauge pressure to confirm its tightness and avoid any leakage during these valve tests.

Each valve tightness test should be held for not less than 15 minutes.

Relief Valve Test

The pressure on gas systems can be reduced after completion of valve tightness test. A service test valve with capacity to discharge working pressure of 133%.

Test for Leakage on Completed Installations: Pressure Systems

The installation, terminal units, theater fittings should be checked for working pressure for 24 hours, to avoid leak. A pipeline of 50 terminal units can have loss up to 0.15 bar (2 psi).

Test for Leakage on Completed Installations: Vacuum Systems

After the initial drying out of the pipeline by the operation of the vacuum plant, the completed vacuum system should then be tested. After initial drying out of pipeline the system should be exhausted to a vacuum of 210 mm Hg absolute.

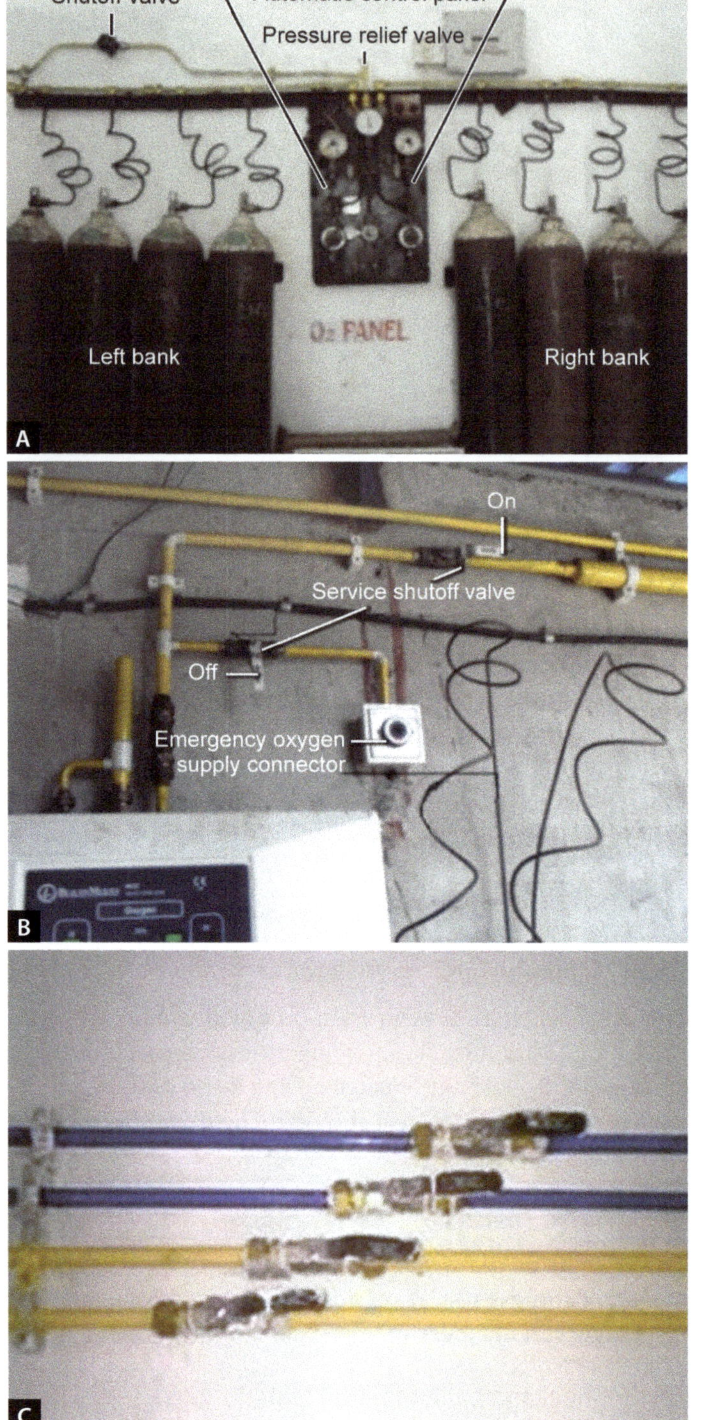

Figs. 17A to C: Pipeline service shut-off valves.

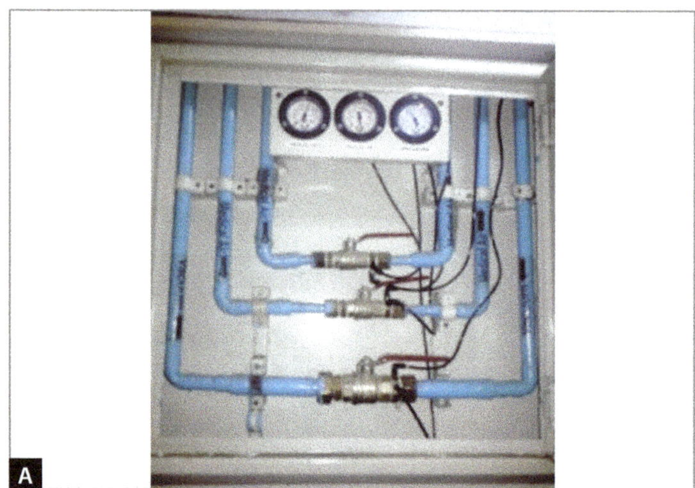

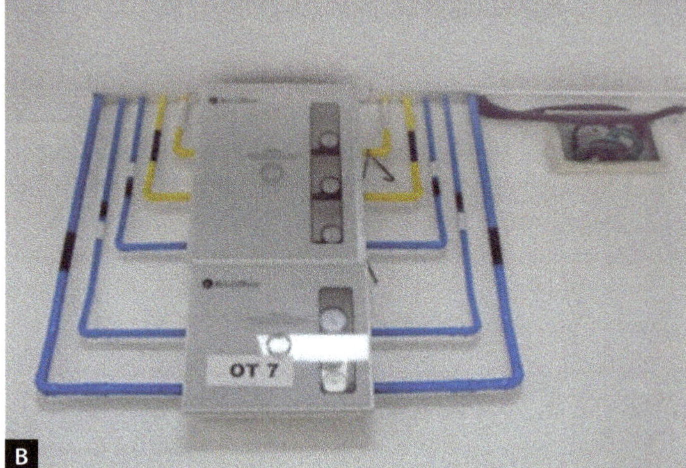

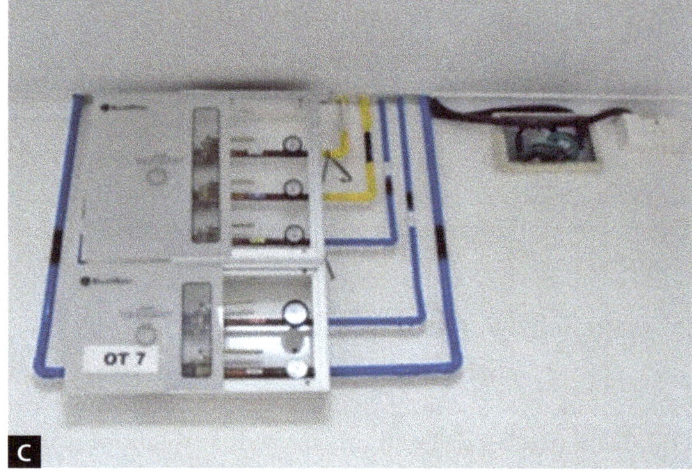

Figs. 18A to C: Pipeline area/zone shut-off valves. (A) Zone shut-off valve; (B) Specific OT—box closed; (C) Specific OT—box opened.

The suggested pressure should be less than 10 mm Hg in 1 hour. This test pressure should be held for 24 hours. A pressure rise in excess of 10 mm Hg per hour normally indicates the need for remedial work and further tests.

Cross-connection

Continuity test to ensure gas specificity at the terminal outlet.

Precommissioning Tests

Before the installation is formally handed over to the user, the following checks and tests should be carried out:

- During the contract period:
    - Pressure test, for leakage in pipelines only
    - Check valve tightness and correct valve zoning
    - Test relief valve operation

- To check for leakage, perform a pressure test
- Ensure smooth mechanical operation and noninterchangeability of each terminal unit of means of test probes
- Ensure for no cross-connections also known as "anticonfusion test" or "continuity test")
- Each terminal unit must be checked for flow rate and pressure
- Check satisfactory operation of manifold changeover valves
- Check satisfactory operation of liquid O_2, compressed air and vacuum plants and all manifolds (including emergency supply panels)
- Alarm signaling system should be in working condition
- Installation system should be purged with air, N_2 and check for cleanliness of system.

At the end, purge the completed installation with the working gas.

Alarms[7]

Master Alarm System[7] (Figs. 19A to C)

A master alarm system monitors the central supply and the distribution system for all medical gas systems. To ensure continuous responsible observation, master signal panels must be located in two separate locations, wired in parallel to a single sensor for each condition. One panel should be in the principal working area of the department responsible for maintaining the system and one or more panels located to assure continuous surveillance during all working hours (e.g., telephone board operator, security office or other continuously staffed location).

Area Alarm Systems[7] (Fig. 19C)

Critical life support areas, such as operating room suites, postanesthesia care units, ICU, coronary care units, etc., must have an area (local) alarm system to indicate if the pressure increases or decreases 20% from normal line pressure. It will be placed downstream of the shut-off valve for the area. Area alarms are sometimes placed in each anesthetizing location.

Local Alarms[7]

Local alarms are installed to monitor the function of the central medical and instrument air systems as well as the vacuum and anesthetic gas scavenging systems. The signals may be located on or in the control panel of the machinery being monitored, within a monitoring device or on a separate alarm panel.

Terminal Units (Wall Outlets, Ceiling Pendants, Bed Head Panels)

The pipeline network which is terminated by a terminal unit can be mounted in a variety of ways to ensure maximum convenience. It may be on the wall or on ceiling or bed head panels.

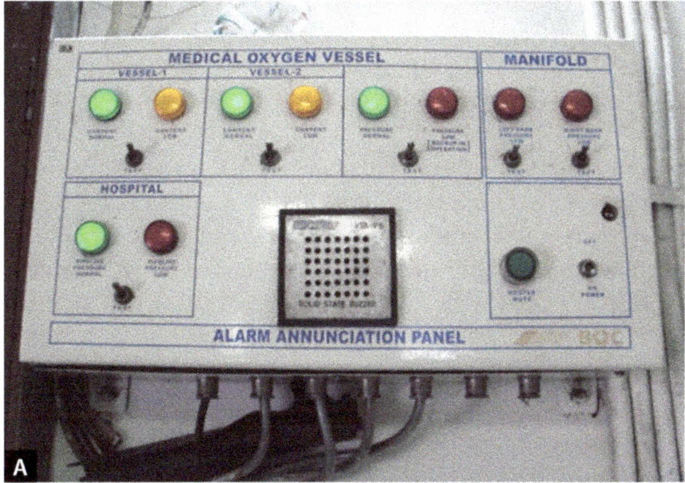

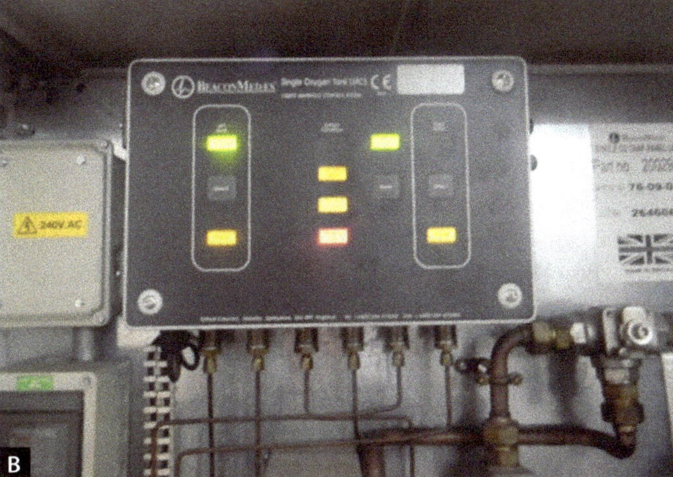

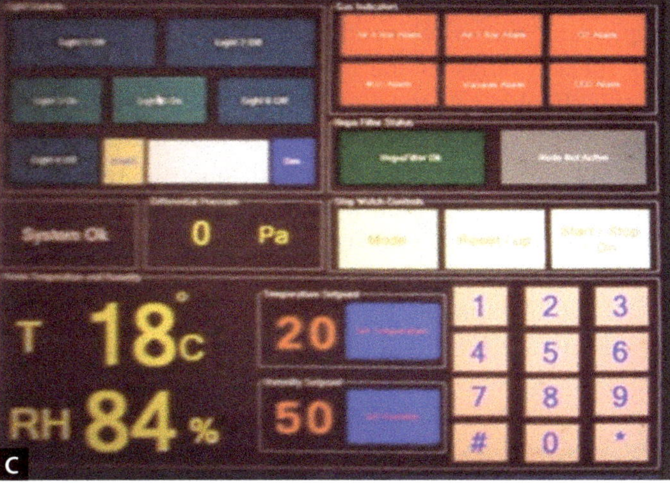

Figs. 19A to C: Alarm systems for central pipelines. (A) Central alarm liquid + manifold; (B) Liquid O_2 alarm panel; (C) Area alarm panel in OT.

Outlets are colored for identification. Instant supply of gas/vacuum can be established by inserting noninterchangeable safety keyed plug connectors into the outlet points. The gas flow shuts off immediately after the plug connector is removed.

Components[7]

Base Block

The base block is the part of a terminal unit that is attached to the pipeline distribution system.

Primary Valve

The primary valve (automatic shut-off valve, self-sealing valve) opens and allows the gas to flow when the male probe is inserted and closes automatically when the connection is broken. This serves to prevent gas loss when the removable component is disconnected. Although often called a check valve, it is not a unidirectional valve and when open will permit flow in either direction. In some terminal units, the face plate and primary valve are an integral unit.

Secondary Valve

The secondary valve (secondary shut-off valve, secondary check valve) is designed so that when the primary valve is removed (e.g., for cleaning or servicing), the gas flow is shut-off. When the primary valve is in place, the secondary valve stays open. With hose booms and pendants incorporating hoses, the secondary valve is fitted at or near the end of the permanent pipe work.

Gas-specific Connection Point (Socket Assembly)

It is incorporated into each terminal unit. It is either part of or attached to the base block. It is the receptor for a noninterchangeable gas-specific connector. The connector may be a threaded DISS or a proprietary (manufacturer-specific) quick connector.

DIAMETER INDEX SAFETY SYSTEM[7]

Diameter index safety system connector consists of a body, nipple, and nut combination. There are two concentric and specific bores in the body and two concentric and specific shoulders on the nipple. The small bore (BB) mates with the small shoulder, and the large bore mates with the large shoulder. To achieve noninterchangeability between different connectors, the two diameters on each part vary in opposite directions so that as one diameter increases, the other decreases. Only properly mated parts will fit together and allow the threads to engage. The American Society for Testing and Materials anesthesia workstation requires that every anesthesia machine have a DISS fitting for each pipeline inlet **(Fig. 20)**.

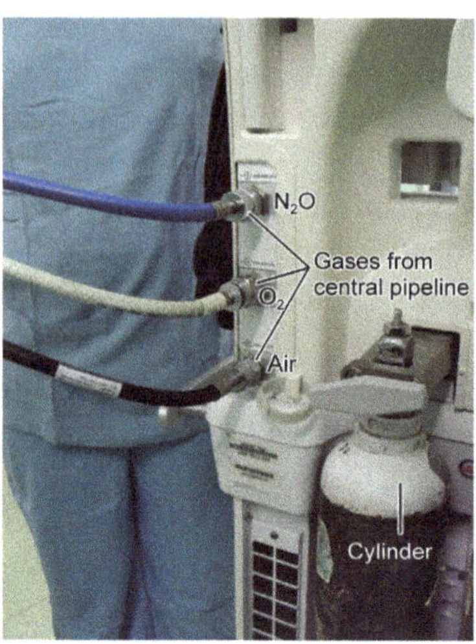

Fig. 20: Diameter index safety system on anesthesia machine.

Quick Connectors

Quick connectors allow apparatus (hoses, flow meters, etc.) to be connected or disconnected by a single action using one or both hands without the use of tools or undue force. Quick connectors are more convenient than DISS fittings but tend to leak more.

Each quick connector consists of a pair of gas-specific male and female components **(Figs. 16A to C)**. A releasable spring mechanism locks the components together. Hoses and other equipment are prevented from being inserted into an incorrect outlet by using different shapes and/or different spacing of mating portions.

Faceplate

The faceplate should be permanently marked with the name and/or symbol of the gas that it conveys. The identifying color will also be present.

Types of Terminal Units[7]

Wall Outlets

Wall outlets **(Fig. 16A)** are simple and well suited where the equipment to be connected is near the wall. However, it leads to personnel tripping over the hoses, difficulty in moving equipment, wear and tear on the hoses.

Ceiling-mounted Hoses

Ceiling-mounted hoses with the terminal unit at the end of the hose may be used. A spring-actuated chain keeps the hose close to the ceiling.

Ceiling Pendants (Fig. 21A)

Rigid or swiveling ceiling pendant in the operation theater will:

- Increase efficiency by keeping medical gas hoses and electrical cables clear of the floor area
- Provide full system compatibility, ensuring complete integration with other products.

Ceiling Columns (Fig. 22B)

Ceiling-mounted columns provide the same services as a pendant but are less versatile with respect to positioning. They can be made retractable by mounting them on tracks. The column can be lowered to attach or detach hoses and then raised to avoid obstruction.

Horizontal Bed Head Panels (Figs. 22A and B)

The bed head panels are ergonomically designed keeping the needs of the ward/ICU/private room in view with desired outlets, electrical sockets and other accessories.

These are extruded aluminum panels, anodized and powder coated with the customer's choice of colors to maintain the esthetics of the hospital.

Flexible Hoses/Flexible Pipelines (Figs. 23A and B)

Flexible hoses extend from terminal units to the anesthesia machine or workstation or other equipment like suction apparatus, ventilators in ICUs. They may be NIQC, DISS or NIST type. They are not part of the piped system but they are important to anesthesiologists.

Noninterchangeable quick connectors/couplers (NIQC)[7,12] commonly used for anesthesia machine at the wall outlets or machine end are known as Schrader probe and Schrader valve **(Figs. 16A to C, 21B and 23A)** and have three components:

1. *Schrader probe:*[7,12] To prevent misconnection to the wrong gas service, the probe for each gas supply has a protruding indexing collar with a unique diameter, which only fits the Schrader socket assembly for the same gas
2. *Flexible hosepipe:*[7,12] Originally, the hoses were made of black reinforced rubber with short lengths of colored sheaths at each end. Modern hoses are color-coded for each gas (oxygen is white; nitrous oxide, French blue; medical air hose, black/white and yellow for vacuum). One end of the hose is fixed with probe which fits to the wall end and at the other end is attached the valve which **(Figs. 1B, 16A to C, and 23)** fits to the probe of a yoke block having pin index system
3. *Yoke block:* It is used to connect pipeline supplies to the machine or to connect the cylinders larger than size E to the machine **(Figs. 1B, 5, 16C, and 23)** with the help of a flexible hose. It is a piece of metal, shaped like a cylinder valve, that is pin indexed and has a port to fit over the nipple of the yoke and it has a conical depression on the other end to fit the tip of the retaining screw into a yoke. It has a connector that fits on a flexible hose of central pipeline system.

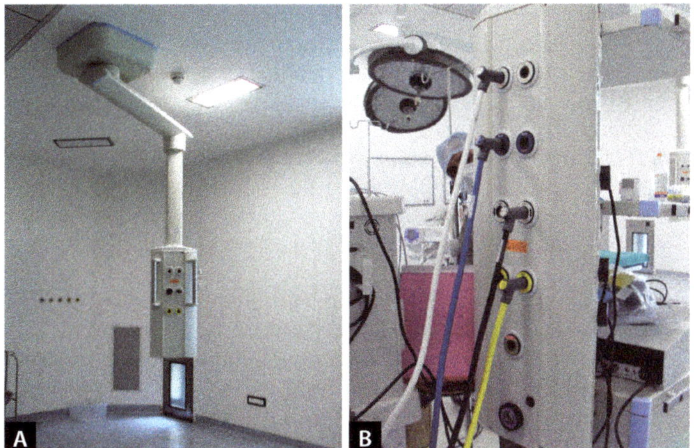

Figs. 21A and B: Terminal units. (A) Ceiling pendant; (B) Ceiling column.

SUCTION AND OXYGEN THERAPY PRODUCTS

Oxygen Flow Meter with Humidifier (Fig. 21B)

Back pressure compensated flow meter will meet strict precision and durability standards. Body is made of brass materials. Humidifier bottle is made of unbreakable polycarbonate material and autoclavable.

Ward Vacuum Unit

Available with 600/2,000 mL jars with safety trap. Jars are made of polycarbonate and are autoclavable. Regulators are available with or without safety trap and will be infinitely adjustable.

Theater Suction Unit

Mobile floor suction unit for operation theater is available in various models as desired by the user: With glass jars, autoclavable polycarbonate jars, regulator with or without safety trap, different types of trolleys having free moving castor wheels.

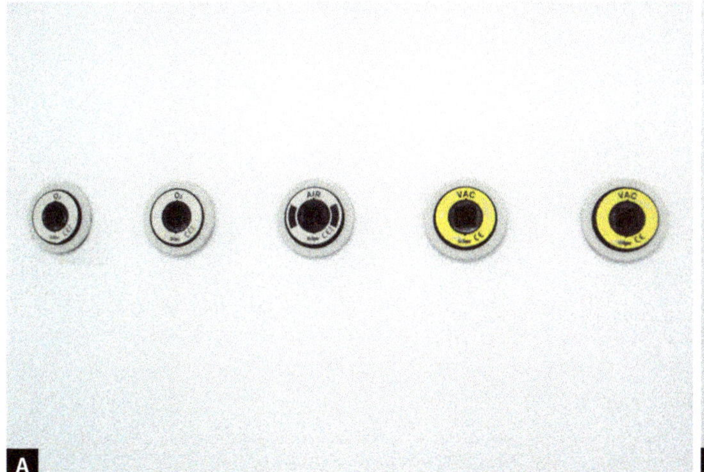

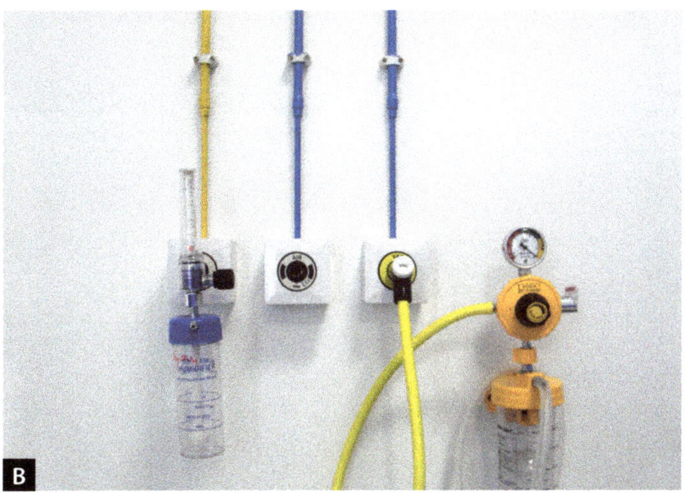

Figs. 22A and B: Terminal units—bed head panels.

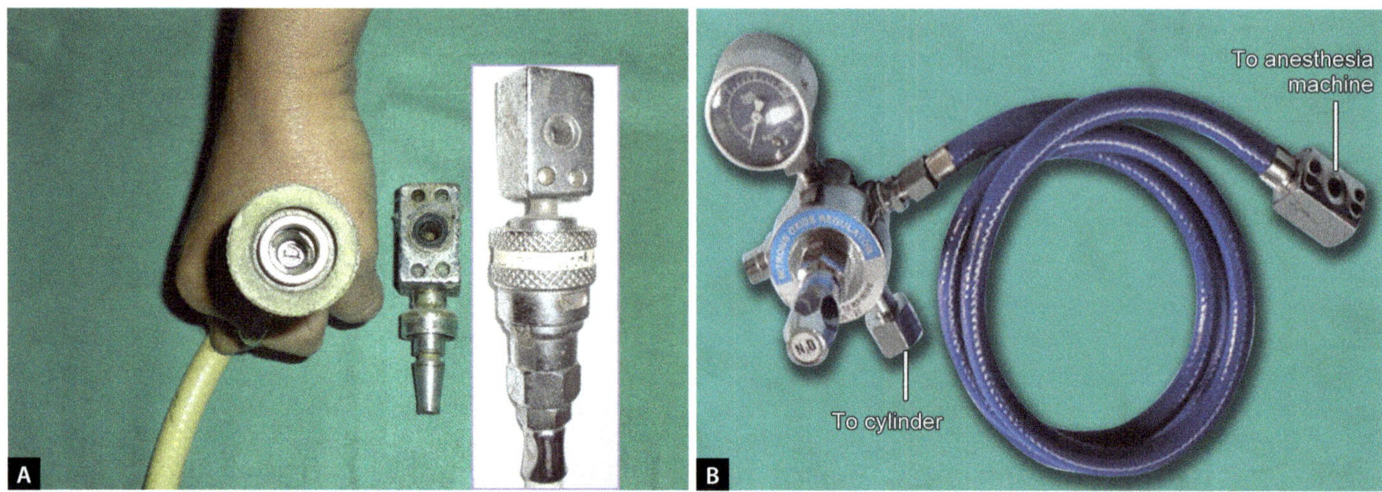

Figs. 23A and B: Flexible hoses. (A) Central line to anesthesia machine; (B) Cylinder to anesthesia machine.

CONCLUSION

Anesthesia practice involves the use of compressed medical gas cylinders and central pipeline gases. There is a possibility of crossover of gas connections, system running out of supply, suffocation, fires, explosions, thermal injuries and so on that can lead to disasters. It is therefore absolutely necessary for the anesthesiologists to understand the design, working principle, and possibilities of hazards related to compressed medical gas cylinders and medical gas central pipeline so as to rectify and prevent mishaps that can jeopardize the safety of patients as well as personal working in operation theaters, ICU, and other areas where these gases are used.

REFERENCES

1. Paul AK. Drugs and Equipment in Anesthesia Practice. New Delhi: Elsevier India Pvt. Ltd.; 2009. pp. 163-76.
2. Gas Cylinders Rules, 2004. DIPP. [online] Available from http://dipp.nic.in/sites/default/files/Gas_cylinder_Rule_2004.pdf. [Last accessed April, 2021].
3. Gas Cylinders Rules, 1981. (2004). Department Of Industrial Policy. [online] Available from dipp.nic.in/English/acts_rules/Acts/Gas_cylinder_Rule_2004.pdf. [Last accessed February, 2014].
4. Medical gas cylinder data chart. [online] Available from http://www.bochealthcare.co.uk/internet.lh.lh.gbr/en/images/cylinder_data_med309965_2011409_54065.pdf. [Last accessed April, 2021].
5. Bureau of Indian Standards (BIS), Division: Mechanical Engineering, Section: Gas Cylinders (MED 16) Gas Cylinders (MED 16)—Mechanical Engineering Division—Public. [online] Available from https://law.resource.org/pub/in/bis/manifest.med.16.html. [Last accessed April, 2021].
6. Gas Cylinders (MED 16)—Mechanical Engineering Division. [online] Available from https://law.resource.org/pub/in/bis/manifest.med.16.html. [Last accessed February, 2014].
7. Dorsch JA, Dorsch SE. Understanding Anesthesia Equipment, 5th edition. Philadelphia: Lippincott Williams & Wilkins; 2007. pp. 26-51.
8. Static and mobile pressure vessels rules, 2016: Draft notification for amendment in SMPV (U) Rules, 2016 and Gas. [online] Available from www.dipp.nic.in/.../draft-notification-amendment-smpv-u-rules-2016-and-gas-cylind. [Last accessed April, 2021].
9. Indian Standards/ISO: Bureau of Indian Standards. [online] Available from www.bis.gov.in/. [Last accessed April, 2021].
10. Lovell T. Medical gases, their storage and delivery. Anaesth Intensive Care Med. 2004;5(1):10-4.
11. International standard iso 7396-1 - SAI Global Store. 2016. [online] Available from https://infostore.saiglobal.com/store/PreviewDoc.aspx?saleItemID=2898755. [Last accessed April, 2021].
12. Sinclair CM, Thadsad MK, Barker I. Modern anaesthetic machines. BJA: CEACCP. 2006;6(2):75-8.

Anesthesia Machine and its Components

SECTION 

The Anesthesia Machine

M Ravishankar, R Sripriya

ABSTRACT

The anesthesia machine has undergone a lot of changes in the last three decades. From being a simple gas delivery system on a tabletop, the machines have become sophisticated complete workstation incorporating all essential components needed to administer anesthesia, monitor and ventilate safely. This chapter on anesthesia machine gives a description of the essential components incorporated in most of the machines, the sequence of arrangement and describes the safety features in the machines. Detailed description of totally electronic advanced anesthesia workstation is included. Recommendations of the safety checkout procedure are appended.

INTRODUCTION

The technological developments in anesthesia system during the last 10 years have been more rapid than most other areas of medical technology. While this progress in the design of anesthesia machine has increased the safety of administering inhalation anesthesia, it contributes to making the system more complex and requires a considerably better education of the operator concerning the equipment. For safe conduct of anesthesia, it is imperative for the anesthesiologist to know the working principles of the anesthesia machine and be able to detect faults if and when they occur. The operator of an anesthesia machine creates an artificial atmosphere to which the patient is exposed and has, therefore, the responsibility to guarantee:

- An oxygen concentration which will prevent hypoxia of the patient
- Satisfactory elimination of carbon dioxide (CO_2)
- Avoidance of accidental administration of excessive anesthetic concentration.

It is absolutely necessary that an anesthesia system be operated under the constant surveillance of a qualified anesthesiologist. Understanding an anesthesia machine will be easier if the gas flow is traced from its source, through the machine, to the patient. The following components are likely to be encountered in sequence:

- Source of gas supply
- Yoke assembly
- Pressure gauge
- Pressure regulators
- Oxygen (O_2) pressure failure safety/warning devices
- Flowmeters
- Oxygen ratio control devices
- Vaporizers
- Common gas outlet
- Breathing systems.

The pressure regulators, flow meters, vaporizers, and breathing systems are discussed separately. The other components will be discussed briefly to give a comprehensive view of the whole machine.

SOURCE OF GAS SUPPLY

The anesthetic gases are usually supplied in cylinders made of molybdenum steel, an alloy **(Table 1)**, which allows the cylinders to be made thinner and lighter for comparable working pressures. Oxygen (O_2), nitrogen (N_2), and air are stored as compressed gas. These do not liquefy at the pressures to which they are filled at 20°C, since their critical temperature is low **(Table 2)**. The quantity of gas inside the cylinder can easily be estimated using a pressure gauge as the quantity is directly proportional to the gauge pressure. In clinical practice, changes in ambient temperature do not affect the pressure significantly.

Nitrous oxide (N_2O), CO_2, and cyclopropane (C_3H_6) liquefy at pressures to which the cylinders are filled at 20°C,

TABLE 1: Components of the alloy.

Component	*Percentage (%)*
Carbon	0.3–0.4
Manganese	0.4–0.9
Silicon (not to exceed)	0.3
Sulfur (not to exceed)	0.35
Phosphorus (not to exceed)	0.35
Molybdenum	0.15–0.25
Chromium	0.8–1.1
Iron	By difference

as the critical temperature of these agents is well above and are therefore stored as liquids. The cylinders are not filled completely but only up to a "filling ratio"

$$\text{Filling ratio} = \frac{\text{Weight of liquid with which it is filled}}{\text{Weight of the water it can hold}}$$

The filling ratio for N_2O and CO_2 is 0.67 in the tropics. The contents of these cylinders can be accurately measured by weighing these cylinders rather than by using a pressure gauge. The pressure gauge will only measure the pressure of the gas (vapor) above the liquid level which will remain constant till all the liquid is converted into (vapor) gas. Thus, the gauge cannot reflect the quantity of gas in the cylinder. If the environmental temperature is above the critical temperature of the gas **(Table 2)**, then the cylinder contents will be fully in gaseous state and the pressure gauge will reflect the quantity of the contents. While using a cylinder of N_2O with a continuous flow of 6 L/min, the cylinder pressure tends to fall mainly due to cooling of the liquid as it vaporizes and the consequent fall in vapor pressure. If the flow is interrupted for a brief period, the gauge will again read full.

Medical gas cylinders are color-coded **(Table 2)** and the name of the gas is also written on the neck of the cylinder. The cylinders are hydraulically tested every 5 years and the year and quarter of testing is recorded by a mark on the neck of the cylinder and valve block. The other markings on the valve block and cylinder **(Fig. 1)** include the number, the name of the owner, the manufacturer and the pressure up to which it can be safely filled. They also show the tare weight (weight of an empty cylinder in kg) for gases, which are stored as liquids.

TABLE 2: Properties of gases.

Gases	*Critical temperature (°C)*	*Color-coding*
O_2	–118.38	Black body with white shoulder
Air	–125	White and black
N_2	–140	Black
N_2O	36.5	French blue
CO_2	31.1	Gray
C_3H_6	124.4	Orange

FLUSH TYPE VALVE FOR CYLINDERS

The medical gas cylinders that can be fixed to the anesthesia machine are provided with a flush type valve. The construction of a flush type pin-index valve is shown in **Figure 2**. The valve has got a tapered screw thread to fit the cylinder, pin-index holes, spindle, gland with a gland nut and an outlet. When the valve is screwed to the cylinder, a fusible material is used to seal the leak between the valve and the cylinder. This material will melt and prevent the risk of an explosion in the event of fire. Occasionally, there is a leak around the spindle of the valve. This can be prevented by gently screwing down the glandnut.

When a cylinder is fitted to the machine, care should be taken to see that the sealing washer (Bodok seal) is present and is in good order to prevent leak between the cylinder and yoke. It is dangerous to use more than one washer because it can override the pin-index system and allow fixation of a wrong cylinder. Also, before fixing the cylinder, the outlet of the valve should be cleared of oil and dust by slowly opening the cylinder and letting out some gas. This is known as "cracking the cylinder". After fitting, the cylinder should always be opened slowly to release the pressure gradually. Sudden opening can produce a shock wave in the pressure gauge and regulator and damage the parts.

Pin-index System

The pin-index system is used in small cylinders that fit directly on to the machine. The cylinder has a flush type valve and the machine has a yoke to accept the valve. The pin-index consists of two pins projecting from the inner surface of the yoke and two corresponding holes in the cylinder valve. There are seven hole positions on the

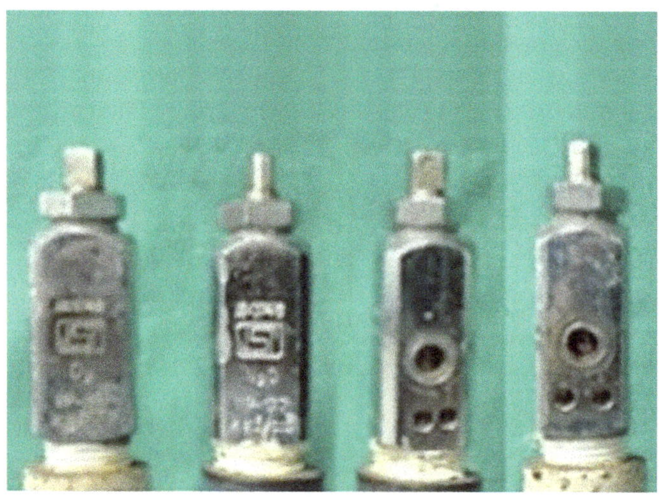

Fig. 1: Markings on flush type valve.

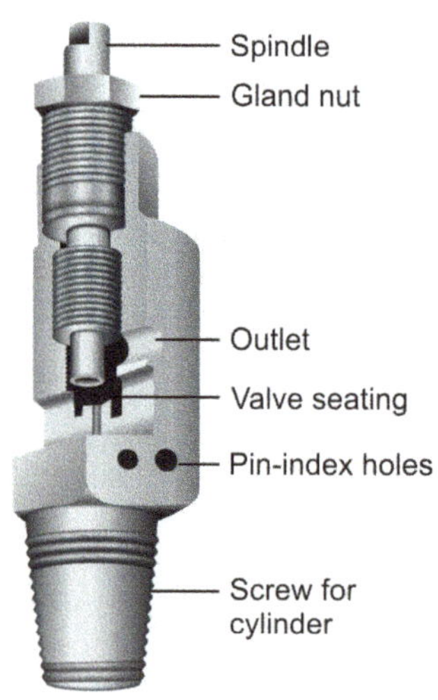

Fig. 2: Construction of flush type valve.

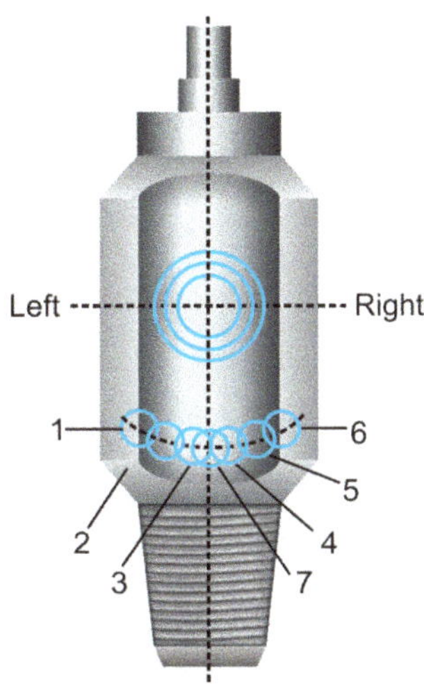

Fig. 3: Pin-index positions.

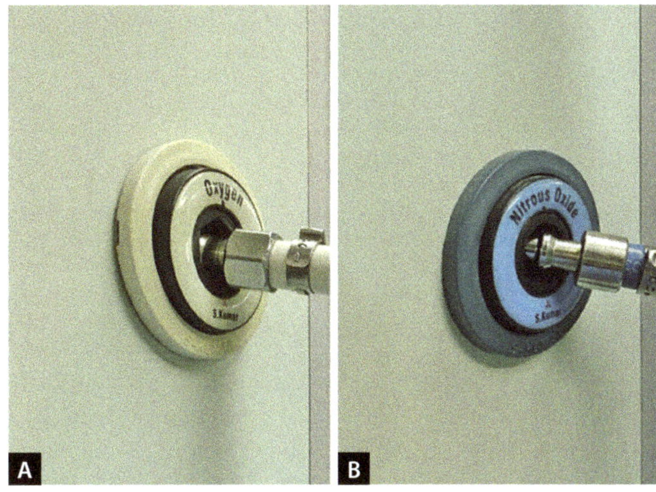

Figs. 4A and B: Quick coupler.

TABLE 3: Pin-index system.

Gas	Index pins
O_2	2–5
N_2O	3–5
C_3H_6	3–6
O_2-CO_2 (CO_2 < 7.5%)	2–6
O_2-CO_2 (CO_2 > 7.5%)	1–6
O_2-He (He > 80.5%)	4–6
O_2-He (He < 80.5%)	2–4
Air	1–5
N_2	1–4
N_2O-O_2 (N_2O 47.5–52.5%)	7

circumference of a circle of 9/16 inch radius centered in the port **(Fig. 3)**. The pins are 4 mm in diameter and 6 mm long. Two pins are assigned for each gas, one on either side of the midline **(Table 3)**. This prevents fixing a wrong gas cylinder into the yoke assembly.

PIPED MEDICAL GASES AND VACUUM SYSTEMS

Piped medical gases and vacuum systems are used in some of the bigger institutions in India. This system allows bulk storage of gases in one place and delivery at constant working pressure through fixed pipelines to the place of utility, using terminal outlets. The terminal outlets are of the Shrader quick coupler type **(Figs. 4A and B)**. Each quick coupler consists of a pair of nonthreaded gas specific male and female components. A releasable spring mechanism locks the components together. The probes (male component) fixed to one end of the flexible pipeline carry an index collar, and the outlets (female component) a groove to accept the collar. Fixation into an incorrect outlet is thus prevented by the use of index collars. There are different shapes and sizes manufactured by different companies. An international standard has not been developed, and hence, it is up to each manufacturer to ensure noninterchangeability between connectors for different gases. The wall outlet and the connector for the flexible pipeline should be from the same manufacturer.

To the other end of the flexible pipeline is attached a yoke block with a pin index. Several accidents have been caused by the connection of the probe for one gas at one end and the yoke block for another gas at the other end of the flexible pipeline. Nearly all these accidents have been caused by the alterations or faulty repairs carried out by incompetent or unauthorized people. To prevent these accidents, the flexible pipelines are also color-coded now and should be serviced by authorized people. The present standard is to fix the flexible pipeline directly to the machine at the special inlet points meant for them using diameter indexed safety system (DISS) screws.

Diameter-indexed Safety System

The DISS, which was developed to provide non-interchangeable threaded connections for medical gas pipelines, consists of a body, nipple and nut combination **(Figs. 5A and B)**. There are two concentric and specific bores in the body and two concentric and specific shoulders on the nipple. The small bore mates the small shoulder and the larger bore mates the large shoulder. To achieve non-interchangeability between different connections, the two diameters of each part vary in opposite directions so that as one diameter increases, the other decreases. Only properly mated parts will allow thread engagement. All machines should have separate inlet for piped gases, with DISS. But in India, it is not followed and the piped gases are fitted to the machine using the yoke block with pin index.

YOKE ASSEMBLY

The hanger yoke assembly supports the cylinder, and connects it to the machine. It has:

- A body, which is the frame work and the supporting structure

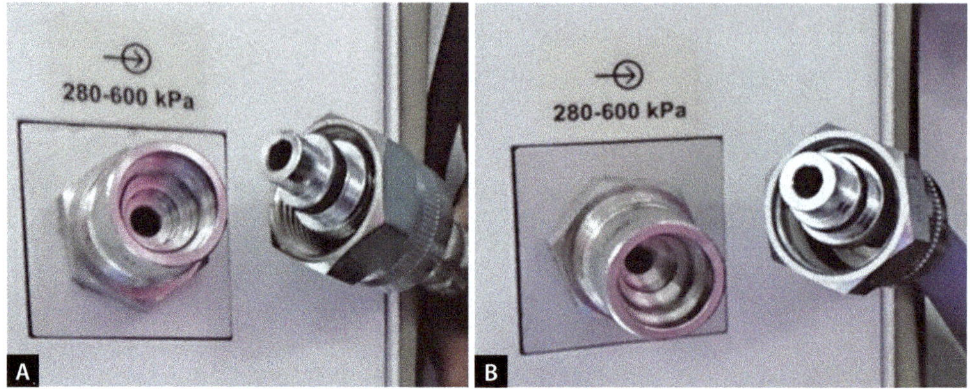

Figs. 5A and B: Diameter indexed safety system.

- The retaining screw, that tightens the cylinder in the yoke
- The index pins, that prevents connection of a wrong cylinder
- A gas seal (Bodok seal) to prevent a leak between the cylinder and the yoke
- A filter, that removes dirt from the gas
- The check valve assembly that ensures unidirectional flow.

Pressure Gauge

All machines have a pressure gauge between the cylinder and the regulator to measure the cylinder pressure. These gauges are usually of Bourdon type **(Fig. 6)**. They consist of a hollow metal tube, bent into part of a circle, connected to the pressure line. The application of pressure to the inside of the tube causes the tube to straighten and this movement is transmitted through a clock work mechanism to the indicator needle. These gauges are used for approximate measurement of high pressure.

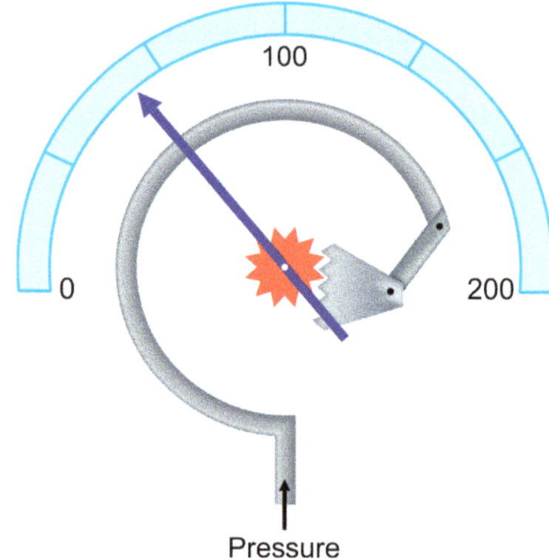

Fig. 6: Bourdon pressure gauge.

OXYGEN PRESSURE FAIL SAFE SYSTEM

This device is designed to prevent delivery of anesthetic gas without O_2 when the O_2 supply fails. This is incorporated at the level of the pressure regulators. The O_2 pressure regulator works as the primary regulator. The output from this regulator controls the secondary regulators or the slave regulators that are located in the N_2O line. In such systems, if the pressure from the O_2 regulator falls, the slave regulator of N_2O will automatically close and will not allow flow of N_2O **(Fig. 7)**. These are two types: one, in which the N_2O regulator will be totally cutoff when the O_2 pressure falls below a critical level; and the other, where the N_2O outlet pressure will also fall proportionate to the fall in O_2 pressure and so the proportional flow will be maintained, though the total flow will fall and finally stop.

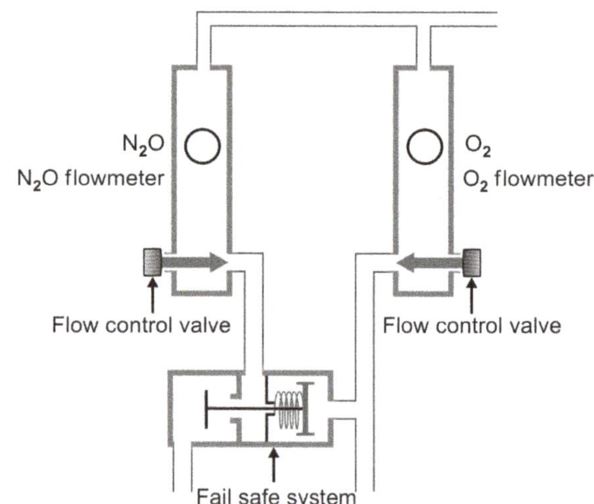

Fig. 7: Slave regulator.

Oxygen Pressure Failure Warning Devices

It is mandatory that in addition to cutting off N_2O flow, there should be an alarm when the O_2 pressure falls, which alerts the anesthesiologist to failing O_2 supply. Devices have been developed which activate an alarm when the O_2 pressure fails. The alarm may be visual, audible or both. With the activation of alarm, the device either cutsoff the N_2O flow or directs the N_2O flow to the atmosphere. The earlier versions of Boyle's machine made by Indian Oxygen Limited (namely the "Boyle basic," "Boyle Tec" and "Boyle Ultima") incorporate a device with a small O_2 tank. This tank is pressurized during normal use. When the O_2 pressure at the source falls, the O_2 from this small cylinder flows through a whistle, incorporated on line, giving rise to an audible alarm for a period of 7–10 seconds. Cessation of the alarm does not mean that the alarm condition has been rectified and measures must be taken to correct it.

The "O_2 pressure fail safe systems" and warning devices control the gas in its associated gas line in response to the pressure in O_2 line. Its safety potential is limited. It will permit administration of hypoxic gas mixtures when the gas flow is erroneously composed with low O_2 flow, the O_2 flow control valve is accidentally adjusted downward, or the O_2 piping system contains a gas other than O_2.

Oxygen Ratio Control Devices

Most modern machines used in all developed countries utilize proportioning systems in an attempt to prevent delivery of a hypoxic mixture. Oxygen and N_2O are interfaced either mechanically or pneumatically so that the minimum O_2 concentration at the common outlet is 25%.

Oxygen Ratio Monitor

Recognizing the limitations of the O_2 pressure fail safe system, the manufacturers of the "Dräger" machine developed a device called oxygen ratio monitor (ORM). It is incorporated at the level of the flowmeter. The ORM consists of a set of linear resistors inserted between the O_2 and N_2O flow control valves and the respective flowmeter. The pressure drop across the resistors is monitored and transmitted via pilot lines to an arrangement of opposing diaphragms. These opposing diaphragms are linked together with the capacity of closing a leaf spring contact and actuating an alarm in the event of O_2 percentage in the mixture of O_2 and N_2O dropping below a certain predetermined value **(Fig. 8)**. The ORM generates an alarm but does not actively control the gas flow. It will not sound an alarm if a hypoxic mixture is administered when the O_2 piping system contains a gas other than O_2.

Oxygen Ratio Monitor Controller

This not only monitors the ratio of O_2 flow and gives an alarm when it falls below 30%, but also reduces the flow of N_2O correspondingly to maintain the ratio. The basic design principles are similar to ORM with the exception that a slave regulator is additionally controlled by the mechanism of opposing diaphragms, which controls the N_2O delivery pressure to the N_2O control valve, and thus, the N_2O flow. The advantage of oxygen ratio monitor controller (ORMC) is its capability to automatically respond to reduction in O_2 pressure or operator error. The disadvantage is that the operator cannot override the function of the device when desired.

Link-25 Control System

Ohmeda anesthesia machines as well as the "Boyle Ultima" machine introduced in India use this Link-25 proportion limiting control device. The heart of the system is the mechanical integration of the N_2O and O_2 flow control valves. It allows independent adjustment of either valve, yet automatically intercedes to maintain a minimum O_2 concentration of 25%. In this system, the N_2O has a gear with 14 teeth which is fixed to the spindle. The oxygen has a gear with 29 teeth which is mounted on the O_2 spindle with threads so that it can float over the spindle. For every 2.07 rotations of the N_2O spindle, the O_2 gear will rotate once. The thread mounting of the O_2 gear allows independent rotation of O_2 flow control valve. The link arrangement is so set, that opening of N_2O will always rotate the O_2 gear, but the gear itself will engage the O_2 control valve spindle only when the proportion of N_2O in the mixture exceeds 75%. The flows in the flowmeters are precisely linked to the rotation by regulating the supply pressure of these gases with secondary regulators situated just before the flowmeter **(Fig. 9)**. The N_2O is supplied at 26 psig and O_2 at 14 psig. This combination of pneumatic and mechanical control maintains the minimum O_2 percentage at 25% whenever a mixture of O_2 and N_2O are used. The O_2 percentage can be independently varied between 25% and 100%.

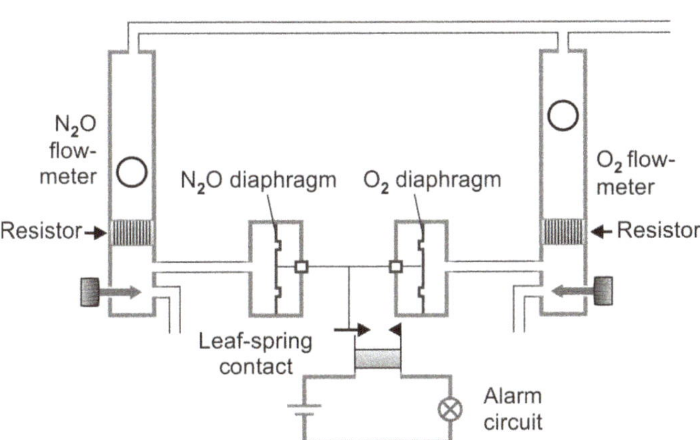

Fig. 8: Oxygen ratio controller.

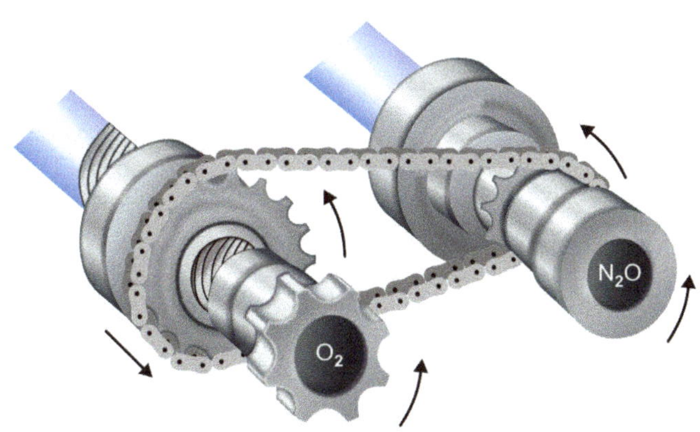

Fig. 9: Link-25 system.

The disadvantage of this system is in the mechanical linkage. If the spindle and the gear are not properly aligned, or if the threads in the spindle undergo wear and tear, the link system is likely to malfunction. Secondly, the proportioning devices can link only O_2 and N_2O. If a third gas like air is included in the flowmeter assembly then it no longer assures a 25% O_2 delivery in the mixture. Most of the modern machines allow an air flowmeter in the flowmeter block.

Other Proportioning Devices

There are many other proportioning devices, such as the Quantiflex®, Ohmeda proportioning system, etc. These devices allow only two gases to be administered, namely O_2 and N_2O. The flow of these gases, are pneumatically and mechanically controlled. Basically, there are two control knobs, one for percentage control and the other for flow control. The flow control knob controls the total flow and the other control maintains the set percentage. The flow of each gas cannot be individually adjusted. These devices are difficult to use with low flow or closed system anesthesia and have not become popular.

Oxygen Analyzer

The use of an oxygen analyzer with an anesthesia system is the single most foolproof measure to prevent delivery of hypoxic mixture to the patients. This is because it is not dependent on pneumatic or mechanical links, but actually measures the O_2 percentage in the gas mixture either by polarographic method or by using a fuel cell. One still has to make sure that the analyzer is working properly and the alarms are set accordingly. These analyzers should be calibrated at regular intervals, preferably with room air to read 21% as we are interested in detecting hypoxia rather than hyperoxia. It must be understood that an O_2 analyzer is most accurate around the concentration which is used for its calibration. The position of the analyzer in the system, whether at the common gas outlet, breathing system or near the endotracheal tube, will depend on the user and the fresh gas flow used.

CONTINUOUS FLOW ANESTHESIA MACHINE

The components of the machine are usually mounted on a table with wheels. It has provision for two cylinders of O_2 and two of N_2O. Each gas cylinder is connected via its yoke to the pressure regulator. There is a pressure gauge before the regulator to read the cylinder pressure. Connections between the yoke, the inlet of the pressure regulator and pressure gauge are made of high pressure metal tubing. This segment is called the high pressure segment of the machine. In machines provided with DISS, the pipeline joins the supply from the cylinders after the pressure regulator; hence, it is in the intermediate pressure segment.

This intermediate pressure O_2 line has branches:

- To the N_2O slave regulator
- O_2 pressure fail-safe valve
- O_2 pressure failure alarm
- To the O_2 flush
- To two outlets for powering ventilators, suction, etc **(Fig. 10)**.

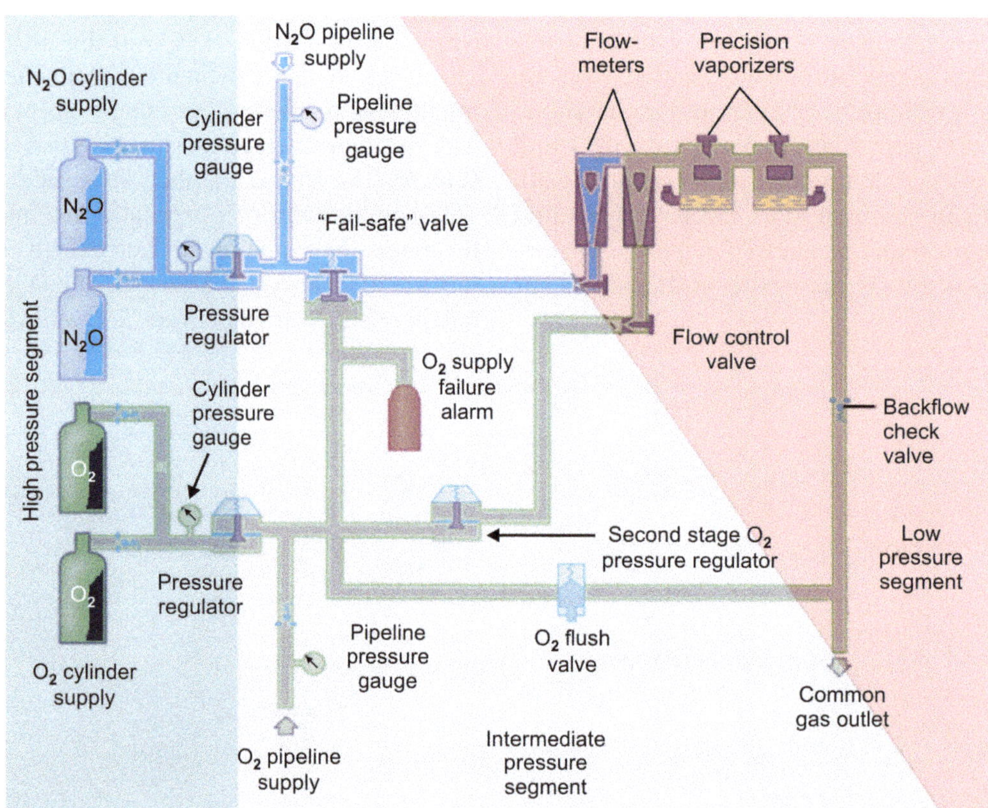

Fig. 10: Schematic diagram of continuous flow anesthesia machine.

The connections in these intermediate pressure metal tubings are made of compression couplings. The metal tubings in the intermediate pressure system can withstand four times the intended pressure.

The pressure regulators in all modern anesthetic machines are preset to 50 psig so that the outlet pressure does not exceed 60 psig at any time. The piped supply of O_2 and N_2O is made at 60 psig. When both cylinder and piped supply are fixed to the machine, the piped supply is preferentially used even if the cylinder is open because the piped pressure is slightly higher than that of the cylinder regulator output.

The N_2O regulators which are slave regulators to O_2, work only when the O_2 pressure is adequate. The outputs of the two N_2O regulators are connected together and to the N_2O flow control valve.

The O_2 and N_2O flow control valves control the flow of gases through the flowmeters. The flowmeters of O_2 and N_2O are mounted together as flowmeter manifold. The anesthesiologist must always note the position of flowmeters before using the machine. For reasons discussed elsewhere, the O_2 may be at the right extreme.

The flowmeter manifold is secured to the back bar of the machine by one or more bolts. That part of the frame of an anesthesia machine, which supports the flowmeters, vaporizers and various other components is known as the back bar. It may consist of a pair of rods or bars. Flowmeters and vaporizers are connected to each other by tapered fittings and are bolted on to the back bar. The fittings between the vaporizers and flowmeters are usually 23 mm cage mount tapers.

The back bar is connected to the common gas outlet with a tubing to which is attached the breathing system. Before the common gas outlet there usually is:

- *A backflow check valve:* It prevents back pressure from being transmitted to the vaporizers
- A relief valve which opens at 5 psig to protect the flowmeters and vaporizers from over pressure when the outlet is obstructed
- A valve to direct the flow toward an auxiliary gas outlet or to a circle system
- *An O_2 flush:* The patient will receive pure O_2 uncontaminated with N_2O, or volatile agent, when it is mounted at this position.

SAFETY MEASURES TO PREVENT DELIVERY OF EXCESSIVE ANESTHETIC CONCENTRATION

There are few situations in which excessive anesthetic concentration can be delivered to the patient. The first is delivery of a fully saturated gas mixture, which is most often the result of liquid anesthetic spilling into the fresh gas delivery system. Nonprecision vaporizers such as the Goldman vaporizer are often used by mounting it in the common gas outlet. They are likely to get accidentally disconnected from the machine, spilling the liquid anesthetic into the breathing system. This is a very dangerous situation and very high concentration of the anesthetic can be inhaled if the vaporizer is connected back to the machine and used. Vaporizers designed in the last 10 years are precision vaporizers which do not allow this to happen as they are mounted on the machine. But the clip on or hook on facility provided with TEC 5 and Dräger 19.3 vaporizers allow them to be dismantled easily, and shifted to another machine. They should be handled upright all the time. Laying the vaporizer on its side, or turning it over will cause the liquid anesthetic to spill into the bypass chamber with the same end result. There is also a danger of delivering high anesthetic concentrations by actuating the O_2 flush if the precision vaporizers are used as "stand alone" vaporizers connected to the common gas outlet.

The second reason that is commonly emphasized for delivery of excessive anesthetic concentration is the pumping effect. This happens when controlled ventilation is used with vaporizers, which are not compensated for back pressure effects and the machine does not have a backflow check valve. The gas pumped back into the vaporizer during intermittent positive pressure ventilation (IPPV) will carry anesthetic vapor and emerge out through the bypass when the pressure is released, thereby, increasing the vapor concentration. This is exaggerated while using low fresh gas flows.

Another dangerous situation is when the vaporizer is filled with a wrong anesthetic agent. For example, methoxyflurane vaporizer filled with halothane or isoflurane will deliver a very high concentration endangering the life of the patient. Another situation when excessive anesthetic concentration can be delivered is, when the carrier gas used is changed from N_2O to air-O_2 or O_2 alone. This is because of the ability of N_2O to dissolve in the liquid anesthetic and get liberated when it is cut off. It is estimated that 100 mL of halothane can dissolve 450 mL of N_2O. This will be released from the liquid when N_2O is cut off, increasing the amount of carrier gas exiting the vaporizing chamber and thereby increasing the vapor concentration.

The following safety measures have been incorporated in modern machines to prevent some of the above mentioned causes:

- Use of backflow check valve before the common gas outlet, so that the fluctuations in pressure during controlled ventilation are not transmitted to the vaporizers
- The construction of the vaporizers has been modified to make them back pressure compensated vaporizers so that both pumping effect and pressuring effects are negated
- The size of the common gas outlet has been changed from 23 mm female to 22 mm male/15 mm female connector to prevent connection of vaporizer to common gas outlet

- Vaporizers with liquid anesthetic inside should be handled carefully without tilting or turning. If the vaporizer is accidentally tipped or laid on its side, it should be emptied and then flushed with a high flow of O_2 with concentration dial turned set to the maximum for at least 10 minutes before using the equipment on patients
- Only one precision vaporizer should be used at any time, so that condensation of liquid anesthetic does not take place into another vaporizer. To prevent simultaneous use of two vaporizers, the contemporary machines are fitted with vaporizers which have a locking mechanism which prevents a second vaporizer to be opened without closing the first one
- Keyed filling devices are available for most new inhalation agents to prevent the use of a wrong volatile anesthetic in a given vaporizer.

SAFETY MEASURES TO PREVENT DEVELOPMENT OF EXCESSIVE PRESSURE ON THE MACHINE AND BREATHING SYSTEMS

To prevent excessive pressures from developing in the machine, pressure relief valves are incorporated into the intermediate pressure system and low pressure system of the machine, and also in the breathing systems connected to the patient.

There is one pressure relief valve after the pressure regulator. If there is a defect in the pressure regulator, the intermediate pressure system is protected from the high pressures by this relief valve, which will release the pressure to the atmosphere with a loud noise, and immediate corrective measures can be taken.

A pressure relief valve situated before the common gas outlet protects the flowmeter and the vaporizers. If there is obstruction to flow at or after the common gas outlet, the pressure in the low pressure system rises and the relief valve will open when the pressure exceeds 300 cmH_2O (in Boyle's machine). This is mainly to protect the flowmeter gaskets and the vaporizers.

All breathing systems have an adjustable pressure limiting (APL) valve which opens the system to the atmosphere. The opening pressure of this valve is adjusted normally according to the breathing system used and its applications. Occasionally, this valve may get stuck and allow development of high pressure. If such an event were to occur, the system should be immediately disconnected from the patient to avoid barotrauma. If the fault cannot be rectified, alternative methods should be used to ventilate the patient and the breathing system should be changed. Some of the APL valves manufactured nowadays vent gases to the atmosphere when the pressure exceeds 60 cmH_2O, even when they are fully closed. Another safety feature in the breathing system is the reservoir bag. Most of these bags can hold ten times the nominal volume and give way when the pressure builds up above 50 cmH_2O.

ADVANCED ANESTHESIA WORKSTATIONS

Over years anesthesia machine has gradually evolved into an integrated multicomponent workstation consisting of electrical, mechanical and pneumatic segments. Many such workstations are available in the market. For the purpose of description and understanding the workstations, the anesthesia integrated system (AISYS) manufactured by GE Medicals is taken up. In the AISYS, most of the components necessary for administration of anesthesia are integrated into one unit **(Fig. 11)**. It consists of the anesthesia machine, vaporizers, ventilator, breathing system, scavenging system, monitors, drug delivery system, suction equipment and a data management system.

The gas delivery system in advanced anesthesia workstations is similar to the basic machines. Gas flows from the high pressure system are reduced to anesthesia machine working pressures by pressure reducing devices, which then goes to the electronic gas mixer, picks up the set vapor from the electronic vaporizer before going to the common gas outlet. The arrangement and functioning of components can be better understood if the gas flow is traced from the source to the patients. Turning the machine's main switch "on" enables the power supply to the electronic control boards. The power strip provided in the back of the machine provides electrical supply to the ventilator and the monitor incorporated in the anesthesia machine. The power supply is provided with a battery backup of two 12 V batteries that can support all the components for up to 90 minutes in case of main power failure. The electrical supply goes to the power controller board which then supplies the display unit board and the anesthesia control board. The system switch that is separate from the main switch enables the electronic components along with the mechanical and pneumatic components.

The interface between the source of gas supply and machine is the same as older machines. The cylinders are connected using pin-index systems and the pipeline

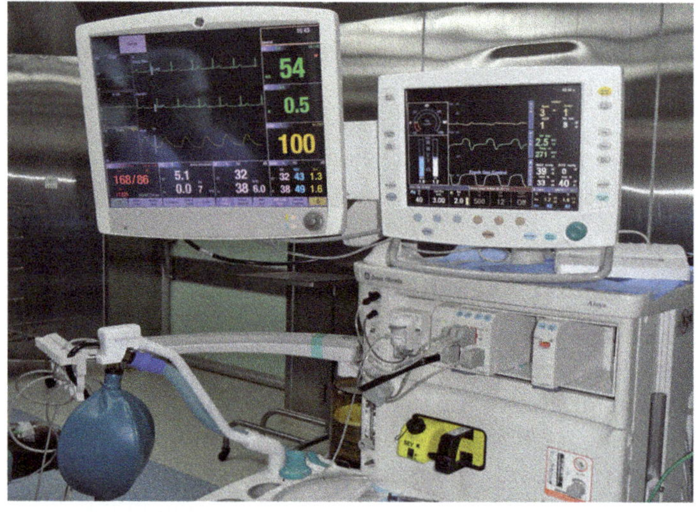

Fig. 11: Advanced anesthesia workstation (Aysis®–GE).

is connected using DISS which is specific for each gas. The pressure at the inlet is monitored with electronic pressure transducers and displayed in the monitor **(Fig. 12)** instead of the pressure gauge. Supply failure alarms are also electronic with a message on the screen and audible alarm to attract attention.

Gas flows from the high pressure system are reduced to anesthesia machine working pressures by pressure reducing devices. The pressure regulators function the same way except for the fact that they are made with no rubber components and does not need servicing for longer periods of time. The metal interconnecting tubings have been replaced with flexible Teflon® tubes with quick fit connectors that withstand high pressures.

The flowmeters are replaced with electronic gas mixer. The flow adjustment utilizes a solenoid valve for each gas. The machine takes an input for total flow and the percentage of O_2 need to be delivered to the patient **(Fig. 13)**. The difference is made up from the second gas, which can be selected from the menu as air or N_2O. Closed-loop flow control is accomplished through a hotwire anemometer in concert with the flow control valves. The mixer response time is 500 millisecond which ensures that it delivers what we want, when we want it. Flow and pressure transducers as well as temperature sensors are used to maintain accuracy.

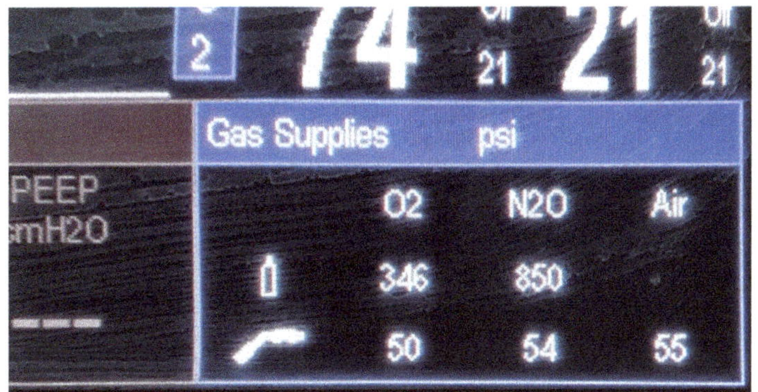

Fig. 12: Cylinder and pipeline pressure displayed on the monitor.

Alternate Oxygen

As a safety backup in case of electronic failure of the gas mixer, the alternate O_2 provides a pneumatic back up O_2 delivery. It activates automatically in case of electronic failure of the gas mixer. It can also be activated manually. The alternate O_2 control is available 20 seconds after the system is turned on **(Fig. 14)**. It can deliver a flow of 0.5–10 L/min through the flowmeter provided for that purpose. 100% O_2 and the selected concentration of agent can be delivered to the patient. However, in case of failure of the electronic vaporizer only O_2 can be delivered.

Electronic Vaporizer

The electronic vaporizer mixes the requested amount of vapor into the fresh gas stream. It has two components:

1. The Aladin™ cassette which holds the liquid.
2. The electronic unit located inside the main unit.

The Aladin™ cassettes are color-coded to identify and magnetically coded for the machine to identify **(Fig. 15)**. The electronic unit identifies the liquid level, temperature of the liquid and the pressure of vapor in the cassette. The display unit will show the agent by name, color, and liquid level. Only one cassette can be fitted to the machine at a time. The cassettes are provided with Quick-fill or Easy-fill system. The Aladin™ cassettes are light weight, maintenance free and provided with cassette overfill, overpressure handling and can be transported in any position.

A subsystem of the anesthesia control board controls the agent delivery. Agent is delivered from the subsystem

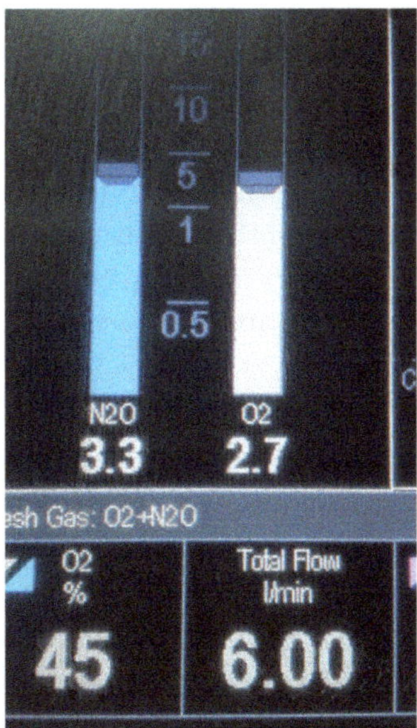

Fig. 13: Electronic flowmeters.

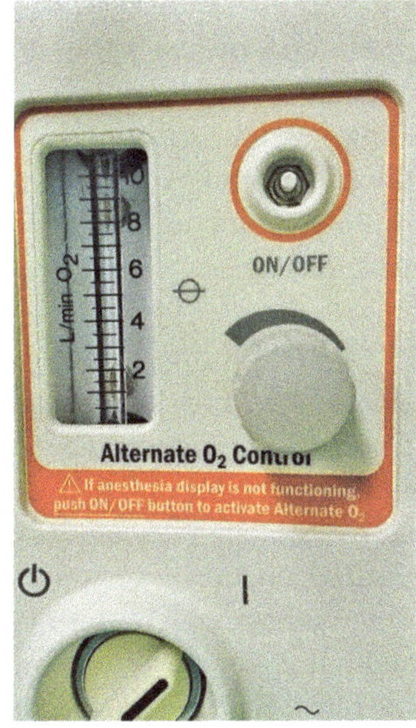

Fig. 14: Alternate O_2 supply. Activates in case of electronic failure.

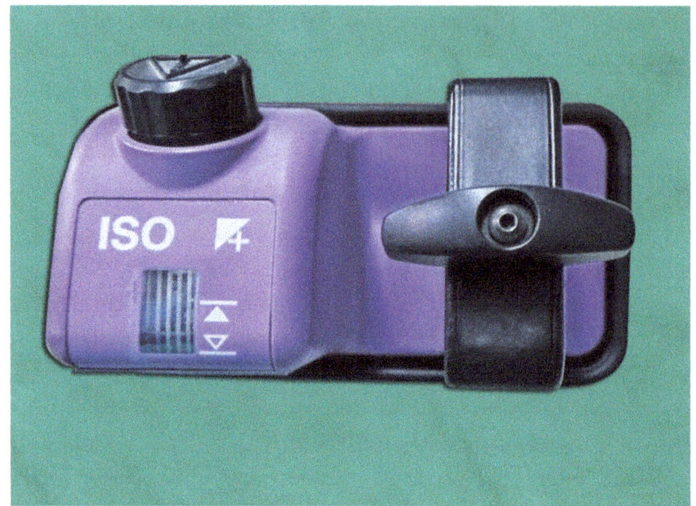

Fig. 15: Electronic vaporizer cassette for isoflurane.

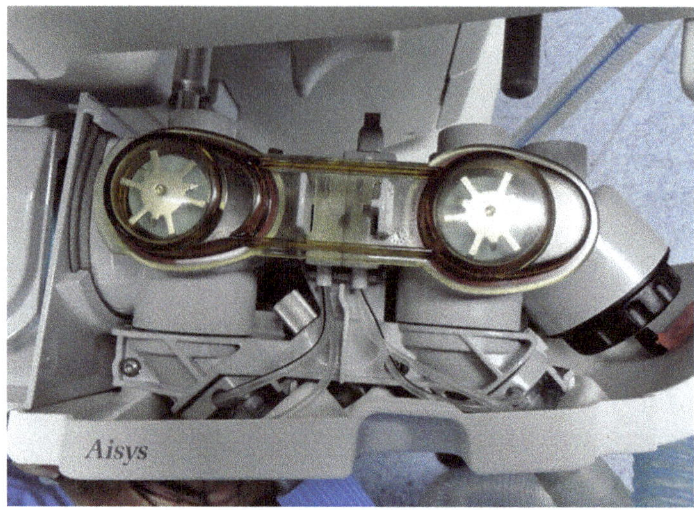

Fig. 16: Flow transducers in both inspiratory and expiratory limbs of the advanced breathing system.

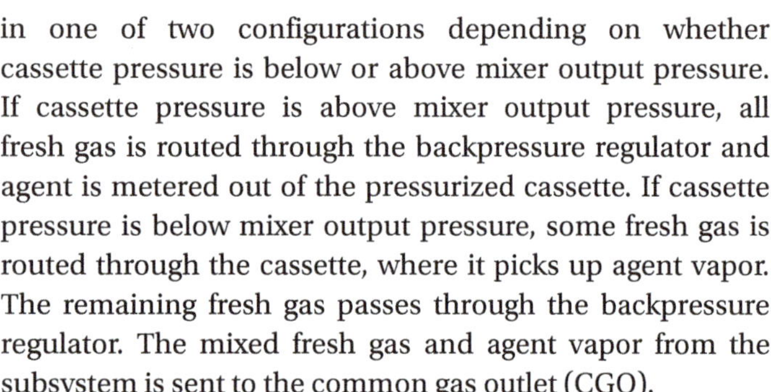

in one of two configurations depending on whether cassette pressure is below or above mixer output pressure. If cassette pressure is above mixer output pressure, all fresh gas is routed through the backpressure regulator and agent is metered out of the pressurized cassette. If cassette pressure is below mixer output pressure, some fresh gas is routed through the cassette, where it picks up agent vapor. The remaining fresh gas passes through the backpressure regulator. The mixed fresh gas and agent vapor from the subsystem is sent to the common gas outlet (CGO).

To meet the requested agent concentration, outflow from the cassette (or flow through the cassette) is controlled with a proportional valve. This means the main subsystem control loop is on cassette flow, not agent concentration directly. If all fresh gas flow is through the backpressure regulator, the control loop depends strongly on mixer reported flow and the cassette flow reading. It depends weakly on reported fresh gas composition, manifold temperature reading, and reported patient airway pressure. If fresh gas flow is split between the cassette and the backpressure regulator, the control loop depends strongly on mixer reported flow, cassette flow reading, cassette pressure reading and cassette temperature reading. It depends weakly on reported fresh gas composition, manifold temperature reading and reported patient airway pressure.

Advanced Breathing System

It has a circuit volume of 2.7 L, delivering rapid wash-in and wash-out times, and fast response. The components are easy to remove and disassemble and fully autoclavable. The dual flow sensing technology (sensors in both inspiratory and expiratory limbs) ensures safe operation **(Fig. 16)**. It is a variable orifice sensor which uses electromechanical technology. It maintains sensitivity and accuracy over a wide range of flow rates. Gas flow is checked 200 times per second to ensure the workstation. is delivering correctly. If water droplets form in any one of the four tubings **(Fig. 16)** the technology used to measure flow (i.e., velocity of sound, VOS) is unable to measure flow. Hence, a heat and moisture exchanger (HME) filter has to be used in low flow anesthesia. A galvanic cell in the inspiratory limb measures O_2 concentration of inspiratory gases. Helium EZ change canister mode seals the breathing circuit when the canister holder is down. Pushing the canister release activates to the EZ change canister mode. The condenser removes water in the system produced from the reaction of CO_2 gas with the absorbent. The condenser is connected between the outlet of the absorber canister and the inlet of the circuit module.

SmartVent Ventilation Technology

Employs fresh gas flow compensation, compensation for compression losses and circuit compliance and for small leakages in the CO_2 absorber, bellows and system. The ventilator can be used to ventilate a wide range of patients from neonates to geriatric. With volume control ventilation (VCV), a minimal tidal volume of 20 mL can be set and with pressure controlled ventilation (PCV), tidal volumes as low as 5 mL can be measured. All the modes in an ICU ventilator are available for intraoperative use as well. A comprehensive view of patient's ventilatory status is displayed and compared in flow, volume and pressure waveforms over time.

Gas Monitoring

Respiratory gas monitoring is via the M-gas module, which is integrated into the machine. The airway module is compact. It measures and displays both the end-tidal and the inspiratory concentrations of the gas concentrations breath by breath **(Fig. 17)**. It is enabled with automatic agent identification system. Helium, CO_2, N_2O and anesthetic agents (AA) are measured by infrared sensor and a paramagnetic sensor is used for O_2 measurement.

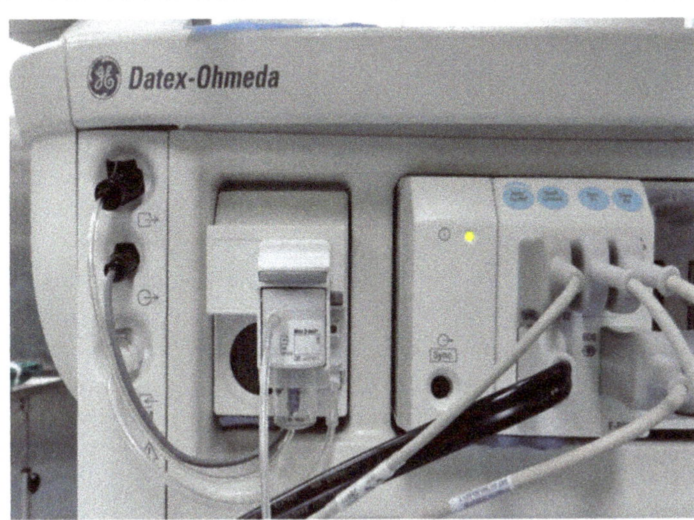

Fig. 17: Gas monitoring module as part of anesthesia machine.

End-tidal Control Mode of Gas Delivery

It is an optional gas delivery mode. The system takes input for the end-tidal oxygen (EtO_2), end-tidal anesthetic concentration (EtAA) and total gas flow values and adjusts the gas composition and total flow to maintain the set target values. The EtAA response time is as quick as 68 seconds ± 28 seconds and settling time of 128 ± 100 seconds. Several safety mechanisms function automatically when entering the end-tidal control (EtC) mode, i.e., the EtC system check, EtC leak check, EtC fresh gas sample check, EtC supervisor and EtC increased flow.

Unique Features of Maquet FLOW-i Anesthesia Machine

The FLOW-i anesthesia delivery system by Maquet is a fully electronically controlled system offering ventilatory precision and a few other safety features. Battery back-up for 90 minutes is provided with rechargeable battery with charging time of 6 hours.

Provision for fixing a pin-indexed cylinder is not standard feature. This optional feature can be ordered separately and fixed permanently. A maximum of two pin-indexed cylinders (O_2/N_2O or O_2/air) can be mounted using a quick release system for docking and release of cylinders. The central pipelines are connected via the DISS. Cylinder pressure is electronically measured.

In FLOW-i, a volume reflector replaces the traditional bellows for ventilation. It has a fixed volume of 1.2 L, no moving parts and is open at both ends. The details of this ventilation system are discussed in Chapter 10. The amount of exhaled gas returning to the patient via the CO_2 absorber is determined by the ratio between the minute volume and the set fresh gas flow. The total system volume (excluding the breathing system) is only 2.9 L. The small system volume allows for fast wash-in and wash-out of anesthetic gases. The volume reflector allows rebreathing of 98% of the exhaled gases.

Electronically controlled gas modules supply the gas mixture (O_2 and air/N_2O) at a dynamic flow needed for high-performance automatic ventilation, or at a constant fresh gas flow during manual ventilation. There are three gas modules (O_2, air, N_2O) to deliver fresh gas, and one reflector gas module (O_2) to drive the volume reflector.

The volume reflector can accurately deliver tidal volumes as low as 5 mL and precisely deliver the set tidal volume even in the presence of high airway pressures and poor lung compliance. In case of leaks, the circuit gets saturated with O_2, thus minimizing the risk of delivery of a hypoxic mixture. An O_2 guard feature automatically increases the FGF and O_2 when the FiO_2 drops below 21%. Another advantage is that the system can deliver the requested breathing gas even in case of leakage, e.g., at the tracheal tube. The volume reflector cannot be emptied like a "bag-in-bottle."

FLOW-i is also equipped to enable the patient to be manually ventilated with oxygen in case the system loses its electrical power (mains and battery backup). The APL valve (max limit of 80 cmH_2O) of the system is also electronic.

In FLOW-i, the automatic gas control (AGC) feature automatically controls the fresh gas flow and anesthetic agent supply in order to achieve the EtAA target within the user set time and maintains the target for the desired time with minimum fresh gas flows (FGF limit of 0.1 L/min to 20 L/min). This is possible because of the use of electronically controlled injection vaporizers. The detailed description of the vaporizer can be found in Chapter 8.

These vaporizers are light weight compared to the conventional vaporizers, can be filled even during usage and desflurane vaporizer need not be heated. Tank liquid level can be visually seen on the vaporizer monitor tube as well as electronically displayed.

Pressure, flow, and gas concentrations to and from the patient are monitored and displayed on a graphical user interface on a control panel. User can set all parameters for the ventilation modes just as in an ICU-ventilator, as well as all gas concentrations, alarm limits, etc., via the graphical user interface.

Disadvantages of Workstations

Potential electrical failure with disruption of mechanical ventilation and gas delivery, display failure, fires and liquid spills have all been reported. Further, they may malfunction or act in a way that the anesthesia provider does not recognize. The anesthesia provider must take time to understand how these workstations function and what needs to be done in case of failure.

Preanesthetic Machine Checkout

The complexities in the machine requires an automated check-out to be carried out before conduct of anesthesia so that functioning of all the individual components are checked.

The machine check takes approximately 8–10 minutes and has to be done at least once in every 24 hours.

SCAVENGING OF ANESTHETIC GASES

The amount of anesthetic gas supplied usually far exceeds the amount necessary for the patient, leading to wastage of gases. The spill of anesthetic gases, such as N_2O and volatile agents, within the closed environment of the operating theater may lead to the chronic exposure of staff with potential adverse consequences on health. Scavenging means collection and disposal of all patient expired or wasted gases used during anesthesia and venting them to the atmosphere away from operation theater. The removal of waste gases is an issue of health and safety. Strict regulations are overseen by bodies, such as the Control of Substances Hazardous to Health (COSHH) in the UK. In USA, the National Institute for Occupational Safety and Health (NIOSH) is responsible for enforcement. In India it has not become mandatory to use scavenging systems in the operating rooms yet.

Scavenging systems generally have four components, which are: (i) collection, (ii) transfer, (iii) receiver, and (iv) disposal. The components can vary in design and function. The collection is usually from the expiratory valve of the breathing system or the exhaust port of the ventilator. The expiratory adjustable pressure limiting (APL) valves in the breathing systems shoulder a jacket as a collecting system **(Figs. 18A to C)**. The outlet of this is 30 mm male connector, which is specific for scavenging. This also prevents misconnection of breathing system components to the scavenging port.

The transfer system is usually a corrugated tube with a connector at both ends. This is a wide bore tubing with 30 mm connector to fit the scavenging ports. The other dimension that is used in scavenging lines is 19 mm connector. 30 mm and 19 mm are the universally recommended diameters for scavenging ports.

Receiving system is the main interface between the collection system and the disposal system and hence a protector of the patient connected to breathing system. It protects the patient from excessive positive or negative pressures. It also acts as a reservoir buffer the peak expiratory flows from the patient circuit.

Receiving systems supplied with Datex Ohmeda machines can be used as passive or active disposal systems. It has two ports for connecting the transfer system tubings and/or connecting a reservoir bag **(Figs. 19A and B)**.

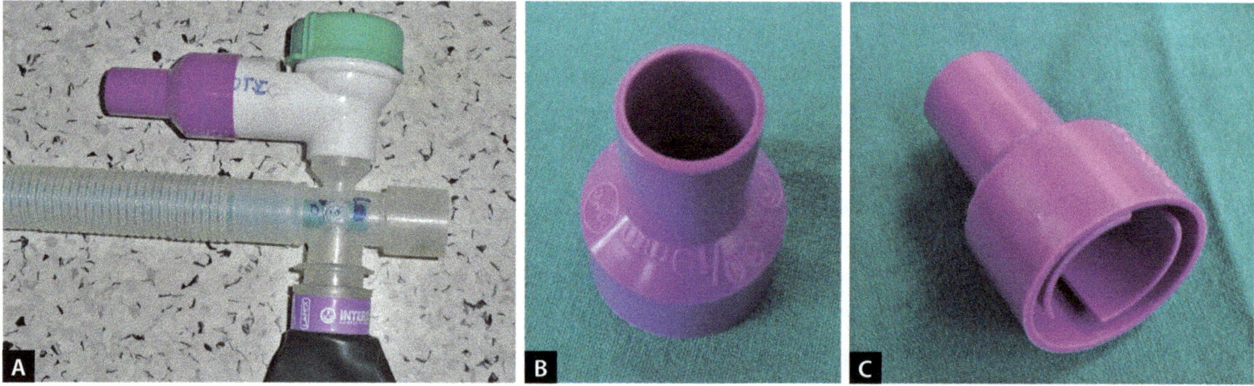

Figs. 18A to C: Connector for scavenging system.

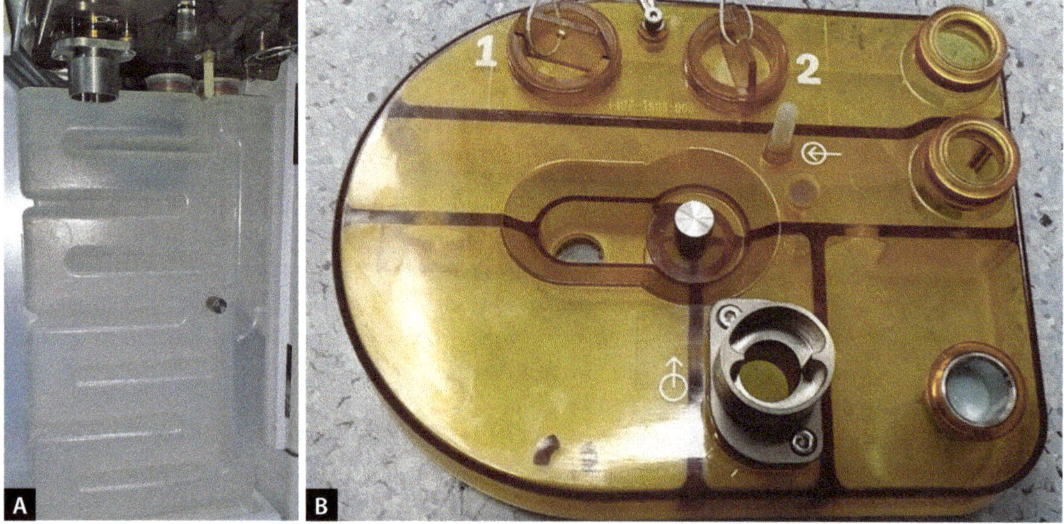

Figs. 19A and B: Receiver system incorporated in Datex Ohmeda machines.

It is mounted under the ventilator exhaust so that the vented gases will be collected directly in the receiver system. There are two other openings in the bottom of the receiver to which is connected a long, wide bore, convoluted tubing system which acts as a reservoir for gases during passive scavenging. There is a unidirectional air intake valve incorporated in the receiver that will come into play during active scavenging so that development of negative pressure will not occur in the receiver.

This receiver can be used either as open or closed. If used as a closed system, a reservoir bag is attached to one of the inlet ports. If used as an open system, the unidirectional valve provides an air-break between the disposal system and the breathing system. The open system relies on an active disposal system to function.

The system may be passive or active depending on the mode of disposal. In passive systems (driven by the patient's expiratory effort), exhaust gases pass along a tube through an outside wall or window and are discharged to the atmosphere. Tubing should be as short and wide as possible to minimize resistance. The outlet should be protected from the elements and should be covered with a mesh to prevent the ingress of insects.

In active systems, a fan or pump in the disposal system draws the anesthetic gases through. On modern anesthetic machines they are designed for use with a central suction system.

CONCLUSION

The outlay of anesthesia machine has been described for a basic machine. The sequence of arrangement of components does not differ from the basic machine to the most advanced machine. Most of the machines used by many people lie in between the basic and the most advanced. The most advanced machine has every control in electronic form mimicking the layout of an intensive care unit (ICU) ventilator. The most commonly used machines are hybrid between the basic and electronic versions. They use electronically controlled ventilators and stand-alone monitors that satisfy minimum monitoring standards. Since there is so much variation, anesthesiologist using the machine should familiarize themselves with the machine and carryout the safety check of the machine before start of the case every day. Recommendations and protocols for checking the machine by different associations are given in the Appendices 1 and 2.

Pressure-reducing Valves (Pressure Regulators)

Vandana V Laheri

ABSTRACT

Medical gases used in anesthesia practice or healthcare facility are supplied under high pressure in the form of cylinders which may be attached to anesthesia machines/workstations or to central manifolds of piped gas supply. The pressure in the cylinders reduces as the cylinders empty. This leads to fall in flow rate. To maintain constant flow with changing supply pressure of cylinders, pressure regulators (pressure-reducing valves) are required to be used. A pressure regulator reduces the high and variable pressure found in a cylinder to a lower, more constant pressure, which is suitable for use. This chapter covers in detail the need for such valves, their design, and the mechanism of working.

INTRODUCTION

Pressure-reducing valves (pressure regulators) are used on anesthesia machines or central pipeline systems to convert the high variable pressure of gas from cylinders (entering into the pressure regulators) to a low constant working pressure (4 bar, 60 psi) of the gas (emerging out from the pressure regulators) so as to prevent damage to the structures of flowmeters, of wall outlets or anesthesia machines, especially the flow control valve needles.

The reducing valves maintain a constant inlet pressure at the level of flowmeter control valves despite the change in cylinder pressure and thereby obviating the need for continuous adjustment of the flowmeter control valves, as the cylinder empties and the pressure drops. Some of the manufacturers incorporate a "nonreturn valve" at the inlet of the reducing valves mounted on anesthesia machines/ workstations. This nonreturn valve prevents refilling of the empty cylinders (still attached to the machine with its valve open) from freshly opened full cylinders and do not allow leakage of gases while changing the empty cylinder.

The anesthesia machine/workstation standard requires a pressure regulator for each gas supplied from cylinders. Without a regulator, it would be necessary to constantly alter the flow control valve to maintain a constant flow through the flowmeter, as the pressure in the cylinder decreases.

PRESSURE REGULATORS (PRESSURE-REDUCING VALVES)

Modern machines have several primary and secondary regulators. Primary regulators reduce high cylinder pressures to the machine working pressure of 4 bar (420 kPa). Some manufacturers adjust the cylinder regulators to just lesser than 420 kPa, which allows the machine to preferentially use pipeline gas. But some regulators weep their cylinder contents; hence, it is important to turn the cylinder off after a machine check. Secondary regulators level out gas delivery. Machine working pressures may vary by up to 20%, especially during periods of peak working hours of hospital. Pressure fluctuations can damage the flowmeter and affect their performance. Secondary regulators set below the anticipated decrease in pressure will make the emergent pressure more uniform.

The pressure-reducing valves function on the principle of balancing of opposing forces acting on the valve-seat area (A_1). Depending on the position of the valve seat (open or closed), the cylinder gas can pass into the chamber of the valve that contains diaphragm, where the pressure gets reduced before emerging through the outlet of the valve. This can be seen and understood from **Figures 1A and B.**[1]

Pressure-reducing valves on anesthesia machine are called "indirect type",[1] because the cylinder pressure (Pc) itself closes the valve seat (A_1), and therefore, the gas from the cylinder cannot pass to the chamber of the valve where the pressure gets reduced, even if the cylinder is open. There are various other forces, which also close the valve seat, e.g., the force of the sealing spring (S_2) and the "reduced pressure (Pr)" itself that acts on the area (A_2) of the "diaphragm" of the reducing valve. The only force that opens the valve seat is the force of the adjusting spring (FS_1). This force (FS_1) is adjustable and can be set by rotating the adjusting screw "in" to increase or "out" to decrease the tension (force) of the adjusting or the main spring (FS_1) and thereby to increase or decrease the "Pr". After setting the pressure, the movement of the adjusting screw, i.e., further compression or relaxation of the spring, can be locked by the locking nut.

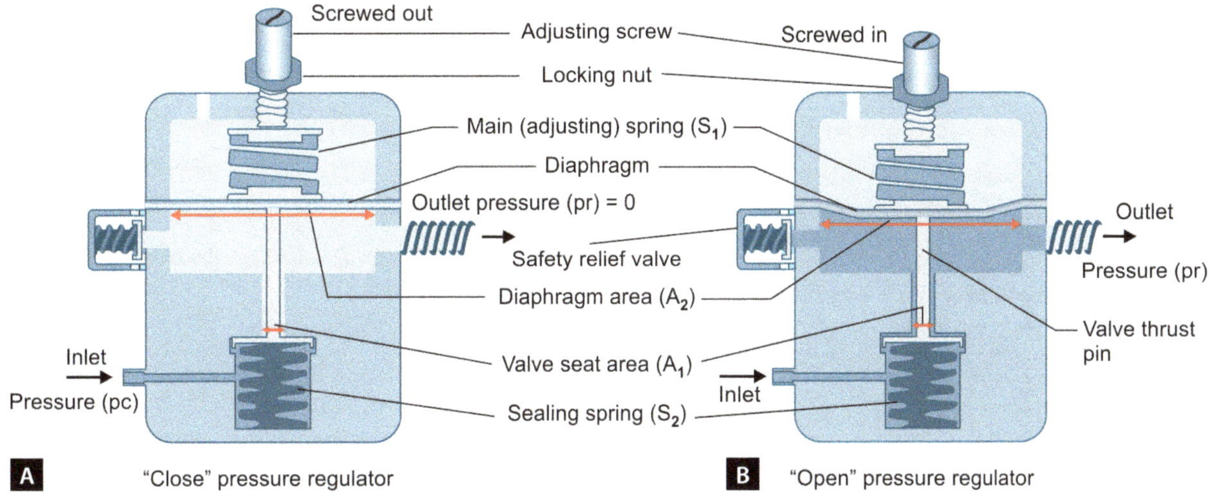

Figs. 1A and B: Schematic diagram of pressure-reducing valve.
Source: Modified from a drawing by Ohmeda.

The "reduced pressure" can be set to the desired value. The service engineer generally does this by using a special kit for adjusting the spring tension (FS_1) and measuring the "reduced pressure" while the machine is not being used on the patient, especially at the time of servicing the machine. These pressure-reducing valves are not permanently set at a fixed pressure during the manufacturing process like Adams valve in which the reduced pressure cannot be altered. These valves are known as "preset" valves because the Pr has to be set by the service person using a tool, and it cannot be altered while the machine is in use.

TABLE 1: Balance of forces acting on valve seat of "preset reducing valve" **(Figs. 1A and B).**

Forces that close the valve seat	=	Force that opens the valve seat
$(Pc \times A_1) + (Pr \times A_2) + FS_2$	=	FS_1
i.e., $(Pr \times A_2)$	=	$(FS_1 - FS_2) - (Pc \times A_1)$
Therefore, Pr	=	$(FS_1 - FS_2)/A_2 - (Pc \times A_1)/A_2$
A_1: Area of the valve seat is small A_2: Area of the diaphragm is large	i.e.,	FS_1 is very large (adjusting spring) FS_2 is very small (sealing spring)
A_2 is much more than A_1 As Pc decreases Pr increases,		$(FS_1 - FS_2)$ is much more than Pc pressure inversion

PHYSICAL PRINCIPLE[1]

Pressure is defined as force acting against an area. Force can be increased either by increasing the pressure or by decreasing the area over which the said pressure is going to act.

A large pressure, Pc (cylinder gas pressure), acting on a small area, A_1, is balanced by a smaller pressure Pr, acting on a large area, A_2 (area of the diaphragm). The force exerted by the higher pressure (Pc) is balanced against the force exerted by the Pr. These types of valves are called direct acting valves. The cylinder pressure acting on area A_1 opens the valve and the reduced pressure acting on Area A_2 closes the valve.

$$Pc \times A_1 = Pr \times A_2 \text{ and } \Delta Pr = \Delta Pc\,(A_1/A_2)$$

However, we are aware that cylinder pressure falls from its "full pressure" to the "atmospheric pressure" as the cylinder becomes empty. This means that as Pc reduces, Pr will also reduce. To make this reduction in Pr negligible, an additional force is introduced by way of using "springs".

The force of the spring is kept large so that the reduction in Pr becomes negligible even if the cylinder pressure drops from full pressure to atmospheric pressure.

On anesthesia machines and central panel of gas manifolds, the situation is reversed. Here, as the Pc decreases, Pr increases. This is because the Pc as well as Pr, both tend to close the valve seat rather than open it. The only force that opens the valve seat for the gases to flow through the valve is the FS_1. This can be very well understood by looking at **Figures 1A and B[1] and Table 1.**

A sealing spring, S_2, is also called a shutoff spring because it closes the valve seat and hence the valve, when the adjusting spring is totally relaxed, i.e., when the adjusting screw is completely screwed out and the cylinder valve is also closed.

When the adjusting screw is totally screwed out, the adjusting spring S_1 is relaxed and the valve is closed. If the cylinder is open, the gas enters the space surrounding the sealing spring, S_2 and the valve seat, A_1 **(Fig. 1A).**[1] Cylinder pressure, Pc, tends to close the valve seat against the nozzle. When the adjusting screw is turned clockwise (screwed in) so that the main spring S_1 exerts a downward force (FS_1) on the diaphragm, the valve thrust pin moves downward, opening the seat **(Fig. 1B).**[1] The gas now enters the chamber under the diaphragm. If the gas flow distal to the pressure reducing valve (i.e., flowmeter on machine) is turned off, gas continues to flow briefly into the space under the diaphragm. Its pressure increases (static increment in Pr), pushing the diaphragm upward until the seat closes against the nozzle, stopping further flow. When the flowmeter is opened, the pressure of the gas under the diaphragm falls, the diaphragm gets pushed

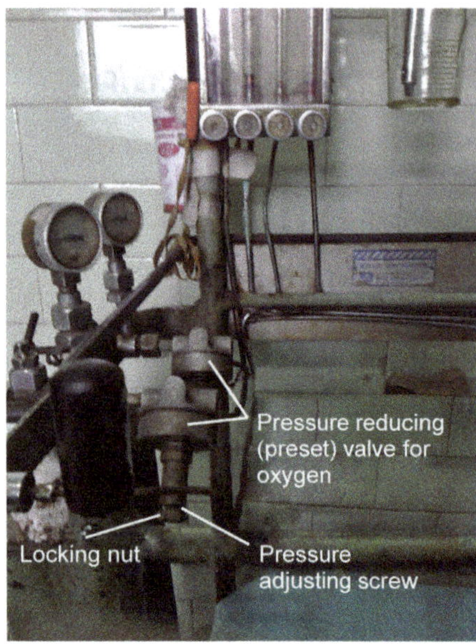

Fig. 2: Pressure reducing (preset) valve on old Boyle machine.

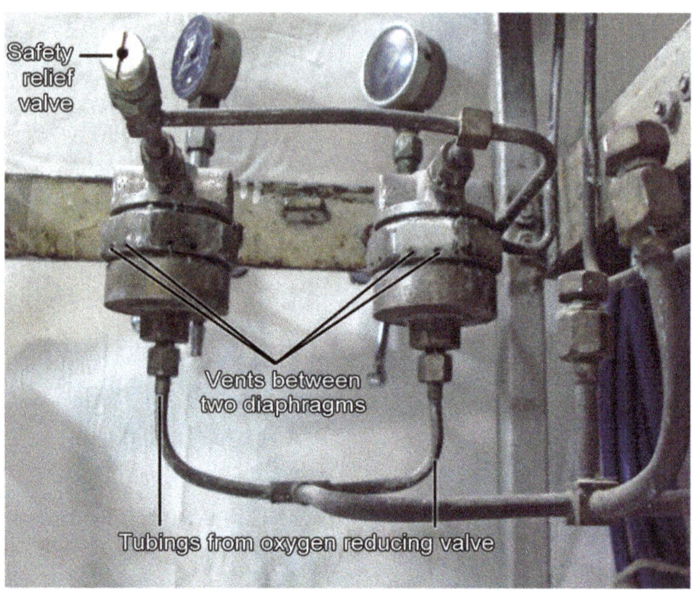

Fig. 3: Master and slave valve on old Boyle machine for N_2O.

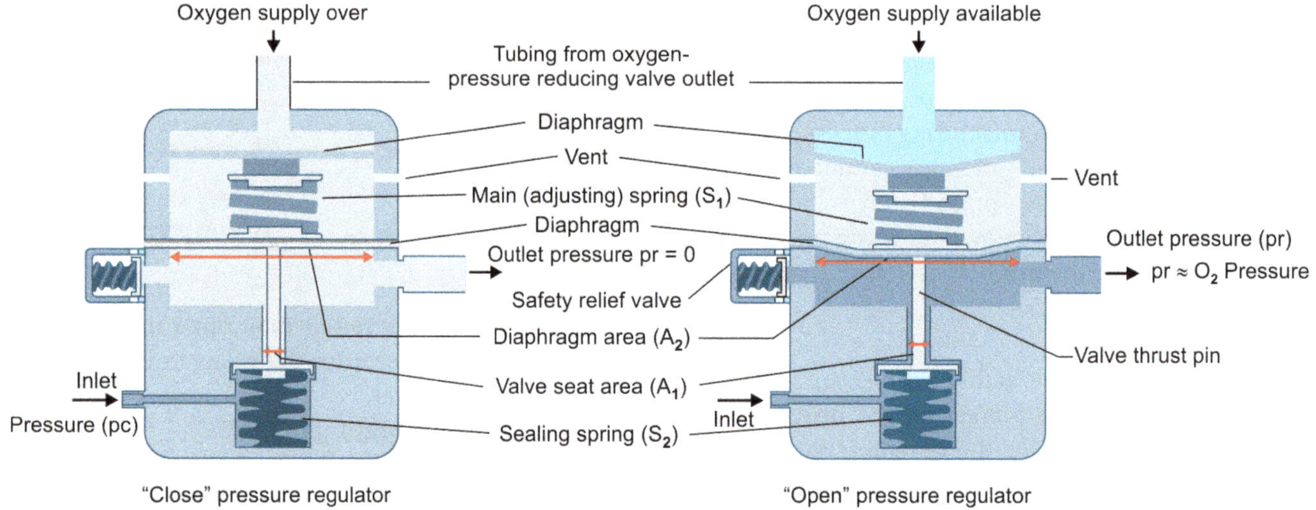

Fig. 4: Schematic diagram of pressure-reducing valve (master and slave).

downward by the spring S_1 and the gas from the valve seat starts flowing into the chamber again till such time that the flowmeter valve is switched off again or the cylinder/central line gets exhausted.

Please note that reducing valves mounted on anesthesia machine (as seen in **Figs. 2 and 3**) are inverted (i.e., upside down in position) as compared to the schematic diagram **(Figs. 1 and 4)**. While setting the Pr, the valves are kept by the service engineer as seen in **Figures 1 and 4**, and then, they are turned down in little slanting position so as to accommodate them in the framework of anesthesia machine.

MASTER AND SLAVE REGULATORS[1] (OXYGEN FAILURE SAFETY VALVE)

In many modern machines, the output pressure (Pr) from outlet of the oxygen-reducing valve replaces the adjusting screw and the adjusting spring (FS_1) of the N_2O-reducing valves via metal tubing **(Figs. 3 and 4)**. This is the only force that opens the valve seat. Therefore, when the oxygen pressure falls, the force that opens the N_2O valve seat also falls and when the oxygen cylinder empties, the force that opens the N_2O valve seat becomes zero and thereby the flow of N_2O is automatically cut off. This is the mechanism of "oxygen failure safety valve".

The valve has three chambers: (i) upper, (ii) middle, and (iii) lower. The upper chamber contains oxygen and the lower, contains N_2O (only if the oxygen is available in the upper chamber). On either side of the middle chamber are the flexible diaphragms. Between the two diaphragms is placed the adjusting spring. The middle chamber is vented to atmosphere by multiple small vents **(Fig. 3)** to prevent mixing of anesthetic gas (N_2O) and oxygen in the event that the diaphragm ruptures or the packing leaks. In the event of malfunction of any of the diaphragms, the vents will bleed, giving a "leaking" sound. The user has to avoid using the machine till the service engineer replaces the diaphragm or the packing.

However, this is not a full proof system against the delivery of a hypoxic gas as one can inadvertently give 100% N_2O at the level of flowmeter control valve. It is possible to switch on N_2O flow control valve without switching on oxygen flow control valve in the event of oxygen central pipeline being connected and having pressure/oxygen cylinder being connected and fully opened. Under this circumstance, 100% N_2O can be delivered to the patient.

SAFETY RELIEF VALVES ON REGULATORS (FIGS. 1, 3 TO 5)

Safety blow-off valves are often fitted on the downstream side of regulators to allow escape of gas if by accident the regulators were to fail and allow a high output pressure. These valves are generally spring loaded, in which case they close when pressure falls again. But if they operate by rupture, then they remain open until repaired by service engineer.

NONRETURN VALVES

Nonreturn valves may be present in the hanger yoke of anesthesia machine or in the pressure-reducing valve. They prevent empty cylinders from being refilled by other cylinders if the empty cylinder is left turned on and the anesthesia machine has dual/double yokes **(Fig. 5A)**.

Pressure regulators can be either adjustable or preset. Adjustable pressure regulator has a means for the user to adjust the "Pr" whereas a tool is required to adjust the Pr in preset regulator.[1]

Both adjustable as well as preset type regulators can be seen on the central panel of piped gas manifold **(Fig. 6)**. The pressure regulators of right bank as well as left bank of the central manifold panel have handles. Moving the handle clockwise will open the valve seat and the gas would flow into the regulator. The more you move the handle clockwise (screw the handle inside the valve) more would be the Pr. One bank is "running" and the other is kept standby, i.e., "reserved". The reduced pressure of "running" bank is set higher (e.g., 100 psi) than that of the "reserved" bank (e.g., 80 psi). The "Pr" of the preset valve which

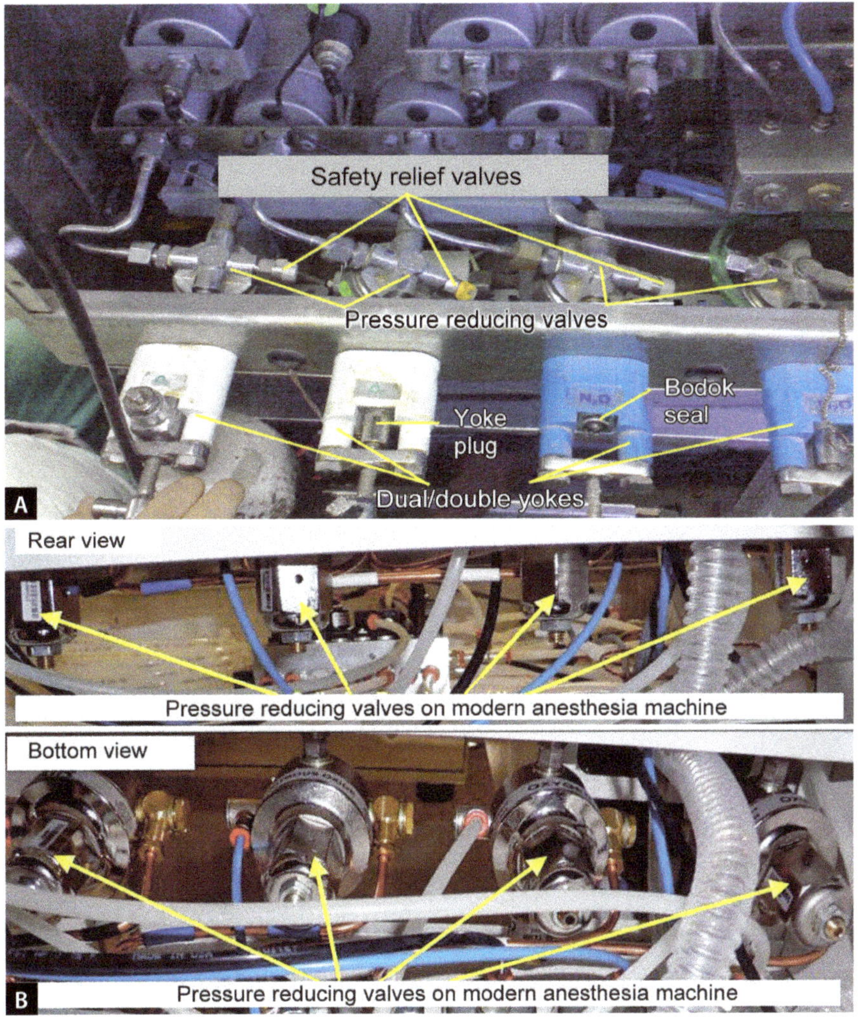

Figs. 5A and B: Pressure-reducing valves on different machines.

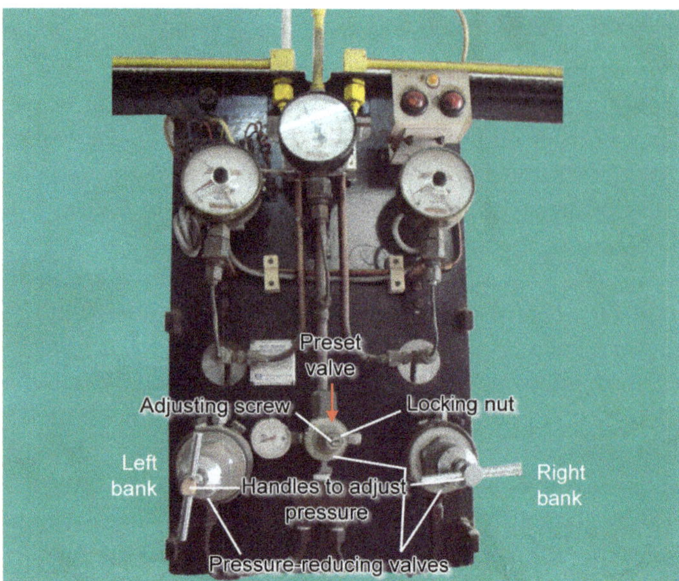

Fig. 6: Pressure-reducing valves in central piped gas manifold panel.

receives gases from both the adjustable pressure regulators is set to the service pressure at (i.e., 55–60 psi). The gases from the "running" bank would be preferentially utilized because the pressure set is higher. Once this pressure falls to the same level as that of "reserved" bank, gases from both the banks would be utilized, simultaneously a visual as well as auditory alarm would sound to alert the operator to switch over the bank and change the cylinders of the nearly empty bank. These types of adjustable pressure regulators are also seen on gas cylinders used in patient care areas or used during transport. The difference is that they can be set by end users whereas those in central manifold room are to be set only by the authorized personnel.

Preset regulators are the ones where the Pr cannot be set by the user as and when needed. "Pr" is adjustable on "preset" regulators; but it requires a tool to adjust the reduced pressure (Pr). Pressure regulators used in anesthesia machines are preset type.

CONCLUSION

Pressure regulators are required to convert high variable pressure of cylinders to low constant working pressure. This avoids damage to the flow control valve and frequent adjustment of flow control valve needed on the flowmeters due to variable input pressure of the cylinders. Pressure regulators used in anesthesia are "indirect-acting pressure regulator" because the components here are arranged in such a way that cylinder pressure tends to close the valve. Pressure increases as the cylinder pressure reduces, but the value of "Pr" mainly depends on the force of adjusting spring (FS_1), which is kept so large that the change in Pr is negligible with change in cylinder pressure. The tension in the spring (FS_1) can be varied by means of the adjustable screw, and in this way, Pr can be varied. For this reason, the main spring is sometimes called the adjusting spring.

REFERENCE

1. Dorsch JA, Dorsch SE. Anesthesia machines. Understanding Anesthetic Equipment, 5th edition. Philadelphia: Wolters Kluwer Health/Lippincott Williams & Wilkins; 2008.

7

CHAPTER

Flowmeters

Preeti G More

ABSTRACT

As oxygen and nitrous oxide are routinely used by the anesthetist, a thorough knowledge about the flowmeters which control the rate of flow of gases is required. Commonly used flowmeters are the conventional or mechanical flowmeters. Electronic flowmeters also have a backup mechanical flowmeter for total fresh gas flow at the common gas outlet. The flowmeter assembly, subassembly, sequence, arrangement, safety features all help in the delivery of safe gases to the patient, which is discussed in this chapter. Proper care and performing checklists will help prevent any malfunction of the flowmeters.

INTRODUCTION

Flowmeter is a device that measures the flow rate of liquid or gas in a closed tube. It is used to control rate of flow of gas and adjust the proportion of gas delivered. The flow rate of gas through a tube will depend on the pattern of flow, whether laminar or turbulent.

The flowmeters used in anesthesia machines help deliver anesthetic gases to the patient. Flowmeters form the low pressure component of the anesthesia machines and are known as rotameters as the "float" rotates with the flow of gases. Rotameter is a variable orifice, constant pressure flowmeter. Flowmeters have been modified, over the years, since the 1920s.

HISTORY

The older flowmeters were wet (water-sight) flowmeters. They were popularly known as water sight feed meters (Bubble flowmeters) as seen in Foregger apparatus, or primitive Boyle's apparatus. The other varieties were the Bourdon tube flowmeter and screen orifice flowmeter.[1] In 1933, Bubble flowmeters were replaced by dry-bobbins or ball-bearing flowmeters. In 1937, rotameters replaced dry-bobbin flowmeters **(Figs. 1A and B)**.

Nowadays, electronic flowmeters are incorporated in newer anesthesia workstations. They have solenoid valves, which controls the flow rate/minute, with a bar (Datex S5) or numerical (Drager) type of display.

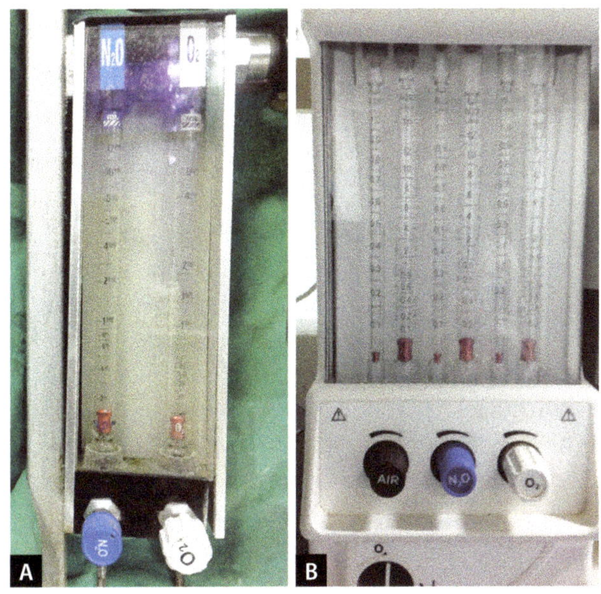

Figs. 1A and B: Different types of flowmeters (rotameters) on anesthesia machines.

THEORY

"Flow" is defined as the quantity of gas (or fluid) passing a point in unit time. The units of flow are in mL/min, L/min, mL/h or L/h. In anesthesia, we talk of flow of gases in mL/min or L/min. Depending on the velocity of the flow, flow can be laminar (at lower velocity) or turbulent (at higher velocity). The flow also depends on the diameter of the tube, the length of the tube and the pressure difference across the tube through which it has to pass. With a given pressure difference across an orifice, flow rate of fluid or gas is proportional to the square of the diameter of the orifice.[2] This pressure difference is a measure of the resistance, which has to be overcome when the gas or fluid is forced or drawn through the tube.

Flow rate also depends on the viscosity (at lower flow rates) and density (at higher flow rates) of the gas itself and whether it passes through a tube or an orifice.

Flow rate through a tube is proportional to the fourth power of the radius.[2] It follows the principle that when flow through a tube is laminar, the flow rate is directly proportional to the pressure gradient across it. When the flow is turbulent, the flow rate is directly proportional to the square root of the pressure gradient.

Laminar flow is directly proportional to pressure gradient across the tube and the radius of the tube and indirectly proportional to the viscosity and the length of the tube. Laminar flow depends on the viscosity and turbulent flow on the density.

Rotameter belongs to a class of meters called variable area meters, which measure flow rate by allowing the cross-sectional area through which the fluid or gas passes to vary, causing some measurable effect.

Most flowmeters (mechanical flowmeters) measure the drop in pressure that occurs when a gas passes through a resistance and correlate this pressure drop to flow.

PHYSICS

For laminar flows, the flow rate of a gas depends on factors as shown below:

- Flow rate = pressure loss/length of the tube × $(\text{diameter})^4$ × 1/viscosity
- Pressure loss = length of tube/$(\text{diameter})^4$ × viscosity × flow rate
- Pressure loss = f × viscosity × length/$(\text{diameter})^4$ × flow rate

These relationships are true only for laminar flows in tubes and is called the Hagen–Poiseuille law, where flow rate (Q) = L/min, pressure loss (P) = mm Hg, length (L) = cm, internal diameter (D) = cm, viscosity (V) relative to that of water = 1, factor f = 6.94×10^{-2}.

In anesthesia machines the flowmeter tubes are not uniform in diameter from bottom to top. They are tapering, with lesser diameter at the bottom and gradually increasing diameter as you go towards the top. Therefore, at low flows the gases pass through a tubular space (since the height of the float is greater than the annular space area between the float and the wall of the tube) and hence viscosity plays a major role whereas at higher flow rates the gases pass through an annular space (since the annular space area between the float and the wall of the tube is greater than the height of float) and hence density plays a major role in determining the flow rate.

The rate of flow of a gas through the flowmeter tube will depend on three factors:[2,3]

1. *Pressure drop across the constriction:* As gas flows around the indicator, it encounters frictional resistance between the indicator and tube wall, and there is loss of energy reflected in a pressure drop.[3] This pressure drop is given by weight of float divided by the cross sectional area of the orifice.
2. *Size of the annular opening:* As the size of the tube varies, increasing from bottom to the top, the annular area varies while the pressure drop across the indicator remains constant for all the positions in the tube. At low flows, the bobbin is at the lower end of the tube, where the diameter of the equivalent channel is smaller than its length. Here the constriction is tubular. As the rate of flow increases the bobbin rises and the diameter of the equivalent channel increases correspondingly, however, the length of the constriction remains constant. When the bobbin reaches topmost, the constriction approximates to an orifice, i.e., the constriction becomes an orifice.
3. *Physical characteristics of the gas:* The viscosity and density of the gases play an important role. When the flow is laminar (generally at lower flows), the rate of flow is inversely proportional to the viscosity of the gas whereas when the flow is turbulent (at higher flows), the rate of flow is proportional to the density of the gas. Different gases used in anesthesia have different velocities, their flow rates under the same conditions vary widely. This fact is of considerable importance when measuring one gas with a rotameter calibrated for another.

The interdependence of flow rates, size of the orifice and pressure difference on each side of orifice is made use of in the design of two main types of anesthetic flow meters:

1. *Variable orifice meters:* In these flowmeters the pressure of the gas on either side of the bobbin remains constant, but the total area of the orifice progressively increases as the flow increases, e.g., rotameter, Coxeter bobbin meter, Heidbrink meter, and Connell meter.
2. *Fixed orifice meters:* In these flowmeters the dimension of the orifice through which the gas flows remains constant, but the pressure of the gas on either side of the orifice is varied, e.g., Bourdon pressure gauge meter **(Figs. 2A and B)**, water depression meter, meter with capillary constriction, Forreger meter, and water-sight meter.

Anesthetic flowmeters are generally one of the following two types:

1. *Dry or bobbin type (variable orifice constant pressure):* In this type there is a constant pressure difference across an orifice or annular space supporting the weight of the bobbin; hence the area of orifice varies with the flow rate of the gas.
2. *Water depression or pressure gauge meter (fixed orifice variable pressure):* In this the pressure difference across an orifice varies with changes in the flow of gas, i.e., size of orifice is constant with pressure difference on either side of it varying with the flow rate of the gas, e.g., water depression or pressure gauge meters.
   - Pressure varies as the square of flow rate[1]
   - P1 – P2 = V2K or
   - P1 = upstream pressure, P2 = downstream pressure, V = velocity of gas, K = a constant for the particular gas being measured.

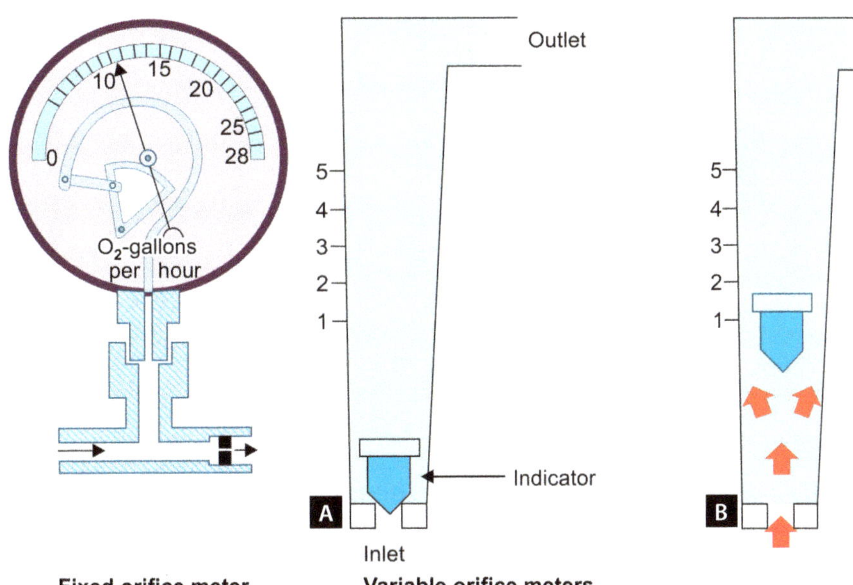

Figs. 2A and B: Fixed and variable orifice flowmeters. (A) No gas flow from the inlet; hence, the bobbin is at the bottom; (B) The gas flow from the inlet and the indicator rising to the top as the flow rate increases.

TYPES OF FLOWMETERS

- Differential pressure
- Variable area
- Inferential
- Positive displacement
- Anemometer
- Ultrasonic
- Fluidic.

Most commonly used flowmeters in anesthesia machines is variable area type.

Variable Orifice Meters (Fixed Pressure Difference)

Principle

In this, the size of the orifice in the flowmeter tube varies with the flow rate. For a given flow rate, the float remains stationary since the forces of differential pressure, gravity, viscosity, density, and buoyancy are balanced. When there is zero flow, the float rests at the bottom of the measuring tube where the maximum diameter of the float is the same as the bore **(Fig. 2A)** of the tube. But when the gas enters the inlet at the base, the float rises and spins on its vertical axis allowing the gas to flow through the annular space between the float and the wall of the flow meter tube **(Fig. 2B)**. The float moves up and down in proportion to gas flow rate such that pressure drop across the float remains constant, higher flows requiring larger annular area than lower flow rates.

Rotameter

It is the type of flowmeters used today in most modern machines. As a gas measuring device, it was patented in Germany in 1908 by Karl Kuppers[2] of Aachen, and used in anesthesia by Maximilian Neu (1910). In 1910, rotameters were used in anesthetic apparatus for measuring flow rates of N_2O and O_2. Magill (1932) used it independently and was further developed by R Salt (1937).[4]

Flowmeter Assembly (Figs. 3A and B)

The flowmeter assembly accurately controls and measures gas flow to the common gas outlet.

It is composed of the flow control valve assembly and the flowmeter subassembly.

The assembly can have direct supply of gases from the pipeline source (50 psig) or from a second stage pressure regulator when cylinders are used.

Flow control valve assembly consists of flow control knobs, needle valve, valve seat, and a pair of valve "stops":[4]

- *Flow control knobs:* They help in controlling the movement of the flow control valve. Flow control knobs when moved anticlockwise will start the gas flow and in clockwise direction will stop it. The gas flow control knobs are touch and color coded (oxygen is large, fluted, projectile knob, white in color, and nitrous oxide is blue in color with fine serrations). At this point the gas pressure is reduced from 15 psi to 5–7 psi.
- *Needle valve:* It is made of a fine pin with a tapered end that fits into a ground metal seat (valve seat). The gas flow can be started, controlled, and stopped by screwing and unscrewing the pin **(Figs. 4A and B)**.
- *Valve seat:* It is a ground metal seat, into which fits the tapered end of the needle valve. Malfunctions in the pin or seat can block the flow of the gas.[5] However, extreme clockwise rotation can damage the needle valve and valve seat.[6] This is prevented with valve "stops".
- *Valve "stops":* It helps prevent damage to the needle valve or seat caused due to extreme clockwise rotation of flow control valve.

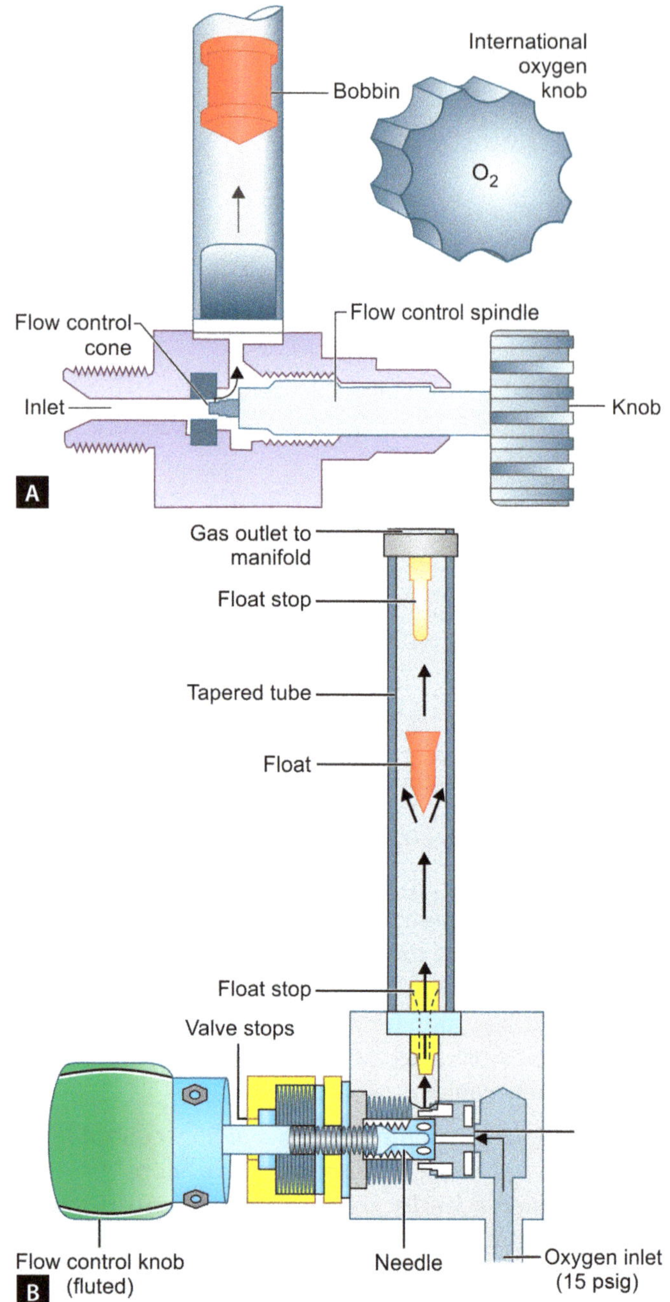

Figs. 3A and B: (A) Flowmeter assembly; (B) Oxygen flowmeter assembly.

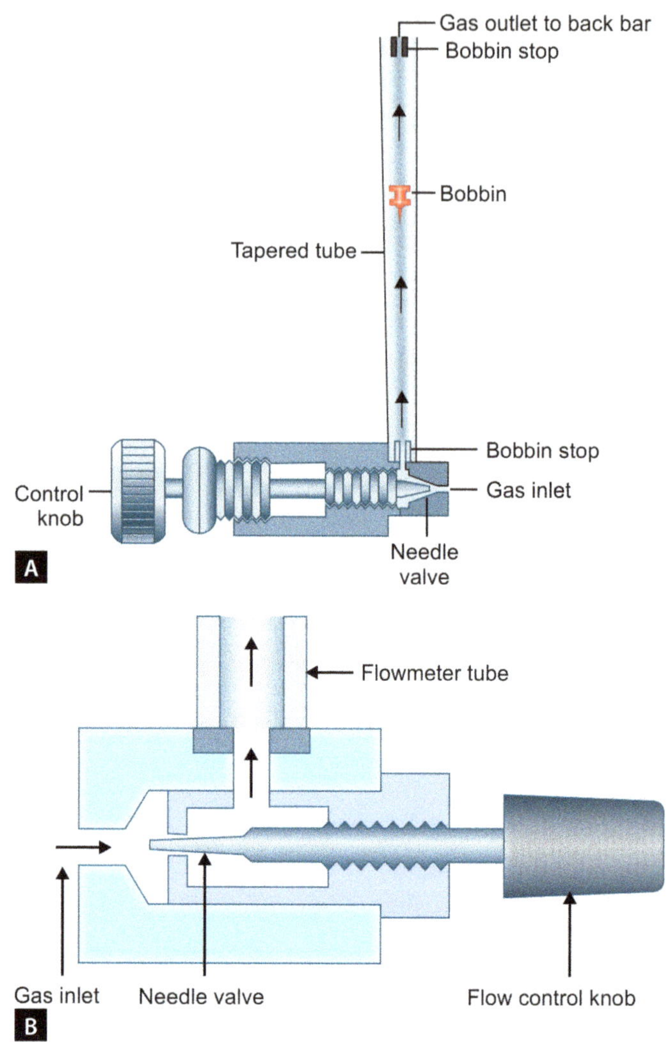

Figs. 4A and B: (A) Flowmeter with a flow control needle valve; (B) Flow control needle valve assembly.

Flowmeter Subassembly (Fig. 5)

It consists of:

- Thorpe's tube with a scale that indicates the flow rate.
- A float or indicator.
- Stop.

Thorpe's Tube

It is made up of Pyrex® glass, transparent, nonconducting material. The length of the tube can vary from 65 mm to 230 mm, differs for different manufacturers of anesthesia machines.

It is conical in shape, tapered vertically with the smallest diameter at the bottom. The tube contains an indicator that is free to move up and down the tube as per increase or decrease in the flow of gas. Some tubes have rib guides, which keeps indicator in the center of the tube. The tubes are contained in a chromium plated metal casing protected by a plastic window. Detachable luminous back plate is provided which illuminates in the dark. Modern machines have flowmeter lights.

The Thorpe's tube is made leak proof and gas tight at top and bottom by "O" rings, neoprene sprockets and washer.

The tube has markings (scale) that will indicate the flow rate of the particular gas. Scale has to be immediately adjacent to the tube[7] and is mostly seen on the right side of the tube. The tube is calibrated for a particular gas that covers flow rates from a few hundred mL/min to more than 10 L/min. Thorpe tube can be single or double tapered. Single tapered tubes have a gradual increase in diameter from bottom to top and are used for lower flows when there are different tubes for high and low flows. Dual taper tubes have two different tapers inside the same tube for fine (low) and coarse (high) flows **(Fig. 6)**.

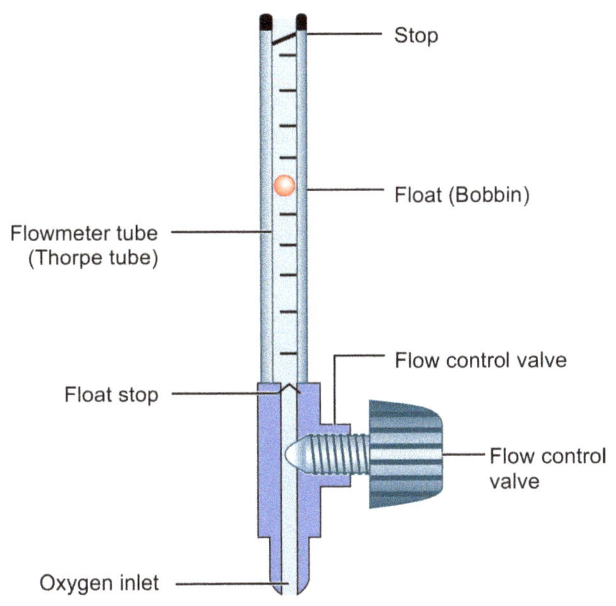

Fig. 5: Oxygen rotameter.

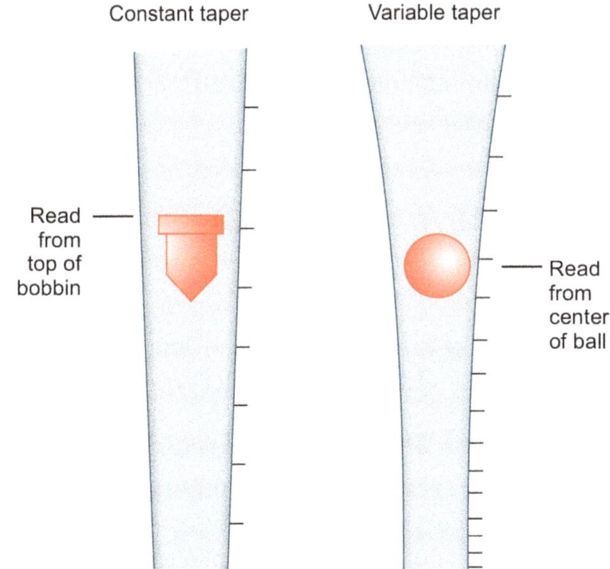

Fig. 7: Rotameters with bobbins.

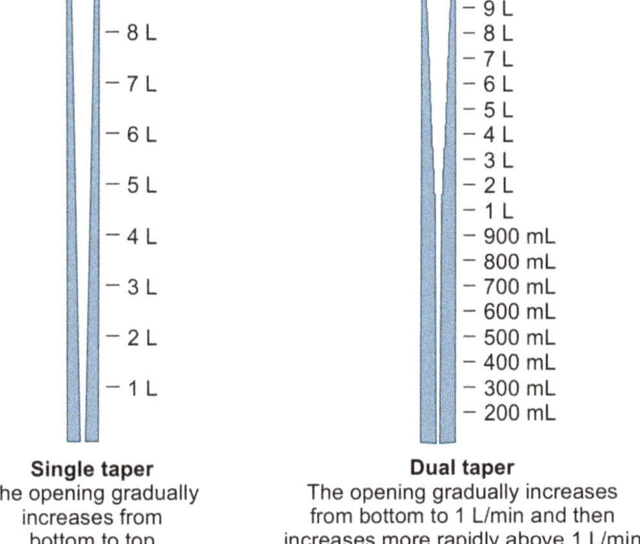

Fig. 6: Flowmeter tubes: Single and dual taper.

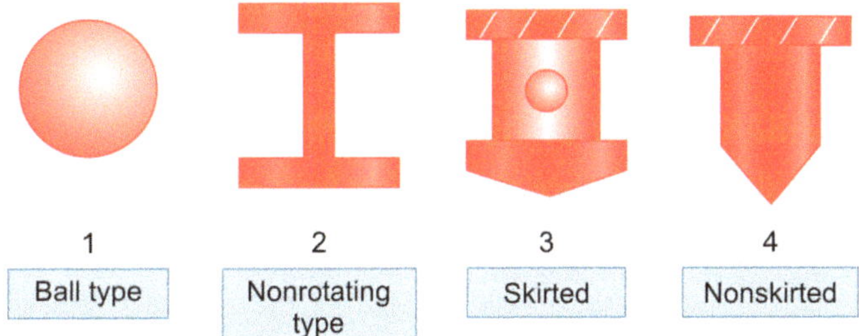

Fig. 8: Reading a flowmeter and different types of bobbins.

The calibrations for different gases are as follows:

- *Oxygen:* Graduated in 100 mL/min, divisions from 100 mL/min to 2,000 mL/min and in 1,000 mL/min divisions from 2,000 mL/min to 5,000 mL/min[8]
- *Nitrous oxide:* Graduated in 1 L divisions from 1 L/min to 10 L/min
- *Carbon dioxide (CO_2):* Graduated in 100 mL/min divisions from 100 mL/min to 2,000 mL/min
- *Cyclopropane:* Graduated in 50 mL/min divisions from 50 mL/min to 750 mL/min divisions
- *Air:* Graduated from 0.05 to 15 L/min.

Indicator (Float or Bobbin)

It is light weight, made of aluminum; hence, it is free to move up and down the tube as per increase or decrease in the flow of gas. It is a free moving device within the tube, if it moves erratically, readings may be inaccurate. It contains antistatic material to prevent sticking to wall of flowmeter.

If there is a leak downstream of the indicator but upstream of the common manifold, a lesser concentration of that gas will appear in the fresh gas flow.[9]

There are two types of indicators:

1. Rotating (rotameters) **(Fig. 7)**
2. Nonrotating
   - Rotating indicators have upper rim, diameter of which is larger than body. Slanted grooves or flutes are cut into the rim so that it rotates freely in the middle of the gas stream. There is often a colored dot on one side of indicator. Reading is taken at upper rim
   - Nonrotating are old, float type are kept at center by flow of gas. Ball float is kept at the center by rib-guides; reading is taken at the center of the ball (i.e., at the maximum diameter of the ball) and has two colors to see the rotations. H-type also there **(Fig. 8)**.[10]

At low flows, the annular-shaped orifice around the float is (relatively) tubular so (according to Poiseuille's law) flow is governed by "viscosity". At high flows (indicated on the wider top part of the float tube), the annular opening is more like an orifice, and "density" governs the flows.

However in ball type indicators, the entire length of the tube the orifice remains orifical and never tubular. Hence, the working of this rotameter will depend on the density of the gas rather than the viscosity.

Stop

It is present at the top; it prevents the float from blocking the outlet and also prevents it from ascending to a point where it cannot be seen.[8]

Hazard: Stop may break off and fall on the indicator, so it can register less flow than is actually occurring.

TEMPERATURE AND PRESSURE EFFECTS

Flowmeters are calibrated at atmospheric pressure (760 torr) and room temperature (20°C).[3] Hence, changes in temperature and pressure (by affecting density and viscosity) of gas affect flowmeter accuracy. In hyperbaric chamber flowmeter will deliver less gas than indicated and with decreased barometric pressure (high altitude) the actual flow rate will be greater than that indicated.

ARRANGEMENT OF DUAL FLOWMETER TUBES

If two flowmeter tubes are present for a particular gas, for high and low gas flows, they can be arranged in:

- Parallel
- Series.

Parallel arrangement has two different tubes with two different control knobs, total flow is the sum of flows shown in the two tubes. This can be hazardous as chances of delivering hypoxic mixture to patient, especially if nitrous oxide flows are high and low flow oxygen has been opened.

In series arrangement only one control knob is present. The gas passes through low flow tube and then into the tube for higher flows **(Fig. 9)**. Total flow is shown by float in high flow tube. Series arrangement is more accurate than parallel.

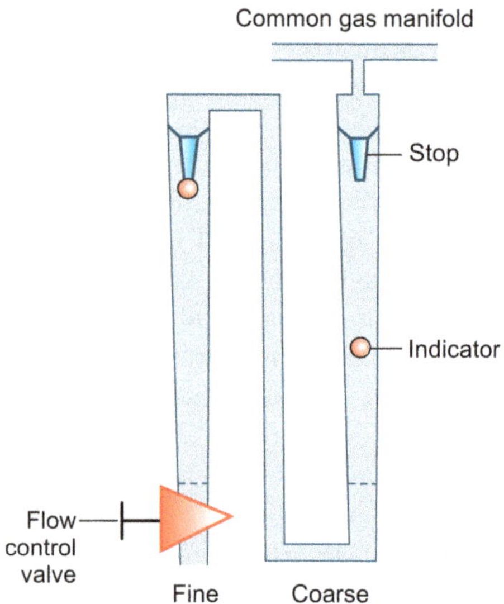

Fig. 9: Flowmeter tubes in series.

Now, with low flow anesthesia delivery systems, flowmeters which accurately measure flows below 1 L/min are used.

In this, two flow meter tubes are used for the same gas, where first tube is calibrated for lower flows from 0–1000 mL/min and the second tube is calibrated for higher flows from 1–10 L/min or more (sequential arrangement) and both are activated from the same flow control valve. This is also called as "cascade" flowmeter tubes.

SEQUENCE OF FLOWMETER TUBES

It is important to prevent delivery of hypoxic gas mixture to the patient, if any leak occurs in any of the flowmeter tubes. Therefore, it is safe to keep oxygen flowmeter downstream of all the gases, otherwise, in case of leaks, oxygen will be selectively lost out from the leak if it is upstream of any of the flowmeter tubes.

If there is a leak downstream of the indicator but upstream of the common manifold, a lesser concentration of that gas will appear in the fresh gas flow.[9]

Figures 10A to D show that in the presence of a flowmeter leak, either at the "O" ring or the glass of the flow tube, a hypoxic mixture occurring is rare if the oxygen flowmeter is downstream of all other flowmeters. Hence, in **Figures 10A and B** are potentially dangerous as a hypoxic mixture can occur as a substantial portion of oxygen flow passes through the leak and all nitrous oxide is directed to the common gas outlet.

In **Figures 10C and D** as the oxygen flowmeter is located downstream, it is safe. Hence, C and D arrangements are safer. A hypoxic mixture is less likely. Drager flowmeters are arranged as in C and Datex Ohmeda flowmeters as in D.

WORKING OF FLOWMETERS

- When the flow control valve is opened the gas enters at the bottom and flows up the tube, the indicator rises up
- The indicator (bobbin) floats freely at a point where the downward force on it (gravity) equals the upward force caused by gas molecules hitting the bottom of the float
- Because the tube is tapered the annular opening around the indicator will increase with height and more gas flows around the float.

It is important to check that the flow control valves are in off position (closed) before starting the machine. If the flow control valves are kept open and the gas supply is restored, the indicator may rise to the top of the tube suddenly and may remain there without anyone noticing it. This may harm the patient if it happens to be gases other than oxygen because inadvertent flow of that gas may contribute to the breathing gases and cause hypoxic gas mixture. Also sudden indicator rise may damage and cause inaccurate reading of the flowmeter.[11]

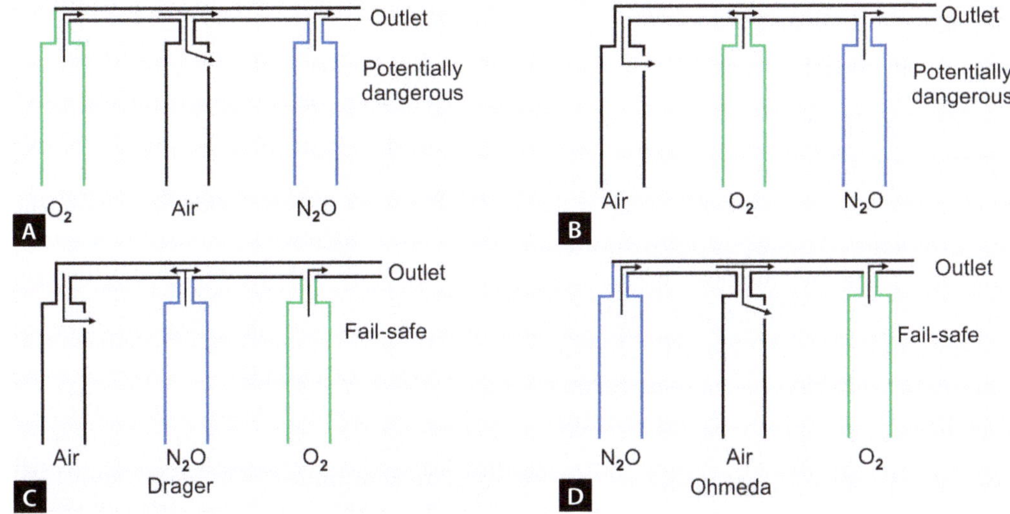

Figs. 10A to D: Sequence of flowmeters.

Variations in Oxygen Flowmeters (Table 1)

Flowmeters on some machines have a "minimum oxygen flow" of 200–300 mL/min. Some newer machines have minimum oxygen flows as low as 50 mL or no minimum oxygen flow at all. Supply pressure is 50 psi on most of the machines. However, Ohmeda has a second-stage regulator which supplies oxygen at 14 psi, and nitrous oxide at approximately 26 psi. This is a component of the fail-safe or hypoxic guard systems (Datex-Ohmeda Link-25 system) in Ohmeda machines.

In Datex-Ohmeda link-25 system **(Fig. 11)** the oxygen flow control-valve is identical to nitrous oxide flow control-valve. Oxygen flow-control valve has a 28-tooth sprocket attached to it whereas nitrous oxide flow-control valve has a 14-tooth sprocket attached to it. Sprockets are linked physically by a chain. When the nitrous oxide flow-control valve is turned through two revolutions, the oxygen flow-control valve revolves once (2:1 ratio). The final flow ratio is 3:1 because the nitrous oxide flow control valve is supplied by approximately 26 psi, whereas the oxygen flow control valve is supplied by 14 psi as mentioned above.

TABLE 1: Different varieties of flowmeters.

Type	*Control*	*Display*	*Example*
Traditional	Mechanical valve	Glass tube	Aestiva, Narkomed 6400
Transitional (hybrid)	Mechanical valve	Electronic	ADU, Fabius®
Electronic	Electronic	Electronic	Aisys®, Avance®

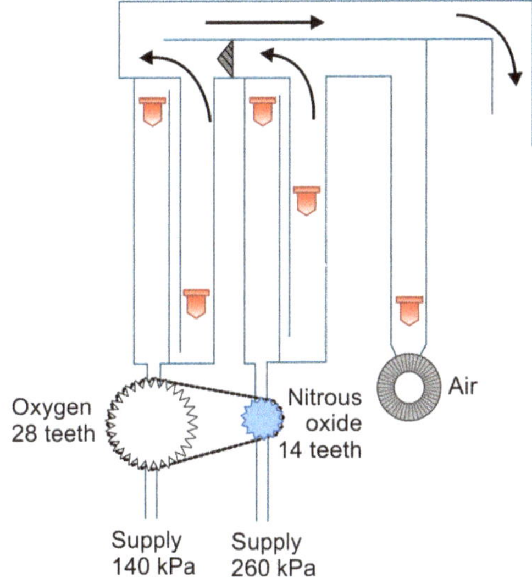

Fig. 11: Safety in flowmeters. Link 25 as seen in Datex–Ohmeda machine.

Traditional Flowmeters

These are the ones that we discussed above, made up of the Thorpe's tube, the flow control knobs with needle valve, indicator or float and valve stops. They have regular mechanical needle valves and glass flow tubes as seen in the Excel, Modulus, Aestiva; and Narkomed 2, 3, 4, and 6000.

Transitional (Hybrid) Flowmeters

Machines with transitional flowmeters have no glass tubes. The flow rate is indicated with a bar graph on a monitor screen. There is a needle valve (so flow can be generated even without electric power) in the ADU and Fabius® GS. Flows are captured electronically as follows—flow from the needle valve is conducted to a small chamber of known volume and held there momentarily by a solenoid valve until the transduced pressure within the chamber reaches a preset limit. This gives a known mass of gas. This cycle is repeated sufficiently often for the desired flow rate to occur, and the number of times the solenoid opens is sensed and can be related to flow. Thus, transitional (and electronic) flowmeters allow automated anesthesia record-keepers to chart fresh gas flows.

Electronic Flowmeters

As in Datex Ohmeda S/5, Drager Fabius® GS have conventional flow control knobs and valves, but have electronic flow sensors and digital displays instead of the glass flow tubes.[12] If electrical failure occurs, there is a pneumatic backup, which maintains delivery of fresh gas.

PROBLEMS WITH FLOWMETERS

- Inaccuracy due to improper assembly and calibration, tube not vertical
- Float or Indicator problems—Damage due to sudden rise at the top due to accidental increase in the flow of gas.[11] It can stick to the tube due to dust and dirt. Bobbin can also stick due to static electric charges caused by friction between the dry gases, rotating bobbin and the nonconducting Thorpe's tube. To prevent this antistatic sprays like Croxtene, Sphirol-H are used to remove the static charges inside the glass tubes
- Leaks in the flowmeter tube
- Using wrong flowmeter when rotameter sequence is altered. This is commonly seen with air and nitrous oxide and hypoxic gas can be delivered[13]
- Inaccuracies in readings at high altitudes and hyperbaric chambers. They under-read at high altitudes (hypobaric) due to reduced gas density and read 30% higher flows in hyperbaric conditions
- Workstations equipped with proportioning systems like oxygen ratio monitor controller (ORMC) and Link 25, need not to be totally "fail-safe" and can still deliver hypoxic mixture if there is a wrong supply of gas other than oxygen, leaks downstream due to broken oxygen flow tube, and improper functioning of second stage regulator, nitrous oxide control valve, and resistors.

SAFETY FEATURES OF FLOWMETERS

Different anesthesia machines incorporate various safety features of flowmeters in their machines as follows:

- *Color and touch-coded flowmeters:* All the needle-valve-control knobs are colored, touch-coded, and clearly marked. The oxygen flow-control knob is touch coded (larger, octagonal profile and protrudes at least 2 mm out more than nitrous oxide knob) and its position is downstream of the block.[14] This minimizes the risk of oxygen leaking from the cracks in other flow meter tubes and also prevents delivery of hypoxic mixture. It is customary in the US for the oxygen flow tube to be on the right of the others, on the left in the UK.[2] In either cases, oxygen always enters the common manifold downstream of other gases. Color code: oxygen is white and nitrous oxide is blue
- Illuminated back helps visualization of the flowmeter block in dim light
- *Hypoxic mixture prevention devices:* These can be mechanical, pneumatic or electronic
  - *Mechanical:* Link 25 proportion limiting control system (Ohmeda) **(Fig. 11)**. A chain link between nitrous oxide and oxygen knobs prevents less than 25% oxygen delivery when nitrous oxide is used. It is a mechanical linkage (chain with a gear ratio of 2:1) between nitrous oxide and oxygen with 14 tooth sprocket on nitrous oxide and 28 tooth sprocket on oxygen to maintain oxygen flow with nitrous oxide.[3,15] An audible alarm sounds to alert the operator that oxygen-nitrous oxide flow ratio has fallen below a preset value
    Another safety feature to prevent the delivery of hypoxic mixture of gases going to the patient when oxygen is placed upstream is the presence of baffles **(Figs. 12A and B)**
  - *Pneumatic [ORMC (Drager)]:* It is a pneumatic oxygen-nitrous oxide interlock system designed to maintain fresh gas oxygen concentration of at least 25 ± 3%. A slave valve that controls the flow of nitrous oxide depending on oxygen flow. Reduction in oxygen pressure are automatically compensated to maintain oxygen concentration of at least 28%[15]
  - *Electronic:* Electronic devices, e.g., Penlon use a paramagnetic oxygen analyzer to continuously sample the gas mixtures from the flowmeters. In this the nitrous oxide gets temporarily shut off when the inspired fraction of oxygen (FiO_2) decreases below 0.25, while an increase in the (FiO_2) will temporarily start the nitrous oxide flow[16]
- Minimum mandatory oxygen flow 250–400 mL/min by inclusion of a resistor in 50 psi pipeline
- Torque required to turn the flow control knobs is high enough to minimize accidental contact
- If oxygen concentration falls below 25%, then battery powered electronic device sounds an audible alarm and nitrous oxide is cut off
- If CO_2 supply is fitted to the anesthesia machine, the flowmeter should be designed to allow a maximum of only 500 mL/min CO_2 to be added to the fresh gas flows so as to avoid hypercarbia.[15]

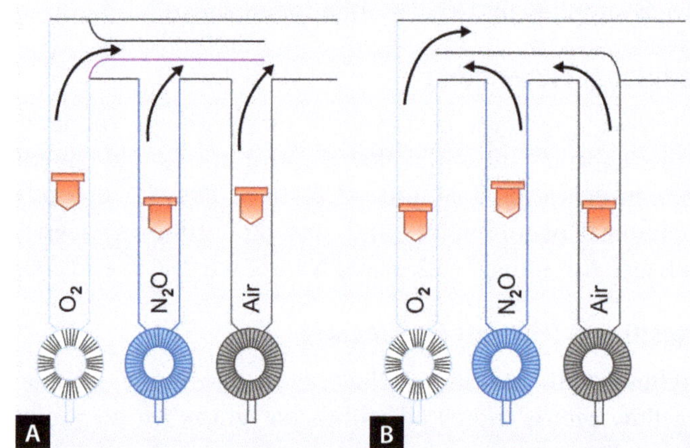

Figs. 12A and B: Safety in flowmeters: Baffles to prevent hypoxic mixture if oxygen is upstream. (A and B) Shows the presence of separate baffles for oxygen so that there is no chance of hypoxic mixture going to the the common gas outlet when oxygen is placed upstream.

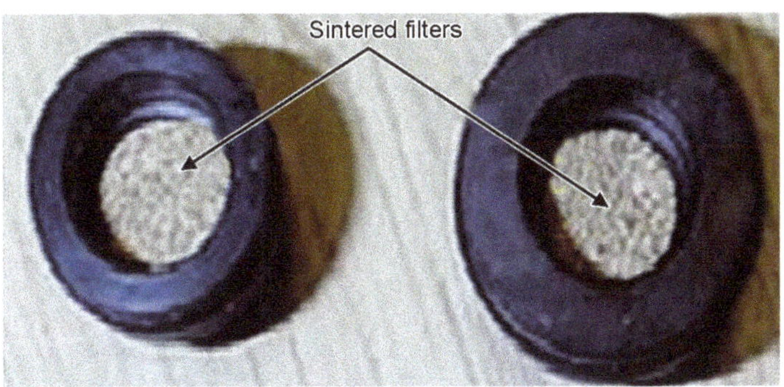

Fig. 13: Sintered filters in flowmeter caps.

Care of flowmeters includes ensuring that:

- Floats spin freely; float does not stick due to dirt or static electricity or back pressure from oxygen flush valve
- Qualified service personnel regularly maintain gas machines and check leaks in flowmeter tubes, replace the sintered filters in the flowmeter tube caps **(Fig. 13)**
- An oxygen analyzer used always
- One never adjusts a flowmeter without looking at it
- One includes flowmeters in visual monitoring sweeps
- One turns flowmeters off before opening cylinders, connecting pipelines, or turning machine "on".[11]

CHECKLIST FOR FLOWMETERS

As per the anesthesia apparatus checkout recommendations,[16,17] flowmeter checklist should include the following:

- Position, color, and touch coding to be checked. Any variation is to be noted
- Adjust flow control knobs to see full range of gas flow
- Bobbin is rotating, not stuck or damaged
- Antistatic spray present
- Oxygen flowmeter is placed downstream
- Radio fluorescent backplate of the flowmeters
- Attempt to create a hypoxic oxygen—nitrous oxide mixture and verify correct changes in flow and/or alarm.

AUXILIARY OXYGEN FLOWMETERS

Auxiliary oxygen flowmeters are separate from the back bar flowmeters and common gas outlet **(Fig. 14)**.[18] It is an optional accessory seen on many models of anesthesia machines.

- They are self-contained having a flow control valve, flow indicator and outlet
- Nasal cannula or other oxygen delivery devices can be attached for the delivery of supplemental oxygen
- It consists of a short tube with a maximum flow of 10 L/min
- It works both on pipeline and cylinder supply of oxygen
- In anesthesia workstations having electronic flow control and measurements (Datex Ohmeda S/5 Avance) auxiliary oxygen flowmeter is conventional (Thorpe's tube) type.

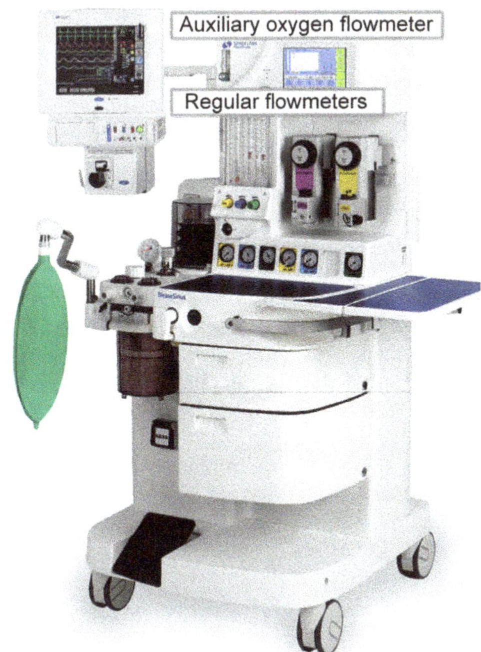

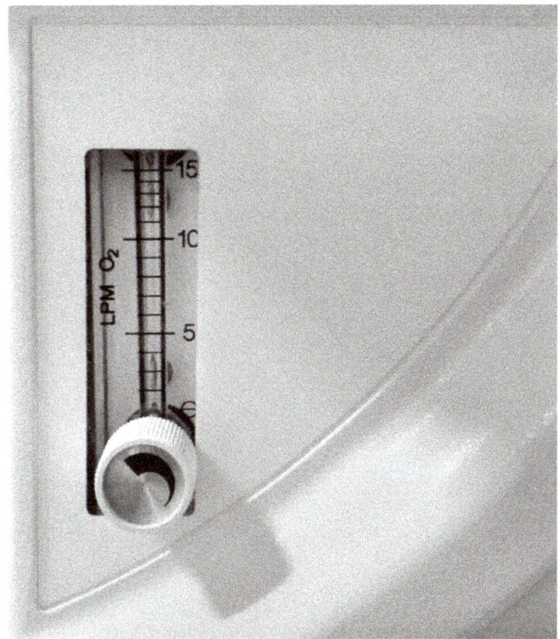

Fig. 14: Auxiliary oxygen flowmeter.

CONCLUSION

Flowmeters are an integral part of the low pressure system in anesthesia machines. The flowmeter assembly accurately controls and measures gas flows to the common gas outlet. Understanding the basic principles, theory, physics, and working of the flowmeters, makes it easy and safe to use. Care of the flowmeters and vigilance while using it will help in safe delivery of gases to the patient.

REFERENCES

1. Dornette WHL, Brechner VL. Instrumentation in Anaesthesiology, 1st edition. Philadelphia: Lea and Febiger; 1959. pp. 153-8.

2. Atkinson RS, Rushman GB, Davies NJH. Lee's Synopsis of Anaesthesia, 11th edition. Oxford: Butterworth-Heinemann Ltd; 1993. pp. 102-3.
3. Dorsch JA, Dorsch SE. Understanding Anaesthesia Equipment, 5th edition. Philadelphia: Lippincott Williams and Wilkins; 2008. pp. 105-10.
4. Barash P, Cullen B, Stoelting R. Clinical Anaesthesia, 5th edition. Philadelphia: Lippincott Williams and Wilkins; 2006. pp. 565-8.
5. Fitzpatrick G, Moore KP. Malfunction in a needle valve. Anaesthesia. 1988;43:164.
6. Hulten P, Boaden RW. Performance of needle valves. Br J Anaesth. 1986;58:919-24.
7. Paul AK. Drugs and Equipment in Anaesthesia Practice, 5th edition. New Delhi: Elsevier; 2005. pp. 215-6.
8. Dudley M, Walsh E. Oxygen loss from rotameter. Br J Anaesth. 1975;47:805.
9. Al-Shaikh B, Stacey S. Essentials of Anaesthesia Equipment, 3rd edition. Edinburgh: Churchill Livingstone; 2007. pp. 21-3.
10. Moon JRA. Rotameter sequence. Anaesthesia. 1996;51:508.
11. Cooper M, Ali D. Oxygen flowmeter dislocation. Anaesth Intensive Care. 1989;17:109-10.
12. Morgan GE, Mikhail MS, Murray MJ. Lange Clinical Anaesthesiology, 4th edition. New York: McGraw Hill; 2008. pp. 55-8.
13. James RH. Rotameter sequence—a variant of read the label. Anaesthesia. 1996;51:87-8.
14. American Society for Testing and Materials. Specifications for minimum performance and safety requirements for components and systems of anaesthesia gas machines (ASTM F-1161-88.). West Conshohocken, PA: ASTM; 1994.
15. Objective Anaesthesia Review: A Comprehensive Textbook for the Examinee, 1st edition. Mumbai: Department of Anaesthesia, Critical Care and Pain (Tata Memorial Centre); 2009. pp. 478-81.
16. American National Standards Institute: Minimum performance and safety requirements for components and systems of continuous flow anaesthesia machines for human use. (ANSI Z79.8-1979). New York: American National Standards Institute; 1979.
17. Association of Anaesthetists of Great Britain and Ireland. Checking Anaesthetic Equipment, 3rd edition. London; 2004.
18. Sinclair CM, Thadsad M, Barker I. Modern anaesthesia machines. Contin Educ Anaesth, Crit Care Pain. 2006;6(2):75-8.

Vaporizers

Anjali A Pingle

ABSTRACT

Volatile anesthetics and, hence, vaporizers form an integral part of current anesthesia practice. Modern vaporizers are compact, safe, and accurate. They are complex feats of mechanical engineering, but are extremely user-friendly. Vaporizer design varies with the properties of each agent. In this chapter, we will look at the factors affecting vaporization and the design modifications incorporated in successive vaporizers. This is followed by descriptions of individual vaporizers in current use, their internal design, filling systems, mounting systems, and safety mechanisms. A brief overview of agents and vaporizers of historical interest is included at the end.

Keywords: Anesthesia machine, anesthesia workstation, anesthetic agent delivery, vaporizers, variable bypass, desflurane vaporizer, dual circuit gas vapor blender, Aladin cassette, injection vaporizer, AnaConDa, historical vaporizers, historical inhalational agents

INTRODUCTION

The use of inhalational anesthetic agents in clinical practice was first demonstrated in 1840s and rapidly became popular all over the globe. Various substances were discovered to have anesthetic properties. Different inhalers were developed for different agents. With time, several of these agents have been rendered obsolete. However, inhalational anesthesia continues to be the mainstay of anesthesia practice.

The agents in current use are highly volatile (high saturated vapor pressures) and very potent (low minimum alveolar concentration). The saturated vapor pressure (SVP) of commonly used volatile anesthetic agents at clinically relevant temperatures is much higher than that needed to produce anesthesia. For example, the SVP of halothane is 243 mm Hg (33% of atmospheric pressure) which is several times higher than its "minimum alveolar concentration (MAC)" of 0.75% (5.7 mm Hg). If halothane is allowed to vaporize freely in the anesthesia delivery system an overdose will result. Hence, a special device is needed to safely and accurately deliver the desired amount of an agent to the patient.

A vaporizer is a device that changes a liquid anesthetic into its vapor and adds a "clinically useful" amount of this vapor to the fresh gas flow (FGF) or the breathing system.

IMPORTANT CONSIDERATIONS IN RELATION TO VAPORIZERS

Vaporizer design is influenced by various physical characteristics of the inhalational agents. All vaporizers take into account the SVP, density, and molecular weight of the agent **(Table 1)** to determine the splitting ratio (ratio of bypass gas to gas going to the vaporization chamber). The potency (MAC) of the agent determines the maximum output that a vaporizer is designed to deliver to achieve an inhalational induction. This is about 3-5 times the MAC.

Definitions

Gas

Any substance above its critical temperature is a gas.

Vapor

A vapor is the gas phase of an agent that is normally a liquid at room temperature and atmospheric pressure.

It is below its critical temperature. It can be liquefied by increasing the pressure.

Critical Temperature

The temperature above which a substance cannot be liquefied, no matter how much pressure is applied, is its critical temperature.

Critical Pressure

The minimum pressure needed to liquefy a substance at its critical temperature is its critical pressure. It is the vapor pressure of a substance at its critical temperature.

Gas Concentration

In anesthesia practice, gas concentration is usually expressed as partial pressure and as volume percent (v/v%).

TABLE 1: Physical characteristics of inhalational agents.

Name	Chemical structure	Formula	Boiling point (°C)	SVP at 20°C (mm Hg)	Blood: gas partition coefficient	MAC in 100% O_2	Molecular weight (g/mole)
Cyclopropane (cycloalkane)	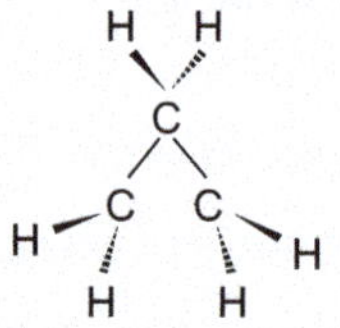 H H C H C C H H H	C_3H_6	32.8	-	0.46	9.2	42
Diethyl ether	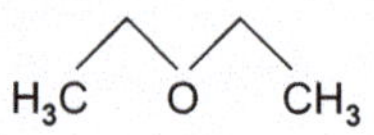 H_3C O CH_3	CH_3CH_2-O-CH_2CH_3	34.6	425	12	1.92	74
Chloroform (chloromethane)	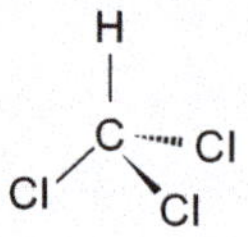 H C Cl Cl Cl	$CHCl_3$	61.2	160	8	0.8	119
Trichloroethylene (chlorinated hydrocarbon)	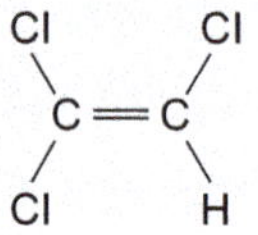 Cl Cl C=C Cl H	$ClCHCCl_2$	872	60	12	0.17	131
Halothane (halogenated hydrocarbon)	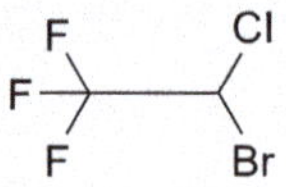 F Cl F F Br	$CF_3CHClBr$	50.2	243	2.54	0.75	197
Enflurane (halogenated ether)	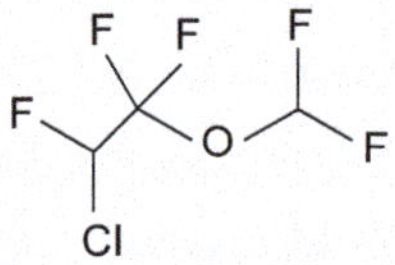 F F F F O F Cl	CHFCl-CF_2-O-CHF_2	56.5	172	1.90	1.63	184
Isoflurane (halogenated ether)	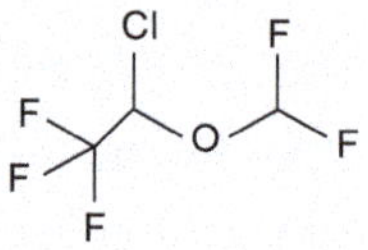 Cl F F O F F F	CF_3-CHCl-O-CHF_2	48.5	184	1.46	1.17	184
Desflurane (fluorinated ether)	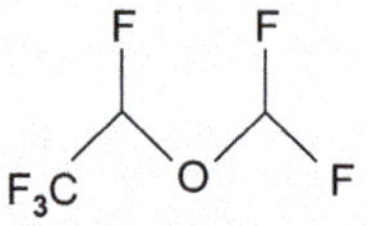 F F F_3C O F	CF_3-CHF-O-CHF_2	22.8	669	0.42	6.6	168
Sevoflurane (fluorinated ether)	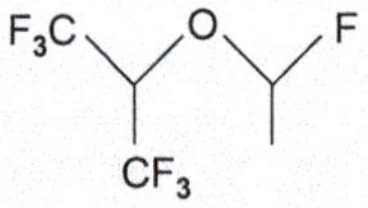 F_3C O F CF_3	$(CHF_3)_2CH$-O-CH_2F	58.5	170	0.69	1.8	200

(SVP: saturated vapor pressure; MAC: minimum alveolar concentration)

Partial Pressure

The molecules of a gas or a vapor in a closed container are in random motion. They strike the walls of the container and generate a pressure. That part of the total pressure due to any one gas in a gas mixture is called the partial pressure of that gas.

Partial pressure is an absolute number and does not change with changes in ambient pressure. The units most commonly used in anesthesia practice are mm Hg, e.g., capnometry.

Dalton's law of partial pressures (1802) states that in a mixture of nonreacting gases, the total pressure exerted is equal to the sum of the partial pressures of the individual gases.

$$P = P_1 + P_2 + P_3 ... + P_n$$

Volume Percent

Volume percent is the number of units of volume of a gas in relation to a total of 100 units of volume for the total gas mixture. In a mixture of gases, the pressure exerted by a gas is proportional to its volume.

$$\frac{\text{Partial pressure}}{\text{Total pressure}} = \frac{v}{v\%}$$

Volume percent is a ratio, and will change with changes in ambient pressure.

In clinical practice, vaporizer dials are marked in v/v%, i.e., volume percent. However, the uptake and anesthetic depth are related to the alveolar and brain partial pressures, respectively. A given partial pressure represents the same anesthetic potency at various ambient pressures.

Saturated Vapor Pressure

Consider a liquid agent in a closed container, the space above the liquid contains air and the agent in vapor phase. At equilibrium, the number of molecules entering and leaving the vapor phase is constant. When the air holds the maximum number of molecules of vapor that it can hold at a given temperature, it is said to be saturated. The maximum partial pressure that can be achieved at any given temperature is called the saturated vapor pressure at that temperature.

If heat is supplied, the kinetic energy and temperature of the system rise. More molecules enter the vapor phase and the partial pressure increases. When SVP equals ambient pressure the liquid boils.

As it is a partial pressure, SVP only changes with temperature and not with changes in ambient pressure.

The saturated vapor pressure is a measure of the volatility of the liquid. Higher SVP denotes greater volatility. Desflurane is very volatile (SVP of 664 mm Hg at 20°C).

Latent Heat of Vaporization

The energy needed to convert a liquid into its vapor at a constant temperature is called the latent heat of vaporization. This heat is drawn from the liquid itself, leading to cooling and a fall in the rate of vaporization. The loss of heat makes the vaporizer output variable. To prevent this, a heatsink is needed.

Specific Heat Capacity

The specific heat capacity is the ability of a substance to retain heat without a rise in temperature. It is the number of calories required to increase the temperature of 1 g of a substance by 1°C. This is applicable in design and construction of vaporizers. Materials used must have a high-specific heat to minimize temperature changes associated with vaporization (water: 4.1813 J/g/K, aluminum: 0.897 J/g/K, copper: 0.385 J/g/K). The water jackets used in the earlier vaporizers have fallen into disuse due to spillage and corrosion.

Thermal Conductivity

Thermal conductivity is a measure of the speed with which heat flows through a substance, e.g., aluminum (204), copper (38.5), stainless steel (16), and bronze (12.5). Metals conduct heat from the atmosphere to the vaporizing chamber when the vaporizer is in use. The wicks are kept in contact with metal walls and coils so that heat lost as a result of vaporization can be replaced quickly as seen in the TEC 5 vaporizer.

The current vaporizers utilize metals like stainless steel, aluminum, and bronze as they have a high-specific heat capacity and high thermal conductivity. The mass of metal acts as a heat sink. Hence, mechanical variable bypass vaporizers are heavy.

HOW MUCH LIQUID DOES A VAPORIZER USE PER HOUR?

This can be determined in two ways:

1. Avogadro's hypothesis (1811)
2. Ehrenwerth and Eisenkraft formula (1993).

Avogadro's Hypothesis (1811)

Avogadro's law states that at constant temperature and pressure, equal volumes of all gases will contain the same number of molecules (6.023×10^{23}, Avogadro's number). This means that at a given temperature and pressure, 1 mole of any gas will occupy the same volume (22.4 L at 1 atm and 0°C, i.e., at standard temperature and pressure, STP).

Consider that,

$$22.4\ \text{L} = 22.4 \times 1{,}000\ \text{mL and } 0°\text{C} = 273\ \text{K}$$

Then,

$$\frac{\text{mL of vapor}}{\text{mL of liquid}} = \frac{\text{Density} \times 22.4 \times 1000}{\text{Molecular weight}} \times \frac{(273 + 21)}{273}$$

Solving this equation for halothane (density is 1.87 and molecular weight is 197 g/mol) 1 mL of liquid will produce:

$$\frac{1.87 \times 22400}{197} \times \frac{(273 + 21)}{273} = 213.7\ \text{mL of vapor}$$

Solving for each agent the values are: halothane—213.7 mL, isoflurane—194 mL, desflurane—194.6 mL, and sevoflurane—164 mL.

Thus, for most commonly used agents, it is about 200 mL of vapor/mL of liquid.

If FGF is 2 L/min and the dialled concentration is 2%:

- mL of vapor used per minute is (2,000 × 0.02) = 40 mL
- mL of vapor used per hour is (40 × 60) = 2,400 mL
- mL of liquid used per hour is (2,400/200) = 12 mL.

Ehrenwerth and Eisenkraft Formula (1993)

- mL of liquid used per hour = 3 × Fresh gas flow (L/min) × dial setting (v/v%)
- If FGF is 2 L/min and the dialled concentration is 2%:
- mL of liquid used per hour = 3 × 2 × 2 = 12 mL.

IDEAL VAPORIZER

The ideal vaporizer should be

- Lightweight, robust, and durable
- Easy to transport
- Corrosion and solvent resistant
- Leak proof
- Economical and safe to use
- Require minimal servicing
- *Accurate over a wide range of:*
  - FGF
  - Liquid agent levels
  - Ambient pressures
  - Ambient temperatures

- *Unaffected by:*
  - Heat loss due to vaporization
  - Pressure changes downstream of the vaporizer
  - Tilting or tipping
- Compatible with vaporizer mounting and interlock systems.

FACTORS THAT AFFECT VAPORIZATION[1]

Temperature

As temperature rises, vaporization increases; hence, SVP increases. When SVP equals the atmospheric pressure, the liquid boils.

Volatility

The more volatile a liquid, the faster it vaporizes and the greater the loss of latent heat of vaporization. As vaporization continues, the liquid cools and the rate of vaporization falls.

Surface Area of the Liquid

The greater the surface area exposed, the greater the rate of vaporization. To achieve saturation of the vaporizer flow, there are various modifications such as, wicks (Rowbotham, TEC vaporizers), lamellae (Aladin™ cassette) or bubbling the agent through the liquid which vastly increases the surface area exposed (copper kettle, Boyle's ether vaporizer).

Gas Flow over the Liquid

If a continuous flow of gas is passed over a liquid the vapor is removed. This will cause a loss of kinetic energy from the system. As the temperature drops, the vaporization will fall unless there is thermocompensation (bimetallic strip in TEC, ether filled bellows in EMO) or supplied heat (TEC 6).

CLASSIFICATION (TABLE 2)

Dorsch and Dorsch classified vaporizers in 1979. As vaporizers, work stations and circuit designs have evolved over time, new terms have come in use and older terms have become obsolete. The classification should be understood in this historical context. The terms used are discussed further in this chapter.

Desflurane vaporizers like the TEC 6 are dual circuit gas vapor blenders. They are difficult to place in the conventional classification system. Also, the injection vaporizer design does not result in loss of latent heat of vaporization from the system as understood conventionally. Rather, the vapor chamber contains an evaporative surface to ensure complete vaporization and to compensate for the evaporative cooling.[7] Thus, though there is electrical heating and electronic monitoring incorporated, injection vaporizers do not strictly fall into the temperature compensated category. So, the author suggests that they may be considered to be vaporizers where temperature compensation is not required or not applicable.

TABLE 2: Classification of vaporizers.

Basis of classification	*Type of vaporizer*	*Examples*
Pressure of fresh gas flow needed	Draw over—fresh gas at atmospheric pressure is drawn through the vaporizer	Goldman, EMO, OMV
	Plenum—pressurized fresh gas source is needed for flow through the vaporizer	Boyle's bottle, TEC series, Dräger vapor 19.1 and 2000, Aladin cassette
Method of vaporization	Flow over without wicks	Goldman
	Flow over with wicks	EMO, OMV, TEC series Dräger vapor series, Aladin
	Bubble through	Copper kettle
	Flow over or bubble through	Boyle's bottle
	Injection	Maquet injector, Dräger DIVA
Method of regulating vaporizer output	Variable bypass	TEC 4,5,7, Dräger vapor 2000 and 19.1
	Measured flow	Copper kettle, Dräger DIVA, Maquet injector
Temperature compensation	Nontemperature compensated	Goldman
	Thermobuffered	EMO, Boyle's bottle with jacket
	Temperature compensated—use a thermostat	TEC 4,5,7, Dräger19.1 and 2000
	Electrically heated Electronically monitored and regulated	Desflurane vaporizers, Aladin cassette, Dräger DIVA, Maquet injector
Agent specificity	Agent specific	TEC, Dräger, desflurane vaporizers
	Multiagent	Goldman, OMV, EMO, Boyle's bottle
Location in the circuit (circle system)	VIC	Goldman
	VOC	Plenum vaporizers

(EMO: Epstein, Macintosh, Oxford; OMV: Oxford miniature vaporizer; VIC: vaporizer inside the circuit; VOC: vaporizer outside the circuit)

Draw-over[1]

The fresh gas (ambient air, with or without oxygen supplementation) is drawn over the liquid in the vaporizer by the patient's inspiratory efforts or negative pressure at the outlet of the vaporizer by mechanical means. Depending on the patient's minute ventilation and respiratory pattern (or minute ventilation generated by mechanical means) the flows vary widely between 0 L/min and 60 L/min in each cycle. Thus, vaporization is primarily affected by the patient's minute volume **(Table 3)**.

These vaporizers are inaccurate and inefficient. The output falls due to two factors: inadequate pick up of vapor at high flows and limitation of the flow splitting valve at low flows.

TABLE 3: Characteristic features of draw-over and plenum vaporizers.

Draw-over	*Plenum*
Patient's efforts are required for functioning of the vaporizer	Gas under positive pressure is required for functioning of the vaporizer
Negative pressure is produced downstream of the vaporizer thus drawing gas through the vaporizer	Positive pressure is produced upstream of the vaporizer, downstream of the flowmeters, so that gas is pushed through the vaporizer
These vaporizers allow bidirectional flow	These vaporizers are meant for unidirectional gas flows
Flow rates can be highly variable as peak inspiratory flow rates (up to 60 L/min) have to pass through it	Flow rates through the vaporizer depend on the flowmeter settings
Resistance to flow is very low so that no respiratory embarrassment occurs at peak inspiratory flow rates	Resistance to flow is higher: 10 cmH_2O at 4 L/min
Can be used as VOC or VIC, e.g., Goldman, OMV, and EMO	Can be only used as VOC and never as VIC, e.g., Boyle bottles, all TEC vaporizers

(VOC: vaporizer outside the circuit; VIC: vaporizer inside the circuit; OMV: Oxford miniature vaporizer; EMO: Epstein, Macintosh, Oxford)

The intrinsic resistance of the vaporizer has to be low so as not to impede the patient's efforts at high flows. Hence, incorporating wicks or baffles is not possible. At very high flows mixing is incomplete and the FGF may not pick up any saturated vapor.

Secondly, it is difficult to design a flow splitting valve, which is accurate over such a wide range of flows. It is designed to present a low resistance at high flow rates. When the flow drops below 4 L/min the resistance is so low that the vaporization chamber with the dense vapor is bypassed altogether and vaporizer output falls significantly.

Plenum[2]

Plenum is a Latin noun (an air filled space in a structure, especially one that receives air from a blower for distribution) (**Table 3**). Here, it refers to the pressurized vaporization chamber. These vaporizers need a pressurized source of FGF to carry the vapor away as their internal resistance is high. They are more accurate as they operate within a smaller range of (0–15 L/min) FGF. The flow does not change with the respiratory cycle. As the flows are lower, there is enough time for saturated vapor to be present in the vaporization chamber at all times. Thus, calibration is more accurate. The pressurized gases are of a similar density as the vapor and mixing is more thorough than in the draw-over vaporizers. The flow resistance across the vaporizer at a flow of 4 L/min is 10 cmH_2O. The amount of vapor delivered depends on the total FGF, which is operator dependent.

Flow-over

The carrier gas passes over the surface of the liquid and carries the vapor molecules.

Bubble Through

The carrier gas is passed through the liquid agent. The bubbles substantially increase the surface area, achieving complete saturation.

Measured Flow

The vaporizer output and the diluent gases are dialled separately. The first such vaporizer was the copper kettle. The fallacy was that, should the diluent gas supply fail, an inadvertent overdose would be delivered. Current measured flow vaporizers are the injector vaporizers which are electronically monitored and will shut down in case of any irregularity. Hence, they are safer in this respect. The best safeguard is anesthesia gas monitoring at the patient end.

Variable Bypass

The variable bypass vaporizer is a flow splitting device. The stream of FGF is split into two by a rotary valve. A very small part enters the vaporizing chamber and most passes through the bypass chamber. Thus, the flow to the vaporizing chamber is a part of the total flow. This is a safety feature. Should the gas supply fail neither carrier gas, nor agent will be delivered to the patient. This eliminated the risk of inadvertent overdose due to diluent gas failure, as seen in the copper kettle vaporizer.

The ratio of bypass flow to vaporizing chamber flow is called the splitting ratio.

$$\text{Bypass flow} = \text{Total flow} - \text{Vaporizer flow}$$

$$\text{The splitting ratio} = \frac{\text{Total flow} - \text{Vaporizer flow}}{\text{Vaporizer flow}}$$

This ratio depends on three factors—the volatility of the anesthetic agent, the temperature, and the dialled concentration.

Consider two agents at a temperature of 22°C and a dial setting of 1%. The more volatile (higher SVP, e.g., isoflurane - 238 mm Hg) the agent the greater the splitting ratio (44:1), that is bypass flow is more. If the agent has a low SVP (sevoflurane–160 mm Hg) the splitting ratio will be lower (25:1) and more carrier gas will pass to the vaporizing chamber.

The thermostat is placed in the bypass chamber, in close proximity to the liquid in the vaporizing chamber and can sense the temperature of the liquid in the vaporizing chamber. A fall in temperature will cause more carrier gas to flow to the vaporizing chamber and vice versa.

The rotary valve is located at the outlet of the vaporizing chamber. It is a variable resistance, which is controlled by the operator.

The output of these vaporizers is determined by the dynamic interaction between two variable resistances—the rotary valve and the thermostat in the bypass chamber.

Injection

The anesthetic agent is injected into the stream of carrier gas and atomizes in the flow. As no vaporization occurs in the chamber containing the liquid there is no loss of heat of vaporization from the system.

Agent Specificity

Modern vaporizers like the TEC and Dräger series are specifically designed for a particular agent, taking into account the physical and chemical properties, especially the SVP. This determines the splitting ratio of the vaporizer. These vaporizers are labeled with the name of the agent, there is color coding and there are filling systems which prevent misfiling with another agent. These are called agent-specific vaporizers. If the wrong agent is filled in a vaporizer a concentration other than that desired will be delivered, resulting in an overdose or in awareness. To prevent this various measures are taken. These are color coding, agent-specific filling systems—keyed fillers, Easy-Fil®, Quik-Fil™ (sevoflurane) and Saf-T-fil™ (desflurane), and automatic detection of the agent used in electronic systems via magnetic sensors—Aladin cassette vaporizers. Agent gas monitors provide an extra layer of safety. The vaporizers that do not possess these features are called nonagent-specific or multi-agent vaporizers.

Location (Table 4)

Draw-over vaporizers can be used within the circuit where the patient's expired gases pass through the vaporizer, e.g., in the inspiratory or the expiratory limb of the circle absorber, known as vaporizer inside the circuit (VIC), or can be mounted on the back bar of anesthesia machine, known

TABLE 4: Characteristic features of vaporizer outside the circuit and vaporizer inside the circuit.

VOC	***VIC***
Most common method of introducing inhalational agent into the breathing system	Not used very commonly
Positioned between flowmeters and CGO or between CGO and breathing system	Positioned in the circle system either in the inspiratory limb or the expiratory limb
Resistance of the vaporizer need not be taken into account	Resistance of the vaporizer has to be very low
Resistance is overdriven by positive pressure of "continuous FGF" and after picking up the anesthetic agent, the gases collect in the reservoir bag from which the patient breathes spontaneously or is manually ventilated	• *If the vaporizer is in the inspiratory limb:* The patient must breathe through the vaporizer during spontaneous breathing (therefore, the patient must work to overcome the resistance) or during controlled breathing the operator overcomes the resistance by pushing gases through the vaporizer • *If the vaporizer is in the expiratory limb:* Whether during spontaneous or controlled breathing the exhaled gases have to pass through the vaporizer and if the resistance to flow is high then there will be expiratory resistance giving rise to increased expiratory work of breathing and in addition, inadvertent PEEP
Factors affecting inspired concentration of inhalational agent: • Performance of the vaporizer in use at the set FGF • Concentration of inhalational agent in exhaled gases • Degree of dilution of FGF with exhaled gases which depends on the MV of the patient. Lower the FGF more difficult it is to predict the inspired concentration of the inhalational agent	*Factors affecting inspired concentration of inhalational agent:* • FGF and dial setting • Efficiency of the vaporizer • Presence of wicks in the vaporizer • Water vapor from exhaled gases may condense on wicks reducing the efficiency of the vaporizer and possibly increasing the resistance to gas flow
Output concentration: Set or lower than set concentration is delivered. As FGF is reduced, two phenomena occur: 1. Exhaled gas coming from the absorber (after CO_2 being absorbed) contains lower concentration of anesthetic agent due to uptake by lung and therefore it dilutes the concentration of inhalational agent when it mixes with FGF and hence delivers lower concentration of agent than the one set on the vaporizer dial 2. At low FGF the efficiency of some of the vaporizers is altered and therefore lower or higher concentrations than the set concentration may be delivered	• *Output concentration:* With recirculating gases vapor is picked up from vaporizers by the gases which already have some vapor of the same inhalational agent, therefore the concentration of vaporized gases is erratic and one should use respiratory gas monitor to know the delivered concentration. Invariably, the delivered concentration is more than the set concentration
• *Spontaneous breathing:* Increasing depth of anesthesia causes fall in minute ventilation. But FGF carrying anesthetic gases remains the same. Thus, there is rise in inspired concentration • *Controlled breathing:* Increase in ventilation dilutes the FGF carrying the anesthetic agent and therefore causes a fall in the inspired concentration	• *Spontaneous breathing:* Excessive depth of anesthesia causes fall in MV which results in decreased flow through the vaporizer and therefore decreased inspired concentration (a safety factor) • *Controlled breathing:* Anesthetic vapor concentration increases with rise in MV
No water vapor can enter the vaporizer	Frequent cleaning, washing and drying required since water vapor from exhaled gases condenses inside the vaporizer chamber

(VOC: vaporizer outside the circuit; VIC: vaporizer inside the circuit; CGO: common gas outlet; FGF: fresh gas flow; PEEP: positive end-expiratory pressure; MV: minute volume)

as vaporizer outside the circuit (VOC). Vaporizer inside the circuit increases the risk of overdose as the output will now also include the vapor in the exhaled gases. When used with other anesthesia circuits, the vaporizers are placed upstream of the bag or bellows. Otherwise the output becomes unreliable.

Plenum vaporizers are placed on the back bar (i.e., as VOC) where the flowmeters are upstream and the bag or bellows and the oxygen flush is downstream.

FACTORS CAUSING VARIATIONS IN VAPORIZER PERFORMANCE AND DESIGN MODIFICATIONS

Temperature

When the vaporizer is in use, the liquid agent cools with time and the vaporizer output will fall. Hence, thermobuffering (water bath with Boyle's bottle) or thermocompensation (TEC—bimetallic strip, invar rod, electropneumatic proportional flow valves in the Aladin™ vaporizer) are employed. The mass of metal in the body of the vaporizer acts as a heat sink. Hence, substances with high-specific heat capacity such as copper, stainless steel, brass (Lease datum, weight 7.5 kg, was 11 kg) or aluminum (Penlon sigma delta, weight 5 kg) are used.

External heat sources may be employed, if the above measures are likely to be ineffective, as is done in the TEC 6 and Dräger D-Vapor® for desflurane.

In the injection vaporizers, the liquid agent atomizes in the vaporization chamber and not in the liquid chamber; hence, the temperature of the liquid does not change and compensation for loss of latent heat of vaporization is not needed. However, electronic temperature regulation is incorporated to prevent "rainout" and ensure complete vaporization.

The thermostats used in most variable bypass, temperature compensated vaporizers are accurate between 15 and 35°C, as these temperatures are encountered most frequently in clinical situations. Beyond this range the output is unreliable.

Flow Rate (Flow Dependence)[3]

When the rate of gas flow affects the concentration at the patient end, it is known as flow-dependence.

At high flows, output falls due to inadequate mixing. At low flows, the pattern of flow becomes turbulent and resistance increases. More gas passes through the bypass chamber and output falls.

This effect is reduced by increasing the surface area and ensuring complete saturation. In the Boyle's bottle, a cowl is lowered, to ensure that all the gas is bubbled through the anesthetic agent. In the "TEC" series, porous Teflon® wicks are used in a helical design. The presence of baffles to divert the gas close to the wicks also improves the efficiency of vaporization.

Backpressure Changes

Pumping Effect (Increased Vapor Output at Low Flows)

This effect applies to plenum vaporizers especially at low flow rates with intermittent positive pressure ventilation (IPPV).

It is more likely if manual ventilation or minute volume divider ventilators (Manley) are used.

The positive pressure at the outlet (downstream) is transmitted to the vapor chamber and the pressure in the chamber rises during inspiration. This drives some saturated vapor retrograde into the inlet path. It enters the bypass when the pressure falls during expiration. The bypass is contaminated with vapor which results in an increased output. This is minimized by increasing the internal resistance of the vaporizer by using baffles, which reduces the back flow into the vaporizing chamber. Other measures to prevent it include an outlet check valve (TEC 4, **Figs. 1A and B**) which maintains constant pressure in the vapor chamber, and long high-resistance inlet pathways (TEC 5) which prevent retrograde flow.[4]

Pressurizing Effect (Decreased Vapor Output at High Flows)

Applies to plenum vaporizers at high flow rates during IPPV and is of minor significance. The positive pressure compresses the carrier gas, thus, concentrating it. When the pressure is released (expiration), volume increases, the gas density falls, and the vapor concentration also falls.

Liquid Levels

If the vaporizer is overfilled, there may be inadequate space for vaporization and the surface area of exposed wicks may be too small to allow complete saturation. Liquid agent may enter the bypass. In the TEC 5 for sevoflurane, if the level of the liquid is too low, the output falls especially with high flows and high dial settings, e.g., during inhalational induction.[4] Liquid level indicators are incorporated. Electronic vaporizers have low liquid level alarms—both visual and audible.

Additives and Agents

Halothane contains 0.01% (w/w) thymol. It is not volatile so accumulates in the vaporizer and the liquid may show yellow discoloration. The development of such discoloration may be used as an indicator that the vaporizer should be drained and cleaned, and the discolored halothane discarded. Current vaporizers do not use cloth wicks so draining is not essential and service intervals are longer. Thymol also causes the movable parts of vaporizers, e.g., dials, to stick.

Anesthetic agents can undergo degradation due to sunlight and are stored in dark brown bottles. In the presence of Lewis acids (metal oxides and metal halides) sevoflurane can be degraded to produce hydrofluoric acid and other toxins. Water prevents the formation of these compounds.

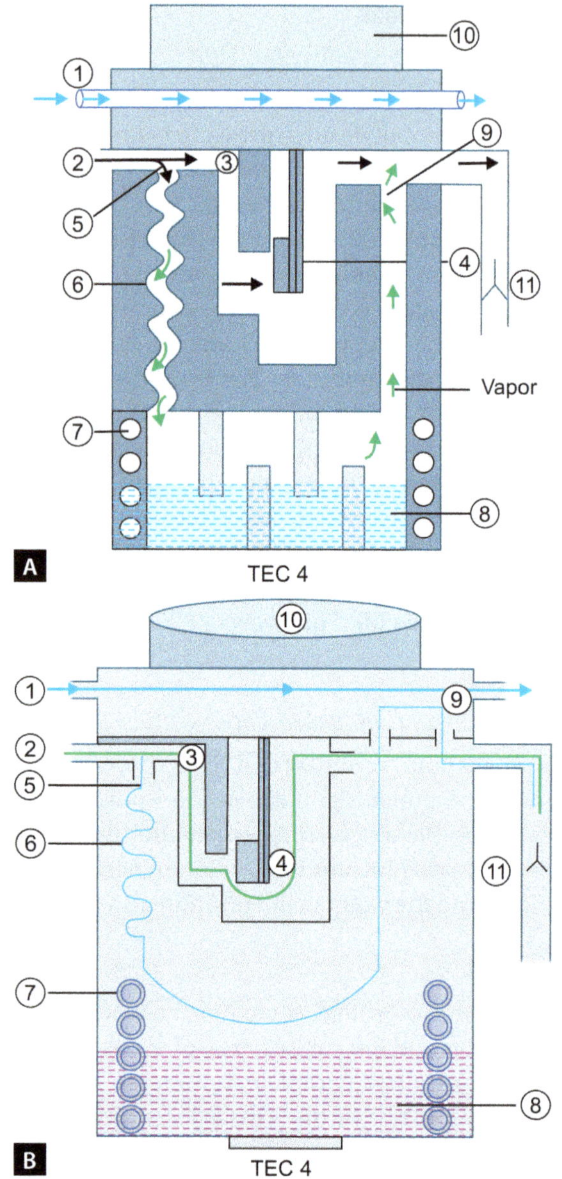

Figs. 1A and B: TEC 4. (A) Schematic diagram; (B) Line diagram. 1. Flow path when vaporizer "off"; 2. Fresh gas flow when vaporizer "on"; 3. Bypass flow; 4. Thermostat; 5. Vaporizing chamber flow; 6. Convoluted path; 7. Teflon wicks with copper nickel spiral; 8. Liquid agent; 9. Vaporizer outlet flow; 10. Concentration control dial; 11. Outlet check valve.

It is added in various proportions by different manufacturers. Some vaporizers may get corroded by the presence of sevoflurane formulations with water.

Carrier Gas Composition

Vaporizers are calibrated with either oxygen or air as the carrier gas by different manufacturers. If nitrous oxide, air, xenon or helium is added to the carrier gas the viscosity and density of the carrier gas will change. This leads to alteration in the performance of the flow splitting valve. Hence, there are changes in vaporizer output. Nitrous oxide dissolves in volatile agents (4.5 mL/mL of liquid agent); hence, output falls in the initial 15 minutes, when nitrous oxide is introduced. During emergence a hypoxic mixture may result as the dissolved nitrous oxide is added to the vaporizing chamber flow. The fall in output is not clinically significant. However, xenon is five times heavier than air and its regular use may potentially result in clinically significant changes in vaporizer output.

Carrier Gas Flow

At both ends of the spectrum, the vaporizer output is lower than the dial settings. When the FGF is low, there is inadequate turbulence to lift the comparatively dense vapor molecules from the surface of the liquid. At high flow rates (such as 15 L/min), the output of most variable bypass vaporizers tends to fall. This is variously attributed to—cooling due to rapid evaporation, incomplete mixing due to rapid flow and inadequate amount of saturated vapor in the vaporizing chamber due to rapid removal.

Effects of Altitude

Variable Bypass Vaporizers

TEC vaporizers are calibrated at sea level (1 atm). Saturated vapor pressure changes only if temperature changes. There is no change if ambient pressure changes. At higher altitudes, the ambient pressure is lower than 1 atm. The SVP now represents a greater percentage of the ambient pressure. The output concentration when measured in v/v% rises. However, the partial pressure of the vapor does not change. The uptake and anesthetic effect depend upon the alveolar and brain partial pressures, respectively. As partial pressure is not altered, there is no change in clinical effect.

There may be slight changes in output due to other factors like:

- The change in density and viscosity of the carrier gas
- The fall in temperature at altitude can cause change in output if beyond the range of the thermostat (18–35°C)
- The fall in temperature causes changes in relative humidity, but aircraft fuselages are pressurized (600 mm Hg) and temperature compensated.

Thus, the TEC vaporizers are inaccurate in volume percent terms when ambient pressure changes, but the clinical effect of this change is negligible. Dial settings need not be changed. MAC values in percentage are inaccurate when using agent monitoring. The values should be displayed as mm Hg or kPa.

Dual Circuit Gas Vapor Blender (TEC 6, Dräger D)

The dual circuit gas vapor blender delivers vapor as a percentage of the FGF. At lower ambient pressures the vaporizer output remains constant when measured as a percentage. Thus, as a device the vaporizer remains accurate. However, the output falls when measured as partial pressure. The output dial needs to be set higher to achieve the same anesthetic effect (manufacturers provide tables for the adjustments required).

MODERN VAPORIZERS

Variable Bypass

TEC 4[5] *(Figs. 1A and B)*

Manufacturer: GE Healthcare, (earlier Datex Ohmeda, still earlier Cyprane), 1983.

Classification: Plenum, variable bypass, flow-over with wicks, temperature compensated, agent-specific models for halothane, isoflurane and enflurane, VOC.

Capacity: 225 mL (of which 100 mL is in wicks).

Filling system: Screw fill or keyed filling systems.

Construction ***(Figs. 1A and B):*** The concentration control dial (10) is at the top. The vaporizing chamber with wicks surrounds the bypass chamber. When the vaporizer is "off," gases pass through a channel at the top of the vaporizer (1). When turned "on," the gases enter the vaporizer (2) and split into the bypass flow (3) which encounters the thermostatic valve (4). As temperature falls, flow is proportionally diverted toward the vaporization chamber (5) to maintain constant vaporizer output.

The fresh gas which enters the vaporization chamber passes through a convoluted passage (6) and enters the bottom of the chamber. There are two concentric wicks (7) which are immersed in the liquid agent. They are separated by a copper nickel helical spacer (7). The fresh gas rises up through the gaps in the helix, picking up vapor on the way. Saturated vapor with the carrier gas leaves the vaporizer through the rotary valve (9) operated by the concentration control dial (10).

Evaluation

- *Flow:* 0.25–15 L/min
- *Temperature:* 18–35°C
- The vaporizer is susceptible to back pressure changes. To overcome the pumping effect, two mechanisms are used. The vaporizer inlet has a convoluted path which increases the length of the inlet. The machine has a one-way check valve (12) inserted at the common gas outlet. This check valve attenuates but does not eliminate the increase in pressure because there is FGF from the flow meters to the vaporizer during inspiration[6]
- Vaporizer output falls at low flows and low dial settings
- The halothane vaporizer contains cotton wicks which may be clogged by thymol. Yearly servicing is needed. Otherwise, 2-year interval is adequate.

Safety features

- Allowable tilt is 180°
- Anti spill mechanism prevents the bypass channel becoming contaminated with liquid
- The vaporizer dial can only be turned on when properly seated and locked onto the back bar.

Disadvantages

- Difficulty in operating single handed
- Frequent service required
- Leakage of agent from drain port
- Can be overfilled if the vaporizer is in "on" position.

TEC 5 (Figs. 2A and B)

Improved design over the TEC 4, particularly ability to operate one-handed, improved performance and 3 yearly service intervals.

Manufacturer: GE healthcare (earlier Datex Ohmeda) in 1989.

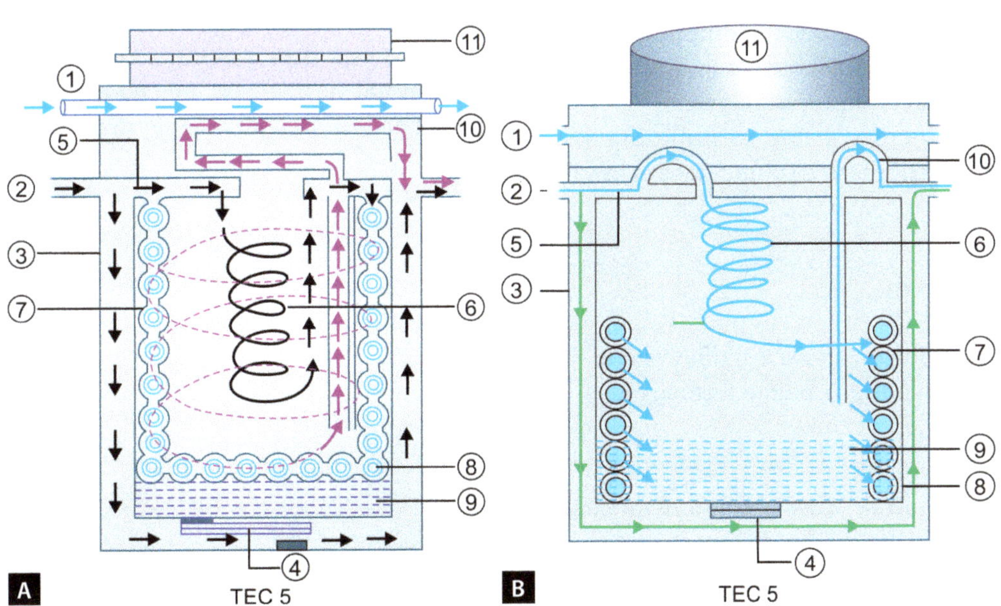

Figs. 2A and B: TEC 5. (A) Schematic diagram; (B) Line diagram. 1. Flow path when vaporizer "off"; 2. Fresh gas flow when vaporizer "on"; 3. Bypass; 4. Thermostat; 5. Vaporizing chamber flow; 6. Helical channel; 7. Porous Teflon® wicks with steel wire spiral; 8. Wick skirt; 9. Liquid agent; 10. Vaporizing chamber outlet through rotary valve; 11. Concentration control dial.

Classification: Plenum, variable bypass, flow-over with wicks, temperature compensated, out of system, agent-specific modules for halothane, isoflurane, enflurane, sevoflurane.

Capacity: 300 mL (225 mL with wet wicks).

Filling system: Funnel fill and keyed filling system.

Construction ***(Figs. 2A and B):*** The control dial (11) is linked to the rotary valve on the top. The gradations from 0% to 1% are finer than earlier models. The control dial is also connected to the locking lever and the dial release. The vaporizer cannot be turned on unless it is locked in position and the dial release is depressed. Single handed, operation is possible. The filling port and liquid level indicator are at the lower left hand corner.

When the vaporizer is "off" the gas passes through the Select-a-tec channel (1). When turned "on," the flow (2) splits into the bypass flow (3) and the vaporizer flow (5). The bypass flow passes along the bottom of the vaporizer past the thermostat—a bimetallic strip (4). As vaporization progresses the liquid cools and more gas is diverted to the vaporization chamber. The gas passes through the central part of the rotary valve via an elongated, helical channel (6) to the center of the wick assembly (7) which is arranged in a concentric double spiral. The wicks are made of teflon® and the wick skirt (8) dips into the liquid. The wicks are held open by a steel wire spiral. Thus, the surface area for vaporization is substantially increased as compared to previous models. The vapor laden gas then passes through the rotary valve to the outlet (10).

Evaluation

- *Flow range:* 0.25–15 L/min
- *Temperature range:* 15–35°C
- Greatest accuracy is at 15-35°C, at 5 L/min with dial settings less than 3%. At flow rates above 10 L/min and with dial settings above 3%, the output falls. Below 15°C the thermostat is unresponsive and output falls. Above 35°C the output is unpredictably high.
- Vaporizer output increases due to pumping effect. When air or nitrous oxide is used output falls at low flows and rises at high flows.

Safety features

- Select-a-tec mechanism
- Keyed filler
- Anti spill up to 180° due to extensive baffle system
- Needs to be locked in position before turning on.

Improvements over TEC 4

- User friendly
- One-handed dial control. Finer gradations of scale at lower dial settings
- Service interval is 3 years
- *Improved accuracy:*
  - Bypass chamber moved to the base contains an improved thermostat—bimetallic strip. Thermostat has better contact with the temperature of the liquid
  - Tubular woven Teflon® wicks and baffle system increase the surface area
  - Helical inlet channel and internal baffle system minimize the pumping effect
- Potential for leaks is minimized
- Capacity has increased from 125 mL to 300 mL so less frequent filling is needed.

TEC 7 (Fig. 3)

Manufacturer: GE Healthcare (earlier Datex Ohmeda) in 2002.

Classification: Plenum, variable bypass, flow-over with wicks, temperature compensated, out of system, agent-specific modules for halothane, isoflurane, enflurane and sevoflurane.

Capacity: 300 mL

Filling system: Wider selection of filler assemblies—funnel filler, Easy-Fil®, Quik-Fil™

Construction: The control dial, linked to the rotary valve is on the top. There are gradations from 0% to 5% for isoflurane and halothane and 0–8% for sevoflurane. The control dial has fine gradations below 1% and is connected to the locking lever. The vaporizer cannot be turned on unless locked in position. The concentration control dial has a release at the back which is depressed before the vaporizer can be turned on. The filling port is at the lower left hand corner, beside which is the liquid level indicator. It contains a prismatic sight glass for easier visibility. An identification label on the back of the vaporizer is seen as the rectangle on the lower right. An anesthesia machine, which uses agent identification technology, will use this label for identification when the vaporizer is mounted on the back bar.

Internal design and mechanics are similar to TEC 5. The external appearance is transformed to match the

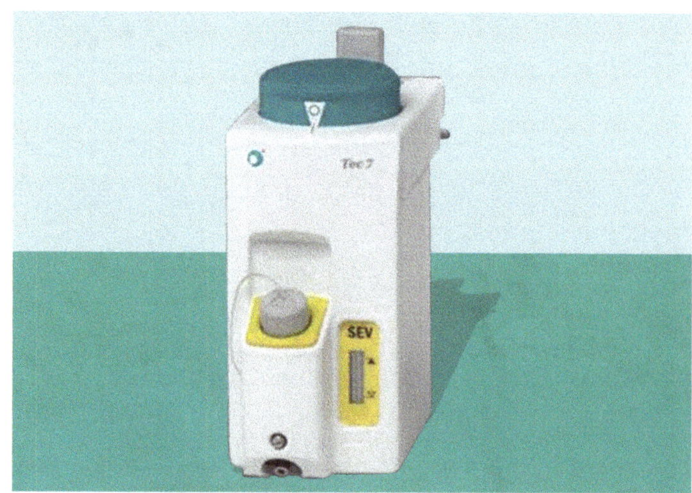

Fig. 3: TEC 7 vaporizer.

workstation. It is white in color with agent identification more obvious.

The vaporizer is coated with Teflon® internally and is made from a single mold thus eliminating the need for seals. These features make it lifetime calibration/maintenance free.

Evaluation: These are similar to the TEC 5. The fall in output, when using carrier gas other than oxygen is exacerbated by low flows and low dial settings. The output may fall up to 20% when low flows with nitrous oxide are used. When the vaporizer is turned on after not being in use for some time, high concentrations of agent may be delivered in the initial 10 seconds.

Hazards: If inverted connect to the scavenging system, set dial to 5% and allow wash out for 5 minutes at a flow of 5 L/min.

AladinTM Cassette (Figs. 4A to C)

Manufacturer: GE Healthcare

Classification: Plenum, variable bypass, acts as an injector when the cassette contains only vapor (see further),[4] flow-over with wicks, electronically temperature compensated, out of system, agent specific, color-coded cassettes for halothane, isoflurane, enflurane, sevoflurane, desflurane (AladinTM 2 cassettes—isoflurane, sevoflurane, and desflurane) weight 2-3 kg depending on the agent module.

Key points: The system integrates electronics with pneumatics, hence, it is very accurate and responsive to rapid changes in FGF or vaporizer dial settings. The design is similar to conventional variable bypass vaporizers, but the factors affecting vaporizer output—flow and composition of carrier gas, temperature and pressure in the vaporizing chamber are sensed and altered electronically (every 200 ms). It is an electronic variable bypass vaporizer which overcomes some limitations of the mechanical variable bypass vaporizers, e.g., can deliver desflurane via the same assembly, end tidal control mode is possible, audible and visual alarms warn of falling liquid level or vaporizer malfunction. However, the system needs electricity or battery back up to be operational.

Capacity: 225 mL

Filling system: Easy-Fil®, Quik-FilTM (sevoflurane only) and Saf-T-filTM (desflurane only).

Construction: This is a vaporizing system which consists of:

- The electronic controls and bypass chamber housed within the anesthesia machine (Aisys, S5 ADU, and Aisys CS[2])
- The AladinTM cassette which contains the liquid and various sensors is a detachable vaporizing chamber. The cassettes for different agents can be slotted into the same system as per operator requirements.

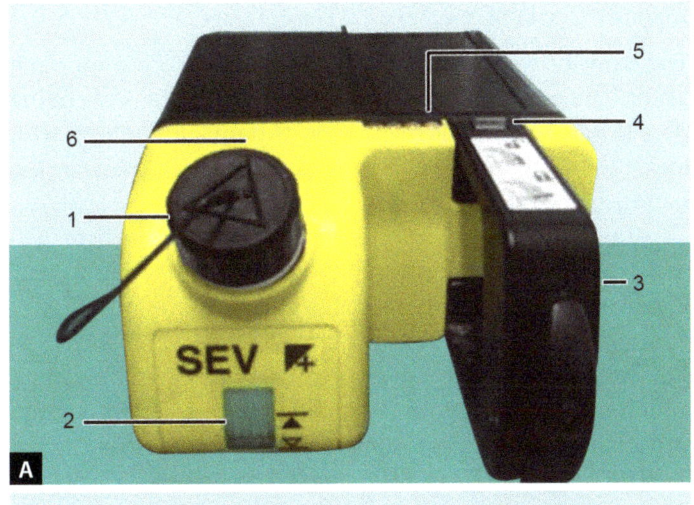

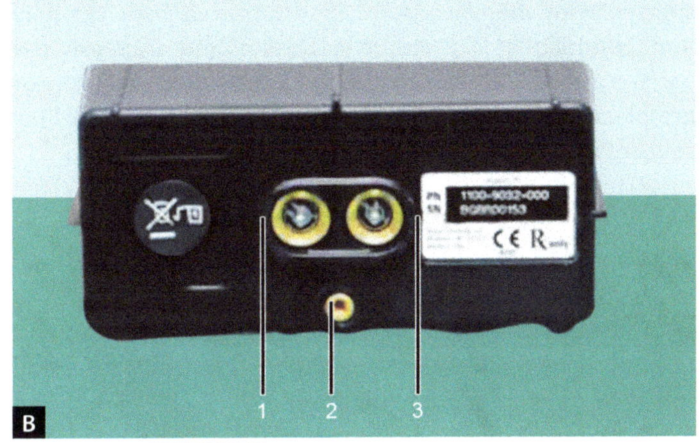

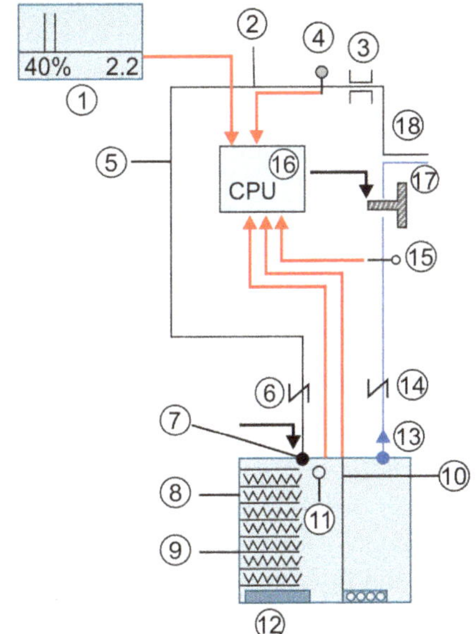

Figs. 4A to C: (A) Aladin™ cassette front. 1. Filling port; 2. Prismatic sight glass; 3. Handle with lock; 4. Handle release; 5. Temperature sensors; 6. Magnetic sensors; (B) Aladin™ cassette back. 1. Inflow port; 2. Temperature sensor; 3. Outflow port; (C) Aladin™ cassette working principle. 1. Electronic flowmeters, agent dial; 2. Bypass flow; 3. Fixed restrictor; 4. Flow sensor—bypass; 5. Vaporizer flow; 6. Electronic inflow check valve; 7. Inlet ball valve; 8. Lamellae of wicking material; 9. Metal baffles; 10. Temperature sensor; 11. Pressure sensors; 12. Invisible magnetic sensor; 13. Outlet ball valve; 14. Electronic outflow check valve; 15. Vaporizer flow sensor; 16. Central possessing unit; 17. Flow control valve; 18. Flow to the patient.

Aladin™ Cassette

The front of the cassette **(Fig. 4A)** is color-coded for each agent. The cassette on the front from left to right has a filling port (1) and prismatic sight glass (2) and the handle with lock (3) which secures the cassette in its slot. Above the handle is the release (4).

Above the filling port are the five magnetic sensors (6) which are read by the machine to identify the agent in use. These are invisible externally. Beside these are four copper temperature sensors (5).

The back of the cassette **(Fig. 4B)** has two ball valves, which act as the inflow (1) and outflow ports (3) for the vaporizing chamber. It also has a temperature sensor (2).

The chamber **(Fig. 4C)** itself consists of a wicking material (8) which is folded into lamellae. These are interspersed with metallic baffles (9) (improved heat capacity and conductivity) to improve mixing and increase the surface area. A pressure sensor (11) and liquid level sensor are placed in the chamber and the outlet contains a flow sensor (15).

The Anesthesia Machine (Fig. 4C)

The bypass channel contains a fixed restrictor (3), proximal to which is the flow sensor (4).

The display screen allows the agent concentration and FGF (1) to be dialled electronically. The central processing unit (CPU) (16) receives input from:

- The concentration control dial
- *Flowmeters:* Carrier gas composition and flow set
- Flow sensors in the bypass channels and vaporizer outflow
- Temperature, pressure and liquid level sensors in the vaporizing chamber.

The CPU (via a control loop) then adjusts the flow control valve (17) in the outlet of the vaporizing chamber to maintain a constant agent output. Electronic control of the flow control valve ensures the accuracy of the vaporizer.

When the system is operational, the FGF passes through the bypass chamber. When the vaporizer flow is dialled by the operator, a small part of the fresh gas flow passes through a mechanical one-way valve and an electronic inflow one-way check valve (6) and enters the cassette by passing through the open mechanical ball valve (7) on the back of the cassette. The inflow valve (6) prevents retrograde flow of vapor into the bypass via the inlet in the case of all agents. This valve is particularly important when desflurane is being used, and the temperature is higher than its boiling point (22.8°C). If this happens, the pressure in the sump rises. When the sump pressure is higher than the bypass pressure, the valve closes and prevents entry of carrier gas into the vaporizing chamber. All the FGF passes through the bypass channel and past its flow sensor. According to the concentration control dial setting, pure desflurane vapor is metered in by the electronically regulated flow control valve. Thus, if all of the desflurane is converted into its vapor there is no flow splitting and the vaporizer acts as an injector type vaporizer. Failure of the inlet check valve will lead to an overdose of the agent. Agent monitoring will alert the user to such an event. A mixing chamber stabilizes the output and reduces the effects of back pressure fluctuations. When the mixer output pressure is greater than the cassette pressure, the system functions as a variable bypass vaporizer. Here, the control loop strongly depends on, mixer reported flow, cassette flow reading, cassette temperature and pressure reading and weakly on FGF composition, manifold temperature and patient airway pressure.

If the cassette pressure exceeds the mixer output pressure, the system functions as an injector vaporizer. Here the FGF passes only through the bypass and not through the cassette. Hence, the control loop depends strongly on the mixer flow.

Please note that, in this case, pure desflurane vapor and not liquid desflurane is added to the FGF. Hence, there is loss of latent heat of vaporization. As we shall see further, this does not occur with injector vaporizers.

Sevoflurane inductions or the use of desflurane as the agent of choice can result in significant loss of latent heat of vaporization and cause cooling. There is a fan under the cassette which becomes operational between 17 and 22°C.

Safety features

- Hypoxia alarm also takes into consideration the desflurane concentration
- The vaporizer can be tilted in any direction. The Aladin cassette is not affected by tipping as the bypass is located in the workstation and cannot be contaminated by the liquid agent
- There is an air vent between the filling port and the vaporizing chamber and during filling, the rising liquid level will eventually block the lower end. The air from the vaporizing chamber can no longer enter the bottle and no more liquid flows into the sump. This prevents over filling
- The liquid level sensor in the sump triggers an audible alarm if the level falls below 10%
- The inlet and outlet check valves are spring loaded valves on the back of the cassette. They allow entry and exit of FGF. They close the entry and exit ports automatically when the cassette is removed or if high pressure or over filling is detected.

Evaluation

- At flows between 0.2 and 8 L/min, the accuracy for all agents is ±10% of the setting or ±3% of the maximum dial setting (whichever is greater). The variability is greater with desflurane up to 13%. At extremes of flow the accuracy decreases. If the FGF composition changes the output is altered automatically to maintain a constant depth. A decrease in ambient pressure will increase the vaporizer output in percentage terms[4]

- Range of ambient temperatures for optimal functioning is 18–25°C.

Hazards

- Overfilling may occur if air enters the bottle. This results in an overdose.
- Leaks may occur if the vaporizer is filled when "on" as the cassette is pressurized.
- If the FGF is very low, the bypass pressure may be lower than that in the vaporizing chamber and the inlet check valve may fail to close. This will allow saturated vapor to enter the bypass channel. This is more likely to occur when desflurane is being used.

Advantages

- Lightweight cassette
- Tilting allowable
- Automatic record keeping and gas usage calculation are possible. Cost of anesthetic agents and gases used per hour is calculated in real time and an accurate bill can be presented.
- On Aisys screen, electronic level sensing and agent identification.
- Vaporizer self-check and diagnosis.
- Electronic control minimizes fluctuations in output due to temperature and pressure variations and adjusts for changes in carrier gas flow rate and composition.

End-tidal control mode allows feedback loop and achieves desired concentration without active intervention by the anesthetist and is more economical.

Maintenance: The cassette surface can be cleaned with a cloth moistened in a mild soap solution. The cassette should be emptied before sending it to a service center.

Desflurane Cassette

Key points: In contrast to the other vaporizers designed for desflurane, the agent vaporizes freely in the cassette without pressurization or heating. The cassette contains a temperature sensor, pressure sensor and liquid level sensor. Below 22.8°C, bypass gas enters the cassette as with other agents. Above the boiling point, the one way check valve closes and vapor is directly injected into the bypass flow. A fan warms the cassette between 17 and 22°C. The system takes into consideration the percentage of desflurane when calculating the fraction of inspired oxygen (FiO_2). Hypoxic alarm is activated if needed.

DUAL CIRCUIT GAS VAPOR BLENDER

TEC 6 (Fig. 5A)

Manufacturer: GE Healthcare ex Ohmeda ex Cyprane, 1993.

Classification: Plenum, dual circuit gas vapor blender, thermo-compensation by supplied heat, agent specific, out of system.

Features of Desflurane which Require a Special Vaporizer

Desflurane is highly volatile (SVP—664 mm Hg) but has moderate potency (high MAC—6%) and low blood gas solubility (B/G-0.42). If used in a conventional bypass vaporizer the output will be unpredictable due to the following three factors:

1. First, as the SVP of desflurane is near the atmospheric pressure (760 mm Hg) large volumes of desflurane vapor (735 mL) will be entrained by 100 mL of carrier gas as compared to the other agents (46 mL and 47 mL for halothane and isoflurane, respectively). To produce a clinically relevant concentration, a very large volume of FGF will be needed. To achieve 6% 12 L/min flows will be needed. For lower concentrations, significantly higher flows, up to 70 L/min are needed. These high flows are not possible with the current workstations.
2. Second, these high flows and rapid vaporization will lead to cooling due to the loss of latent heat of vaporization. The temperature fluctuations are beyond the range of the thermostats used in conventional mechanical variable bypass vaporizers in common use. The rate of vaporization will fall. Thus, vaporization will be unpredictable.
3. Third, due to the unpredictable vaporizer output and the low blood gas solubility of desflurane, any fall in vapor concentration will expose the patient to the risk of awareness.

Comparison with Variable Bypass Vaporizers

The variable bypass vaporizers incorporate two variable resistances, the interaction of which determines vaporizer output. The first is the manually controlled, operator dialled, variable resistance—the flow splitting valve. This is controlled by moving the concentration control dial. The second resistance is the thermostat in the bypass chamber (bimetallic strip, liquid filled bellows, invar rod) which changes the proportion of the flow going to the vaporization chamber.

The TEC 6 has a fixed resistor in the FGF circuit, which generates a "working pressure". This is sensed by the pressure transducer and balanced electronically and pneumatically between both circuits. The second variable resistance (thermostat) is replaced by the agent pressure regulating valve, which is controlled electronically.

Capacity: 450 mL

Filling system: Saf-T-Fil. Please refer to filling systems, see further.

Mounting: Compatible with Select-a-tec. The vaporizer should be mounted on the extreme right-hand side (downstream) on the back bar as its power cord may interfere with the seating of the other vaporizers.

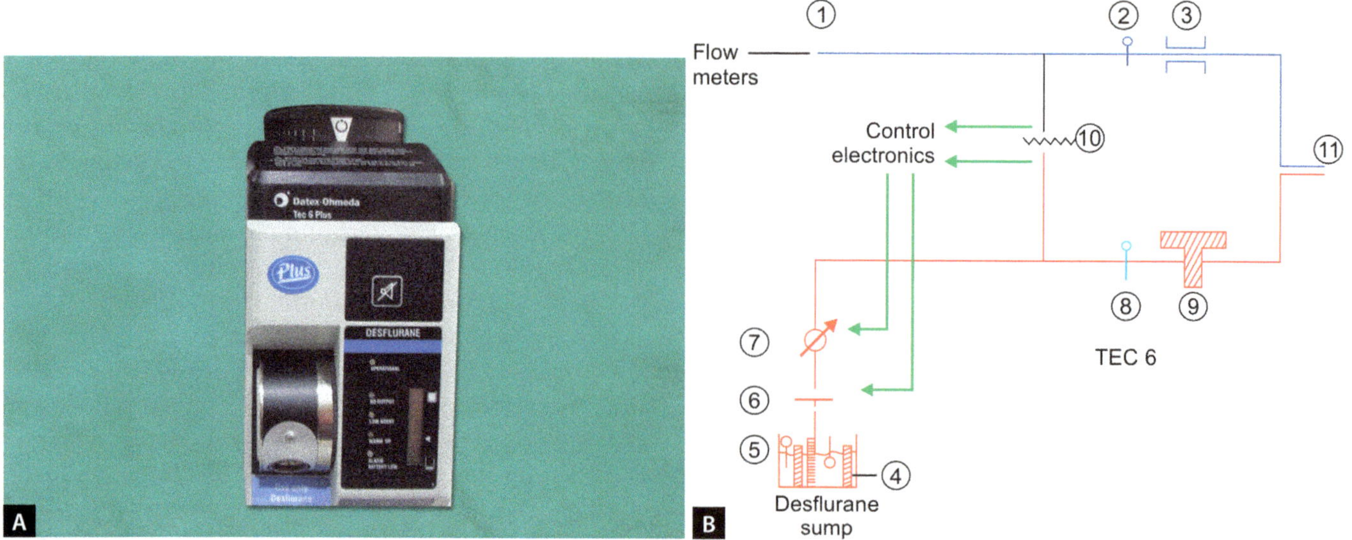

Figs. 5A and B: TEC 6. (A) Vaporizer; (B) Working principle. 1. FGF/vaporizer inlet; 2. Pressure sensor/FGF; 3. Fixed resistor; 4. Heating element; 5. Desflurane sump assembly; 6. Sump shut-off valve; 7. Pressure regulating valve; 8. Vapor circuit pressure sensor; 9. Variable resistor—concentration control dial; 10. Differential pressure transducer; 11. Vaporizer outlet. (FGF: fresh gas flow)

Construction[4] ***(Fig. 5B):*** It is slightly larger than other TEC vaporizers. The concentration control dial is at the top and dial settings are from 0% to 18%. A release must be activated for dialing above 12%. Battery (9 volts, for alarms and LED), power cord and drain port are at the bottom. The filling port is at front left and admits only desflurane bottles. The sump (5) at the bottom contains two heating elements (4), filling port, drain port and temperature, pressure and agent level sensors. The agent level sensor measures capacitance.

The vaporizer performs a self-test when switched on. It becomes operational 5–10 minutes after switching on. This is the time taken for heating desflurane. The liquid agent in the sump is heated to 39°C, and the unit is pressurized to 1,500 mm Hg (nearly 2 atm absolute). This is because at 39°C the SVP rises to 1,500 mm Hg. When operational temperature is attained the shut-off valve (6) opens and operational LED lights up. When switched on the vaporizer is warm to touch.

The fresh gas flow (1) enters the vaporizer and encounters the fixed resistor (3). This generates a back pressure which is sensed by the pressure sensor (2). This pressure in the gas circuit is called the working pressure and is balanced by the pressure transducer (10). The control electronics measures the changes in temperature and vapor pressure in the vapor circuit or changes in the fresh gas flow rate. This information is then used to balance the pressure in the two circuits. The agent vapor pressure is electromechanically balanced by altering a variable resistor—agent pressure regulating valve (7).

Thus, the concentration delivered by the TEC 6 depends only on the ratio of FGF through the fixed restrictor to the agent vapor flow through the variable resistor, which depends on the concentration dial setting (9). If the dial is turned up, the resistance to desflurane flow decreases and more agent is delivered. If the FGF is turned up, the back pressure at the fixed resistor increases and the control electronics increase the desflurane flow, thus maintaining the ratio constant. The two circuits are separate until they merge just proximal to the vaporizer exit (11).

The vaporizer can be filled while in use and when warming up, but the flow should be less than 8 L/min at a dial setting of less than 8%. This is to minimize the risk of awareness as the MAC of the agent is high and blood gas solubility is low. Turning the vaporizer off during filling will lead to a rapid fall in agent partial pressure.

Alarm systems (TEC 6 plus has audible alarms): When misfilled, the vaporizer detects malfunction and shuts off. The display panel is on the front right. The lag period between dysfunction detection and alarm activation is 10 seconds, except for tilt. The LEDs and their significance are:

- *Amber LED warm-up mode:* Initial warm-up period after switching on
- *Green LED operational mode:* Operating temperature reached, short tone sounds
- *Red LED no output alarm:* LED flashes and an auditory alarm of repetitive tones sounds if the vaporizer is not able to deliver vapor. This happens if:
  - Agent level less than 20 mL
  - Tilting the vaporizer more than 10°
  - Power failure
  - An internal malfunction
- *Amber LED low agent:* Less than 50 mL, audible alarm
- *Amber LED alarm battery low:* No audible alarm.

Level indicator is an LCD, visible when powered. It displays 50–425 mL. Arrow indicates refill mark at 250 mL.

Evaluation

- *Flow:* 0.2–10 L/min
- *Temperature:* 18–30°C

Electricity consumption is low. The battery must be replaced annually.

Hazards

- Vapor may leak into the fresh gas when the vaporizer is off
- The bottle may be dropped when released under pressure
- If the machine uses fresh gas decoupling, special software needs to be installed
- The vaporizer should be placed such that its power cord does not cause problems with the seating and mounting of other vaporizers.

Maintenance

- Service interval is 1 year
- Can be wiped with a damp cloth.

MEASURED FLOW INJECTOR VAPORIZERS

Principle

The liquid agent is held in a separate pressurized chamber and is injected into the carrier gas flow. An injector assembly is used which causes a fine spray of liquid droplets to enter the carrier gas in a pulsed manner. The vaporization is monitored electronically. The rate of injection is regulated electronically to achieve the concentration set by the anesthetist. As vaporization does not occur in the liquid chamber there is no loss of heat of vaporization from the system as understood conventionally. Thermostats, heat sinks and heating elements are not needed.

The vapor chamber contains an evaporative surface to ensure complete vaporization, prevent condensation (rain out) of the vapor as it encounters the cold diluent gas and to compensate for the evaporative cooling.[7] Thus, though there is electrical heating and electronic monitoring incorporated, injection vaporizers do not strictly fall into the temperature compensated category. So, the author suggests that they may be considered to be vaporizers where temperature compensation is not required or not applicable.

This vaporizer design leads to the following advantages as well. As the liquid agent cannot spill into the vaporization chamber, these vaporizers are not vulnerable to tipping. As with the dual circuit gas vapor blender, these vaporizers can be filled while in use, but agent delivery ceases while filling is in progress.

Maquet Injection Vaporizer[7,8]

Manufacturer: Maquet Critical Care AB, Getinge Group, Sweden, 2013.

Classification: Plenum, measured flow, injector, out of system, agent-specific modules for isoflurane, desflurane, sevoflurane. Weight—3.2 kg.

Capacity: 300 mL

Filling system:

- Isoflurane—Key fill (Maquet)
- Sevoflurane—Quik fill (Abbott) and Key fill (Maquet)
- Desflurane—Saf-T-Fil (Baxter)

Construction and Working Principle (Fig. 6)

This electronic injector vaporizer is designed to work with the FLOW-i System patented by Maquet (2011). The vaporizer modules are available for Isoflurane (0–5%), Desflurane (0–18%), Sevoflurane (0–8%). At a given time, two modules can be slotted on the FLOW-i via the docking valve (1). Externally, the lid, filling port, liquid level indicators—float and LEDs are visible (7). The low and medium priority alarms sound if the liquid level falls to 10% and 5%, respectively. The modules are checked during the system checkout (leaks and function), hence there is no need for calibration. There is no concentration control dial. The agent concentration is set electronically via the workstation display. The vaporizers can be refilled while still slotted in the machine and with one in use. Unlike the dual circuit gas vapor blender for desflurane the vaporizer does not need to be heated up before use.

The vaporizer lid has a filling port which is equipped with a sensor and a safety fill valve (3) as the liquid containing chamber is pressurized. If the lid is open the vaporizer will be deactivated. The vaporizer contains two chambers—the liquid agent container (6) and the vaporizing chamber (14). The driving gas (4) enters the liquid container after passing through a docking valve (1). The docking valve will close and seal off the liquid chamber when the module is disconnected. The driving gas pressure is 120 kPa. This pressurizes the container and forces the liquid (6) through the injector assembly (11). It also minimizes the evaporation of the agent within the chamber. From the container the liquid passes through a transducer (9) which senses the liquid pressure and then through a safety valve (10) which is close to the injector. The safety valve is closed when the vaporizer or the entire system is turned off or is in standby. The safety valve will stop the delivery of liquid agent to the injector in case of vaporizer malfunction. In the vaporization chamber (14) the liquid is forced through a nozzle plate (12) to form a fine spray, which causes the agent to vaporize. This process is monitored by the optical injection detector (13). The liquid is injected in pulses of varying duration (2–10 ms for isoflurane and sevoflurane, and 5–10 ms for desflurane), depending on the set and measured concentrations. Each pulse volume is 0.8 mL of liquid agent per ms. Thus, 1.6–8 mL of isoflurane or sevoflurane and 4–8 mL of desflurane can be injected in each pulse. The maximum speed of injection is 10 m/sec. The vaporization chamber has two temperature sensors (15). A heating foil (16) along the wall opposite the injector maintains the temperature at 47°C for isoflurane and sevoflurane and at 37°C for desflurane to ensure complete vaporization. There is a

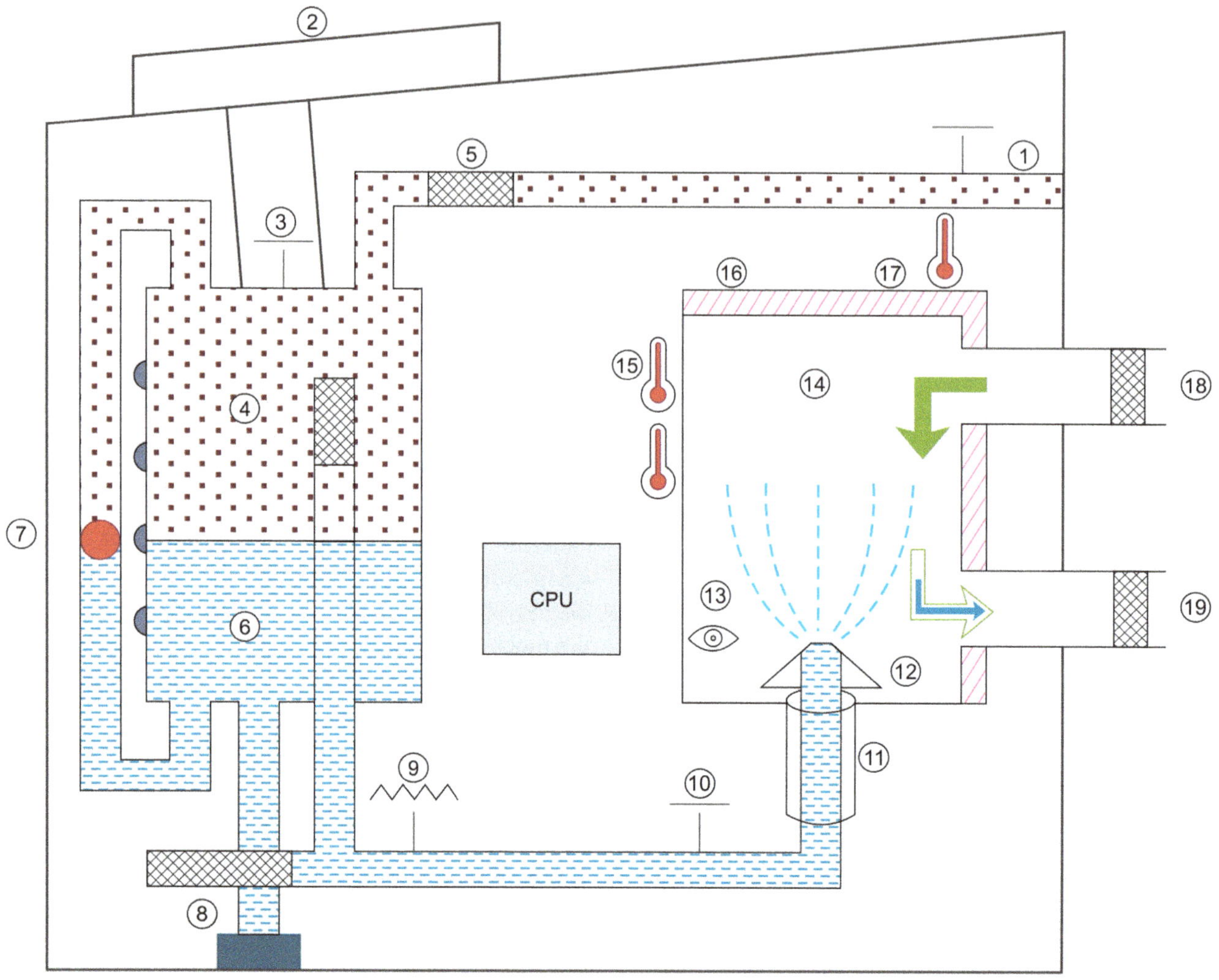

Fig. 6: Maquet Injector Vaporizer Working principle. 1. Docking valve, entry of vaporizer drive gas; 2. Vaporizer lid with filling port; 3. Safety fill valve; 4. Driving gas; 5. Driving gas filter; 6. Liquid agent container; 7. Liquid level indicator; 8. Sintered glass liquid agent filter and drain plug; 9. Liquid agent pressure transducer; 10. Safety valve; 11. Injector assembly; 12. Nozzle plate; 13. Optical injection detector; 14. Vaporizing chamber; 15. Vaporizing chamber temperature sensor; 16. Heating foil; 17. Heating foil temperature sensor; 18. Fresh gas inlet; 19. Fresh gas outlet.

temperature sensor for the heating foil as well (17). The heating foil is switched off at 140°C. Fresh gas enters the vaporization chamber (18) and exits carrying the agent (19). The vaporizer output is monitored by an Anesthesia Agent Gas Monitor downstream of the vaporizer. The data from the lid sensors, liquid level sensors, temperature sensors, optical sensors and pressure transducer is integrated in the CPU. The vaporizer output is altered by changing the duration of the pulses. The amount of agent injected depends on the desired concentration set and the fresh gas flow. The injector assembly oscillates, giving rise to a high sound. The vaporizer is designed to minimize this sound. Alarms are activated and the vaporizer switched off if the vaporization chamber temperature exceeds 60°C or the heating foil temperature exceeds 170°C.

Dräger Direct Injection of Vapor Anesthetic[1,9,10]

Manufacturer: Dräger Medical

Classification: Plenum, measured flow, injector, agent-specific module, out of system.

Needs electricity and a separate air supply, principle similar to fuel injector in automobile engines.

The Direct Injection of Vapor Anesthetic (DIVA®) is purpose built to be used in conjunction with the Dräger Zeus® anesthetic work station. It has two sections, a plug in vaporizing module which is agent specific and a built in gas supply module which is incorporated in the anesthesia work station. The vaporizing module has a filling device, a storage tank, a capacitance level gauge and an overpressure relief valve. The storage tank can be filled during use as the pressure is relieved by solenoid valves and the chamber can be opened without any leak. The agent from the storage tank enters the pump tank. The pump tank is pressurized to 2.4 bar by air and the liquid enters the metering tank where it vaporizes.

The machine uses a closed loop feedback control. It monitors the pressure of the agent in the vaporizing chamber, the FGF and the target expired agent concentration. The FGF composition, desired FiO_2 and end-tidal agent concentration are set by the user on the touch screen.

The machine then injects enough vapor to attain these values. It uses various modes. The "uptake mode" allows quantitative closed-system anesthesia as it closely follows the uptake of the agent by the patient and replaces only that which is utilized.

Low Flow Techniques: Advantages of Measured Flow Vaporizers

The currently used mechanical variable bypass vaporizers (TEC series, Drager Vapor 19 and 2000) are flow splitting devices designed to deliver a clinically acceptable concentration at the outlet. This involves the use of high flows to achieve safe concentrations of volatile agents. Electronic variable bypass vaporizers (Aladin cassette with ADU) work on the same principle of flow splitting and the use of high flows, but use electronic monitoring and regulation for greater accuracy and reliability.

In the past few years, low flow anesthesia is increasingly being practiced. If the fresh gas flows are low, the carrier gas passing through a variable bypass vaporizer will carry very little anesthetic vapor (in mL) to the outlet, even at the highest dial settings. Hence, vaporizer output will fall. At FGF of 6000 mL/min and at a dial setting of 2%, 120 mL/min of sevoflurane vapor is delivered to the circuit. If the flow is decreased to 600 mL/min the vaporizer output will fall to 12 mL/min. If the dial setting is increased to the maximum 8%, the output will be 48 mL/min. This will get diluted in a much larger volume (circuit and patient's lungs). Thus, the time taken to change the FGF composition during low flows is very long (long time constants). Rapid changes in the depth of anesthesia are not possible when using variable bypass vaporizers and low flows. This is a significant disadvantage.

There are two instances during a case when a large amount of vapor is required to be delivered within a short period of time. The first is at induction, when agent uptake in the tissues is high. The second instance is when a rapid increase in the depth of anesthesia is required during the case (a second surgical incision). To deliver the large amounts of vapor the system must revert to high flows which results in loss of gas from the system which is wasteful, uneconomical and results in theater pollution. If an electronic variable bypass vaporizer system is using a Target Control Mode (which closely follows the patient uptake) and the set target is increased, the system will try to attain the new target in less than 2 minutes. If the change is large, the FGF is increased and the solenoid valve is opened increasing the vaporizer output. If the change is small the FGF is kept constant and only the solenoid valve is opened.

The injector type vaporizers overcome this problem by increasing the amount of vapor directly added to the carrier gas without any change in the carrier gas flow. This allows a rapid increase in the depth of anesthesia. This is possible because the amount of vapor added is metered in separately and is independent of the carrier gas flow. When using metabolic flow, the amount of sevoflurane needed to be delivered by the vaporizer to attain an end-tidal concentration of 2% in a volume of 6 L comprising the functional residual capacity of the patient (2,000 mL) and the circuit volume (4,000 mL) may be as high as 40%. This can only be achieved by injectors. The use of anesthetic agent and gas monitoring (AGM) downstream to the vaporizer prevents unsafe concentrations from being delivered.[9]

However, if a rapid decrease in the depth of anesthesia is required it is only possible by increasing the FGF, whether a variable bypass or injector type vaporizer is used.

NEW INHALED ANESTHETIC DELIVERY SYSTEM

These are systems which deliver volatile anesthetic for out of operation theater locations, primarily for ICU sedation, also useful in severe bronchospasm and status epilepticus. There are two such systems. The AnaConDa is described in detail below. The Mirus system developed by Pall Medical, Germany is the first reflection system to administer desflurane as well as isoflurane and sevoflurane. It administers the agent during early inspiration, reuses 90% of the exhaled agent, monitors ventilation parameters as well as end tidal concentration and offers an automatic target control mode.[13]

AnaConDa® (Anesthetic Conserving Device)[1,11] (Figs. 7A and B)

Manufacturer: Sedana Medical, Uppsala, Sweden, 2004.

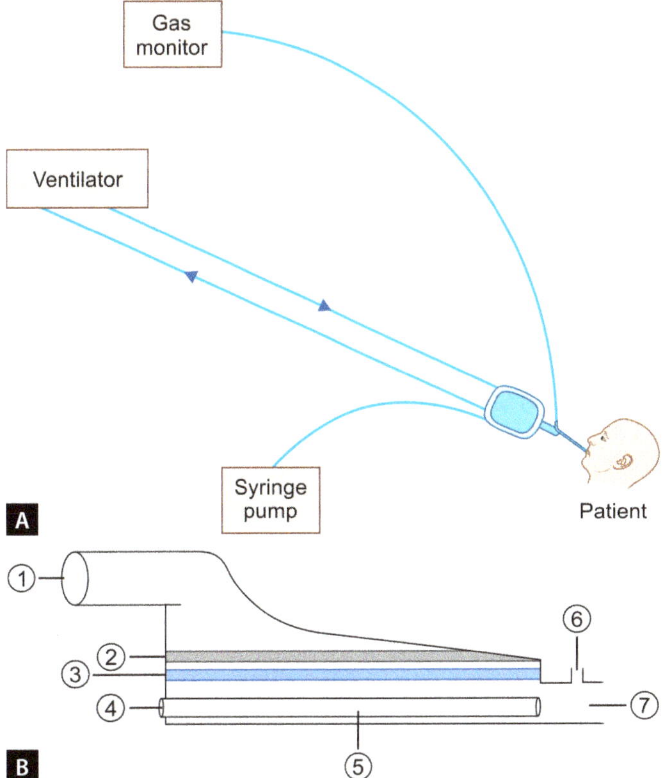

Figs. 7A and B: AnaConDa. (A) Setup; (B) Cross-section. 1. Ventilator Y-piece; 2. Carbon fibers; 3. Bacterial filter; 4. For the syringe pump; 5. Liquid vapourizes; 6. Gas sampling port; 7. To the patient airway.

Agents: Sevoflurane, Isoflurane.

It is a modified bacterial filter or heat and moisture exchanger (HME) placed between the catheter mount (7) and Y piece (1, it is an oval device which allows laminar flow). It is disposable, must be replaced every 24 hours or if clogged by secretions. In addition to the hemodynamic monitoring in the ICU patient, anesthesia gas monitoring is essential when using this system.

Construction: It is available in two sizes, 50 mL for patients below 50 kg weight and tidal volumes from 200 to 350 mL, 100 mL for patients above 50 kg and tidal volumes of 350–1,200 mL. It contains a layer of activated carbon fibers (2) in addition to the bacterial filter (3). The liquid anesthetic is supplied via a syringe pump to the patient's side of the fibers (4). The syringes are specifically designed and have a keyed system which is unique for the syringe and adaptor such that no other syringe fits. The liquid instantly vaporizes (5) in the flow and is delivered to the lungs during inspiration. During expiration, 90% of the exhaled volatile anesthetic molecules condense on the surface of the activated carbon fibers and is adsorbed. The molecules are released again during the next inspiration. As a result, the AnaConDa® can be considered to be a disposable vaporizer. The device increases the physiological dead space as carbon dioxide is reflected as well. This is a limitation to using low tidal volume ventilation in ARDS patients.

Differences with Conventional Vaporizers

- Anesthetic concentration is adjusted through the infusion of the liquid anesthetic
- The vaporization depends on the rate at which the infusion is run and not the fresh gas flow rate, onset is slower
- Anesthetic agent consumption with the AnaConDa® is constant and independent of the circuit and FGF.

FILLING SYSTEMS

The American Society for Testing and Materials International (ASTM) machine standard recommends, but does not require, that a vaporizer designed for a single agent be fitted with a permanently attached, agent-specific device to prevent accidental filling with the wrong agent. These systems reduce the air pollution associated with filling and draining of vaporizers.

Draw-over Vaporizers (Fig. 8)

Most of the older vaporizers (Goldman, Boyle's bottle) consist of a channel and a glass chamber which contains the liquid agent. The chamber can be unscrewed from the back bar or gas channel and liquid poured in the unit. Draining is recommended after use and during transport. After draining the vaporizer, excess liquid is decanted into its container. This may be added to the wrong container. Thus, leading to misfilling during subsequent use. The filling and draining ports are common sites of leak if not tightened properly.

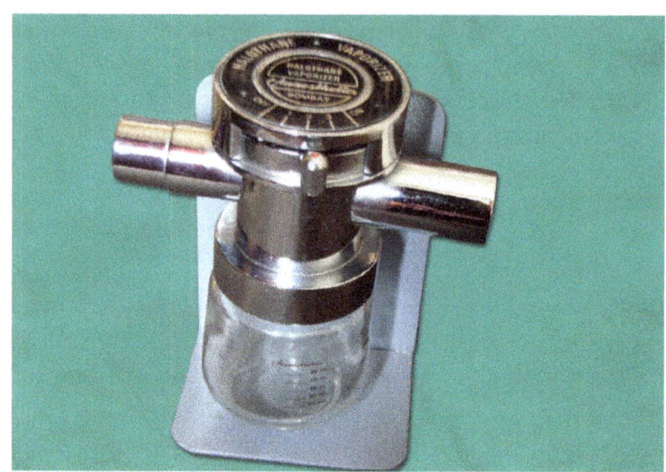

Fig. 8: Goldman vaporizer.

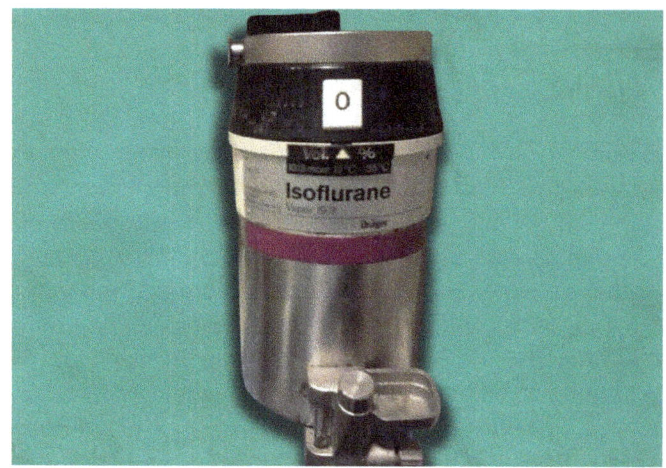

Fig. 9: Screw fill system.

The hazards are filling the wrong agent, overfilling and environmental pollution. To overcome these hazards, there has been progressive improvement in design. When ordering a vaporizer, it is possible to choose the filling system.

Screw Fill (Fig. 9)

The early plenum vaporizers had a filling port at the bottom, and a liquid level indicator—sight glass. The screw threaded stopper is unscrewed, agent filled and stopper replaced. The filling should stop when the level reaches the recommended maximum on the indicator.

Key Fill Systems (Figs. 10A to C)

Agent Specific

Manufacturer: Earlier Cyprane, now GE Healthcare.

The Fraser Sweatman pin safety system is based on color coding for agents (red—halothane, orange—enflurane, violet—isoflurane, yellow—sevoflurane, and blue—desflurane). The various parts are made to align and fit into each

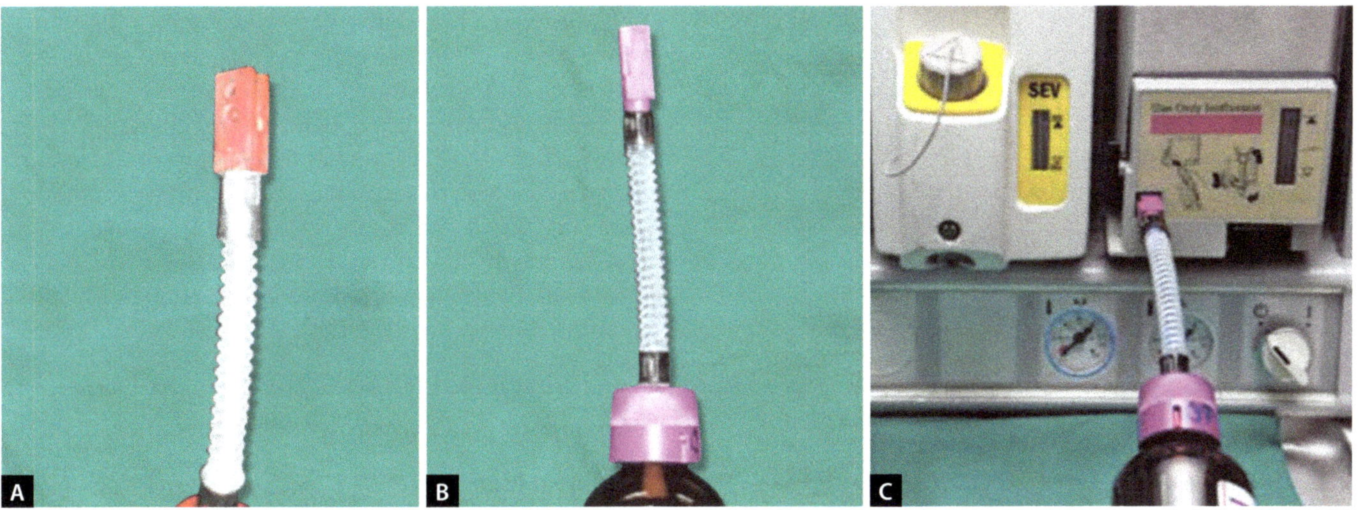

Figs. 10A to C: Key fill system. (A) Halothane; (B) Isoflurane; (C) Isoflurane key filler with vaporizer.

other like a key in a lock. The design of the projections and the slots they fit in are unique for each individual agent. It has three parts:

1. The bottle with neck collar
2. The adaptor
3. The vaporizer filling port
   i. The bottle has a color-coded label and neck collar. The collar has two projections
   ii. The adaptors are also color-coded. The bottle end has two notches which fit the size and placement of the projections on the neck of the corresponding agent bottle. The distal end has a groove which aligns with the ledge in the filler port. The larger hole is for anesthetic agent, and the smaller hole is for air. These are connected by a corrugated tube which allows the bottle to be held higher or lower than the port.
   iii. The vaporizer has a colored stripe on it. The filling port has a ledge which corresponds to the adaptor and is agent specific.

These ports are seen on the TEC 5. The locking lever for the filling device is at the bottom on the left. The lever for filling-draining is at the base, below the sight glass. The bottle adaptor is inserted into the port and the locking lever is pulled down to hold it in place. When filling, the bottle is lifted up, and the filling-draining lever is pulled forward. After the sump is filled, filling-draining lever is returned to the closed position and the bottle is lowered. The locking lever is pushed upward and the bottle is removed. When draining the same sequence is followed, but the bottle is lowered rather than lifting it up.

Vaporizers should be filled only when securely locked on the back bar. This avoids tilting and overfilling and minimizes leaks.

Easy-Fil[4] (Fig. 11)

The system is manufactured by GE healthcare. The principle is similar to the key-fill system. It is easier to use. The port on the vaporizer has been modified with corresponding modification to the distal end of adaptor. The filler channel and the bottle adaptor have grooves and ridges which align with each other. Each agent has a unique combination.

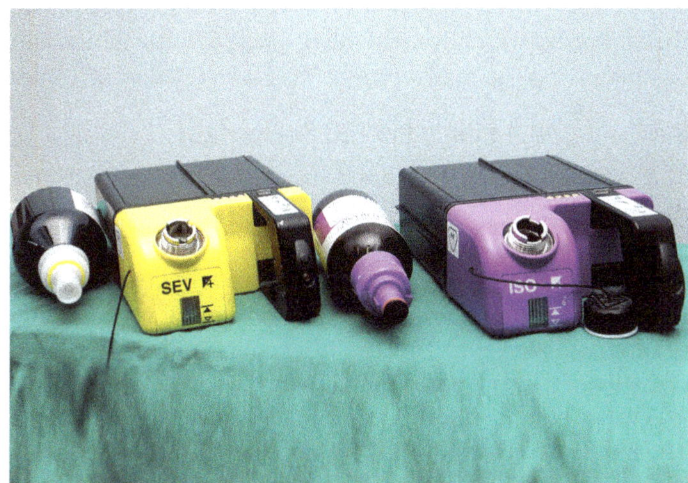

Fig. 11: Easy-Fil system.

The bottle collar remains the same. The corrugated tubing has been dispensed with. It is provided with the TEC 7.

All the above filling systems can lead to misfilling if the wrong agent is decanted into the agent-specific bottle. To prevent this, the following systems have evolved.

Quik-Fil[2,4] (Fig. 12A)

Abbott Laboratories produces sevoflurane bottles which are sealed and the agent-specific filling device is fitted permanently on to the neck with a tamper proof crimped metal seal. The bottle is opened and inverted onto the filling port. A valve opens when a slight pressure is applied on the bottle and the agent enters the vaporizer. This prevents spilling and minimizes pollution.

The sealed bottles ensure that the liquid contained in the bottle is definitely the one displayed on the label. The bottle

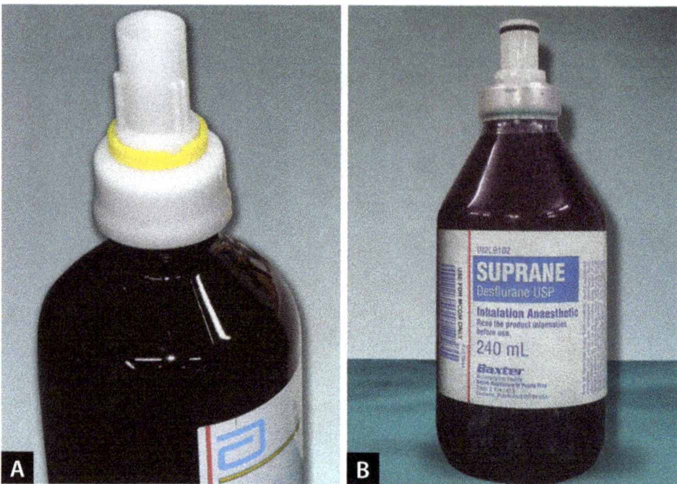

Figs. 12A and B: (A) Quik-Fil; (B) Saf-T-Fil™.

is made of plastic. So it is unbreakable as compared to the earlier bottles which were made of glass. A bottle which can be opened may be inadvertently filled with the wrong liquid.

Saf-T-Fil: ™2,4 Filling the TEC 6 (Fig. 12B)

The system is manufactured by Baxter Healthcare for desflurane.

The desflurane bottle has a filler nozzle which fits into the filler port of TEC 6. The nozzle is crimped onto the neck of the bottle to ensure that the bottle will contain only desflurane. The vaporizing chamber contains desflurane at a pressure of nearly 2 atm. The "O" ring on the nozzle prevents leak of pressurized desflurane vapor from the vaporizer. The bottle is inverted and the nozzle is pushed onto the spring loaded aperture of the port. The contents enter the vaporizer. The LCD display indicates the level. When filling is complete the bottle is returned to the starting position. The spring then ejects the filler nozzle. As the liquid in the bottle enters the sump of the vaporizer it is replaced by the desflurane vapor. When the bottle is removed from the filling port, the pressure inside it is high until the vapor condenses to liquid and the bottle may shatter. Hence, the bottle is made of glass and is coated with plastic to prevent injury to the bystanders if the bottle shatters.

The vaporizer can be filled while in use. If the vaporizer has been removed from the back bar and a tilt is present, overfilling can occur. The shut-off valve prevents the liquid from leaving the sump.

DRAINING THE VAPORIZERS

This is undertaken prior to transport or storage. In the case of halothane, draining may be recommended more frequently if cotton wicks are used.

The hazards associated with draining are leaks, environmental pollution, misfilling of emptied agent in wrong bottle, the problem of disposing the liquid agent drained—sevoflurane and desflurane. Hence, the procedure should be undertaken only when essential.

The funnel fill systems have a draining plug which is removed and the filling port is opened to allow for the entry of air and both should be closed securely when done. The keyed filler system has been discussed above. The rest of the systems have a screw at the bottom of the vaporizer which needs to be released and a drain adaptor fitted to the drain port site. It is recommended that if the agent cannot be returned to the bottle, as with bottles with seals and crimps, the container should be left in an area outside the operation theater.

VAPORIZER MOUNTING SYSTEMS

The mounting systems can be permanent or detachable.

Permanent Mounting

The permanent mounting systems require tools to remove or install a vaporizer on the anesthesia machine. There is less physical damage to vaporizers and fewer leaks. The problems with permanent mounting are inadequate number of mounting locations to accommodate all the vaporizers that are likely to be needed. If there is a malfunction and the vaporizer needs to be exchanged, it cannot be removed easily especially with a case underway.

Detachable Mounting (Figs. 13A and B)

Here the vaporizers can be mounted or removed without using tools. They are standard on most new anesthesia machines. Each manufacturer has slight differences in configuration but the basic principle remains the same. The Select-a-tec system is seen in machines by GE and a similar system from Dräger Medical is widely used.

The Select-a-tec system (first seen on TEC 4) consists of a pair of port valves for each vaporizer position. **Figure 13A** shows the internal structure and the green channel is the path of gas flow when there is no vaporizer mounted on the back bar. The port valve has O-rings **(Fig. 13B)**. If missing or misaligned, these are common sites of vaporizer leaks. Each vaporizer has a mounting bracket which contains two plungers (spindles), which fit over the port valves. A seal is formed between the vaporizer and the port valves due to the weight of the vaporizer and the O-rings. On the back of each vaporizer is a locking lever.

Before mounting a vaporizer, the control dial must be turned off and the locking lever should be unlocked. The adjacent vaporizer must be turned off. The vaporizer is placed onto the mounting system and locked in position.

After a vaporizer has been mounted:

- Look at the tops of the vaporizers, they should be at the same height and level with each other
- Try to lift the vaporizer. If it can be moved without unlocking, it is improperly positioned
- It should be possible to turn on only one vaporizer at a time
- The anesthesia machine must be checked for leaks with each vaporizer in both the "ON" and "OFF" position.

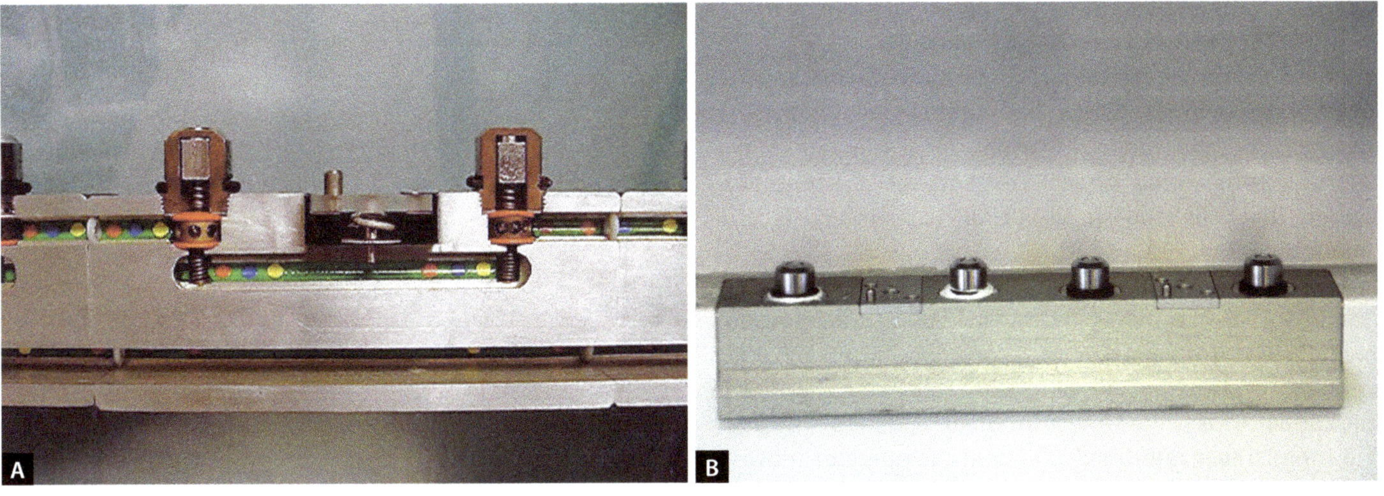

Figs. 13A and B: (A) Select-a-tec system; (B) Dräger mounting system.

When the vaporizer is turned on, the two plungers move downward and open the port valves allowing fresh gas to enter the vaporizer. When the vaporizer is turned off, the port valves remain closed and the FGF passes through the back bar without entering the vaporizer.

To remove the vaporizer from the machine, the vaporizer is turned off and the locking lever is unlocked. The vaporizer is lifted off the manifold.

The Dräger Medical mounting system is shown in **Figure 13B**. It has a slightly different configuration. Certain Dräger vaporizers display a "T" (travel) position on the concentration control dial. These are the Vapor® 2000 vaporizer and the Dräger D vaporizer for desflurane. These vaporizer dials must be in the "T" **(Fig. 14)** position before they can be unlocked from the machine. These vaporizers have valves which in the "T" position, isolate the vaporizing chamber and prevent liquid agent from passing into the bypass channel and contaminating it if the vaporizer is tilted when it is not mounted on the machine. This ensures that the vaporizers are not affected by tilting/tipping.

Advantages

- More compact anesthesia machine as fewer mounting locations needed
- Replacement is possible during a case
- If malignant hyperthermia is a potential problem, the vaporizers can be removed altogether.

Disadvantages

- Partial or complete obstruction to gas flow can occur due to misalignment
- Potential for leaks is high, a common leak source is an absent or damaged O-ring or if the locking lever is unlocked
- Awareness can occur if there is failure to deliver agent vapor to the fresh gas due to problems with the mounting system

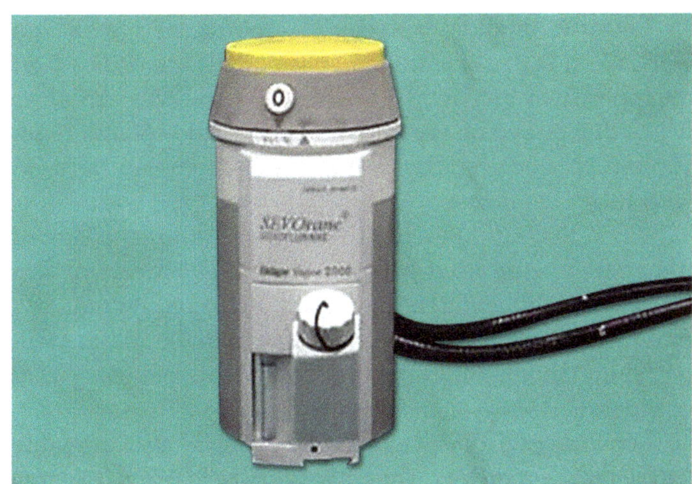

Fig. 14: Dräger Vapor® 2000 "T" position.

- If something is pushed under the vaporizer, so that it slightly lifts off the O-ring, a leak may result when the vaporizer is turned "ON"
- Miscellaneous instruments placed on the vaporizer—syringes for cuff inflation—may interfere with the locking and concentration dials and cause leaks or render the vaporizer nonfunctioning.

The mounting systems may vary among manufacturers and there may be no compatibility between machines and vaporizers produced by different manufacturers.

VAPORIZER EXCLUSION SYSTEMS

If two vaporizers are used simultaneously the vaporizer downstream can be contaminated by the agent used in the upstream vaporizer. This will make the output of the downstream vaporizer unpredictable. Hence, vaporizers should never be used in series.

The vaporizer exclusion systems ensure that only one vaporizer is in use at a given time. These systems work by rendering the concentration control dials of adjacent vaporizers inoperable. These should be checked with the anesthesia apparatus checkout procedure.

The Select-a-tec system (Datex-Ohmeda/GE) is used on several machines. When the vaporizer dial release is unlocked and the vaporizer turned on a pin moves two extension rods which project out and the concentration control dials of the neighboring vaporizers become inoperable **(Figs. 15A and B)**.

The Dräger vaporizers have a vapor exclusion system which consists of notches on the back of the concentration control dials. If a vaporizer is turned "on," a pin occupies the notch of the adjacent vaporizers rendering the dial in operational. This is the Dräger Interlock® I system.

In the Dräger Interlock® II system the operator moves a rod to release the concentration control dial of the vaporizer to be used. This locks the dial of the other vaporizer in place **(Fig. 16)**.

Both the interlock systems incorporate devices which work when the concentration control dials are situated on the top of the vaporizer. They will not function if a vaporizer with a dial placed on the front is in use (Penlon Sigma Delta vaporizer). However, the Select-a-tec system can be used with such a vaporizer.

When buying vaporizers, it is important to be aware of the system being used with the current vaporizers. If two vaporizers with different vaporizer exclusion systems are mounted on the back bar of a machine both the systems will be nonfunctional and it will be possible to use vaporizers in series.

For example, the Select-a-tec system is also available with Dräger vaporizers. Thus, it is possible to use a Dräger D vaporizer on a GE machine along with TEC vaporizers, while being sure that the vaporizer exclusion system is fully functional.

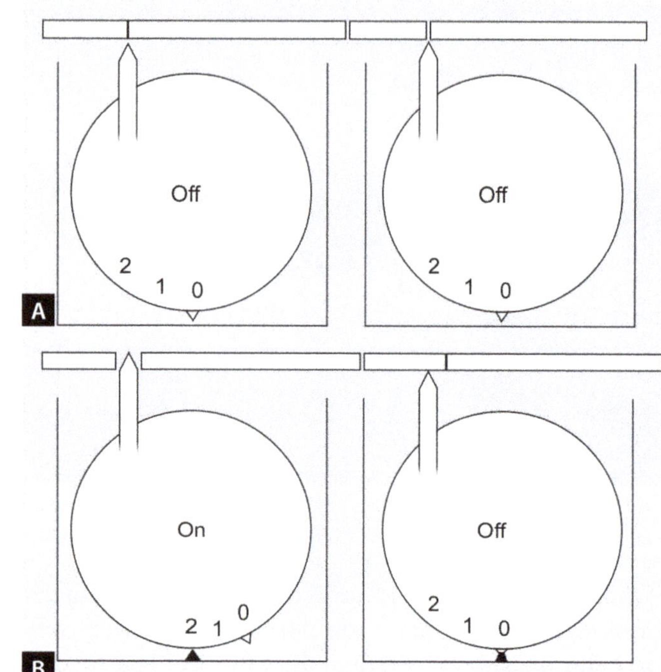

Figs. 15A and B: Select-a-tec interlock system. (A) When both vaporizers are off; (B) When the first vaporizer is turned on.

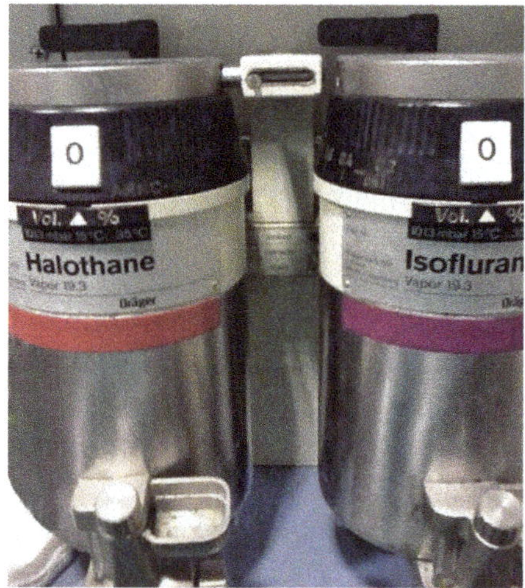

Fig. 16: Dräger Interlock® II system.

CALIBRATION AND SERVICING OF VAPORIZERS[1]

Each vaporizer is individually calibrated in the factory using a computer and refractometer. The accuracy is influenced by the agent used, the temperature compensation mechanism, the splitting valve and the flow dynamics within the vaporizer. The vaporizer is filled with the agent and stored at 23°C for 4 hours. A control dial with a unique serial number is then attached and rotated over a range of flows. The output is measured by a refractometer. A calibration scale is etched on the dial. The dial is reattached and calibration reconfirmed.[1] In clinical practice, vaporizer dials are marked in v/v%, i.e., volume percent and vaporizers are calibrated at sea level.[7]

The vaporizers should be serviced as per manufacturer recommendations. These are usually at 3–5-year intervals. Halothane vaporizers may need more frequent servicing due to the use of thymol. Each part of the vaporizer is numbered before dismantling, it is then reassembled and calibration confirmed after each service. Some vaporizers may be life time service free like the Aladin™ cassette and the Maquet injector vaporizer module which is checked by the CPU daily or the TEC 7 which has a Teflon® coating.

HAZARDS

Misfilling[12]

As the vaporizers in use today are concentration calibrated, any mistake in filling the vaporizer will lead either to an overdose or to awareness. If a highly volatile agent is used in a vaporizer for an agent with low volatility it will lead to increased output and vice versa. Consider two commonly used agents **(Table 5)**. If isoflurane is filled in a vaporizer meant for sevoflurane an overdose will result as the vaporizer chamber flow is greater in a sevoflurane vaporizer. In practice, it is likely, that a correctly filled vaporizer is then erroneously topped up by the wrong agent. The volatile

TABLE 5: Splitting ratios for various agents at 22°C.			
Dialled percentage	***Halothane (SVP – 243 mm Hg)***	***Isoflurane (SVP – 238 mm Hg)***	***Sevoflurane (SVP – 160 mm Hg)***
1%	46:1	44:1	25:1
2%	22:1	21:1	12:1
3%	14:1	14:1	7:1

agents do not react with each other but affect each other's rate of vaporization. The MAC of the resultant mixture is difficult to predict and major errors in agent delivery can occur. The use of an Anesthetic AGM downstream to the vaporizer provides an early warning in case of such a mishap.

Misfilling is an unlikely occurrence in the currently used vaporizers due to agent-specific filling systems. If misfilling occurs the vaporizer should be drained completely and flushed until no agent is detected at the outlet. The vaporizer should be returned to the manufacturer for cleaning and servicing.

Tipping

Tipping or tilting a vaporizer may cause liquid agent to enter the bypass channel. If the liquid comes in contact with lung tissue it may cause irreversible tissue damage. A more likely outcome is an overdose as 1 mL of liquid produces 200 mL of vapor. If the vaporizer is tipped it should be disconnected from the system and flushed with oxygen at high flows and low dial settings until no agent is detected at the outlet. If AGM is not available the manufacturer's instructions in the vaporizer manual should be followed. Some manufacturers suggest that if tilted a vaporizer should be flushed with oxygen at 5 L/min for 5 minutes.

Tipping is unlikely when permanent mounting is in use. If detachable mounting is used, vaporizers should be turned off completely when removed from the machine and placed such that no tilting is possible.

The following vaporizers are not affected by tipping. The Aladin™ cassettes are not affected by tipping as the bypass for the fresh gas is contained in the work station and cannot be contaminated by liquid agent when the cassette is removed from the machine. The agent modules of the injection vaporizers—Dräger DIVA and the Maquet Injector type vaporizer have separate liquid containers and vaporization chambers, hence liquid agent cannot contaminate the diluent gas. The Dräger® 2000 and Dräger Vapor D (only in the "T" position) are not affected by tipping as in the "T" position a valve becomes operational and completely seals off the vaporization chamber from the bypass chamber preventing contamination of the bypass channel.

Leaks

The two most common sites of leaks are an improperly closed filling port and the O-rings if the vaporizer is wrongly seated. Leaks are most likely during filling or draining. Leaks may cause the bag or bellows to collapse and may result in awareness.

Overfilling

Overfilling can occur if the vaporizer is tilted. This will lead to loss of surface area available and decrease vaporization.

No Output

The lack of output will cause awareness. The most common cause is an empty vaporizer. A malfunction will cause electronic vaporizers to shut down automatically. Spare vaporizers should be available in an emergency.

Reversal of Flow

Flow reversal occurs if there is misalignment of parts after servicing. This will lead to increased output.

Projectile

In the magnetic resonance imaging suite (MRI), vaporizers should be firmly secured to the back bar. Very few vaporizers contain ferromagnetic material and are generally safe to use in this setting. However, if ferromagnetic material is present, the vaporizer may act as a projectile.

SAFETY FEATURES OF VAPORIZERS

- Clear color-coding indicator on the vaporizer and agent bottle
- Agent-specific filling systems with sealed bottles
- Agent level indicators
- Mounting systems with interlock to prevent simultaneous use of two vaporizers
- Filling port is low to avoid overfilling
- Electronic vaporizers have audiovisual alarm systems which detect malfunction—tilting, low agent and low temperature
- Agent monitoring allows detection of misfilling, overdose and low output. The use of this monitor prevents incidences of accidental awareness.

Sequence of Vaporizers

Vaporizers should not be used simultaneously. However, when vaporizers are permanently mounted on the back bar and there is no interlock, it is possible to accidentally turn on two vaporizers simultaneously. The danger being that over a period of time, the vapor from the upstream vaporizer will condense and contaminate the downstream vaporizer. Hence, the order in which they are mounted becomes important.

- The more volatile agents (highest SVP) are placed downstream.
- The more potent agents are placed downstream so that an overdose is unlikely during subsequent use, even if contamination occurs.
- Placing agents which have toxic byproducts downstream prevents contamination of other vaporizers.

AGENTS AND VAPORIZERS OF HISTORICAL INTEREST

Cyclopropane (Trimethylene)[13]

- First synthesized by August von Freund in 1882
- Stored in an orange cylinder as a liquid at a pressure of 5 bar. It has its own flowmeter.
- Very explosive
- Quick induction, cardio stable
- Preferred for children and the elderly
- Respiratory depressant
- Vagotonic and ventricular dysrhythmias noted.

Diethyl Ether[13]

- Prepared by Valerius Cordus who called it sweet oil of vitriol
- WE Clarke used it clinically for anesthesia but did not publish the results
- WTG Morton on October 16, 1846, did a live demonstration of ether
- Flammable in air and explosive in oxygen
- High blood gas solubility—wide therapeutic range
- Slow induction and recovery
- Maintains blood pressure, less arrhythmogenic
- Initially increase in respiration but then decreases as the anesthesia deepens
- Bronchial muscle and skeletal muscle relaxant.

Chloroform[13]

- Introduced to clinical practice by JY Simpson
- Decreases blood pressure gradually
- Sudden cardiac arrest during lighter plane of anesthesia may be due to ventricular fibrillation or vagal inhibition
- Delayed liver damage from first to third day after anesthesia.

Trichlorethylene[13]

- Introduced by CL Hewer in 1941.
- Nonflammable, nonirritant, no cardiorespiratory depression.
- Analgesic—surgery and labor (0.5%).
- Very potent hence very cheap.
- Tachypnea, dysrhythmias, postoperative nausea and vomiting (PONV).
- Phosgene is produced with soda lime. It is a potent nerve poison, especially affecting cranial nerves, cures trigeminal neuralgia.

OPEN DROP METHOD

Folded Handkerchief

Used for chloroform.

Schimmelbusch Mask with Bellamy Gardner Bottle[14] (Figs. 17A and B)

The Schimmelbusch Mask (1890) is a wire frame mask used with a suitable drop bottle like the Bellamy Gardner bottle (1908). It was the most common drop bottle in use.

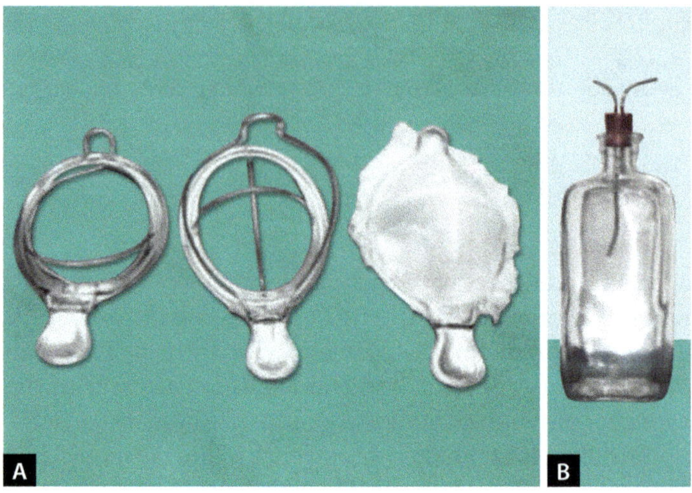

Figs. 17A and B: (A) Schimmelbusch mask; (B) Bellamy Gardner bottle.

The dropper consists of a red rubber stopper with two metal tubes. The longer tube dips into the liquid and the shorter acts as an air vent allowing air to enter the bottle. It can be used for chloroform or a mixture.

The Schimmelbusch mask is a wire frame mask with a gutter to collect excess liquid agent, over which gauze or lint is applied and the agent is dropped by a drop bottle. The agent vaporizes as the patient breathes to-and-fro through the mask. The mask is a loose fit to allow air dilution. This is especially important in the case of chloroform or ethyl chloride where overdose may occur due to inadequate dilution. For ether, 16 layers of gauze are used and the entire face covered. For chloroform, 12 layers of gauze or one layer of lint is used and only half of the mask is used. The rest of the face is covered with a split gamgee to protect the eyes.

Ogden Inhaler[14]

It is similar to the above masks with an upright wire cage around the periphery. Gamgee is wrapped around the cage to increase the concentration by decreasing air dilution.

DRAW-OVER VAPORIZERS

KEM Bottle (Fig. 18)

Classification: Draw-over, flow-over without wicks, non-temperature compensated, multiple agents.

Designed by Dr Paluel J Flagg, American Anesthesiologist to deliver ether. He is the author of the "Art of Anaesthesia" and "Art of Resuscitation". The Flagg's can, was first described in 1919. A Flagg Airway was attached to one end of a rubber tube and the other end was attached to the open spout of an ether can. The top of the can had several holes punched-in to allow air entrainment. The can was held in one hand to warm the ether and help vaporization. During use, the patient's nose was kept closed to prevent air dilution. It was used in the field during World War I (WWI) and the Spanish Civil war when compressed gases were not available. In 1929, the Flagg's can, was adapted for use in KEM Hospital, Mumbai. This adaptation is known as the KEM bottle.

It consists of a glass bottle with a metal lid. The lid has two metal tubes—one for the entry of air and the other is connected to the endotracheal tube by a length of rubber tubing. There is also a port for adding oxygen.

Goldman (Fig. 8)

Classification: Draw-over, variable bypass, flow-over, non-temperature compensated, multiple agents—halothane, isoflurane, noncalibrated, VIC/VOC.

Manufacturer: BOC, 1959, adapted from Leyland fuel pump.

Capacity: 30 mL

Originally designed for administering halothane, by Victor Goldman for dental anesthesia in intermittent flow machines. The Goldman can be used in the circle system due to low internal resistance. When used as VIC, concentration may exceed 3%. Output is very variable. Now Mark IV is available.

Advantages: Small, simple, inexpensive, portable and user friendly.

Output can be increased by wiping away water of condensation from the surface or wrapping with warm gamgee.

Rowbotham

Similar to Goldman, modified with steel wire-gauze wick.

Oxford Miniature Vaporizer[14] (Fig. 19)

Classification: Draw-over, variable bypass, flow-over, non-temperature compensated, but buffered, multiple agent—Ether, Trilene, Halothane (detachable scales for each).

Manufacture: Penlon

Capacity: 30 mL

Advantages: Portable, multiagent, robust, and minimal servicing.

- The maximum output is between 2 and 4% with halothane between 0 and 30°C, and higher above this.
- Made from stainless steel, resistant to corrosion, body also acts as a heat sink.
- Stainless steel mesh wicks increase the output but do not significantly increase resistance.
- Thermobuffering is achieved with a water bath (heat sink) with ethylene glycol as antifreeze. The dial may stick due to thymol.
- The Oxford miniature vaporizer (OMV) is reasonably accurate over a wide range of flow rates and tidal volumes.
- Performs very well at small tidal volumes, and is suitable for pediatric anesthesia.
- In spontaneously breathing pediatric patients, the OMV should be used as part of a continuous flow system (plenum).

Epstein Macintosh Oxford Ether Inhaler (Fig. 20)

Classification: Draw-over, variable bypass, flow-over, non-temperature compensated, but buffered, multiple agent—designed for diethyl ether (40 mL when full) but does not have an agent-specific filling system, EMOtril is designed for trichloroethylene, level compensated.

Manufacturer: Owen Mumford, developed by the Nuffield Department of Anesthetics, Oxford in 1956. Dr HG Epstein, Dr R Macintosh.

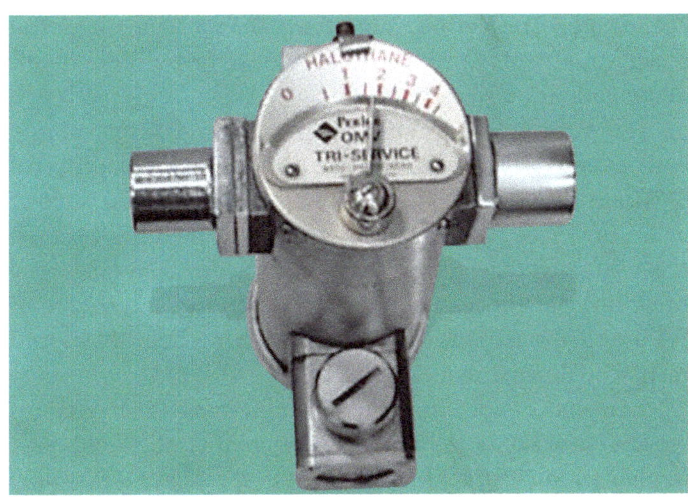

Fig. 19: Oxford miniature vaporizer.

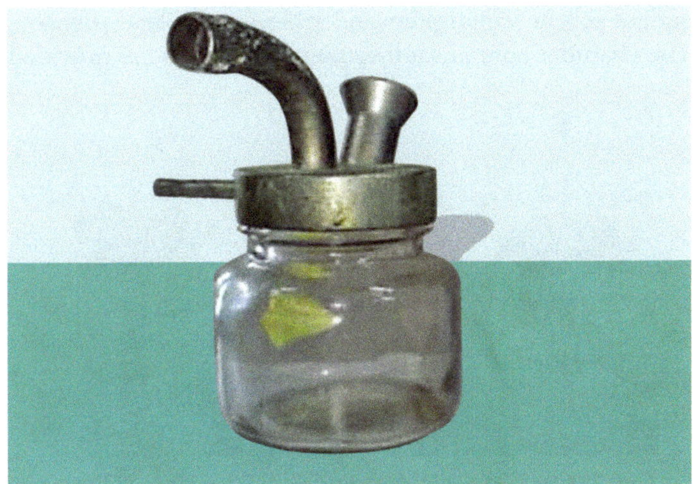

Fig. 18: KEM Bottle (adaptation of Flagg's can).

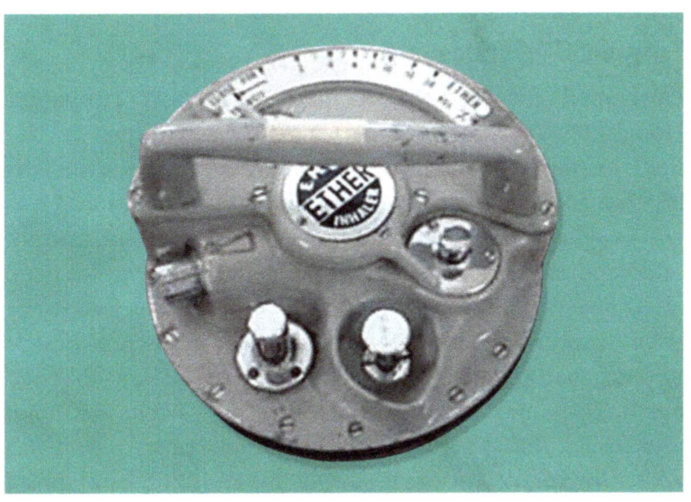

Fig. 20: Epstein Macintosh Oxford ether inhaler.

Advantages: Rugged, portable, reliable, independent of the need for pressurized gas, field ready, safe in the hands of a relatively inexperienced anesthetist.

Construction: The vaporizer consists of three parts: a bypass chamber, a mixing chamber and a vaporizing chamber. The vaporizing chamber is annular in shape and its walls are lined with cloth wicks. A control lever with a transit lock, determines the amount of air flowing through the vaporizing chamber and the bypass channel. The vaporizing chamber is surrounded by a water bath (1250 mL) for thermo-buffering. The water bath can be emptied for transport. There is a temperature indicator (works between 15 and 30°C), which changes form black to red. Cold water can be added if the temperature rises. Too cold or hot water should never be added due to the risk of explosion with ether. Water at room temperature should be used.

The thermostat is a small metal bellows containing liquid ether (in some cases Freon gas) attached to a spindle. The thermostat is fitted at the outlet of the vaporizing chamber below an orifice. As the temperature increases, the bellows expand. This pushes a plunger into the orifice and decreases the flow out of the vaporizing chamber. Cooling has the opposite effect.

Operation: The other important factor affecting the concentration of the vapor leaving the vaporizer is the depth of the patient's respiration.

The vaporizer is calibrated from 2 to 20% by volume with an accuracy of ± 0.75% at the 8% setting between 13 and 32°C and 4–12 L/min. The vaporizer was designed to be used as a draw-over vaporizer with an Oxford inflating bellows. It is calibrated for intermittent flows as with a spontaneously breathing patient. Inaccurate if placed between a source of IPPV and the patient. Oxford self-inflating bellows should be placed downstream when used.

The entire Epstein, Macintosh, Oxford (EMO) setup weighs over 10 kg, limiting its potential for field use. In plenum mode, the EMO only begins to perform reasonably accurately with flow rates around 10 L/min, and is therefore not ideal for pediatric use with a T piece.

Triservice Apparatus

Developed for the British defense services (Brigadier Houghton, Whiston Hospital), can be airdropped in the field by parachute, without the oxygen cylinder, weighs 25 kg. It consists of the Laerdal manual resuscitator and two OMVs. They have three folding legs to keep them upright and capacity is increased to 50 mL each. They can be used alternately to allow quick switchover between agents or used in series with halothane or ether for induction though not for maintenance. There are different scales for each agent. The vaporizers are drained after use. Wicks are metal and hence nonabsorbent. At O-position contents will not spill if inverted. The heat sink is a water bath containing ethylene glycol as antifreeze.

PLENUM VAPORIZERS

Boyle's Ether Vaporizer (Figs. 21A to C)

Manufacturer: BOC, 1920s

Classification: Plenum, variable bypass, flow-over and/or bubble through, nontemperature compensated, multiple agents—ether, trichloroethylene, chloroform, methoxyflurane, and VOC.

Construction: It is a glass bottle with a copper lid which contains a bypass channel, lever and plunger. Copper is an anticatalyst which prevents decomposition of ether. The "U" shaped inlet tube within the vaporizer and the cap of the plunger are made from unplated copper.

It is filled with 270 mL (half full, 10 ounces) liquid diethyl ether to allow room for vaporization. If Trilene or Chloroform is used, only 1 cm depth of liquid is used as they are more potent. When the plunger is depressed, the cowl descends and the gas bubbles through the agent. This allows the maximum rate of vaporization but the temperature of the system falls. As the temperature and vaporization fall the patient can awaken. A water bath may be used for thermo-buffering.

The ether bottle fell out of use due to flow dependence.[3]

Copper Kettle

Classification: Plenum, measured flow, bubble through, non-temperature compensated but has heat sink, VOC, multiple agents—originally designed for chloroform, then ether, halothane and isoflurane.

Manufacturer: Dr Lucien E Morris (1914–2011) in 1952.

Principle: A small precise volume of carrier gas is completely saturated with the anesthetic agent and a predetermined amount is added to the FGF. This differs from the percentage v/v% of the total gas flow which is used in other vaporizers. Every time the FGF is changed the vaporizer setting has to be manually changed. This system requires continuous close attention and modification.

Construction: There is a separate oxygen flowmeter for flow to the kettle. The oxygen passes through a sintered diffuser and is broken up into multiple small bubbles. This increases the surface area for vaporization and achieves complete saturation. The chamber contains a thermometer. Charts are provided

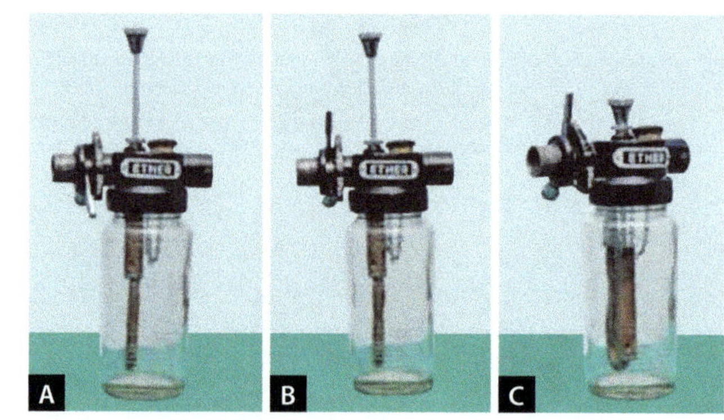

Figs. 21A to C: Boyle's ether vaporizer. (A) Off; (B) On—flowover; (C) Plunger depressed—bubble through.

for flows required for a given concentration. The computation and adjustment are done by the operator. For ether, the original heat sink was an entire table top made of copper. For halothane, a glass container is used.

This flow is then added to the diluent gas flow which is regulated with a separate set of flowmeters.

$$\text{Percentage vapor flow} = \frac{\text{Partial pressure of the anesthetic}}{\text{Atmospheric pressure}} \times 100$$

Disadvantages

- Foaming may occur.
- If the diluent gas flow falls suddenly, the patient will get an overdose of anesthetic (32% halothane, 32% isoflurane).

Siemen's KION® Vaporizer[15] (Fig. 22)

Principle: If a small amount of volatile agent is added to the FGF, ensuring its complete vaporization, there would be no need for a separate vaporization chamber with compensation for loss of latent heat of vaporization.

Manufacturer: Siemens in 1980s, for use with the Siemen's 900D ventilator.

Classification: Plenum, concentration calibrated injector, no thermocompensation needed, VOC, agent specific—halothane, isoflurane, and enflurane.

Capacity: 125 mL

Filling system: Agent specific system with different collars and port adaptors for each agent.

Construction: The concentration control dial (5) is above the agent reservoir (9) and the liquid level indicator. The filling port is to the left. On the right is the on-off valve (4) which has a release device which needs to be operated before turning on the vaporizer. The fresh gas (1), flows to the bellows (2)

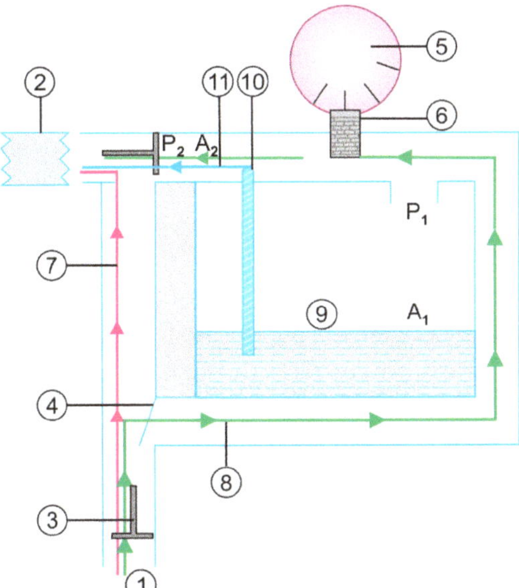

Fig. 22: Siemen's KION® vaporizer. 1. Fresh gas flow; 2. Bellows; 3. Bellows valve; 4. Vaporizer on-off valve; 5. Concentration control dial; 6. Variable resistance throttle valve; 7. Flow to bellows; 8. Flow to vaporizer; 9. Liquid agent; 10. Injector nozzle; 11. Vaporizer outlet.

when the bellows need refilling. This is controlled by the bellows valve (3).

When the vaporizer on-off valve is "ON", the FGF enters the vaporizer. The concentration control dial adjusts a throttle valve (variable resistance) (6) placed in the path of the gas flow. This generates a backpressure (P_1) which is transmitted to the surface of the liquid (A_1) in the reservoir. This generates a pressure (P_2) which forces liquid anesthetic up the capillary to the injector nozzle (10) (A_2) into the path of the gas flowing to the bellows. The liquid quickly vaporizes in the moving gas stream.

$$P_1 A_1 = P_2 A_2$$

Both A_1 and A_2 remain constant. Hence, when P_1 rises, P_2 rises and more liquid is forced through the nozzle and converted into vapor. There is no energy lost from the reservoir; hence, no thermocompensation is needed.

CONCLUSION

Vaporizer technology has evolved as new agents and new anesthesia delivery systems have come into use. In the interests of accuracy and patient safety, some agents, techniques and devices have become obsolete. Most of the systems in use today, confirm to American Society for Testing and Materials standards. They range from rudimentary draw-over vaporizers to electromechanical devices which are so accurate that they make "quantitative closed-system anesthesia delivery" possible.

This wide array of vaporizers allows versatility, safety, and accuracy when practicing the art of anesthesia under varied conditions.

REFERENCES

1. Davey AJ, Moyle TB. Ward's Anesthetic Equipment, 6th edition. Philadelphia: WB Saunders, Elsevier; 2012.
2. The Merriam-Webster Dictionary, 11th edition. Merriam-Webster, Inc; 2010.
3. Davis PD, Parbrook GD, Kenny GN. Basic Physics and Measurement in Anaesthesia, 4th edition; 2003.
4. Dorsch JA, Dorsch SE. Understanding Anesthesia Equipment's, 5th edition. Lippincott Williams & Wilkins; 2008.
5. Davey AJ, Moyle TB. Ward's Anaesthetic Equipment, 5th edition. Philadelphia: WB Saunders Elsevier; 2010.
6. Miller RD. Miller's Anaesthesia, 7th edition. Churchill Livingstone; 2010.
7. Miller RD. Miller's Anaesthesia, 8th edition. Churchill Livingstone; 2015.
8. https://www.accessdata.fda.gov/cdrh_docs/pdf10/K102182.pdf
9. Young J, Kapoor V. Principles of anaesthetic vaporizers. Anaesth Intensive Care Med. 2010;11(4):140-3.
10. Baum JA. New and alternative delivery concepts and techniques. Best Pract Res Clin Anaesthesiol. 2005;19(3):415-28.
11. Soro M, Badenes R, Garcia-Perez ML, et al. The Accuracy of the anesthetic conserving device (AnaConDa©) as an alternative to the classical vaporizer in anesthesia. Anesth Analg. 2010; 111(5):1176-9.
12. Longnecker DE, Anesthesiology, 2nd edition. McGraw Hill; 2012
13. Nicholas JH, Davies MA, Jeremy N. Lee's Synopsis of Anaesthesia, 13th edition. Philadelphia: Elsevier; 2005.
14. Davey AJ, Moyle TB. Ward's Anaesthetic Equipment, 2nd edition. Philadelphia: WB Saunders Elsevier; 2003.
15. Dorsch JA, Dorsch SE. Understanding Anaesthesia Equipments, 4th edition: Lippincott Williams & Wilkins; 2006.

Anesthetic Breathing Systems

M Ravishankar, R Sripriya

ABSTRACT

During the initial phase of development of anesthesia, the attention was mainly diverted to administering a single agent, and apparatus were developed to suit the purpose. Magill and Rowbothom were the forerunners in development of a simple anesthetic gas delivery system popularly known as the "Magill's circuit".

With introduction of cyclopropane, the explosive nature of the agent prompted Waters to develop the "to and fro" canister and use it for closed system anesthesia. As there was no proper definition for a breathing system, there were many classifications before the present classification came into existence.

The breathing systems were classified according to the method used for CO_2 elimination as:

- Breathing systems with CO_2 absorber and
- Breathing systems without CO_2 absorber.

Each was further subdivided into unidirectional flow and bidirectional flow systems. The fresh gas flow requirements for effective elimination of CO_2, for the partial rebreathing systems, when used during spontaneous breathing and controlled ventilation, are discussed in detail. The way to use the closed system for low flow anesthesia has been detailed.

INTRODUCTION

Since the introduction of diethyl ether as an anesthetic in 1846, the specialty of anesthesia has come a long way. In the initial phase, the attention was mainly diverted to administering a single agent, and apparatus were developed to suit the purpose. The reintroduction of nitrous oxide in 1868, and facility to store it in cylinders, created an interest in administering a combination of agents to anesthetize patients. Any resemblance to a breathing system was developed by Barth (1907), using his valve with a nitrous oxide cylinder, a reservoir bag, and Clover's inhaler. Different positions of the lever in the valve allowed complete rebreathing to completely breathing from the atmosphere. Developments of Boyle's machine (1917) and mastering of endotracheal intubation with a soft red rubber single lumen tube by Magill and Rowbothom were the forerunners for development of a simple anesthetic delivery system by Magill popularly known as the "Magill's circuit". Cyclopropane was introduced into clinical practice in 1929. The explosive nature of the agent prompted Waters to develop the "to and fro" canister and use it for closed system anesthesia. Brian Sword in 1936 introduced the circle system. The Ayre's T-piece was introduced in 1937, Epstein-Macintosh, Oxford (EMO) inhaler in 1941, and Minnitt's "gas and air" apparatus with demand valve in 1949.

With the introduction of many breathing systems, attempts were made to classify them in the 50s and 60s, but lack of a proper definition leads to more confusion than clarity.

DEFINITION

A breathing system is defined as an assembly of components, which connect the patient's airway to the anesthetic machine creating an artificial atmosphere, from and into which the patient breathes.

It primarily consists of:

- A fresh gas entry port or delivery tube through which the gases are delivered from the machine to the system
- A port to connect it to the patient's airway
- A reservoir for gas, in the form of a bag or a corrugated tube to meet the peak inspiratory flow requirements
- An expiratory port or valve through which the expired gas is vented to the atmosphere
- Flow directing valves and carbon dioxide absorber if total rebreathing is to be allowed, and
- Corrugated tubes for connecting these components.

REQUIREMENTS OF A BREATHING SYSTEM

The components when assembled should satisfy certain requirements: some essential, others desirable.

Essential

The breathing system must
- Deliver the gases from the machine to the alveoli in the same concentration as set and in the shortest possible time
- Effectively eliminate carbon dioxide
- Have minimal apparatus dead space and
- Have low resistance.

Desirable

Desirable requirements are on follows:
- Economy of fresh gas
- Conservation of heat
- Adequate humidification of inspired gas
- Light weight
- Convenience during use
- Efficiency during spontaneous as well as controlled ventilation (efficiency is determined in terms of CO_2 elimination and fresh gas utilization)
- Adaptability for adults, children and mechanical ventilators
- Provision to reduce theater pollution.

CLASSIFICATION OF BREATHING SYSTEMS

There are numerous classifications of breathing systems, many of them are irrelevant as they do not define a breathing system. Different researchers classified the same system under different headings, adding to confusion.[1] McMohan in 1951 classified them as open, semiclosed, and closed taking the level of rebreathing into account as follows:
- *Open:* No rebreathing
- *Semiclosed:* Partial rebreathing
- *Closed:* Total rebreathing.

Dripps et al. have classified them as insufflation, open, semiopen, semiclosed, and closed taking into account the presence or absence of reservoir, rebreathing, CO_2 absorption, and directional valves.[1] The ambiguity of the terminology used as open, semiopen, semiclosed and closed allowed inclusion of apparatus that are not breathing systems at all into the classification.

To overcome this problem, Conway[2] suggested that a functional classification be used and classified according to the method used for CO_2 elimination as:
- Breathing systems with CO_2 absorber
- Breathing systems without CO_2 absorber.

DM Miller[3] in 1988 widened the scope of this classification so as to include the enclosed afferent reservoir system.

A new breathing system called "the maxima"[4] has been designed by Miller in 1995, and to include it in the classification,[5] the enclosed afferent reservoir systems have been grouped under "displacement afferent reservoir" systems. The classification suggested in **Table 1** is a partial modification of Miller.[3]

TABLE 1: Classification of breathing systems.

Breathing systems without CO_2 absorption	*Breathing systems with CO_2 absorption*
• Unidirectional flow – Nonrebreathing systems – Circle systems • Bidirectional flow – Afferent reservoir systems - Mapleson A - Mapleson B - Mapleson C - Lack's system – Enclosed afferent reservoir systems - Miller's (1988) – Efferent reservoir systems - Mapleson D - Mapleson E - Mapleson F - Bain's system – Combined systems - Humphrey ADE[6]	• Unidirectional flow – Circle system with absorber • Bidirectional flow – To and fro system

BREATHING SYSTEMS WITHOUT CO_2 ABSORPTION

Unidirectional Flow

Nonrebreathing Systems

They use nonrebreathing valves, and there is no mixing of fresh gas and the expired gas.

Functional analysis: When the patient takes a breath, the inspiratory unidirectional valve opens and the gases flow into the patient's lungs **(Figs. 1A and B)**. The expiratory unidirectional valve closes the expiratory port during spontaneous breathing. During controlled ventilation, the reservoir bag is squeezed and the inspiratory unidirectional valve itself closes the expiratory port. At the start of expiration, the inspiratory unidirectional valve returns back to position and expiration takes place through the expiratory port, opening the expiratory valve.

The fresh gas flow (FGF) should be equal to the minute ventilation (MV) of the patient. These systems satisfy all four essential requirements, but are not very popular because of the following reasons:
1. FGF has to be constantly adjusted and is not economical.
2. There is no humidification of inspired gas.
3. There is no conservation of heat.
4. They are not convenient as the bulk of the valve has to be positioned near the patient.
5. The valves can malfunction due to condensation of moisture and lead to complications.

Circle systems: These systems are designed with a CO_2 absorber as an essential component of the system. To use it without absorber is uneconomical, as it needs an FGF more than the alveolar ventilation.

The essential components of the circle without absorber are:
- Fresh gas entry
- Two unidirectional valves

- Two interconnecting tubing (inspiratory, expiratory)
- Y-piece to connect to the patient
- Reservoir bag (RB) and
- A relief valve.

The arrangement of the components is shown in **Figure 2**.

The effect of arrangements of various components in the effective elimination of CO_2 and fresh gas economy when used with high flows were analyzed by Egar and Ethans.[7] A short description is given below.

Fresh gas inlet is usually placed between the RB and the inspiratory unidirectional valve **(Fig. 2)**. In this position (FGF), during spontaneous breathing, FG flows through the inspiratory unidirectional valve to the patient. This valve closes during exhalation due to backpressure and fresh gas flows in a retrograde direction into the reservoir bag. Exhaled gas predominantly the dead space gas will also reach the RB.

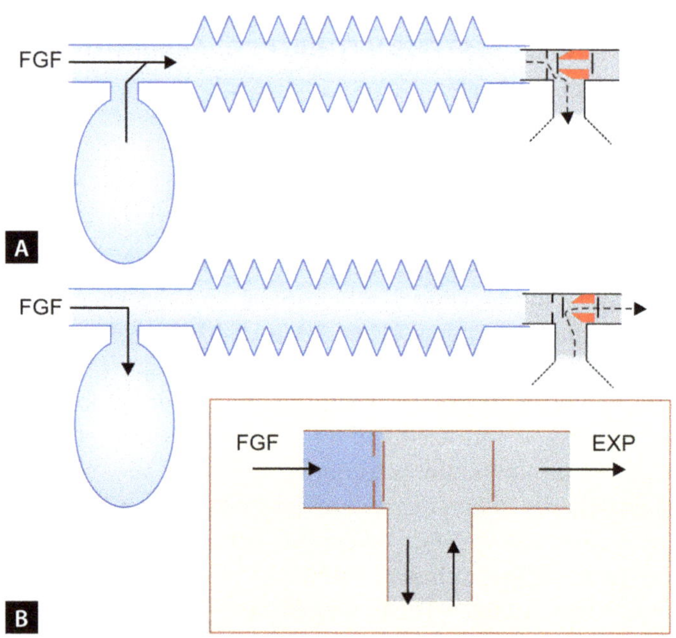

Figs. 1A and B: Nonrebreathing systems. (A) Inspiration; (B) Expiration. (FGF: fresh gas flow; EXP: expiration)

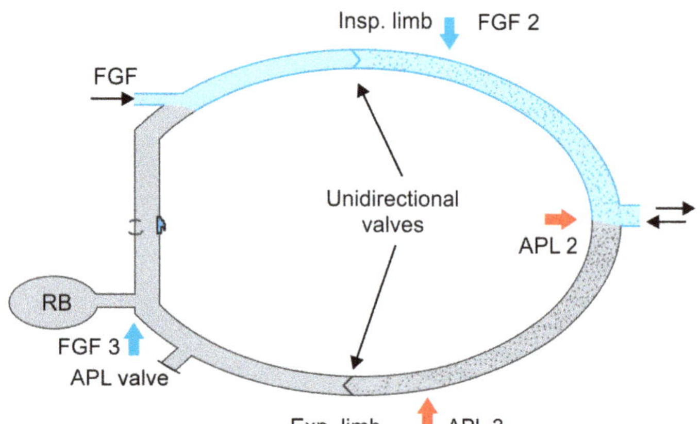

Fig. 2: Circle system without absorber. (FGF: fresh gas flow; APL valve: adjustable pressure-limiting valve; Insp: inspiration; Exp: expiration)

Once the RB is full, the adjustable pressure-limiting (APL) valve opens and the expiratory gas flowing in the expiratory limb is vented to atmosphere. The flow will be unidirectional to the patient but bidirectional between the FG entry and RB. CO_2 elimination is likely to be satisfactory if FGF is more than the alveolar ventilation.

Keeping the FG entry downstream of inspiratory unidirectional valve (FGF 2) will reflect changes in the fresh gas composition more rapidly to the patient but during exhalation, fresh gas mixes with exhaled gas and escape though the APL valve without reaching the patient. This results in poor economy of fresh gas. It needs much higher FGF for CO_2 elimination. Placing the fresh gas inlet just upstream of the RB (FGF 3) does not add any advantage, as it will prevent dead space gas from entering the RB but will be advantageous if the APL valve is positioned at the "Y" piece (APL 2) of the system.

During controlled ventilation, the APL valve has to be partly closed and the gas venting takes place during inspiration when the RB is squeezed. This leads to loss of FG through the APL valve if it is positioned downstream of the expiratory unidirectional valve. CO_2 elimination could be better if the APL valve is positioned upstream (APL 3) of the expiratory unidirectional valve.

Detailed discussion beyond this in present context is not essential.

Bidirectional Flow

Systems with bidirectional flow are extensively used. These systems depend on the FGF for effective elimination of CO_2. Understanding these systems is most important as their functioning can be manipulated by changing parameters like FGF, alveolar ventilation, apparatus dead space, etc. We will analyze these in detail.

Fresh Gas Supply

Fresh gas flow forms one of the essential requirements of a breathing system. If there is no FGF into the system, the patient will get suffocated. If the FGF is low, most systems do not eliminate CO_2 effectively, and if there is an excess flow there is wastage of gas. So, it becomes imperative to specify optimum FGF for a breathing system for efficient functioning.

"If the system has to deliver a set concentration in the shortest possible time to the alveoli, the FGF should be delivered as near the patient's airway as possible."

Elimination of Carbon Dioxide

The following may be taken as an example for better understanding of CO_2 elimination by the bidirectional flow systems. Normal production of CO_2 in a 70 kg adult is 200 mL/min, and it is eliminated through the lungs. Normal end-tidal concentration of carbon dioxide ($EtCO_2$) is 5%.

Hence, for eliminating 200 mL of CO_2 as a 5% gas mixture, the alveolar ventilation has to be:

$$\frac{200 \times 100}{5} = 4{,}000 \text{ mL}$$

This 4,000 mL or 4 L is the normal alveolar ventilation. Any breathing system connected to an adult's airway should provide a minimum of 4 L/min of CO_2 free gas to the alveoli for eliminating CO_2. If the alveolar ventilation becomes less than 4 L/min, it would lead to hypercarbia. If the alveoli are ventilated with 5 L/min of a gas containing 1% CO_2, or 8 L/min of a gas containing 2.5% CO_2, it could still eliminate 200 mL of CO_2 per minute from the alveoli. It may be construed as 4 L CO_2 free gas and 1 L of gas with 5% CO_2 in the first instant and as 4 L of CO_2 free gas and 4 L of gas with 5% CO_2 in the second instant. In effect, 4 L of alveolar ventilation with CO_2 free gas is provided in both cases.

Apparatus Dead Space

It is the volume of the breathing system from the patient-end to the point up to which to and fro movement of expired gas takes place. In an afferent reservoir system with adequate FGF, the apparatus dead space extends up to the expiratory valve positioned near the patient **(Figs. 3A to C)**. If the FG enters the system near the patient-end as in an efferent reservoir system, the dead space extends up to the point of FG entry. In systems where inspiratory and expiratory limbs are separate, it extends up to the point of bifurcation. The dynamic dead space will depend on the FGF and the alveolar ventilation. The dead space is minimal with optimal FGF. If the FGF is reduced below the optimal level, the dead space increases and the whole system will act as dead space if there is no FGF. Increasing the FGF above the optimum level will only lead to wastage of FG.

Subclassification of Bidirectional Flow Systems

Mapleson[8] did a theoretical analysis of the fresh gas requirements of the semiclosed systems available at that time. It is only proper to refer to it as "Mapleson systems" as he gave a nomenclature as A, B, C, D and E for easy identification as per their construction. For better understanding of the functional analyses, they have been classified as:

- Afferent reservoir system (ARS)
- Enclosed afferent reservoir systems (EARS)
- Efferent reservoir systems (ERS)
- Combined systems.

The afferent limb is that part of the breathing system, which delivers the fresh gas from the machine to the patient. If the reservoir is placed in this limb as in Mapleson A, B, C and Lack's systems, they are called afferent reservoir systems.

The efferent limb is that part of the breathing system, which carries expired gas from the patient and vents it to the atmosphere through the expiratory valve or port. If the reservoir is placed in this limb as in Mapleson D, E, F and Bain's systems, they are called efferent reservoir systems.

Miller and Miler[9] have described enclosed afferent reservoir system.

AFFERENT RESERVOIR SYSTEMS

The Mapleson A, B and C systems have the reservoir in the afferent limb and do not have an efferent limb **(Fig. 4)**. Lack system has an afferent limb reservoir and an efferent limb through which the expired gas traverses before being vented into the atmosphere **(Fig. 5)**. This limb is coaxially placed inside the afferent limb. "These AR systems work efficiently during spontaneous breathing provided the expiratory valve is separated from the reservoir bag and FGF by atleast one tidal volume of the patient and apparatus dead space is minimal." They do not function efficiently during controlled ventilation. If the FGF is close to the expiratory valve as in Mapleson B and C, the system is inefficient both during spontaneous and controlled ventilation. The efficiency is determined in terms of CO_2 elimination and FGF utilization.

Mapleson[8] has analyzed these bidirectional flow systems using mathematical calculations. He made a few basic assumptions while analyzing breathing systems. These are:

- Gases move enbloc. They maintain their identity as fresh gas, dead space gas and alveolar gas. There is no mixing of these gases
- The RB continues to fill up, without offering any resistance till it is full
- The expiratory valve opens as soon as the reservoir bag is full and the pressure inside the system goes above atmospheric pressure
- The valve remains open throughout the expiratory phase without offering any resistance to gas flow and closes at the start of the next inspiration.

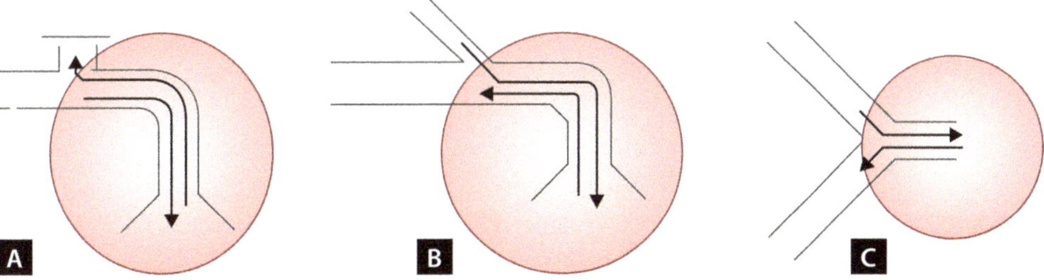

Figs. 3A to C: Apparatus dead space. (A) Magill system; (B) Efferent reservoir (ER) system; (C) Circle system.

Mapleson 'A' or Magill's System

Functional Analysis

Spontaneous breathing: The system is filled with fresh gas before connecting to the patient. When the patient inspires, the fresh gas from the machine and the reservoir bag flows to the patient, and as a result the reservoir bag collapses **(Fig. 6A)**. During expiration, the FG continues to flow into the system and fill the reservoir bag. The expired gas, initial part of which is the dead space gas, pushes the FG from the corrugated tube into the reservoir bag and collects inside the corrugated tube **(Fig. 6B)**. As soon as the RB is full, the expiratory valve opens and the alveolar gas is vented into the atmosphere **(Fig. 6C)**. During the expiratory pause, alveolar gas that had come into the corrugated tube is also pushed out through the valve, depending on the FGF. The system is filled with only fresh gas and dead space gas at the start of the next inspiration when FGF is equal to the alveolar ventilation **(Fig. 6D)**. All the alveolar gas and dead space gas are vented through the valve and some FG also escapes, if the FGF is higher than the minute ventilation. Some amount of alveolar gas will remain in the system and lead to rebreathing with an FGF less than the alveolar ventilation. This has been confirmed theoretically and experimentally by many investigators.[8,10] The system functions at maximum efficiency, when the FGF equals the alveolar ventilation, the dead space gas (which has not taken part in gas exchange) is rebreathed and utilized for alveolar ventilation.

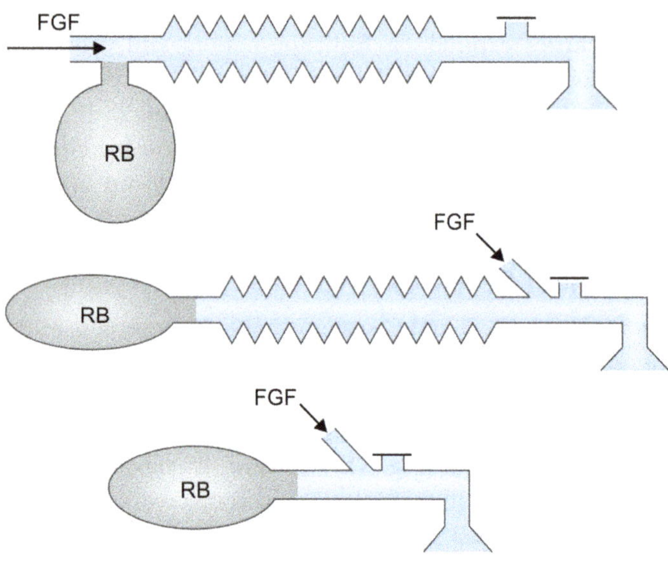

Fig. 4: Afferent reservoir systems. Mapleson A, B and C. (FGF: fresh gas flow; RB: reservoir bag)

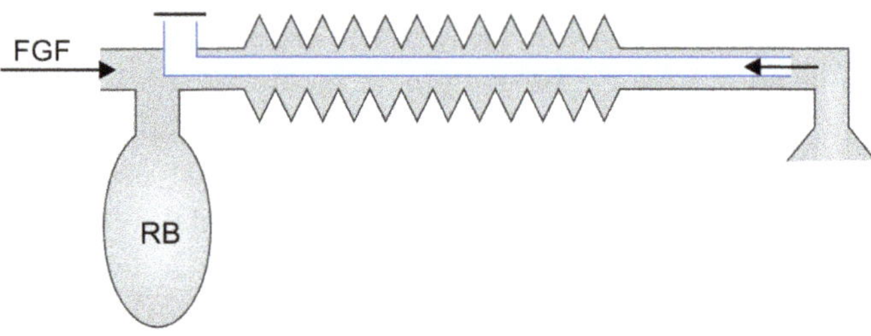

Fig. 5: Lack's system. (FGF: fresh gas flow; RB: reservoir bag)

Controlled ventilation: To facilitate intermittent positive pressure ventilation (IPPV) the expiratory valve has to be partly closed. During inspiration, the patient gets ventilated with FG and part of the FG is vented through the valve **(Fig. 7A)** after sufficient pressure has developed to open the valve. During expiration, the FG from the machine flows into the RB and all the expired gas (i.e., dead space gas and alveolar gas) flows back into the corrugated tube till the system is full **(Figs. 7B and C)**. During the next inspiration, the alveolar gas is pushed back into the alveoli followed by the FG. When sufficient pressure is developed, part of the

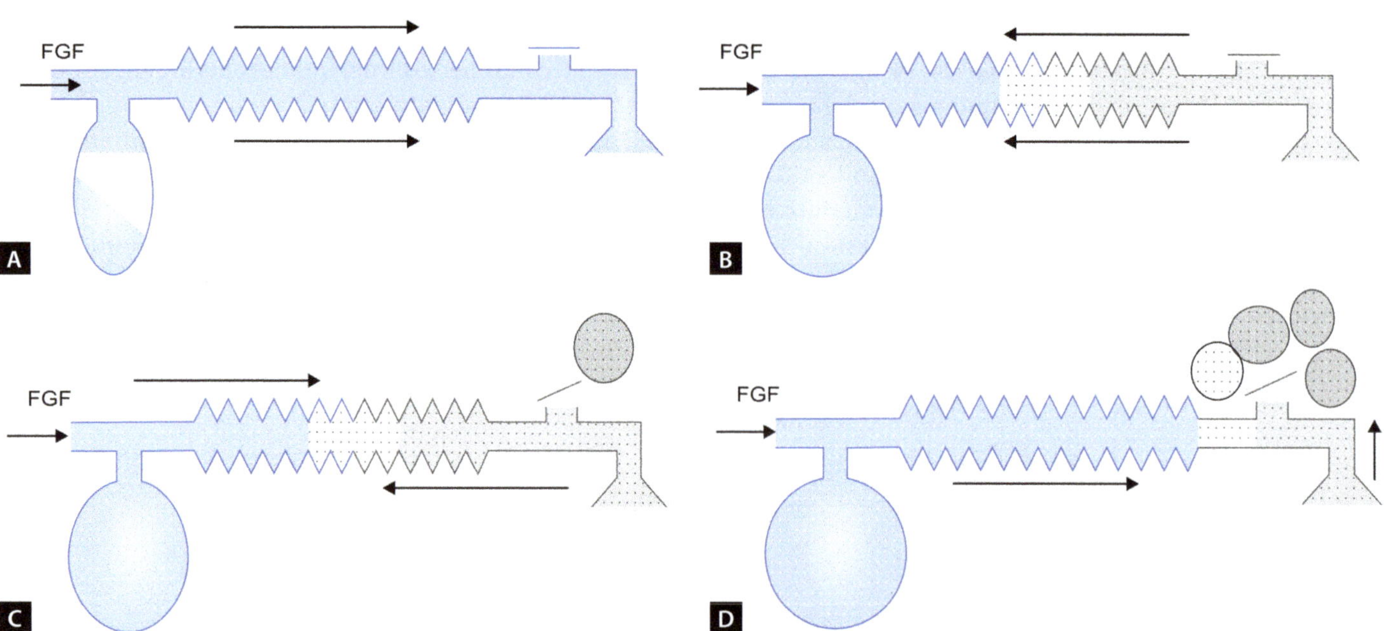

Figs. 6A to D: Afferent reservoir systems: Spontaneous breathing. (A) Inspiration; (B) Early expiration; (C) Late expiration; (D) Expiratory pause. (FGF: fresh gas flow)

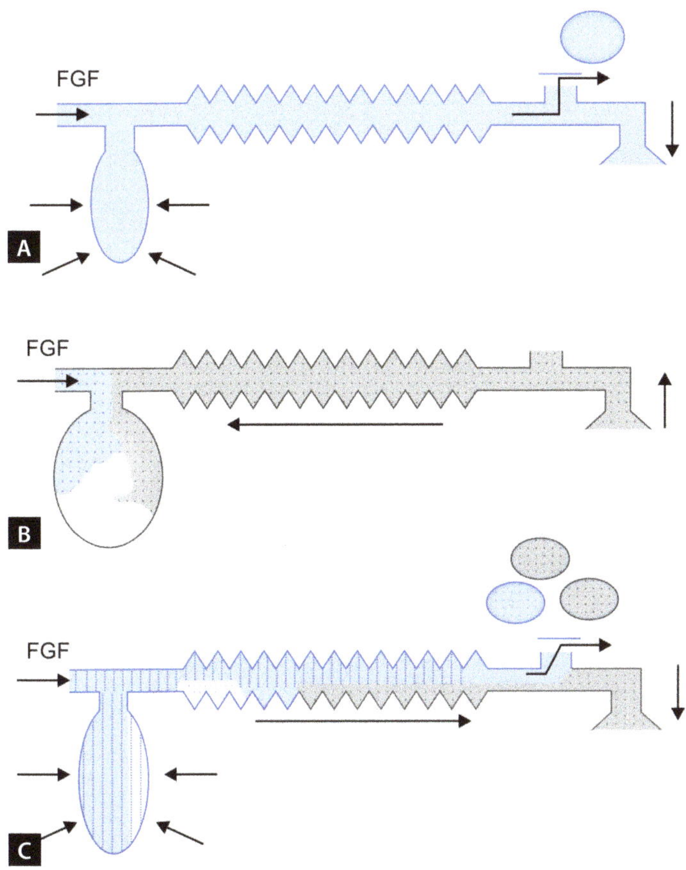

Figs. 7A to C: Afferent reservoir systems. (A) Inspiration; (B) Expiration; (C) Next inspiration. (FGF: fresh gas flow)

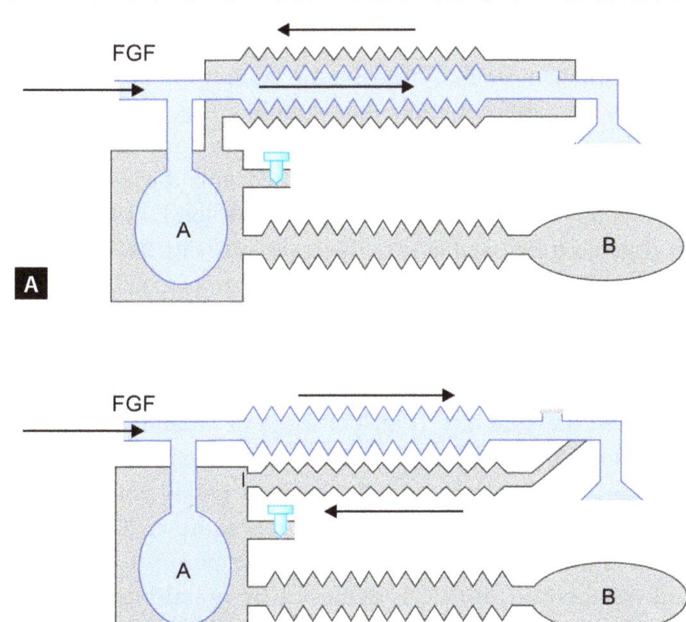

Figs. 8A and B: Enclosed afferent reservoir system. (A) Whole system enclosed; (B) Only reservoir enclosed. (FGF: fresh gas flow)

expired gas and part of the FG escape through the valve **(Fig. 7C)**. This leads to considerable rebreathing, as well as excessive waste of fresh gas. Hence, these systems are inefficient for controlled ventilation.

Lack's System

This system functions like a Mapleson A system both during spontaneous and controlled ventilation. The only difference is that the expired gas instead of getting vented through the valve near the patient is carried by an efferent tube placed coaxially and vented through the valve placed near the machine end **(Fig. 5)**. This facilitates easy scavenging of expired gas.

Mapleson B and C Systems

In order to reduce the rebreathing of alveolar gas and to improve the utilization of FG during controlled ventilation, the FG entry was shifted near the patient. This allows a complete mixing of FG and expired gas. The end result is that these systems are neither efficient during spontaneous nor during controlled ventilation.

Enclosed Afferent Reservoir Systems

This has been described by Miller and Miller.[9] The system consisted of a Mapleson A system enclosed within a non-distensible structure **(Fig. 8A)**. It may also be constructed by enclosing the RB alone in a bottle and connecting the expiratory port to the bottle with a corrugated tube and a one way valve **(Fig. 8B)**. To the bottle is also attached a reservoir bag and a "variable orifice" for providing positive pressure ventilation.

Functional Analysis

During spontaneous ventilation, the gas is vented from the system in a manner which is identical to the Mapleson A system. In this mode, the variable orifice is kept widely open to allow free communication to the atmosphere. In controlled ventilation, the reservoir bag "B" is squeezed intermittently and the variable orifice is partly closed to allow building-up of pressure in the bottle. The pressure thus developed closes the expiratory valve, and squeezes the enclosed afferent reservoir and the patient gets ventilated. The expiration takes place in a manner similar to that described during spontaneous ventilation when the pressure is released in reservoir "B". Hence, this system should function efficiently during spontaneous and controlled ventilation with an FGF equivalent to alveolar ventilation. The fresh gas requirement and the utilization of this system has been investigated by a group of investigators from Manchester[11-13] and a group from Wales[14] under the guidance of Mapleson. They have reported varying figures for utilization as 82%, 93% and 74%, respectively.[11,12,14] The reasons for this lesser percentage of utilization have been quoted as faulty methodology for calculation,[15] resistance offered by the reservoir bag and tubing and early opening of the unidirectional valve during expiration,[14] etc. Though the fresh gas requirement is higher than the alveolar ventilation in this system as shown by the above studies, it is still more efficient than the Bain's system for controlled ventilation.

Efferent Reservoir Systems

The Mapleson D, E, F and Bain's systems have a 6 mm tube as the afferent limb that supplies the FG from the machine. The efferent limb is a wide-bore corrugated tube to which the reservoir bag is attached and the expiratory valve is positioned near the bag. In Mapleson E system, the corrugated tube itself acts as the reservoir **(Fig. 9)**. In Bain's system, the afferent and efferent limbs are coaxially placed **(Fig. 10)**.

All these ER systems are modification of Ayre's T-piece. This consists of a light metal tube 1 cm in diameter, 5 cm in length with a side arm **(Fig. 11)**. Used as such, it functions as a nonrebreathing system. Fresh gas enters the system through the side arm and the expired gas is vented into the atmosphere and there is no rebreathing. The dead space is minimal as it is only up to the point of FG entry and elimination of CO_2 is achieved by breathing into the atmosphere. FGF equal to peak inspiratory flow rate of the patient has to be used to prevent air dilution.

In an attempt to reduce FGF requirements, ER systems are constructed with reservoirs in the efferent limb. The functioning of all these systems is similar. "These systems work efficiently and economically for controlled ventilation as long as a volume equivalent to at least one tidal volume of the patient separates the FG entry and the expiratory valve." They are not economical during spontaneous breathing.

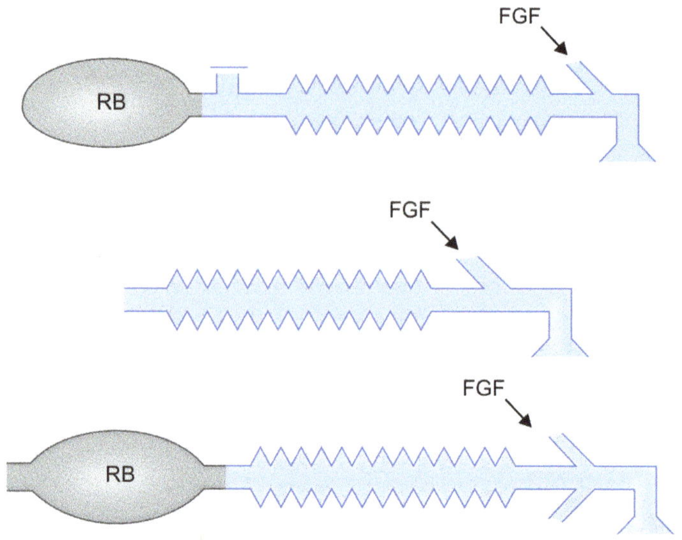

Fig. 9: Efferent reservoir systems. Mapleson D, E, and F. (FGF: fresh gas flow; RB: reservoir bag)

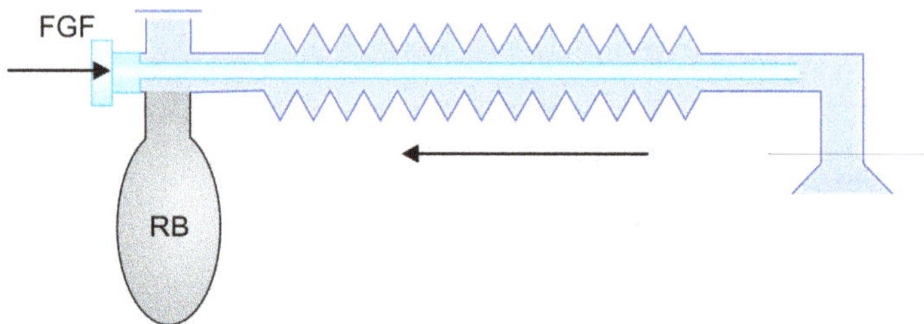

Fig. 10: Bain's system. (FGF: fresh gas flow; RB: reservoir bag)

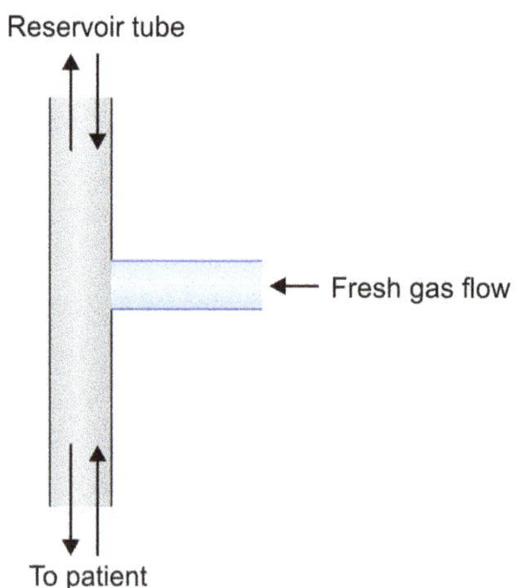

Fig. 11: Ayre's T-piece.

Functional Analysis

Spontaneous respiration: The breathing system should be filled with FG before connecting to the patient. When the patient takes an inspiration, the FG from the machine, the reservoir bag and the corrugated tube flow to the patient **(Fig. 12A)**. During expiration, there is a continuous FGF into the system at the patient end. The expired gas gets continuously mixed with the FG as it flows back into the corrugated tube and the reservoir bag **(Fig. 12B)**. Once the system is full the excess gas is vented to the atmosphere through the valve situated at the end of the corrugated tube near the reservoir bag. During the expiratory pause the FG continues to flow and fill the proximal portion of the corrugated tube while the mixed gas is vented through the valve **(Fig. 12C)**. During the next inspiration, the patient breathes FG as well as the mixed gas from the corrugated tube **(Fig. 12D)**. Many factors influence the composition of the inspired mixture. They are FGF, respiratory rate, expiratory pause, tidal volume and CO_2 production in the body. Factors other than FGF cannot be manipulated in a spontaneously breathing patient. It has been mathematically calculated and clinically proved[8,16] that the FGF should be at least 1.5–2 times the patient's minute ventilation in order to minimize rebreathing to acceptable levels.

Controlled ventilation: To facilitate IPPV, the expiratory valve has to be partly closed so that it opens only after sufficient pressure has developed in the system. When the system is filled with fresh gas, the patient gets ventilated with the FGF from the machine, the corrugated tube and the reservoir bag **(Fig. 13A)**. During expiration, the expired gas continuously gets mixed with the fresh gas that is flowing into the system at the patient end. During the expiratory pause the FG continues to enter the system and pushes the mixed gas towards the reservoir **(Fig. 13B)**. When the next inspiration is initiated, the patient gets ventilated with the gas in the corrugated tube, i.e., a mixture of FG, alveolar gas and dead space gas **(Fig. 13C)**. As the pressure in the system increases, the expiratory valve opens and the contents of the reservoir bag are discharged into the atmosphere.

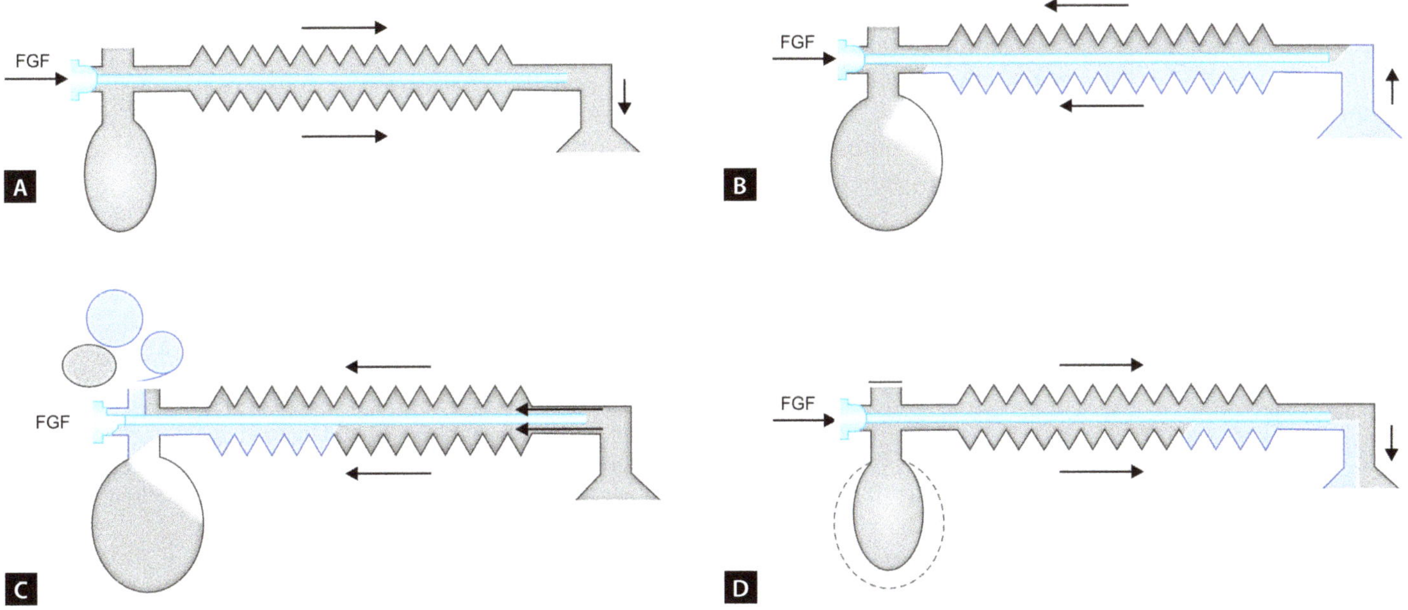

Figs. 12A to D: Efferent reservoir system: Spontaneous breathing. (A) Inspiration; (B) Early expiration; (C) Expiratory pause; (D) Next inspiration. (FGF: fresh gas flow)

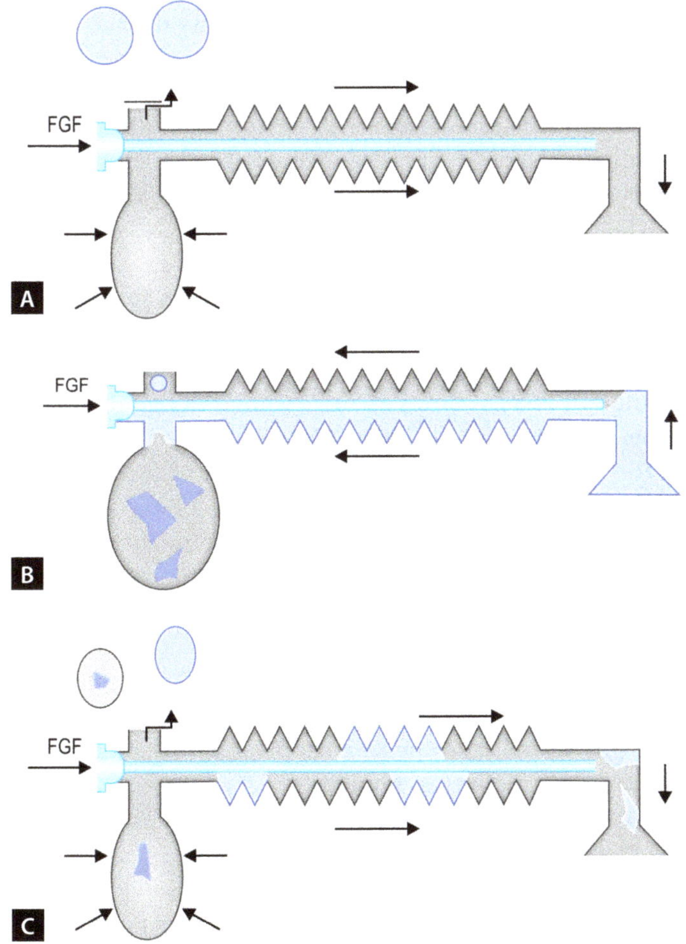

Figs. 13A to C: Efferent reservoir system: Controlled ventilation. (A) Inspiration; (B) Expiration; (C) Next inspiration. (FGF: fresh gas flow)

Factors that influence the composition of gas mixture in the corrugated tube with which the patient gets ventilated are the same as for spontaneous respiration, namely FGF, respiratory rate, tidal volume and pattern of ventilation.

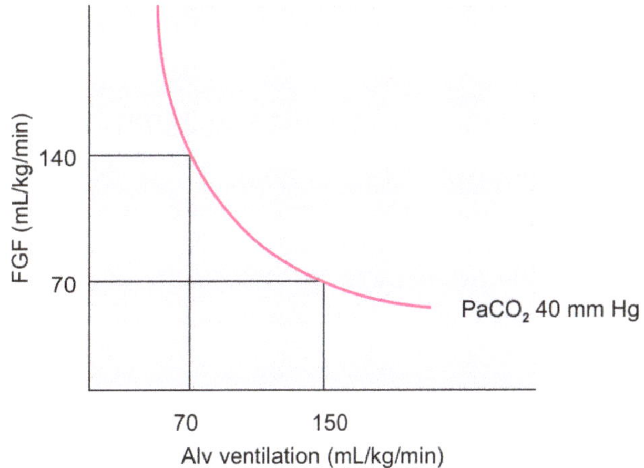

Fig. 14: Relationship between fresh gas flow (FGF) and alveolar ventilation. (FGF: fresh gas flow; Alv: alveolar)
Source: Rose DK, Froese AB. The regulation of PaCO2 during controlled ventilation of children with a T-piece. Can Anaesth Soc J. 1979;26: 104-13.

The only difference is that these parameters can be totally controlled by the anesthesiologist and do not depend on the patient. Using a low respiratory rate with a long expiratory pause and a high tidal volume, most of the FG could be utilized for alveolar ventilation without wastage.

Analyzing the performance of these systems during controlled ventilation, two relationships have become evident (i) when FGF is very high the partial pressure of carbon dioxide in the blood ($PaCO_2$) becomes ventilation dependent (as during spontaneous respiration) and, (ii) when the minute volume exceeds the FGF substantially, the $PaCO_2$ is dependent on the FGF.[17] Combining these influences a graph can be constructed as shown in **Figure 14**. An infinite number of combinations of FGF and minute ventilation can be chosen to achieve a desired $PaCO_2$. One can use a high FGF and a normal minute volume of

70 mL/kg to achieve a normal $PaCO_2$ of 40 mm Hg. This is uneconomical and leads to low humidity and heat loss. Alternately, an FGF equivalent to the predicted minute volume, i.e., 70 mL/kg can be chosen and the patient ventilated with at least twice the predicted minute volume, i.e., 140 mL/kg. Here, a deliberate controlled rebreathing is allowed in order to maintain normal $PaCO_2$ along with high humidity, less heat loss and greater economy of fresh gas. Combinations between these two extremes can also be used. It is important to remember that using a low FGF with normal minute ventilation, can lead to hypercarbia; a moderate FGF and hyperventilation, can lead to hypocarbia.

Combined Systems

To overcome the difficulties of changing the breathing systems for different modes of ventilation, Humphrey designed a system called Humphrey ADE,[18] with two reservoirs, one in the afferent limb and the other in the efferent limb. While in use, only one reservoir will be in operation and changing the position of a lever can change the system from ARS to ERS. It can be used for adults as well as children. The functional analysis is the same as Mapleson A in ARS mode and as Bain in ERS mode. It is not yet widely used.

BREATHING SYSTEMS WITH CO_2 ABSORPTION

Systems so far described have relied on FGF for effective elimination of CO_2. Any desire to economize on FGF by allowing a total rebreathing, should be accompanied by removal of the expired CO_2 by chemical absorption. The systems designed for these purpose are again classified as:

- Unidirectional flow
  - Circle system
- Bidirectional flow
  - To and fro system

Design of Circle Systems

The essential components of the circle system are:

- A CO_2 absorbent canister
- Two unidirectional valves
- Fresh gas entry
- Y-piece to connect to the patient
- Reservoir bag
- Adjustable pressure relief valve and
- Low resistance interconnecting tubing.

The arrangement of the components is shown in **Figure 15.**

For efficient functioning of the system the following criteria should be fulfilled.

- There should be two unidirectional valves on either side of the reservoir bag
- APL valve should be positioned in the expiratory limb only
- The FGF should enter the system proximal to the inspiratory unidirectional valve.

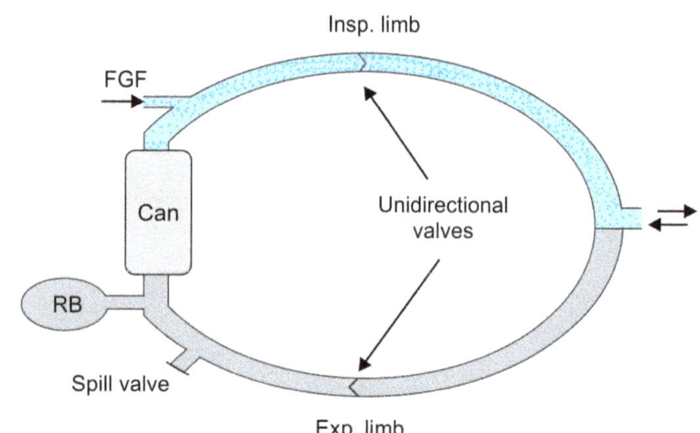

Fig. 15: Schematic diagram of a circle system. (FGF: fresh gas flow; RB: reservoir bag; Insp: inspiration; Exp: expiration)

Functional analysis: During inspiration the FG along with the CO_2 free gas in the RB flow through the inspiratory limb and inspiratory unidirectional valve to the patient. No flow takes place in the expiratory limb as the expiratory unidirectional valve is closed by backpressure transmitted to the valve. During expiration the inspiratory unidirectional valve closes and the expired gas flows through the expiratory unidirectional valve in the expiratory limb to the CO_2 absorbent canister and to the RB. The CO_2 is absorbed in the canister. The FGF from the machine continues to fill the reservoir bag. When the reservoir is full the APL valve opens and the excess gas is vented to atmosphere. By selecting a suitable position for the APL valve, the expired gas can be selectively vented when the FGF is more than the alveolar ventilation. To facilitate controlled ventilation the APL valve has to be partly closed and the excess gas is vented during inspiration. The gas flow pattern is similar to that described above.

The advantages and disadvantages of the various arrangements of the components were analyzed by Eger and Ethans.[7] The relative positions of the components of the circle system are of particular importance to the functioning of the system only when the FGF is high, the gas components of the system unmixed and CO_2 absorber not used. When the FGF is reduced below the alveolar ventilation, the CO_2 absorber is a must as the gas in the system become more uniformly mixed, and the relative position of the system's components become less important.

Low Flow Anesthesia

The technique of reusing the expired gas for alveolar ventilation after absorption of CO_2 can be traced to the very beginning of anesthesia when Dr John Snow used caustic potash to absorb CO_2 from the expired gas. This concept was considerably simplified by the introduction of "To and Fro" system by Waters and the circle system by Brian Sword, which utilized sodalime for absorption of CO_2. It reigned supreme in the early half of this century when expensive and explosive agents like cyclopropane were utilized. The introduction of nonexplosive agents like halothane and plenum vaporizers that performed optimally only in the presence of higher flows, resulted low flow anesthesia becoming less popular. With the added knowledge of the disadvantages of using high percentages of O_2 for prolonged periods and the necessity to use a second gas to control the percentage of oxygen, coupled with the complexities involved in the calculation of uptake of anesthetic agents during the closed circuit anesthesia, made this technique even less popular.[19] However, the awareness of the dangers of theater pollution with trace amounts of the anesthetic agents and the prohibitively high cost of the new inhalational agents, have helped in the rediscovery of low flow anesthesia.

Baker,[20] in his editorial had classified the FGF used in anesthetic practice into the following categories:

Metabolic flow	:	About 250 mL/min.
Minimal flow	:	250–500 mL/min.
Low flow	:	500–1000 mL/min.
Medium flow	:	1–2 L/min.

For most practical considerations, utilization of a fresh gas flow less than 2 L/min may be considered as low flow anesthesia.

Equipment: The minimum requirement for conduct of low flow anesthesia is a circle system with efficient CO_2 absorber and leak not exceeding 200 mL.

Monitoring

Inspired O_2 concentration should be monitored at all times if N_2O is used in more than 65% concentration, as one of the adjuvant gas. $EtCO_2$ monitoring seems to be necessary to ensure proper functioning of the absorber. If monitoring of end tidal anesthetic concentration is available, the administration of low flow anesthesia becomes very easy.

Concerns during Low Flow Anesthesia

- Is there a risk of delivery of hypoxic mixture?
- What is concentration of agent in the inspired gas?
- Sevoflurane—Can it be used?
- Changing agent concentration as and when required—Is it possible?
- How will be the recovery when used for prolonged period?

Delivery of hypoxic mixture: The dynamics of closed system should be understood clearly to dispel this concern. During inspiration the flow takes place through the inspiratory unidirectional valve to the patient. During expiration, the gas mixture from the lung flows through the expiratory limb and expiratory unidirectional valve to the RB. It does not flow back through the inspiratory limb as the inspiratory unidirectional valve closes due to backpressure. During next inspiration, the gas mixture in the RB flows through the sodalime canister where the CO_2 is removed and through the inspiratory unidirectional valve. During the process it gets mixed with the FG flowing from the machine **(Fig. 16)**. As the FGF is in the range of 500–1000 mL, and the total minute ventilation in the range of 4–5 L, the gas coming from the RB where the oxygen percentage is equal to the expired oxygen percentage determines the composition of the gas breathed in. If the expired oxygen percentage is maintained above 25%, then there is no chance of delivering a hypoxic mixture to the patient.

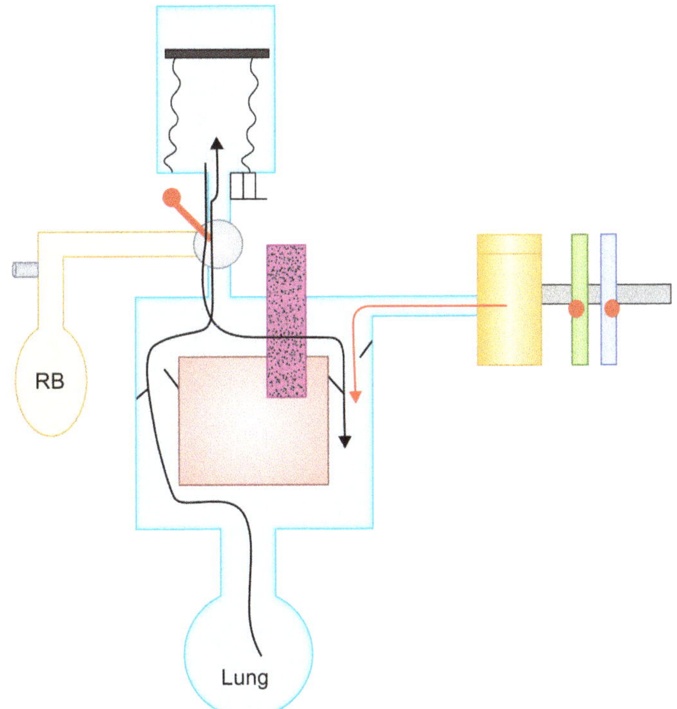

Fig. 16: Dynamics of gas flow in circle system. (RB: reservoir bag)

Uncertain agent concentration: The explanation is same as above as the mass of volatile agent is less in the FG delivered, and the inspired gas is always a mixture of FG and the gas from the RB, the concentration of gas in the inspired mixture will always be less than the dial setting. Other factors like alveolar ventilation, cardiac output and blood gas solubility will determine the alveolar concentration. Hence, it is imperative to have knowledge of uptake and distribution to reasonably predict the agent concentration in the alveoli in the absence of agent monitoring. Still, regimens suggested by experts after carrying out studies can satisfactorily be used. Computer simulations like the Gas Man® can enhance the practice to a greater extent.

Sevoflurane—Can it be used?: This should not be a concern now, as it has been consistently shown that with the use of absorbents that does not contain KOH and NaOH, the concentration of compound A and methanol are considerably less. Such absorbents are now available in India and can safely be used.

Changing agent concentration as and when required—Is it possible?: With less soluble agents like desflurane and sevoflurane, it is possible to change concentration in the alveoli by increasing the flow as well as the agent concentration to higher levels for a short period of time. The flow can be reduced to low flow after a minute. It can be better understood using the Gas Man® simulations.

How will be the recovery when used for prolonged period?: If the FGF is increased to 6–8 L at the end of surgery, the washout of agent will be similar to using high gas flows through out the case. The pattern of recovery will be similar for less soluble agents.

Suggested Technique

The patient may be induced and intubated using intravenous agents and connected to circle system with CO_2 absorber. Start with a total FGF of 100 mL/kg for initial 10 minutes, N_2O to O_2 ratio of 60:40 along with 1.5% isoflurane or 3% sevoflurane. FGF can be reduced to 300 mL/min of N_2O and 300 mL/min of O_2 at the end of 10 minutes without changing the dial setting of 1.5% isoflurane or 3% sevoflurane for the rest of the period. This will maintain the anesthetic depth of 1–1.2 MAC. Combining it with a narcotic agent will ensure steady state anesthesia. If the agent is cut off 10 minutes before end of surgery without changing the gas flow and resort to high flow of oxygen 8 L/min at the end of surgery, the patients will recover smoothly in 7–9 minutes time.

A number of advantages have been demonstrated for low flow systems.

- *Economy:* The FGF could be reduced to as low as 500–1000 mL.
- *Humidification:* In the low flow system, once the equilibrium has been established, the inspired gas will be fully saturated with water vapor.[21]
- *Reduction of heat loss:* In addition to conserving water the low flow system will also conserve heat. The CO_2 absorption is an exothermic reaction and the system may actively assist in maintaining body temperature.
- *Reduction in atmospheric pollution:* The loss from the system will equal the FGF minus the CO_2 that is absorbed; hence, the reduction in atmospheric pollution.

The technique has potential disadvantages:

- A greater knowledge of uptake and distribution is required.
- Real danger of hypercapnia may result from
  - An inactive absorber
  - Incompetent unidirectional valves and
  - Incorrect use of absorber bypass, necessitating $EtCO_2$ monitoring as mandatory.

Bidirectional Flow Systems

The Waters "to and fro" system is valveless and conveniently portable. It has been widely used in the past and now is only of historical importance and hence not discussed.

REFERENCES

1. Dorsch JA, Dorsch SE. Breathing Systems II. In: Dorsch JA, Dorsch SE (Eds). Understanding Anaesthesia Equipment, 2nd edition. Baltimore: Williams & Wilkins; 1984.
2. Conway CM. Anaesthetic breathing systems. Br J Anaesth. 1985;57:649-57.
3. Miller DM. Breathing systems for use in anaesthesia. Evaluation using a physical lung model and classification. Br J Anaesth. 1988;60:555-64.
4. Miller DM. An enclosed efferent afferent reservoir system: the Maxima. Anaesth Intensive Care. 1995;23:284-91.
5. Miller DM. Breathing systems reclassified. Anaesth Intensive Care. 1995;23:281-3.
6. Miller DM, Palm A. Comparison in spontaneous ventilation of the Maxima with the Humphrey ADE breathing system and between four methods for detecting rebreathing. Anaesth Intensive Care. 1995;23:296-301.
7. Eager EI, Ethans CT. The effects of inflow, overflow and valve placement on economy of circle system. Anesthesiology. 1968;29:93-100.
8. Mapleson WW. The elimination of rebreathing in various semiclosed anaesthetic systems. Br J Anaesth. 1988;26:323-32.
9. Miller DM, Miller JC. Enclosed afferent reservoir breathing systems. Description and clinical evaluation. Br J Anaesth. 1988;60:469-75.
10. White DC, Calkins J. Anaesthetic machine and breasting apparatus. In: Nunn JF, Utting JE, Brown BR (Eds). General Anaesthesia, 5th edition. London: Butterworths; 1989. pp. 428-56.
11. Droppert PM, Meakin G, Beatty PC, et al. Efficiency of a new afferent reservoir breathing system during controlled ventilation. Br J Anaesth. 1991;66:638-42.
12. Meakin G, Jennings AD, Beatty PC, et al. Fresh gas requirements of an enclosed afferent reservoir breathing system during controlled ventilation in children. Br J Anaesth. 1992;68:43-7.
13. Beatty PC, Meakin G, Healy TE. Fractional delivery of fresh gas: a new index of the efficiency of semiclosed breathing systems. Br J Anaesth. 1992;68:474-7.
14. Tham EJ, Davies R, Slade JM, et al. Efficiency of breathing systems A and D in the Carden Ventmasta ventilator. Br J Anaesth. 1993; 71:741-6.
15. Ravishankar M, Chatterjee S. Fractional utilisation of fresh gas by breathing systems without carbon dioxide absorption. Br J Anaesth. 1993;71:706-7.
16. Ward CS. Anaesthetic Equipment: Physical Principles and Maintenance, 2nd edition. London: WB Saunders; 1985.
17. Rose DK, Froese AB. The regulation of $PaCO_2$ during controlled ventilation of children with a T-piece. Can Anaesth Soc J. 1979;26:104-13.
18. Humphrey D. A new anaesthetic breathing system combining Mapleson A, D and E principles. A simple apparatus for low flow universal use without carbon dioxide absorption. Anaesthesia. 1983;38:361-72.
19. Baum JA, Aitkenhead AR. Low flow anaesthesia. Anaesthesia. 1995;50:37-44.
20. Baker AB. Low flow and Closed Circuits. Anaesth Intensive Care. 1994;22:341-2.
21. Kleemann PP. Humidity of anaesthetic gases with respect to low flow anaesthesia. Anaesth Intensive Care. 1994;22(4):396-408.

Anesthesia Ventilators

Anila D Malde

ABSTRACT

Modern anesthesia ventilators are classified depending on drive mechanism, circuit design, type of bellows, and modes. Bellows in a box is the most commonly used design. Ascending bellows are preferred over descending bellows as disconnection or leak can be easily made out. Tidal volume (VT) discrepancy, excessive pressure, and disconnection are the most commonly encountered problems. Fresh gas compensation and fresh gas decoupling (FGD) have solved the problems to a certain extent. With the FGD, descending bellows have returned into practice. Piston based design, volume reflector, turbine technology, accuracy of delivery of small VTs, closer location of flow sensor, suitability of low flow system, and availability of multiple modes including spontaneous ones are some of the advanced features. Pressure, volume monitoring, graphic analysis, and appropriate setting of alarm limits can make anesthesia ventilators quite safe.

INTRODUCTION

The ventilator on the modern anesthesia workstation serves as a mechanized substitute for the manual squeezing of the reservoir bag of the circle system, the Bain's circuit, or another breathing system. In most contemporary machines, ventilator replaces the reservoir bag in the breathing system. It may be connected to the breathing system by a bag/ventilator selector valve **(Fig. 1)**. On some newer workstations, turning the bag/ventilator selector switch to the ventilator position or a mode selection switch turns ON the ventilator. On other ventilators, there is an ON-OFF switch.[1,2]

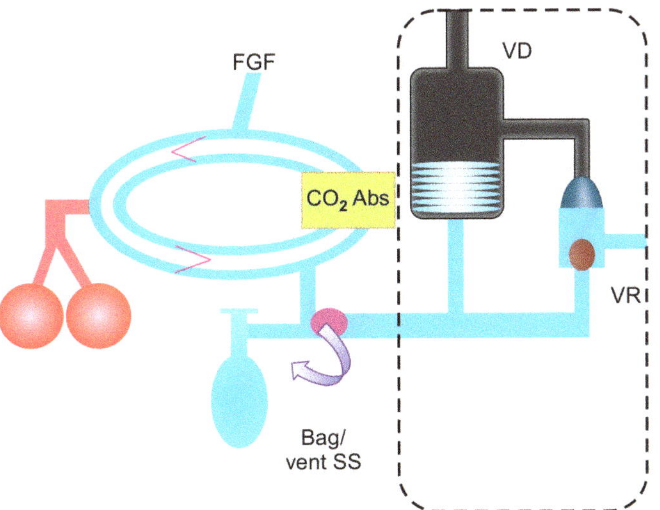

Fig. 1: Classic circle system with bag/ventilator selector switch. (Bag/vent SS: bag/ventilator selector switch; CO_2 Abs: carbon dioxide absorber; FGF: fresh gas flow; VD: ventilator driving gas; VR: ventilator relief valve or spill valve)

Classification of anesthesia ventilators is mentioned in **Box 1**.

BOX 1: Classification of anesthesia ventilators.[1,2]

- Power source
  - Compressed gas
  - Electricity
  - Both
- Drive mechanism and circuit designation
  - *Double-circuit ventilators with bellows:* A driving force such as pressurized gas compresses a component analogous to the reservoir bag known as the ventilator bellows. The bellows then in turn delivers ventilation to the patient
    - Driving gas
      - 100% oxygen in the Datex-Ohmeda 7000, 7800, 7100, and 7900
      - Oxygen and air through a venturi device in the North American Dräger AV-E and AV-2+
      - User selectable compressed air or oxygen in some newer pneumatic anesthesia workstations
  - Piston-driven single-circuit ventilators
  - Reflector
  - Turbine
- Bellows
  - Ascending (standing) bellows ascend during the expiratory phase
  - Descending (hanging) bellows descend during the expiratory phase
- Modes
  - Volume-controlled mode (VCV)
  - Pressure-controlled mode (PCV)
  - Synchronized intermittent mandatory ventilation mode (SIMV)
  - Pressure support mode (PSV)
  - PSV-Pro
  - PCV with volume guarantee
- Inspiratory phase
  - Time triggering
    - Timing device
      - Fluidic timing device in older pneumatic ventilators
      - Solid-state electronic timing device in contemporary electronic ventilators
  - Pressure triggering (adjustable) in more advanced ventilation modes, such as SIMV, and pressure-support mode

BAG IN A BOTTLE, DOUBLE CIRCUIT ANESTHESIA VENTILATOR[1-4]

It has bellows in a box design. The components are driving gas, bellows, bellows housing, spill valve, drive gas exhaust valve, ventilator hose, and positive end-expiratory pressure (PEEP) valve. The bellows assembly consists of a rubber or latex-free material bellows in a clear rigid plastic enclosure and inside of the bellows is connected to the breathing system. The pressurized oxygen or air from the ventilator power outlet (45–50 psig) is routed to the space between the inside wall of the plastic enclosure and the outside wall of the bellows. The ventilator contains its own pressure-relief (pop-off) valve, called the spill valve. The pressure of the anesthesia provider's hand is replaced by the driving gas pressure that compresses the bellows **(Fig. 2)** and during inspiration, the driving gas flows between the bellows and its housing. The force of the driving gas compresses bellows and the gases inside the bellows pass to breathing system. At the same time, a side stream of the driving gas closes the spill valve (disc valve in Datex Ohmeda ventilator or ball valve of the Dräger ventilators). Thus, during inspiration, the gases are not allowed to pass out through spill valve **(Fig. 3)**. During expiration, the bellows re-expands as breathing system gases and fresh gas flow into it **(Fig. 4)**. The driving gas is vented to atmosphere through the exhaust valve and after the bellows is fully expanded, excess gas from the breathing system is vented through the spill valve. The bellows refill first because a weighted ball or similar device is incorporated into the base of the ventilator relief valve. This ball produces 2–3 cm water of back pressure; therefore, spill valve opens only after the bellows fills completely and the pressure inside the bellows exceeds the pressure threshold of the "ball valve." This design causes all ascending bellows ventilators to produce 2–3 cm water pressure of PEEP within the breathing circuit when the ventilator is in use.

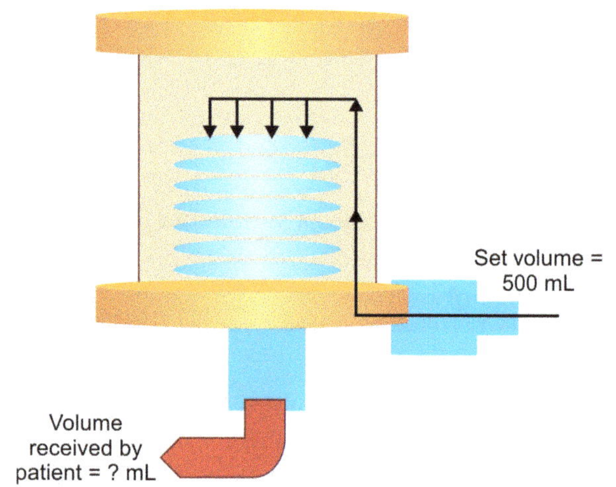

Fig. 2: Bellow-based ventilator depicting compression-induced loss.

Adding PEEP decreases the VT delivered, with the effect greater with small VTs. On newer ventilators with integral PEEP, ventilation may be better maintained.

Most contemporary electronic ventilators have an ascending bellows design. Examples include the Dräger Medical AV-E, AV-2+, the Datex-Ohmeda 7000, 7800, and 7900 series **(Table 1)**. Very few ventilators have descending bellows design **(Figs. 5 and 6)**. Out of the two configurations, the ascending bellows is generally safer. An ascending bellows will not fill if a total disconnection occurs **(Fig. 7)**. However, the bellows of a descending bellows ventilator will continue its upward and downward movement despite a patient disconnection. The driving gas pushes the bellows upward during the inspiratory phase.

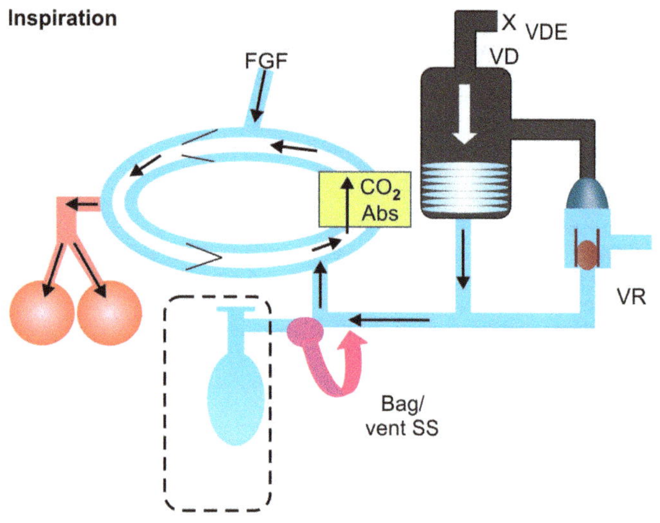

Fig. 3: Inspiratory phase of gas flow in a traditional circle system with an ascending bellows ventilator. (FGF: fresh gas flow; CO_2 Abs: carbon dioxide absorber; Bag/vent SS: bag/ventilator selector switch; VD: ventilator driving gas; VR: ventilator relief valve or spill valve; VDE: ventilator drive gas exhaust valve; X: ventilator drive gas exhaust valve in closed position)

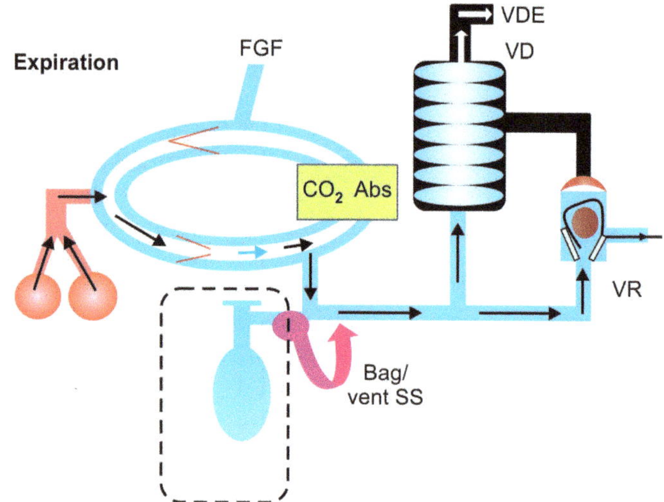

Fig. 4: Expiratory phase of gas flow in a traditional circle system with an ascending bellows ventilator. (FGF: fresh gas flow; CO_2 Abs: carbon dioxide absorber; Bag/vent SS: bag/ventilator selector switch; VD: ventilator driving gas; VR: ventilator relief valve or spill valve; VDE: ventilator drive gas exhaust valve)

TABLE 1: Differences between Datex-Ohmeda versus Dräger AV-E ventilator.[5]

	Datex-Ohmeda	***Dräger AV-E***
Driving gas	100% O_2	Air/O_2 mixture
Leak (hole) in the bellows will lead to	O_2 enrichment	Decrease in the FiO_2
Economy	O_2 consumption is high as the driving gas is a little greater than the set minute ventilation	Economizes on the use of compressed O_2
Bellows excursion	Bellows empties only the set tidal volume (VT) into the circuit	Bellows is emptied completely during inspiration, as VT is determined by setting the expansion limit of the bellows
Graduation markings on the bellows	From 0 mL at the top to 1,600 mL at the bottom of the bellows housing, as the VT is displaced from the bellows by a metered volume of compressed O_2 during inspiration	The bellows is graduated from 0 mL below to 2,000 mL at the top of the housing
The decrease in patient VT on application of positive end-expiratory pressure (PEEP)	More significant with the models 7000 and 7810 as bellows empties only the set VT into the circuit. Bellows has a capacity of 1,600 mL, the compression volume in the circuit at end inspiration is greater than in the Dräger AV-E ventilator system by a volume of (1,600 mL -VT)	Less effect because the bellows empties completely during each inspiration. Compression volume loss will be just determined by VT
The circuit pressure relief ("pop-off") valve	• In 7000 and 7800 series ventilators, the circuit pressure relief ("pop-off") valve is flush-mounted inside the bellows. The design does not use a relief valve pilot line and is, therefore, not vulnerable to the effects of this line kinking • In ADU workstation, the ventilator pressure relief valve is visible but there is a direct rather than a pilot tube connection to the driving gas circuit	Pressure-relief valve is controlled via an external relief valve pilot line, which is a short length of plastic tubing. Kinking/occlusion during inspiration causes it to remain closed thereafter and excess gas cannot leave the anesthesia circuit resulting in barotrauma. If the tubing is occluded during exhalation, during the next inspiratory cycle, pressure cannot be transmitted through to the valve to hold it closed. Patient circuit gas can then leak out to the scavenging system rather than entering the patient circuit, resulting in hypoventilation
Pressure-relief valve in the driving gas circuit	• Present • Preset to 65 cmH_2O in 7000 models • Adjustable in the 7900 series	• Absent in most of the original AV-E ventilators • Dräger pressure limit control valve, with variable relief pressure settings, is available and may be retrofitted to standing bellows versions of these ventilators, thereby providing a pressure limit. • It is now standard with the more recent model, the Dräger AV 2+

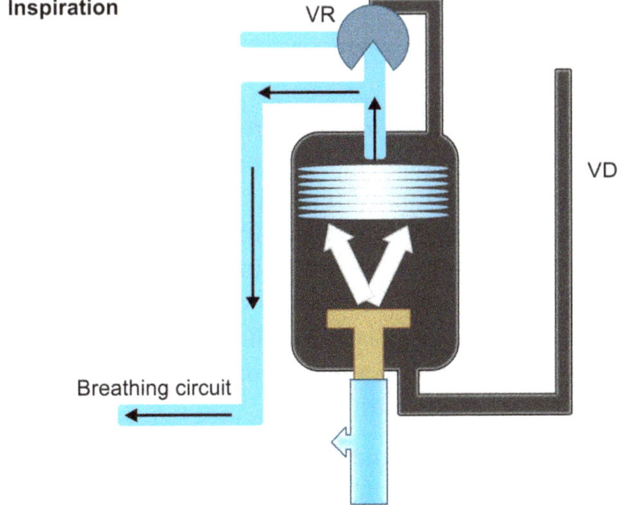

Fig. 5: Inspiratory phase of gas flow in a traditional circle system with a descending bellows ventilator. (VD: ventilator driving gas; VR: ventilator relief valve or spill valve. Not shown in the diagram is ventilator drive gas exhaust valve)

Fig. 6: Expiratory phase of gas flow in a traditional circle system with a descending bellows ventilator. (VD: ventilator driving gas; VR: ventilator relief valve or spill valve. Not shown in the diagram is ventilator drive gas exhaust valve)

During the expiratory phase, room air is entrained into the breathing system at the site of the disconnection because gravity acts on the weighted bellows **(Figs. 8 and 9)**. The disconnection pressure monitor, and the volume monitor may be fooled even if a disconnection is complete. Some contemporary anesthesia workstation designs have returned to the descending bellows to integrate FGD (Dräger Medical Julian and Data scope Anestar).

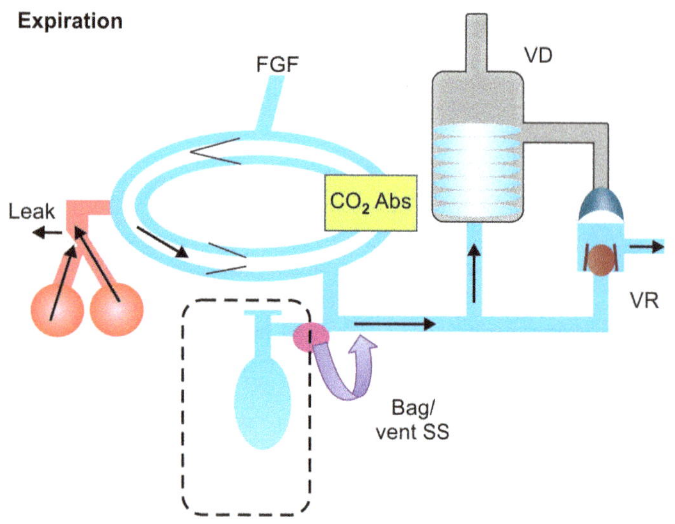

Fig. 7: Expiratory phase of gas flow in a traditional circle system with an ascending bellows ventilator with leak at Y piece. Note that bellows fail to rise to top. (FGF: fresh gas flow; CO_2 Abs: carbon dioxide absorber; Bag/vent SS: bag/ventilator selector switch; VD: ventilator driving gas; VR: ventilator relief valve or spill valve)

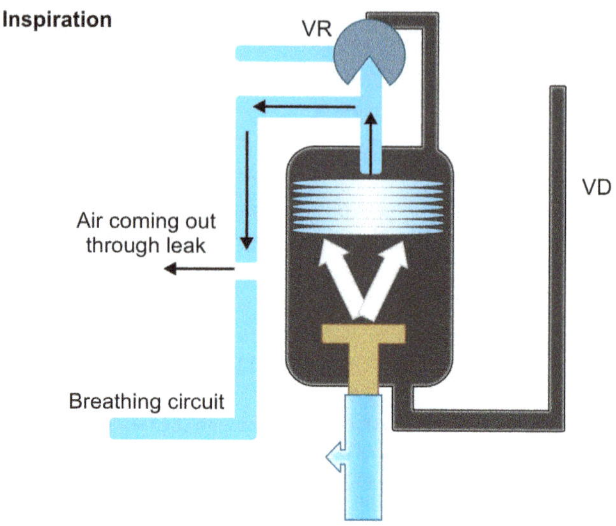

Fig. 9: Inspiratory phase of gas flow in a traditional circle system with descending bellows ventilator. There is a major leak in the patient end of the breathing circuit. Gases passing to atmosphere through the leak site. (VD: ventilator driving gas; VR: ventilator relief valve or spill valve. Not shown in the diagram is ventilator drive gas exhaust valve)

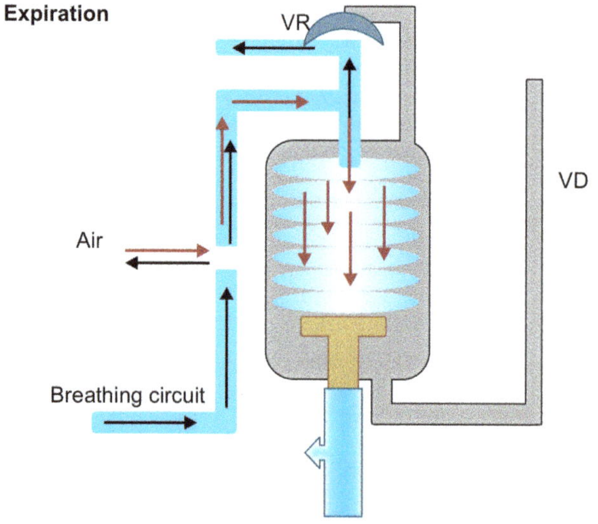

Fig. 8: Expiratory phase of gas flow in a traditional circle system with a descending bellows ventilator. There is a major leak in the patient end of the breathing circuit. Air entrainment through the leak site. (VD: ventilator driving gas; VR: ventilator relief valve or spill valve. Not shown in the diagram is ventilator drive gas exhaust valve)

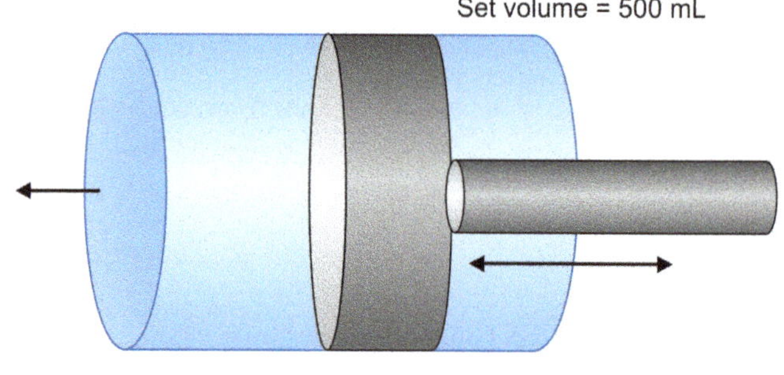

Fig. 10: Piston ventilator with accurate delivery of tidal volume.

PISTON-DRIVEN SINGLE-CIRCUIT VENTILATORS

A computer-controlled stepper motor is used instead of compressed drive gas to actuate gas movement in the breathing system. In these systems, rather than having dual circuits with patient gas in one and drive gas in another, a single patient gas circuit is present. The piston operates much like the plunger of a syringe to deliver the desired VT or airway pressure to the patient **(Fig. 10)**.

Following are the advantages:

- Ability to deliver accurate VTs to patients with very poor lung compliance and to very small patients. During volume-controlled ventilation the piston moves at a constant velocity whereas during pressure-controlled ventilation the piston moves with decreasing velocity
- Sophisticated computerized controls can provide advanced types of ventilatory support such as synchronized intermittent mandatory ventilation (S-IMV), pressure-controlled ventilation (PCV), and pressure support-assisted ventilation, in addition to the conventional control mode ventilation
- There is no need of driving gas.

Disadvantage: As with the bellows, the piston fills with gas from the breathing circuit. To prevent generation of significant negative pressure during the downstroke of the piston, the circle system configuration must be modified. The ventilator must also incorporate a negative-pressure relief valve (Dräger Fabius GS) or can terminate the piston's downstroke if negative pressure is detected (Dräger Narkomed 6400).

VOLUME REFLECTOR

The volume reflector is a device in Maquet FLOW-i anesthesia workstation.[3] It is a coiled, 3.6 m plastic channel of 1.2 L capacity, which acts as reservoir for exhaled gases **(Figs. 11 and 12)**. It is "in circuit" during both automatic and manual modes of ventilation. The reflector gas module is a solenoid-controlled oxygen flow source which serves as the driving force for controlled ventilation. During inspiration, the reflector gas module acts like a piston pushing the exhaled gas from the volume reflector, through the carbon dioxide absorber to the patient. Both the fresh gas and the reflector gas modules work together in a coordinated manner to control gas flow and pressure, so that set VT is achieved, and desired oxygen and anesthetic concentration are maintained. The gas modules use feedback loop-controlled, solenoid-actuated, pneumatic valves like servo-controlled ICU ventilator.

In the spontaneous mode of ventilation, the reflector gas module is disabled. The patient breathes in and out of the volume reflector, and circuit pressure is controlled by the operator adjustable adjustable pressure limiting (APL) valve.

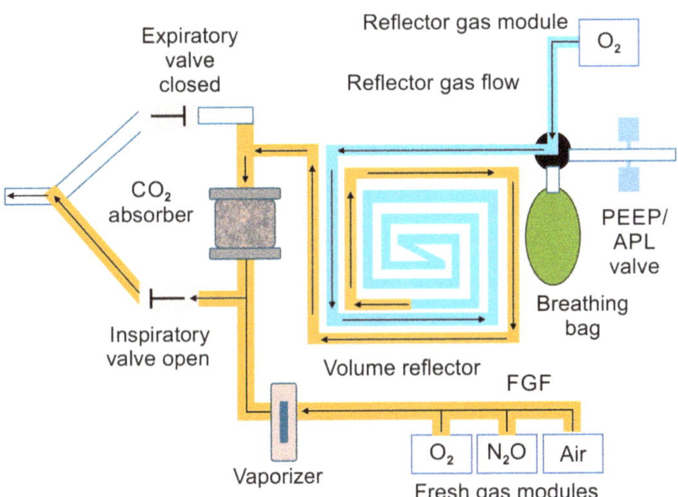

Fig. 11: Maquet FLOW-i anesthesia workstation breathing circuit and gas supply system during inspiration. (PEEP: positive end-expiratory pressure; APL: adjustable pressure limiting; FGF; fresh gas flow)

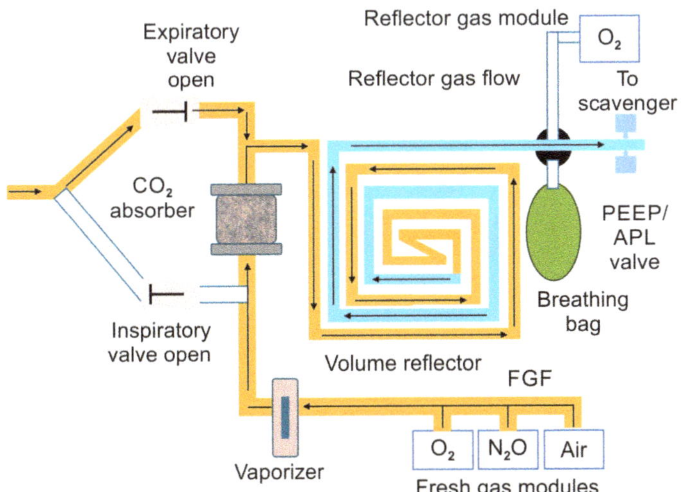

Fig. 12: Maquet FLOW-i breathing circuit and gas supply during exhalation in a controlled ventilation mode. (PEEP: positive end-expiratory pressure; APL: adjustable pressure limiting; FGF; fresh gas flow)

The FLOW-i system can compensate for breathing system leaks by increasing reflector gas module flow. The operator is informed if this occurs. However, in this case, dilution of anesthetic gas occurs as reflector gas module provides only 100% oxygen.

TURBINE VENTILATORS (DRÄGER PERSEUS)[6]

TurboVent 2 on Perseus A500 (Dräger) is a compressor/blower. It is run by electric motor. Like a super powerful hair dryer, during inspiration, it rapidly (in milliseconds) increases the rotation speed to reach the set inspiratory pressure. It generates inspiratory flow quickly, (180 L/m which is highest among current anesthesia ventilators). Thus they are well-suited to deliver patient triggered breaths. It spins at a low rate during expiration also. This maintains PEEP, and also a flow of 0.6 L/m though the breathing circuit, improving mixing of gases in the circuit, and reducing the work of breathing of any small spontaneous breaths.

The data from pressure and flow sensors are electronically controlled.

The ventilation pressure and flow during inspiration and expiration are attained by means of the turbine and the Pmax/PEEP flow valve in the breathing system.

Advantages:

- Because of availability of peak inspiratory flow as high as 180 L/min, it responds efficiently to patient trigger similar to high-end ICU respirators
- Work of breathing as low as on ICU respirators
- Allows spontaneous breathing during ventilation at any time, thereby providing all ventilation modes commonly used in intensive care
- It can be used in wide range of patients from neonates to adults.

PROBLEMS ASSOCIATED WITH ANESTHESIA VENTILATORS AND THEIR SOLUTIONS

Tidal Volume Discrepancies[3-5]

The large discrepancies between the set and actual VT can occur because of following reasons.

Tidal Volume Gain is because of Ventilator-fresh Gas Flow Coupling

In most anesthesia workstations, gas flow from the anesthesia machine into the breathing circuit is continuous and independent of ventilator activity. During the inspiratory phase of mechanical ventilation, the ventilator relief valve is closed, and the breathing system's adjustable pressure limiting valve ("pop-off" valve) is most commonly out of circuit. Therefore, the patient's lungs receive the volume from the bellows plus that from the flow meters.

Gain due to excessive fresh gas flow (FGF) can be calculated as per following formula:

$$\text{Tidal volume gain per breath (mL)} = \frac{\text{FGF (mL/min)} \times \text{I:E ratio (\%)}}{\text{Respiratory rate per minute}}$$

For example, if fresh gas flow rate is set at 6 L per minute, I: E ratio is 1:2 and respiratory rate is 10 per minute

Then

$$\text{Tidal volume gain per breath (mL)} = \frac{6{,}000 \text{ (mL/min)} \times 33 \text{ (\%)}}{10 \text{ per minute}} = 200 \text{ mL}$$

This is in addition to ventilator output.

The increasing fresh gas flow increases the VT, minute ventilation, and peak inspiratory pressure. To avoid problems with ventilator-fresh gas flow coupling, airway pressure and exhaled VT must be monitored closely, and excessive fresh gas flows must be avoided.

The inappropriate activation of the oxygen flush valve during the inspiratory phase can result in barotrauma and/or volutrauma because excess pressure and volume may not be able to be vented from the circle system.

Tidal Volume Loss

The breathing circuit compliance, gas compression, leakage in anesthesia machine, breathing circuit, and patient's airway causes VT loss.

The compliance of breathing circuit is 5 mL/cmH_2O and 100 mL of VT is lost if inspiratory pressure is 20 cmH_2O. Therefore, stiffer pediatric circuit with smaller compliances of 1.5–2.5 mL/cmH_2O are preferred. Compression losses, normally about 3%, are due to gas compression within the ventilator bellows and in the breathing circuit (15 mL if set tidal volume is 500 mL).

Gas sampling for capnography and anesthetic gas measurements represents additional losses unless the sampled gas is returned to the breathing circuit, as occurs in some machines.

The VT discrepancies can be detected by placement of spirometer. The inspiratory and expiratory VTs can be measured in advanced ventilators. The compliance and compression losses are apparent if spirometer is placed at the Y connector in the breathing circuit.

Several mechanisms have been built into newer anaesthesia machines to reduce tidal volume discrepancies.

Fresh Gas Compensation[3-5]

During the initial electronic self-checkout, some machines measure total system compliance and subsequently adjust the excursion of the ventilator bellows or piston; leaks may also be measured but are usually not compensated.

Methods of Modulation

Feedback adjustment: The VT delivered at inspiratory valve is measured by flow sensor for first few breaths. Subsequently it adjusts metered drive gas flow to compensate VT loss due to compression of gases in ventilator, its circuit and absorber system. However, loss in the patient's circuit is not compensated.

The system also compensates for gas gains because of anesthesia machine fresh gas flow. Thus, the user-set VT is delivered to the patient circuit even when fresh gas flow, respiratory rate, or I: E ratios are altered.

Pre-emptive adjustment: In Datex-Ohmeda/5 ADU, a D-lite flow sensor continually measures fresh gas and vaporizer flow and subtracts this amount from the metered drive gas flow **(Fig. 13)**.

The Dräger Perseus,[6] unlike other Dräger workstations, has no FGD valve and FGF inlet is placed between turbine and inspiratory unidirectional valve **(Fig. 14)**. The blower draws inspiratory volume from the manual breathing bag as well as from fresh gas flow. Fresh gas flow is not diverted

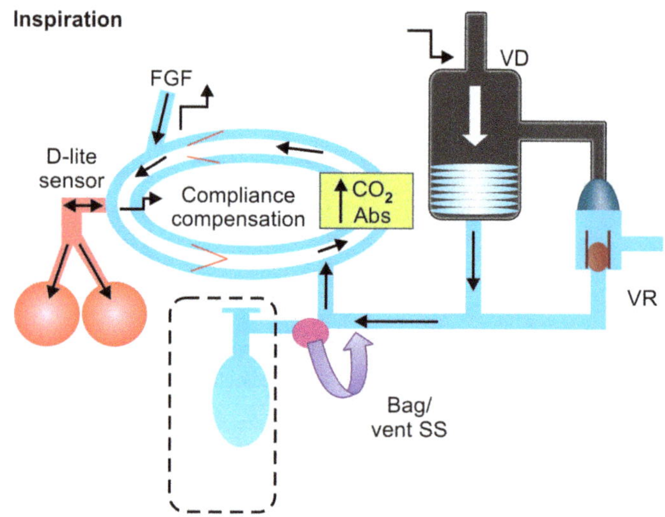

Fig. 13: Diagrammatic representation of Datex-Ohmeda/5 ADU with D-lite sensor showing continuous measurement of compliance, fresh gas flow, and adjustment of driving gas accordingly. (FGF: fresh gas flow; CO_2 Abs: carbon dioxide absorber; Bag/vent SS: bag/ventilator selector switch; VD: ventilator driving gas; VR: ventilator relief valve or spill valve)

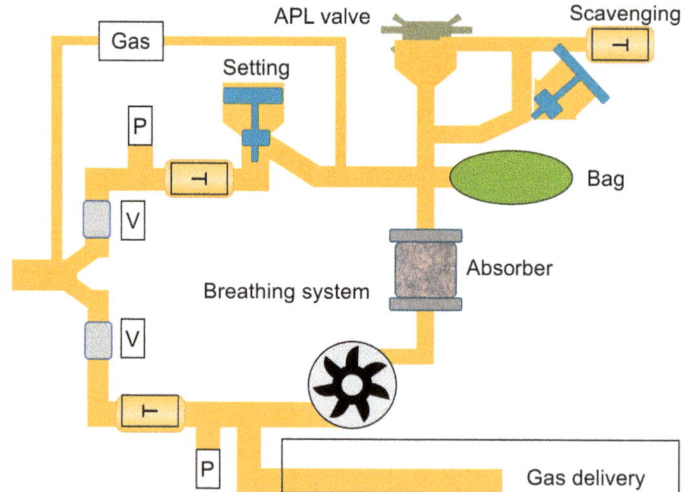

Fig. 14: Perseus breathing circuit. (APL: adjustable pressure limiting)

to the reservoir bag during inspiration (as in Apollo or Fabius), but is added to VT during inspiration.[6] Information from flow and pressure sensors is utilized to control turbine speed and the Pmax/PEEP valve, which stops inspiration when the desired VT and inspiratory time (Ti) are reached. In the Perseus, the manual breathing bag empties during inspiration (like a bellows), and fills during expiration.[6]

Fresh Gas Decoupling[5,7]

There are two ways of decoupling fresh gas flow and VT:

1. Stop the fresh gas flow during inspiration. Machines that use electronic control of gas flow (Dräger Julian) can decouple fresh gas flow from the VT by delivery of fresh gas flow only during exhalation
2. Divert the fresh gas flow during inspiration (Data scope Anestar, Dräger Fabius GS and Narkomed 6400). During the inspiratory phase **(Figs. 15 and 16)** the fresh gas via the fresh gas inlet is diverted into the reservoir bag by a decoupling valve that is located between the fresh gas source and the ventilator circuit. The reservoir bag serves as an accumulator for fresh gas until the expiratory phase begins. During expiratory phase **(Figs. 17 and 18)**, the decoupling valve opens, allowing the accumulated fresh gas in the reservoir bag to be drawn into the circle system to refill the descending bellows or piston ventilator chamber. Since the ventilator exhaust valve also opens during expiratory phase, excess fresh gas, and exhaled patient gases can escape to the scavenging system.[5,7]

Current fresh gas decoupled systems are designed with either piston-type or descending bellows-type ventilators. Since the bellows in either of these types of systems refills under slight negative pressure, it allows the accumulated fresh gas from the reservoir bag to be drawn into the ventilator for delivery to the patient during the next ventilator cycle. Conventional ascending bellows ventilators, which refill under slight positive pressure, cannot be used with FGD.

The newer hanging bellows which are used with FGD lacks an internal weight, and senses when the bellows do not

Fig. 15: Inspiratory phase gas flows of a circle system with descending bellows and fresh gas decoupling. (–ve pr. relief valve: negative pressure relief valve; VDG: ventilator drive gas)

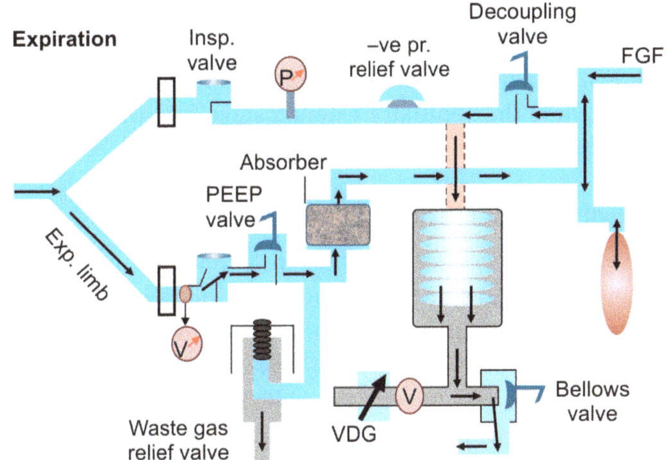

Fig. 17: Expiratory phase gas flows of a circle system with descending bellows and fresh gas decoupling. (–ve pr. relief valve: negative pressure relief valve; VDG: ventilator drive gas)

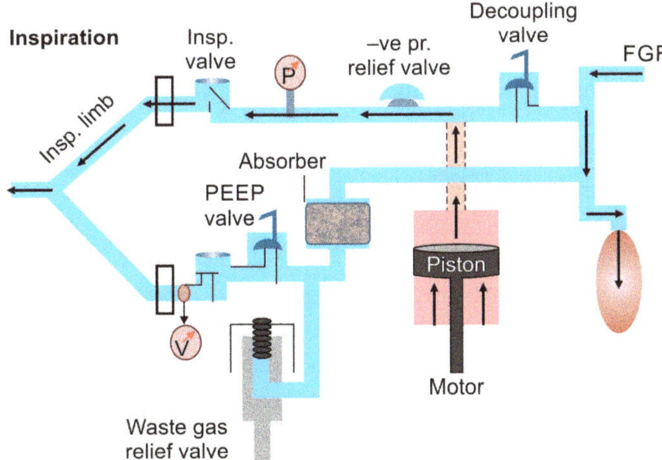

Fig. 16: Inspiratory phase gas flows of a circle system with piston ventilator and fresh gas decoupling. (–ve pr. relief valve: negative pressure relief valve)

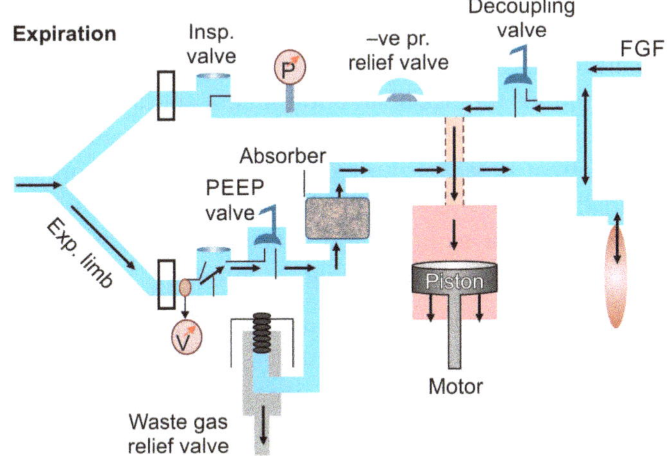

Fig. 18: Expiratory phase gas flows of a circle system with piston ventilator and fresh gas decoupling. (–ve pr. relief valve: negative pressure relief valve)

return to the full "down" position. One needs to rely more on the pressure and capnography waveforms as opposed to the bellows. Water may gather in the descending bellows leading to reduction in VT and infection. This can be prevented by heating the absorber head.

In workstations without FGD, the reservoir bag is out of circuit during mechanical ventilation. In machines with FGD, reservoir bag is in circuit and inflates during inspiration and deflates during expiration.

Exception is Dräger Perseus, where the manual breathing bag moves during mechanical ventilation, but in a direction opposite to Apollo/Fabius. Here, the circuit differs from Apollo in two aspects: (i) it lacks a decoupling valve and (ii) the Pmax/PEEP valve is moved from proximal (upstream) of the expiratory unidirectional valve, to downstream from it.[6]

Advantage of Fresh Gas Decoupling

Decreased risk of barotraumas and volutrauma: With a traditional circle system, increases in fresh gas flow from the flow meters or from inappropriate use of the oxygen flush valve may contribute directly to VT, which if excessive, may result in pneumothorax or other injury. Since systems with FGD isolate fresh gas coming into the system from the patient while the ventilator exhaust valve is closed, the risk of barotrauma is greatly reduced.

Disadvantage of Fresh Gas Decoupling

Generation of negative pressure: In a fresh gas decoupled system, the bellows or piston refills under slight negative pressure. If the volume of gas contained in the reservoir bag plus the returning volume of gas exhaled from the patient's lungs is inadequate to refill the bellows or piston, negative patient airway pressures could develop.

To prevent generation of significant negative pressure during the downstroke of the piston, the circle system configuration must be modified. The ventilator must also incorporate a negative-pressure relief valve (Dräger Fabius GS) or can terminate the piston's downstroke if negative pressure is detected (Dräger Narkomed 6,400). Introduction of a negative-pressure relief valve to the breathing circuit may introduce the risk of air entrainment and the potential for dilution of oxygen and volatile anesthetic concentrations if the patient breathes during mechanical ventilation and low fresh gas flows. System should have high priority audible and visual alerts to notify the user that fresh gas flow is inadequate and room air is being entrained.

Reliance on the reservoir bag as accumulator: Fresh gas decoupling system such as seen on the Narkomed 6000 series relies on the reservoir bag to accumulate the incoming fresh gas. If the reservoir bag is removed during mechanical ventilation, or if it has a significant leak from poor fit on the bag mount or a perforation, room air may enter the breathing circuit as the ventilator piston unit refills during expiratory phase. This may potentially result in awareness, hypoxia and pollution of the operating room.

Excessive Positive Pressure[3-5]

Causes

- Incorrect settings on the ventilator
- Ventilator malfunction. In the Dräger AV-E, the ventilator pressure-relief valve is controlled via an external relief valve pilot line, a short length of plastic tubing. Kinking this tubing can cause ventilator malfunction. Occlusion during inspiration, when the valve is being held closed, causes it to remain closed thereafter and excess gas cannot leave the anesthesia circuit. Consequently, pressure in the circuit rises and, if not relieved, could result in barotrauma
- *Sticking of spill valve:* Ventilator relief valve incompetency can result from a disconnected pilot line, a ruptured valve, or from a damaged flapper valve. A ventilator relief valve stuck in the closed or partially closed position can produce either barotrauma or undesired PEEP
- Excessive suction from the scavenging system can draw the ventilator relief valve to its seat and close the valve during both the inspiratory and expiratory phases. In this case, breathing circuit pressure escalates because excess anesthetic gas cannot be vented
- Coupling of fresh gas flow
- *Use of the oxygen flush valve during the inspiratory cycle of a ventilator:* As the ventilator spill valve will be closed and the APL valve is excluded, there will be transfer of oxygen (600–1000 mL/s) and circuit pressure to the patient's lung.
- High gas pressure to patient's airway can be transmitted by a leak in the ventilator bellows resulting in pulmonary barotrauma which will be indicated by rise in inspired oxygen concentration (if oxygen is the sole pressurizing gas).

Effects

- Increase the risk of pulmonary barotrauma (e.g., pneumothorax)
- Hemodynamic compromise during anesthesia.

Prevention

- Fresh gas compensation
- Fresh gas decoupling
- High-pressure alarm
- *Factory preset inspiratory pressure safety valve:* The piston driven Fabius GS, and few others have this valve that opens at a preset airway pressure such as 75 cm of water pressure to minimize the risk of barotrauma
- *Pressure limiters:* On workstations equipped with adjustable inspiratory pressure limiters such as the Datex-Ohmeda S/5 ADU, Aestiva, Dräger Medical's Narkomed 6000 series, 2B, 2C, GS and Fabius GS,

maximal inspiratory pressure may be set by the user to a desired peak airway pressure. An adjustable pressure relief valve will open when the predetermined user-selected pressure is reached. However, user must preset the appropriate "pop-off" pressure. If the setting is too low, insufficient pressure for ventilation may be generated, resulting in inadequate minute ventilation; if set too high, the excessive airway pressure may still occur, resulting in barotrauma.

Control Assembly and Power Supply Problems

The control assembly can be the source of both electrical and mechanical problems.

Disconnection of the Breathing Circuit and Leaks

A common source of leaks with older absorbers is failure to close the APL (pop-off) valve on initiation of mechanical ventilation. The bag or ventilator switch on contemporary absorbers helps minimize this problem.

Preexisting, undetected leaks can occur in compressed, corrugated, disposable anesthetic circuits. To detect such a leak preoperatively, the circuit must be fully expanded before the circuit is checked for leaks.

VENTILATION MODES

Volume and pressure-controlled mode are described in **Table 2**.

Other Modes

Other modes which are available are:[6]

- *SIMV-PSV:* Synchronized intermittent mandatory ventilation mode with volume-control breaths plus pressure support
- *SIMV-PC:* Synchronized intermittent mandatory ventilation mode with pressure-control breaths plus pressure support
- *Pressure support:* With laryngeal mask airway (LMA), spontaneous (unassisted) breathing is usually kept. To keep LMA in place, one must maintain deep plane of anesthesia, which may cause respiratory depression. Here, PSV mode is quite useful
- *PSV-Pro:* Pro is short for "protect," meaning that after 10–30 seconds of apnea the mode will revert to PCV. If the patient begins breathing again, the ventilator will switch back to PSV-Pro
- *PC-VG:* Means pressure controlled with volume guarantee, it has both pressure control mode and through volume guarantee control of arterial CO_2
- *VC-CMV-AF:* Autoflow applies the set VT with the minimum pressure required. If resistance or compliance changes, the pressure adapts gradually, by automatic adjustment of inspiratory pressure and flow. AF may be applied in any volume-controlled mode.[6]
- *PC-BIPAP:* Means pressure control-biphasic positive airway pressure, in which patient can breathe spontaneously

TABLE 2: Differences between volume and pressure-controlled modes.[6]

	Volume control	***Pressure control***
Frequency of use	Most commonly used	Less commonly used
Preset parameter	Tidal volume	Inspiratory pressure at a level above PEEP
Flow pattern	Constant	Decelerating
Pressure	Accelerating	Constant
Variable parameter due to changes in resistance and compliance of the breathing system and the patient	Pressure	Tidal volume
Effect of addition of PEEP	Decreases the tidal volume delivered, with the effect greater with small tidal volumes. On newer ventilators with integral PEEP, ventilation may be better maintained	Reduction in tidal volume
Effect of closed system suctioning	Significant rise in airway pressure when the catheter is inserted and low airway pressure during suctioning	Less intrinsic PEEP during catheter insertion and less sub atmospheric pressure during suctioning than during VCV
Advantages or Indication	Preset tidal volume delivery	• In patients with lung injury or during single-lung ventilation, PCV may improve oxygenation and produce greater VT than volume control VCV because of the decelerating flow pattern that delivers gas to the alveoli early during inspiration • It may be useful if there is an airway leak (e.g., uncuffed tube, supraglottic airway device, bronchopleural fistula). However, if there is a large leak, the cycling pressure limit may not be reached, causing a prolonged inspiration
Disadvantage	The inspiratory phase may be terminated before the tidal volume has been delivered if the peak airway pressure reaches the set pressure limit.	Appropriate VT delivery may not occur unless proper inspiratory time or I: E ratio are set

(PEEP: positive end-expiratory pressure; VCV: volume-controlled mode; VT: tidal volume; PCV: pressure-controlled mode) at wish with specified number of mandatory breaths. The mandatory breaths are synchronized with breathing attempts. The pressure difference between PEEP and Pinsp, the lung mechanics, and breathing effort of patient results in VT. The VT and MV may vary with change in resistance and compliance. During spontaneous breathing at PEEP level, the patient can be supported using PS[6]

- *PC-APRV:* Means pressure control-airway pressure release ventilation, the spontaneous breathing of patient at upper pressure level "Phigh" which is maintained for the duration "Thigh", i.e., time at high pressure. Here, for active expiration and elimination of CO_2, the pressure is reduced for short time. The alteration between two level of pressure is time cycled and machine triggered. The pressure difference between Plow and Phigh and lung mechanics results in to expiration of VT.[6]

MONITORING[6]

Pressure Monitoring

- Peak inspiratory pressure provides an indication of dynamic compliance
- Plateau pressure mirrors static compliance.

An increase in both peak inspiratory pressure and plateau pressure implies an increase in VT or a decrease in pulmonary compliance. An increase in peak inspiratory pressure without any change in plateau pressure signals an increase in airway resistance or inspiratory gas flow rate.

Many anesthesia machines graphically display breathing-circuit pressure. The shape of the breathing-circuit pressure waveform can provide important airway information.

Respiratory Volume Monitors

Volume monitors measures exhaled VT, inhaled VT, minute volume, or all three. They are useful in detecting disconnections. The user should bracket the high and low threshold volumes slightly above and below the exhaled volumes. For example, if the exhaled minute volume of a patient is 8 L/min, reasonable alarm limits would be 6–10 L/min.

- Many Datex-Ohmeda ventilators are equipped with volume monitor sensors that use infrared light/turbine technology. These volume sensors are usually located in the expiratory limb of the breathing circuit and thus measure exhaled VT. With the older infrared type sensors, exposure to a direct beam of light from the overhead surgical lighting could cause erroneous volume readings as the surgical beam interferes with the infrared sensor
- In the case of the Datex-Ohmeda S/5 ADU, the D-Lite® spirometry connector is placed at or near the level of the patient connection and permits measurement of both inhaled and exhaled volumes and pressures
- Datex-Ohmeda Aestiva, Aespire, and other workstations that incorporate the 7100 ventilators or 7900 Smart Vent. These systems generally utilize differential pressure transduction technology to determine inhaled and exhaled volumes as well as to measure airway pressures
- The Dräger Medical Narkomed 6000 series 2B and GS workstations commonly use an ultrasonic flow sensor located on the expiratory limb
- Other systems from Dräger measure exhaled volume using "hot wire" sensor technology. With this type of sensor, a tiny array of two platinum wires is electrically heated to a high temperature. As gas flows past the heated wires, they tend to be cooled. The amount of energy required to maintain the temperature of the wire is proportional to the volume of gas flowing past it. This system has been associated in at least one report with accidental development of a fire in the breathing circuit.

TYPICAL VENTILATOR ALARMS

- High pressure
- Pressure below threshold for 15–30 seconds (apnea or disconnect)
- Continuing high pressure
- Sub-atmospheric pressure
- Low tidal or minute volume
- High respiratory rate
- Reverse flow (may indicate incompetence of expiratory unidirectional valve in the breathing circuit)
- High PEEP
- Low oxygen-supply pressure

APNEA/DISCONNECT ALARMS

Apnea/disconnect alarms may be based on the following:[6]

- *Chemical monitoring (lack of end tidal carbon dioxide):* Some contemporary anesthesia workstation designs have returned to the descending bellows to integrate FGD (Dräger Medical Julian and Datascope Anestar). An essential safety feature on any anesthesia workstation that utilizes a descending bellows is an integrated CO_2 apnea alarm that cannot be disabled while the ventilator is in use
- *Mechanical monitoring:*
  - Failure to reach normal inspiratory peak pressure. Various anesthesia workstations and ventilators have different locations for the airway pressure sensor. An audible or visual alarm threshold pressure alarm limit may be preset at the factory or adjustable. The operator should set the pressure alarm limit to within 5 cm water of the peak inspiratory pressure
  - Failure to sense return of VT on a spirometer
  - Failure of standing bellows to fill during mechanical ventilator exhalation
  - Failure of manual breathing bag to fill during mechanical ventilation (machines with FGD—the Julian, Fabius GS, Narkomed 6,000)
- *Electronic:* Failure of the hanging bellows to fill completely (the "garage door" electronic eye sensor on the Julian).

Most modern anesthesia ventilators also have integrated spirometers and oxygen analyzers that provide additional alarms. Though several disconnection monitors exist, the most important monitor is a vigilant anesthesiologist monitoring breath sounds, chest wall excursion, and mechanical monitors.

Up to late 1980s, anesthesia ventilators were mere supplements to the anesthesia machine. However, they have a central role in newer anesthesia workstations. Differences between old and new anesthesia ventilators are enumerated in **Table 3**. Though many advanced ICU-style ventilation features have also been integrated into anesthesia ventilators, some fundamental differences in ventilation parameters and control systems remain.

SALIENT MODERN FEATURES[6]

Piston Ventilator System (Apollo, NM 6000 and Fabius GS)

Advantages:

- Quiet
- No PEEP
- Precise VT delivery
  - Compliance and leak compensation
  - Fresh gas decoupling
- Rigid piston design leading to less compliance losses compared to a flexible standing bellows compressed by driving gas
- Transducer for compliance and leak measurement is near the piston unlike a bulky, costly sensor close to the patient's airway (D-Lite sensor on the ADU).
- No need of driving gas and hence more economic.

Disadvantages of the piston design:

- Quiet (less easy to hear regular cycling)
- In many workstations, piston is not visible and, therefore, disconnections or spontaneous respiratory efforts cannot be easily made out
- Potential for negative end expiratory pressure.

Accuracy at Lower Tidal Volumes

Modern anesthesia ventilators provide smaller VTs (Narkomed 6,000: 10–1400, Fabius GS: 20–1,400, Apollo: 20–1,400, Aestiva: 20–1,500, ADU: 20–1,400). However, one should substitute a pediatric circuit for VTs less than 200 mL, use smaller filters, and a pediatric D-Lite sensor on the ADU.

Location of Flow Sensor

In the Aestiva flow sensors was placed between the disposable corrugated breathing circuit limbs and the absorber head. It compensates VTs for fresh gas flow, loss of compliance, internal leaks of machine, and absorber head, but not in breathing hoses.

The GE D-lite sensor is placed distal to Y-piece on ADU, to compensate leaks, compliance loss upto the Y piece. However, it becomes bulky, causing difficulty in mask ventilation. Sensor is exposed to more exhaled moisture.

The Narkomed 6000 tests compliance and leaks of all components upto the Y-piece via a pressure transducer within the internal circuitry near the bellows. Here the sensor is relatively protected from moisture.

Suitability for Low Flows

Features of low flow ventilators are:

- Testing of compliance and leak
- Leak detection is automatic
- Compensation or decoupling of fresh gas
- Absorber head are warmed

TABLE 3: Old versus new anesthesia ventilators.[1]

Old	New
Could not provide high inspiratory pressures or flows	High inspiratory pressures and flows can be delivered
For positive end-expiratory pressure (PEEP), a PEEP valve had to be added in the anesthesia breathing system. Some of these valves were imprecise, not variable, and could be misconnected	Newer anesthesia ventilators have an integral PEEP valve
User had to manually enable the low-pressure alarm when the ventilator was turned ON	Turning the ventilator ON involves fewer steps and automatically enables the low airway pressure alarm
May have been necessary to close the adjustable pressure limiting valve and/or turn the bag/ventilator switch when turning on the ventilator	Adjustable pressure limiting valve is out of circuit when ventilator with ascending bellows is in use
Separate models or different bellows assemblies were required for adult and pediatric patients	Same bellows assemblies required for adult and pediatric patients
The delivered VT was affected by fresh gas flow	The delivered tidal volume is not affected by fresh gas flow. Either there is fresh gas compensation or fresh gas decoupling
The delivered tidal volume was affected by breathing system compliance	The delivered tidal volume is not affected by breathing system compliance
Only single volume control mode	Several ventilatory modes
Less flexibility in tidal volume delivery	Improved flexibility so that the ventilator can deliver volumes for a wide range of patients from the smallest child to the largest adult

- Low volume absorber heads canisters such as Appollo-1500 mL; NM 6,000–1,500 mL; Fabius 1500 mL; and ADU-750 mL
- Electronic detection of bellows not filling (Julian)
- Low flow wizard is an electronic monitor that gives indications when fresh gas flow is excessive or too low by monitoring gas volume passing through the scavenger. It is available in Apollo and NM 6000 machines.

Lung Protective Ventilation

Atelectasis during general anesthesia can lead to post-operative pulmonary complications (PPCs). Prophylactic lung protective ventilation (LPV) includes use low tidal volumes (VT), moderate PEEP, and recruitment maneuvers (RMs). Lung RMs are intended to open collapsed alveoli by applying transient increases in transpulmonary pressure. In Aisys CS2, Avance CS2, and Carestation 600 series, lung RMs have been automated. They are referred to as Vital Capacity and Cycling under the Procedures key. Vital capacity (single-step RM) is the manual "bag squeezing" or vital capacity (VC) method of applying and holding a set inflation pressure for a specific duration of time. Cycling (multistep RM) is an automated, programmable feature employing an incremental increase in airway pressure and/or PEEP. The pulse pressure variation (dPP) and systolic pressure variation (SPV) are clinical decision tools that may help to predict hemodynamic instability induced by PEEP and the application of RMs. Perseus A500 workstation from Dräger has similar features.

Many features of anesthesia ventilators are suitable for many situations.

CONCLUSION

Modern anesthesia ventilator is one of the most important and complicated part of newer anesthesia workstations. Though technical aspects are quite different, it can provide accurate and wide range of tidal volumes plus multiple modes like ICU ventilators.

REFERENCES

1. Dorsch JA, Dorsch SE. Anesthesia ventilators. In: Understanding Anesthesia Equipment, 5th edition. Philadelphia: Wolters Kluwer, Lippincott Williams and Wilkins; 2008. pp. 310-71.
2. Morgan GE. Mikhail MS, Murray MJ. The anesthesia machine. In: Clinical Anesthesiology, 4th edition. USA: McGraw-Hill Companies; 2006.
3. Venticinque SG, Andrews JJ. Inhaled anesthetic delivery systems. In: Miller RD (Ed). Miller's Anesthesia, 8th edition. Philadelphia: Saunders, An imprint of Elsevier Inc; 2015. pp. 752-820.
4. Riutort KT, Brockwell RC, Brull SJ, et al. The anesthesia workstation and delivery systems. In: Barash PG, Cullen BF, Stoelting RK, et al (Eds). Clinical Anesthesia, 6th edition. Philadelphia: Lippincott Williams & Wilkins; 2009. pp. 644-94.
5. Eisenkraft JB. Anesthesia delivery system. In: Longnecker DE, Brown DL, Newman MF, et al (Eds). Anesthesiology. New York: Mc Graw Hill Medical; 2008. pp. 767-820.
6. Abromovich A. Fresh gas decoupling minimizes complexity. APSF Newsletter. 2005;20:35.
7. Dosch MP, Tharp D. The anesthesia gas machine. Anesthesia gas machine> components & systems> delivery> ventilators. [Revised March 2016]. [online] Available from http://healthprofessions.udmercy.edu/programs/crna/agm/. [Last accessed May, 2021].

Airway Equipment

SECTION 5

Face Masks

Naina P Dalvi, Nazmeen I Sayed

ABSTRACT

The ability to hold the mask and to administer positive pressure ventilation through the mask is a basic skill that all anesthesia providers must master. This chapter discusses the structure of face mask in great detail. It also describes different modifications of face masks with their uses.

INTRODUCTION

Face mask was basically invented to administer anesthesia. They are made up of such a shape that they will comfortably fit over the patient's nose and mouth with minimal leak and without undue force.

In 1890, Schimmelbusch **(Fig. 1)** invented a mask for the delivery of anesthetics to surgical patients. It was primarily designed for ether and chloroform anesthesia. Both ether and chloroform can cause irritation if they come into contact with the patient's skin, so Schimmelbusch designed a metal mask, over which gauze could be stretched and secured. The mask was placed over the patient's mouth and nose, and anesthetic agent was applied to the gauze, allowing the patient to inhale the anesthetic as they breathed normally.[1]

Bellamy Gardner face mask **(Fig. 2)** for inhaling ether had hinged wire mesh covered with double layer of wool fabric held in place by lever.[2]

Yankauer face mask **(Fig. 3)** had mesh and removable spiral wire collar holding down a piece of gauze onto which agents such as ether or chloroform was applied.

Ochsner wire framed face mask **(Fig. 4)** was an adult size mask in which collar to hold lint in place was missing.

The present day face mask helps in delivering oxygen and other gases without putting any invasive airway in the patient's mouth. It is also useful in administering

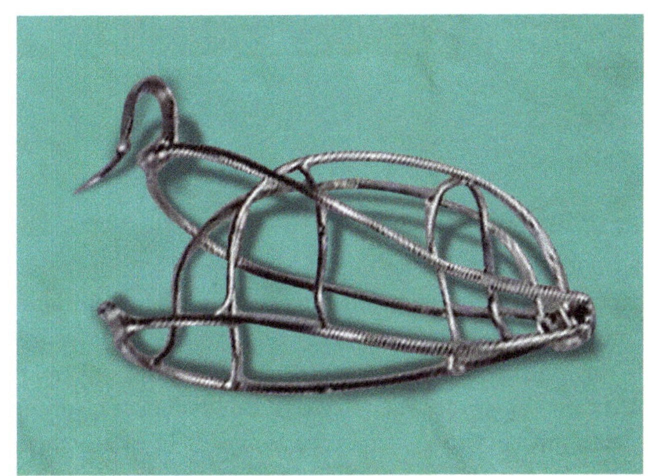

Fig. 2: Bellamy Gardner mask.

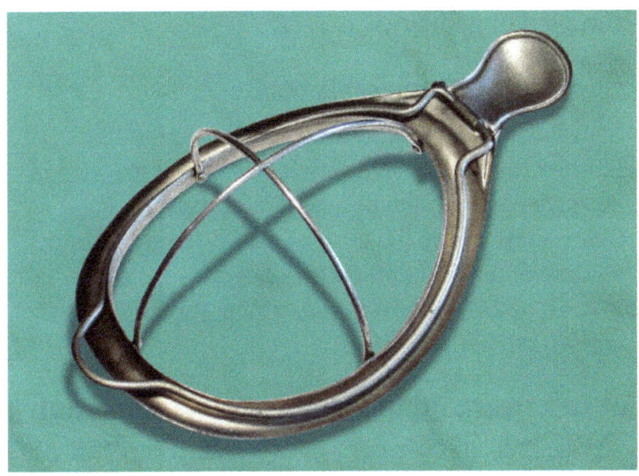

Fig. 1: Schimmelbusch mask.

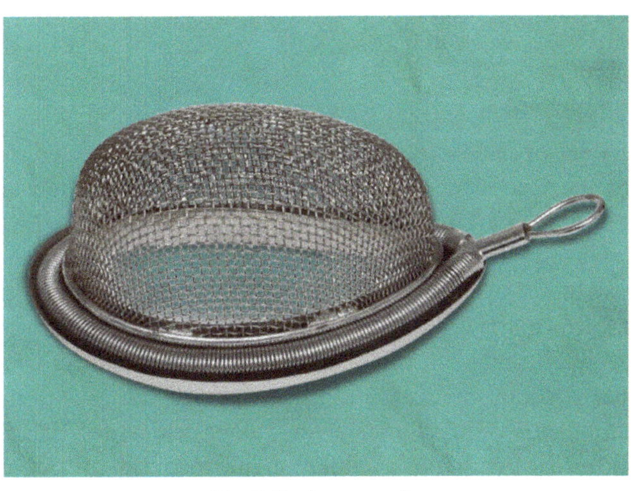

Fig. 3: Yankauer mask.

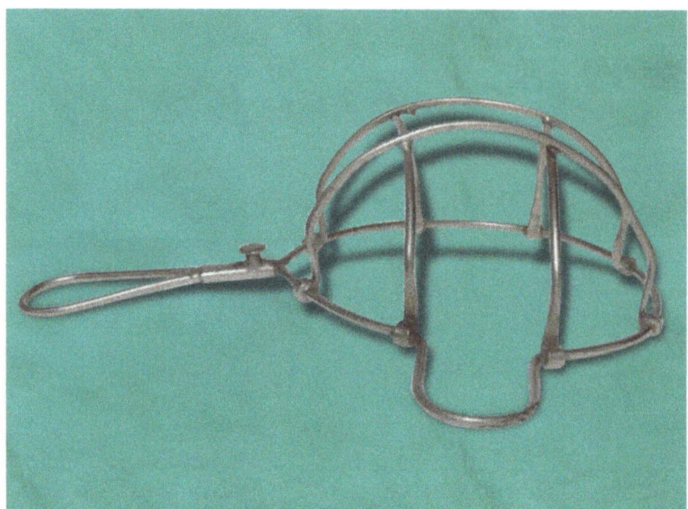

Fig. 4: Ochsner mask.

noninvasive positive pressure ventilation for treatment of respiratory failure.

FACE MASKS

The face mask is made up of different materials like black rubber, clear plastic, an elastomeric material, or a combination of these. In this era of disposable equipment, most of the anesthetists prefer using disposable plastic masks. It consists of three parts:

1. The body.
2. The edge.
3. The mount.[3,4]

Body or Dome

The body or dome is the main part of the mask. It is made up of black rubber, neoprene, plastic, and polycarbonate or silicone rubber. The transparent body made of polycarbonate or plastic allows monitoring of respiration by the appearance of condensation during exhalation. It also helps in detecting vomitus, secretions, blood or lip color during anesthesia. It is better accepted by a conscious patient and less threatening to the small children. Some masks have a malleable wire stiffener in the body so as to fit the mask to the face.

Edge or Seal

The edge or seal is the part of the mask that comes in contact with the face. The edge may be anatomically shaped and fitted with a cuff or flap. The cuff or cushion is inflated with air so as to have a good fit on face when pressure is applied, whereas a flap is a soft pliable extension of the body that conforms to the contour of the face and gives a good seal.

A good seal or fit is essential for positive pressure ventilation without gas leak and to prevent air dilution during spontaneous ventilation. Old edentulous or bearded patients may have difficult mask ventilation due to lack of proper seal around the mask. Few of the options are to leave dentures in place during mask ventilation to avoid sunken cheeks and to use a bigger mask held firmly with two hands, respectively. Reusable masks with a cuff have a small filling tube with a cap to regulate the degree of inflation of the cuff.

Mount or Connector

The connector or mount or collar is on the top of the body of mask and on opposite side from the seal. It is thicker than body of the mask and has 22 mm internal diameter. Some anesthesia masks are supplied with a ring having hooks for attachment of a head harness. Head harness is helpful as it allows the anesthetist to keep both hands free during anesthesia with inhalational agents and during noninvasive ventilation in the intensive care units.

A perfect fit of the mask is achieved by anatomically shaping the body of the mask, by the use of an air filled cuff with a soft cushion or by a soft pliable flap that fits the anatomy of the face.

The face mask and its adaptor normally constitute the major part of the mechanical dead space. The dead space within the body of the facemask is nonsignificant in adults but may constitute 30% or more of the tidal volume of neonates and infants. It can be decreased by using a smaller mask, by increasing pressure on the mask and by inflating the cushion of the mask with more air. Several different designs like Rendell-Baker or Laerdal masks help to minimize the apparatus dead space by allowing a good fit.

Masks are available in variety of sizes and shapes depending on patient's age and size. The sizes available are 0, 1, 2, 3, 4, and 5. Face masks are of two types:

1. Reusable masks **(Fig. 5)**.
2. Disposable masks **(Fig. 6)**.

Advantages of Disposable Masks[5]

- Transparent hence can observe vomitus, secretions, blood or lip color during anesthesia
- Use of inert plastic prevents risk of allergy
- Avoids the cost of sterilization
- Scented variety of disposable mask is more readily accepted by patient.

Disadvantages of Disposable Masks

- Material is cheaper and may be of lower quality
- Limited range of designs and sizes available
- Sizes may not equate between manufacturers
- Some masks may have a poor quality seal due to fixed volume of the air filled cuffs
- Poor fit of the mask may cause ulceration on the areas of face due to high pressure.

MASK STRAPS OR HEAD HARNESS (FIGS. 7A AND B)

A mask strap consists of thin strips arranged in a circle with two or four projections. The head rests in the circle, and the straps attach around the mask. The masks have connector to which these straps are attached. Mask straps are used to hold the mask firmly on the face. Vigilant supervision is needed when harness is attached for hands free ventilation

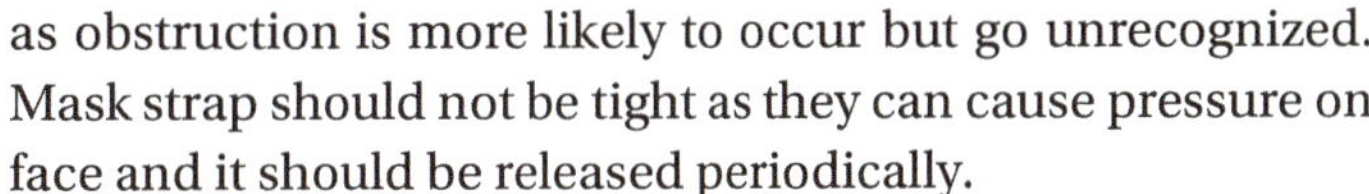

as obstruction is more likely to occur but go unrecognized. Mask strap should not be tight as they can cause pressure on face and it should be released periodically.

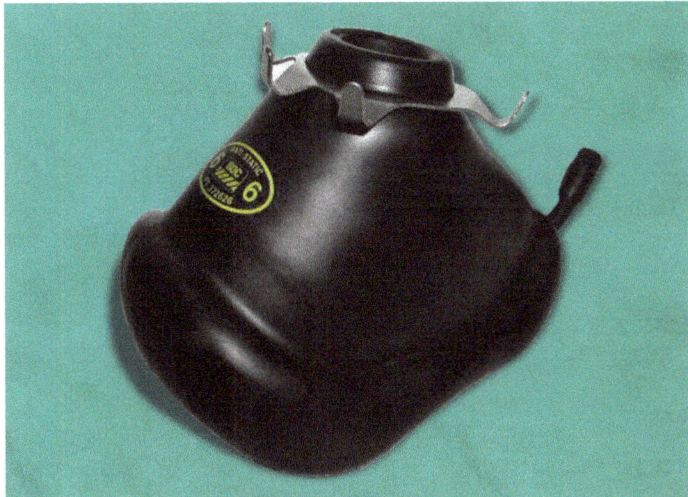

Fig. 5: Reusable mask.

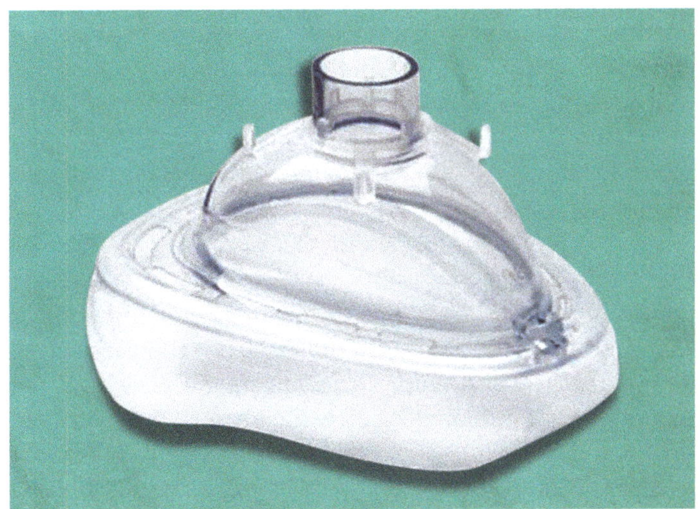

Fig. 6: Disposable mask.

SPECIFIC MASKS

Rendell-Baker-Soucek Mask[6]

The Rendell-Baker-Soucek (RBS) mask **(Fig. 8)** was designed, using well-known dental principles, so that "the mask fits the face as a denture fits the palate". It has a triangular body due to which, this mask has low dead space. The excellent fit obtained provides an airtight seal without the need for apneumatic cuff, which always increases the dead space. The minimal dead space in the masks (4 cc in size 1 and 8 cc in size 2) when used with the new partitioned adapter makes it feasible to anesthetize quite small babies. Rendell-Baker-Soucek mask may have a pacifier too. Hence, this mask is useful in pediatric patients. This mask can be used for the patient with a tracheostomy.[7]

Endoscopic Masks[8]

An endoscopic mask is specifically designed to allow mask ventilation during endoscopic procedures **(Fig. 9)**. It has an elastic diaphragm with a 3 mm diameter opening designed for the passage of a fiberoptic bronchoscope. This technique allows the anesthesiologist to assist ventilation during periods of shallow breathing or desaturation. The endoscopy mask permits the delivery of a higher concentration of oxygen to the patient than a nasal cannula. Positive pressure ventilation can be employed when necessary.

Scented Masks[9]

To make preoxygenation and inhalation anesthesia more acceptable, scented masks have come into practice. They mask the odors of inhalational agents. The scent may be incorporated into the mask during manufacturing or can be applied by the user later.

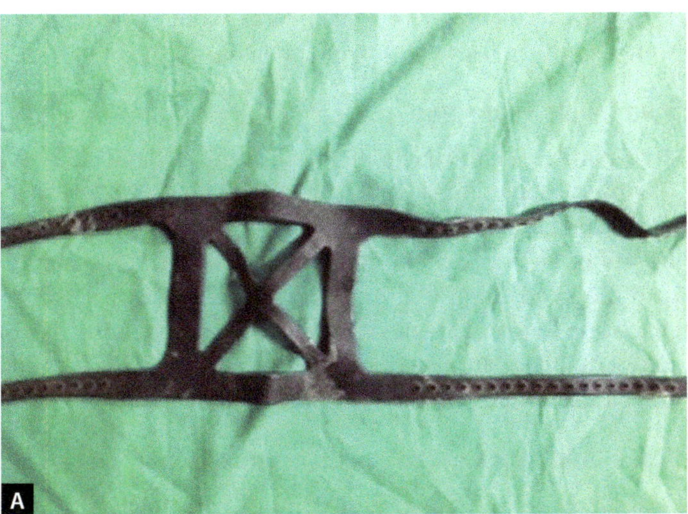

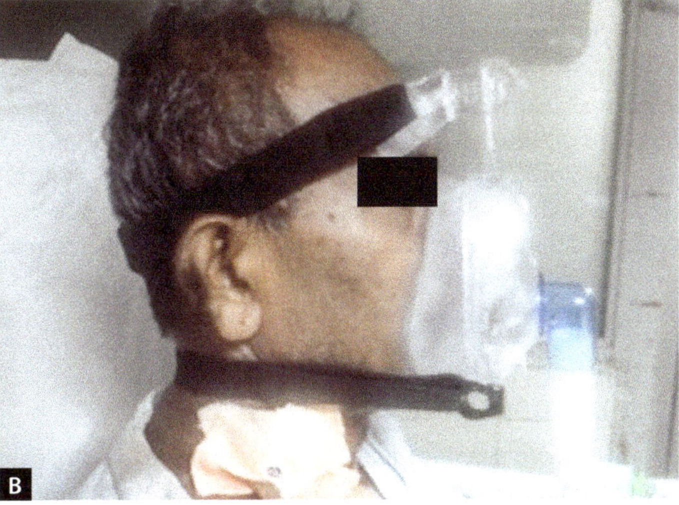

Figs. 7A and B: Disposable mask. (A) Head harness; (B) Harness applied to patient.

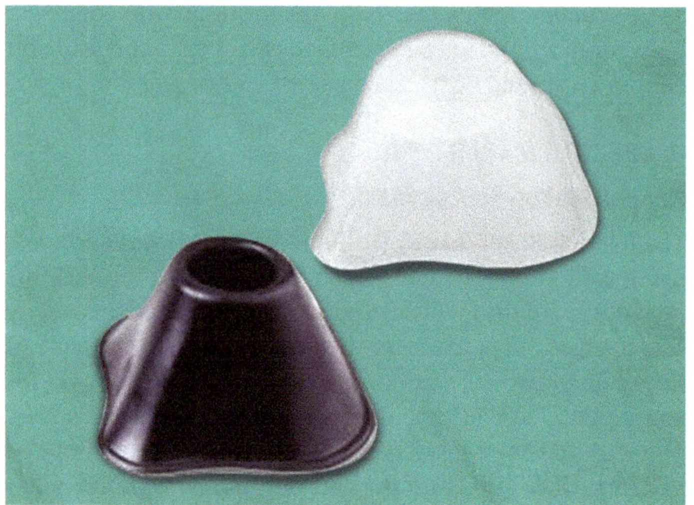

Fig. 8: Rendell-Baker-Soucek mask.

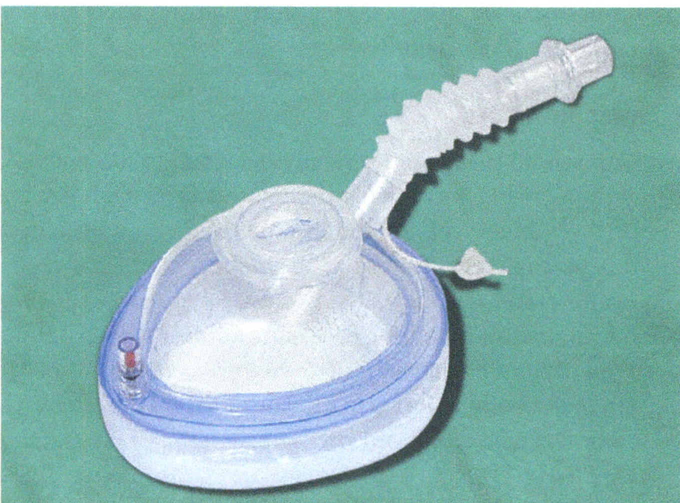

Fig. 9: Endoscopic mask.

Dental Masks or Dental Inhalers

Dental masks are smaller than usual masks as they are designed to fit the nose only. They allow complete access to the mouth during dental procedures.

Masks for Noninvasive Positive Pressure Ventilation or Continuous Positive Airway Pressure (Fig. 10)

These masks are made of plastics and soft silicone rubber similar to anesthesia face masks, but are of better quality for more comfort and tolerability. They may cover the mouth and nose or just the nose for nasal continuous positive airway pressure. These masks may have additional ports for valves and airway manometry. They have attachment for harness to keep the mask comfortably on the patient's face.

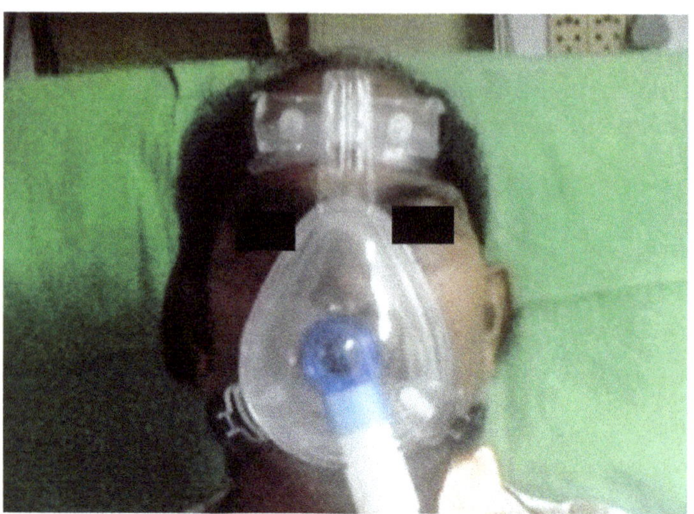

Fig. 10: Continuous positive airway pressure mask.

TECHNIQUES FOR FACE MASKS APPLICATION (VIDEO 4)

An appropriate size face mask is important for a tight seal on the patient's face allowing good mask ventilation. An ill-fitting mask will demand more pressure on patient's face leading to cramps in the hands of the user after some time. An inadequate seal will cause air dilution during spontaneous respiration and inadequate gas exchange during controlled ventilation. This may lead to awareness in spontaneously breathing patients due to air dilution, hypoxia or hypercarbia due to inadequate ventilation in those on controlled ventilation and more consumption of gases as well as increased pollution of operation room environment in spontaneous or controlled breathing.

There are several methods of holding a mask to maintain an open airway and a tight seal.

One-hand Technique

In one-hand technique **(Fig. 11)**, the thumb and index finger of the left hand are placed on the mask body to press mask downward. The remaining three fingers are placed on the mandible with little finger below the angle of the mandible (to lift the mandible for proper fitting) avoiding the soft tissue. This is known as "E-C technique" where thumb and index fingers form alphabet C and remaining three fingers form alphabet E. Additional downward pressure, if needed is then exerted by the anesthetist's chin on the mask. Care should be taken to prevent pressure on the eyes.

Two-hands Technique

Two-hands method **(Fig. 12)** is used for difficult airway.[10] The thumbs and index fingers are placed on either side of the mask body. Remaining fingers of both the hands are placed on either side under the mandible. The mandible is lifted and the head extended. In case of inadequate seal, chin is placed on the mask to exert more downward pressure. In case of two-hand technique, second person is needed to ventilate the patient while the airway is maintained by first person.

Mask Ventilation of the Tracheostomy Stoma

A RBS or other pediatric size mask can be used over a tracheotomy stoma.[7] The mask is placed around the stoma

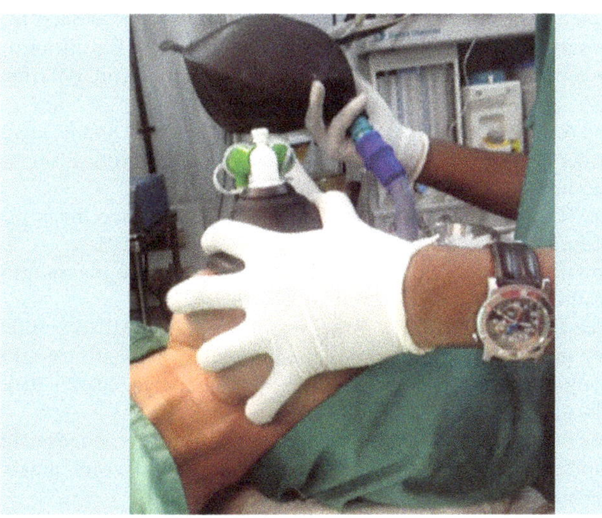

Fig. 11: One-hand mask holding technique.

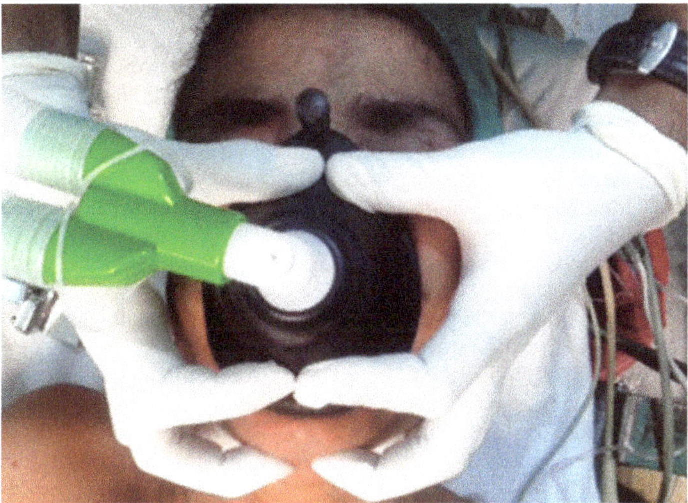

Fig. 12: Two-hands mask holding technique.

in a reverse manner with the nasal portion pointing in a caudal direction and apex resting on the suprasternal notch. Patient can be then ventilated.

Difficult Face Mask Ventilation

In approximately 5–6% of patients receiving general anesthesia, the mask ventilation is found to be difficult. Following are few of the conditions, where we expect difficult mask ventilation:[11]

- *Edentulous patients:* The sagging cheeks and resorption of alveolar process creates gap between face and mask. Insertion of an oral airway, leaving the patient's dentures in place or packing the cheeks with gauze pieces will improve the mask ventilation
- *Facial burns:* Loss of skin due to burns leaves lots of bare and fragile area over face making mask slippery. Keeping gauze piece between face and mask will help
- Male patients have higher incidence of difficult mask ventilation
- Bearded patient
- Obese patients, history of snoring
- Sometimes in anticipated difficult intubation, e.g., higher Mallampati classification, receding mandible, micrognathia, etc.

Advantages of Face Masks

- Minimal occurrence of sore throat
- Less anesthetic depth than using a supraglottic device or endotracheal tube
- Economical method to manage the airway for short duration.

Disadvantages of Face Masks

- Mask holding keeps one person occupied all the time
- Considering the leak around the mask in case of ill-fitting mask, higher fresh gas flows are often needed[12]
- In remote location anesthesia like computed tomography scan and magnetic resonance imaging, mask ventilation is difficult
- Mask ventilation cannot be used for long duration as it is tiresome to continuously hold the mask
- It is difficult to maintain airway with mask and requires lot of manipulations. In such cases laryngeal mask airway is a good option **(Video 4)**.

COMPLICATIONS[3,4]

Skin Allergy

Reaction to the material of mask can cause dermatitis exactly around the area of contact between the mask and skin. Chemical used for sterilization of reusable masks can cause allergic reaction or if rubber is a component of a face mask, a serious reaction can occur in the patient with latex allergy.[13,14]

Nerve Injury[15]

Pressure from a mask or mask strap and jaw thrust for a long time may result in pressure injury to underlying nerves. The mask should be removed from the face periodically so as to avoid continuous pressure on one particular area. In such procedures, supraglottic airway (SGA) device or endotracheal intubation should be considered.

Gastric Inflation

The chances of gastric inflation are more with masks than with SGA device when used for positive pressure ventilation. It is advisable to use inspiratory pressure below 20 cmH_2O.

Eye Injury and Skin Necrosis

A face mask inadvertently placed on an open eye can give rise to corneal abrasion. Pressure on the medial angles of the eyes and supraorbital margins during mask holding for long time can cause eyelid edema, chemosis of the conjunctiva, pressure on the supraorbital nerve, corneal injury, and rarely blindness.[16] Chemicals used for sterilization of masks can cause corneal irritation and ulceration. Similarly, undue pressure on face to keep a tight seal can cause skin ulceration and necrosis.[17]

Cervical Spine Movement[18]

Mask ventilation moves the cervical spine more than SGA or tracheal intubation. This may be of significance in the patient with an unstable cervical spine injury.

Environmental Pollution

Mask ventilation is associated with greater operating room pollution with anesthetic gases than when a tracheal tube or SGA is used.

User Fatigue

Holding a mask onto the face for long time may result in operator fatigue.

Jaw Pain

Postoperative jaw pain is more common after mask anesthesia than when an SGA device is used.

CONCLUSION

Face mask is a basic equipment needed for airway management; hence knowledge about the different types and sizes of masks, their uses in different situations, advantages and disadvantages of one over the other will help anesthetist manage airway well.

REFERENCES

1. The Wood Library Museum. (2013). Schimmelbusch mask. [online]. Available from http://woodlibrarymuseum.org/museum/item/58/schimmelbusch-mask. [Last accessed February, 2014].
2. Bhargava AK. Early devices for inhalation of Ether and Chloroform. Indian J Anaesth. 2003;47(3):176-7.
3. Dorsch JA, Dorsch SE. Face masks and airways. In: Dorsch JA, Dorsch SE (Eds). Understanding Anesthesia Equipment, 5th edition. Philadelphia: Lippincott Williams and Wilkins; 2007.
4. Diba A. Airway management devices. In: Davey AJ, Diba A (Eds). Ward's Anaesthetic Equipment, 5th edition. London: Elsevier Saunders; 2005.
5. Diaz JH. A new transparent disposable plastic face mask for children and adults. Anesthesiology. 1993;78(6):1195-6.
6. Rendell-Baker L, Soucek DH. New paediatric face masks and anesthetic equipment. Br Med J. 1962;1(5293):1690.
7. McGrath BA, Bates L, Atkinson D, et al. Multidisciplinary guidelines for the management of tracheostomy and laryngectomy airway emergencies. Anaesthesia. 2012;67(9):1025-41.
8. Rauch RY, Brener CE. Airway management for paediatric esophagogastroduodenoscopy using an endoscopy mask. Anaesth Analg. 2003;96(1):303-4.
9. Hinkle AJ. Scented masks in pediatric anesthesia. Anesthesiology. 1987;66(1):104-5.
10. Adnet F. Difficult mask ventilation. An underestimated aspect of the problem of the difficult airway? Anesthesiology. 2000;92(5):1217-8.
11. Langeron O, Masso E, Huraux C, et al. Prediction of difficult mask ventilation. Anesthesiology. 2000;92(5):1229-36.
12. McDouall SF, Campbell RC, Tasker RC. Clinical alert: failure in face mask seal as a consequence of incorrect face mask assembly. Br J Anaesth. 2003;91(6):924-5.
13. McKinstry LJ, Fenton WJ, Barrett P. Anesthesia and the patient with latex allergy. Can J Anaesth. 1992;39(6):587-9.
14. Weiss ME, Hirshman CA. Latex Allergy. Can J Anaesth. 1992;39(6):528-32.
15. Bhuiyan MS, Chapman M. Mental nerve injury following facemask anaesthesia. Anaesthesia. 2006;61(5):516-7.
16. Munn KA, Williams RT, Shafto CM. Transient unilateral blindness following general anaesthesia: Case report. Can Anaesth Soc J. 1978;25(5):433-5.
17. Smurthwaite GJ, Ford P. Skin necrosis following continuous positive airway pressure with a face mask. Anaesthesia. 1993;48(2):147-8.
18. Brimacombe J, Keller C, Kunzel KH, et al. Cervical spine motion during airway management: as cinefluoroscopic study of the posteriorly destabilized cervical vertebrae in human cadavers. Anesth Analg. 2000;91(5):1274-8.

Laryngoscopes

Naina P Dalvi, Nazmeen I Sayed

ABSTRACT

Laryngoscope, an instrument used to visualize the larynx, is to the anesthetist what the oxygen is to a living being. This essential topic is covered in detail in this chapter. Beginning from a brief history this chapter describes the basic structure of laryngoscope and then goes ahead to describe its essential modifications till date. "Video laryngoscopes" the latest invention requiring equal attention is covered in another chapter.

INTRODUCTION

Laryngoscope is an instrument used to visualize the larynx and surrounding structures either by displacing the soft tissue away from the line of vision or by optical aids. The main purpose of a laryngoscope is to aid the intubation. Laryngoscopes, by bringing the esophagus and larynx under view, are helpful in passing the nasogastric tube, oral suctioning, throat packing, and removing oral foreign body.

Tracheal intubation with metal tubes was practiced in 1880s by physicians William Macewen and Joseph O'Dwyer using fingers as a guide to treat subglottic edema due to diphtheria[1] **(Fig. 1)**. Larynx was first visualized by Manuel Garcia, a singer, who used an indirect mirror to visualize the cord movement during singing.[2] Many mirror based instruments were invented by otolaryngologists to visualize the larynx. But a rigid laryngoscope design that is still popular among the ear, nose, and throat (ENT) surgeons for direct laryngoscopy was described by Caveliar Jackson around 1907. Jackson laryngoscope has a "U" shaped handle with a straight blade and "O" shaped flange **(Fig. 2)**. The laryngoscope had a battery based external light source. In 1913, Janeway designed the "L" laryngoscope with straight blade and batteries within the handle. Enumerable modifications of the straight blade were then introduced, but the design that persists is the Miller's modification of straight blade introduced in 1941. Laryngoscopy in this era was performed by lifting the epiglottis. This type of laryngoscopy is a struggle in adults and so no design of straight blade was satisfactory. Relief came when Sir Robert Macintosh introduced his curved blade in 1943, the Macintosh blade, and described the indirect method of epiglottis lift to expose the larynx. Macintosh blade has no substitute for laryngoscopy in normal patients and has undergone negligible changes since first introduced. Macintosh blade was not the answer for anterior larynx or difficult intubation. The era of indirect laryngoscopy in anesthesia started with the Siker mirror laryngoscope and then by prisms introduced by Huffman.

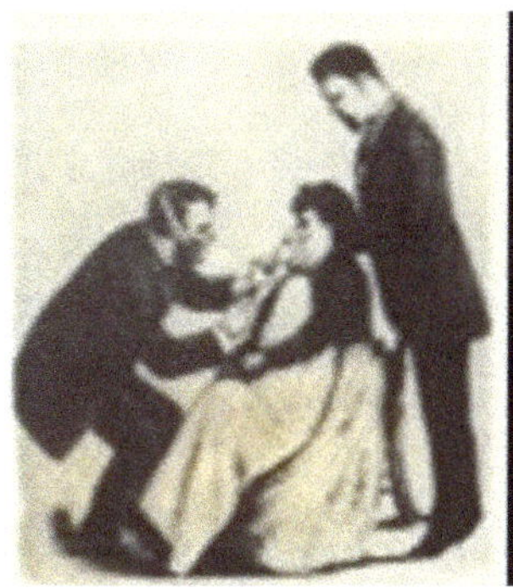
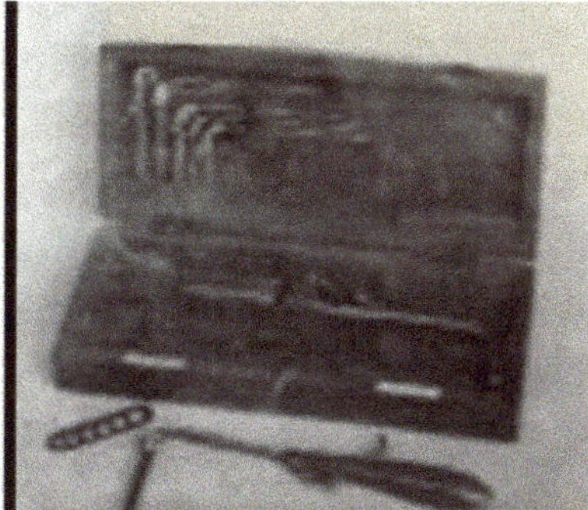

Fig. 1: Blind tactile intubation with metal tube by Joseph O'Dwyer.

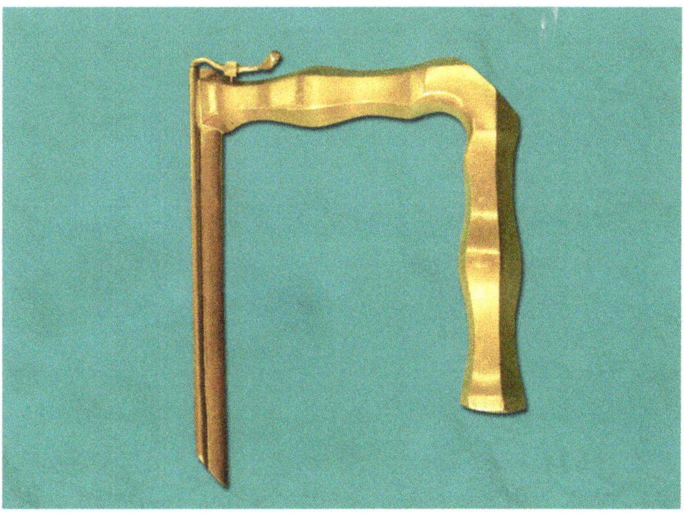

Fig. 2: Caveliar Jackson laryngoscope.

VARIOUS PARTS OF LARYNGOSCOPE

A laryngoscope consists of a detachable blade and a handle. The blade is attached to the handle by a "hinge" type of joint.

Blade

Blade is that portion of the laryngoscope that is introduced in the mouth. It has a tongue, flange, base, web, light source and a tip **(Figs. 3 and 4)**.

- The tongue or spatula is that portion of the blade which is used to swipe the tongue aside and depresses lower jaw for visualization of the larynx. Depending on the shape of the tongue or spatula, the blades are classified as straight or curved
- The flange accommodates the tongue and keeps it away from the line of vision. The flange, web and tongue decide the cross-sectional shape of the blade
- The portion of the blade that connects the tongue and the flange is called the web or the vertical part

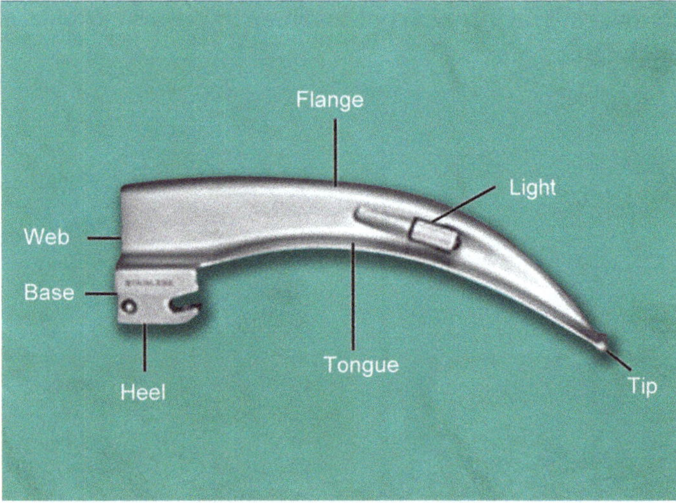

Fig. 3: Parts of curved blade.

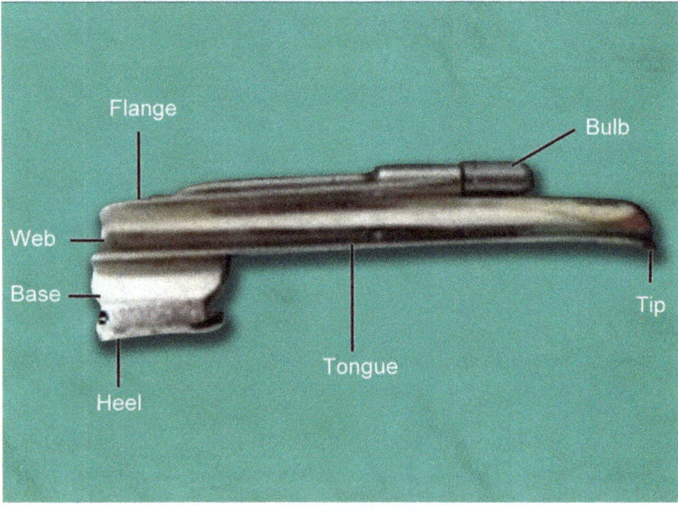

Fig. 4: Parts of straight blade.

- Tip is the most distal part of the blade that is used to lift the epiglottis either directly or indirectly by upward traction or "hooking the vallecula"
- The part of the blade that contacts the handle is called the base. The slot on the base helps in hinging the handle
- The lowermost part of the base is the heel. Heel contains small metal ball that provides the contact for the handle
- The light source is either an incandescent bulb or a fiberoptic channel with a halogen or xenon bulb in the handle **(Fig. 5)**. Light can be measured at a number of points:[3]
  - *At its source:* Luminous flux, measured in lumens
  - *At the surface receiving the light that is being illuminated:* Illuminance measured in lux. A minimum illumination of 700 lux at a distance of 20 mm has been suggested in a draft standard for laryngoscopes from the International Organization for Standardization (ISO). The proposed standard of 700 lux may possibly be too bright. Factors such as light distribution and laryngoscope design also need to be considered and maintained as they may have considerable effect on light requirements. A laryngoscope with an adjustable light output may be the answer to provide every anesthetist's illumination needs[4]
  - *By looking at the amount of light re-emitted from a surface in a given direction:* Luminance measured in candela per square meter (cd/m^2). During direct laryngoscopy, perception of the surface brightness of the larynx depends on light transmitted back to the laryngoscopist's eyes from the surface of the larynx; this is the luminance. The luminance of the larynx is dependent, in turn, on both the illuminance and the light reflected from the tissues. The minimum required luminance for effective laryngoscopy is 100 cd/m^2.

The sizes of blades to be used in patients given by ISO standards **(Table 1)**.[5]

Handle

The part of the laryngoscope that is held in the hand is called the handle. Handles are striated to give a firm grip and harbor the batteries. Contact area on the handle comes in contact with the metal ball on the heel of the blade when the blade is hinged to the handle, thus completing the electrical circuit that powers the bulb. They also harbor the halogen bulb in laryngoscopes with fiberoptic illumination. Stubby handles are used in obese patients or parturient to avoid the large breast. Pencil handles are used in pediatric patients. Fiberoptic handles have a green band **(Fig. 6)**.

Patil Syracuse handle is an adjustable handle where in the blade can be locked in four positions making different angles with the handle (180°, 135°, 90°, and 45°) **(Fig. 7)**.[6]

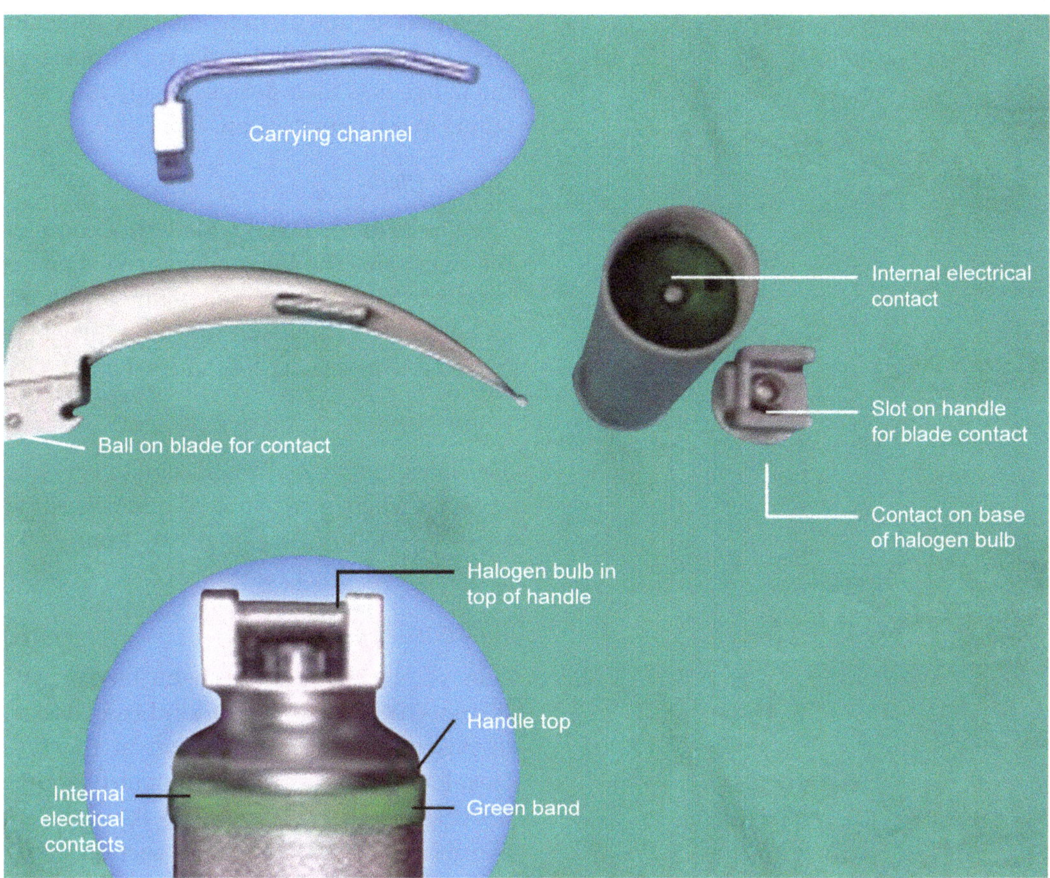

Fig. 5: Fiberoptic light source.

TABLE 1: The sizes of blade and their uses.

Size	*Patient type*
000	Small premature infant
00	Small premature infant
0	Neonate
1	Small child
2	Child
3	Adult
4	Large adult
5	Extra-large adult

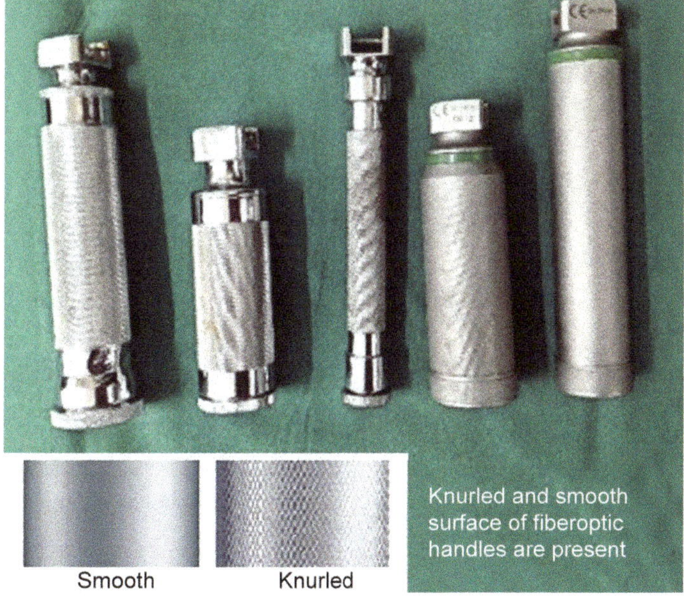

Fig. 6: Types of handle.

Using a Howland lock on any conventional laryngoscope can reduce the blade angle to 45° **(Fig. 8)**.

TYPES OF LARYNGOSCOPES (TABLE 2)

Laryngoscopes with Straight Blades

Laryngoscopy before introduction of Macintosh laryngoscope was by the blade being introduced from the center of the mouth and lifting the epiglottis directly. Thus, in the initial years of history laryngoscope blades were straight blades as they gave more room for intubation.

The basic design of the straight blade consists of a straight tongue, a flange that curves to the right and a curved tip to lift the epiglottis. The tongue, web and flange together formed a channel that was used for unobstructed vision directly up to the larynx. This channel was used to pass the endotracheal tube (ETT).

"The larger the curve the better the insertion of tube" was the opinion held in the 1930s and 1940s. But later it was realized that broad bases at the proximal end caused dental damage,[7] so the height of blades were successively reduced. As the ETT is introduced through such channels

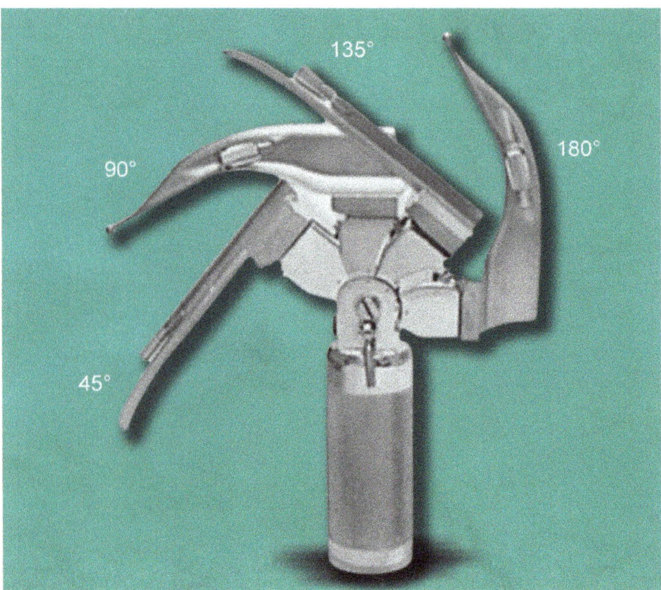

Fig. 7: Patil Syracuse handle.

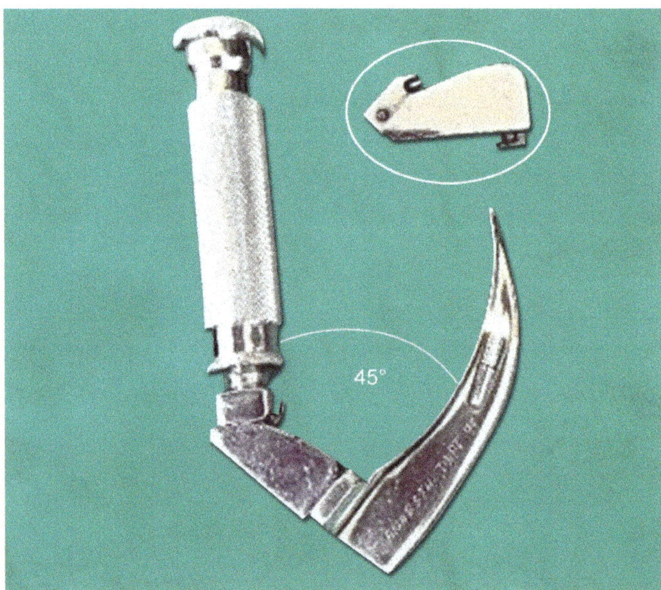

Fig. 8: Howland lock.

TABLE 2: Types of laryngoscope.

Rigid	
• Direct-classified on the bases of the blade type	
Laryngoscopes with straight blade	Guedel, Wisconsin, Miller, etc.
Laryngoscopes with curved blade	Macintosh, Bizzarri-Giuffrida, etc.
Laryngoscopes with features of both blades	Cardiff, Dorges
Laryngoscopes for special purpose	Flexitip, Polio, Oxiport, Tull, etc.
• Indirect	
Prisms	Belscope, Trueview, Huffman prism
Optical	Bullards, UpsherScope, Augustine Scope
Optical stylet type	Bonfil's retromolar, Shikani's intubating stylet
Video laryngoscopes	Berci DCI, C-Mac, Glidescope, etc.
Flexible	
Fiberoptic bronchoscope	–

the larynx is out of sight causing difficulty in intubation. So the large right sided curve was progressively reduced and the flange was then designed only to keep the tongue from falling in the line of vision.

Guedel Blade

The flange of the Guedel blade is a complete "U" turned to the right side. The tongue is placed at an angle of 72° to the handle to allow lifting the epiglottis without using the teeth as a fulcrum. The distal tip has a 10° curve. Guedel blade is available in sizes 1, 2, 3, and 4 **(Fig. 9)**.

Flagg Blade

The Flagg blade is straight with a very slight curve at the distal tip, a light source placed quite distally and the C-shaped cross-section tapering gradually from its proximal to distal end. It is available in sizes 0, 1, 2, 3, and 4 **(Fig. 10)**.

Wisconsin Blade

One of the popular straight blades of 1930s was the Wisconsin type. The Wisconsin blade, designed by University of Wisconsin Anesthesiologists at the Wisconsin General Hospital in Madison, is a straight blade with a flange that widens distally and curves to the right. This curve forms two-thirds of circle in cross-section. The tip is widened to help lift the epiglottis. Wisconsin blade is available in sizes 2, 3, and 4 with newer versions having fiberoptic lights **(Fig. 11)**.

The whitehead modification of Wisconsin blade has a reduced flange and is open proximally and distally **(Fig. 12)**.

Wis-Foregger is a modification of the Wisconsin blade with a flange that expands towards the distil end. The distil part is wider with slight right curve **(Fig. 13)**.

Wis-Hipple blade is a modification of Wisconsin blade meant mainly for infants. The semicircular channel is present but the flange is more parallel to the spatula and is less curved. It is available in sizes 00, 0, 1, and 1.5 **(Fig. 14)**.

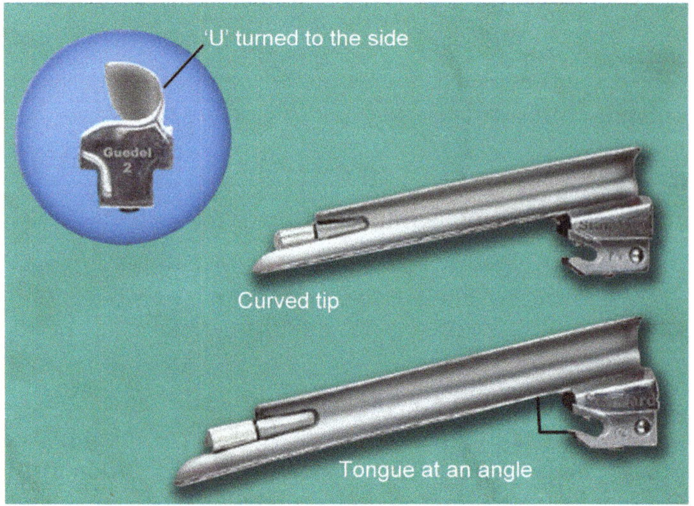

Fig. 9: Guedel blade.

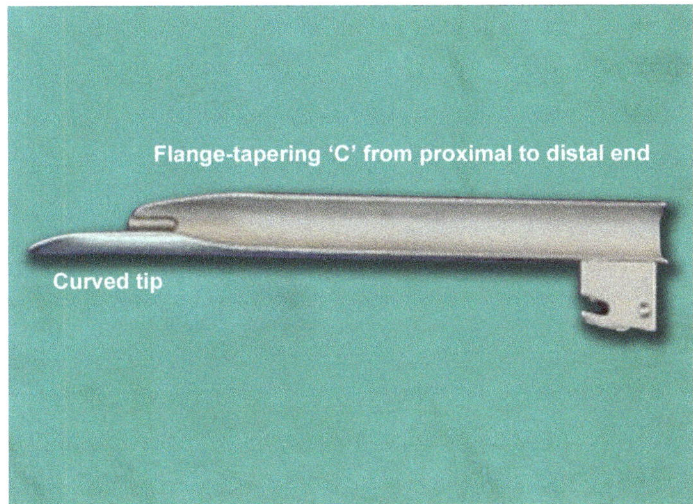

Fig. 10: Flagg blade.

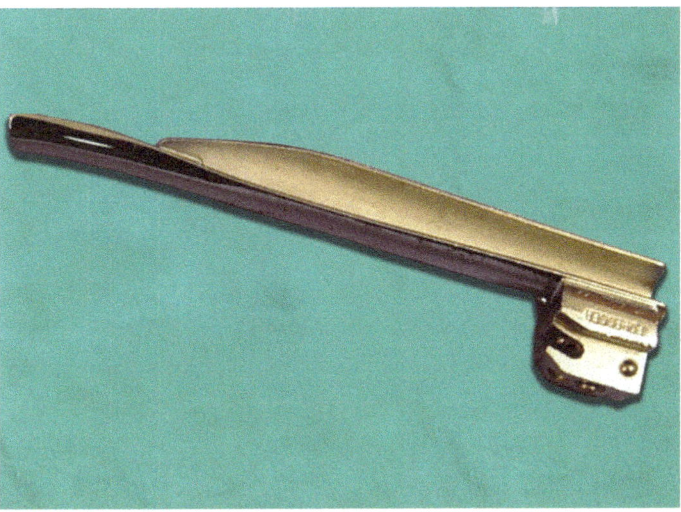

Fig. 13: Wis-Foregger blade.

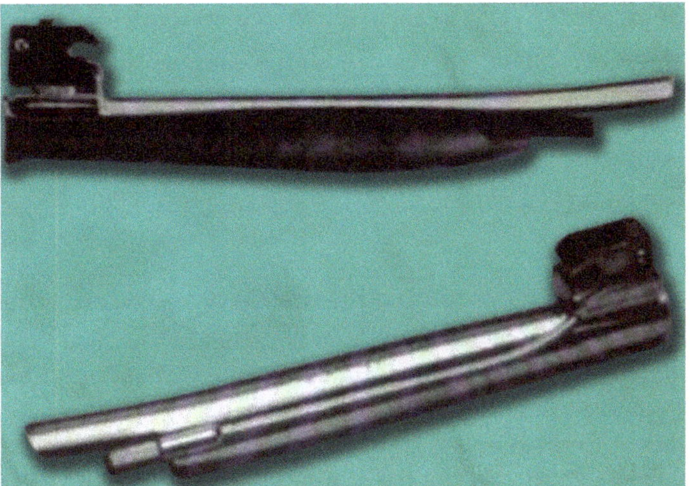

Fig. 11: Wisconsin blade.

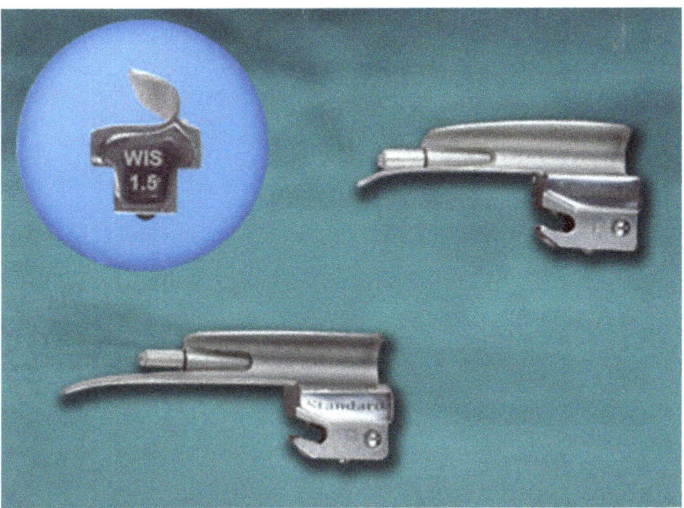

Fig. 14: Wis-Hipple blade.

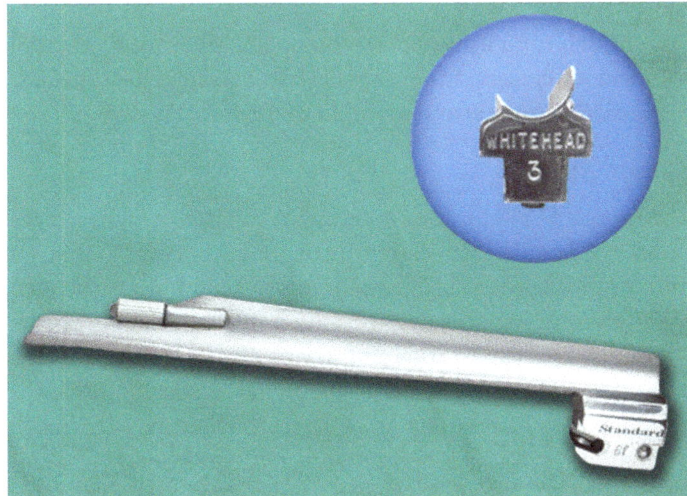

Fig. 12: Whitehead modification of Wisconsin blade.

Miller Blade

In 1941, Sir Robert A Miller modified the existing straight blade to form the Miller's blade which was meant for both adult and pediatric patients.[7] This blade was longer than the old straight blades and only one size was available for all patients except infants. It was shallow at the base and narrower at the tip. The distal 2 inch of the blade was curved upwards to allow lift of epiglottis. For better light the bulb was placed distally close to the tip. Flange was "C" shaped. Like in other straight blades, the tongue, web and the flange were to form a channel for visualizing the larynx and passing the tube **(Fig. 15)**.

Disadvantage of Miller blade is that the light source would disappear under the tongue[8] and the tongue tends to bulge in front of the blade.

Present Miller's blade has undergone the following modifications **(Fig. 16)**:

- In 1946 Miller described the pediatric modification of his adult blade.[9] This blade could be inserted anterior or posterior to the epiglottis. Miller sizes available now are 00, 0, 1, 2, 3, and 4
- Flange height has been reduced and the flange is less curved and forms a compressed "D" when seen longitudinally

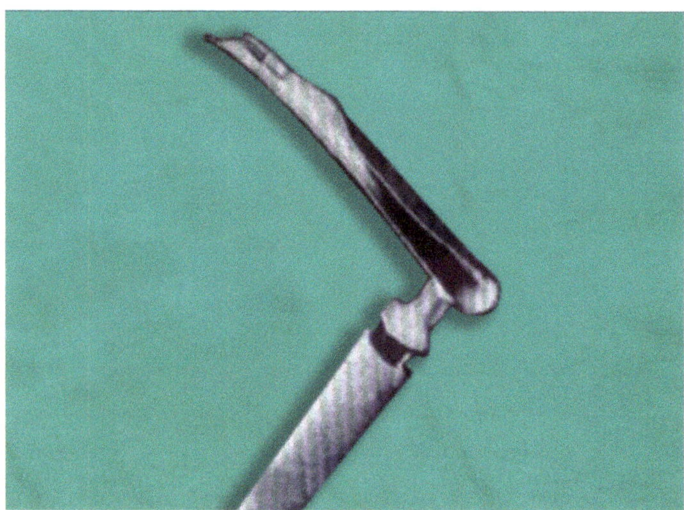

Fig. 15: Original Miller blade.

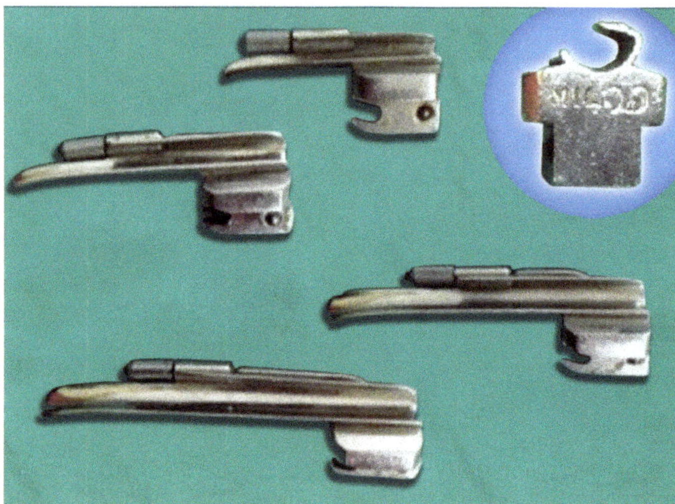

Fig. 16: Present day Miller's blade.

- The tongue is straighter
- The channel formed by the tongue and the flange is no longer meant for introducing the ETT. The tube is inserted from the angle of the mouth
- Miller blades with fiberoptic light source are available. Some of these blades have the bulb protected by the flange **(Fig. 17)**.

Miller's blade still forms the prototype of straight blade in the present era as it is inseparable from infant and difficult pediatric intubation. It forms a part of the armamentarium of pediatric difficult airway algorithm of American Pediatric Association.[10] Advantage being—

- Curved tip of the straight blade is ideal for elevation of the floppy infant epiglottis. Attempts to lift the epiglottis directly with the smooth rounded tip of the Macintosh blade causes the epiglottis to slip out
- Better vision with a straight blade when compared to curved blades in anterior larynx (e.g., infant larynx and micrognatia)[11,12]
- Narrow based straight blade occupy less space than the curved blades.

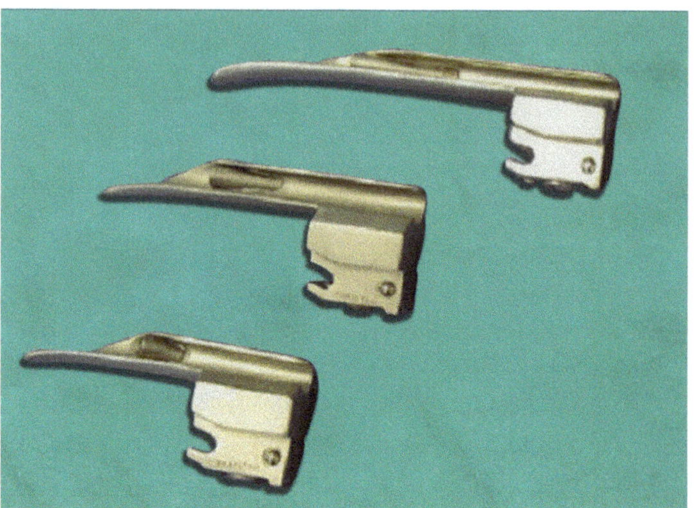

Fig. 17: Miller's blade: Bulb protected by flange.

Snow Blade

In 1962, Dr John Snow introduced a slimmer and smaller version of the Miller blade which was 15 mm in width and height and 162 mm in length. The distal one inch is curved upwards and has a rounded peak at the tip to lift the epiglottis **(Fig. 18)**.[13]

Phillips Blade

The Phillips blade designed by Dr Otto C Phillips in 1972 combines the features of Jackson and Miller blade. The shaft of the Jackson blade was maintained for easy ETT insertion. Thus the blade has a large "C" shaped large channel for tube insertion and a small curved tip to lift epiglottis efficiently. The curved tip of miller blade helps lifting the epiglottis. The light bulb is in the left **(Fig. 19)**.[12]

Schapira Blade

Dr Max Schapira introduced a blade in 1973 with a minimal web and no flange. This blade also had a deeper curve distally to cradle the tongue and sweep it to the left **(Fig. 20)**.[14]

Seward Blade

The Seward blade has a straight tongue which curves upwards distally. The flange proximally curves to the left and forms a reverse "Z" shape in cross-section with the web and tongue. Towards the rounded tip, the flange curves slightly to the right protecting the bulb. The Seward blade was designed to be used in neonatal resuscitation. It is suitable for children up to 5 years of age and for nasal intubation. It has an adult sized light bulb for a brighter vision **(Fig. 21)**.[9]

Robertshaw Blade

One of the few blades used in infants and children is the Robertshaw blade. The distinguishing feature of this blade is that the step is deviated to the left and it has a minimal flange curving to the right. These flange tappers smoothly

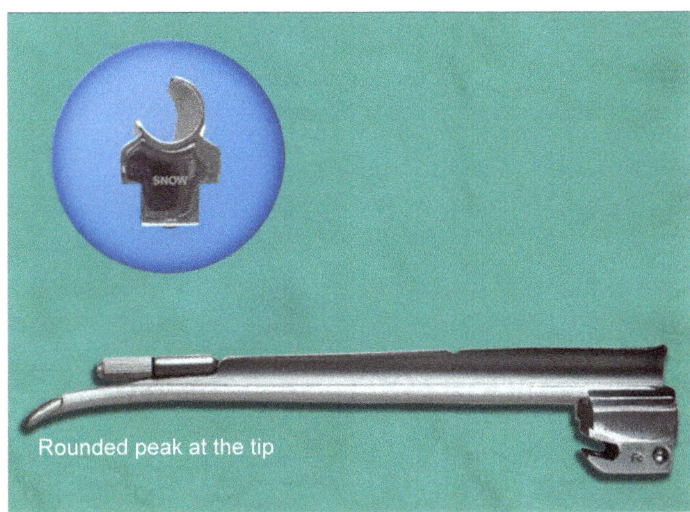

Fig. 18: Snow blade.

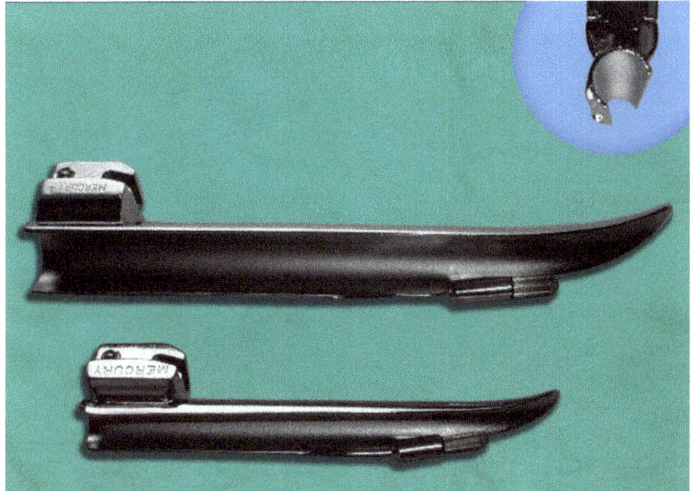

Fig. 19: Phillips blade.

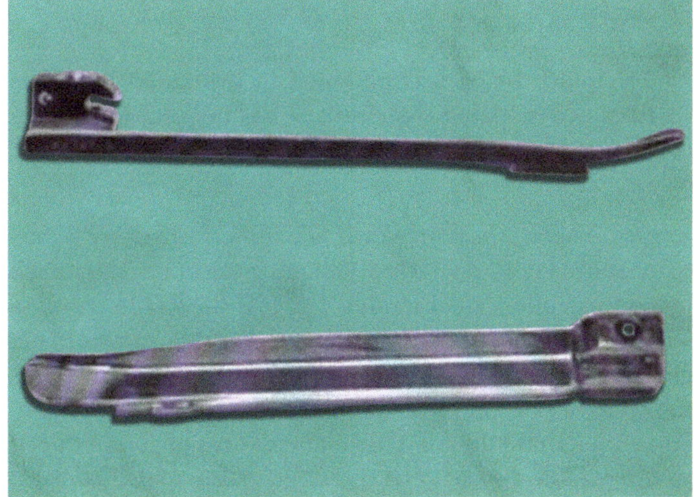

Fig. 20: Schapira blade.
Source: Schapira M. A modified straight laryngoscope blade designed to facilitate endotracheal intubation. Anesth Analg. 1973;52(4):553-4.

to the tip. Thus the channel of the straight blades is lost in this model. The vertical height is also reduced so the lateral wall is obliterated. Thus Robertshaw blade provides

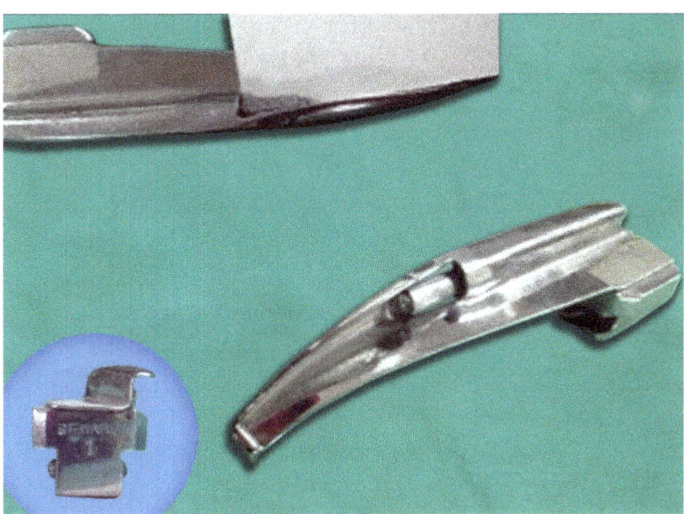

Fig. 21: Seward blade.

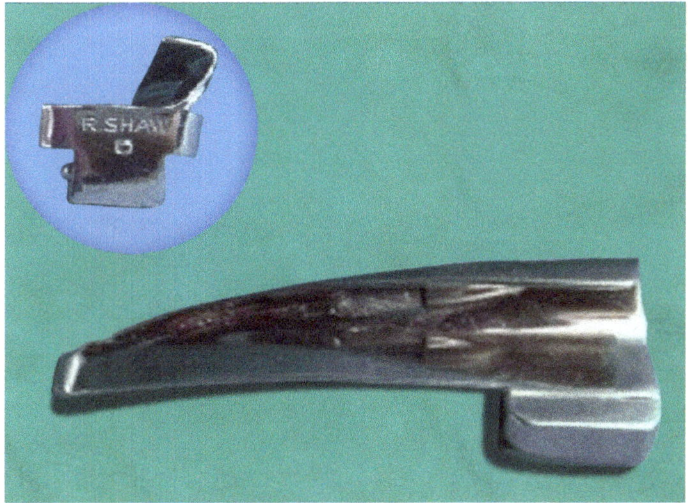

Fig. 22: Robertshaw blade.

binocular vision.[9] The light source is well protected from the tongue inside the vertical step. The straight tongue has a gentle curve near the tip and this blade is used to lift the epiglottis indirectly **(Fig. 22)**.

Cranwall Blade

The Cranwall blade has a curved tip like a Miller blade. There is a reduced flange to decrease the potential for damage to the upper teeth **(Fig. 23)**.

Oxford Blade

The Oxford or Bryce-Smith blade is a straight blade in which the flange and the web form a U-shape and the flange gradually tapers distally with the distal 2–5 cm being open. Though meant for neonates, it can be used for children up to 3 years. The broad proximal flange helps prevent the upper lip from obscuring the view and also potentially helps in difficult cleft-palate situations. The light is well protected in the web to the right of the flange. Green line version is available **(Fig. 24)**.

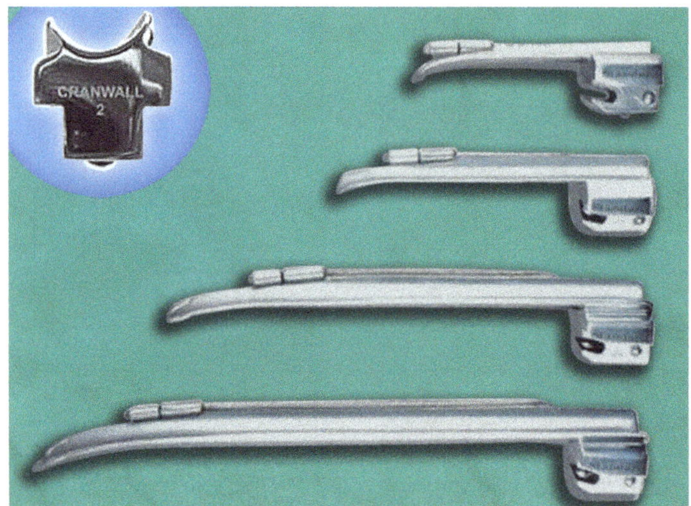

Fig. 23: Cranwall blade.

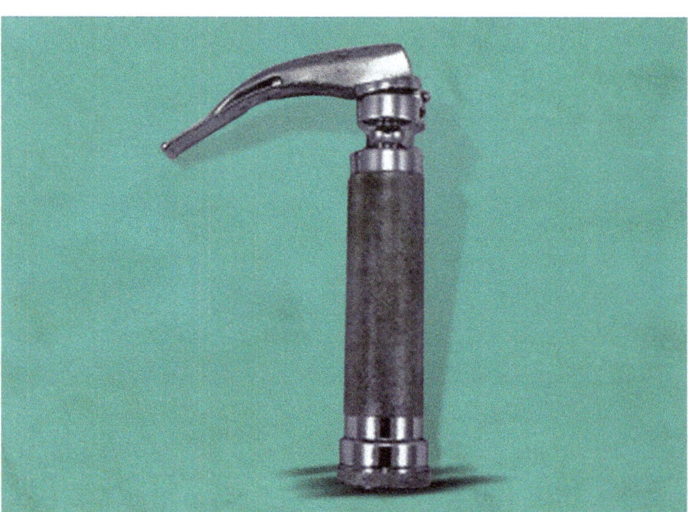

Fig. 25: Original Macintosh blade.

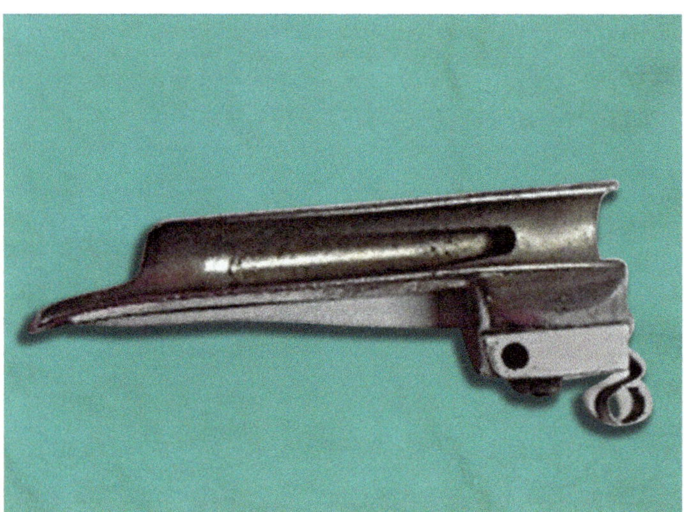

Fig. 24: Oxford blade.

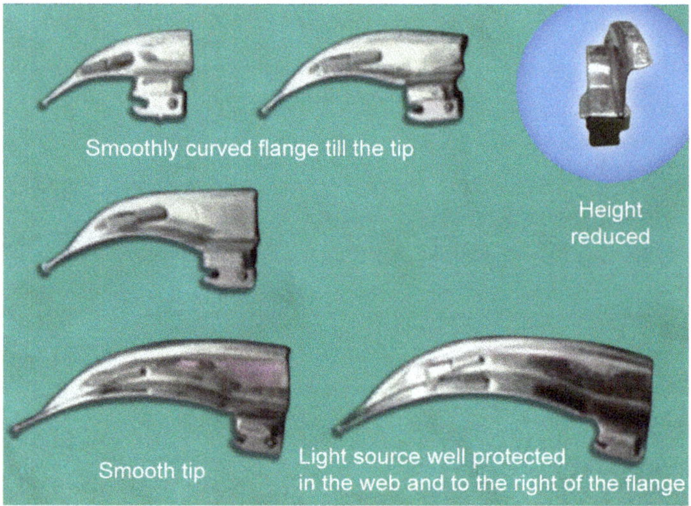

Fig. 26: English Macintosh blade.

Laryngoscopes with Curved Blade

Macintosh Curved Blade

Sir Robert Reynolds Macintosh in 1943 during a tonsillectomy surgery noticed how easily the Boyle Davis mouth gag lay open the larynx. The same day he got the mouth gag soldered to a handle. Thus the Macintosh curved blade was invented. Macintosh blade was shorter than the existing blades so that the tip finished just before the epiglottis. Initially this blade had various types of curves as Macintosh was of the opinion that the curve did not matter but the length had to be short enough just to reach the epiglottis. Later, the curve of the Macintosh blade was settled to match the anatomical curve of the Magill's ETT.[15]

Macintosh blade has a curved spatula, the vertical height is raised and the flange is turned to the left. The tongue, web and the flange form a reverse "Z" in cross-section. The tip is smooth and rounded **(Fig. 25)**. Versions with fiberoptic light source are also available.

Macintosh blade was patented in two countries. Thus we have two models of Macintosh, the "English" Macintosh or the E-Mac and the "American" MacIntosh or the A-Mac.

English Macintosh: Longworth Scientific Instrument Company (now Penlon) in 1958 shifted from brass Macintosh blade to stainless steel model. The less malleable stainless steel resulted in changes in the standard Macintosh blade giving rise to the "E-Mac" or English Macintosh.[15] Thus the straight portion of the flange was reduced to a smooth curve right up to the tip. The height of the flange is reduced so the blade is longer than the original Macintosh blade to improve vision in anterior larynx. Size 0, 1, 2, 3, 4, and 5 are available **(Fig. 26)**.

American Macintosh: A-Mac still retains the original shape of standard Macintosh. The flange is higher than E-Mac and is straight proximally to provide more space. The curved flange ends proximal to the tip **(Fig. 27)**.

But compared to A-Mac, E-Mac has better laryngoscopic view.[16]

Reduced flange Macintosh: It is a modification of Macintosh blade, where the proximal flange is reduced to avoid dental injuries **(Fig. 28)**.

Improved vision Macintosh: Improved vision Macintosh has a concave tongue in the midportion to allow better vision **(Fig. 29)**.

Left-handed Macintosh: Mirror-image version of the Macintosh blade exists for use with the right hand in which the flange is on the opposite side. Potential uses include laryngoscopy of patients in the right lateral decubitus position, or with right-sided facial or oropharyngeal abnormalities, and procedures in which the ETT should be located on the left side of the mouth.

Bizzarri-Giuffrida Blade

The Bizzarri-Giuffrida blade (flangeless Macintosh) is named after its two inventors Dr Joseph G Giuffrida and Dr Dente V Bizzari.[17] The vertical part of Macintosh blade is removed and only a small part of the flange protecting the bulb is left. This blade was designed to be used in patients with limited mouth opening, buck teeth, and anterior larynx. The slimness of the blade allows easy insertion and manipulation of the blade in such difficult intubation **(Fig. 30)**.

Choi Double-angle Laryngoscope

Choi in 1990s described a double-angled blade **(Fig. 31)**.[18] Choi intended to design a blade eliminating the drawbacks of both Macintosh and Miller blade. Thus the flange of Macintosh blade is removed and the straight tongue is given two incremental angles—proximal 20° and distal 30°. The spatula and tip are wide and flat so that tongue or epiglottis can be lifted easily. The light source lies along the left edge of the blade between the two angles and is protected by the minimal flange. The double-angled blade can be used to lift the epiglottis directly or indirectly. It is commercially available in one adult and one pediatric size.

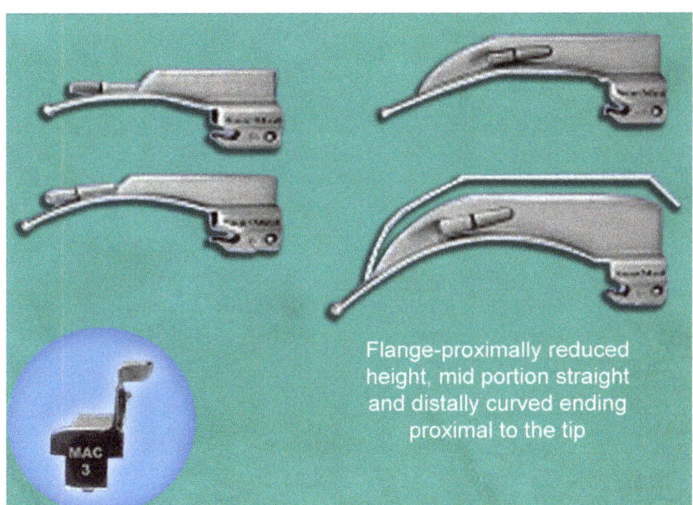

Fig. 27: American Macintosh.

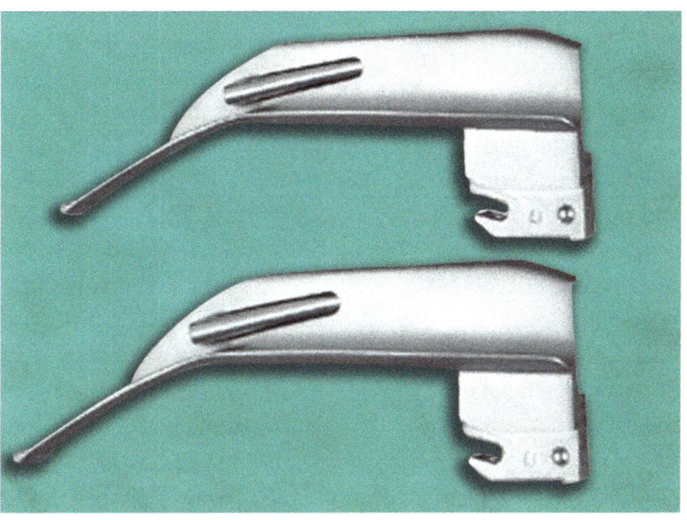

Fig. 29: Improved vision Macintosh blade.

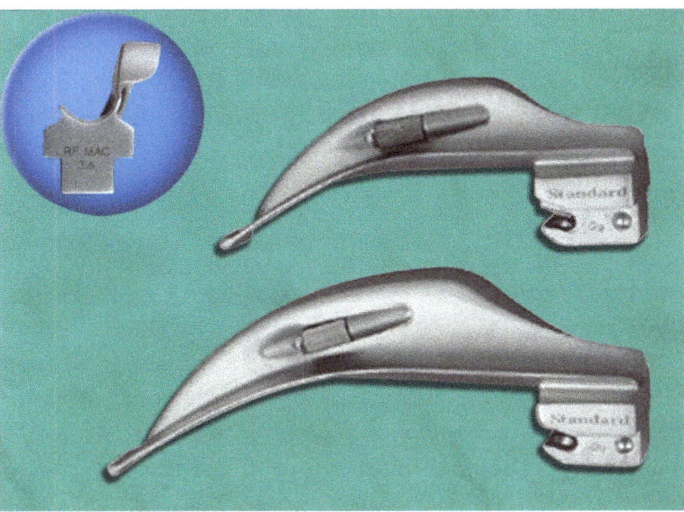

Fig. 28: Reduced flange Macintosh blade.

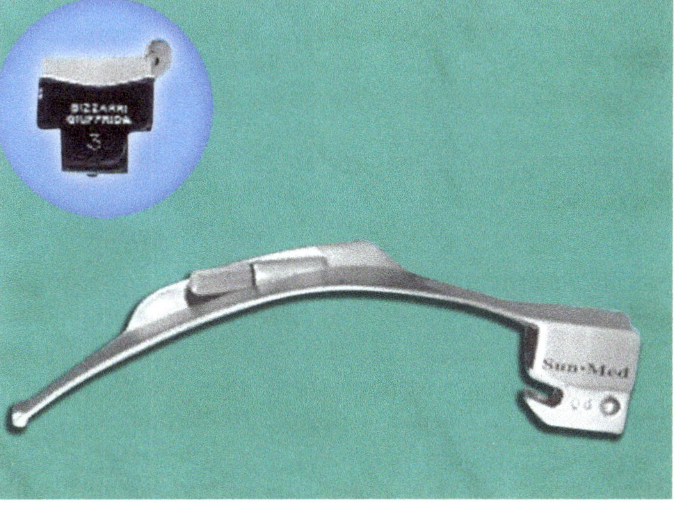

Fig. 30: Bizzarri-Giuffrida blade.

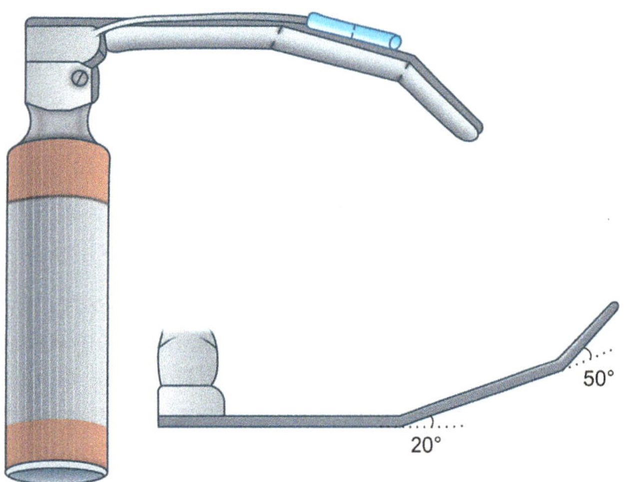

Fig. 31: Choi double-angle laryngoscope.
Source: Choi JJ. A new double-angled blade for direct laryngoscopy. Anesthesiology. 1990;72:576.

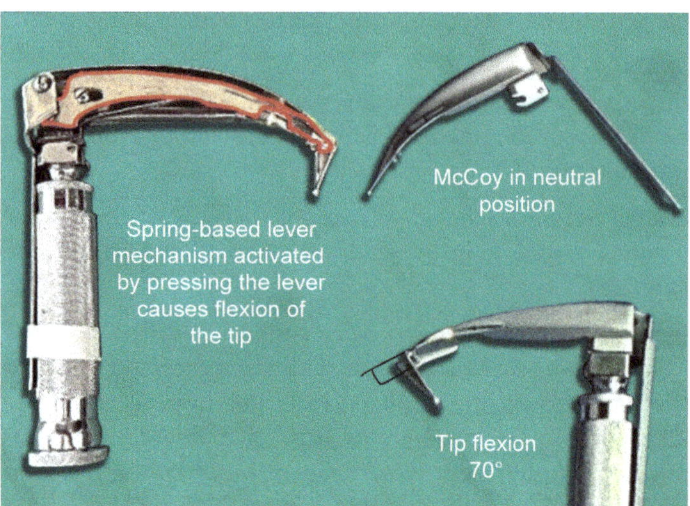

Fig. 32: McCoy blade.

McCoy Blade

The McCoy blade [Corazzelli-London-McCoy (CLM) blade] is a flexible tip blade that has a hinged tip controlled by the lever. When the lever is pressed towards the handle, 2.5 cm of the distil tip is flexed by 70°.[3] This blade is called by various names such as Flipper, Flex-tip, levering laryngoscope blade and articulating laryngoscope blade. McCoy blade is a modification of Macintosh blade available in sizes 1, 2, 3, and 4. Greenline version of McCoy laryngoscopes are available. This blade is inserted and used as the normal curved blade with the tip lying in the vallecula. When the lever is activated the tip flexes and elevates the epiglottis furthermore, thus improving the Cormack and Lahane laryngoscopic grade. McCoy blade forms a part of the difficult intubation trolley. McCoy blade with bougie has been used to successfully intubate Cormack and Lahane grade IV patients. Due to minimal cervical manipulation, the blade has been preferred in the unstable cervical spine.[19,20] The head extension required for laryngoscopy and the stress response to laryngoscopy are less with the McCoy blade than with the Macintosh blade **(Fig. 32)**.[21,22]

Flexi-tip is available with the Seward straight blade in size no. 1 for pediatric use **(Fig. 33)**.[11]

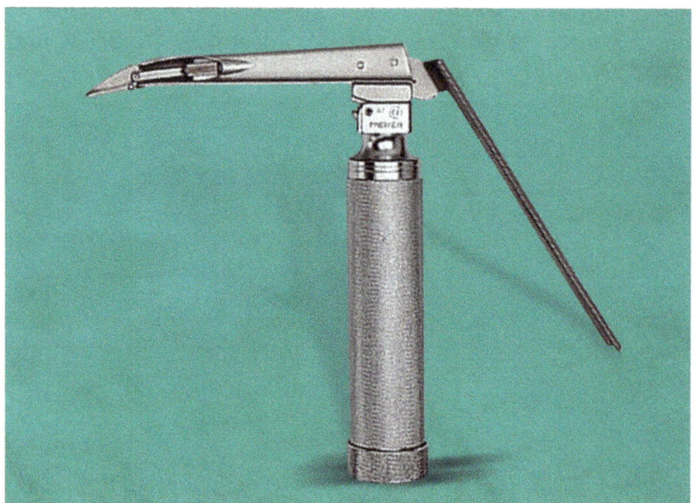

Fig. 33: Flexi-tip with Seward straight blade.

Laryngoscopes with Features of both Straight and Curved Blade

Cardiff Blade

Cardiff blade was designed with features of both straight and curved blade in order to have a universal blade for children of all age groups. This blade is meant to lift the epiglottis indirectly as most anesthetists are comfortable with this method of laryngoscopy. The proximal 6 cm of the tongue and flange are straight and form a reverse "Z" in cross-section. The web and flange are attenuated distally so that the terminal part continues as a curved spatula, narrowing at the tip. It terminates with a thickened, transverse bead. The blade when opened makes an angle of 85° with the handle. A miniature halogen bulb is embedded in the web. The proximal straight part provides more space and ensures laryngeal view when the ETT is introduced. The 85° angle allows gentle indirect lift of the epiglottis instead of forceful leverage **(Fig. 34)**.[9]

Dorges Blade

Similar effort to have a universal blade in adults and children resulted in the introduction of the Dorges universal laryngoscope. The blade is mainly straight with a slightly curved distal end, enabling its use by direct or indirect elevation of the epiglottis. It tapers gradually from the heel to 11 mm at its tip, corresponding to the width of a Macintosh 2 blade tip. The working length of 125 mm, however, is between those of Macintosh 3 and 4 blades. Similarly, the lower profile 15 mm reverse Z-shaped vertical step and

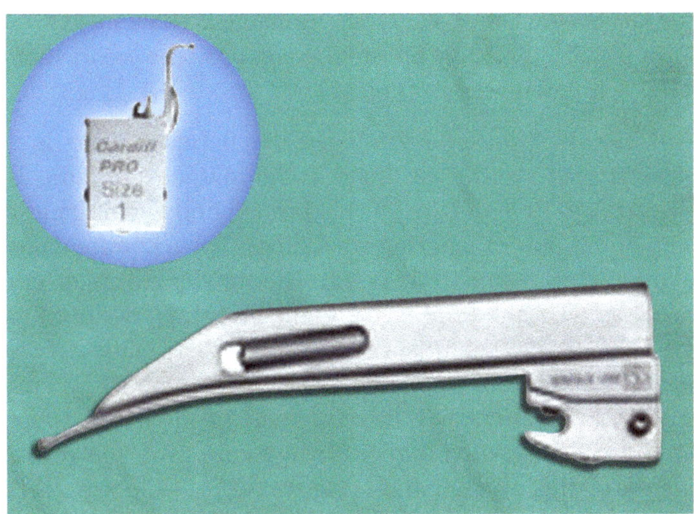

Fig. 34: Cardiff blade.

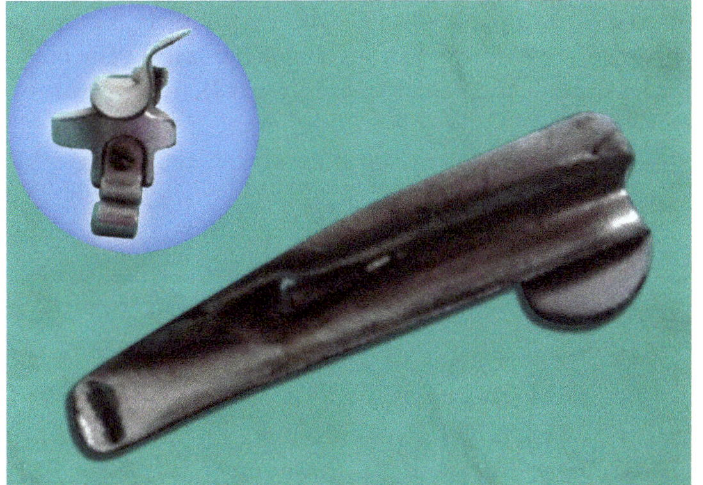

Fig. 35: Soper blade.

flange may facilitate the blade's insertion in limited mouth opening situations. Two (10 kg and 20 kg weight) markings on the front and rear of the blade serve as a rough guide for insertion depth when using the blade in the pediatric patient more than 10 kg.[3]

Soper Blade

Originally described as a modification of Macintosh, but is essentially a straight blade with a slight distal curve. Like in the Macintosh, the step and the flange form a reverse Z in cross-section. A transverse slot in the distal tip is provided to help lift the epiglottis **(Fig. 35)**.

Blades with Special Functions

Oxiport Blade

A channel for oxygen insufflation is present in the Oxiport blade which comes in the Miller or Macintosh profile **(Fig. 36)**.

Tull (Suction) Laryngoscope

Laryngoscope with a suction port that extends down to the handle and has a finger controlled valve to operate.

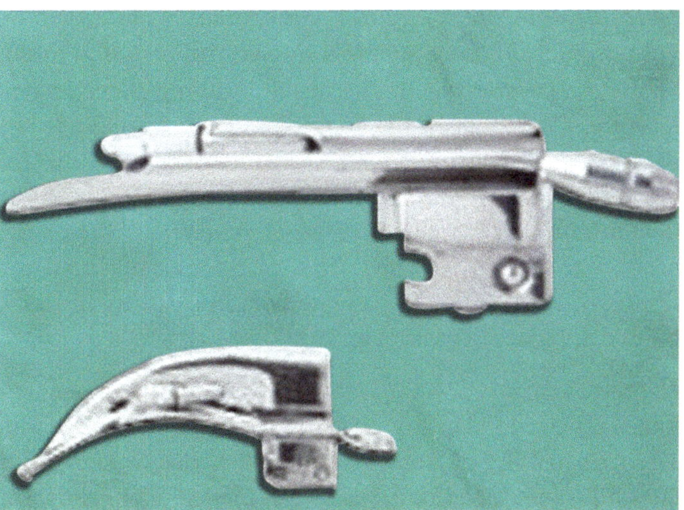

Fig. 36: Oxiport blade.

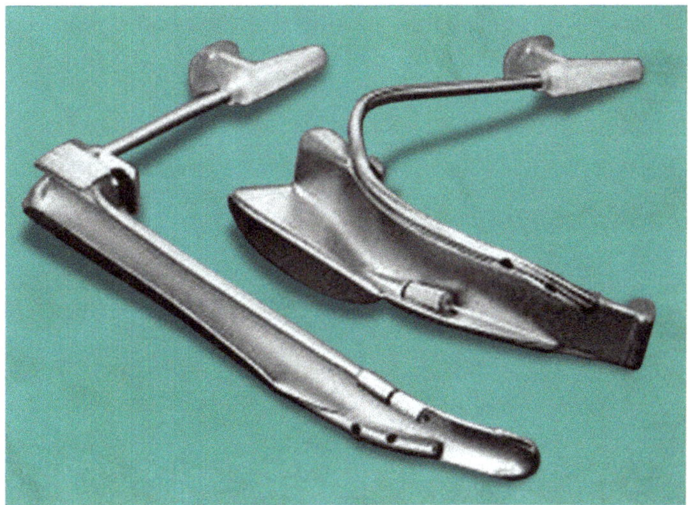

Fig. 37: Tull (suction) laryngoscope.

This laryngoscope also comes in both Miller and Macintosh profile **(Fig. 37)**.

Polio Blade

A modification of Macintosh curved blade described by Dr Foregger in 1954 is a special blade meant for intubation of patients in "iron-lung" ventilators. The blade makes an obtuse angle with the handle and thus does not impinge on the chest plate of the respirator during intubation.[23]

The use of this blade has also been described in obese patients with large breast, in kyphoscoliosis with barrel chest, in patients with restricted neck movements due to cervical collar **(Fig. 38)**.[24]

Rigid Indirect Laryngoscopes

Prisms Type

Prisms refract light to bring the laryngeal view in the line of vision. Thus prisms are a form of indirect laryngoscope. Mirror prism was used by Siker in his laryngoscope in 1965. Huffman designed a prism made of Plexiglass® in 1968. Belscope is a laryngoscope based on prisms mechanics.

Siker laryngoscope: A mirror laryngoscope described by Ephraim S Siker has a stainless steel mirror attached to the blade in a copper jacket. The distal portion is three inches long and at an angle of 135° to the 2½ inch proximal portion of the blade. The mirror gives an inverted image of the larynx. The copper jacket conducts the patient's endogenous heat minimizing fogging. Because of the curve of the blade, a styleted ETT is required. This blade was invented for difficult laryngoscopy in patients with buck teeth, anterior larynx and macroglossia **(Fig. 39)**.[25]

Huffman's prisms: John P Huffman, a research nurse anesthetist replaced the mirror prism by Plexiglass® (acrylic glass). The prism was cut, sanded, and polished to an angle of 30° and was clipped to a Macintosh blade.[26] The refraction provided by the prism brought the larynx and tip of a tracheal tube into the line of vision.

Prisms are available in different sizes and can be attached to the blades by metal clips **(Fig. 40)**. The image is right side up.

The Prismview™ blades are available in Macintosh A or E profile. The optically polished prism provides a refraction of 30° without inversion **(Fig. 41)**.

Belscope: Bellhouse CP designed the Belscope. This is a straight blade with a 45° bend at the midpoint. A lamp is placed 2 cm from the tip. The blade has a horizontal shallow step and a pair of tapering steel lungs that accommodates a prism just before the bend. The acrylic prism is cut at 62° angle at the front face and the rare surface is used to view the image. The prism is detachable. The blade comes in three sizes from tip to the angle i.e., 6.7 cm, 8 cm, and 9.3 cm. The angulated Belscope can be used for direct laryngoscopy or for indirect laryngoscopy with the prism in case of difficult intubation **(Fig. 42)**.[27]

Viewmax®: Viewmax® blade has a detachable metal channel, attached to the Macintosh blade, with an optical lens at the tip and an eye piece distally. The lens refracts the image 20° anteriorly for better viewing in anterior larynx. The blade comes in adult and pediatric sizes **(Fig. 43)**.

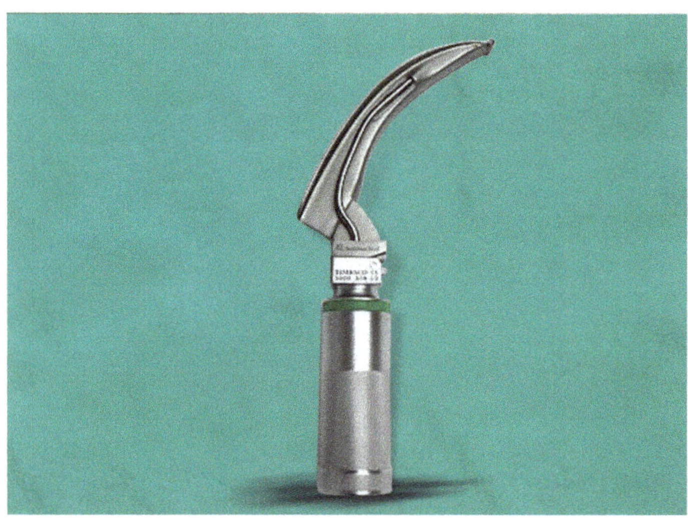

Fig. 38: Polio blade.

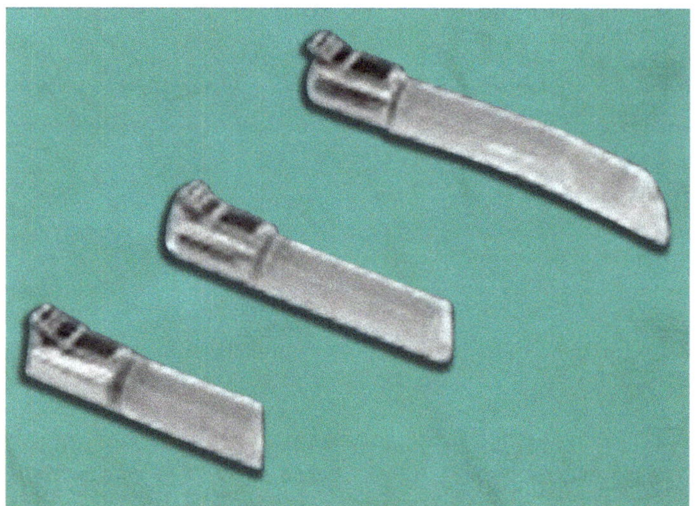

Fig. 40: Prisms.

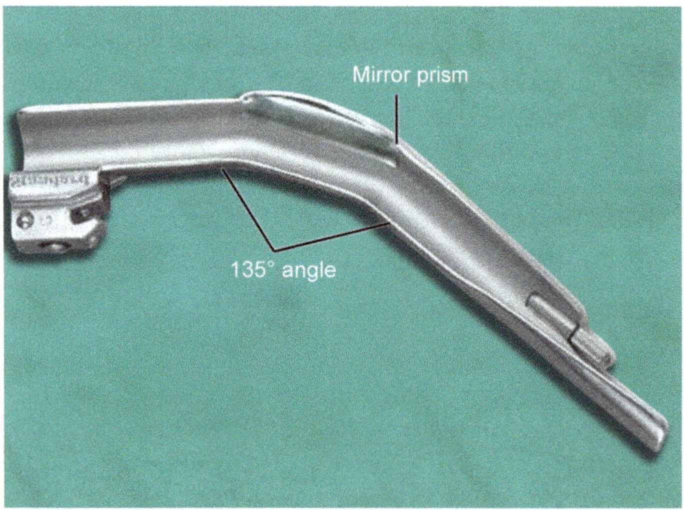

Fig. 39: Siker laryngoscope.

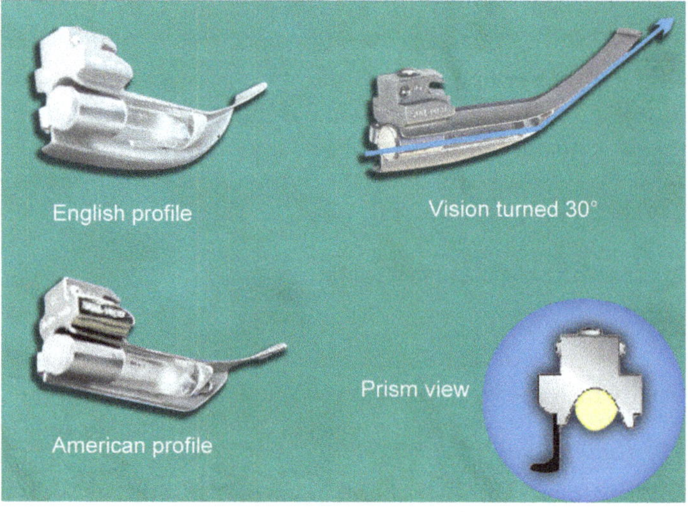

Fig. 41: Prismview™ laryngoscope.

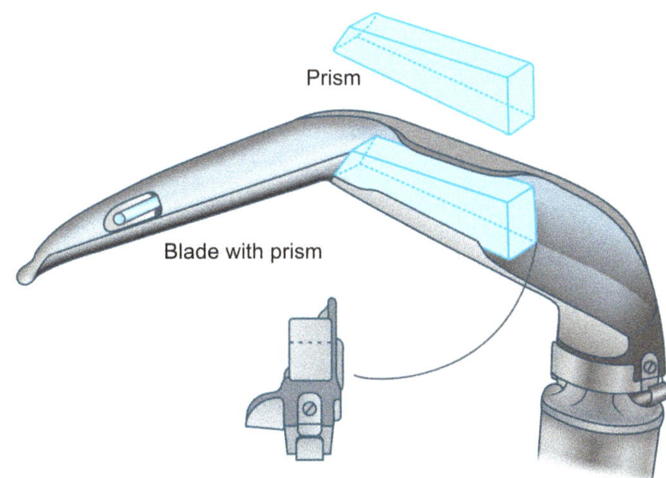

Fig. 42: Belscope laryngoscope.

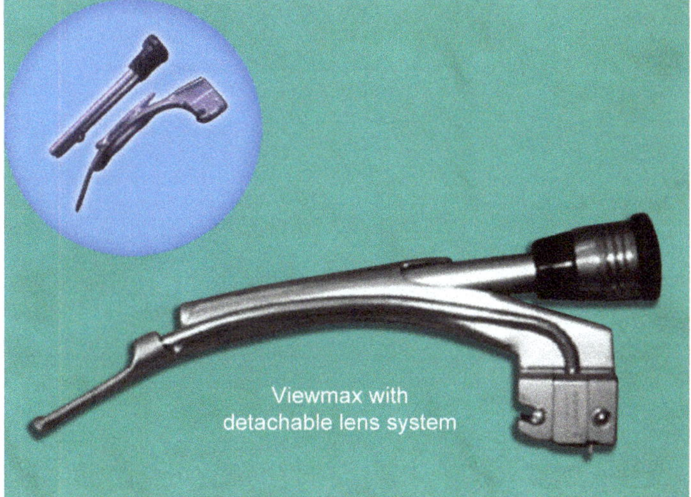

Fig. 43: Viewmax® blade.

Rigid Indirect Fiberoptic Laryngoscopes (Optical)

After introduction of science of fiberoptic in medical field in 1930s, an array of fiberoptic laryngoscopes were designed, first rigid then flexible. Now fiberoptic bundles could be used to visualize the glottis. As the larynx is not under direct vision, these laryngoscopes are called "indirect". The basic structures of an indirect rigid fiberoptic laryngoscope are:

- Three channels, two fiberoptic channels for light and image bundles and a working channel
- Anatomically curved thin blade
- An eye piece with diopter adjustment for image viewing either directly or by a camera source on the monitor. This eyepiece is an extension of the fiberoptic viewing channel
- Handle.

The rigid fiberoptic indirect laryngoscopes are:

- Bullard laryngoscope
- UpsherScope laryngoscope
- Augustine Scope™
- WuScope.

Bullard Intubating Laryngoscope

The Bullard laryngoscope, designed by Dr Roger Bullard is the prototype of rigid indirect laryngoscopes **(Fig. 44)**. Bullard laryngoscope comes in three sizes:[28]

1. Pediatric (newborn to 2 years)
2. Pediatric long (2–10 years)
3. Adult.

Bullard laryngoscope has an anatomical curved blade posterior to which run the above mentioned three channels **(Fig. 45)**. The thickness of the blade is 0.64 cm. The pediatric blade has a width of 1.3 cm while the adult blade has a width of 2.5 cm. The internal radius of curvature is 0.74 inch and 1.32 inch in pediatric and adult blade respectively. The blade curves up to 90°. A disposable plastic blade tip extender can be used to extend the length of the Bullard laryngoscope blade tip. Designed to aid in picking up the epiglottis in larger patients, this device clicks firmly to the metal blade tip. The extender may remain in the mouth after removal of the blade; hence it is necessary to inspect the blade and the extender after withdrawal.

The working channel splits proximally to into two parts: (i) a part with a luer-lock and (ii) another for the stylet. In the pediatric version the second part accepts the Bullard intubating mechanism **(Fig. 46)**.

The Bullard intubating mechanism is a thumb-lever activated forceps that allows the operator both to advance the intubating forceps (and attached ETT) into the larynx and to release the ETT when properly positioned.[29]

The luer-lock part can accept a syringe for local anesthetic instillation or attachment of oxygen tubings.

A working channel extends to the tip. It can be used for suction, oxygen insufflation, administration of local anesthetics or saline, passage of epidural catheter or passage of an airway exchange or jet ventilation catheter.[30]

The channel for illumination has a conventional battery harboring handle attachment. An adopter and handle for high illumination light source is optionally provided. The handle and the eyepiece are at 45° angle.

The light bundle begins 2 mm from the tip. Proximally they end at the eyepiece. The eyepiece has diopter adjustment and can be connected to a camera source.

UpsherScope Laryngoscope

It differs from the Bullard laryngoscope in having a J-rather than L-shaped blade, which is narrower and more rounded in profile. The blade has a "C" shaped tube guiding channel open towards the right on the posterior aspect. Located along with the tube channel are two fiberoptic channels, one for operator viewing and one for illumination. The blade is curved 60°. The C-shaped tube channel and the fiberoptic bundles end 1 inch from the tip of the blade. The power source is a conventional battery handle. The proximal part has also the eyepiece with diopter adjustment which can be attached to a snap on camera. This tube channel can take an

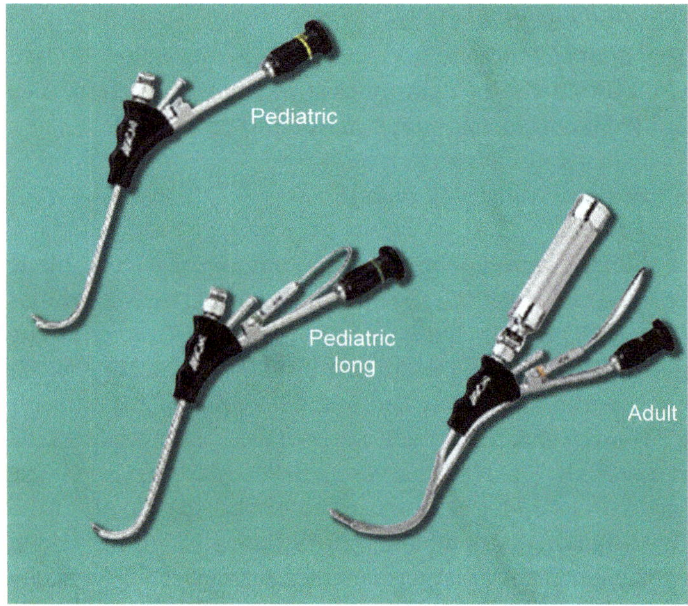

Fig. 44: Different sizes of Bullard laryngoscope.

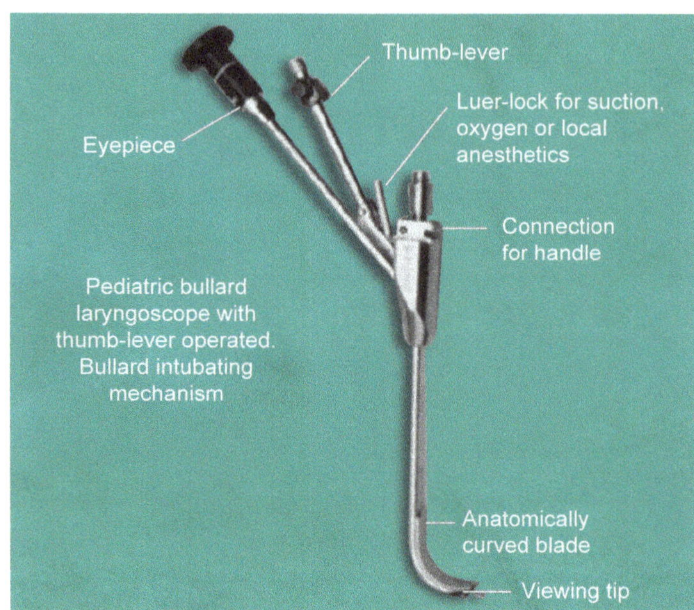

Fig. 46: Bullard laryngoscope: Pediatric version.

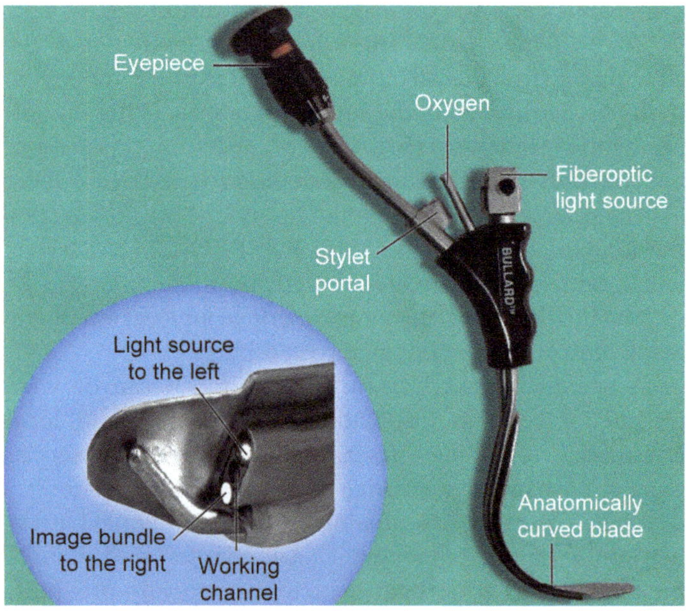

Fig. 45: Parts of Bullard laryngoscope.

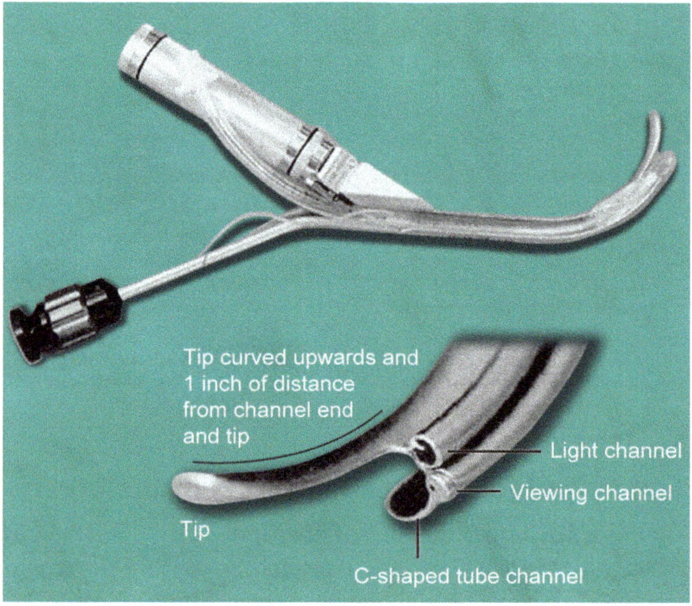

Fig. 47: UpsherScope laryngoscope.

ETT up to 8.5 mm internal diameter. UpsherScope comes in only one adult size **(Fig. 47)**.[31]

Two reasons might account for the limited usefulness of the UpsherScope. First, the blade shape does not match airway anatomy in all patients. The angle of the blade curvature, and especially that of tube channel, is 60° often resulting in a restricted view of the larynx. Second, as the fiberoptic bundles end 1 inch from the tip, the blade tip is not seen entirely during intubation causing difficulty in lifting the epiglottis.

Augustine Scope™

Like the UpsherScope, the Augustine Scope has a tube channel and fiberoptic image and light channels and does not have a working channel, but the tube channel is lateral to the blade tip and the tip has modifications for easy lift of epiglottis. Two bulbous protrusions are present on either side of a middle indentation of the tip. When the leading edge is placed in the vallecula, the middle indentation straddles the hypoepiglottic fold in the vallecula and the protrusions lie in the recesses of the vallecula. Traction brings the cords in view. A metallic epiglottis flap is also present that lifts the epiglottis as the tube is advanced. The Augustine has an inbuilt light source with battery pack and an eyepiece.[32] This scope is not commercially available **(Fig. 48)**.

WuScope

The WuScope designed by Dr Tzu-Lan Wu, is a combination of rigid laryngoscope and a flexible fiberscope. It is also called "combination intubating device".[33]

The rigid blade part consists of a handle, main blade and a bivalve element. All the three parts have to be assembled and then attached to the fiberscope body. The main blade and the bivalve element have corresponding grooves that when attached form two passageways: (i) The fibercord passageway and (ii) a larger ETT passageway. Both these pieces are "arc" shaped. This assembly is then attached to the cone-shaped handle. The axis of the handle and blade are at 110°. An oxygen channel is present alongside the fibercord passageway. The vertical height of the assembled blade is 16–18 mm and thus requires a mouth opening of at least 20–25 mm.

Two sizes are available: (i) an adult size and (ii) an extra-large adult size. Adult size can take a tube up to 8.5 mm and the extra-large adult blade takes up to 9.5 mm and is meant for patients more than 70 kg **(Fig. 49)**.

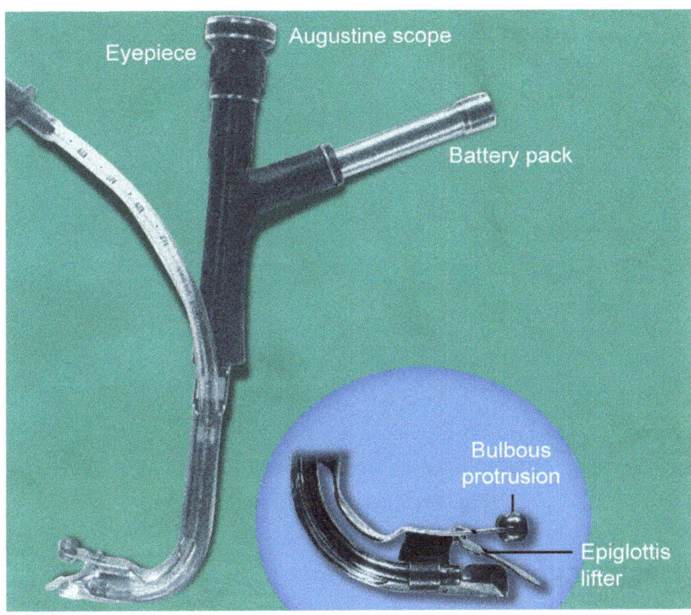

Fig. 48: Augustine scope laryngoscope.

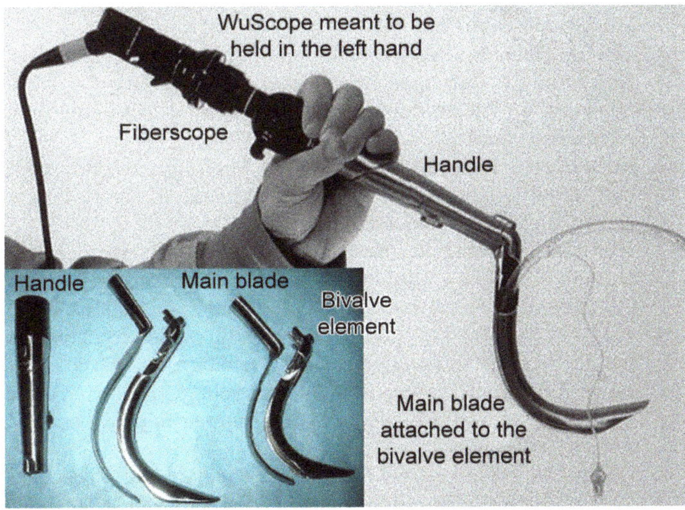

Fig. 49: WuScope laryngoscope.

Technique of Use

As the image bundles in the indirect laryngoscopes directly face the larynx, the alignment of the airway axis is not required. Thus intubation with these scopes is in the neutral position.

The handle is held parallel to the patient and the blade is introduced in the mouth and curved along the tongue till the vallecula is visualized. The handle should now be perpendicular to the patient. The epiglottis may be lifted by "scooping" mechanism of the blade as in the Bullard and UpsherScope. Once the larynx is under vision, the ETT is advanced either through the tube channel as in the UpsherScope and Augustine Scope or over a catheter as in the WuScope or over a stylet as in Bullard laryngoscope.

The ETT tip can also be guided in the larynx using a flexible tip stylet.[34]

The quality of the image may get affected by the condensation of warm expired gases on the lens. An antifogging method is always necessary in an indirect laryngoscope. The common antifogging methods used are:

- Immersion of the fiberoptic end of the blade in warm water at temperature 40–50° prior to use
- Use of antifogging solution
- Use of oxygen at 6–8 L/min from the working channel.[35]

Advantages

- The blade can be used to lift the epiglottis and the image bundles then face the larynx directly. Thus, indirect laryngoscopes are useful in visualizing around the corners in difficult intubation. Indirect rigid laryngoscopes have been used in morbid obesity, tonsillar hypertrophy, Treacher Collins syndrome in pediatric patients[36-38]
- As alignment of oral, pharyngeal and tracheal axis is not required, there is minimal cervical movement with these laryngoscopes[39]
- The working channel is an advantage. Blood and secretions can be suctioned and clarity of image maintained. Local anesthetics can be instilled and oxygen supplemented
- The traction for laryngoscopy is minimal thus well tolerated by patients for awake intubation
- Bullard laryngoscope having a blade thickness of only 0.64 mm can be introduced with ease in restricted mouth opening
- Nasal intubation is also possible with Bullard laryngoscope
- Double lumen tubes have been inserted with Bullard laryngoscope and WuScope.

Disadvantages

- Bulky devices and as in case of WuScope time to assemble the scope is present

- Though larynx is under vision, introducing the ETT may require blade adjustment and take time
- Minimum mouth opening of 20-25 mm required in all indirect scopes except Bullard laryngoscope
- A learning curve is present; experience increases the success of intubation
- Expensive and may not be available everywhere.

Optical Intubating Stylets

Stylet with fiberoptic cable in the stainless steel body are called as optical intubating stylets, optical stylets, intubating fiberoptic stylets, stylet laryngoscopes, or visual scopes. This is the modified version of intubating stylet. Because of the image bundle in the distal tip, the larynx can be visualized as the ETT is railroaded over it.[5]

The Bonfils Retromolar Intubation Fiberscope[40]

This optical stylet was first described by Bonfils in 1983 that used it to intubate children with Pierre Robin syndrome. The Bonfils Retromolar Intubation Fiberscope is a rigid, straight fiberoptic device with a 40° curved tip. It is 40 cm long. The 40° angle permits targeted intubation. It has 110° angle of view. A handle with an eyepiece is provided at the proximal end which can be connected to a camera. It can be used with an external light source or a battery handle. It comes in three sizes—an adult size with outer diameter of 5 mm and two pediatric sizes with 3.5 mm and 2 mm outer diameter **(Fig. 50)**.

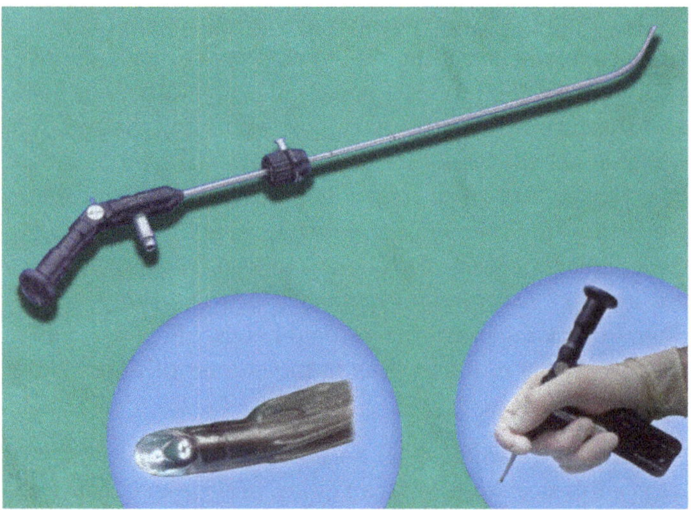

Fig. 50: Bonfils retromolar fiberscope.

Shikani Optical Stylet[3]

Shikani first described the Shikani Optical Stylet in 1999. It is a stainless steel malleable stylet. It comes in a preformed J-shape that can be bent at the tip. It has a handle, eyepiece, adjustable tube stop, and integral port for insufflating oxygen through the tracheal tube. The adult-size Shikani can accommodate various ETT sizes 5.5-9.0 mm, and the pediatric version supports ETT sizes 3.5-5.0 mm **(Fig. 51)**. Video laryngoscope discussed elsewhere.

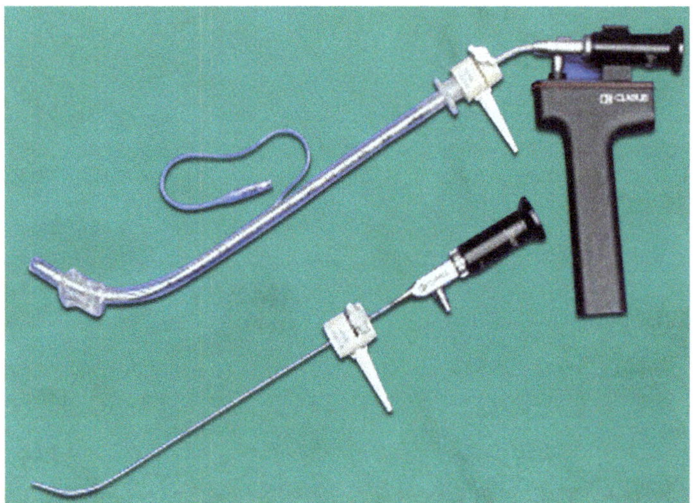

Fig. 51: Shikani optical stylet.

CONCLUSION

Going through history, we realize that innumerable laryngoscopes have been invented; some have probably been used only by the inventors. The design that stood the test of time is the Macintosh curved blade for most patients and Miller straight blade for infants. But these blades also have their limitations and cannot be called laryngoscopes for difficult intubation. For difficult intubation, the aid of optics is necessary to "look around the corners". These indirect laryngoscopes have a learning curve. So the authors feel that to master laryngoscopy, sufficient number of direct laryngoscopy and adequate practice with indirect laryngoscopes in normal patients will bring the best result in situation of a difficult intubation.

REFERENCES

1. Rosenberg H, Axelrod JK. The introduction and popularization of endotracheal intubation into anesthesia practice. Bull Anesth Hist. 2003;21(4):1-6.
2. Jahn A, Blitzer A. A short history of laryngoscopy. Log Phon Vocol. 1996;21:181-5.
3. Law JA, Hagberg CA. The evolution of upper airway retraction: New and old laryngoscope blades. In: Hagberg CA (Ed). Benumof's Airway Management, 2nd edition. Philadelphia: Mosby Elsevier; 1996.
4. Malan CA, Scholz A, Wilkes AR, et al. Minimum and optimum light requirements for laryngoscopy in paediatric anaesthesia: A manikin study. Anesthesia. 2008;63:65-70.
5. Dorsch JA, Dorsch SE. Laryngoscopes. In: Dorsch JA, Dorsch SE (Eds). Understanding Anesthesia Equipment, 5th edition. Philadelphia: Lippincott Williams and Wilkins; 2007.
6. Patil VU, Stehling LC, Zauder HL. An adjustable laryngoscope handle for difficult intubations. Anesthesiology. 1984;60:609.
7. Miller RA. A new laryngoscope. Anesthesiology. 1941;2:317-20.
8. Bruin G. The Miller blade and the disappearing light source. Anesth Analg. 1996;83:888.
9. Doherty JS, Froom SR, Gildersleve CD. Paediatric laryngoscopes and intubation aids old and new. Pediatr Anesth. 2009;19(1): 30-7.

10. Difficult Airway Society. Paediatric Difficult Airway Guidelines. [online] Available from www.das.uk.com/content/pediatric-difficult-airway-guidelines. [Last accessed February, 2014].
11. Walker RW, Ellwood J. The management of difficult intubation in children. Pediatr Anesth. 2009;19(1):77-87.
12. Phillips OC, Duerksen RL. Endotracheal intubation: A new blade for direct laryngoscopy. Anesth Analg. 1973;52:691-8.
13. Snow JC. Modification of laryngoscope blade. Anesthesiology. 1962;23:394.
14. Schapira MA. Modified straight laryngoscope blade designed to facilitate endotracheal intubation. Anesth Analg. 1973;52: 553-4.
15. Scott J, Baker PA. How did the Macintosh laryngoscope become so popular? Pediatr Anesth. 2009;19(1):24-9.
16. Asai T, Matsumoto S, Fujise K, et al. Comparison of two Macintosh laryngoscope blades in 300 patients. Br J Anaesth. 2003;90(4):457-60.
17. Bizzarri DV, Giuffrida JG. Improved laryngoscope blade designed for ease of manipulation and reduction of trauma. Anesth Analg. 1958;37:231-2.
18. Choi JJ. A new double-angle blade for direct laryngoscopy. Anesthesiology. 1990;72:576.
19. Gabbott DA. Laryngoscopy using the McCoy laryngoscope after application of a cervical collar. Anaesthesia. 1996;51: 812-4.
20. Laurent SC, de Melo AE, Alexander-Williams JM. The use of the McCoy laryngoscope in patients with simulated cervical spine injuries. Anaesthesia. 1996;51:74-5.
21. McCoy EP, Mirakhur RK, McCloskey BV. A comparison of the stress response to laryngoscopy. The Macintosh versus the McCoy blade. Anaesthesia. 1995;50:943-6.
22. Sugiyama K, Yokoyama K. Head extension angle required for direct laryngoscopy with the McCoy laryngoscope blade. Anesthesiology. 2001;94:939.
23. Weeks DB. A new use of an old blade. Anesthesiology. 1974; 10:200-1.
24. Lagade MRG, Poppers PJ. Revival of the polio laryngoscope blade. Anesthesiology. 1982;57:545.
25. Siker ES. A mirror laryngoscope. Anesthesiology. 1956;17:38-42.
26. Huffman J, Elam JO. Prisms and fiberoptics for laryngoscopy. Anesth Analg. 1971;50:64-7.
27. Bellhouse CP. An angulated laryngoscope for routine and difficult tracheal intubation. Anesthesiology. 1988;69:126-9.
28. Shulman GB, Connelly NR, Gibson C. The adult Bullard laryngoscope in paediatric patients. Can J Anaesth. 1997;44: 969-72.
29. Borland LM, Casselbrant M. A new indirect oral laryngoscope (pediatric version). Anesth Analg. 1990;70:105-8.
30. D'Alessio JG. The Bullard laryngoscope as jet ventilator. Anesth Analg. 1995;81:435.
31. Fridrich P, Frass M, Krenn CG, et al. The UpsherScope™ in routine and difficult airway management: A randomized, controlled clinical trial. Anesth Analg. 1997;85:1377-81.
32. Krafft P, Krenn CG, Fitzgerald RD, et al. Clinical trial of a new device for fiberoptic orotracheal intubation [Augustine Scope]. Anesth Analg. 1997;84:606-10.
33. Wu T, Chou H. A new laryngoscope: the combination intubating device. Anesthesiology. 1994;81:1085-7.
34. Cooper SD, Benumof JL, Ozaki GT. Evaluation of the Bullard laryngoscope using the new intubating stylet: comparison with conventional laryngoscopy. Anesth Analg. 1994;79:965-70.
35. Crosby ET. Techniques using the Bullard laryngoscope. Anesth Analg. 1995;81:1314-5.
36. Cohn AI, Hart RT, McGraw SR, et al. The Bullard laryngoscope for emergency airway management in a morbidly obese patient. Anesth Analg. 1995;81:872-3.
37. Andrews SR, Mabey MF. Tubular fiberoptic laryngoscope (WuScope) and lingual tonsil airway obstruction. Anesthesiology. 2000;93:904-5.
38. Harea J. Bullard laryngoscope proven useful in difficult intubations in children with Treacher Collins. Anesth Analg. 2004; 98:1809-18.
39. Smith CE, Pinchak AB, Sidhu TS, et al. Evaluation of tracheal intubation difficulty in patients with cervical spine immobilization fiberoptic (WuScope) versus conventional laryngoscopy. Anesthesiology. 1999;91:1253-9.
40. Thong SY, Wong TG. Clinical uses of the Bonfils retromolar intubation fiberscope: A review. Anesth Analg. 2012;115:855-66.

Tracheal Tubes

Naina P Dalvi

ABSTRACT

The gold standard for securing the airway is tracheal intubation. In the modern era of supraglottic airways (SGAs), an endotracheal tube (ETT), once placed, offers both reliability and protection that few, if any, SGA can currently provide.

Since William MacEwen, a surgeon in 1878, described endotracheal intubation for the first time, lot of research has been carried out regarding the structure of endotracheal tubes and it is still ongoing. Depending on the specific requirement, newer and newer modifications in the tubes are being done for patient's benefit.

This chapter describes the structure of an ETT in great detail, along with the technique of intubation and its different modifications. It also comments on the various technical aspects of ETTs as anesthetists use them routinely. Also different newer tubes with their specific indications are also touched upon.

INTRODUCTION

The endotracheal tube (ETT) (intratracheal tube, tracheal catheter) is a device that is inserted through the larynx into the trachea to convey gases and vapors to and from the lungs.[1] A cuffed endotracheal tube, isolates the trachea from esophagus and protects the lungs from inhalation of foreign material. It permits surgical access during head and neck surgery.[2]

Vesalius in 1542 described successful intermittent blowing into a reed placed in the trachea of an animal with an open thorax.[3] In 1667, Robert Hooke, at the Royal Society in London, ventilated a dog for over an hour a pair of bellows tied into the trachea. This led to the concept of artificial respiration by intubation of the trachea.

In 1871, Friedrich Trendelenburg came up with a cuffed catheter which looked similar to the present ETT, which was passed through a tracheostomy to prevent soiling of the lungs during operations on the upper airway.[4]

William MacEwen, a surgeon in 1878 placed a metal tube by manual palpation through the mouth into the trachea and used chloroform to anesthetize the patient for resection of a tumor at the base of the patient's tongue. It was the first time that "endotracheal anesthesia" was born.

IW Magill and ES Rowbotham, anesthetists with British Army during War of 1914–18, brought the concept of "insufflation anesthesia" during head and neck surgery. The uncuffed rubber tube was passed blindly through the nose into the trachea. This technique was followed in United Kingdom for many years.

In 1941, Gillespie, in endotracheal anesthesia, mentioned that, "an experienced worker should be able to intubate all but the most difficult cases in 10 minutes. The beginner will often require 30."

Dorrance in 1910 and then Guedel and Waters in 1928 described the cuffed rubber orotracheal tube to be used during general anesthesia for securing airway. But it was used routinely only after 1950s.[4]

A cuffed tracheal tube, once placed, provides the perfect protection for the lungs and the tube is the least likely device to be dislodged. It is the most preferred way of securing airway in most of the places **(Video 5)**.

ENDOTRACHEAL TUBE DESIGN

An ETT is described in following parts **(Fig. 1)**:

- Patient end
  - Bevel
  - Murphy eye
- Curve of tube
- Markings on the tube
- Tracheal tube material
- Tube size
- Tube cuff
- Machine end.

The Patient or Distal End

It is inserted into the trachea. It has a bevelled tip **(Fig. 2)**.

Bevel

Bevel is a slanted portion at the distal end which faces to the left when the tube is held in anatomical position. This is because the tube is usually introduced from the right, and the larynx is easier to visualize with the bevel facing to

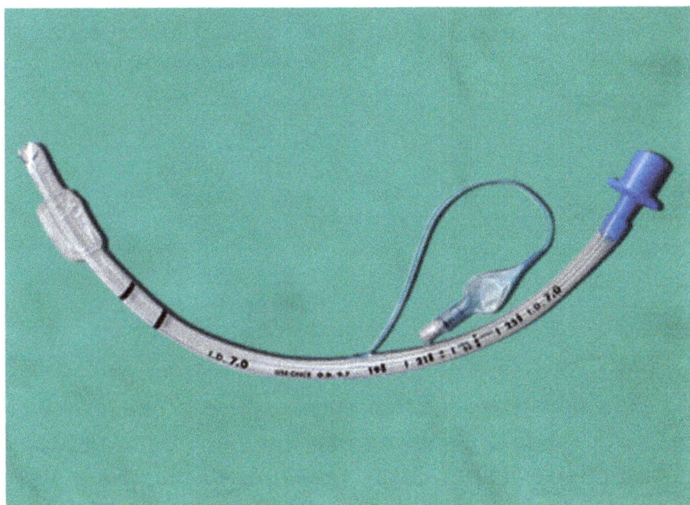

Fig. 1: Cuffed endotracheal tube.

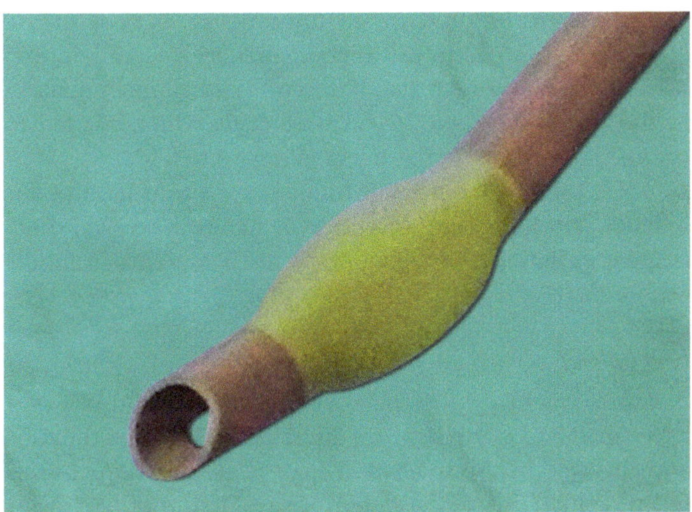

Fig. 2: Bevel and Murphy eye.

the left. The angle of the bevel is the acute angle between the bevel and the longitudinal axis of the tracheal tube and it is about 38 ± 10°. The bevel facilitates insertion and allows the tip of the tube to be seen passing between the vocal cords. Also, bevel reduces nasal morbidity during nasotracheal intubation.

Murphy Eye

Murphy eye is a hole in the wall opposite the bevel. A tube with Murphy eye is known as Murphy type tube.[5]

Advantages: In case of blockage of bevel, it provides a secondary port for gas movement in and out of the tube.

Disadvantages: Forceps, tube exchangers, and fiberscopes may get caught in it. Sometimes, secretions may accumulate in the eye.

Tracheal tubes lacking the Murphy eye are known as Magill's type tubes. If a Murphy eye is not present, the cuff is usually placed closer to the tip. This may decrease the risk of inadvertent bronchial intubation.

Curve

An orotracheal tube has a preformed curve approximately matching the anatomical curve of the airway. This preformed curve makes intubation easier. A typical tracheal tube is shaped like an arc of a circle with a radius of curvature of 140 ± 20 mm.

Markings on the Tube

Typical tracheal tube markings are situated on the bevelled side of the tube above the cuff. They are

- The word oral or nasal or oral/nasal
- *Tube size:* Tracheal tube size is either in millimeters [internal diameter (ID)] or French scale size (three times the external diameter in millimeters). The tubes size 6 mm and smaller show the external diameter in millimeters. Because of variations in wall thickness, tubes having the same ID may have different external diameters. In cuffed tubes, it is mentioned on the pilot balloon or between the cuff and the takeoff point of the inflation tube and for uncuffed tubes, the size marking is toward the patient end
- The name or trademark of the manufacturer or supplier
- A longitudinal line of radiopaque material runs throughout the length of tube for confirmation of the correct placement from an X-ray
- A transverse black line is made few centimeters proximal to the cuff. It indicates the distance that the tube should be placed in trachea so that the mark is just visible above the larynx. This is to prevent the tube remaining too out or the tube going too in inside the larynx
- The distance from the tip of the bevel is marked in centimeters on the tube
- A cautionary note such as "Do not reuse" or "Single use only" if the tube is disposable
- *Markings describing implant testing and Conformité Européenne (CE) markings:* The type of plastic used in the construction of tracheal tubes is tested to make sure that it is nonirritant. Four samples of the plastic, under sterile conditions, are planted under the paravertebral muscle of anesthetized rabbits along with two samples of Reference Standard Negative Control plastic for 70–144 hours. The implant sites are then examined for signs of inflammation. Tubes earlier had a test number (Z79-IT), which denoted the test method decided by the Z79 Toxicity Subcommittee of the American National Standards Institute set up in 1968 in the USA. Conformité Européenne marking now denotes compliance with the essential requirements of the medical devices directive.

Tracheal Tube Material

Tracheal tubes are mainly made up of red rubber or polyvinyl chloride (PVC). Some are made up of natural latex or silicone rubber.

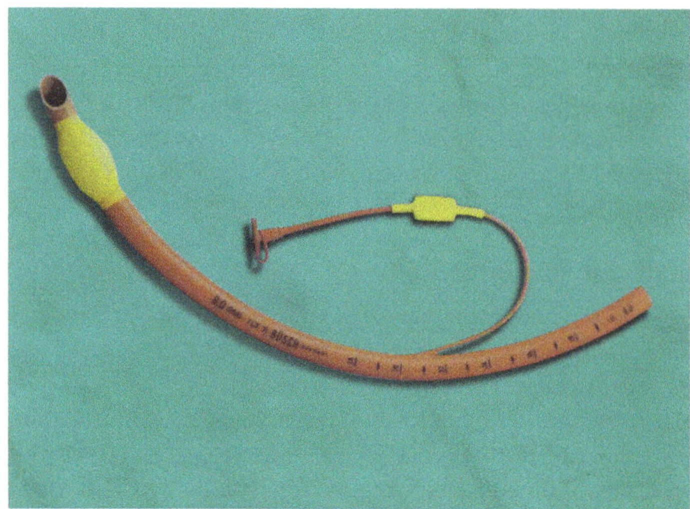

Fig. 3: Cuffed red rubber tube.

Red Rubber or Natural Latex (Fig. 3)

Advantages: It can be reused repeatedly after cleaning and sterilizing after every use. It makes the tube adequately rigid and less traumatic.

Disadvantages: As it is opaque, cleaning of the lumen may not be proper. Repeated sterilization makes the tube soft and kinkable. The latex material is potentially allergenic and irritant. Cuffs are thick and require high intracuff pressures to inflate them.

Polyvinyl Chloride

Advantages: It is relatively inexpensive. It is compatible with tissues, less kinkable and nonirritant. They are disposable hence allow single patient use thus preventing transmission of infection. They are presterilized. As the material is usually clear, foreign bodies and blockages are seen and can be cleaned.

Disadvantages: Polyvinyl Chloride tubes do not have the elasticity of rubber and are relatively rigid. Hence, they can be difficult to insert sometimes and can be traumatic.

Silicone Rubber (Polymethylsiloxane)

Siliconized plastic refers to a PVC material incorporated with a very small amount of silicone oil to form a surface monolayer with no trace of latex in it. It decreases the surface adhesion. It is opaque and pearlescent. It is significantly expensive, but it withstands autoclaving and therefore can be reused.

Tube Size

Adults

Previously, the widest diameter tracheal tube, that would pass easily through the narrowest part of the airway, was the correct size so as to reduce the resistance to gas flow and minimize the work of breathing.

TABLE 1: Approximate size of the tube as per age.

Age	*Tube size internal diameter in mm*
10–14 years	7.0–7.5
7–10 years	6.5–7.0
4–6 years	5.5–6.5
1–4 years	4.5–5.5
6–12 months	4.5–5.0
1–6 months	4.0–4.5
Neonates	2.5–3.5

Currently, there is a trend towards use of much smaller diameter tubes. It is proven that the diameter of the tube does not determine airway pressures distal to it unless the tube is very narrow[6] and small tubes are easier to insert and reduce the trauma of intubation. Only if the tube is too small, a high cuff pressure will be needed to achieve a seal, increasing pressure on the mucosa. In case of use of larger tubes, there are higher chances of cord injury, hoarseness and sore throat. If the cuff is too large in relation to the tracheal lumen, it will have folds when inflated to occlusion. Aspiration may occur along those folds.

Ideal tube in the average adult is a 7.5 mm ID tube for females and an 8.5 mm ID tube for males. However, there is great variation in sizes and shapes of trachea in adults **(Table 1)**.

Children

Pediatric tracheal tubes have been uncuffed and use of a tube small enough to leave an audible leak between the tube and the wall of the trachea at high peak airway pressures (20–25 cmH_2O) is still standard. In children, the narrowest part of the airway is the cricoid ring. A small degree of edema in the pediatric airway will reduce the lumen of the trachea considerably (1 mm of circumferential swelling reduces the diameter of the adult airway by less than 10% and that of an infant by as much as 30%) and may lead to respiratory compromise.

The following formulae can be of use for selecting the proper size tube in children.

Uncuffed Tubes

- *For children below 6 years:* Age in years/3 + 3.5
- *For children older than 6 years:* Age in years/4 + 4.5
- ID—internal diameter = Age in years/4 + 4 (modified Cole formula) for children above 2 years
- ID—internal diameter = 3 mm for those 3 months of age and younger
- ID—internal diameter = 3.5 mm for those from 3 months to 9 months of age
- ID—internal diameter = (Age in years + 16)/4 over 9 months of age
- External diameter is the same width as the distal phalanx of the little finger approximately.

Cuffed Tubes

- ID—internal diameter in mm = Age/4 + 3 (Khine formula)
- A tube 0.5–1 mm smaller than that calculated for an uncuffed tube.

Tracheal Tube Cuffs

A cuffed tracheal tube has an inflatable sleeve near the patient end of the tube. When this cuff is inflated with desired volume of air, it seals the space between the tube and the tracheal wall. It has an inflation tube connecting pilot balloon to the cuff. The pilot balloon has a one way inflation valve. In tubes which do not have inflation valve, cuff inflation is maintained by applying a clamp to the external inflation tube or by applying a plug in its free end.

Cuff types: Depending on the pressure needed to inflate the cuff, it is divided into low volume, high pressure cuff and high volume and low pressure cuff **(Fig. 4)**.

Low Volume, High Pressure Cuff

The red rubber tube cuffs were made of a relatively low compliance thick rubber. These cuffs required a high pressure to distend them and were relatively low volume (high pressure low volume cuffs). These cuffs inflate in a circular shape rather than conforming to the shape of the trachea.

The low volume, high pressure cuff has a small diameter at rest and a low residual volume (the amount of air that can be withdrawn from the cuff after it has been allowed to assume its shape with the inflation tube exposed to atmospheric pressure). It has a small area of contact with the tracheal wall and distends and deforms the trachea to a circular shape.

In order to achieve enough contact with the tracheal wall and a good seal, relative overinflation was required, with the result that the high pressure within the cuff was transmitted to the tracheal wall. This readily led to a reduction of mucosal pressure to critical levels (capillary perfusion pressure is usually about 35 mm Hg) could lead to mucosal ischemia, development of tracheal scarring and tracheal stenosis in case of prolonged use.

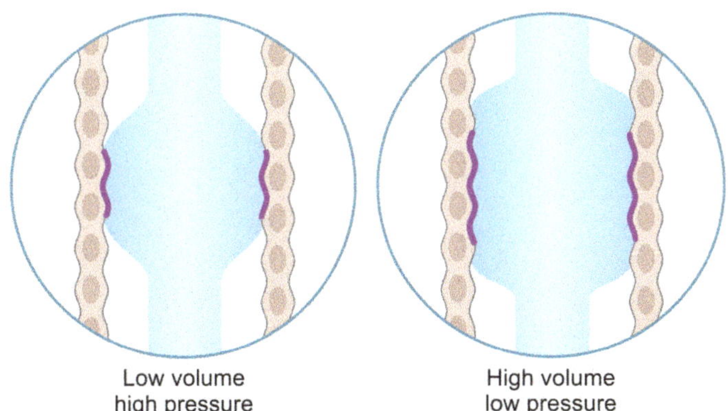

Fig. 4: Low volume, high pressure and high volume, low pressure cuff.

Advantages

- Better protection against aspiration
- Better visibility during intubation than low pressure cuffs
- Lower incidence of sore throat
- They are less expensive.

Disadvantages

Ischemic damage to the tracheal wall mucosa following prolonged use.

High Volume, Low Pressure Cuff

A high volume, low pressure cuff is made from a thin inelastic material (PVC) and has a large resting volume and diameter. As this cuff has a thin wall, it seals the trachea without stretching the tracheal wall. As the cuff is inflated, the area of contact becomes larger and the cuff adapts itself to the tracheal surface. There is a large area of contact between the cuff and tracheal wall before full inflation of the cuff. The pressure within the cuff can therefore be kept much lower and can achieve a seal with minimal risk of occluding mucosal blood flow.[7]

Advantages

It is possible to measure and regulate the pressure exerted on the tracheal mucosa, as the intracuff pressure closely approximates the pressure on the tracheal wall. Thus lesser cuff related complications following prolonged intubation.

Disadvantages

- It may be more difficult to insert, as the cuff may obscure the view of the tube tip and larynx
- Greater incidence of sore throat unless the cuff is specially designed so that the tracheal contact area is small
- It may not effectively prevent fluid from leaking into the lower airway even at cuff pressures as high as 60 cmH_2O, more with spontaneous respiration than intermittent positive pressure ventilation (IPPV), continuous positive airway pressure (CPAP), etc.
- A number of small folds (microfolds) remain in the cuff even after good seal and create small channels (microchannels) running the length of the cuff. These channels may contribute to the causation of ventilator-associated pneumonia (VAP) by allowing passage of infective pharyngeal contents beyond the cuff
- When nitrous oxide is used, it will diffuse into the cuff. This added volume will increase the pressure on the tracheal mucosa
- Any cuff can be overfilled or the volume and pressure can increase during use, resulting in high intracuff and tracheal wall pressures.[7]

Foam Cuff

The foam cuff is made up of polyurethane foam and comes with bigger diameter and residual volume. The cuff is deflated by applying suction and when the negative pressure is released, the cuff expands.

When in place in the trachea, the amount that the foam expands determines the pressure exerted laterally on the tracheal wall and it is inversely proportional to each other. The more the foam expands, the lower the pressure. It provides a good seal at a low tracheal wall pressure, when used according to the appropriate size.

Lanz Cuff

The Lanz cuff comprises of a latex pilot balloon inside a transparent plastic sheath and has a pressure regulating valve between the balloon and the cuff. The pilot balloon is designed to maintain an intracuff pressure of 20–25 torr at end expiration.

The pressure regulating valve permits gas flow from the balloon to the cuff and vice versa. This prevents gas leak around the cuff during positive pressure ventilation and nitrous oxide related cuff pressure rise. It eliminates the need to measure cuff pressure. It may not give good seal in patients requiring high airway pressures. If the balloon is compressed or overinflated, the intracuff pressure will rise.

Cuff Pressure

An optimal cuff pressure will give a good seal without compromising the blood supply of trachea. The recommended pressure on the lateral tracheal wall is between 18 and 25 mm Hg in normotensive adults.

Leak test is performed to measure the pressure exerted by the cuff of the tracheal tube on the tracheal mucosa. The valve on the breathing circuit is closed partially. The bag is squeezed with increasing pressure till an audible leak is detected around the tube. The airway pressure at which the audible leak is recorded is the pressure exerted by the tube in the tracheal mucosa.

In children, lower pressure should be used to prevent tracheal ischemia.

The intracuff pressure and volume of a cuff inflated with air rise when nitrous oxide is administered for long time.[8] The rate of diffusion depends on the permeability of cuff material, the surface area of cuff exposed to nitrous oxide and partial pressure of nitrous oxide. When nitrous oxide administration is discontinued, the pressure in the cuff decreases rapidly.

Intracuff pressure monitoring can be done manually either by palpation over the larynx or palpation of the pilot balloon. It can be measured by connecting the inflation tube to the pressure transducer of a monitor or direct measurement with a manometer **(Fig. 5)**.

Cuffed versus Uncuffed Tube (Fig. 6)

Cuffed tubes are routinely used in adults and uncuffed tracheal tubes are preferred in young children. In recent years, cuffed tracheal tubes have been used more often in small children.

Advantages of cuffed tubes include decreased risk of aspiration; ability to use high inflation pressures and low fresh gas flows, accurate monitoring of end-tidal gases, tidal volume. Disadvantage of using a cuffed tube in children include the need to choose a slightly smaller tube. It will increase resistance and work of breathing; inadvertent over inflation of the cuff will result in excessive mucosal pressure and the risk of injury to the vocal cords. Relatively small amounts of inflated air lead to rapid increases in cuff pressure and volume.

Tube Length

The minimal tube length is fixed as per American Society for Testing and Materials/International Organization for Standardization (ASTM/ISO) standard which increases as ID increases. Many available tubes are longer than the minimum required by the standard and can be shortened as per requirement.

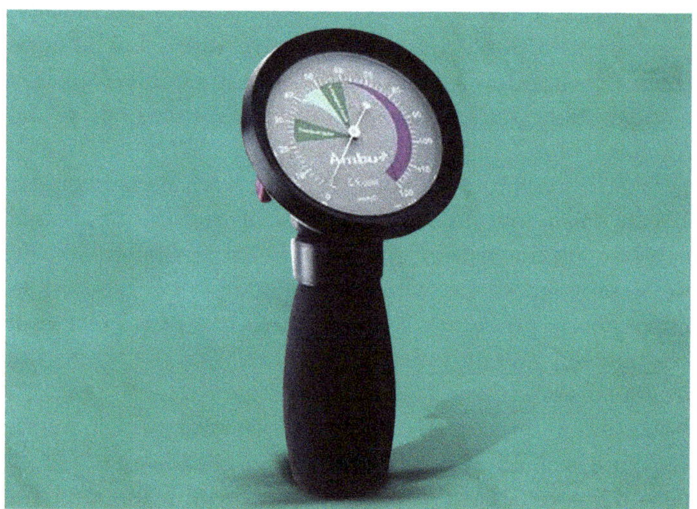

Fig. 5: Cuff pressure manometer.

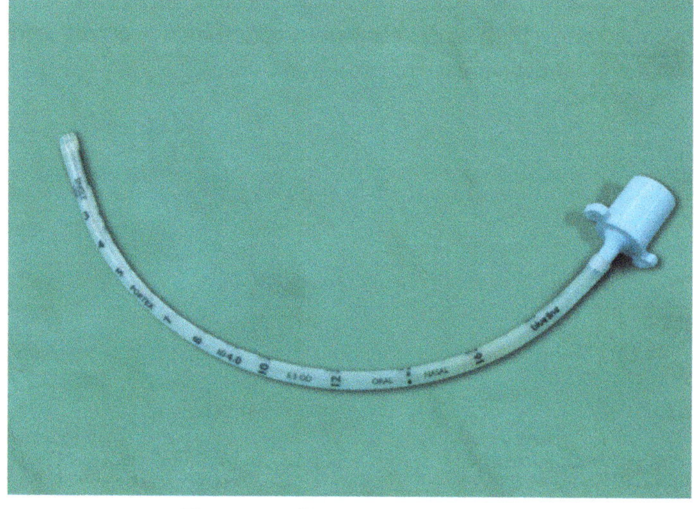

Fig. 6: Uncuffed endotracheal tube.

The Machine or Proximal End

It receives the connector and projects from the patient. The tracheal tube connector is made of plastic or metal. The size of patient end of the connector is designated by the ID of this end in millimeters. The machine end of the connector has a 15 mm male fitting. The connector should be of the same size as the tube. The most commonly used connectors are the straight and 90° curved (right angle).[9]

Endotracheal connectors can be curved or straight. Their one end connects to the tube and other end connects to the catheter mount. In case of disposable tubes, universal connectors or adaptors are fitted with the tube. The curved connectors are Magill's connectors (oral and nasal), Rowbotham connectors, Nosewothy connectors, etc. **(Fig. 7)**.

Catheter mounts are made up of metal tube or plastic tube. It adapts the endotracheal tubes with the breathing circuit and minimizes the movement of the tube in trachea **(Fig. 8)**.

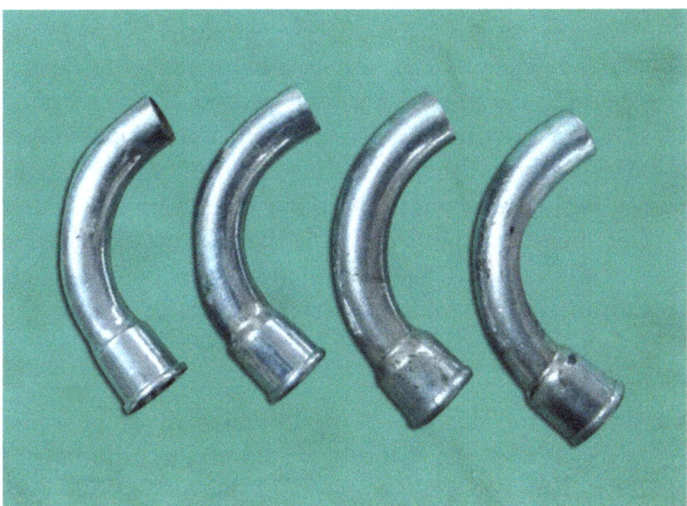

Fig. 7: Magill's oral connectors.

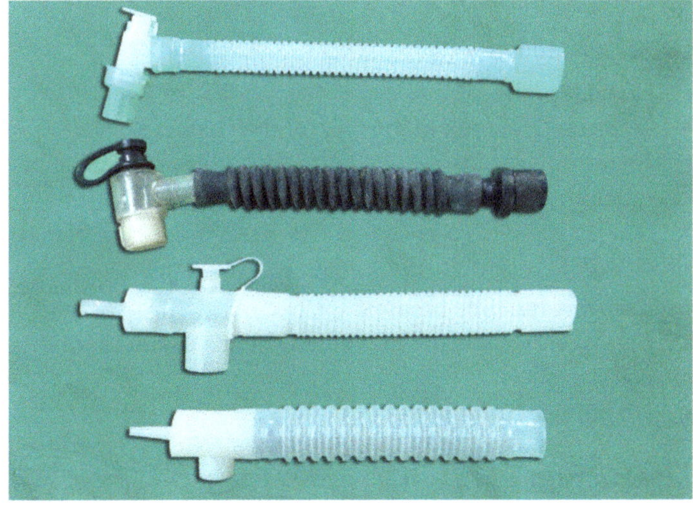

Fig. 8: Catheter mounts.

ENDOTRACHEAL INTUBATION

Indications

Surgical Indications

- Patients for surgery who are full stomach
- Patients requiring IPPV
- All head and neck procedures with compromised airway
- Surgery for a long time also nonsupine position
- Abdominal, thoracic, neurosurgical procedures
- Double lumen tubes for intrathoracic surgery.

Nonsurgical Indications

- Cardiopulmonary-cerebral resuscitation
- Conscious or semiconscious patients unable to protect the airway
- Inadequate or gasping respiration
- Tracheobronchial toilet for retained secretions.

Contraindications

No absolute contraindications, but difficult intubation in
- Severe airway trauma
- Cervical spine injury
- Aneurysm of arch of aorta
- Laryngeal edema.

TECHNIQUES OF ENDOTRACHEAL INTUBATION (VIDEO 5)

Before insertion, the tube should be examined for defects such as cracks, holes and for obstructions. The cuff, if present, should be inflated and the syringe removed to check for leaks in the inflation valve. The cuff should be inspected to make certain that it inflates evenly and does not cause the tube lumen to be reduced. After the sterile wrapping is opened, the tube should be handled only at the connector end.

Orotracheal Intubation

Patient is given "morning air sniffing" position (Chevalier Jackson position), i.e., extension at atlanto-occipital joint and flexion of neck (atlanto axial joint) by keeping a pillow below the neck. This position brings the oral, pharyngeal and laryngeal axis in one line thus facilitating the visualization of vocal cords on direct laryngoscopy **(Fig. 9)**.

In case of suspected cervical spine injury, laryngoscopy is done with stabilization of spine in a neutral position.[10]

For oral intubation, only the cuff should be lubricated. After opening the mouth with right hand, introduce the laryngoscope into the right side of mouth. The tongue is taken to the left along the blade. The blade is passed in till the tip lies in glossoepiglottic fold. After lifting the laryngoscope in the direction of handle, the glottis will be seen. Once vocal cords are seen, it is easy to insert the tube. The tube should be introduced into the right corner of the mouth and directed toward the glottis with the bevel parallel to the vocal cords.

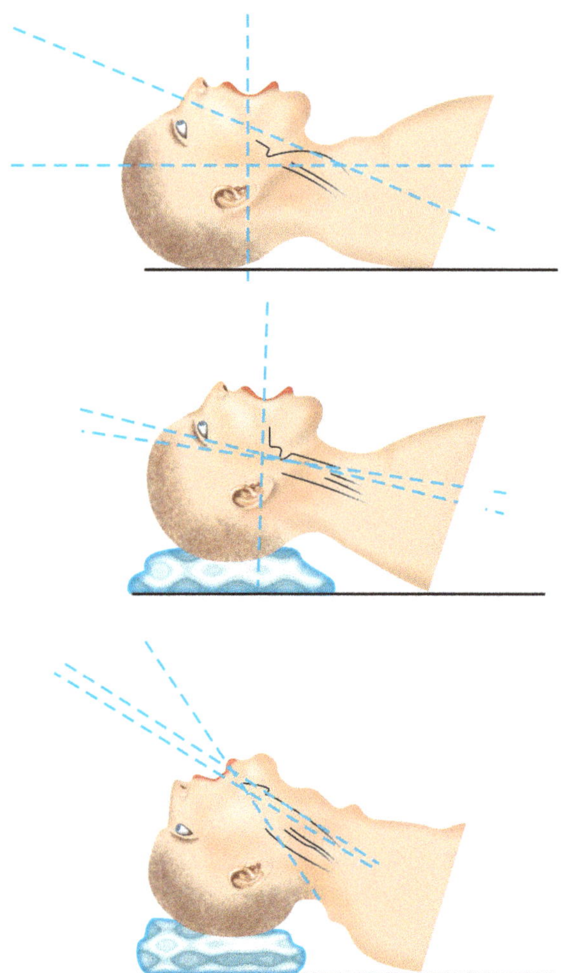

Fig. 9: Position for endotracheal intubation.

Advantages

- It can be performed quickly and easily than nasal intubation
- It allows use of a wider and shorter tube than for nasal intubation.

Disadvantages

- The possibility of oropharyngeal complications
- Oral intubation is usually not well tolerated by the conscious patient
- Significant cervical spine motion may be associated with direct laryngoscopy
- A bite block, rolled gauze, or oral airway should be placed between the teeth to prevent the patient from biting the tube.

Other techniques of orotracheal intubation are blind oral intubation and digital intubation.

Blind Oral Intubation

A blind oral technique is performed with the head flat, then tilted back in maximum extension. Pressure is applied to the cricoid cartilage with one hand while the tracheal tube with stylet in it is introduced into the mouth with the other, following the curve of the tube. The tube is advanced till the tube is felt advancing into the trachea. Manipulation of larynx is needed as this is a blind procedure. Capnography can be used in spontaneously breathing patient.

Digital Technique

In a digital (tactile) technique, the mouth is opened, fingers of one hand are used to push the tongue away and the other hand is used to put the tube in the trachea. The intraoral hand is used to guide the tracheal tube tip.

Nasotracheal Intubation

The tube should be thoroughly lubricated along its entire length with a sterile, water soluble lubricant. The cuff should be fully deflated. The patency of the nostril is checked. Preferably vasoconstrictor drops are put in the nose. When the tube is inserted, the bevel opening should face laterally. It should be advanced along to the floor of the nose while slightly lifting the tip of the nose. The tube should be pulled cephalad as it is passed posteriorly until it contacts the posterior pharyngeal wall.

After the tube is in the pharynx, laryngoscope is introduced. The position of the larynx is manipulated by flexing or extending the neck or external pressure on the larynx. Magill's forceps can be used to grasp the tip and direct it through cords avoiding damaging the cuff. If the tip passes through the vocal cords but cannot be negotiated further, then the tube is directing the tip into the anterior wall of the larynx. The intubation is then possible with slight withdrawal of tube and flexion of neck.

Indications

- Surgical procedures involving the oral cavity, oropharynx, and face where an oral tube would obstruct the view of the surgeon
- Surgery for fractured mandible, temporomandibular joint ankylosis, intraoral pathology
- Neck injury or cervical spine disease.

Contraindications

- Coagulopathy
- Suspected fracture at the base of the skull
- Nasal polyps, abscesses, foreign bodies, and possibly epiglottitis.

Advantages

- Securing the tube is easier
- Less of cervical spine movement hence useful in trauma cases
- No biting of tube.

Disadvantages

- Intubation usually takes longer

- A size smaller than oral tracheal tube is accepted, resulting in increased resistance
- Severe bleeding may occur to injury to nasal septum or turbinates
- High incidence of bacteremia, sinusitis, and otitis.

Blind Nasal Intubation

This technique is useful in patients where intubation is difficult or mouth opening is not adequate. It may be performed under general or local anesthesia. In a spontaneously breathing patient, the tube is inserted through the nostril and patient's breath sounds are used to guide placement. When the breath sounds are maximum, the tube is gently pushed in trachea during inspiration. Capnometer can be attached to the tube and end-tidal CO_2 is used as a guide.

Blind nasal intubation needs flexion or extension of the head or manipulation of the larynx by external pressure. It does require some experience and expertize. Sometimes, partially inflation of the cuff helps to elevate the tip from the posterior pharyngeal wall and center it. The cuff is deflated before the tube is advanced into the trachea. The blind technique may be useful when direct laryngoscopy or fiberoptic intubation would be difficult.

Depth of Insertion

- The tube is advanced until the mark at the proximal end of the cuff lies at the vocal cords
- The tube tip should be inserted not more than 1 cm past the cords in children under 6 months, not more than 2 cm past the cords for patients up to 1 year, and not more than 3–4 cm past the cords in larger patients
- The tube is fixed at the anterior incisors at 23 cm in adult males and at 21 cm in females.[11] In nasaotracheal intubation, 5 cm more is added to this length
- The approximate length can be estimated by aligning the proximal end of the cuff externally at the level of the cricoid cartilage and angling the tube anteriorly toward the level of angle of mouth

A number of formulae have been developed in children, including the following:

For oral intubation:

- According to Lau et al, 2006[12]
  - Above 1 year, length in centimeters = Age/2 + 13 cm
  - Below 1 year, length in centimeters = Weight (in kg)/ 2 + 8 cm
- Length in centimeters = Height (in cm)/10 + 5 cm
- *Rule of 7-8-9:* Infants weighing 1 kg are intubated to a depth of 7 cm at the lips, 2 kg infants to a depth of 8 cm, and 3 kg infants to a length of 9 cm.

For nasotracheal intubation:

- L = (S × 3) + 2, where L is the length in centimeters, and S is the ID of the tube in millimeters
- According to Lau et al, 2006[12]
  - Above 1 year, length in centimeters = Age/2 + 15 cm
  - Below 1 year, length in centimeters = Weight (in kg)/ 2 + 9 cm.

Confirmation of Correct Placement of Tube

Tube placement in trachea can be confirmed clinically or with the help of special equipment.

- Clinical confirmation (primary confirmation)
  - Direct visualization of tube passing through vocal cords
  - Moisture of exhaled gases in the lumen of tube if tube is transparent
  - Palpation of tube over trachea
  - Bilateral chest movement
  - Bilateral air entry on auscultation of chest
  - *Feel of the reservoir bag:* Movement of the reservoir bag with the patient's spontaneous respiratory efforts
- Confirmation with equipment (secondary confirmation)[13]
  - *Pulse oximeter:* Good patient color or adequate pulse oximeter readings confirm tracheal placement
  - *Capnometer:* Exhaled CO_2 monitoring is the most reliable method of detecting endotracheal intubation. The classic capnograph will confirm correct placement of tube. Bronchospasm, cardiac arrest, no pulmonary embolism may give false negative CO_2 levels. Exhaled gases forced into the stomach during mask ventilation, CO_2 as a byproduct of antacids or from ingestion of carbonated beverages will show irregular capnograph; but the CO_2 levels will rapidly diminish with repeated ventilation
  - *Esophageal detector device:* The esophageal detector device **(Figs. 10A and B)** consists of a large syringe or selfinflating compressible bulb attached to the tracheal tube using an adaptor. The plunger is withdrawn, or the compressed bulb is released. If the tube is in the trachea, gas from the patient's lungs will fill up the syringe or inflate the compressed bulb without resistance. However, if the tube is in the esophagus, apposition of the esophageal walls around the tube tip will cause a negative pressure or resistance. It is used immediately after tube placement, prior to delivering the first breath.
    The bulb may not re-expand rapidly morbidly obese or pregnant patient, patients with bronchospastic disease, pulmonary edema, and upper or lower airway obstruction. Incompetent gastroesophageal junction (obesity, pregnancy) may show false positive result
  - *Colorimetric end-tidal CO_2:* A chemical (colorimetric) detector **(Fig. 11)** consists of a pH sensitive indicator which changes color when exposed to carbonic acid that is formed as a product of the reaction between

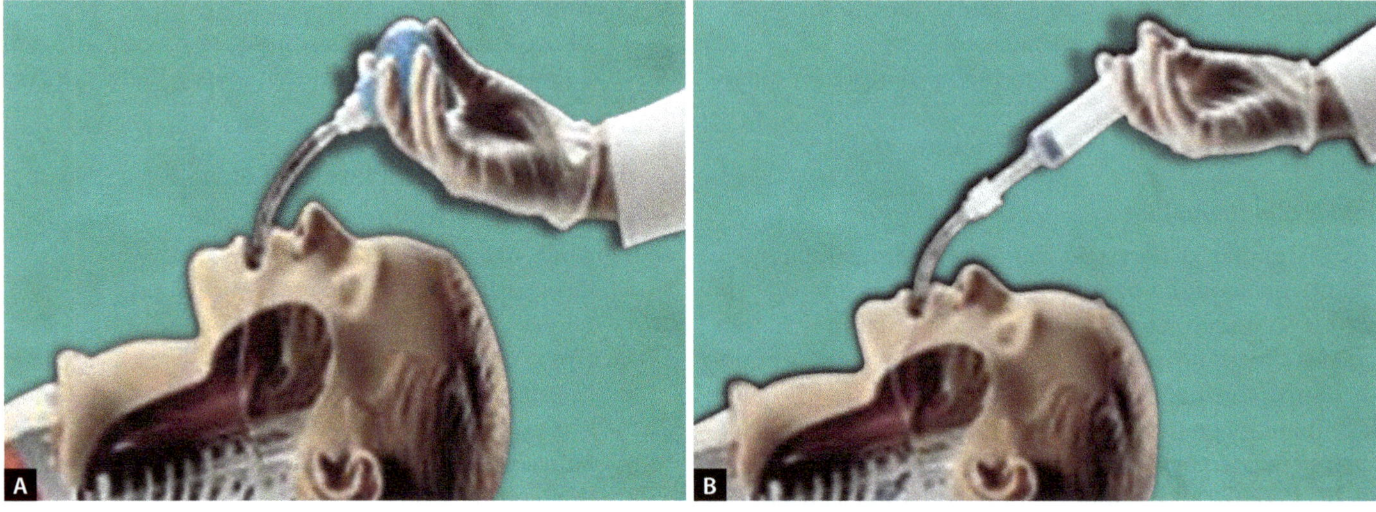

Figs. 10A and B: Esophageal detector device.

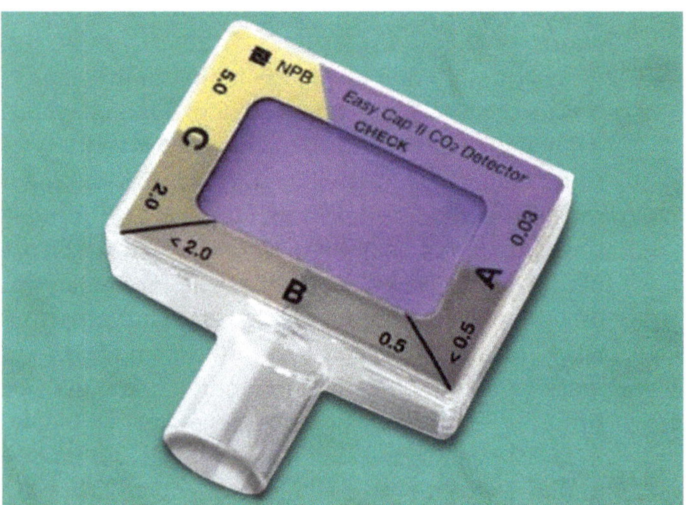

Fig. 11: Colorimetric CO_2 detector.

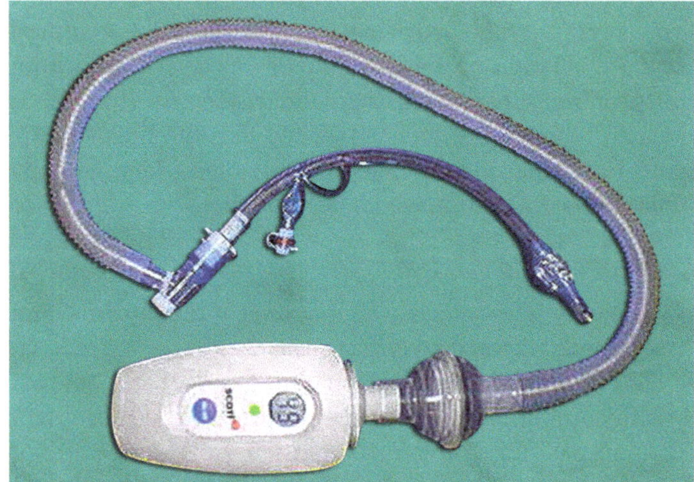

Fig. 12: Sonomatic confirmation of the tracheal intubation (SCOTI).

CO_2 and water. The device can be placed between patient and the breathing system or resuscitation bag. The color chart on the dome is designed to be read under fluorescent light. A hydrophobic indicator in a colorimetric device shows a color change from blue to green to yellow when exposed to CO_2

- *Chest X-ray:* Placement of tube can be confirmed by tracing the radio opaque marker on the tube. Chest radiography is time consuming and expensive
- *Sonomatic confirmation of the tracheal intubation (SCOTI)*[14] ***(Fig. 12)****:* It is a lightweight battery powered, sonomatic device which emits sound waves into the tube and analyzes the reflection. It provides guidance into the trachea and gives alarm if tube going in esophagus
- *Fiberscopic view:* The tracheal rings can be visualized by using a fiberscope. This is a reliable method but requires special instrumentation, skill, and time
- *Tracheal illumination:* A lighted intubation stylet through the tube will illuminate the anterior neck though trachea. It may not be so in obese or burns contracture patients
- *Pressure and flow-volume loops:* Appropriate pressure volume loops will confirm tracheal placement of tube.

Tube is then fixed with adhesive tape or commercially available tube holder. In case of bearded patients or facial burns, it can be secured with a tube tape or umbilical tape. If the tube is not well fixed, either accidental extubation or endobroncheal advancement of tube can occur.

A high pressure cuff should be inflated with the minimal amount of gas that will cause it to seal against the trachea at peak inspiratory pressure. With a low pressure, high volume cuff, the cuff should be inflated to a pressure of 18–25 mm Hg at end-expiration in adults. In children, still lower pressures are advised. Cuff pressure should be measured by manometer and adjusted frequently.

COMPLICATIONS OF INTUBATION

Trauma

Intubation is often associated with trauma to the structures in the upper and lower airways. Hematomas, contusions, lacerations, vocal cord avulsions, and fracture of larynx and rarely arytenoid cartilage dislocation also can be seen.

Nasal intubation may cause abrasion or laceration of the nasal mucosa, nasal septal injury and dislodgement of adenoid, nasal polyps, or turbinates. Rare cases of tracheal, bronchial, pharyngeal, esophageal and laryngeal perforation can occur.

Esophageal Intubation

Esophageal intubation is a dreadful complication and should be diagnosed fast. Recognition and prompt correction are necessary to prevent dire consequences. Mostly in chidren and in the obese patient, recognizing esophageal intubation is difficult as it closely resembles tracheal intubation. Auscultation of chest is not complete without epigastric auscultation. The abdomen can be observed for gastric distention. We may see gastric contents in the tube.

Inadvertent Bronchial Intubation

Inadvertent bronchial intubation is seen commonly with emergency intubations and in pediatric patients. The incidence was higher with use of Ring-Adair-Elwyn (RAE) tubes. Usually, it is a right endobronchial intubation as right main bronchus is more straight. It can lead to atelectasis in the nonventilated lung and hyperinflation and barotrauma in ventilated lung.

Bronchial intubation can occur intraoperatively during suctioning, change of position of patient's head or patient repositioning. It is recommended that tube position is confirmed regularly after repositioning. Placing the cuff just below the vocal cords in children and a few centimeters past the vocal cords in adults will prevent endobronchial intubation.

Foreign Body Aspiration

During intubation, a variety of materials that can cause blockage and can be aspirated into the trachea may cause problems. That involves teeth, adenoid or nasal tissue during its passage. A portion of a cuff or tip of tube from Murphy eye may separate out.

Careful inspection of equipment before use will help to avoid introduction of foreign bodies. Similarly, tube should be examined after extubation for missing parts.

Foreign body aspiration should be suspected whenever obstructive signs or symptoms appear. The patient's airway should be searched immediately and bronchoscopy done if needed.

Tracheal Tube Obstruction

Obstruction can be partial or complete and more common in infants and small children.

Causes

- *Biting:* It is seen in lighter planes of anesthesia. Adequate depth of anesthesia and a bite block or oral airway will prevent biting of tube
- *Kinking:* Kinking of tube is a frequent cause of tracheal tube obstruction. Kinking occurs due to change in head position, flexion of the neck, shifting from one side of the mouth to other. At times, tubes are made with thin sidewalls. Kinking sometimes occurs at the distal part of the connector. The tip of a tube may fold, causing obstruction
- *Material in the lumen of the tube:* A tracheal tube may be obstructed by dried secretions, blood, pus, tumor, or dried up lubricant. Foreign bodies like tooth, rubber from a mask, an inflation valve, small part of an intravenous (IV) set, an IV needle, glass ampoule, part of a nasogastric tube, caps from syringes are some of the rare foreign bodies which may obstruct the trachea
- *Cuff problems:* If the tube cuff inflates eccentrically, i.e. in one direction, it may displace the bevel from the centre of the trachea and impinge against the tracheal wall. Over inflation of the cuff may cause compression of the tube lumen. Cuff deflation will solve the problem
- *External compression or displacement:* The aorta or the thyroid gland may cause the bevel to lie against the tracheal wall or compress the tube. A nasogastric tube or suction catheter knotted around the tube or a nearby surgical retractor can cause compression. Sometimes pharyngeal abscess like Ludwig's angina may cause compression of the tube
- *Change in body position:* A shift in body position may cause the tracheal tube to become obstructed.

Prevention of Obstruction

- Use of transparent tubes for early detection of material blocking the lumen
- Use of a Murphy type tube
- A flexometallic tube for surgery of head and neck
- Careful use of lubricants
- Placing a bite block securely between the molar teeth
- Maintenance of adequate level of anesthesia
- Careful examination of tube before use for patency of the lumen and functioning of cuff.

Treatment

High inspiratory pressures and an increase in the difference between peak and plateau airway pressure with volume-controlled ventilation or reduced tidal volume during pressure-controlled ventilation will indicate tube obstruction. Pressure volume loops and the capnograph with increased slope will confirm the diagnosis.

- Altering the patient's head position or deflation of the cuff

- Laryngoscopy to check for kinking of tube
- Passing a suction catheter or stylet down the tube
- Endotracheal suction to remove clotted blood or mucus
- Check equipment between the breathing system and the tracheal tube.

Aspiration

During long-term intubation, secretions seeping around the tracheal tube cuff are the most important risk for pneumonia. Higher incidence with low pressure cuffs, uncuffed tubes, and spontaneous ventilation is seen. Retained pharyngeal secretions can also lead to aspiration.

During extubation, give head low and lateral position before cuff deflation, and deflate the cuff during positive airway pressure to blow material collected above the cuff into the pharynx.

Leaks

A leak will cause inadequate ventilation and may lead to aspiration. A torn cuff uncuffed tube or defect in the tube may make it impossible to inflate the cuff. A leak despite cuff inflation with excess of air may suggest protrusion of the cuff above the vocal cords. A laser beam can perforate the cuff. If the nasogastric tube has inadvertently passed into the trachea alongside the tracheal tube, then there will be considerable leak of gases.

When a leak is present, laryngoscopy should be performed. In case of damaged cuff or tube, it should be changed. If the cuff is above the vocal cords, it should be deflated and the tube advanced further. In case of uncuffed tube, pharyngeal packing is done to control the leak.

Difficult Extubation

Failure of deflation of cuff is the most common cause of difficult extubation. It is due to the problems of inflation tube like biting of the inflation tube by the patient, inadvertent cutting of inflating tube or the inflating tube getting entangled with a nasogastric tube. In surgical procedures near the tube, there is a risk of the tracheal tube or inflation tube getting transfixed to adjacent tissues.

Cuff can be deflated by cutting the inflation tube. If the cuff still remains inflated, the tube should be pulled out up to the vocal cords and then can be deflated with a needle inserted through the cricothyroid membrane or can be punctured under vision with laryngoscopy. If the tube is surgically fixed to adjacent tissues, surgical re-exploration may be required.

Unintended Extubation

It is commonly seen in smaller patients and in patients with burns. Neck extension or lateral head rotation and prone position or upper airway swelling can dislodge the tube. If the cuff is at or just above the vocal cords, this may cause the tube to move farther out of the trachea. Sometimes, removal of a surgical drape over the tracheal tube may result in unintended extubation. The tube should be well secured. If the securing tape becomes wet, it should be replaced. Pulling on the tube should be avoided.

Postoperative Complications

Sore Throat

Sore throat is a common postoperative complication seen commonly in females, head and neck surgeries, prone position, prolonged ventilation and with use of larger tubes and with use of high pressure cuff. Preoperative inhalation of a steroid or gargling with sodium azulene sulfonate, inflating the cuff with a lidocaine or saline solution are some of the ways to reduce incidence of sore throat.[15] Lignocaine spray and cricoids pressure during intubation increase the incidence of sore throat.[16]

Hoarseness

Hoarseness may be decreased by using tubes with low pressure cuffs, smaller tubes, and lubrication with lidocaine jelly. Hoarseness increases with difficult and long intubation.[16]

Neurologic Injuries

Trigeminal, lingual, buccal, and hypoglossal nerve palsies.

Upper Airway Edema

Edema may occur anywhere along the path of the tube, including the tongue, uvula, epiglottis, aryepiglottic folds, vocal cords, and the retroarytenoid and subglottic spaces. Even mild degree of laryngeal edema (postintubation croup or inflammation, acute edematous stenosis, stridor, and subglottic edema), especially in the young child, may produce a significant reduction in the internal cross-sectional area. It is most commonly seen after surgery involving the head and neck and with increased duration of intubation. It may manifest any time during the first 48 hours after extubation. The symptoms may range from hoarseness or croupy cough to respiratory obstruction.

Intubation should be atraumatic, and adequate anesthetic depth and/or good muscle relaxation should be maintained to prevent tube movement. Head movement should be kept to a minimum.

Vocal Cord Dysfunction, Ulcerations

Vocal cord paralysis and paresis is seen and mostly resolves spontaneously, usually within days or weeks. Ulcerations (erosions) of the larynx and trachea increase with the duration of intubation. If the ulcer is superficial, regeneration to normal epithelium occurs relatively quickly. If the ulcer is very deep, scar tissue may form.

Vocal Cord Granuloma

Incidence is between 1 in 800 and 1 in 20,000 and more common in women. It occurs due to trauma, infection, excessive cuff pressure or prolonged intubation.

Patient may be asymptomatic or have persistent hoarseness, pain or discomfort in the throat, chronic cough, etc. Strict voice rest in patient with persistent hoarseness may prevent the development of a granuloma.

Latex Allergy

While most tracheal tubes are made from PVC, some laser tubes are made from latex-containing rubber.

Infection

A high incidence of sinusitis and otitis is seen. Pneumonia in case of prolonged intubation is fairly common.

Tracheal Stenosis

Tracheal stenosis is more common with long-term intubation.[17]

SPECIAL TUBES

Cole Tube (Fig. 13)[18]

Cole tube is used in emergency neonatal resuscitation. It is an uncuffed oral tube with a patient end with smaller diameter than the rest of the shaft. It has a shoulder at the junction of narrow patient end and broad proximal end. This shoulder prevents inadvertent bronchial intubation and also provides airtight seal. The size of Cole tube is same as the ID of patient end.

The resistance offered by the Cole tube is more than that of a comparable tube of constant lumen and can cause trauma to the larynx and tracheal ring dilatation if the shoulder forced into the larynx.[19] It cannot be used for nasal intubation. But Manczur et al. proved that the resistance by Cole tube is much lesser than the same sized usual endotracheal tube of same diameter.[20] There are chances of blockage of tube with secretions due to narrow patient end.

Microcuff Endotracheal Tubes (Fig. 14)

It is a cuffed tube specially designed for children. It consists of a short, ultra-thin polyurethane cuff located away from the subglottic area. The cuff effectively seals the tracheal wall at pressures as low as 10 cmH_2O and fills the gap between the tube and the tracheal wall without folds. The cuff is inflated with 0.1 mL air at a time continuously measuring the cuff pressure. The ultra-thin polyurethane cuff (10 µm) allows tracheal sealing at low pressures and provides a uniform and complete surface contact with minimal formation of cuff folds. Uninflated, the cuff adds only a minimal amount to the external diameter of the tracheal tube. Shortened cuffs and the elimination of a Murphy eye allow a more distal position of the upper cuff border, thereby reducing the risk of pressure being applied to the cricoid ring and adjacent mucosa.[21]

Ring-Adair-Elwin Tube

This tube is named after its inventors, Ring, Adair, and Elwin. Ring-Adair-Elwin (RAE) tube has a preformed bend with a marking at the bend so as to facilitate surgery on head and face.[22]

Oral or South Polar Ring-Adair-Elwin Tube (Fig. 15A)

The external portion of the oral version is bent at an acute angle so that when in place, it rests on the patient's chin with the connector on chest and the proximal tube passes down the chin away from the face, thus improving surgical access in cleft lip, palate, and nasal surgeries.

Nasal or North Polar Tube (Fig. 15B)

The nasal version has a cephalic curve so that when in place the outer portion of the tube is directed over the patient's forehead. This helps to reduce pressure on the nares.

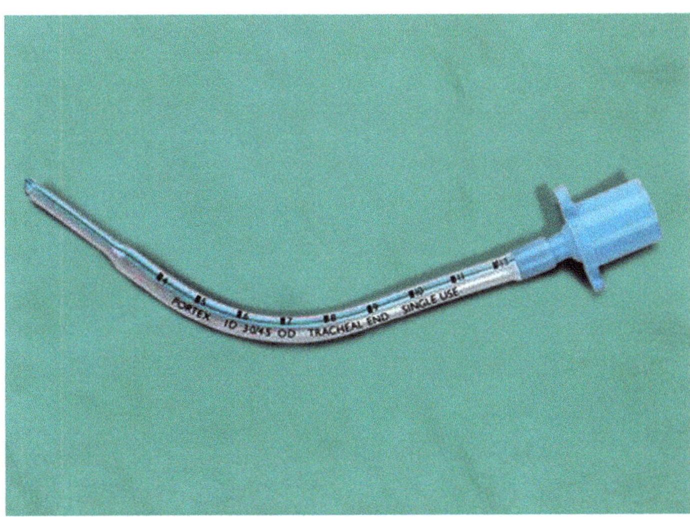

Fig. 13: Cole tube.

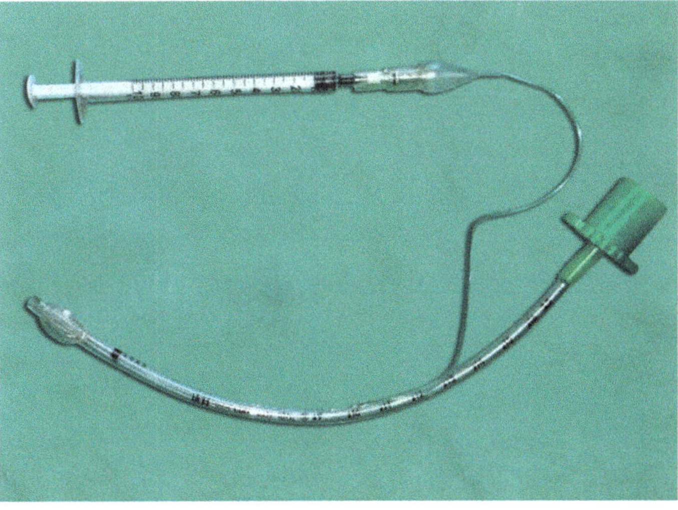

Fig. 14: Microcuff endotracheal tube.

The nasal version is bent where it exits the nose so that the part with connector passes upwards to the forehead. It is used for surgeries on the lower face, mandible and floor of mouth.

The nasal and oral versions are available in various sizes and in cuffed and uncuffed versions. Uncuffed RAE tubes are shorter than cuffed RAE tubes and oral tubes are shorter than nasal tubes. As the diameter increases, the length and distance from the distal tip to the curve also increases. In an appropriate size tube, when the mark at the bend is at the teeth or nares, the tube is satisfactorily positioned in the trachea in most of the cases. While selecting the tube, patient's height and weight should be considered along with age as a smaller size tube may not reach below the glottis.

Advantages

- These tubes are easy to secure and reduce the risk of accidental extubation
- The curve of tube helps to place the circuit away from the surgical field
- The long length may make them useful for insertion through a supraglottic airway device
- The nasal tube may be useful for oral intubation of patients who are to be in the prone position.

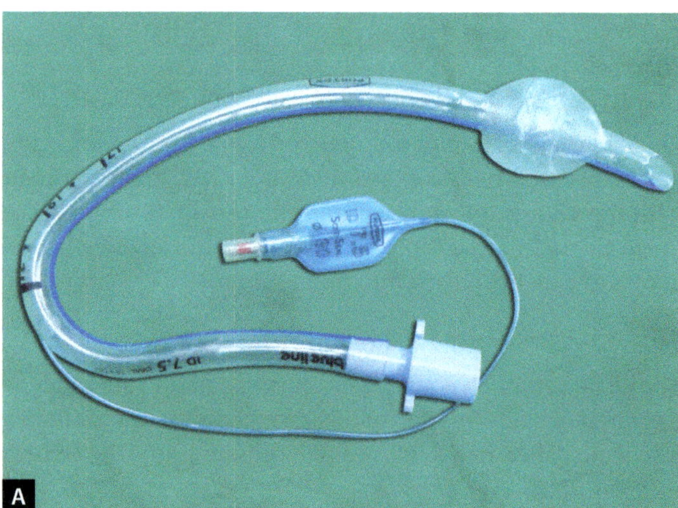

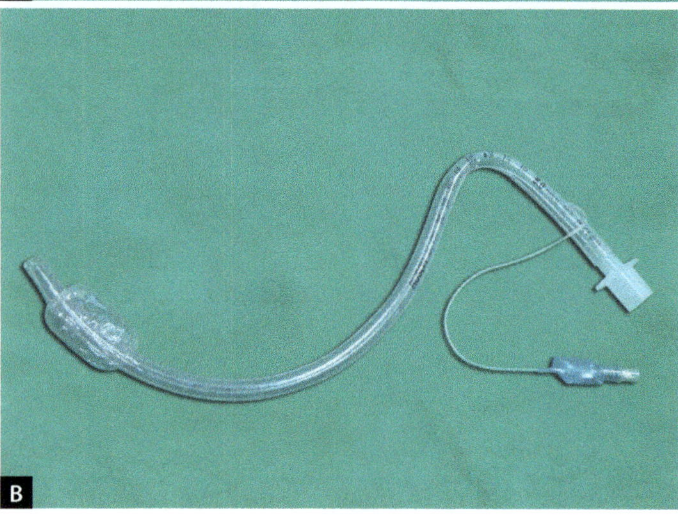

Figs. 15A and B: (A) South polar tube; (B) North polar tube.

Disadvantages

- There is a difficulty in passing a suction catheter through them
- These tubes offer more resistance than comparably sized conventional tubes
- Since they are designed to fit the average patient, a tube may be either too long or too short for a given patient
- As patients inevitably vary in size the tube may be too long for a given patient leading to the tip entering the bronchus, especially in smaller children
- Sometimes, with the trend of using smaller calibre tubes, a chosen RAE tube may be too short to reach below the glottis, increasing the risk of inadvertent extubation.

Flexometallic Tubes (Figs. 16 and 17)

The flexometallic (spiral embedded, armored, reinforced, wire reinforced) tube is made up of rubber, PVC, or silicone and has a metal or nylon spiral wound reinforcing wire within the wall of the tube which makes it flexible and nonkinking. The reinforcing spiral will not stretch to accommodate a connector so the tubes cannot be cut to a shorter length than supplied. The ISO connectors are therefore usually bonded at production to a non reinforced part of the tube. These tubes are usually supplied at a length of 30 cm or greater for an ID of 5.0 mm and above.

Advantages

- The primary advantage of these tubes is resistance to kinking and compression, hence, useful in head and neck surgery, where head and neck is rotated or flexed
- The portion of the tube outside the patient can be angled away from the surgical field without kinking, making it useful for surgery in patient with tracheostomy, for submental intubation, and retromolar positioning
- It may pass more easily over a fiberscope than a conventional tube.

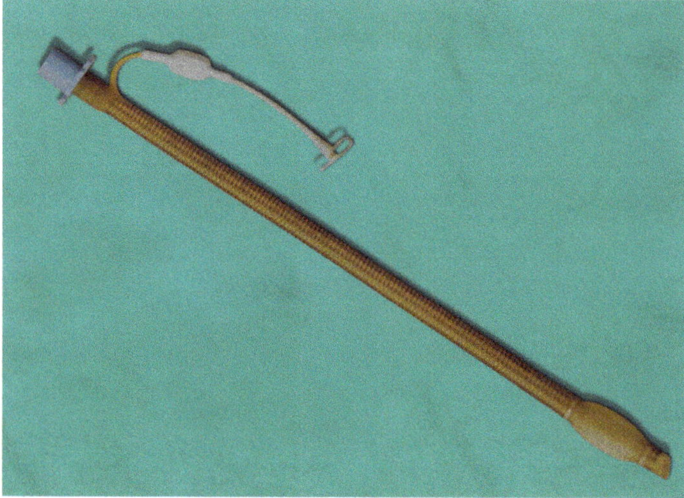

Fig. 16: Rubber flexometallic tube.

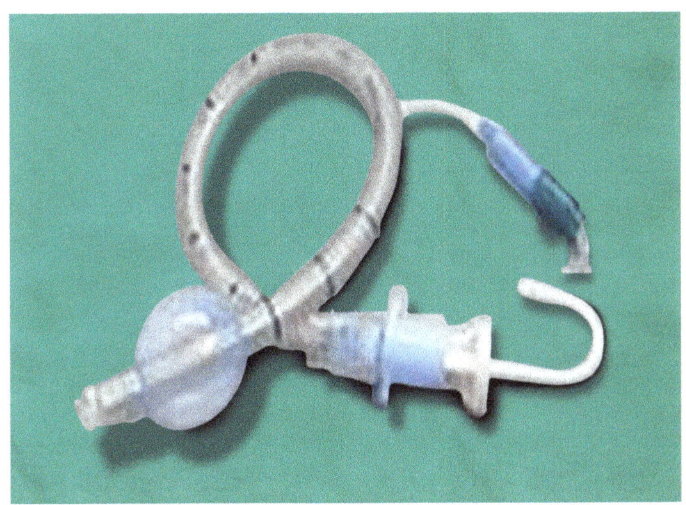

Fig. 17: Polyvinyl chloride flexometallic tube.

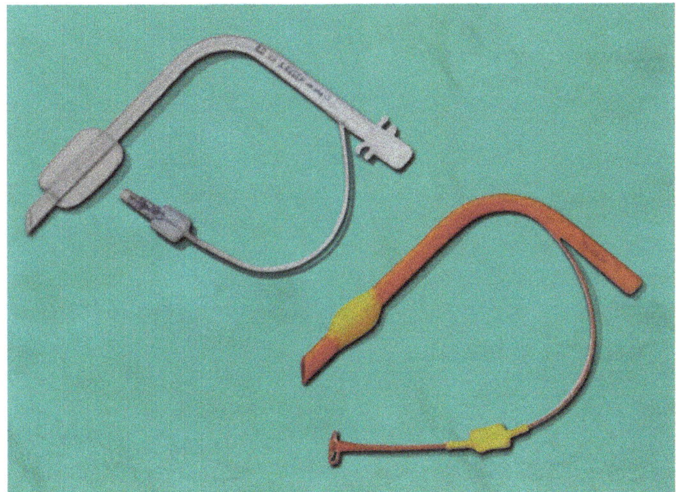

Fig. 18: Oxford tube.

Disadvantages

- A forceps and/or a stylet will often be needed for intubation and it may rotate on the stylet during insertion
- It is difficult to pass the tube through the nose
- Reinforced tubes have a thicker wall and therefore we get a smaller ID for a given outer diameter (OD)
- Because of the spiral, these tubes cannot be shortened. The elastic recoil force may increase the tendency to unintentional extubation
- Repeated sterilization makes the tubes sticky and soft mainly at the junction of the start of the spiral and the connector and can cause kinking at this junction
- The elastic recoil force may increase the incidence of accidental extubation hence throat pack and proper fixation of tube is must
- The tube does not have Murphy eye, hence may result in obstruction if the bevel abuts the wall of the trachea
- The metal wire spiral may obscure radiological imaging in some cervical spine surgery.

Oxford Tube (Asslop's Tube) (Fig. 18)[18]

It is an L-shaped tube made up of red rubber. It may be cuffed or uncuffed. The ID is uniform throughout the tube but the thickness of the tube wall varies. A portex tube may be better than red rubber tube in terms of kinking and resistance.[23]

Advantages

- As the proximal portion of tube is thicker than the tracheal part, a bigger tube can be passed through the trachea
- The thicker wall at the lips prevents compression by the mouth gag in cleft lip or palate surgery
- It also can be used in prone position surgeries like posterior fossa surgery and cervical spine surgery, etc.

Disadvantages

- All sizes are not available
- The bevel situated posteriorly may abut against tracheal wall during flexion of head
- The tube, because of its acute curve offers greater resistance and difficult to suction
- The distance from the bevel to curve is fixed; hence to avoid endobronchial intubation a proper size tube must be used.

Microlaryngeal Tracheal Surgery Tube (Fig. 19)[9]

The microlaryngeal tracheal surgery tube (MLT or LTS) is available with an ID of 4, 5, or 6 mm, but an adult sized length and high volume low pressure cuff (same as on a standard 8 mm ID tube). This helps to keep the tube centered in the trachea. Sometimes it may have a yellow-colored cuff.

Advantages

- For microlaryngeal surgery and for patients with narrow airway where a normal sized tracheal tube cannot be inserted
- The small tube diameter provides better visibility and access to the surgical field
- Its length allows it to be used for nasal intubation and intubation via a laryngeal mask airway (LMA) or other supraglottic airway device.

Disadvantages

- Narrow diameter may lead to resistance to exhalation hence obligates controlled ventilation and a long expiratory phase should be used to allow complete expiration
- This type of tube is not safe for use with lasers
- Due to their flexibility they can be difficult to insert unless Magill's forceps is used.

Tehran Tube (Fig. 20)

The upper airway makes a curve with its convexity following the natural lordosis of the cervical vertebrae.

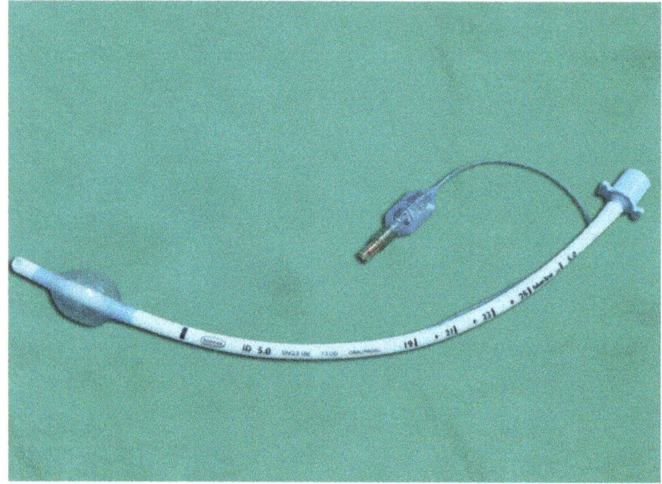

Fig. 19: Microlaryngeal tube.

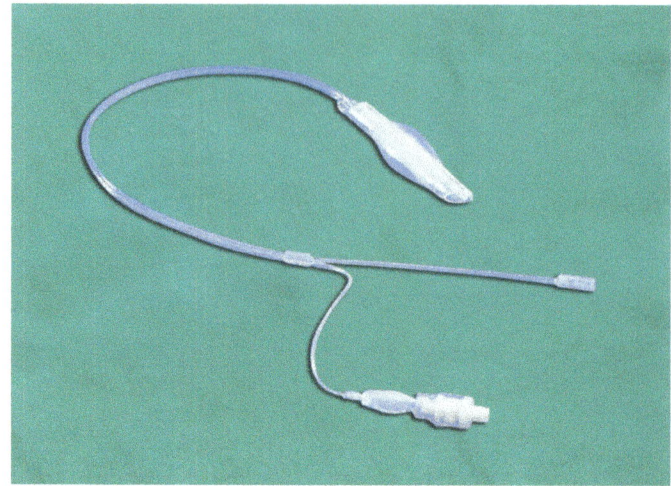

Fig. 21: Carden tube.

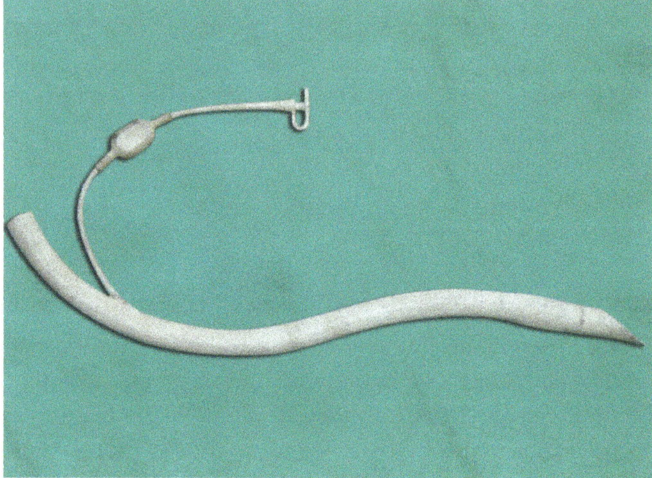

Fig. 20: Tehran tube.

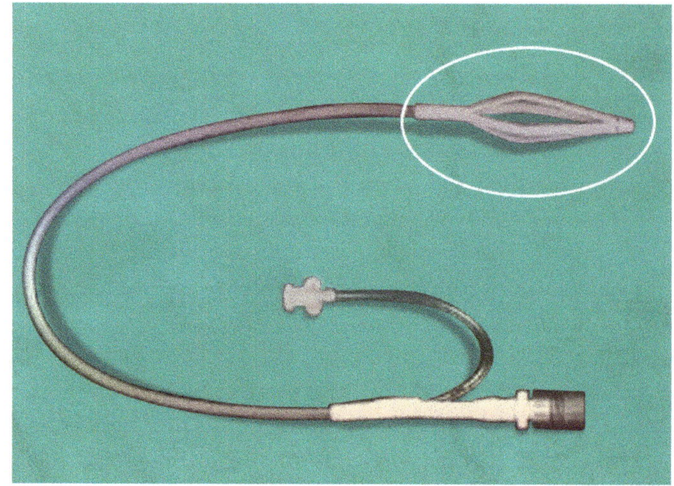

Fig. 22: Hunsaker Mon-Jet ventilation tube.

This interferes with the introduction and satisfactory positioning of a nasal endotracheal tube. To overcome this difficulty, a double curved, S-shaped Tehran tube for nasal intubation was developed. It is a reusable tube made up of silicone. It is very useful for blind nasal intubation.[24]

Carden Tube (Fig. 21)

This tube was developed to facilitate microsurgery of the larynx. It is rarely used now. It comprises a shortened cuffed tracheal tube that sits wholly below the glottis attached to a long catheter for insufflation of gas and a long pilot tube for the cuff. It may be inserted by grasping the tube with Magill's forceps and placing it under direct vision. Alternatively, the Carden tube and an uncut plain tube, just wide enough to fit inside it, are threaded onto a stylet. This assembly is introduced through the larynx. The cuff of the Carden tube is inflated, the stylet is withdrawn and anesthesia is maintained in the usual manner through the plain tube.

Hunsaker Mon-Jet Ventilation Tube (Fig. 22)

The Hunsaker tube is laser resistant tube with OD of 3 mm. It is used for subglottic jet ventilation. It has a separate lumen for monitoring airway pressure and respiratory gases. The patient end has a basket shaped distal extension designed to center the tube. It is used to administer one-lung ventilation. It is compatible with carbon dioxide, neodymium-yttrium aluminum-garnet (Nd-YAG), and argon lasers.

Laryngectomy Tube (Fig. 23)

Laryngectomy tube is designed to be inserted into a tracheotomy. It is "J" shaped and needs to be straightened while insertion. The tip may be short and/or without a bevel to avoid advancement into a bronchus. This allows the part of the tube external to the patient to be directed away from the surgical field.

The short distance between the cuff and distal tip of the tube may cause the bevel to abut the tracheal wall.

Endotrol Tube (Fig. 24)

The Endotrol tube has a pull ring loop (trigger) that is connected to the tip of the tube with a cable embedded in the tube. Pulling the trigger decreases the tube's inside radius and moves the tip anteriorly.

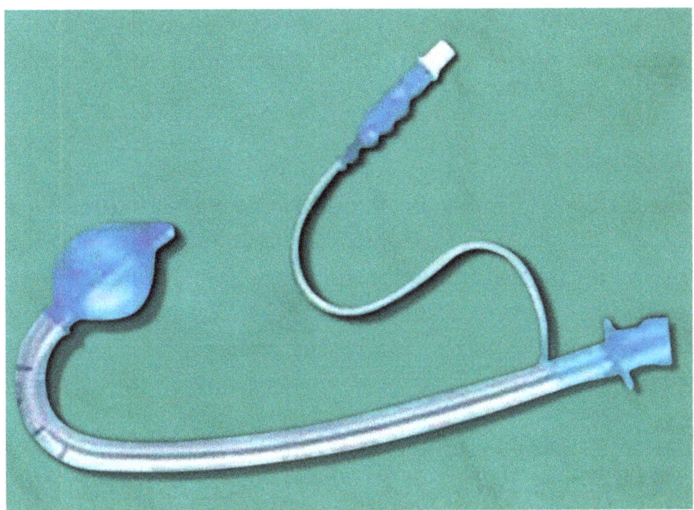

Fig. 23: Laryngectomy tube.

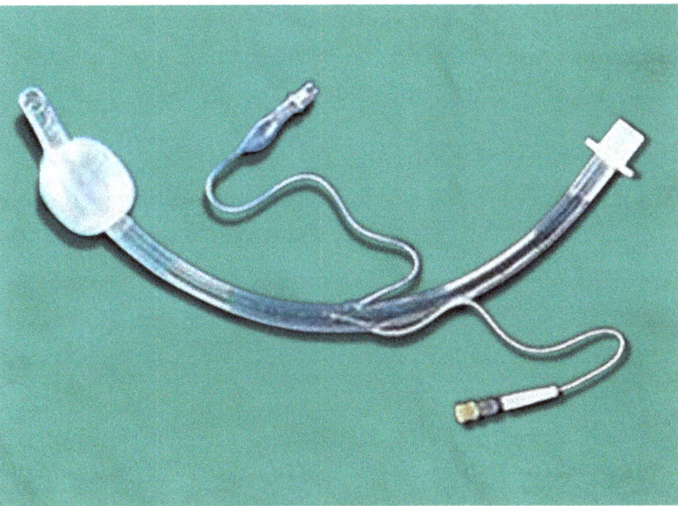

Fig. 24: Endotrol tube.

The Endotrol tube has been used for blind nasal intubation and intubation using a laryngoscope mainly in patient's where cervical spine injury is suspected.

EndoFlex® Tube (Fig. 25)

The EndoFlex® tube is designed to aid intubation when the patient has an anterior larynx. Pulling the white bar toward the connector causes the tube to flex at the cuff and the tip to move anteriorly.

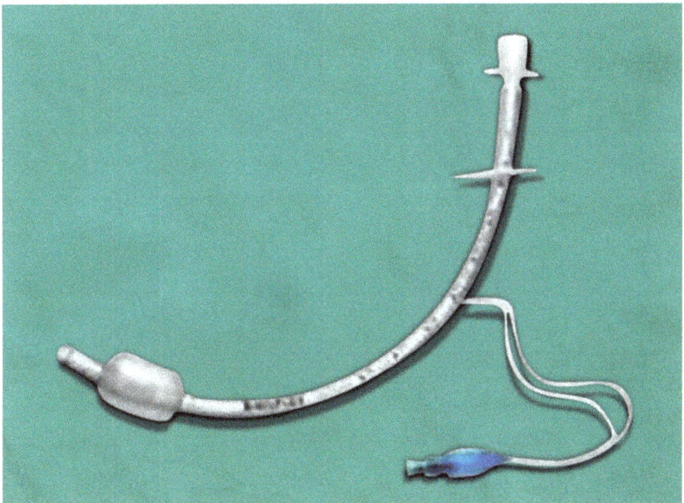

Fig. 25: EndoFlex® tube.

Parker Flex-Tip® Tube (Fig. 26)

The Parker Flex-Tip® tube has a "hooded" curved, flexible tapered tip that points toward the center of the distal lumen on the concave surface of the tube so that the bevel faces posteriorly during insertion. The tube is available in a variety of shapes with and without a cuff. There are Murphy eyes on the right and left sides of the tube and has a very thin cuff. This tube is easier to advance over a flexible endoscope than a conventional tube.

Electromyogram Reinforced Tracheal Tube (Fig. 27)

This tube is designed to monitor recurrent laryngeal nerve electromyogram (EMG) activity during surgery. The tube is wire reinforced and has four stainless steel electrodes above the cuff. The electrodes are connected to a monitor.

Intubating Laryngeal Mask Airway Tracheal Tube (Fig. 28)

The intubating laryngeal mask airway (ILMA) tracheal tube is designed to be inserted through the intubating laryngeal mask but can be used separately. It is a straight, wire reinforced silicone tube with a blunt tip, short bevel, and Murphy eye. It has a high pressure, low volume cuff. It is reusable and can be autoclaved. It is available in sizes 6, 6.5, 7, 7.5, and 8.

This tube is preferred than a PVC tube to advance over a fiberscope during both oral and nasal intubation. It has been used for submental intubation.

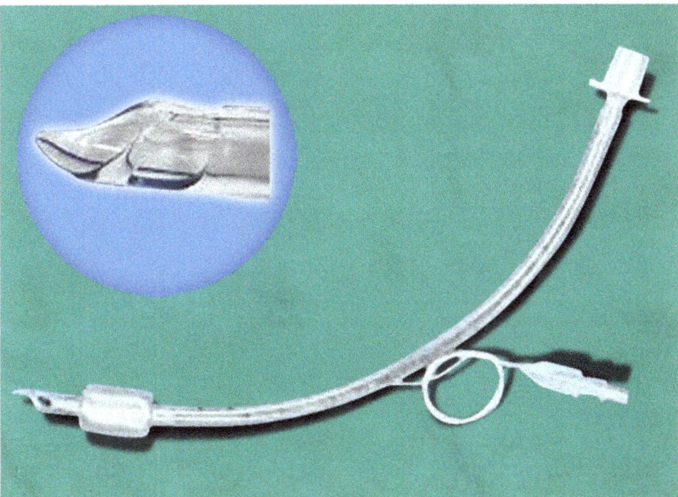

Fig. 26: Parker Flex-Tip® tube.

The disadvantages of this tube are eccentric cuff inflation, deformity of spirals due to biting, leaks and the tip folding during insertion. This tube should be used with caution if prolonged intubation is anticipated because of the high pressure cuff. Cuff inflation should be limited to the minimum volume that seals the trachea. It is a magnetic resonance imaging (MRI) compatible tube.

Hi-Lo Evac® Tube (Fig. 29)

The Hi-Lo Evac® tube incorporates a dedicated channel that can be used to clear secretions below the vocal cords but above the cuff. Results were mixed when using this tube to prevent or delay pneumonia. The lumen may become blocked by secretions.

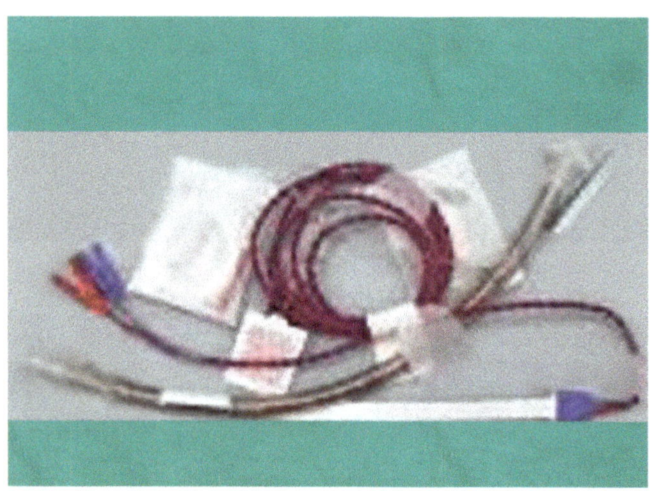

Fig. 27: Electromyogram reinforced tracheal tube.

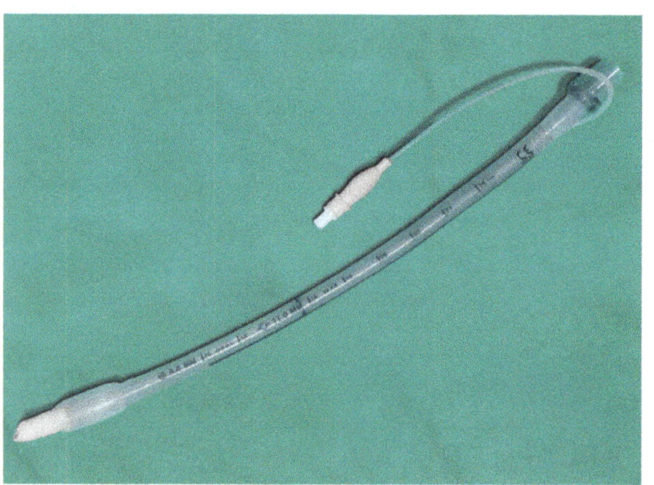

Fig. 28: Intubating laryngeal mask tracheal tube.

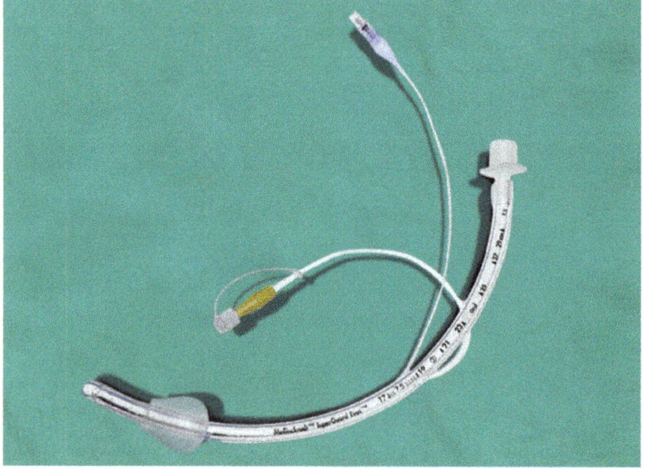

Fig. 29: Hi-Lo Evac® tube.

Hi-Lo Jet Tube

The Hi-Lo Jet tube is an uncuffed tube with an additional lumen that can be used for jet ventilation, monitoring airway pressure, sampling respiratory gases, administering local anaesthetics, or irrigating the airway. One problem with the tube is that a suction catheter may bind in the small tracheal tube lumen.

Laryngotracheal Instillation of Topical Anesthesia (Fig. 30)

It has an additional small-bore channel incorporated within the concave surface of the tube. Ten small holes at the distal 13 cm of the tube allow the injected medication to be sprayed both above and below the cuff. It can provide a smooth emergence from anesthesia without coughing in most cases.

Double Lumen Tubes

They are used for lung isolation in thoracic surgeries. It is discussed in the Chapter 14.

Laser-resistant Tubes[1]

Conventional tracheal tubes of either plastic, silicone or rubber may be damaged by the carbon dioxide, potassium titanyl phosphate (KTP) or Nd-YAG laser beam. These materials burn more fiercely in the presence of oxygen or nitrous oxide than in air and are easily ignited by a direct or indirect strike from the laser beam. The resultant fire can produce serious upper airway burns and severe distal inhalation injury. A number of tracheal tubes have been designed to be used for laser surgery. Though these tubes are laser resistant but may catch fire if the laser power is too great or the laser application too long.

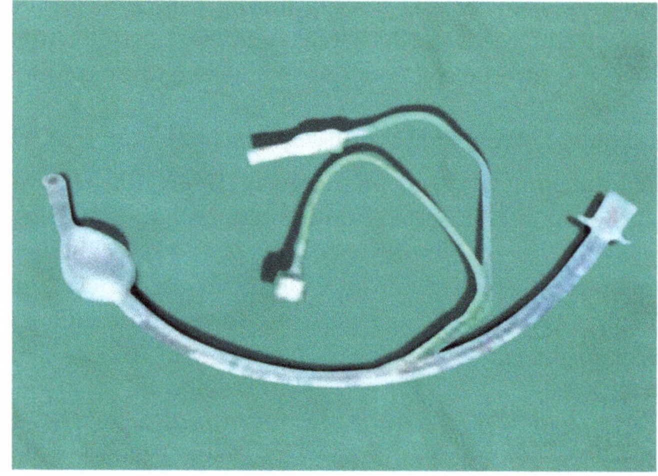

Fig. 30: Laryngotracheal instillation of topical anesthesia.

Laser-Shield II Tube (Fig. 31)

The Laser-Shield II is made from silicone with an inner aluminium wrap and an outer teflon coating. The cuff is not laser resistant and contains methylene blue crystals. It should be inflated with water or a saline solution. The part of the tube distal to the cuff is also unprotected. Moist cottonoids are used for wrapping the cuff through out the procedure. It is designed for use with CO_2 and KTP lasers. Exposure of the unprotected parts of the tube proximal and distal to the cuff can result in rapid combustion.

Laser-Flex Tracheal Tube (Fig. 32)

The Laser-Flex tube is a stainless steel tube with a smooth plastic surface and a matte finish to reflect a laser beam. It is designed for use with CO_2 and KTP lasers. The wall of the tube is thicker than that of most other tubes. It has two PVC cuffs and a Murphy eye. The two cuffs have separate inflation tubes that run along the inside of the tube. The distal cuff is filled followed by the proximal cuff. The distal cuff can be used if the proximal one is damaged by the laser. Small uncuffed tubes are also available. The cuffs should be filled with saline colored with methylene blue. The Laser-Flex tube is somewhat stiff and has a rough surface. The double cuff adds to the time of intubation and extubation. The large external diameter can be a problem in small patients.

Sheridan Laser Tracheal Tube (Fig. 33)

The Sheridan laser tube is a red rubber tube wrapped with copper foil tape and then wrapped with a water absorbent fabric. Moist radiopaque pledgets are placed above the cuff. It is designed for use with a CO_2 or KTP laser. It has high pressure cuff.

Norton Tube (Fig. 34)

The Norton tube is a reusable, flexible, spiral wound metal tube with a stainless steel connector and thick walls. The exterior of the tube has a matte finish to decrease

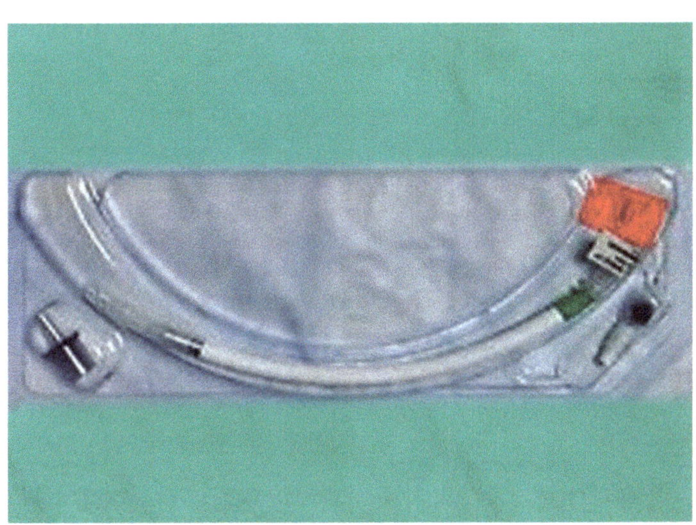

Fig. 31: Laser-Shield II tube.

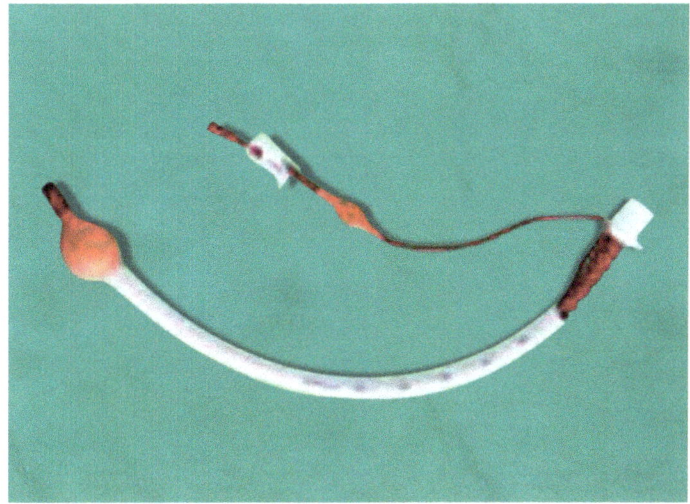

Fig. 33: Sheridan laser tube.

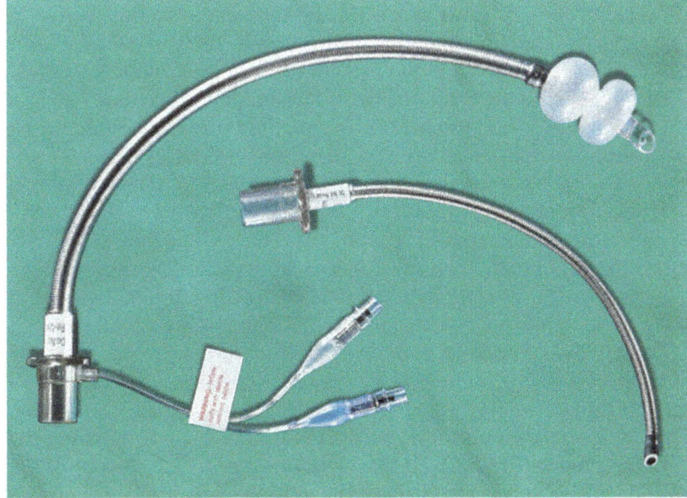

Fig. 32: Laser-Flex tube.

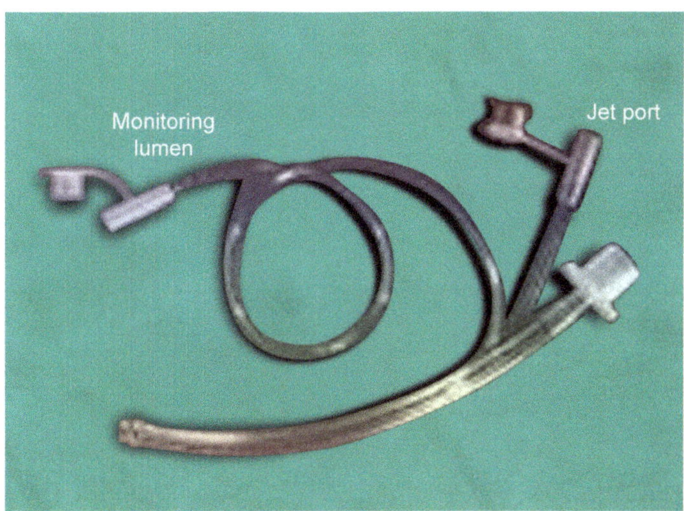

Fig. 34: Norton tube.

reflection of the laser beam. It has no cuff. A separate cuff may be attached, or packing around the tube can be used to achieve a seal. Studies show this tube is acceptable for use with KTP, Nd-YAG, and CO_2 lasers. The tube's exterior is somewhat rough and may have sharp edges that could cause tissue damage. The large external diameter and stiffness can make surgical exposure difficult.

Bivona Fome-Cuff Laser Tube (Fig. 35)

The Bivona Fome-Cuff laser tube has an aluminium and silicone spiral with a silicone covering. It has a self-inflating cuff of a polyurethane foam sponge with a silicone envelope. The cuff should be filled with saline during use. The inflation tube runs along the exterior of the tube and is colored black so that it can be positioned away from where the laser will be used. It is marketed for use with the CO_2 laser. When burned, the silicone covering forms an ash that is left in the trachea, hence high incidence of sore throat has been noted with this tube.

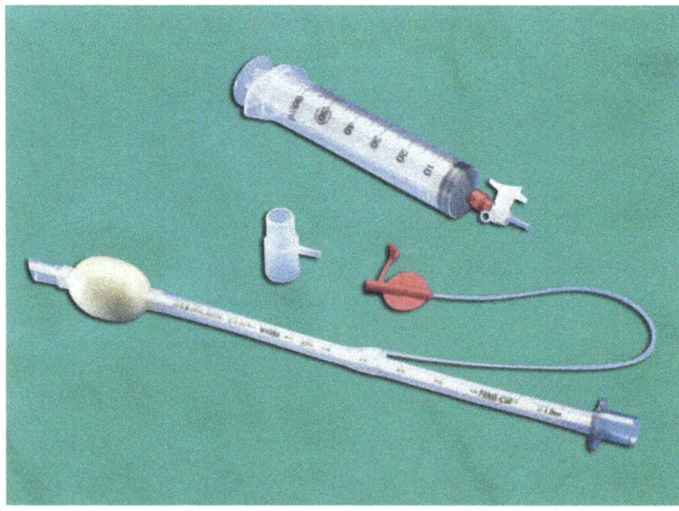

Fig. 35: Bivona Fome-Cuff laser tube.

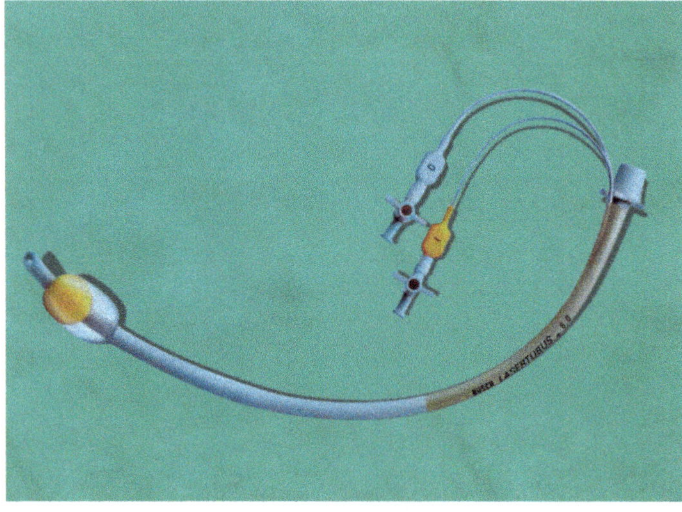

Fig. 36: Lasertubus™.

Lasertubus™ (Fig. 36)

This tube is made of white rubber and has a cuff-within-a-cuff design. If the outer cuff is perforated by the laser beam, the trachea will still be sealed by the inner cuff. The manufacturer recommends that the inner cuff be filled with air and the outer cuff with water or saline. The shaft above the cuff is covered by a corrugated silver foil, which is covered by a Merocel® sponge that should be moistened with saline before use. This tube is recommended for use with argon, Nd-YAG, and CO_2 lasers. Bending the tube in the area above the sponge covering can predispose the tube to kinking.

CONCLUSION

Endotracheal intubation is a gold standard for intubation. It is mandatory for every anesthesiologist to be aware of its indications, contraindications and complications along with the equipment used for it. Endotracheal tubes are available in different sizes, materials and characteristics depending on their indications in different types of surgery variable age group. In depth knowledge of endotracheal tubes is beneficial.

REFERENCES

1. Dorsch JA, Dorsch SE. Tracheal tubes. In: Dorsch JA, Dorsch SE (Eds). Understanding Anesthesia Equipment, 5th edition. Philadelphia: Lippincott Williams & Wilkins; 2007.
2. Khan RM. Conventional laryngoscopy and tracheal intubation/extubation (Adult and pediatric). In: Khan RM, Maroof M (Eds). Airway Management, 4th edition. Hyderabad: Paras Medical Publisher; 2011.
3. Vesalius A. De Humanis Corporis Fabrica, 1st edition. Basel: Octavo; 1542. p. 658.
4. Diba A. Airway management devices. In: Davey AJ, Diba A (Eds). Ward's Anaesthetic Equipment, 5th edition. London: Elsevier Saunders; 2005.
5. Forestner JE. Frank J, Murphy MD, CM, 1900–1972: His life, career, and the Murphy eye. Anesthesiology. 2010;113(5):1019-25.
6. Branson RD. Endotracheal tubes and imposed work of breathing: What should we do about it, if anything? Crit Care. 2003;7(5):347-8.
7. Seegobin RD, Van Hasselt GL. Endotracheal cuff pressure and tracheal mucosal blood flow: endoscopic study of effects of four large volume cuffs. Br Med J (Clin Res Ed). 1984;288(6422):965-8.
8. Al-Shaikh B, Jones M, Baldwin F. Evaluation of pressure changes in a new design tracheal tube cuff, the Portex Soft Seal, during nitrous oxide anaesthesia. Br J Anaesth. 1999;83(5):805-6.
9. Paul AK. Endotracheal equipments. In: Paul AK (Ed). Drugs and Equipments in Anaesthetic Practice, 3rd edition. New Delhi: BI Churchill Livingstone; 1998.
10. Mayglothling J, Duane TM, Gibbs M, et al. Emergency tracheal intubation immediately following traumatic injury: An eastern association for the surgery of trauma practice management guideline. J Trauma. 2012;73(5):S333-40.
11. Sitzwohl C, Langheinrich A, Schober A, et al. Endobronchial intubation detected by insertion depth of endotracheal tube, bilateral auscultation, or observation of chest movements: randomised trial. BMJ. 2010;341:c5943.
12. Lau N, Playfor SD, Rashid A, et al. New formulae for predicting tracheal tube length. Paediatr Anaesth. 2006;16(12):1238-43.

13. Kulkarni A, Chatterjee A. Endotracheal tubes, double lumen tubes and combitube. In: Kulkarni AP, Divatia JV, Patil VP, Gehdoo RP (Eds). Objective Anaesthesia Review: A Comprehensive Textbook for the Examinees, 3rd edition. New Delhi: Jaypee Brothers Medical Publishers (P) Ltd.; 2013.
14. Petroianu G, Maleck W, Bergler W, et al. Sonomatic confirmation of tracheal intubation using the SCOTI. Prehosp Disaster Med. 1997;12(2):149-53.
15. Rao M, Snigdha, Alai T, et al. Instillation of 4% lidocaine versus air in the endotracheal tube (ETT) cuff to evaluate post intubation morbidity-a randomized double blind study. J Anesth Clin Sc. 2013;2:19. [online] Available from http://dx.doi.org/10.7243/2049-9752-2-19. [Last accessed February, 2014].
16. Maruyama K, Sakai H, Miyazawa H, et al. Sore throat and hoarseness after total intravenous anaesthesia. Br J Anaesth. 2004;92(4):541-3.
17. Suskeviciene I, Bukauskas T, Karbonskiene A, et al. Challenges in the management of acquired tracheal stenosis: A case report. Acta Medica Lituanica. 2012;19(3):154-9.
18. Deshpande S. Endotracheal tubes. In: Despande S (Ed). Anaesthesia: Drugs, Equipments, ECG and X-rays, 1st edition. Hyderabad: Paras Medical Publishers; 2002.
19. Hatch DJ. Tracheal tubes and connectors used in neonates-dimensions and resistance to breathing. Br J Anaesth. 1978;50(9):959-64.
20. Manczur T, Greenough A, Nicholson GP, et al. Resistance of pediatric and neonatal endotracheal tubes: influence of flow rate, size, and shape. Crit Care Med. 2000;28(5):1595-8.
21. Weiss M, Dullenkopf A, Bottcher S, et al. Clinical evaluation of cuff and tube tip position in a newly designed pediatric preformed oral cuffed tracheal tube. Br J Anesth. 2006;97(5):695-700.
22. Ring WH, Adair JC, Elwyn RA. A new paediatric endotracheal tube. Anaesth Analg. 1975;54(2):273-4.
23. West MR, Jonas MM, Adams AP, et al. A new tracheal tube for difficult intubation. Br J Anaesth. 1996;76(5):673-9.
24. Tashayod M. A new double-curved endotracheal tube for nasal intubation. Br J Anaesth. 1967;39(10):823-6.

Double Lumen Tubes and Bronchial Blockers

Vijaya P Patil, Bhakti D Trivedi, Madhavi D Desai

ABSTRACT

The lung isolation techniques are required not only to facilitate surgical exposure in many thoracic and sometimes other surgeries like spine surgeries; but also in nonsurgical situations like pulmonary hemorrhage, or whole lung lavage. This chapter will discuss various indications, and devices available for lung isolation in current clinical practice, various techniques of lung isolation, merits and demerits of each isolation device and choice of device in various situations.

INTRODUCTION

The lung isolation techniques are mainly employed to facilitate surgical exposure for procedures in the thoracic cavity. This has advantages such as to prevent contamination of the contralateral lung in cases of massive bleeding or presence of abscess; to achieve effective ventilation in patients with bronchopleural fistula requiring mechanical ventilation and for independent lung ventilation in intensive care unit (ICU) for patients with unilateral parenchymal lung injury. The various sizes of double lumen tubes and variety of endobronchial blockers (EBBs) are available for the same purpose.

HISTORY OF LUNG ISOLATION

In 1931, Gale and Waters used cuffed rubber endotracheal tube (ETT) inserted into the bronchus for thoracic procedure for the first time.[1] In 1935, Archibald used rubber EBB positioned by radiography to achieve lung isolation. In following year Sir Ivan Magill used rubber EBB that could be accurately positioned under direct vision using a rigid endoscope passed down the blocker tube's lumen. This was followed by introduction of double-lumen bronchial tubes (DLTs) by Gebauer and later Carlen's and thus started the era of lung isolation.

HISTORY OF DOUBLE LUMEN TUBES

The left-sided DLTs were introduced for the first time in 1939 by Gebauer; which were designed for bronchospirometry. However, this tube had a single channel for inflation of both tracheal as well as bronchial cuffs. An year later, Zavod introduced a similar double lumen tube with two separate channels for inflation of individual cuffs.[2] In 1949, Carlen's, a clinical physiologist reported lung separation with a similar DLT, which was also primarily meant for bronchospirometry; but this tube had a hook to secure it in correct position **(Fig. 1A)**.[1] In 1960, White introduced right-sided version of Carlen's DLT which also had carinal hook. At the same time, realizing problems associated with carinal hook; in 1959, Bryce-Smith designed a left-sided DLT without a carinal hook. One year later Bryce-Smith along with Salt and White made right-sided DLT with a slotted bronchial cuff; which was also without carinal hook.

The previous DLTs had two main drawbacks, namely difficult placement and high airway resistance that restricted their use. In 1962, Roberts Shaw made the red rubber DLT, which had wide lumens and a molded curvature to reduce kinking and improve gas flow during one lung ventilation **(Fig. 1B)**. This tube became the prototype of the modern day DLT.

These tubes provided main modality for lung separation until disposable, polyvinyl chloride (PVC) double lumen tubes of the Robert Shaw design were introduced in 1980s. The rubber tubes have thick wall, and therefore, lesser internal to external diameter ratio. Also, these tubes have low volume-high pressure cuff subjecting tracheal and bronchial mucosa at risk of pressure necrosis.

New PVC double lumen tubes **(Fig. 1C)** are thin-walled and have larger internal to external diameter ratios as compared with rubber DLTs. Their transparent material allows observation of moisture during ventilation and the presence of secretions or blood in either lumen. They are also less irritant and therefore, can be retained in body for longer time. The tracheal as well as bronchial cuffs of these tubes are high volume-low pressure. All these properties reduce the danger of ischemic pressure damage to the airway mucosa. With more and more indications for lung isolation, new tube designs continue to come in the market. There are short DLTs for patients with tracheostomy **(Fig. 1D)**. The new Silbroncho tube has distal 5.1–5.8 cm portion wire-reinforced to maintain tip angulation at 45° **(Fig. 1E)**. Wire enforcement prevents obstruction and kinking from mediastinal compression when the tube is positioned in the dependent lung. They are available in both right- and left-sided versions in 33, 35, 37, and 39 Fr sizes.

Viva Sight DLT is manufactured in a left-sided version, in sizes 35, 37, 39, and 41 Fr **(Fig. 1F)**. Its shape is identical to that of other commonly used DLTs. It has a camera embedded at the distal end of its tracheal lumen and can be connected to an external monitor with a video cable. This helps in real-time visualization of the intubation. It has an extra side-port attached to flush the camera lens with saline. The confirmation of intubation is like with any other DLTs (the carina should be clearly visible and the upper

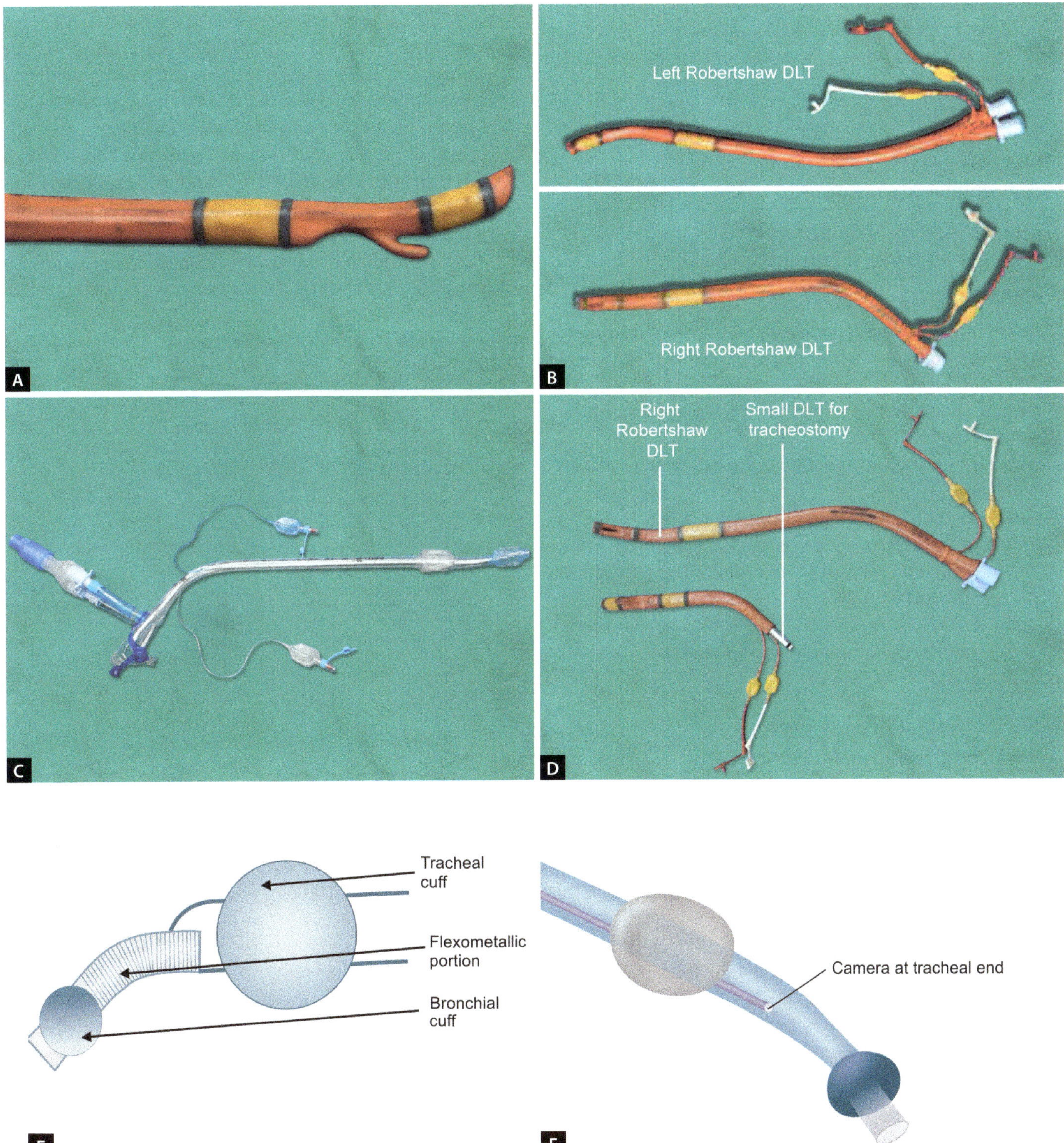

Figs. 1A to F: (A) Carlen's double lumen tube; (B) Robertshaw double lumen endotracheal tube; (C) Left double lumen tube (polyvinyl chloride); (D) Small for tracheostomy; (E) Silbroncho double lumen endotracheal tube; (F) VivaSight double lumen tube.

edge of the bronchial cuff seen in the main-stem bronchus). The proposed advantage is reduction in the need of fiberoptic bronchoscopic confirmation during DLT placement however current literature doubts this.[3] Another advantage is that it allows real time monitoring of the tube placement throughout the surgery. The downside of this is overheating and melting on the distal portion of the tube due to the heat generated by camera light.[3]

All modern double lumen bronchial tubes except VivaSight are either right- or left-sided and they all have:

- Longer bronchial lumen entering one of the bronchus with a cuff
- Shorter tracheal lumen with a cuff
- Preformed curve to facilitate entry into the bronchus
- Malleable stylet
- Radiographic marker along the length of the tube.

INDICATIONS FOR THE USE OF LUNG SEPARATION TECHNIQUES

In Operation Room

- *Before anesthetizing a patient with massive intrapulmonary bleed:* Open surgery or interventional radiologic procedures
- Patients with bronchiectasis and lung abscess undergoing surgeries for same
- Surgeries for major bronchopleural or bronchoesophageal fistula repair
- Major bronchial disruption or trauma repair
- Unilateral lung lavage for pulmonary alveolar proteinases
- *Video-assisted thoracoscopic procedures:* Lung resections and esophageal surgeries
- Open thoracic surgeries of esophagus, spine surgeries those require transthoracic approach, and minimally invasive cardiac surgeries.

In Intensive Care Unit

- Unilateral parenchymal injury
  - Aspiration
  - Pulmonary contusion
  - Pneumonia
- Single lung transplant (postoperative complications)
- Bronchopleural fistula needing mechanical ventilation.

SELECTING SIZE OF DOUBLE LUMEN BRONCHIAL TUBE

There is no absolutely accurate method for selecting the correct sized tube. The age, gender, height, or weight are relatively poor predictors of airway size. The selection of a DLT based on these criteria often results in a tube that is either too large or too small.

Following tips are suggested:

- *Based on sex and height of patients:* Size 35 Fr is recommended for females of height less than 160 cm, 37 Fr for females of height more than 160 cm, 37 Fr for males of height less than 170 cm, and 41 Fr for males of height more than 170 cm.[4]
  One can also use a formula based on height to decide optimal depth of insertion for left-sided DLTs.
  Depth of insertion in cm (at incisors) = 12 + patient height (cm)/10.
  Studies have shown that in small below average Asian population, DLT size cannot be predicted from the height[5] and hence alternative methods need to be used.
  Brodsky and Lemmens[6] based on their vast experience of 1170 left-sided DLT placements; found that the average depth of left DLT placement in a 170 cm, tall man or woman was 28–29 cm, with a change of approximately ± 1.0 cm for each 10 cm, change in height.
- *Based on radiological studies:* Regarding the selection of the proper size of DLT, all studies have focused on the left-sided DLT, in part due to the infrequent use of the right-sided DLT. Direct measurement of bronchial width by X-ray chest **(Fig. 2)**[7] or chest computed tomography (CT) scan **(Fig. 3)**[8] is a better way to select a DLT.

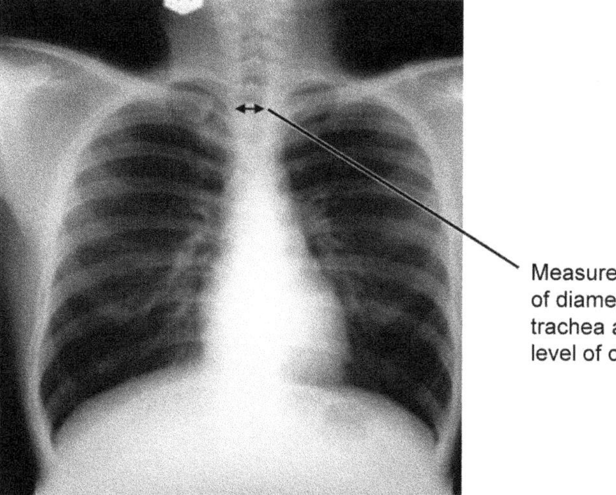

Fig. 2: X-ray-guided measurement of tracheal width.

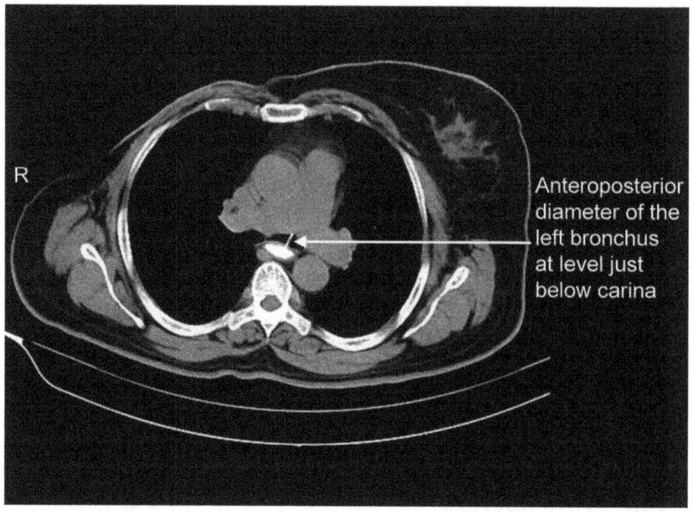

Fig. 3: Computed tomography-guided measurement of left bronchus.

Unfortunately, the left main bronchus is not visible on as many as 25–50% of chest radiographs. When the bronchus cannot be directly measured, tracheal width can be used to estimate left-bronchial width.[9] The diameter of the left bronchus is directly proportional to the diameter of the trachea. If tracheal width (WT) is known, left bronchial width (WLB) in millimeters can be calculated as:

$$WLB = (0.4 \times WT) + 3.3 \text{ or}$$

Predicted left bronchial width = WT (mm) × 0.68.[10]

INSERTION TECHNIQUE

There are two ways of placing the DLT:

1. *The "blind" technique:* Polyvinyl chloride DLTs are straight with curve only at bronchial tube level and have malleable stylet to retain memory of curve.
   - The DLT is inserted with concavity facing anteriorly (tip directed upwards) and rotated by 90° towards the bronchus to be intubated after bronchial cuff (distal cuff) passes through vocal cords
   - After the tube passes through glottis, remove the stylet to avoid trauma to airway. Advance the tube while keeping 90° rotation towards the side to be intubated until moderate resistance is felt; this depth is usually 28–30 cm in a normal adult. Avoid using excess force while inserting the tube to prevent airway damage
   - Connect the DLT to the anesthesia circuit, inflate the tracheal cuff and auscultate chest for breath sounds as well as confirm presence of end-tidal CO_2 on the capnogram
   - Take note of the peak airway pressures now
   - Clamp the fresh gases to tracheal lumen and open the port of tracheal lumen. Inflate the bronchial cuff gradually until no air entry is detected on the contralateral lung and no air leak is felt at the tracheal opening during ventilation
   - Auscultate the lung to ensure that there is good air entry at the apex and base of the lung unilateral, and there is no air entry in the contralateral lung
   - Note peak airway pressures. In an adult with normal lungs, rise in peak airway pressure for same tidal volume should not be more than 8–12 cmH_2O
   - Ventilate both lungs again
   - Clamp fresh gas flow inlet of bronchial lumen and start tracheal ventilation. Confirm unilateral air entry by auscultation and unilateral chest expansion
   - Note the peak airway pressures again. If there is larger airway pressure rise, or reduced air entry it suggests that either the bronchial cuff is causing obstruction by herniation across the carina or tube is far too in and tracheal lumen has entered the bronchus
   - Deflate the bronchial cuff and auscultate. If there is no difference in air entry or if there is no change in airway pressures on deflation of the cuff, it suggests that the tracheal portion of the tube is endobronchial, and the tube should be slightly withdrawn. However, if on deflation of bronchial cuff, air entry improves and airway pressure comes down, it suggests probable herniation of bronchial cuff and tube needs to be pushed further into the bronchus
   - After clinical confirmation of placement of tube, insert fiberoptic bronchoscope (FOB) down the tracheal lumen and visualize carina. At this point, one should be able to see the carina in front and the blue cuff of endobronchial tube in the main bronchus **(Fig. 4A)**. Refer to **Video 10** for bronchoscopic confirmation of DLT.
   - Next, insert FOB down the bronchial lumen and visualize secondary carina **(Fig. 4B)**. In addition, in right-sided tube, confirm opening of the right upper lobe bronchus against hole in the endobronchial portion of tube. Refer to **Video 10** on orientation of bronchoscopic view.
   - Any mal positioning of the tube can be visualized and corrected under FOB guidance. **Figure 4C** shows herniation of bronchial cuff in to the trachea. This DLT needs to be advanced into the left bronchus.

     "Head Turn" maneuver: Another major problem while inserting left DLT by blind method is entry of tube in right main bronchus. If left DLT enters right main stem bronchus repeatedly; deflate both cuffs, withdraw the tube into the trachea. Turn patient's jaw toward the left shoulder while bending the right ear to the right shoulder and then advance the tube. This maneuver was proposed by Brodsky and in his study, this "head turn" maneuver was successful in 208 of the 269 (77.4%) patients.[6]
2. *The "direct vision" technique:* Another reliable method of DLT placement is by using FOB.
   - Insert the DLT through the glottis with direct laryngoscopy, rotate it 90° to the side of endobronchial tube, and advance it till the proximal edge of the tracheal cuff is just beyond the vocal cords so that the tip of the bronchial lumen is supracarinal
   - With inflation of tracheal cuff, initiate ventilation of both lungs and confirm tube placement by auscultation and capnometry
   - Place FOB through the bronchial lumen and advance until the carina and main stem bronchi are clearly identified
   - Advance the FOB into the desired main stem bronchus and after deflation of the tracheal cuff, slide the DLT over FOB until its bronchial lumen comes into view beyond the tip of the FOB.

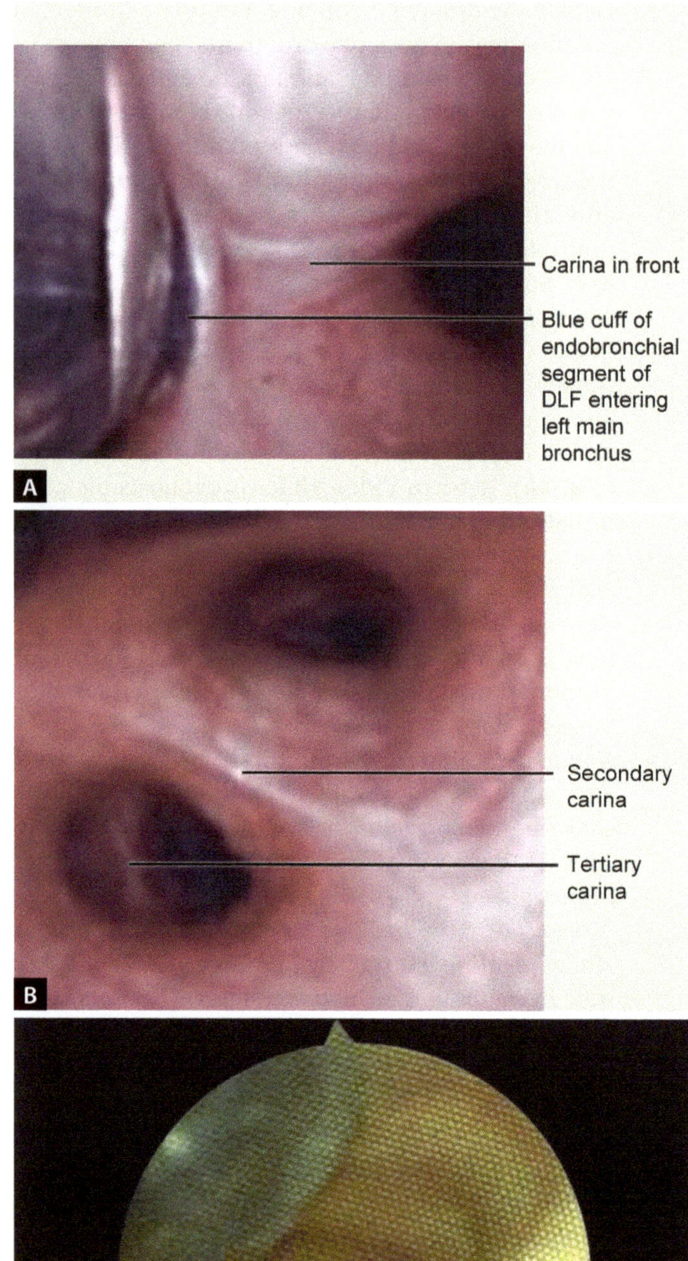

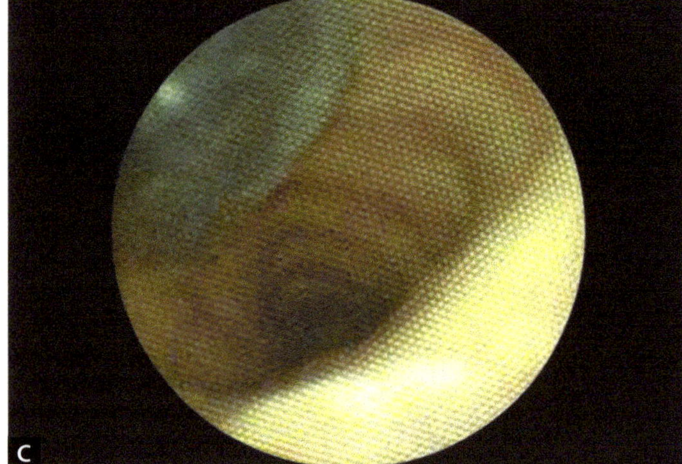

Figs. 4A to C: (A) Fiberoptic view through tracheal lumen; (B) Secondary carina; (C) Left double lumen endotracheal tube bronchial cuff herniation into trachea; needs to be advanced further to the bronchus.

Whether DLT is inserted blindly or under vision, monitoring of the position of tube is necessary when the patient's position is changed from supine to lateral decubitus because displacement can occur in up to 32% of cases.[11] The distal displacement is more common than proximal displacement. Movements of 16–19 mm of a left double lumen tube and 8 mm of a right double lumen tube can compromise functional lung separation in an adult.[12]

Advantages of Double Lumen Tubes

- Easier to position
- Can be positioned without bronchoscopy
- Less time is required to position as compared with EBB
- More rapid lung collapse, as compared with EBB
- Less likely to be displaced as compared with EBB
- Allows either lung to be ventilated, collapsed, and re-expanded
- Each lung can be suctioned adequately
- Each lung can be inspected with a bronchoscope
- Continuous positive airway pressure (CPAP) can be easily applied to operated lung
- Enables independent lung ventilation in ICU.

Disadvantages of Double Lumen Tubes

- It may be impossible to place a DLT in a patient with a difficult airway
- The large size and design of DLTs can cause airway damage during insertion, prolonged use, and removal
- There can be a problem in proper placement especially if the tracheal or bronchial anatomy is severely distorted
- Lesions within the trachea, like tumors, are relative contraindications to DLT placement
- If patient's condition necessitates mechanical ventilation postoperatively, changing a DLT to a single-lumen ETT at the end of surgery can be hazardous
- Intubated patient from ICU coming for a surgery requiring lung isolation would require change of single-lumen ETT to a DLT, which can be dangerous in patients who are fluid resuscitated and have airway edema, those with cervical spine injuries, difficult airways, and in those that cannot tolerate periods of apnea
- Double-lumen tubes are manufactured in limited sizes 28, 35, 37, 39, and 41 Fr and are often too big for most of pediatric patients
- Lumens of DLTs are narrow as compared to single lumen tube.

Method of Sterilization

All current double lumen tubes are disposable; recommended for single use.

BRONCHIAL BLOCKERS

In 1935, Archibald used a rubber bronchial blocker to facilitate lung surgeries first time in history.[1] Since then a variety of balloon tipped catheters have been used as bronchial blockers including Fogarty embolectomy catheter, Foley catheter and even Swan Ganz catheter. However, problem with these devices are many, and include difficult placement due to their lack of directing mechanism,

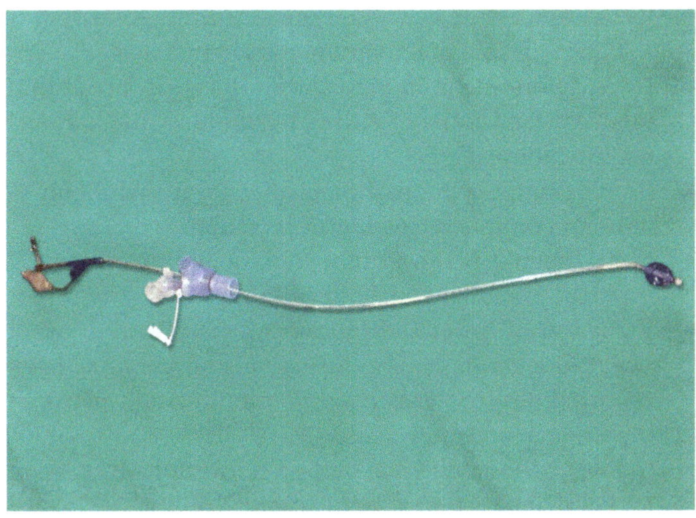

Fig. 5: Coopdech endobronchial blocker.

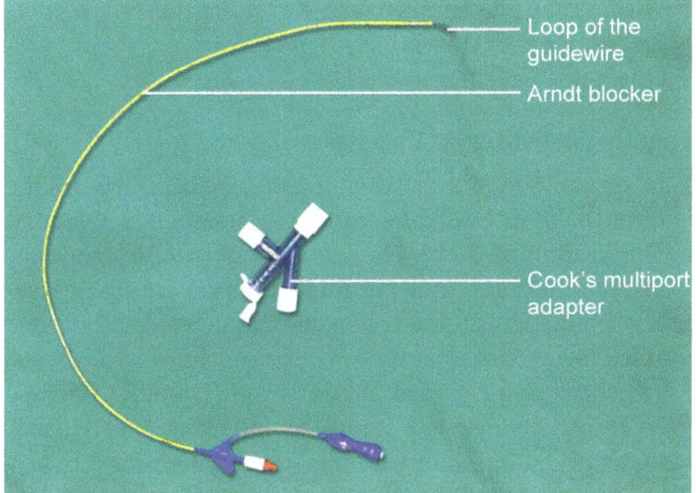

Fig. 6: Arndt endobronchial blocker.

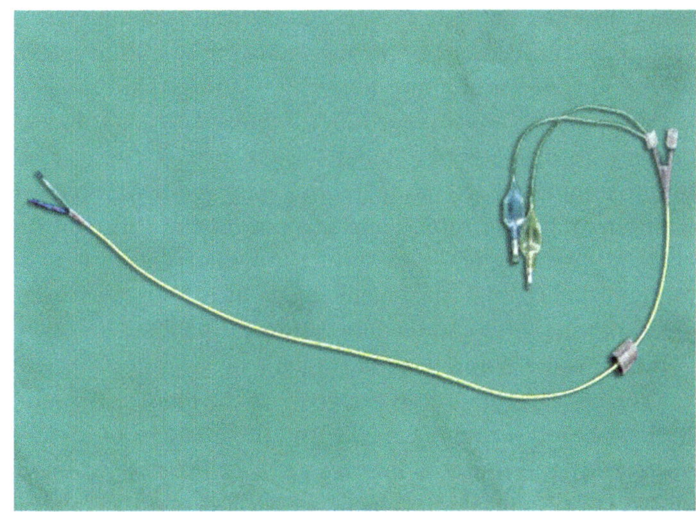

Fig. 7: EZ endobronchial blocker.

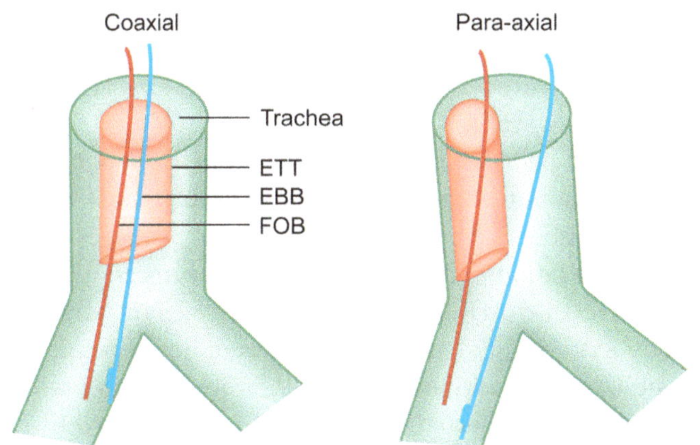

Fig. 8: Types of placement of endobronchial blockers. (ETT: endotracheal tube; EBB: endobronchial blocker; FOB: fiberoptic bronchoscope)

inability to perform suction or oxygen insufflation due to lack of lumen and poor occlusion of bronchus due to the high pressure-low volume spherical-shaped cuff. To overcome these problems, a combined endotracheal tube and bronchial blocker, the Univent tube, was introduced in the 1980s.[13] Recently, several blockers have become available like Coopdech **(Fig. 5)**, Cohen, Arndt **(Fig. 6)**, and EZ blocker **(Fig. 7)**. Bronchial blockers can overcome many of the previously discussed disadvantages and contraindications of DLT use.

Technique of Insertion

Coaxial Placement

In the classically described method, first intubate the trachea with a single lumen tube, and confirm the placement by auscultation and capnography. Introduce the EBB through the lumen of the ETT. Insert the FOB with external diameter of 4.00 mm or less (depending on size of ETT) along the EBB through the endotracheal tube and then place EBB under vision into the main stem bronchus of the lung to be collapsed. This is called coaxial placement **(Fig. 8)**. Inflate the balloon with 4–5 mL of air under direct vision. When EBB is correctly positioned, FOB examination will show that the proximal or outer surface of the inflated balloon is located just below the tracheal carina, usually around 5 mm inside the desired bronchus. Once adequate initial placement is achieved, the balloon of the EBB should be deflated before turning patient into lateral decubitus to prevent dislodgement (inflated EBB balloon can easily pop out of bronchus while changing position), except when indication for lung isolation is protecting normal lung from getting contaminated, in which case balloon should be kept inflated while giving position.

Paraxial Placement

Alternately, blockers can also be inserted along the side of single lumen tube (paraxial placement) which can be done with patient awake or under anesthesia. In awake technique,

EBB is inserted through the vocal cords under FOB guidance and placed in desired bronchus followed by either awake intubation or intubation under anesthesia. Alternately, patients can be anesthetized first, followed by insertion of blocker through cords under vision up to the carina (approximately 26–28 cm in adults), followed by intubation with single lumen tube. Final position of the EBB can be adjusted by using FOB through ETT. Pediatric sized FOB is required for coaxial placement needs of EBB; but paraxial positioning of EBB can be done using adult FOB with outer diameter of 6–6.5 mm in adult **(Fig. 8)**.

The coaxial insertion is preferred as the blocker remains well anchored through the ETT and the chances of its free movement and mucosal injuries are less. Because of small airway size, coaxial placement of a blocker may not be always possible in small children. Thus, paraxial placement of Arndt EBB or Fogarty is often practiced in children.[14]

Advantages of Blockers

- Unlike double lumen tubes, EBB adds no further complexity to intubation
- Offers a distinct advantage in the intubation of difficult upper airways
- Useful in pediatric patients in whom the tracheobronchial size may not accommodate even the smallest double lumen tube
- Lung isolation in distorted neck (e.g., burns contracture, postradiation) and tracheobronchial anatomy (by extraluminal tumors or thoracic aortic aneurysm etc.), where positioning of DLT is difficult or impossible
- EBB can be inserted through DLT intraoperatively as a rescue method in case of failed lung isolation using DLT
- Repositioning is possible in lateral decubitus, if the blocker is malpositioned after giving position for thoracotomy
- Rupture of the tracheal cuff during intubation is not an uncommon problem when using DLTs, which, on occasion, requires the use of multiple DLT tubes. This problem is not seen with the use of EBB
- EBB can be used when ETT is already in place (oral, nasal, tracheostomy)
- Not necessary to change ETT if postoperative ventilation required
- Allows selective lobar blockade
- Useful for patients requiring nasotracheal intubation.

Disadvantages of Blockers

- Tedious final placement after intubation
- Final placement to achieve adequate lung isolation takes little longer than DLT insertion and requires bronchoscopic guidance
- Difficult to place when bronchoscopic visualization is limited by massive hemoptysis
- EBBs cannot be used when the side of the bleeding is unknown in case of intrapulmonary hemorrhage
- Dislodgement is more common with bronchial blockers than in DLTs during positioning and surgical manipulation of lung
- By blocking up the pathological side, it is difficult to monitor continued bleeding or secretions
- Lung collapse is slower though final quality of surgical exposure is similar with both DLTs and EBBs
- Inclusion of bronchial blocker or distal wire loop of Arndt blocker in stapler during lung surgery has been reported and requires good communication between the surgeon and anesthetist
- Inflated balloon may slip in trachea causing blockade of ETT and obstruction to ventilation
- Due to very narrow suction channel suctioning of blood or thick secretions is difficult
- Bronchial blockers present the potential risk of perforating a bronchus or lung parenchyma
- Sizes not available for children less than 1 year.

Fogarty Endovascular Catheter

It is available in 2–9 Fr sizes. It has a high-pressure, low-volume balloon and does not have a lumen for suction or application of CPAP. Though they are not designed for bronchial blockade they are traditionally used. The placement is difficult as there is no guiding mechanism but only a stylet.

In children for coaxial placement; the smallest tracheal tube recommended is 4.5 mm ID for using 5 Fr Fogarty catheter and 4 mm internal diameter (ID) ETT for 2 Fr and 3 Fr Fogarty catheters with a fiberscope of less than 2 mm external diameter. Before the availability of Marraro DLT, this was the only possible method of lung isolation in infants. In adults, the 8 Fr catheter can be placed through 7 mm or 8 ID ETT using a fiberscope of 3.4/3.7 mm external diameter. For coaxial placement, Fogarty catheter needs to be inserted through the Cook's multiport adapter so that patient can be ventilated.

Arndt Wire-guided Endobronchial Blocker

This is the first independent bronchial blocker. It is available in 5 Fr and 7 Fr with high volume-low pressure spherical cuff and 9 Fr with spherical and elliptical cuffs **(Table 1)**. Spherical balloon is designed for right main stem bronchus to avoid the blockade of the opening of right upper lobe to ensure complete deflation of right bronchus. It is also used for selective lobar blockade. Elliptically-shaped cuff fits better into the left main-stem bronchus because of its elongated shape. The catheter has 1.4 mm central channel which contains a nylon guidewire with loop that projects out from the distal tip. The Arndt blocker with fully deflated cuff and the FOB are introduced through the multiport connector. The mechanical ventilation can be continued throughout

TABLE 1: Characteristics of commonly used endobronchial blockers.

	Arndt	*Coopdech*	*EZ*	*Fogarty*
Size (French)	5, 7, 9	9	7	2–9 Fr
Balloon shape and color	• 5, 7—spherical • 9—spherical and elliptical • All cuffs blue	• Small spindle-shaped, blue • Rectangular, blue	• Spherical • One cuff green and other blue	Spherical, transparent
Cuff characteristic	High volume-low pressure	High volume-low pressure	High volume-low pressure	Low volume-high pressure
Murphy eye	Present in 9 Fr	Absent	Absent	Absent
Center channel	Present	Present	Present	Present
Smallest ETT for coaxial use	• 4.5 (5 Fr) using FOB <2 mm • 7.0 (7 Fr) using FOB <3 mm • 8.0 (9 Fr) using FOB 3.4 mm	• 7.0 (9 Fr) using FOB <3 mm • 8.0 (9 Fr) using • FOB 3.4 mm/3.7 mm	7.0 (7 Fr) using FOB <3 mm	• 4 (2 and 3 Fr) and • 4.5 (5 Fr) using FOB <2 mm
Guidance mechanism	Nylon wire-loop coupled with FOB	Preformed bend at tip	Natural curve at bifurcation	Stylet

(ETT: endotracheal tube; FOB: fiberoptic bronchoscope; Fr: French)

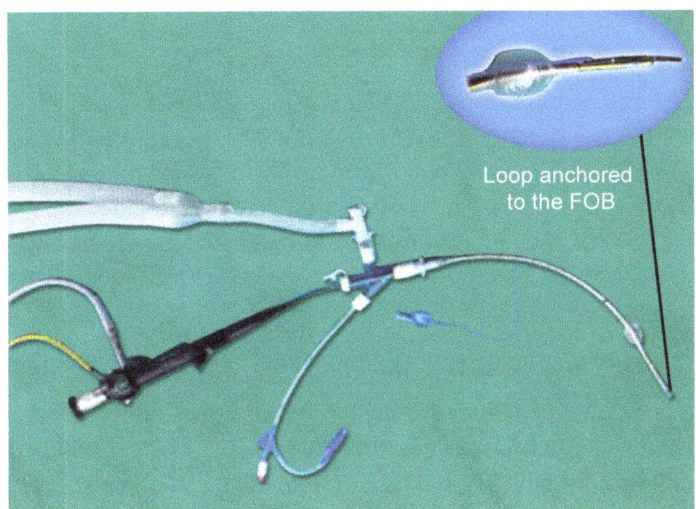

Fig. 9: Arndt blocker.

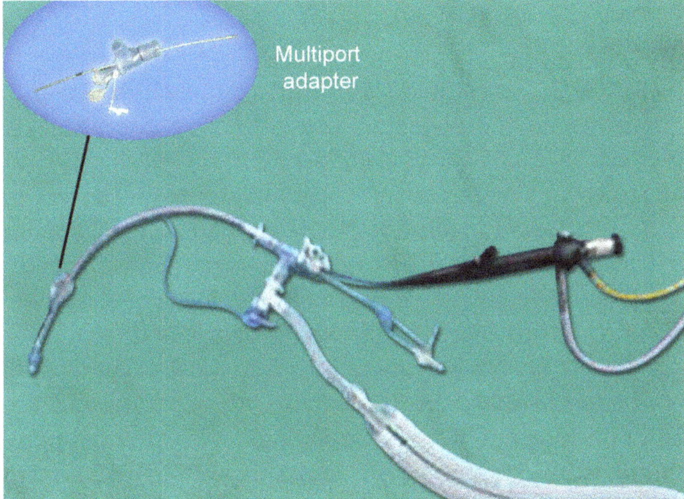

Fig. 10: Coopdech endobronchial blocker tube.

the placement, using a breathing circuit attached to the third (horizontal) port of the adapter. The wireloop of the Arndt blocker is coupled with the FOB and serves as a guide to introduce the blocker into desired bronchus **(Fig. 9)**. Once the deflated cuff is below the entrance of the bronchus, the FOB is withdrawn, and the cuff is fully inflated with 2–3 mL of air for selective lobar, or 5–8 mL of air for bronchial blockade. After the patient is turned to the lateral decubitus position, bronchoscopic confirmation of the position is mandatory. Refer to **Video 10** for Arndt blocker insertion.

In case after changing the patient position, one needs to reposition blocker, the guidewire loop cannot be reinserted in 5 Fr and 7 Fr. Hence, it is advisable not to withdraw the wireloop till the blocker position is reconfirmed after patient positioning.

Coopdech Blocker

The blocker kit contains blocker and the joint connector incorporated with blocker; which is functionally same to Cook's multiport connector **(Fig. 10)**. It is a 9 Fr, 60 cm blocker; available in two types: (i) type A (without autoinflator) and (ii) type B (with autoinflator device). Each type is available in rectangular and spindle-shaped cuffs. In type B Coopdech blocker; air is injected in the autoinflator balloon in advance before introducing the blocker through ETT. Once the blocker tip reaches the target place; the operator presses the autoinflator button which features a one touch structure. The valve opens by pressing the button and directs the accumulated air from the autoinflator to the pilot balloon.

Thus, operator can inflate the balloon by pressing the autoinflate button while still performing bronchoscopy. Refer to **Video 10** for insertion of Coopdech blocker. The FOB and the Coopdech blocker are inserted through multiport connecter till carina is seen. Then the blocker is advanced into the desired bronchus and the cuff is inflated **(Fig. 11)**.

After placement of any of the EBB, disconnect the ETT from the anesthesia circuit and apply continuous suction to the blocker channel to deflate the lungs. Then inflate cuff of the blocker and resume ventilation through the ETT. This ensures adequate deflation of the nonventilated lung.

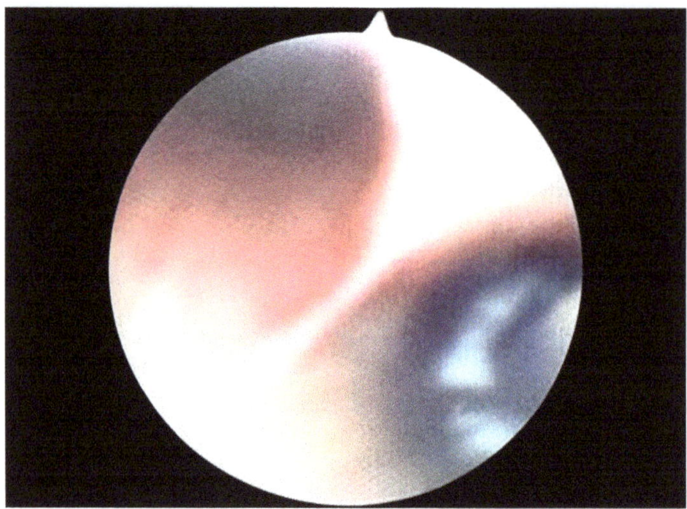

Fig. 11: Bronchial blocker in right main bronchus.

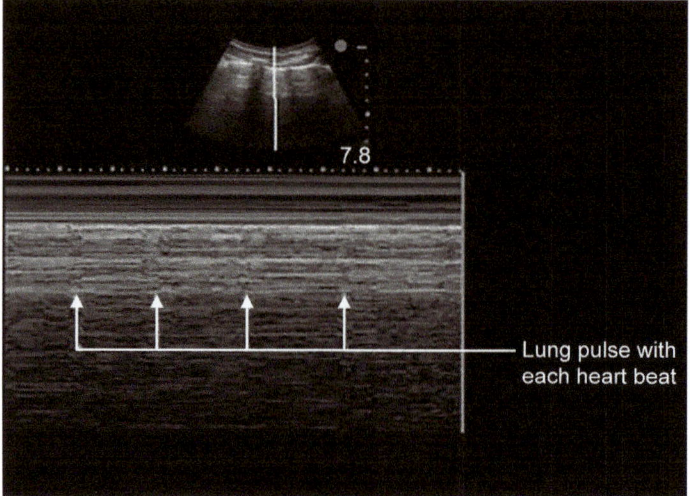

Fig. 12: Lung pulse.

EZ Blocker

It is a 7 Fr 75 cm catheter, has a bifurcation at its distal end. It has green cuff on one limb and blue on another **(Fig. 7)**. Intubate as usual with an endotracheal tube (ET) size 7.0 mm or larger attach the EZ-multiport adapter to the machine end of ETT. And confirm depth of intubation leaving 4 cm between distal tip of the ET tube and the carina using FOB, to allow sufficient space for the deployment of the bifurcated tips. Now insert EZ blocker through the adapter into the ETT. As the blocker emerges through the distal end of the endotracheal tube, the bifurcated cuffs separate and are naturally directed into the left and right main stem bronchi. Confirm blocker placement and orientation by inflating and deflating individual cuffs using FOB. The advantage is cuff inflation can be performed on the side desired to be collapsed, just before lung isolation, which minimizes the need to manipulate the catheter after placement and reduces the potential for the cuffs to become dislodged.

Method of Sterilization

All EBBs are disposable; recommended for single use.

ROLE OF ULTRASONOGRAPHY IN LUNG ISOLATION

After positioning of DLT or EBB, ultrasound of the chest can be done to assess collapse of the lung. In the absence of lung inflation there is no movement between parietal and visceral pleura (lung slide). Hence, absent lung slide confirms absent air entry on the nonventilated side and thus correct lung isolation. However, in presence of adhesions between parietal and visceral pleura, the nonventilated lung may not collapse despite achieving good isolation. Therefore, absence of lung slide confirms the isolation; but may not guarantee complete collapse of the nonventilated lung.

The "lung pulse" **(Fig. 12)** is a dynamic ultrasound sign described as the association of absent lung sliding along with heart rhythm perception at pleural line; it is used in early diagnosis of complete atelectasis.

LUNG ISOLATION IN PEDIATRIC PATIENTS

The lung isolation in children is challenging owing to their small airway size and unavailability of very small DLT, and therefore, endobronchial intubation with single lumen tube was the commonly practiced method in children. The Fogarty embolectomy catheter was often used in very small children for lung isolation in children until Arndt blocker was introduced.

Marraro Pediatric Bilumen Tube (Fig. 13)[15]

It is a DLT specially designed for infants and neonates. It is a single use PVC tube made of two separate uncuffed tubes of different lengths fused together. The tracheal tube is shorter and is attached to the longer bronchial tube along its whole length. It is a thin walled, kink resistant, light weight, thermosensitive tube, which confers to the child's trachea-bronchial anatomy. The bronchial tube has an oval opening "Murphy's eye" to prevent exclusion of the upper right lobar bronchus in case of selective right bronchial intubation. Both the lumens are circular in cross-section along the whole length to facilitate the introduction of a suctioning catheter and to perform bronchial aspiration. There is a radiopaque line running along the entire length of the tube. A disposable metal stylet (of the length of the longer tube) is used to intubate to maintain the shape of the bi-lumen tube. The tube has universal connectors so that it is easily linked to anesthesia machine or ventilators. Since the transverse diameter of the tube is larger than AP diameter, it is positioned perpendicular to the vocal cords.

The caliber suggested for Marraro Pediatric Bilumen tube are described in **Table 2**.

Disadvantages of Marraro Tube

- Tracheal, carinal and bronchial trauma can occur while introduction of the tube
- It can be easily obstructed due to secretions, due to its narrow caliber

- Dislocation of the tube is easy
- It offers more resistance to airflow due to its long and narrow lumen.

Other various possible options available in pediatric patients are described in **Table 3**.

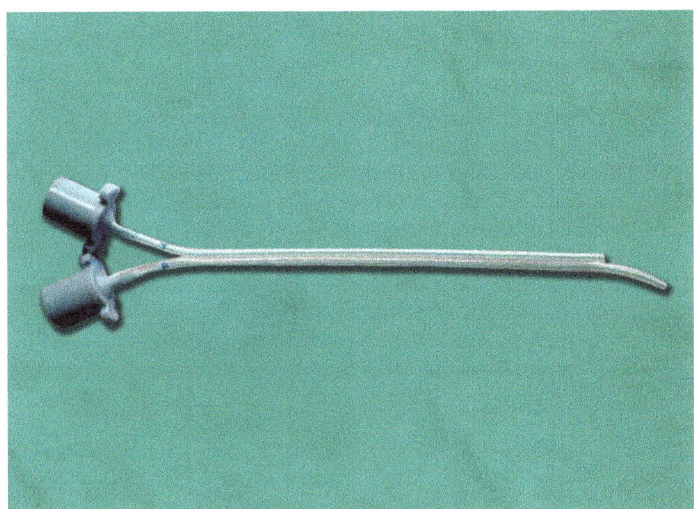

Fig. 13: Marraro Bilumen tube.

TABLE 2: Marraro Pediatric Bilumen tube.

Age	*Caliber suggested*
Premature baby (1400–2500 g)	2 + 2
Newborn (2500–4000 g)	2.5 + 2/2.5 + 2.5
1 month	2.5 + 2.5
6 months	3 + 2.5
12 months	3.5 + 3

TABLE 3: Other methods of pediatric lung isolation.

Method	*Remarks*
Arndt 5 Fr blocker	• Smallest tracheal tube recommended for use with this pediatric bronchial blocker is 4.5 mm ID, which requires a fiberoptic scope of less than 2.0 mm coaxial placement for limiting the use of this technique in infants[16] • 2.2 mm or 2.8 mm scope may be used with larger tracheal tubes
DLT	• Smallest size available 26 Fr. Corresponds to 8.7 mm outer diameter. Therefore, limits the use in children more than 8-year-old or more than 30 kg in weight
Univent blocker	• The smallest univent tube has a large outer diameter (8 mm OD) and narrow inner diameter (3.5 mm ID) limiting its use to an older age group
Fogarty endovascular catheter	• Size 2, 3, 5 Fr are used in children • Smallest tracheal tube possible is 4.5 mm ID for using 5 Fr Fogarty catheter and 4 mm ID ETT for 2 Fr and 3 Fr Fogarty catheters with a fiberscope of less than 2 mm external diameter
Endobronchial intubation with single lumen tube	• May provide partial lung isolation if uncuffed tube is advanced in the contralateral bronchus • Intraoperative suction of the surgical lung is not possible

(DLT: double lumen tube; OD: outer diameter; ETT: endotracheal tube; ID: internal diameter; Fr: French)

Airway Trauma during Use of Double Lumen Endotracheal Tube or Bronchial Blocker

The recent meta-analysis showed that the incidence of sore throat was significantly more with DLTs. The incidence and severity of airway injury was significantly less in EBB which included bronchial and vocal cord redness, edema, and hematoma, vocal cord thickening, erythema, and granuloma. The frequency of mal positioning was associated more with EBB. The quality of lung collapse and time taken for collapse were comparable with both DLT and EBB.[17]

The incidence of sore throat and vocal cord injuries were reduced by thermal softening of DLTs by dipping them in saline at 40°C for 10 minutes.[18]

WHAT TO USE WHEN

The decision to use which technique for lung isolation depends on clinical setting as no technique is perfect as we have seen above. Surgery on patients with massive intrapulmonary hemorrhage or drainage of copious secretions will be best managed with DLT; whereas lung isolation for patients with difficult airway, patients requiring nasotracheal intubation or for surgeries like esophagectomies where indication is just lung separation, as well as in small children, EBB would be a technique of choice.

CONCLUSION

Double lumen endotracheal tubes and bronchial blockers have been found to be clinically equivalent in terms of performance in providing lung collapse for patients with normal airways. Until recently, use of DLTs had been the method of choice for separating the lungs in most adult patients, however with familiarity of bronchial blockers use of blockers is increasing steadily. Each device provides advantages depending upon the case, such as absolute lung separation with a double-lumen endotracheal tube or the use of a bronchial blocker in a difficult airway for a patient requiring lung isolation. No matter what method of separating the lungs is chosen, there is a real need for the immediate availability of a small-diameter fiberoptic bronchoscope with a suction port to confirm correct position of device and rule out malposition which can occur anytime during surgical procedure.

REFERENCES

1. American Society of Anesthesiologists: Practice guidelines for management of the difficult airway: An updated report. Anesthesiology. 2003;98:1269-77.
2. Leiner G, Liebrel J. The technique of bronchospirometry. Dis Chest. 1950;17(5):578-83.
3. Saracoglu A, Saracoglu KT. VivaSight: a new era in the evolution of tracheal tubes. J Clin Anesth. 2016;33:442-9.
4. Slinger PD, Campos JH. Anesthesia for Thoracic Surgery. Miller's Anesthesia, 7th edition. Philadelphia: Churchill Livingstone; 2009.
5. Yasumoto M, Higa K, Nitahara K, et al. Optimal depth of insertion of left-sided double lumen endobronchial tubes

cannot be predicted from body height in below average-sized adult patients. Eur J Anaesthesiol. 2006;23:42-4.

6. Brodsky JB, Lemmens HJ. Left double lumen tubes: clinical experience with 1,170 patients. J Cardiothorac Vasc Anesth. 2003;17:289-98.
7. Brodsky JB, Mackey S, Cannon WB. Selecting the correct size left double lumen tube. J Cardiothorac Vasc Anesth. 1997;11: 924-35.
8. Eberle B, Weiler N, Vogel N, et al. Computed tomography-based tracheobronchial image reconstruction allows selection of the individually appropriate double lumen tube size. J Cardiothorac Vasc Anesth. 1999;13:532-7.
9. Brodsky JB, Macario A, Mark JB. Tracheal diameter predicts double-lumen tube size: a method for selecting left double lumen tubes. Anesth Analg. 1996;82:861-4.
10. Brodsky JB, Lemmens HJ. Tracheal width and left double lumen tube size: a formula to estimate left-bronchial width. J Clin Anesth. 2005;17:267-70.
11. Inoue S, Nishimine N, Kitaguchi K, et al. Double lumen tube location predicts tube malposition and hypoxemia during one lung ventilation. Br J Anaesth. 2004;92:195-201.
12. Benumof JL, Partridge BL, Salvatierra C, et al. Margin for safety in positioning modern double-lumen endotracheal tubes. Anesthesiology. 1987;67:729.
13. Campos JH. An update on bronchial blockers during lung separation techniques in adults. Anesth Analg. 2003;97:1266-74.
14. Watson CB. Lung isolation for surgery: state of the art. Anesthesiology News Guide to Airway Management. www.anesthesilogynews.com; 2009. pp. 75-89.
15. Pediatric Intensive Care Unit. [online] Available from www.picu.it. [Last accessed February, 2014].
16. Wald SH, Mahajan A, Kaplan MB, et al. Experience with the Arndt paediatric bronchial blocker. Br J Anaesth. 2005;94:92-4.
17. Ana CS Bennett K, Alston RP, Adams G, et al. A Comparison of the Efficacy and Adverse Effects of Double-Lumen Endobronchial Tubes and Bronchial Blockers in Thoracic Surgery: A Systematic Review and Meta-analysis of Randomized Controlled Trials. J Cardiothorac Vasc Anesth. 2015;129:955-66.
18. Seo JH, Cho CW, Hong DM, et al. The effects of thermal softening of double-lumen endobronchial tubes on postoperative sore throat, hoarseness and vocal cord injuries: a prospective double-blind randomized trial. Br J Anaesthesia. 2016;116(2):282-8.

15

CHAPTER

Cricothyrotomy: Emergency Surgical Airway of Choice

Vijaya P Patil

ABSTRACT

In all difficult airway algorithms, cricothyrotomy is the lifesaving procedure and is the final "cannot intubate, cannot oxygenate, previously known as cannot ventilate cannot intubate (CVCI)" option, whether in prehospital, emergency department, intensive care unit, or operating room patients. It is a safe, quick, and temporary way to provide oxygenation and ventilation when conventional methods are unsuccessful. A correctly performed cricothyrotomy may be lifesaving in a CVCI situation and every practicing anesthesiologist should have experience with cricothyrotomy. The purpose of this chapter is to highlight the various ways of performing cricothyrotomy and options of ventilation through cricothyrotomy.

INTRODUCTION

Surgical airway is defined as creation of an airway by opening of trachea by surgical means so that patient can be ventilated and oxygenated. This approach is used in life-threatening difficult airway scenarios.

The American Society of Anesthesiologists[1] task force on management of the difficult airway defined a difficult airway as the clinical situation in which a conventionally trained anesthesiologist experiences difficulty with face mask ventilation, difficulty with tracheal intubation, or both. Many difficult airway societies across the world have their own guidelines about how to manage difficult airway situations. In all of these algorithms, cricothyrotomy is the lifesaving procedure, and is the final CICO (cannot intubate, cannot oxygenate) option in hypoxic patient, whether in prehospital retrieval situation, emergency department, intensive care unit (ICU), or operating room patients. The increased use of rescue ventilation devices, particularly the laryngeal mask airway (LMA), and combitude has dramatically reduced use of cricothyrotomy in the emergency setting making it infrequently done procedure. In record of National Emergency Airway Registry project of 6,000 intubations in emergency department, incidence of cricothyrotomy was 0.9%.[2]

Emergency surgical airway approach mainly consists of two techniques—needle cricothyrotomy and surgical cricothyrotomy; both of which use cricothyroid membrane to access airway.

Why Use Cricothyroid Membrane?

Cricothyroid space is readily felt between the thyroid above and the cricoid below with the membrane between them. It is much easier to make a quick opening at this point than it is in the trachea below, as it is most superficial structures (overlying the cricothyroid membrane include only skin, subcutaneous tissue, and thin fascial layers) and is held steady in place by the cartilage above and below it. This space is relatively avascular as it is crossed by only a small branch of the superior thyroid artery, the cricothyroid branch which is quite small and easily controllable.

ANATOMY OF CRICOTHYROID MEMBRANE (FIG. 1)

The cricothyroid membrane can usually be found approximately 1–1.5 fingerbreadths (2–3 cm) below the thyroid cartilage prominence in the midline of the neck in adults. In infants and young children, where thyroid prominence is not well-developed, following the tracheal rings superiorly to locate prominence of cricoid cartilage is better option.

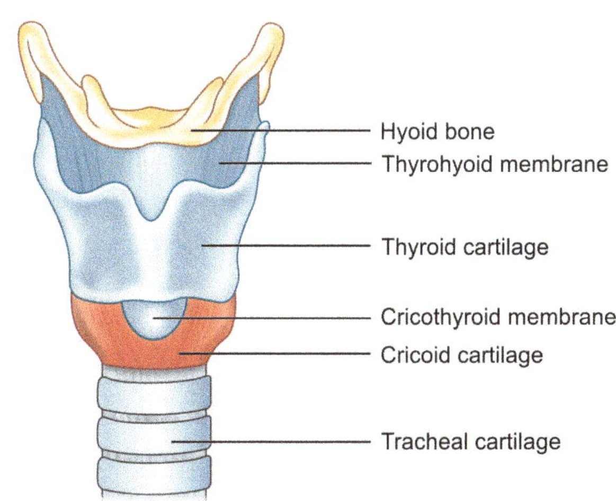

Fig. 1: Anatomy of anterior neck.

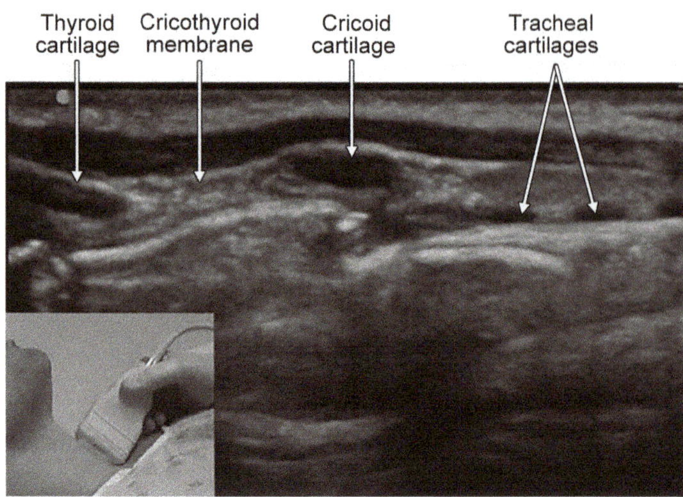

Fig. 2: Ultrasound of anterior neck.

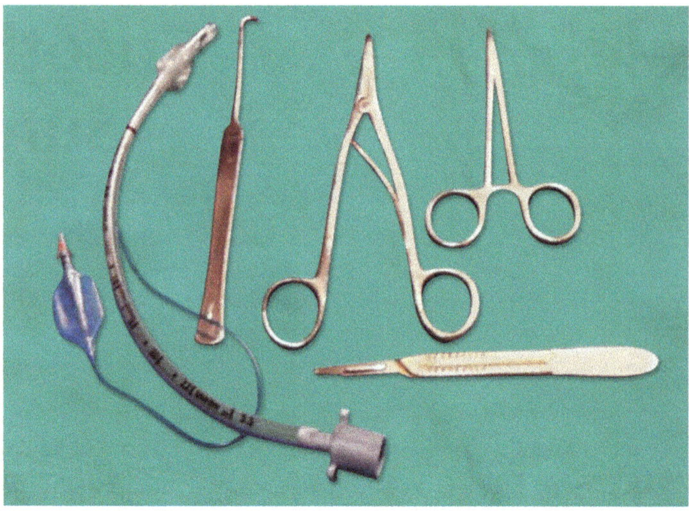

Fig. 3: Equipment for surgical cricothyrotomy.

The cricothyroid arteries and veins usually cross the membrane in upper third portion and come from the sides, hence, cricothyrotomy should be attempted in the central, lower portion of the membrane to avoid bleeding. In adult cadaveric study by Bennett and colleagues the size of the cricothyroid membrane was found to be around 13 mm (8–19 mm) superoinferiorly, and 12 mm (9–19 mm) side to side.[3] Important anatomical structures, which are very close to cricothyrotomy site are the thyroid gland with its vessels, large vessels of the neck and vocal cords which are located around a centimeter away from membrane superiorly.

ROLE OF ULTRASOUND

In the current era of point of care management, ultrasound has gained significant importance. It can be used successfully for identification of cricothyroid membrane, especially in patients with difficult anatomy. On ultrasound of anterior neck in sagittal section, thyroid, cricoid, and tracheal cartilages are seen as homogenous hypoechoic structures. Cricothyroid membrane appears as hyperechoic band linking the larger oblong hypoechoic thyroid and more round cricoid cartilages as seen in **Figure 2**. Ultrasound has shown to help identify cricothyroid membrane accurately and quickly even in emergency situation[4] and thus aid in front of neck access.

TECHNIQUES

Surgical Cricothyrotomy

It can be performed using two basic approaches, one approach uses Seldinger technique, i.e., dilator over guidewire. The other approach uses direct percutaneous placement of small sized endotracheal tube (ETT) without guidewire (surgical cricothyrotomy).

Standard Surgical Cricothyrotomy

Generally this procedure is done in semi-urgent scenario.

Equipment ***(Fig. 3)***

- Skin disinfectant
- Scalpel with number 11 stab blade
- 5.0/6.0 no. cuffed ETT
- Tracheal hook
- Tracheal dilator
- Artery forceps, 1% lignocaine with adrenaline and surgical drapes.

Procedure

1. Hyperextend the neck if no contraindications. This will make larynx and cricothyroid membrane prominent. Quickly clean the site with disinfectant, and if time permits, drape and infiltrate skin, and subcutaneous tissue with 1% lignocaine with adrenaline
2. Perform laryngeal handshake **(Figs. 4A to C)**. Laryngeal handshake is a term coined by Dr. Richard Levitan. This involves grasping the larynx with the index finger and thumb of nondominant hand at level of hyoid bone, sliding down over thyroid laminae and further down over cricoid cartilage. This helps one to identify the three dimensional structure of larynx. On identification of cricoid cartilage, larynx is stabilized by the thumb and middle finger, and the index finger is used to palpate the cricothyroid membrane
3. Incise the skin vertically in midline around 2 cm
4. Identify the membrane
5. Incise cricothyroid membrane in horizontal direction around 1 cm in lower half portion to avoid bleeding
6. Insert the tracheal hook and apply gentle upward and cephalad traction on inferior aspect of thyroid cartilage
7. Insert the dilator or artery forceps to dilate the space and insert 6.0 no. cuffed ETT. Inflate the cuff, cut tube to appropriate length and secure with tape after confirming proper endotracheal placement.

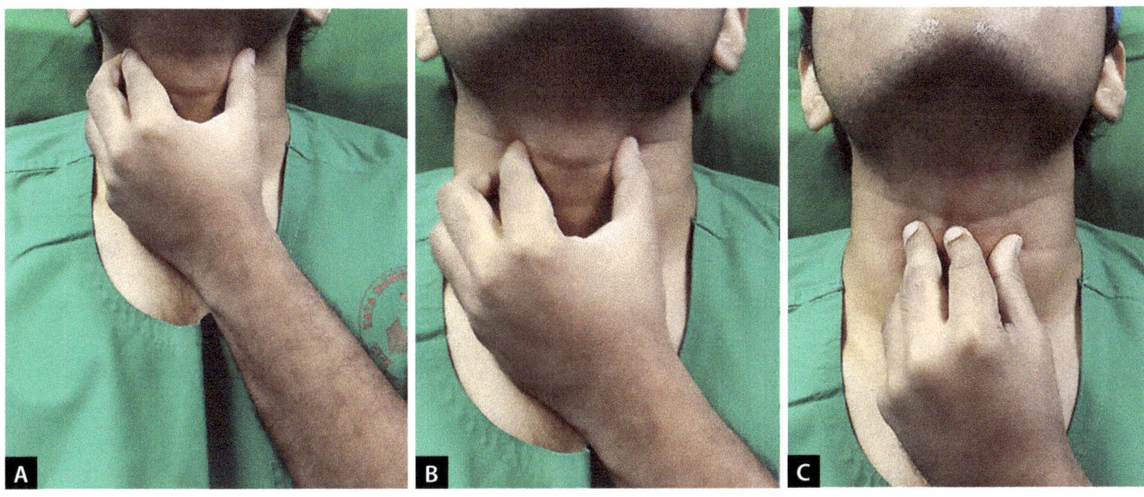

Figs. 4A to C: Laryngeal handshake.

Modifications of Surgical Technique

To cut short the time of procedure in emergency, standard surgical technique has been modified.

Rapid four-step technique

1. Initial steps of positioning and stabilization are same as described previously
2. Make a horizontal stab incision using 11 number blade through the skin and cricothyroid membrane. Take care so that only tip of the blade enters the trachea to avoid damaging posterior wall
3. Keep the blade in place and insert tracheal hook or artery forceps in the hole created so as not to loose the tract from skin to trachea. Place an artery forceps or dilator if present through the incision and open the membrane perpendicular to direction of incision. Alternatingly, one can also reverse scalpel, place handle into incision and rotate 90° to hold lumen open
4. Pass a small ETT number 5.0/6.0 through the opening, inflate the cuff, and cut to an appropriate length.

Quick three-step emergency cricothyrotomy

This modification has been described by Allan Macintyre in Military Medicine[5]

1. First step of positioning and stabilization are same as described previously
2. In the second step, after taking stab incision through skin and cricothyroid membrane, rotate the scalpel through 90° angle with sharp edge pointing caudally, the elastic bougie is placed into the defect, and advanced it until resistance is appreciated indicating entry into the right main stem bronchus
3. In third step, cuffed ETT is passed over the elastic bougie ensuring that bevel of ETT tube is horizontally lined up with cricothyroid incision. Apply gentle pressure while advancing the ETT through the cricothyroid membrane. As the bevel of the ETT is passing through the membrane, it opens the defect, allowing placement of the larger ETT. Once the ETT cuff has entered the trachea, remove the elastic bougie, and inflate the ETT cuff.

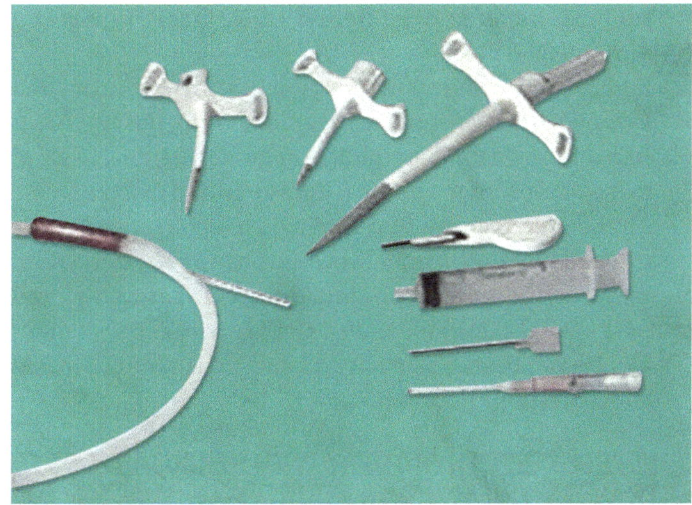

Fig. 5: Melker emergency cricothyrotomy set (Seldinger technique).

This three-step airway procedure requires only three items, namely, a scalpel, an ETT, and an elastic bougie.

Seldinger Technique

This technique is used with commercial cricothyrotomy sets **(Figs. 5 and 6)**.

Many commercial cricothyrotomy sets are available in market and their contents are almost same which comprise of locator needle, guidewire, scalpel, and small cuffed or uncuffed tracheostomy tube with dilator [3–6 mm inner diameter (ID)]. The procedure is similar to central venous cannulation.

Procedure

1. Initial steps are same as for surgical techniques
2. After locating cricothyroid membrane, take a small horizontal incision in skin and subcutaneous tissue
3. Insert locator needle attached to saline filled syringe at 45° directed caudally. After loss of resistance, apply gentle

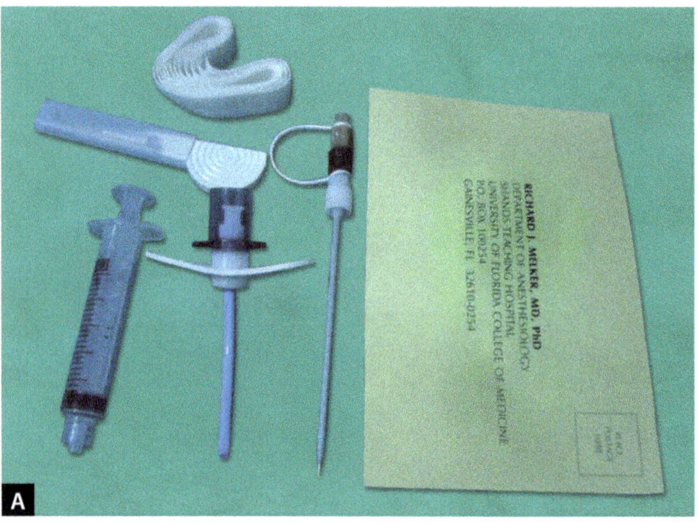

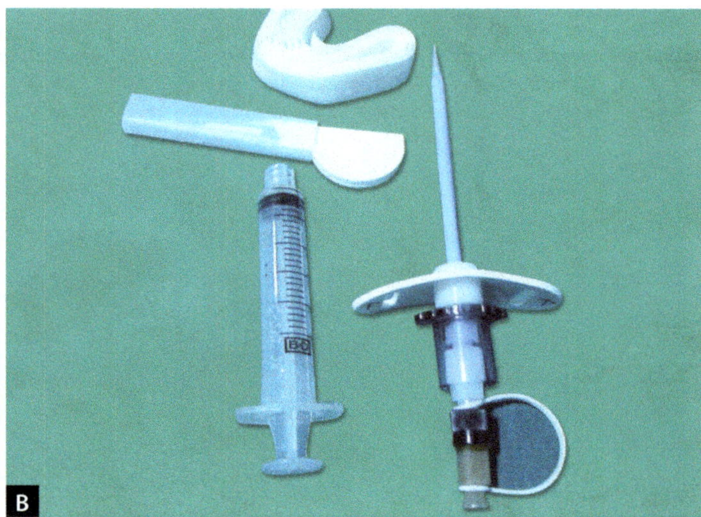

Figs. 6A and B: Melkar's cannula over needle set.

suction to confirm aspiration of air freely indicating intratracheal placement of tip

4. Remove the syringe and insert guidewire into the trachea
5. Remove the needle and leave guidewire in place
6. Insert tube dilator assembly over guidewire. Insertion of this assembly may require a little force and twisting
7. All the time confirm that guidewire can be moved freely to avoid bending of guidewire and false passage creation.
8. Remove the guidewire and dilator, inflate cuff, and perform bag mask ventilation. Confirm correct placement of tube by chest expansion and end-tidal carbon dioxide concentration ($EtCO_2$) trace.

NEEDLE CRICOTHYROTOMY WITH PERCUTANEOUS TRANSTRACHEAL VENTILATION

Needle cricothyrotomy involves passing a large bore intravenous cannula through the cricothyroid membrane. This technique was originally used for passive transtracheal oxygenation in the 1950s. It provides a temporary secure airway to oxygenate and ventilate a patient in severe respiratory distress in CVCI (cannot ventilate cannot intubate) situations. The delivery of oxygen to the lungs through a catheter inserted through cricothyroid membrane into the trachea using a high pressure gas source is called percutaneous transtracheal ventilation (PTV) and it can sustain life for a longer period of time than passive transtracheal oxygenation alone. This procedure can be done in any primitive setup very rapidly without any sophisticated equipment and one can achieve adequate oxygenation within seconds. Also, this is the procedure of choice in pediatric age group (<12 years) where cricothyrotomy is not possible due to anatomical limitations.

But, the disadvantages of this procedure are—there is risk of aspiration, there is no complete control of airway, and one cannot perform suction. Also there is high risk of failure because of kinking, malposition, or displacement of these narrow bore cannulae.

Equipment

- Oxygen flowmeter
- Oxygen source at 50 psi (wall/oxygen cylinder with pressure reducing assembly)
- Standard oxygen tubing with side hole cut near the end
- Intravenous cannula: 16- to 18-gauge for infants and young children and 12- to 16-gauge for adults and adolescents
- Three-way stopcock
- 3 mL syringe with plunger removed with 7.5 mm ET connector (bag-valve-mask connector) or 3.0 mm ID ETT connector attached directly to the cannula (bag-valve-mask connector)
- Sanders jet injector when planning transtracheal jet injection.

Technique

1. Initial steps are same as for surgical technique
2. Attach saline filled syringe to cannula. Insert through skin and cricothyroid membrane into trachea at a 45° angle, caudally. A "pop" would be felt as the cannula enters the trachea
3. Confirm intratracheal placement by free aspiration of air. If in doubt, remove and reinsert the cannula
4. Once you are sure of catheter placement, withdraw the needle and advance catheter in trachea full length so that hub rests on skin
5. Attach any assembly of choice (mentioned in equipment) and ventilate with bag-valve-mask assembly or attach modified oxygen tubing and begin ventilation using at least 50 psi oxygen supply at a ratio of 1:4.

Ventilating with Cricothyroid Cannula

There are three techniques of ventilation—either using bag-valve assembly, ventilating with modified oxygen tubing, or jet ventilation.

1. *Using bag-valve assembly* **(Fig. 7)**:
   - Take a 2 mL syringe and remove its plunger. Attach syringe to the cannula hub. Attach 7.5 mm universal ETT connector to the barrel of syringe. Attach bag-valve assembly with oxygen and start ventilating
   - Alternatively, one can use 3.5 mm ID ETT connector for same purpose. Here there is no need to attach syringe to cannula but directly attach tube connector to cannula and use bag-valve assembly to ventilate
   - Ventilate at ratio of 1:4. Guide your ventilation with chest rise
   - One can deliver a tidal volume (TV) of 500 mL in 5 seconds using this technique as shown by Marr,[6] however, one has to take into account compliance of lung parenchyma and degree of upper airway obstruction. Ventilation with this assembly is quite inadequate especially with patent upper airway.
2. *Using modified oxygen tubing:* Cut a side hole near the end of standard oxygen tubing. Attach this tubing to 50 psi oxygen source and begin ventilation by intermittently opening and closing the side hole. Alternatingly, one can use stopcock interposed between cannula and oxygen tubing for the same purpose. Do not use common gas outlet of anesthesia machine as the pressure reducing valve at back bar will open at 40–60 kPa (5.8–8.7 psi).
3. *Performing jet ventilation* **(Fig. 8)**: This should be avoided in children for the risk of barotrauma. Attach jet ventilation assembly to 50 psi oxygen source (wall/ machine) with adjustable regulator so that pressure can be titrated to the lowest effective pressure required to deliver desired TV. Since the gas flow through 14 G catheter at 50 psi is 1,600 mL/s, adequate TV is delivered in less than 1 second for normally compliant lung. Keep a longer time for expiration. Since expiration will occur through upper airway, it is important to ensure that upper airway is patent before doing jet ventilation to avoid barotrauma. Avoid jet ventilation where upper airway patency is in doubt and in children below 5 years. In these cases prefer bag connector assembly for ventilation.

High pressure oxygen delivery systems are optimal to provide effective ventilation through the relatively narrow catheters used for PTV to overcome the resistance of narrow cannula compared to low pressure systems like bag-valve assembly. When ventilating through needle cricothyrotomy one has to ensure proper exhalation especially when patency of upper away is in doubt. In these situations, the critical aspect is not lung inflation but lung deflation. Exhalation of 500 mL via a 14 G cannula would take at least 30 seconds.[7] Delivering further breaths without allowing full expiration will inevitably lead to barotraumas. However, in cases of incomplete obstruction the amount of exhalation through the upper airway may be greater than expected and inflation via a cannula might be safe if administered with care. Safety of jet ventilation can be further improved by using an automated jet ventilator with end expiratory pressure monitoring linked to a pause function.[8] One has to keep in mind that the application of PTV should be considered as a rescue and temporary maneuver while a more secure permanent airway is being established at the earliest opportunity.

Needle cricothyrotomy is contraindicated in:
- Laryngeal injury with known damage to cricoid cartilage (laryngeal fracture)
- Tracheal rupture
- Tracheal transection with distal tracheal retraction into the mediastinum.

COMPARISON OF DIFFERENT TECHNIQUES

Time Taken for Procedure and Complications

There is a learning curve for performing this procedure and in the study by Eisenburger,[9] both techniques of surgical versus Seldinger cricothyrotomy showed poor performance (success rate of 70% with surgical as against 60% with

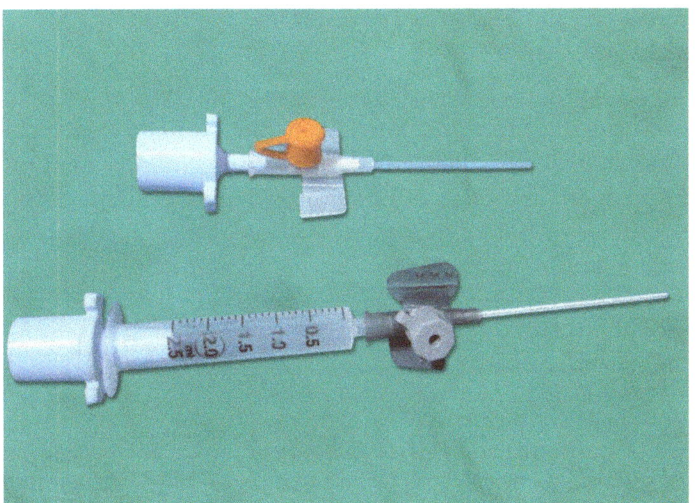

Fig. 7: Cannula cricothyrotomy assembly for bag-valve ventilation.

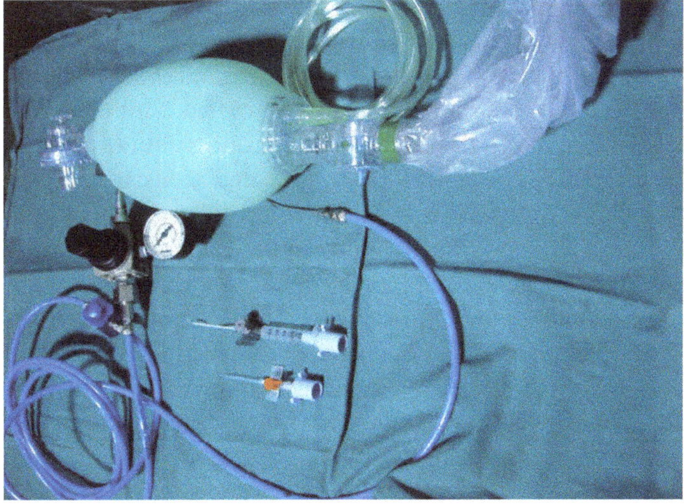
Fig. 8: Equipment for percutaneous transtracheal ventilation.

Seldinger technique) in the hands of inexperienced ICU physicians. Study performed in mannequins by Wong and coworkers showed that minimum five cricothyrotomies should be performed to do successful cricothyrotomy in 40 seconds.[10]

Cadaveric study by Mutzbauer et al. showed a longer time for procedure and higher incidence of bleeding and cartilage damage in surgical cricothyrotomy as against needle cricothyrotomy.[11] Fikkers and colleagues documented almost similar findings where they found catheter-over-needle technique quick, safe and reliable over guidewire technique using mini-tracheostomy set.[12] However, study by Schober and colleagues recorded exactly opposite findings in their study in inexperienced healthcare personnel, where anatomical-surgical techniques showed a higher success rate, a faster tracheal tube insertion time and a lower complication rate compared with puncture techniques, suggesting that they may be the techniques of choice in emergencies.[13] Toye and Weinstein[14] suggested that cricothyrotomy via the Seldinger technique damaged the tissues less than a surgical technique.

Study by Mariappa showed 100% success rate with Seldinger technique using Melker set as against surgical technique which showed 55% success with median time for procedure less than 60 seconds in both groups.[15] It also showed tendency toward more damage to posterior tracheal wall with surgical technique as against Seldinger technique. Vadodaria and coworkers have recorded 100% success rate with Seldinger study using Melker kit in plastic model.[16] In the study by Schaumann et al. comparing Seldinger technique versus surgical technique there was no difference in two techniques regarding time taken to location of membrane, however, surgical technique took significantly longer time for puncture as well as establishment of ventilation (98.7 ± 58.3 versus 119.2 ± 61.2 and 108.6 ± 59.5 versus 136.6 ± 66.3, respectively).[17]

Quality of Ventilation

Craven, et al. looked at quality of ventilation using various cricothyrotomy devices which compared a 13G Ravussin cannula (needle cricothyrotomy cannula), a 4 mm QuickTrach®, a 6 mm Melker, and a cuffed 6 mm tracheal tube to ventilate the model lung. Authors found that the 6 mm cuffed tracheal tube provided consistent good ventilation independent of upper airway resistance followed by the Ravussin with jet ventilation and the Melker with a standard anesthetic circuit. The cannula with jet ventilation provided excellent ventilation with a patent upper airway, but with complete upper airway obstruction, ventilation was impossible. The Melker device which had uncuffed tube provided good ventilation with moderate to complete airway obstruction, but with open upper airway minute volume delivery was suboptimal. The 4 mm QuickTrach® provided poor ventilation unless the airway was occluded.[18] This study very clearly shows importance of lung compliance, type of cricothyrotomy device and state of upper airway while considering adequacy of ventilation.

ROLE OF TRACHEOSTOMY IN EMERGENCY

In all "difficult airway algorithms" cricothyrotomy is the life-saving procedure and is the final CVCO option. From literature, emergency cricothyrotomy seems to be an infrequent and uncommon procedure and becoming rarer still with LMA and combitude use. Success of any procedure depends on experience of operator. Obviously the rule is "do what you can do best". Surgeons experienced in performing surgical tracheostomies might opt out for tracheostomy in desperate situations and might be more successful. There have been case reports suggesting even percutaneous tracheostomies might be the technique of choice in experienced hands, but that cannot be generalized.[19-21] It should be kept in mind that an emergency tracheostomy is a far more complex operation than cricothyrotomy.

Advantages of Cricothyrotomy over Tracheostomy that makes it the Procedure of Choice in Emergency Situations

Cricothyrotomy is technically simple, has low complication rates, can be performed at bedside, does not need neck hyperextension, there are less chances of esophageal injury, and virtually no chance of pneumothorax or major arterial damage.

COMPLICATIONS OF CRICOTHYROTOMY

- Potentially life-threatening failure to establish an airway
- Subcutaneous emphysema
- Bleeding
- Risk of aspiration in needle cricothyrotomy and use of uncuffed tube
- Inadequate ventilation mainly with the use of needle cricothyrotomy.

CONCLUSION

Cricothyrotomy is technique of choice in CVCI situations; however, this procedure is relatively rare. Nonetheless, every physician dealing with airway should be trained for this. From literature there is enough evidence to suggest that Seldinger technique is better in terms of high success rate with fewer complications.

REFERENCES

1. American Society of Anesthesiologists: Practice guidelines for management of the difficult airway: An updated report. Anesthesiology. 2003;98:1269-77.
2. Sagarin MJ, Barton ED, Chng YM, et al. Airway management by US and Canadian emergency medicine residents: a multicenter analysis of more than 6,000 endotracheal intubation attempts. Ann Emerg Med. 2005;46(4):328-36.

3. Bennett JD, Guha SC, Sankar AB. Cricothyrotomy: the anatomical basis. J R Coll Surg Edinb. 1996;41(1):57-60.
4. Mallin M, Curtis K, Dawson M, Ockerse P, Ahern M. Accuracy of ultrasound-guided marking of the cricothyroid membrane before simulated failed intubation. Am J Emerg Med. 2014;32: 61-3.
5. MacIntyre A, Markarian MK, Carrison D, et al. Three-step emergency cricothyroidotomy. Mil Med. 2007;172(12): 1228-30.
6. Marr JK, Yamamoto LG. Gas flow rates through transtracheal ventilation catheters. Am J Emerg Med. 2004;22(4):264-6.
7. Ryder IG, Paoloni CC, Harle CC. Emergency transtracheal ventilation: assessment of breathing systems chosen by anaesthetists. Anaesthesia. 1996;51(8):764-8.
8. McLeod AD, Turner MW, Torlot KJ, et al. Safety of transtracheal jet ventilation in upper airway obstruction. Br J Anaesth. 2005; 95(4):560-1.
9. Eisenburger P, Laczika K, List M, et al. Comparison of conventional surgical versus Seldinger technique emergency cricothyrotomy performed by inexperienced clinicians. Anesthesiology. 2000;92(3):687-90.
10. Wong DT, Prabhu AJ, Coloma M, et al. What is the minimum training required for successful cricothyroidotomy? A study in mannequins. Anaesthesiology. 2003;98(2):349-53.
11. Mutzbauer TS, Munz R, Helm M, et al. Emergency cricothyrotomy—puncture or anatomical preparation? Peculiarities of two methods for emergency airway access demonstrated in a cadaver model. Anaesthesist. 2003;52(4):304-10.
12. Fikkers BG, van Vugt S, van der Hoeven JG, et al. Emergency cricothyrotomy: A randomised crossover trial comparing the wire-guided and catheter-over-needle techniques. Anesthesia. 2004;59(10):1008-11.
13. Schobera P, Hegemannb MC, Schwartea LA, et al. Emergency cricothyrotomy-a comparative study of different techniques in human cadavers. Resuscitation. 2009;80(2):204-9.
14. Toye FJ, Weinstein JD. Clinical experience with percutaneous tracheostomy and cricothyroidotomy in 100 patients. J Trauma. 1986;26(11):1034-40.
15. Mariappa V, Stachowski E, Balik M, et al. Cricothyroidotomy: comparison of three different techniques on a porcine airway. Anaesth Intensive Care. 2009;37(6):961-7.
16. Vadodaria BS, Gandhi SD, McIndoe AK. Comparison of four different emergency airway access equipment sets on a human patient simulator. Anaesthesia. 2004;59(1):73-9.
17. Schaumann N, Lorenz V, Schellongowski P, et al. Evaluation of Seldinger technique emergency cricothyroidotomy versus standard surgical cricothyroidotomy in 200 cadavers. Anesthesiology. 2005;102(1):7-11.
18. Craven RM, Vanner RG. Ventilation of a model lung using various cricothyroidotomy devices. Anaesthesia. 2004;59(6):595-9.
19. Klein M, Weksler N, Kaplan DM, et al. Emergency percutaneous tracheostomy is feasible in experienced hands. Eur J Emerg Med. 2004;11(2):108-12.
20. Ben-Nun A, Altman E, Best LA. Emergency percutaneous tracheostomy in trauma patients: An early experience. Ann Thorac Surg. 2004;77(3):1045-7.
21. Schlossmachera P, Martineta O, Testudb R, et al. Emergency percutaneous tracheostomy in a severely burned patient with upper airway obstruction and circulatory arrest. Rescuscitation. 2006;68(2):301-5.

Supraglottic Airway Devices

Sheila N Myatra, Jeson R Doctor

ABSTRACT

A new era in airway management was marked with the introduction of the laryngeal mask airway (LMA) Classic™ more than 35 years ago. Supraglottic airway devices (SADs) are devices, which are intermediate between a facemask and an endotracheal tube (ETT), having their advantages and disadvantages over each of them. They can be used to ventilate patients electively as also in an emergency. Some SADs can also be used as a conduit for intubation. With the continuous evolution of SADs, newer devices have been designed, which have improved safety and efficacy and have revolutionized airway management.

INTRODUCTION

The supraglottic airway devices (SADs) are used to ventilate the patients above the level of the vocal cords. For years, airway management is emphasized largely on successful tracheal intubation. The development of the laryngeal mask airway (LMA) in 1981 marked a paradigm shift, changing the focus of airway management, from intubation to oxygenation and ventilation. The SADs are an intermediate between a facemask and an endotracheal tube (ETT). The main advantages of these devices are that they are less invasive for the respiratory tract, better tolerated by patients with increased ease of placement, improved hemodynamic stability, less sore throat, and less coughing. They provide hands-free airway and easier placement even by inexperienced personnel along with a relatively secure airway.

FEATURES OF AN IDEAL SUPRAGLOTTIC AIRWAY DEVICE[1]

- An SAD must efficiently seal the upper airway during spontaneous and positive pressure ventilation
- It should have low resistance to respiratory gas flow
- It should protect the subglottic airway from upper airway secretions and gastric contents
- It should have a low incidence of airway morbidity and adverse events
- The shape, material, cuff volume, and cuff position should be such that it is easily accepted by the oropharynx.

ADVANTAGES AND DISADVANTAGES OF SUPRAGLOTTIC AIRWAY DEVICE

Advantages of Supraglottic Airway Device over an Endotracheal Tube

- Insertion of an SAD may be less stimulating to the sympathetic nervous system than direct laryngoscopy and placement of a semirigid ETT into the trachea, thereby decreasing the risk of adverse cardiovascular events in patients with coronary artery disease
- An SAD is tolerated at lighter levels of anesthesia than an ETT
- The incidence of postoperative sore throat is also significantly less in patients receiving an SAD as compared to an ETT (17%—as against 45% for ETT)
- SAD typically does not require neuromuscular blockade, thereby avoiding any associated morbidity and side effects of the medication or its antagonists
- Insertion of an SAD requires minimal training, it does not require a laryngoscopy and so it can be easily inserted by a nonclinical or paramedic staff during cardiopulmonary cerebral resuscitation (CPCR)
- It is a rescue device in a complete ventilation failure scenario (CVF) situation
- It can be easily inserted in patients with a cervical spine injury without movement and displacement of a cervical spine.

Disadvantages of Supraglottic Airway Device over an Endotracheal Tube

- It is not a definitive airway (a tube in trachea) and so it does not provide absolute protection against aspiration. It is not recommended for electively securing an airway in patients who are not adequately fasting, have delayed gastric emptying, history of gastroesophageal (GE) reflux, etc.
- It cannot be recommended for use in patients with poor lung compliance because of the lower seal pressures as compared to an ETT. If the pressures required for ventilation are high, it can lead to dislodgment of the SAD and gastric insufflations

- It is not a choice for restricted mouth opening or upper airway abnormality. An awake fiberoptic bronchoscope (FOB)-guided intubation would be preferred.

ADVANTAGES OF SUPRAGLOTTIC AIRWAY DEVICE OVER A FACE MASK

- Hands-free maintenance of the airway preventing fatigue of the operator
- More secure and reliable means of maintaining the airway
- Lower chances of gastric insufflations.

DISADVANTAGES OF A SUPRAGLOTTIC AIRWAY DEVICE OVER A FACE MASK

Incidence of sore throat is higher (17% for SAD as against 3% for face mask).

INDICATIONS FOR THE USE OF SUPRAGLOTTIC AIRWAY DEVICES

- *Elective ventilation:* The SADs can be used as an alternative to mask anesthesia in the operating room or in place of an ETT for short and elective surgical procedures under general anesthesia. Relative indication in professional singers is to avoid complications of endotracheal intubation and damage to the vocal cords
- *Difficult airway:* It should be an integral component of the difficult airway cart for both anticipated and unanticipated difficult airway. It forms an integral part of the All India Difficult Airway Association (AIDAA) 2016 guidelines for the management of unanticipated difficult intubation (Step 2) in Adults, Pediatrics, Obstetrics, and in the intensive care unit (ICU)[2-5]
  - As a rescue device during failed intubation or ventilation
  - In a patient who cannot be intubated, but can be ventilated as an alternative to bag-mask ventilation, as it is easier to maintain
  - In a patient who cannot be intubated or ventilated (CVF), LMA insertion can be attempted while preparing for cricothyrotomy
- *Cardiac arrest:* Since 2000, American Heart Association guidelines for CPR proposed the LMA for airway management as an acceptable alternative to intubation during cardiac arrest
- *Conduit for intubation:* The SADs can be used as a conduit for intubation when intubation is unsuccessful. The AIDAA 2016 guidelines for the management of unanticipated difficult tracheal intubation, do not recommend blind intubation through the supraglottic device (SGD). The intubation through the supraglottic airway should always be under vision using an FOB with or without the use of an Aintree catheter
- *As a bridge to extubation:* According to the AIDAA 2016 extubation guidelines, whenever deep extubation is to be performed in a normal airway, the ETT tube can be replaced with an SGD either behind the ETT (Bailey's maneuver) or after removal of the ETT.[6]

CONTRAINDICATIONS TO SUPRAGLOTTIC AIRWAY DEVICE USE

- Any patient at risk of aspiration—not adequately fasting, intestinal obstructions, patients undergoing emergency surgery
- Patients with obstruction in upper airway such as tumor, abscess, edema and/or hematoma
- Patient with restricted mouth opening—trismus
- Patient with disrupted upper airway, facial or upper airway trauma, and burns-following caustic ingestion
- Patients who are morbidly obese, more than 14 weeks pregnant, have received prior opioids medication or any condition associated with delayed gastric emptying
- Patients with stiff lungs, i.e., reduced lung compliance/ increased resistive work of breathing, such as pulmonary fibrosis and status asthmaticus. SADs form a low-pressure seal around the laryngeal inlet and ventilating patients with these conditions may require higher pressure and so the ventilation may be inadequate due to inadequate tidal volume delivery. Also, gastric insufflation may occur as ventilation is delivered at higher pressure and gases may leak around the cuff as the sealing pressure is low (LMA Classic™—20 cmH_2O).

With newer safer SAD devices, which provide higher sealing pressure like the LMA ProSeal™ and Supreme™, Auragain, and i-gel use in conditions like obesity, stiff lungs laparoscopic surgery, etc., may be relative contraindications today.

Mnemonic for Contraindications

- *RODS:*
  - Restricted mouth opening
  - Obstruction in upper airway
  - Disrupted upper airway, e.g., trauma, intraoral burns following caustic ingestion
  - Stiff lung (poor compliance).

CLASSIFICATION OF SUPRAGLOTTIC AIRWAY DEVICES

Supraglottic devices can be classified using the Millers classification **(Table 1)**.

Supraglottic devices are alternatively classified into generations:

1. *First generation:* Only with an airway tube and a seal pressure of 20 cm of water
2. *Second generation:* With a gastric channel/port for the drain tube, a seal pressure of more than 30 cm of water and a bite block.

In addition to the second generation SAD's, a few have proposed the use of the terminology third generation

TABLE 1: Classification of supraglottic airway devices (Miller's classification).[7]

	Cuffed perilaryngeal sealers		Cuffed pharyngeal sealers		
	Without directional sealing	*With directional sealing*	*Without esophageal sealing cuff*	*With esophageal sealing cuff*	*Cuff less preshaped sealers*
Devices	• LMA™ • ILMA • Soft Seal® LM • Ambu LM	PLMA	Cobra-PLA™	• LT • LTS • Combitube	• SLIPA • I-gel • Baska® Mask

(LMA: laryngeal mask airway; ILMA: intubating laryngeal mask airway; LM: laryngeal mask; PLMA: ProSeal™ laryngeal mask airway; LT: laryngeal tube; LTS: laryngeal tube suction; SLIPA: streamlined liner of the pharynx airway)

SAD in which the mask seal improves with each positive pressure breath, e.g., Baska mask. However, the use of this nomenclature of third generation is debatable.[8,9]

PERILARYNGEAL SEALERS (TABLE 1)[7]

Laryngeal Mask Airway[1,10]

The LMA was invented by Dr Archie Brain in 1983. It has been in clinical use since 1988.

Laryngeal Mask Airway Classic™[1,10]

The LMA Classic™ **(Fig. 1)** is an important development in airway management. Initially, it was available in Europe in 1988 and in 1992 in USA after approval from Food and Drug Administration (FDA) for clinical use.

It is a "bowl-shaped" mask surrounded by an oval, inflatable, silicone cuff designed to seal around the laryngeal inlet and to prevent obstruction to epiglottis there are two elastic bars across the bowl aperture. It is in continuation with a curved, wide-bore tube that can be connected to a self-inflating (e.g., Ambu) bag or a ventilatory circuit.

It is available in sizes 1–6, designed to fit most from neonates to adults and is reusable up to 40 times and is sterilized by steam autoclaving **(Table 2)**.

A card is available to keep track of the number of uses. LMA cuff should be completely deflated prior to autoclaving. Thoroughly wash the cuff and airway tube in warm water using a dilute (8–10% v/v) sodium bicarbonate solution until all visible foreign matter is removed. And following this the LMA can be sent for autoclaving after deflating the cuff completely.

Once LMA is placed in oropharynx, cuff is inflated enough so that airway leak pressure is between 20 and 25 cmH_2O. In case of misplacement of LMA, there is low airway leak pressure, it will not serve purpose of prevention of leak instead will cause pressure ischemia of pharynx and postoperative sore throat. The adjustment of LMA either by withdrawing or reinserting will correct low airway pressure leak. The LMA Classic™ was made for general anesthesia with spontaneous ventilation. It can be used with peak airway pressure between 20 and 25 cmH_2O for pressure support ventilation.

The maximum intracuff pressure inside the silicon cuff of an LMA is recommended to be less than 60 cmH_2O,

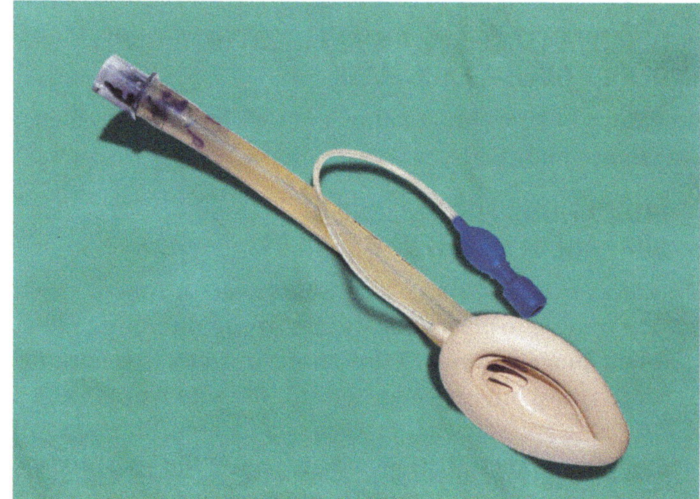

Fig. 1: Laryngeal mask airway classic.
Courtesy: J Doctor, SN Myatra. Department of Anaesthesia, Critical Care and Pain, Tata Memorial Hospital, Mumbai.

TABLE 2: Laryngeal mask airway sizes and cuff inflation volumes.[10]

Weight (kg)	*LMA size*	*Air inflation volume (mL)*
<5	1	4
5–10	1.5	7
10–20	2	10
20–30	2.5	14
30–50	3	20
50–70	4	30
70–100	5	40
>100	6	50

which is the perfusion pressure of the pharyngeal mucosa. Any pressure exceeding this pressure will lead to injury of the pharyngeal mucosa and higher incidence of postoperative sore throat.

Preuse checks: The following tests should be carried out prior to use of an LMA:

- The interior of the airway tube should be inspected to ensure that it is free from blockage or loose particles. If any cuts or indentations are found, discard the device
- Holding at each end flex the airway tube to increase its curvature up to but not beyond 180°. Should the tube kink during this procedure, discard the device

- Deflate the cuff fully. Reinflate the device cuff with a volume of air 50% greater than the maximum inflation value for each size
  - Size 1: 6 mL
  - Size 1½: 10 mL
  - Size 2: 15 mL
  - Size 2½: 21 mL
  - Size 3: 30 mL
  - Size 4: 45 mL
  - Size 5: 60 mL
  - Size 6: 75 mL
- Examine the cuff for leaks, herniation, and uneven bulging. The shape of blue inflation pilot balloon should be elliptical not spherical at 50% over inflated balloon
- The airway connector should fit tightly into airway tube
- The discoloration of airway tube affects visibility of fluid in tube
- To secure attachment to cuff and balloon gently pull the inflation line
- Probe gently two flexible bars into the mask aperture to confirm the damage. The epiglottis may obstruct airway, if aperture bars are not intact. In case of damaged aperture bars avoid using mask.

Preinsertion preparation: The LMA cuff should be deflated completely to create the stiff thin leading edge, necessary to wedge the tip behind the cricoid cartilage. The back of the cuff should be lubricated prior to insertion. It is advisable to use water-soluble lubricant such as K-Y jelly, as other lubricants may block the aperture. The silicon-based lubricants may degrade LMA components and lignocaine lubrication can delay the return of the protective reflexes in addition may possibly provoke an allergic reaction of surrounding structures.

Method of insertion:

1. *Standard insertion method:*
   - For LMA insertion, anesthesia must be deep enough and should be done following induction agent and a muscle relaxant
   - A standard head and neck position as for normal tracheal intubation is maintained during insertion of LMA
   - Hold LMA like pen with the index finger placed anteriorly at the junction of the cuff and tube. Now press the tip up against the hard palate before pushing further into the pharynx
   - Using the index finger, push the mask backward still maintaining pressure against the palate
   - Maintain the index finger pressure backward against the posterior pharyngeal wall to avoid collision with the epiglottis. Now insert index finger fully into the mouth for complete insertion. Now hold tube with other hand while withdrawing the finger from the mouth
   - The black line on tube must face the upper lip. Now inflate the cuff without holding the tube with the recommended volume of air to allow the LMA to position itself correctly and obtain a low-pressure seal. Do not overinflate the cuff
   - Hold the tube to prevent displacement and connect it to gas supply. To confirm correct placement gently inflate lungs
   - Now insert a bite-block to prevent form biting and damage to LMA, and tape the device to ensure that the proximal end of the airway tube is pointing caudally. When correctly placed, the tube should be pressed back into the palate and posterior pharyngeal wall.
2. *Thumb insertion method:* It is suitable for patients where access to the head from behind is difficult or impossible such as during cardiopulmonary resuscitation.

Now LMA is held with the thumb in the position occupied by the index finger. The tip of the mask is pressed against the front teeth and the mask is pressed posteriorly along the palate with the thumb. As the thumb reaches nears the mouth, the fingers are stretched forward over the patient's face and advance the thumb to its fullest extent. The pushing action of the thumb against the hard palate serves to press the head into extension by maintaining neck flexion for head support. Lastly, push the tube into its final position using the other hand before removing thumb.

When appropriately positioned, the distal tip of the silicone cuff rests against the upper esophageal sphincter, the sides of the cuff in the pyriform fossa and the upper part of the cuff against the tongue base.

Maintaining the airway:

- The dislodgment or incorrectly placed LMA can cause obstruction. The correct placement of LMA is confirmed by auscultation and when in doubt reinsert the LMA
- It may mimic a bronchospasm, if there is malposition of the mask tip into the glottis
- Do not move the device in the pharynx in a light plane of anesthesia
- Bite-block must be kept in place till the device is removed
- Once reflexes are fully returned then only deflate the cuff
- Air may be withdrawn from the cuff during anesthesia to maintain a constant intracuff pressure (ideally about 60 cmH_2O).

Before removal confirm following:

- The assembly of LMA with bite-block kept in situ till return of consciousness
- Do thorough oral suction and confirm restoration of swallowing reflexes
- Deflate the cuff completely just prior to removal, although partial deflation can be recommended to assist in the removal of secretions. Some people also recommend removal of the LMA without deflation.

Complications:

- The most common complication is postoperative sore throat. Cuff malposition or excessive cuff pressure may be exacerbated by incorrect mask size, prolonged surgery, and use of nitrous oxide. Simply monitoring the cuff pressure intraoperatively (and evacuating air to maintain constant cuff pressure) was shown to reduce the incidence of postoperative sore throat
- The other adverse events reported are arytenoid dislocation, trauma to the pharyngeal cavity, airway edema, tongue edema, rarely hypoglossal nerve injury, tongue numbness secondary to lingual nerve injury, tongue macroglossia, recurrent laryngeal nerve injury, inferior alveolar nerve injury, and vocal cord paralysis. The nerve injuries are probably due to malposition of LMA or excessive intracuff pressure; which causes compression of nerves and/or blood vessels
- Laryngeal spasm may occur, if the patient becomes too lightly anesthetized during surgical stimulation or if bronchial secretions irritate the vocal cords during emergence from anesthesia. If laryngeal spasm occurs, do not remove the LMA, but treat the cause. Only remove the device when airway protective reflexes are fully competent.

Laryngeal Mask Airway Unique™[1,10]

The LMA Unique™ **(Fig. 2)** was among the first single-use equivalents of the original, reusable SADs. The development of this device was motivated by concerns about the transmission of infectious agents, especially prions, by residual proteinaceous material found on autoclaved airway management equipment. The LMA Unique™ is a disposable, sterile version of the LMA Classic™, is available in five sizes, and has clinical applications and performance similar to those of the LMA Classic™.

Fig. 2: Laryngeal mask airway unique.
Courtesy: J Doctor, SN Myatra. Department of Anaesthesia, Critical Care and Pain, Tata Memorial Hospital, Mumbai

Laryngeal Mask Airway Classic Excel™[1,10] *(LMA North America, Inc.)*

The LMA Classic Excel™ **(Fig. 3)** improves on the LMA Classic™ with the addition of an epiglottic elevating bar and removable connector to facilitate introduction of an ETT through the LMA after placement. It has an increased angle, which aids intubation. The LMA Classic Excel™ is available in sizes 3–5 and accommodates ETTs up to size 7.5; it is reusable up to 60 times.

Laryngeal Mask Airway Flexible™

The LMA Flexible™ **(Fig. 4)** combines the original LMA cuff design with a narrower, longer, and wire-reinforced flexible airway tube.

It has long and narrow airway tube, this makes intubation impossible; however, its flexibility and extra length allow it

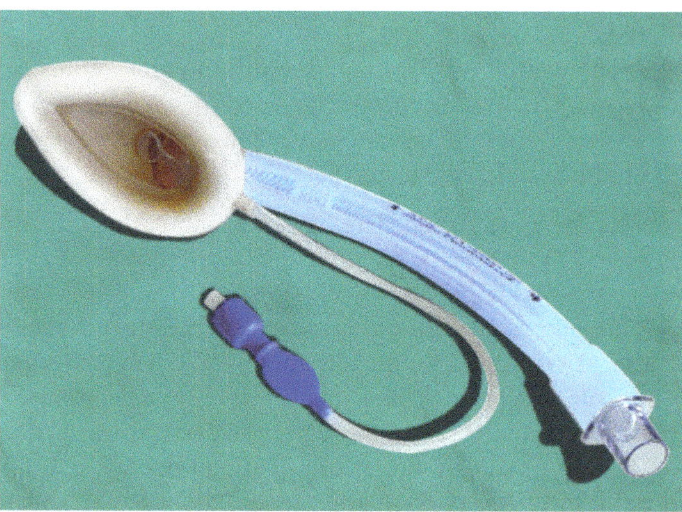

Fig. 3: Laryngeal mask airway classic excel.
Courtesy: J Doctor, SN Myatra. Department of Anaesthesia, Critical Care and Pain, Tata Memorial Hospital, Mumbai.

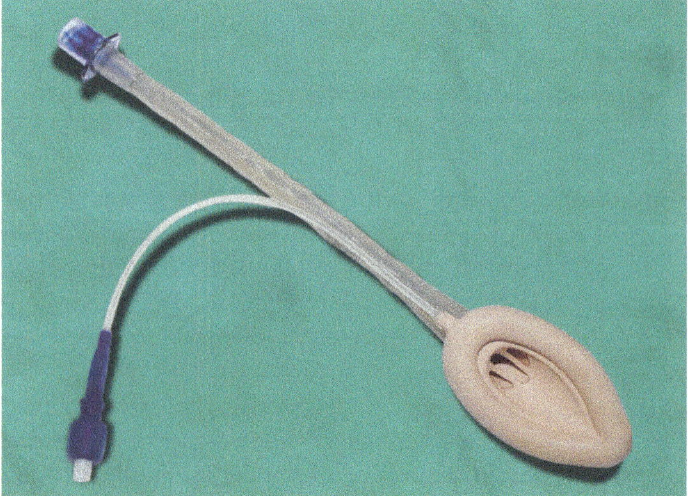

Fig. 4: Laryngeal mask airway flexible.
Courtesy: J Doctor, SN Myatra. Department of Anaesthesia, Critical Care and Pain, Tata Memorial Hospital, Mumbai.

to position away from surgical field without displacement of cuff. Hence, it is popular with ear/nose/throat and maxillofacial or dental surgeries. They are available in sizes 2-6 and are reusable and disposable.

Intubating Laryngeal Mask Airway/LMA Fastrach™[1,10,11]

The FastTrack intubating LMA (FT-LMA) **(Fig. 5)** was first developed by Dr A Brain in 1997 in response to difficulties found when attempting to insert an ETT blindly into the trachea through the LMA Classic™. A study shows the success rate for blind intubation was 96.5%. Intubation under fiberoptic scope guidance was possible in those who failed blind intubation.[12]

The FT-LMA is an intubating laryngeal airway intended to provide both ventilation and the consistent ability to pass an ETT blindly into the trachea.

Compared with the Classic™ Laryngeal Mask Airway (cLMA), the primary distinguishing features of the FT-LMA include:

- An anatomically curved rigid airway tube
- An integrated guiding handle
- An epiglottis-elevating bar (replacing the standard cLMA vertical aperture bars) **(Fig. 6)**
- A guiding ramp built into the floor of the mask aperture.

Together, these features allow optimal alignment of the mask aperture with the glottic opening and provide a conduit for ETT passage. FT-LMAs are available in sizes 3, 4, and 5. There are reusable and disposable versions available **(Table 3)**.

Insertion technique of intubating laryngeal mask airway (ILMA):

- Select device of appropriate size
- Deflate the cuff
- Apply water-soluble lubricant to posterior surface
- Ensure proper head and neck position—neutral, single pillow, and minimal extension
- The ILMA is introduced in the oral cavity holding the rigid handle parallel to the patient's chest. Glide the mask along the palate till the straight part of the rigid tube is parallel to the chin, thereafter rotate the rigid handle directing toward the patient's nose till it cannot be advanced any further
- Inflate cuff as per manufacturer's recommendation, so that intracuff pressure does not exceed 60 cmH_2O
- Rotate device gently in the sagittal plane until ventilation is optimized.

Chandy maneuver consists of two steps. The first step is rotating the LMA in coronal and sagittal plane in an attempt to find a position that offers least resistance to ventilation. The second step consists of grasping the handle firmly and use it to draw the LMA forward 2-5 mm in a lifting action without levering on the teeth. This maneuver increases seal pressure and aligns the axes of the trachea and FastTrack™ endotracheal tube (FETT) and facilitates blind intubation.

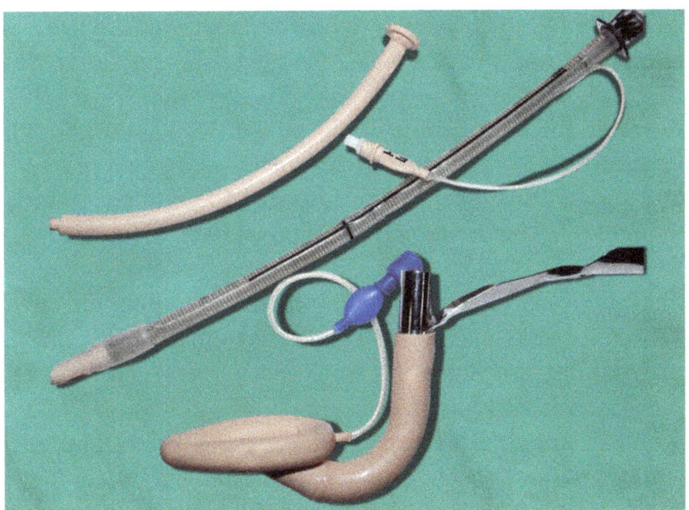

Fig. 5: FastTrack intubating laryngeal mask airway (FT-ILMA).
Courtesy: J Doctor, SN Myatra. Department of Anaesthesia, Critical Care and Pain, Tata Memorial Hospital.

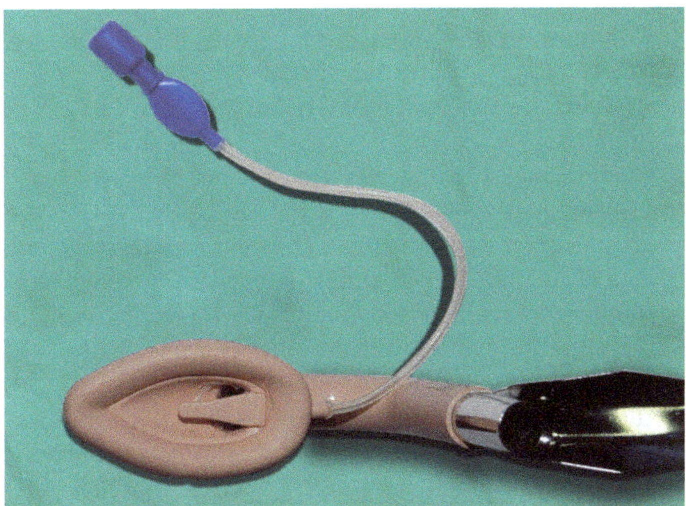

Fig. 6: Laryngeal mask airway FastTrack epiglottis elevating bar.
Courtesy: J Doctor, SN Myatra. Department of Anaesthesia, Critical Care and Pain, Tata Memorial Hospital, Mumbai.

TABLE 3: Laryngeal mask airway FastTrack™ sizes and inflation volumes.[10,11]

Size	*Weight (kg)*	*Cuff inflation volumes (mL)*
3	30–50	20
4	50–70	30
5	70–100	40

Intubation through the ILMA: Laryngeal mask airway FETT is a wire-reinforced cuffed ETT with an internal diameter of 8.0 mm and can be passed through the ILMA. The ETT has a transverse line at 15 cm, which coincides with the epiglottic elevating bar in the elliptical cuff of the ILMA. It is recommended to use this tube with the ILMA. Using the conventional ETT through the ILMA is not recommended and can lead to laryngeal trauma. Prior to insertion, lubricate the FETT well, and fit the connector. The LMA FETT also has a longitudinal black line on the tube, and the tube is introduced with this line facing the rigid handle of the ILMA. The FETT should not be introduced beyond the 15 cm mark. Now grip the LMA handle firmly and lift (without levering) it forward by a few millimeters, this increases the seal pressure and optimally aligns the tracheal and FETT axes (the Chandy maneuver). The mask may sometimes have a tendency to flex and the FETT can then pass in the esophagus rather than the trachea, this is avoided by the Chandy maneuver. Thereafter, advance the FETT gently beyond the 15 cm mark; at this point, it is lifting the epiglottic elevating bar **(Fig. 7)**. Advance the FETT further using clinical judgment. Inflate the FETT and attach it to the breathing circuit to check and confirm endotracheal position using capnography.

It is recommended to remove the ILMA following insertion of FETT, as it can lead to pharyngeal edema and increased mucosal pressure because of the rigid steel tube in the ILMA. If the ILMA has to be kept in situ, the cuff of the ILMA should be deflated to a pressure of 20–30 cmH_2O.

- Administer 100% O_2 for few minutes and then disconnect the FETT and the breathing circuit
- Deflate the ILMA completely but keep the FETT cuff inflated
- Remove the ETT connector and ease the LMA FastTrack™ out by gently swinging the handle caudally. Use the stabilizing rod to keep the ETT in place while removing the LMA FastTrack™ until the tube can be grasped at the level of the incisors. Remove the stabilizing rod and gently unthread the inflation line and pilot balloon of the ETT
- Replace the ETT connector and reconfirm the position of the ETT by capnography.

Indications of use of ILMA:

- Anticipated and unanticipated difficult intubations
- Suspected or confirmed cervical spine injury.

An FOB can also be used for intubation through the FETT and ILMA. (This technique is recommended by the AIDAA 2016 Airway Guidelines for the management of unanticipated difficult intubation).

Laryngeal Mask Airway ProSeal™ [1,10]

The LMA ProSeal™ **(Fig. 8)** has four main components—(1) mask, (2) inflation line with pilot balloon, (3) airway tube, and (4) drain tube.

The mask is designed to conform to the contours of the hypopharynx, with its lumen facing the laryngeal opening. It has a main cuff that seals around the laryngeal opening and the larger sizes also have a rear cuff (dorsal cuff), which helps to increase the seal. This softer and revised cuff arrangement (dorsal cuff) is responsible for the higher seal pressures of 30 cmH_2O for the LMA ProSeal™.

There is an inflation line terminating in a pilot balloon and valve attached to mask inflation and deflation. A red plug is also fitted to the valve assembly to allow residual air in the mask to be vented during autoclaving. It prevents expansion of the cuff when left open during steam autoclaving. The plug must be detached before autoclaving and replaced before clinical use. Some older LMA ProSeal™ devices may not have a red plug fitted.

A drain tube passes lateral to the airway tube and traverses the floor of the mask, opening at the mask tip opposite the upper esophageal sphincter. This tube prevents inadvertent gastric insufflations and allows for blind insertion of orogastric tubes even without use of Magill's forceps. The position of the drain tube inside the cuff prevents the epiglottis occluding the airway tube thereby eliminating the need for aperture bars.

The airway tube is wire reinforced to prevent collapse and terminates with a standard 15-mm connector. This double tube arrangement along with the drain tube securely

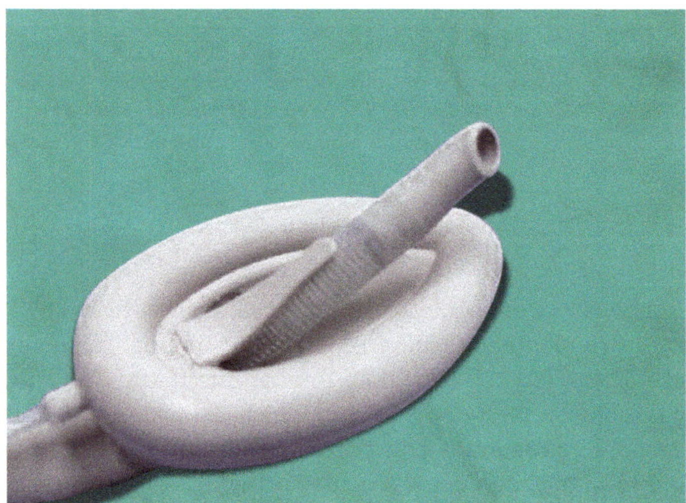

Fig. 7: Intubation through intubating laryngeal mask airway.
Courtesy: J Doctor, SN Myatra. Department of Anaesthesia, Critical Care and Pain, Tata Memorial Hospital, Mumbai.

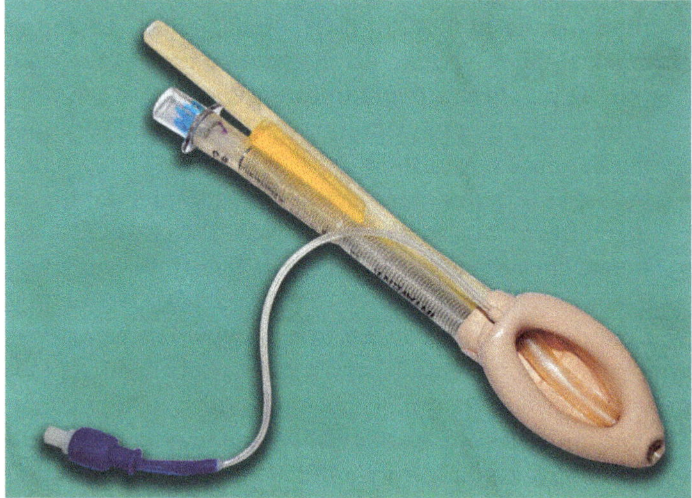

Fig. 8: Laryngeal mask airway proseal.
Courtesy: J Doctor, SN Myatra. Department of Anaesthesia, Critical Care and Pain, Tata Memorial Hospital, Mumbai

anchors the LMA and reduces the likelihood of mask rotation. A built-in bite-block (except size 1) reduces the danger of airway obstruction or tube damage. The LMA ProSeal™ size 1 also differs from the other sizes in that it has a relatively larger drain tube (8 Fr).

A malleable introducer tool is available in adult and pediatric sizes to aid insertion, if it is desirable to avoid placing a finger in the patient's mouth. It is supplied in the recommended curvature for immediate use.

A location strap (introducer strap) for the introducer is present at the junction of the mask and the two tubes. It can also accommodate the index finger or thumb for manual insertion.

A dedicated deflation device (Cuff-Deflator) is available to aid complete deflation for successful sterilization, optimum insertion, and positioning in the patient.

All components are latex free.

The Laryngeal Mask Company recommends that the LMA ProSeal™ be used a maximum of 40 times before being discarded.

It is available in sizes 1, 1.5, 2, 2.5, 3, 4, and 5.

Methods of insertion are described below:

- Introducer technique **(Video 7)**
- Digital insertion technique **(Video 7)**
- Thumb insertion technique
- Bougie-guided through the drain tube with a pharyngoscopy **(Video 7)**
- 180° rotation technique **(Video 7)**.

Laryngeal Mask Airway Supreme™[1,10]

The LMA Supreme™ **(Fig. 9)** is a sterile single use supraglottic airway management device. The anatomically-shaped airway tube is elliptical in cross-section and ends distally at the laryngeal mask. Intubation is not possible with LMA Supreme™ due to the elliptical shape of the airway tube.

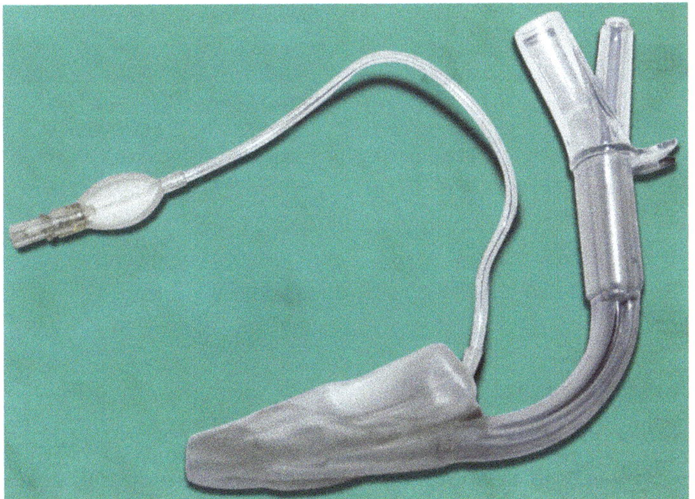

Fig. 9: Laryngeal mask airway supreme.
Courtesy: J Doctor, SN Myatra. Department of Anaesthesia, Critical Care and Pain, Tata Memorial Hospital, Mumbai.

There are two lateral grooves in the airway tube to prevent the airway tube kinking when flexed.

The inflatable cuff is designed to conform to the contours of the hypopharynx, with the bowl and the mask facing the laryngeal opening. The cuff has molded fins, which prevent epiglottis from obstructing the airway lumen. The tip of the cuff is reinforced to prevent it from folding during insertion. Attached to the mask is a cuff inflation line terminating in a pilot balloon and one-way check valve for mask inflation and deflation.

The drain tube opens as a separate port proximally and continues distally along the anterior surface of the cuff bowl, passing through the distal end of the cuff to communicate distally with the upper esophageal sphincter. The drain tube may be used for the passage of a well-lubricated gastric tube to the stomach for evacuation of gastric contents. It may also be used as a monitor of correct positioning of the LMA. If it is correctly positioned at the upper esophageal sphincter then a pressure on the suprasternal notch will cause the meniscus of 1–2 mL of jelly in the drain tube to move up and down (suprasternal notch test).[10] Similar movement will also be observed during intermittent positive pressure ventilation (IPPV) **(Video 7)**.

The LMA Supreme™ can be easily inserted without the need for digital or introducer tool guidance and enough flexibility to permit the device to remain in place, if the patient's head is moved in any direction. A built-in bite-block prevents tube damage and obstruction by patient biting.

The LMA Supreme™ also has a new fixation system, which prevents proximal displacement. This enhances the seal of the distal end around the upper esophageal sphincter.

All components are latex free.

The LMA Supreme™ is supplied sterile and for single use only.

It is terminally sterilized by ethylene oxide gas.

It is available in sizes 1–5. It also provides a seal pressure of 30 cmH_2O like the ProSeal™ LMA.

Tests for correct placement of an SGD:

- Visual assessment of depth of insertion
- Unobstructed inspiratory and expiratory flow—adequate chest rise, no audible leak, and expired tidal volume should match set tidal volume or peak pressure
- Suprasternal notch tap test (in devices with a gastric channel)
- Gel displacement test
- Passage of gastric tube or polyvinyl chloride (PVC) catheter through drain tube
- Soap bubble test
- Thread test
- Fiberoptic bronchoscopy through the SGA and Brimacombe grading of view of the glottic inlet—gold standard.

Laryngeal Mask Airway CTrach™[1]

The LMA CTrach™ **(Fig. 10)** system is a new system for airway management and endotracheal intubation. It is based on the ILMA (LMA FastTrack™) system with two in-built fiberoptic channels, one to convey light from and the other to convey the image to the viewer. This fiberoptic system is sealed and robust, and the CTrach™ can be autoclaved. The CTrach™ has an epiglottis elevating bar, which elevates the epiglottis during passage of the ETT through the CTrach™ into the larynx. A rechargeable battery is provided for up to 30 minutes of continuous use. A charger cradle for recharging the viewer is included in the system.

The LMA CTrach™ system is indicated as a device for achieving and maintaining an airway in both anticipated and unexpected difficult intubation situations.

The manufacturing and marketing of the LMA CTrach™ has been stopped.

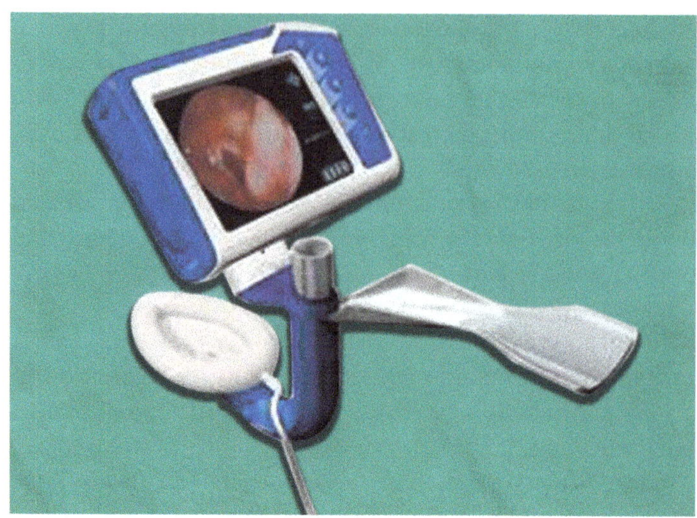

Fig. 10: Laryngeal mask airway CTrach.
Courtesy: J Doctor, SN Myatra. Department of Anaesthesia, Critical Care and Pain, Tata Memorial Hospital, Mumbai.

LMA Protector™[10]

The LMA Protector™ **(Fig. 11)** is one of the most advanced second generation supraglottic airway devices. It combines a pharyngeal chamber and dual gastric drainage channels, designed specifically to divert gastric content away from the airway. Direct intubation using visual guidance is possible through the device. The phthalate free silicone cuff has shown to reduce the incidence of sore throat and achieve higher seal pressures as compared to the PVC cuffs. The second seal technology is provided by the elongated cuff which facilitates an upper esophageal seal. In addition, the device has a cuff pilot technology with an integrated color-coded cuff pressure indicator, which enables continuous cuff pressure monitoring at a glance. It is available in 3 sizes **(Table 4)**.

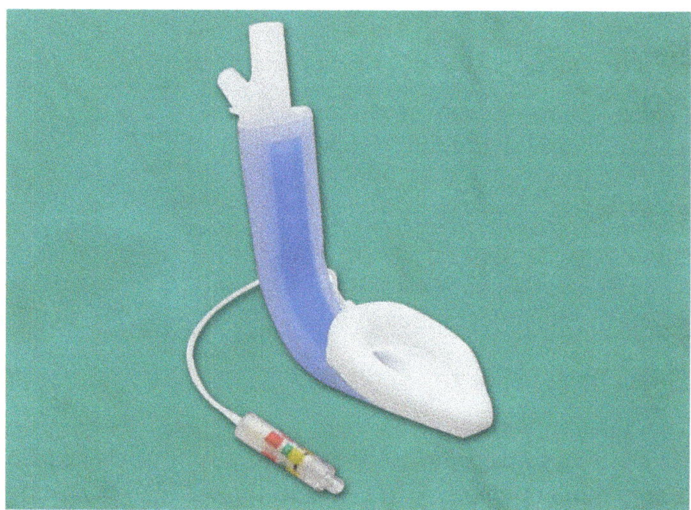

Fig. 11: Laryngeal mask airway (LMA) protector.
Courtesy: Teleflex Incorporated.

Laryngeal Mask Airway Gastro™ Airway[10]

Laryngeal mask airway Gastro™ airway **(Fig. 12)** is the first laryngeal mask specifically designed to enable clinicians to manage the patient's airways during an endoscopic procedure. It facilitates direct endoscopic access via an integrated endoscope channel and allows the clinician to monitor end-tidal carbon dioxide for patient safety. The device has a separate endoscopic channel to allow the passage of an endoscope under direct vision **(Table 5)**. An adjustable strap and holder maintain the device in position during the procedure. An integrated bite block reduces the risk of damage to the airway tube and the endoscope in case the patient tries to bite. The phthalate free silicone cuff has been shown to reduce the incidence of sore throat and achieve higher seal pressures as compared to PVC cuffs. In addition, the device has a cuff pilot technology with an integrated color-coded cuff pressure indicator, which enables continuous cuff pressure monitoring at a glance.

TABLE 4: Laryngeal Mask Airway Protector™ sizes.

Airway size	*Patient weight (kg)*	*Maximum size of orogastric-tube (Fr)*	*Maximum size of endotra-cheal tube*	*Maximum in-tracuff pressure (cmH_2O)*
3	30–50	16	6.5	60
4	50–70	18	7.5	60
5	70–100	18	7.5	60

Ambu Laryngeal Masks[13]

Ambu Aura Once™ Disposable Laryngeal Mask

- It has built-in anatomical correct curve, which is easy for atraumatic insertion **(Fig. 13)**
- Reinforced tip resists folding over during insertion and plugs the upper esophageal sphincter

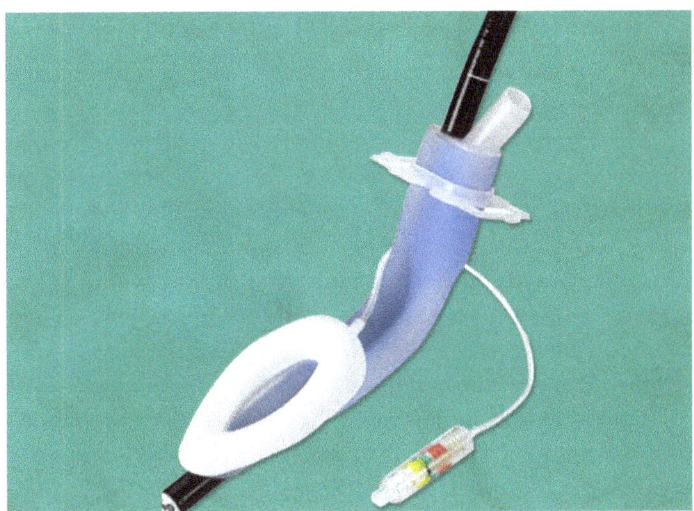

Fig. 12: Laryngeal mask airway (LMA) Gastro™.
Courtesy: Teleflex Incorporated.

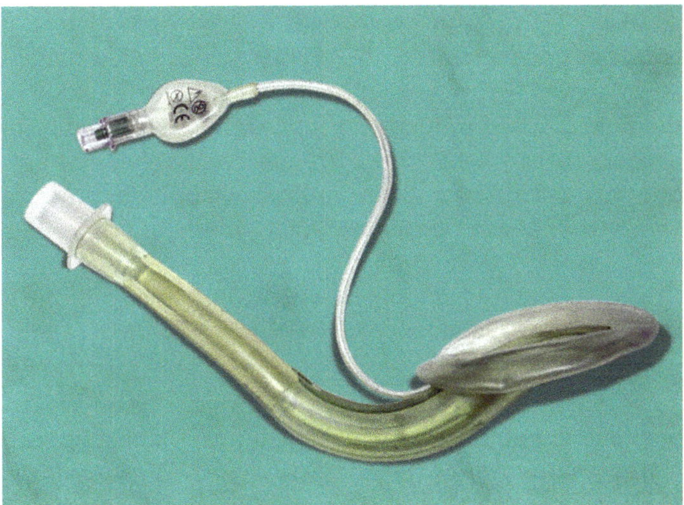

Fig. 13: Ambu laryngeal mask.
Courtesy: J Doctor, SN Myatra. Department of Anaesthesia, Critical Care and Pain, Tata Memorial Hospital, Mumbai.

TABLE 5: Laryngeal mask airway Gastro™ sizes.

Airway size	*Patient weight (kg)*	*Maximum intracuff pressure (cm of water)*	*Maximum size of endoscope (outer diameter in mm)*
3	30–50	60	14
4	50–70	60	14
5	70–100	60	14

- Cuff and airway tube molded as single unit for extra-safety—no separation
- The surface has an easy glide texture to ease insertion
- The cuff is extra-soft, which ensures the best possible seal and least mucosal pressure
- Pilot balloon identifies mask size and provides precise tactile indication of degree of inflation
- The ergonomically-shaped airway tube has firm grip during insertion
- The convenient depth marks assist for monitoring of correct position
- It comes in sterile package and ready for use
- Available in eight sizes—1, 1.5, 2, 2.5, 3, 4, 5, and 6.

Ambu Aura I™ Disposable Laryngeal Mask

Intubating capability using standard ETT.

Ambu Auragain™ Disposable Laryngeal Mask

Integrated gastric access and intubation capability in an anatomically curved single-use device.

Ambu Auraflex™ Disposable Laryngeal Mask

The flexible airway tube is reinforced with kink-free wire, which eliminates the risk of airway tube occlusion.

Ambu Aurastraight™ Disposable Laryngeal Mask

Has a straight airway tube without a preformed curve.

Ambu Aura40™ Reusable Laryngeal Mask

Autoclavable, and can be reused 40 times. Has a preformed curve like the Aura Once. Has a color-coded pilot balloon.

Air-Q/Intubating Laryngeal Airway

This was developed by Dr Daniel Cook and introduced in 2004. The air-Q/ILA is available as a disposable (air-Q) or nondisposable (ILA) device **(Fig. 14)**. This is used either as an SAD, or as conduit for tracheal intubation. It has an elliptical, cuffed mask with a curved airway tube a detachable connector. The unique features that make it suitable for tracheal intubation are a shorter shaft than the cLMA with a wide lumen for intubation, no aperture bars in the mask, a removable connector and a keyhole-shaped distal airway tube to direct a tracheal tube toward the larynx. If ventilation is inadequate with this device, the "Klein maneuver" can be performed. This corrects the downfolding of the epiglottis using a jaw thrust and an up-down maneuver of the ILA.

For tracheal intubation, the ET is advanced to a depth of 12–15 cm, so that the tip of the tube is close to the air-Q/ILA opening. The ET is then introduced into the trachea blindly or with the aid of an FOB. After intubation, the ILA can also be left in place as a bridge to extubation. Success of blind intubation is higher with use of a flexible reinforced ET. (The AIDAA 2016 Airway Guidelines do not recommend blind intubation through an SAD).

The list of the other laryngeal mask like devices includes:

- Sheridan® laryngeal mask (Teleflex Medical)
- Portex® Soft Seal® laryngeal mask (Smiths Medical)
- Ultra CPV and Ultra Flex™ CPV (AES Inc.).

PHARYNGEAL SEALERS (TABLE 1)

Cobra Perilaryngeal Airway[14]

It is a cuffed pharyngeal sealer without an esophageal balloon. The Cobra perilaryngeal airway (CobraPLA™) **(Fig. 15)** consists of a breathing tube with a distal circumferential inflatable cuff proximal to the ventilation outlet. It is named so because of the widened distal part resembles the hood of the Cobra. When properly positioned, the Cobra head sits over glottis and seals off the hypopharynx. This distal part prevents soft tissue collapse and allows positive pressure ventilation. A soft flexible grill placed anteriorly prevents epiglottis from downfolding. The grill allows passage of an ETT when required. A ramp present within this head, which directs the ventilation or a blindly passed ETT into the glottic aperture.

It has a circumferential cuff, which rests in the hypopharynx at the vallecula. When inflated, it lifts the base of the tongue exposing the glottic aperture, and also seals the airway.

The CobraPLA™ is available in eight sizes according to the weight and size of the patient including adult and pediatric sizes **(Table 6)**.

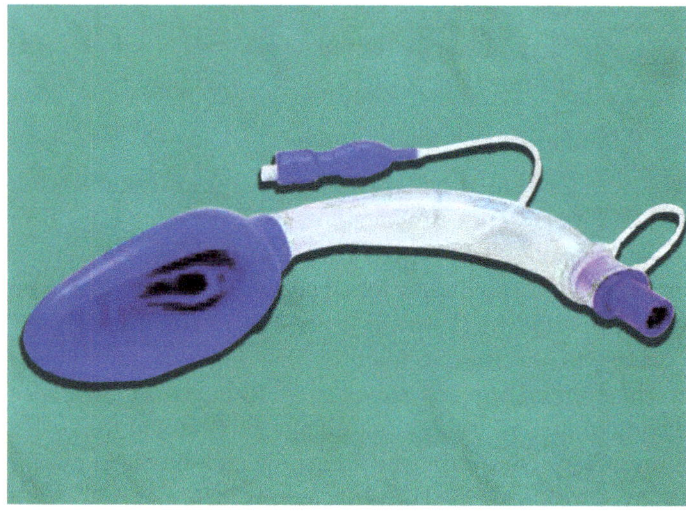

Fig. 14: Air-Q intubating laryngeal airway.
Courtesy: J Doctor, SN Myatra. Department of Anaesthesia, Critical Care and Pain, Tata Memorial Hospital, Mumbai.

Laryngeal Tube[1,15] and Laryngeal Tube Suction[15]

These are cuffed pharyngeal sealers with an esophageal balloon.

The laryngeal tube (LT) **(Fig. 16)** is a silicon reusable airway tube provided with two cuffs (pharyngeal and esophageal), a single balloon for inflation of both the cuffs and a color-coded 15-mm universal connector.

The airway tube is short and has a blind tip. It also has markings to indicate the adequacy of placement. When correctly positioned, the black markings on the airway tube should be at the incisors of the patient.

The proximal cuff lies in the hypopharynx and separates the laryngopharynx from the nasopharynx and the oropharynx. The proximal cuff is protected by a bend located in a "V" dent of the pharyngeal cuff. With cuff inflation, soft tissue is deflected from this opening, helping to maintain a patent airway. The distal cuff lies in the upper esophagus. Both cuffs are high volume and low pressure to avoid ischemic damages and permit a good seal. A wedge-shaped block closes the tip of the tube, thus diverting the ventilation to the trachea. The cuffs should be inflated, with the aid of the laryngeal cuff pressure gauge, to 60 cmH_2O. Due to a single inflation line, both cuffs will inflate simultaneously.

TABLE 6: CobraPLA™ sizes, cuff volumes, and endotracheal tube sizes.[14]

Cobra size	*Weight (kg)*	*Cuff volume (mL)*	*ETT size*
½	>2.5–5	<8	3
1	5–10	<10	4.5
1½	10–15	<25	4.5
2	15–35	<40	6.5
3	35–70	<65	6.5
4	70–100	<70	8
5	100–130	<85	8
6	>130	<85	8

(ETT: endotracheal tube)

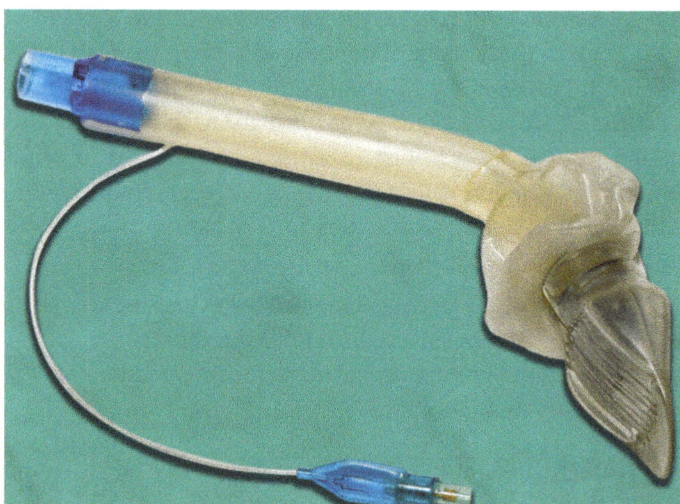

Fig. 15: Cobra perilaryngeal airway.
Courtesy: J Doctor, SN Myatra. Department of Anaesthesia, Critical Care and Pain, Tata Memorial Hospital, Mumbai.

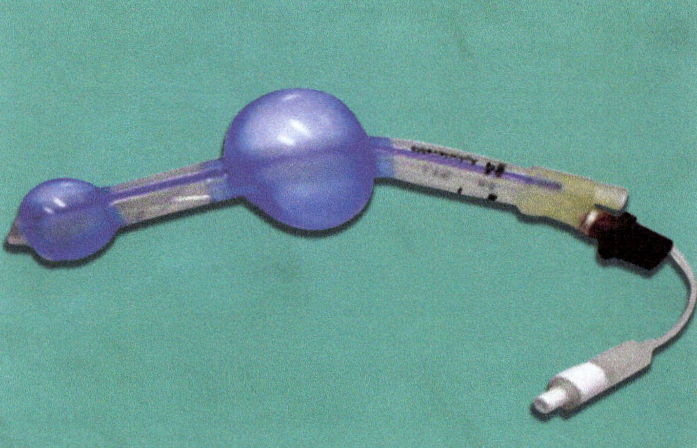

Fig. 16: Laryngeal tube.
Courtesy: J Doctor, SN Myatra. Department of Anaesthesia, Critical Care and Pain, Tata Memorial Hospital, Mumbai.

The LT and laryngeal tube suction (LTS) have an accompanying syringe, which has color-coded markings (of the same color as the universal connectors of the LT) to inflate the two cuffs of the LT with predetermined quantity of air.

Three-side eyelets on each side allow improved collateral ventilation in cases where the epiglottis obstructs the main ventilation orifice.

The LTS is double lumen silicon version of the LT. The additional lumen is situated behind the lumen for ventilation. This lumen is for insertion of gastric tube allowing suction of gastric contents. The suction port opens distally at the esophageal end distal to the esophageal cuff.

The LT and the LTS are available in disposable and reusable versions. The reusable version is designed to be reused up to 50 times. Laryngeal tube size selection is based on the patient's weight for infants and children and height for adults **(Table 7)**.

Esophageal–Tracheal Combitube[1]

It is a cuffed pharyngeal sealer with an esophageal balloon.

The Combitube **(Fig. 17)** is a disposable, double-lumen tube that has two balloons, two tubes, and two separate inflation lines.

TABLE 7: Laryngeal tube and laryngeal tube suction sizes and color coding.[15]

Size	*Patient*	*Patient weight*	*Color-code*
0	Newborn	<5 kg	Transparent
1	Child	5–12 kg	White
2	Child	12–25 kg	Green
2.5	Child/adult	125–150 cm	Orange
3	Adult	<155 cm	Yellow
4	Adult	155–180 cm	Red
5	Adult	>180 cm	Purple

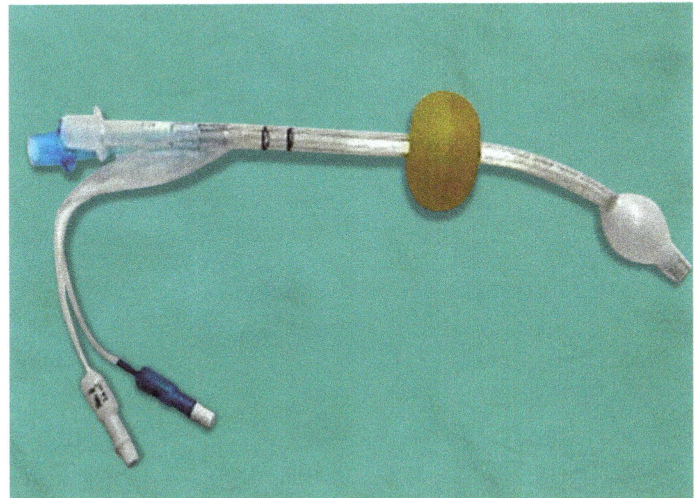

Fig. 17: Combitube.
Courtesy: J Doctor, SN Myatra. Department of Anaesthesia, Critical Care and Pain, Tata Memorial Hospital, Mumbai.

It has a large proximal oropharyngeal balloon (beige) and a distal white esophageal (or tracheal) balloon. The oropharyngeal balloon requires 85–100 mL for inflation and the esophageal balloon requires 12–15 mL for inflation. There are eight ventilatory holes between the cuffs, and a single ventilatory port at the distal tip. Lumen 1 (blue proximal connector) goes to ventilation holes between balloons, while lumen 2 (clear proximal connector) runs completely through to distal tip. There are two black lines on the tube, which are depth indicators for insertion of the Combitube.

There is ventilation with the Combitube regardless of whether the distal tip is in the esophagus (common) or in the trachea (rare). When the Combitube is in the trachea, it functions like a conventional ETT when the distal cuff is inflated. When the distal tip is in the esophagus, the distal cuff seals the esophagus against regurgitation of gastric contents, and a gastric tube can be placed through the esophageal lumen. The eight ventilatory holes between the two cuffs can be used to ventilate the patient.

The Combitube enters the esophagus in greater than 95% of cases, the ventilation is through lumen 1 (blue connector) via supraglottic holes located between balloons. Rarely, the Combitube enters the trachea—if this occurs, ventilation of the lungs will only occur through lumen 2.

The Combitube is available in two sizes—37 F and 41 F. The 41 F is recommended for patients taller than 152 cm and 37 F is recommended for shorter patients. However, the Combitube is recommended for use only in patients taller than 4.5 feet.

Contraindications:

- Hiatus hernia
- Esophageal pathology
- Caustic ingestions
- Patients shorter than 4.5 feet
- Intact gag reflex.

It is seldom used outside of the prehospital and emergency setting, as it does not allow for long-term airway control. With the availability of better airway gadgets especially better SGAs role of Combitube even in prehospital setting has declined.

Easy Tube®

The Easy tube® **(Fig. 18)** is a disposable, polyvinyl chloride, and latex-free SAD. It has a double-lumen and is similar in design to the Combitube. It enters the esophagus in most cases. Easy tube® is more user friendly, has a better fiberoptic view, and a shorter time to achieve an effective airway than Combitube.

CUFFLESS PRESHAPED SEALERS (TABLE 1)

Streamlined Liner of the Pharynx Airway[14,16]

The streamlined liner of the pharynx airway (SLIPA) **(Fig. 19)** is a latex-free slipper-shaped device. It is a cuffless preshaped sealer made of stiff medical grade thermoplastic material to facilitate easy insertion. After insertion, it warms up to body temperature and softens, improving the seal and comfort. It has two components—a stem and a chamber.

The chamber is hollow and boot shaped having a capacity of 50 mL to accommodate secretions and stomach contents preventing aspiration. The chamber consists of three parts—(1) toe, (2) bridge, and (3) heel. The toe sits at the upper end of esophageal opening, the bridge comes to rest at the vallecula, and the heel of SLIPA fits in the nasopharynx. The bridge has two lateral bulges, which occupy the pyriform fossa of the larynx. These prevent downfolding of the epiglottis in front of glottic opening.

The stem is connected to the chamber at one end and has a 15-mm universal connector to fit the breathing system at the other. The universal connector is color coded for the size.

Streamlined liner of the pharynx airway is available in six adult sizes—47, 49, 51, 53, 55, and 57 **(Table 8)**. These sizes correspond to the maximal transverse diameter (in mm) of the bridge. The best way of selecting SLIPA of the correct size is to see the distance between two cornu of the thyroid cartilage and selecting a size that will match the width of the bridge.

The production of the SLIPA has been stopped and it is no longer available.

i-gel[17]

The i-gel **(Fig. 20)** airway is a cuff less, sterile, and latex-free SAD. It is made of a soft and gel-like transparent medical grade thermoplastic elastomer. It is designed to create a noninflatable anatomical seal of the pharyngeal, laryngeal, and perilaryngeal structures while avoiding the compression trauma that can occur with inflatable SADs.

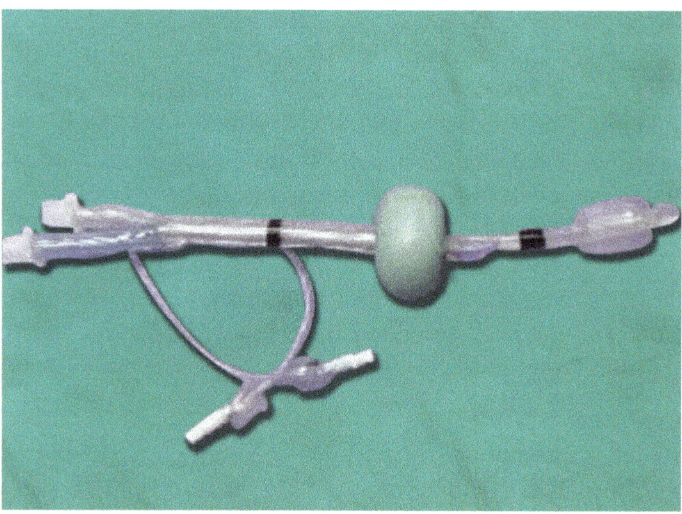

Fig. 18: Easytube.
Courtesy: J Doctor, SN Myatra. Department of Anaesthesia, Critical Care and Pain, Tata Memorial Hospital, Mumbai.

TABLE 8: Streamlined liner of the pharynx airway (SLIPA) sizes and color-coding.[16]

SLIPA size	*Patient*	*Correspond-ing LMA size*	*Color*	*Height and range*
47	Very small female	–	Green	152 cm (145–160 cm)
49	Small female	3	Blue	160 cm (152–168 cm)
51	Medium female	4	Yellow	168 cm (160–175 cm)
53	Large female/ small male		White	173 cm (163–182 cm)
55	Medium male	5	Red	182 cm (173–193 cm)
57	Large male		Orange	190 cm (180–200 cm)

(LMA: laryngeal mask airway)

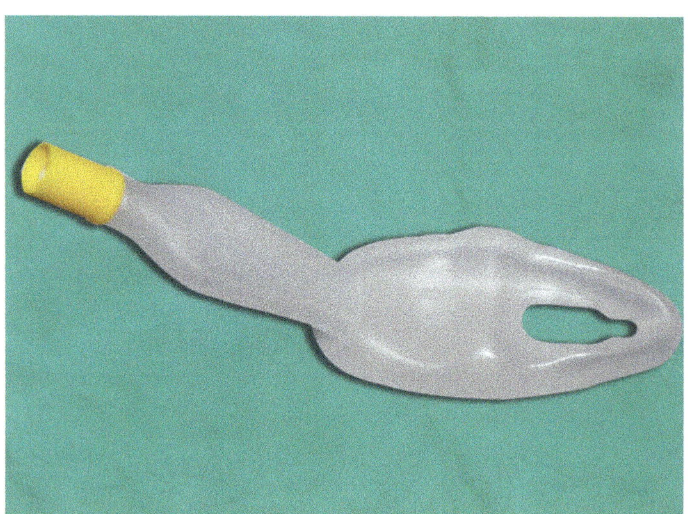

Fig. 19: Streamlined liner of the pharynx airway.
Courtesy: J Doctor, SN Myatra. Department of Anaesthesia, Critical Care and Pain, Tata Memorial Hospital, Mumbai.

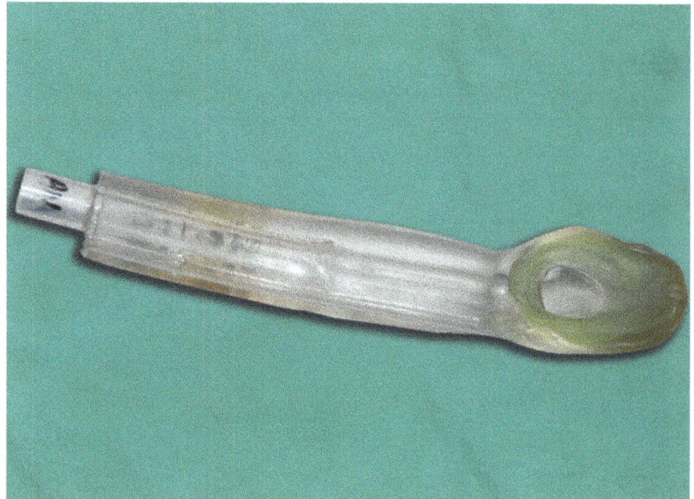

Fig. 20: I-gel.
Courtesy: J Doctor, SN Myatra. Department of Anaesthesia, Critical Care and Pain, Tata Memorial Hospital, Mumbai.

It consists of a noninflatable cuff, an integrated gastric channel (except size 1), an epiglottic rest, and a buccal cavity stabilizer with an integrated bite block and a universal 15-mm connector.

The soft noninflatable cuff fits snugly onto the perilaryngeal framework, mirroring the shape of the epiglottis, aryepiglottic folds, pyriform fossa, perithyroid, pericricoid, posterior cartilages, and spaces. The tip of the cuff lies in the proximal opening of the esophagus and isolates the esophageal opening from the laryngeal inlet. It also houses the opening of the gastric channel. The cuff ensures that the blood flow to the laryngeal and perilaryngeal structures is maintained and reduces the possibility of any neurovascular compression.

The epiglottic rest at the proximal end of the cuff helps prevent the epiglottis from downfolding or obstructing the distal opening of the airway. It rests at the base of the tongue, and also prevents the device from moving upward out of position and the tip from moving out of the upper esophagus.

An integrated gastric channel can provide an early indication of regurgitation, facilitates venting of gas from the stomach, and allows for the passing of a nasogastric tube to empty the stomach contents. Size 1 i-gel does not have a gastric channel. The gastric channel runs through the device from its proximal opening at the side of the flat connector wing to the distal tip of the noninflatable cuff.

The buccal cavity stabilizer has a widened, elliptical, and laterally flattened cross-sectional shape. This shape provides good vertical stability and axial strength on insertion eliminating the potential for rotation and malposition. It has a standard round airway channel and a separate gastric channel. The firmness and curvature allows the device to be smoothly inserted by grasping the proximal end of the device.

The functions of innovative connector are as follows:

- Standard 15-mm connection for anesthetic system or for patient
- In case of entry for the gastric channel, the 15-mm connection is independent and is located on the right-hand side of the connector wing. Not applicable to size 1 i-gel
- The distal part of connector can be bite block, which runs through the center of the proximal part of the buccal cavity stabilizer
- The V-shaped junction of the distal tip of the body of connector reduces the risk of kinking
- The integral part of bite block marked with horizontal black line acts as guide for correct positioning also signifies optimum position of teeth with device *in situ* (not applicable to the pediatric sizes)
- The information such as size and recommended weight is on bite block **(Table 9)**.

TABLE 9: i-gel sizes.[17]

i-gel size	*Patient size*	*Patient weight (kg)*	*Size of ETT (mm)*	*Size of nasogastric tube (Fr)*
1	Neonate	2–5	3	N/A
1.5	Infant	5–12	4	10
2	Small pediatric	10–25	5	12
2.5	Large pediatric	25–35	5	12
3	Small adult	30–60	6	12
4	Medium adult	50–90	7	12
5	Large adult	90+	8	14

(ETT: endotracheal tube)

Elisha Airway Device[18]

The Elisha airway device (EAD) **(Fig. 21)** is made of latex-free medical-grade silicone. It has three separate channels for ventilation, intubation, and gastric tube insertion. The ventilation channel (VC) and the intubation channel (IC) are side by side with a partitioning wall between them, but they join at the ventilation outlet situated in front of the laryngeal inlet. The VC has a standard 15 mm connector located on the proximal end of the device. The IC allows passage of an 8.0 mm internal diameter (ID) ETT for blind or fiberoptic-guided intubation. The gastric tube channel (GTC) is a separate channel and located in the distal end of the device. The EAD has two high-volume and low-pressure balloons—a proximal balloon that seals the oropharynx and nasopharynx, and a distal balloon that seals the esophagus. Both balloons are inflated through a single pilot port with 50 mL of air, to maintain an intraballoon pressure of approximately 70 cmH_2O.

Baska® Mask Airway[19]

The Baska® mask **(Fig. 22)** is a newer SAD similar to the LMA. It is available in single use disposable as well as multiple use versions (sterilized by autoclaving—70 uses).

It has a noninflatable cuff that is continuous with the airway channel and thus gets inflated with positive pressure ventilation, reducing chances of gastric insufflation, and aspiration. Positive pressure ventilation improves the cuff seal.

The Baska® mask has a distal opening that sits in the upper esophagus, and the dorsal surface of the cuff is made in a way that it directs any oropharyngeal contents such as secretions toward the side channels to which suction can be attached. It comes with an elbow connector for suctioning.

The tube also has an in-built bite-block, reducing the risk of patients' biting the airway.

Anterior to the cuff, there is a hand-tab attached which allows manipulation by manually curving the mask during insertion.

It is always inserted in the neutral position. At the proximal end, there are loops which help in fixation of the mask.

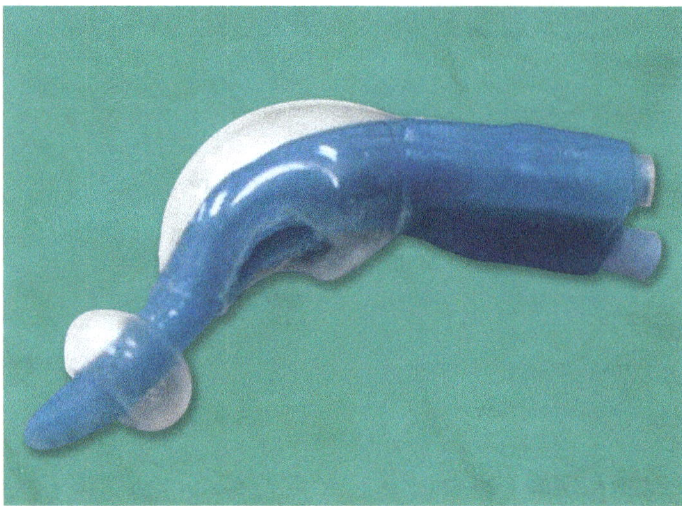

Fig. 21: Elisha airway device.
Courtesy: J Doctor, SN Myatra. Department of Anaesthesia, Critical Care and Pain, Tata Memorial Hospital, Mumbai.

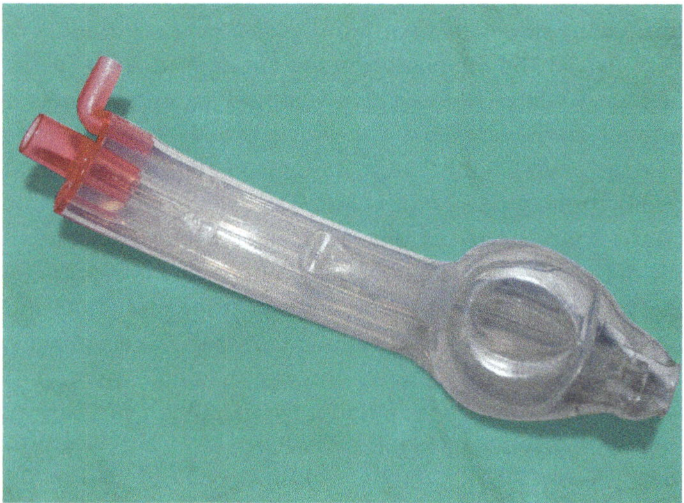

Fig. 22: Baska mask airway.
Courtesy: J Doctor, SN Myatra. Department of Anaesthesia, Critical Care and Pain, Tata Memorial Hospital, Mumbai.

It comes in four sizes that have color coded 15-mm connecters: sizes 3—green, 4—yellow, 5—red, 6—blue. The pediatric sizes are under development.

Other SADs like the cuffed oropharyngeal airway (COPA) and the pharyngeal airway express (PAX) are no longer manufactured.

SUPRAGLOTTIC AIRWAY DEVICES IN SPECIAL SITUATIONS

Laryngeal Mask Airway in Prone Position

The use of the Classic™ LMA in the prone position is controversial, but the ProSeal™ LMA (ProSeal™ LMA) may be more suitable, as it forms a better seal and provides access to the stomach. A retrospective audit done by Brimacombe JR et al. has suggested that the insertion of and maintenance of anesthesia with the ProSeal™ LMA in the prone position is feasible only by experienced users.[20]

Laryngeal Mask Airway in the Obstetric Patient

The LMA is a part of the difficult airway algorithm for the obstetric difficult airway. When tracheal intubation has failed, ventilation with mask and cricoid pressure or with an LMA or SAD should be considered for maintaining an airway and ventilating the lungs. The AIDAA 2016 guidelines for the management of unanticipated difficult intubation in Obstetrics recommend the use of a second generation SGD with the release of cricoid pressure during insertion of the SGD.[3]

Laryngeal Mask Airway in Cardiopulmonary Cerebral Resuscitation

Supraglottic airways that have been studied in cardiac arrest are the LMA, the esophageal-tracheal tube (Combitube) and the LT or King LT. When prehospital providers are trained in the use of advanced supraglottic airways (SGD), they have replaced the Combitube.

Laryngeal Mask Airway in Obesity

The LMA is contraindicated in grossly or morbidly obese patients because of the increased risk of regurgitation and the requirements for high-airway pressure ventilation.[21] However, it is indicated for airway rescue in emergency situations and the ProSeal™ LMA may be used as a temporary ventilatory device before laryngoscope-guided tracheal intubation.[22]

Laryngeal Mask Airway in Laparoscopy

The LMA ProSeal™ and Supreme™ offers a cuff that allows a higher seal pressure than the LMA Classic™, and a drain tube that allows venting of the stomach contents, and blind insertion of standard gastric tubes. All these factors are designed to reduce gastric insufflation, regurgitation, and subsequent pulmonary aspiration. These properties of the LMAs (LMA ProSeal™ and LMA Supreme™) and i-gel offer greater protection regarding aspiration pneumonitis. Since 2002, several clinical studies have recommended their use for laparoscopic surgery.[23] Only SAD devices, which offer higher seal pressures and the provision for passing gastric tubes should be recommended for use in laparoscopic surgery.

INTUBATION THROUGH SUPRAGLOTTIC AIRWAY DEVICE

Supraglottic airway device can facilitate tracheal intubation in patients with a difficult intubation. The AIDAA 2016 guidelines for the management of unanticipated difficult tracheal intubation, do not recommend blind intubation through the SGD. Intubation through the supraglottic airway should always be under vision using an FOB with or without the use of an Aintree catheter.

Blind Intubation

If the SAD is perfectly positioned, the aperture lies against the glottic inlet, and making blind tracheal intubation possible. However, the success rate is low and variable and hence the ILMA (described earlier) was designed. In most SADs, the long length and narrow diameter of the shaft, fixed 15-mm adapter, and mask aperture bars make blind tracheal intubation difficult and removal of the SAD over the ETT challenging. Larger ETT can be used with the air-Q, as it has a shaft with larger internal diameters and a removable connector. This is not recommended by the AIDAA 2016 guidelines for the management of unanticipated difficult tracheal intubation.

One-step Fiberoptic-assisted Intubation

The average distance of the LMA grille to the vocal cords is 3.5 cm, and leaving only 4.5 cm of tube length beyond the vocal cords. Hence, there is a chance of inflating the cuff of the ETT in the larynx increasing the possibility of laryngeal nerve damage. Both success rate and safety of intubation are highest when the intubation is done under vision using a fiberscope. The ETT is threaded over the fiberscope, which is then passed through the glottis opening into the trachea and then the ETT is railroaded into the trachea over the fiberscope. After tracheal intubation, the fiberscope is removed. The ILMA though designed for blind intubation, has an intubation failure rate, however, of 3–4% due to poor alignment of the epiglottis elevating bar. Fiberoptic guidance can increase the success rate to 100%.[12]

Two-step Fiberoptic-assisted Intubation

This technique uses an Aintree intubating catheter (Cook Medical), which is passed over a fiberoptic scope, which is passed through the SAD into the trachea. The SAD and FOB are then removed, leaving only the Aintree catheter in the trachea. This serves as a bougie to guide the ETT into the trachea. Oxygen delivery can be continued through the hollow Aintree catheter and may increase the safety of the technique. The advantage of this technique is that since the ETT is passed over the catheter and not through the SAD; hence, there are no limitations to the size or type of the ETT that can be used unlike previous methods described.

SUPRAGLOTTIC AIRWAY DEVICE AS A BRIDGE TO EXTUBATION

Upper airway obstruction and hypoxemia may be commonly seen during extubation from general anesthesia in deeper planes before return of airway reflexes. On the other hand during an "awake" extubation, the patient has regained full airway reflexes and this can sometimes result in severe coughing, and adverse hemodynamic changes. SADs can provide a wonderful bridge to facilitate a smooth transition from deep anesthesia to awake intubation. The ETT is replaced with an SAD, while the patient is still in deep anesthesia. The SAD provides a stable and patent airway during emergence from anesthesia, which is helpful in situations where manipulation of the patient's head and neck or pressure from facemask application might harm the patient or the surgical result.

According to the AIDAA 2016 extubation guidelines, whenever deep extubation is to be performed in a normal airway the ETT tube can be replaced with an SGD either behind the ETT (Bailey's maneuver), railroading of an SGD over a tube exchanger passed through the ETT or after removal of the ETT.[6]

CONCLUSION

A new era of airway management was marked with the introduction of the cLMA more than 30 years ago. With improvements in design, which enhanced both safety and efficacy of the SAD, most of the earlier absolute contraindications for its use, are only relative today. SADs have not only enhanced airway management during elective surgery, but are a boon during difficult airway management and CPR. There are very few randomized controlled trials comparing different SADs in patients with difficult airways. Most of the safety data comes from extended use rather than high-quality evidence. Hence, claims of efficacy and particularly safety of specific devices must be interpreted with caution. Proper patient selection, attention to size selection, appropriate placement, and maintenance of an intracuff pressure will certainly help to enhance the safety and efficacy during SAD use. The SGD has become an integral part of various difficult airway algorithms across the globe.

REFERENCES

1. Luba K, Cutter TW. Supraglottic airway devices in the ambulatory setting. Anesthesiol Clin. 2010;28:295-314.
2. Myatra SN, Shah A, Kundra P, et al. All India Difficult Airway Association 2016 guidelines for the management of unanticipated difficult tracheal intubation in adults. Indian J Anaesth. 2016;60:885-98.
3. Ram Kumar V, Dinesh E, Shetty SR, et al. All India Difficult Airway Association 2016 guidelines for the management of unanticipated difficult tracheal intubation in obstetrics. Indian J Anaesth. 2016;60:899-905.
4. Pawar DK, Doctor JR, Raveendra US, et al. All India Difficult Airway Association 2016 guidelines for the management of unanticipated difficult tracheal intubation in Paediatrics. Indian J Anaesth. 2016;60:906-14.
5. Myatra SN, Ahmed SM, Kundra P, et al. The All India Difficult Airway Association 2016 guidelines for tracheal intubation in the Intensive Care Unit. Indian J Anaesth. 2016;60: 922-30.
6. Kundra P, Garg R, Patwa A, et al. All India Difficult Airway Association 2016 guidelines for the management of anticipated difficult extubation. Indian J Anaesth. 2016;60: 915-21.
7. Miller DM. A proposed classification and scoring system for supraglottic sealing airways: a brief review. Anesth Analg. 2004;99:1553-9.

8. Cook TM. Third generation supraglottic airway devices: an undefined concept and misused term. Time for an updated classification of supraglottic airway devices. Br J Anaesth. 2015;115:633-4.
9. Miller DM. Third generation supraglottic airways: is a new classification needed? Br J Anaesth. 2015;115:634-5.
10. Teleflex Inc. (2020). LMA. [online] Available from http://www.lmana.com. [Last accessed December, 2020].
11. Gerstein N, Braude DA, Hung O, et al. The FastTrack intubating laryngeal mask airway: an overview and update. Can J Anaesth. 2010;57:588-601.
12. Ferson DZ, Rosenblatt WH, Johansen MJ, et al. Use of the intubating LMA-FastTrack in 254 patients with difficult-to manage airways. Anesthesiology. 2001;95:1175-81.
13. Ambu A/S. (2017). Ambu. [online] Available from http://www.ambu.com. [Last accessed November, 2017].
14. Hooshangi H, Wong D. Brief review: the Cobra perilaryngeal airway (CobraPLA) and the streamlined liner of pharyngeal airway (SLIPA) supraglottic airways. Can J Anesth. 2008;55: 177-85.
15. VBM Medizintechnik GmbH. (2017). VBM. [online] Available from http://www.vbm-medical.de. [Last accessed November, 2017].
16. SLIPA. (2016). Streamlined Liner of the Pharynx Airway. [online] Available from http://www.slipa.com. [Last accessed November, 2017].
17. Intersurgical Ltd. (2017). Intersurgical complete respiratory systems. i-gel. [online] Available from http://www.i-gel.com. [Last accessed November, 2017].
18. Vaida S, Gaitini D, Ben-David B, et al. A new supraglottic airway, the Elisha Airway Device: a preliminary study. Anesth Analg. 2004;99:124-7.
19. Baska Mask. (2017). Baska Mask. [online] Available from http://baskamask.net. [Last accessed November, 2017].
20. Brimacombe JR, Wenzel V, Keller C. The proseal laryngeal mask airway in prone patients: a retrospective audit of 245 patients. Anaesth Intensive Care. 2007;35:222-5.
21. Brimacombe JR, Brain AI, Berry A. The Laryngeal Mask Airway: A Review and Practical Guide. London: WB Saunders; 1997.
22. Keller C, Brimacombe J, Kleinsasser A, et al. The Laryngeal Mask Airway ProSeal™ as a temporary ventilatory device in grossly and morbidly obese patients before laryngoscope-guided tracheal intubation. Anesth Analg. 2002;94:737-40.
23. Beleña JM, Núñez M, Gracia JL, et al. The Laryngeal Mask Airway Supreme™: safety and efficacy during gynaecological laparoscopic surgery. South Afr J Anaesth Analg. 2012;18:143-7.

Nonrebreathing Valves

Prerana N Shah

ABSTRACT

Nonrebreathing valves, as the name implies, prevent rebreathing of the gases by ensuring unidirectional flow of gases. Their use is mostly restricted to manual resuscitation as most anesthesiologists use circle absorber system. The role of nonrebreathing valves has been highlighted in clinical situation where it plays vital role during maintenance of anesthesia and provides stability to circulatory, respiratory, and neurological system. It ultimately ensures safe intraoperative period.

INTRODUCTION

Nonrebreathing valves (NRV) ensure unidirectional flow of gases. During inspiration, gases flow exclusively into the patient port, while during exhalation, they vent out through the expiratory port.[1]

VALVE TERMINOLOGY

- *Valve body assembly:* It is the housing with associated internal parts
- *Valve body:* It is the housing for valve body assembly
- *Valve seat/seating:* It is the surface with a partially or completely obstructed opening
- *Valve inlet:* Fresh gas enters the valve through the inlet and is usually a 22-mm male connection
- *Patient port:* It is the part attached to mask or endotracheal tube (ETT) or supraglottic device. It is usually a 15-mm female connection with a concentric 22 mm male connector
- *Exhalation port:* It is the channel through which exhaled gases escape to atmosphere or scavenging system after having passed through valve.

VARIOUS TYPES OF NONREBREATHING VALVES

- *Positional:* This type of NRV must remain horizontal as it requires gravity to close it completely
- *Nonpositional:* It is closed by elastic tension of rubber or by spring
- *Flap:* It has a movable part made of flexible material and is secured at its centre or its edge
- *Fish mouth:* It is a special type of flap valve in which two flaps approximate at midpoint
- *Disk:* It has movable part that is flat and made of plastic or metal. It is held on its seat by gravity or spring disk
- *Mushroom:* It has a hollow balloon-like structure that occludes the opening when inflated
- *Relief valve:* It is an optional valve but recommended to vent the excess gas to atmosphere.

Classification

Nonrebreathing valve can be classified depending upon the type of respiratory function and the position.

Depending on the Type of Respiratory Function

The patient exerts a negative pressure which is transmitted to the inside of the valve during spontaneous ventilation. However, during controlled respiration, a positive pressure exists inside the valve during inspiration.

Valves designed for spontaneous respiration, e.g., Stephen Slater valve: During inspiration, the negative pressure exerted by the patient closes the exhalation port. During exhalation the pressure in the valve increases and gas escapes through the exhalation port. If this valve is to be used for controlled ventilation, it is essential to close the exhalation port with a finger during inspiration.

Valves designed for controlled respiration, e.g., (artificial mandatory breathing unit) AMBU resuscitation valve: In this type of valve, a rise in pressure opens the inlet and closes the exhalation port. If the patient is allowed to breathe spontaneously, room air through the exhalation port will be inspired. Hence, it cannot be useful for general anesthesia.

*Valves designed for both spontaneous and controlled ventilation **(Fig. 1)**:* Ruben valve, AMBU E, and Lewis Leigh valve can be used for both spontaneous and controlled ventilation. The exhalation port is closed and the inlet opens during inspiration with either controlled or spontaneous respirations. Only dual purpose valves are used during anesthesia.

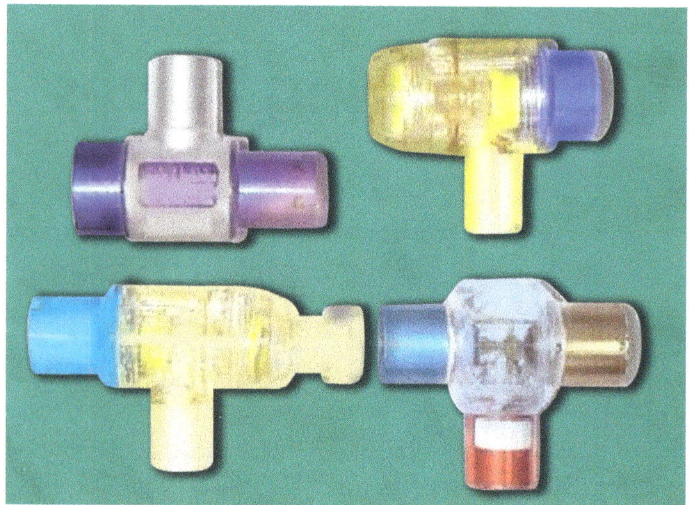

Fig. 1: Ruben, artificial mandatory breathing unit and Mitchell valve.

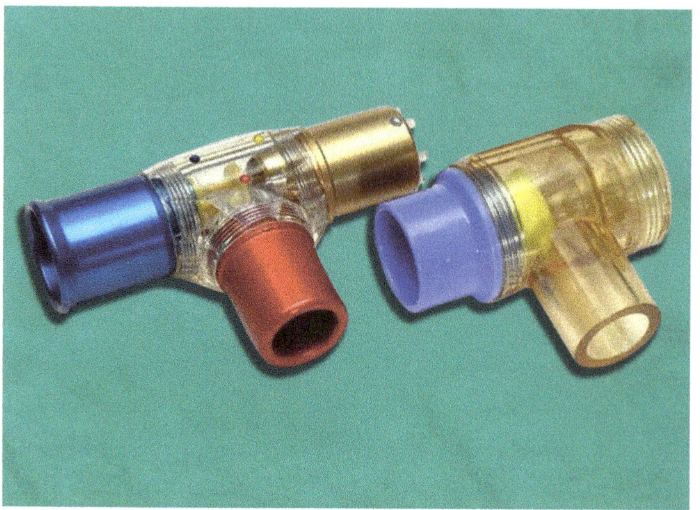

Fig. 2: Ruben and artificial mandatory breathing unit E2.

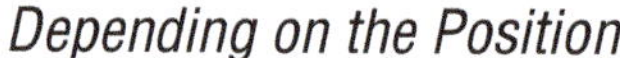

Depending on the Position

Positional valve: It works on gravity.

Nonpositional: It is not dependant on any position, e.g., flap valve, fish mouth valve, disk type.

Aga-poly valve: It is used with Sanjivani manual resuscitation bag for giving general anesthesia. It has inspiratory limb, expiratory limb, patient end and vaporizer end. It has a dead space of about 7–8 mL and has low resistance. It is available as simple poly valve to be used with ventilator and revivator valve with oxygen attachment.

AMBU E, AMBU Hesse, AMBU E2 can be used as dual purpose valves.

AMBU valve: It is available in various variants and is used for controlled ventilation. It is commonly used with AMBU resuscitation bag **(Fig. 2)**.

It is made of metal or plastic material. It has a movable yellow plastic disk that is held in place by a spring. A locating pin centers the disk.

When the AMBU resuscitation bag is squeezed, the force of the gas pushes the disk to close the exhalation port, thus allowing the inhalation. During exhalation the pressure on the inlet side of the disk falls and the spring pushes the disk to close the inlet, thereby allowing the exhaled gases to pass through the exhalation port. During spontaneous ventilation, the interior of disk does not move and the patient inhales atmospheric air.

When reassembling it after disassembling for cleaning, the guide pin must be inserted through the appropriate channel.

AMBU E valve: The unidirectional flow of gases is controlled by two labial flap valves one each for inhalation and exhalation. It can be used for both spontaneous and controlled respiration. It is made up of transparent plastic. The inlet end is blue colored.

During spontaneous respiration the negative pressure during inspiration closes the valve at the expiratory port and the fresh gases flow in through the inspiratory port. During expiration, the valve at the inspiratory port closes and the valve at the expiratory port opens so as to allow the expired gases to be vented to the atmosphere. The valve at the expiratory port prevents inhalation of the downstream gases during spontaneous ventilation. When AMBU E is used for controlled ventilation, higher amount of gases are required to produce a complete expiratory seal. If the flows are not high, the seal may be incomplete allowing some of the inspiratory gas to pass straight across the valve. Hence, lower tidal volumes are delivered. It has a dead space of 10 mL. It cannot be used with resuscitators that do not produce initial high surge of gas required to produce an effective seal.

AMBU E2 valve: It contains single unidirectional valve with no valve at the expiratory end. It can be used for spontaneous and controlled respiration. The negative pressure created by the patient during spontaneous inspiration opens the inspiratory port. It also draws air from the expiratory port. The result is that a mixture of fresh gas and air is inhaled. During controlled respiration the positive pressure from bag, the expiratory port is occluded by inspiratory valve, so that fresh gases pass to the patient. During expiration, the inspiratory port closes and exhaled gases pass through the expiratory port to the atmosphere. It has a dead space of 10 mL.

AMBU Hesse valve: It is similar to AMBU E valve, but is slightly larger in size. It can be used for both spontaneous and controlled respiration. It has an inspiratory leaf, an expiratory leaf and a mushroom valve. When used for controlled ventilation, small increase in pressure within the self inflating bag due to manual compression expands the elastic mushroom valve that completely occludes the expiratory port. Further compression of the bag opens the inspiratory leaf valve, forcing gas from the bag into the inspiratory port thus providing inspiratory flow. At the beginning of exhalation phase the self inflating bag starts to re-expand. The reduced pressure within causes the mushroom valve to collapse and the inspiratory leaf valve to close, sealing the bag off from the main valve. The exhaled gases then leave the system through the expiratory port via the expiratory leaf valve.

During spontaneous breathing, the negative pressure produced by the patient during inspiration causes the expiratory leaf valve to close, sealing the expiratory port. This ensures that the inspired gas is drawn from the bag and not from the ambient air through the expiratory port. It has a dead space of 14 mL.

AMBU valves can be disassembled for cleaning and the parts may be boiled, autoclaved or gas sterilized.

Fink valve: It can be used for both spontaneous and controlled ventilation. It comes as either straight or right angle valve. The valve body is made of metal. It has a flexible diaphragm above exhalation port. The pressure tube from inlet side of inspiratory flap valve can communicate to atmosphere through a top vent over diaphragm. It has an adjusting knob at top connected to rotating disk.

During spontaneous ventilation, the knob is turned clockwise. During inspiration, negative pressure exerted by patient opens inhalation flap and closes exhalation flap. On exhalation, inspiratory valve is closed by exhaling gases.

During controlled ventilation, knob is turned counter clockwise maximally. When the bag is squeezed, pressure in inlet increases and the diaphragm is pushed downwards on the exhalation flap. Gases flow to the patient through the inhalational flap. During exhalation, pressure at the inlet decreases, inhalation flap closes, diaphragm moves upward, exhalation flap opens and gases pass to atmosphere. The valve can be gas sterilized after disassembling and washing the parts.

Frumin valve: It can be used for spontaneous or controlled ventilation. It has 90° and 180° models. It has a clear plastic body with rubber or silicon inspiratory flap valve and inflating rubber mushroom valve which covers exhalation port. Pressure channel connects inlet with cavity of mushroom valve.

During controlled ventilation, pressure on mushroom and common chamber is same during inspiration but as mushroom's surface area is more than expiratory valve seat, gases do not pass out through the expiratory port. As pressure at inlet drops mushroom deflates and gases pass to atmosphere.

During spontaneous respiration, inspiratory flap is pulled open to draw fresh gas.

The valve can be gas sterilized after disassembling and washing the parts. It helps in determining the true dead space-to-tidal volume ratios.[2]

Laerdal valve: It can be used for spontaneous and controlled ventilation. It has a clear plastic body and contains a rubber inspiratory fish mouth valve with a circular flange. A circular exhalation flap valve occludes the exhalation port. It is available in three sizes, i.e. adult, child and infant. All sizes have 23 mm external diameter expiratory port and 22 mm external diameter or 15 mm internal diameter inspiratory port to minimize misconnections.

During spontaneous respiration the fish mouth valve opens and allows the gas to pass to the patient during inspiration. Almost simultaneously the outer disk portion of the valve is pushed against the apertures in the valve body, thus sealing the expiratory port. The exhalation flap prevents the room air from being inhaled through the exhalation ports. During exhalation, the fish mouth valve closes, preventing rebreathing into the bag. It also lifts the outer disk shaped portion of the expiratory apertures thus allowing exhaled gases to escape.

During controlled ventilation the pressure at the inlet opens the fish mouth valve and pushes the exhalation ports during inspiration. This allows the fresh gases to pass to the patient and prevents its loss through the exhalation ports. During exhalation the valve functions the same as with spontaneous respirations.

The child and infant valves have overpressure safety valves built into the inspiratory port and are set to blow off at a pressure of 45 cmH_2O. If needed, the safety valve can be over-ridden by finger pressure or a lock clip over the valve. It has a dead space of 7 mL.

The valve can be disassembled to clean or repair broken parts. It can be cleaned with chemical solutions, boiling or autoclaving.

Lewis-Leigh inflation (Sanjivani) valve **(Fig. 3)**: It can be used for spontaneous or controlled ventilation. It has a clear plastic body with a chimney which may be rotated 90°. This changes the position of the exhalation valve seat at the bottom of the chimney. A disk type valve is located at the top of the exhalation chimney. The rubber flap valve can seat either on the ridge of the body or on the lower end of the chimney. When the chimney is rotated counterclockwise the flap valve is prevented from seating on the chimney but not on the ridge. This valve is a modification of the Digby Leigh valve. The Digby Leigh valve had a simple disk type exhalation valve instead of the chimney. It was necessary to close the exhalation valve with the finger when controlled or assisted ventilation was used.

During inspiration, the flap valve moves away from its seat on the body and closes the base of the chimney. The disk valve in the chimney prevents air from being drawn into the valve during spontaneous ventilation. Gas hence flows to the patient. At the end of inspiration, when the pressure in the system returns to atmospheric, the flap valve returns to its resting position over the fresh gas inlet.

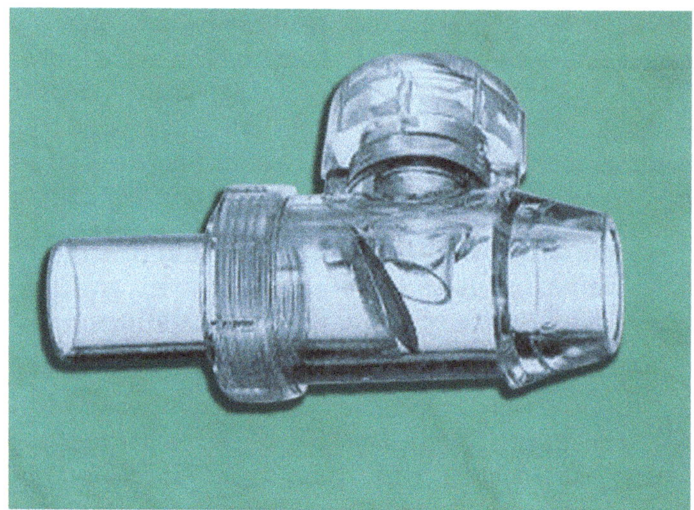

Fig. 3: Lewis-Leigh valve.

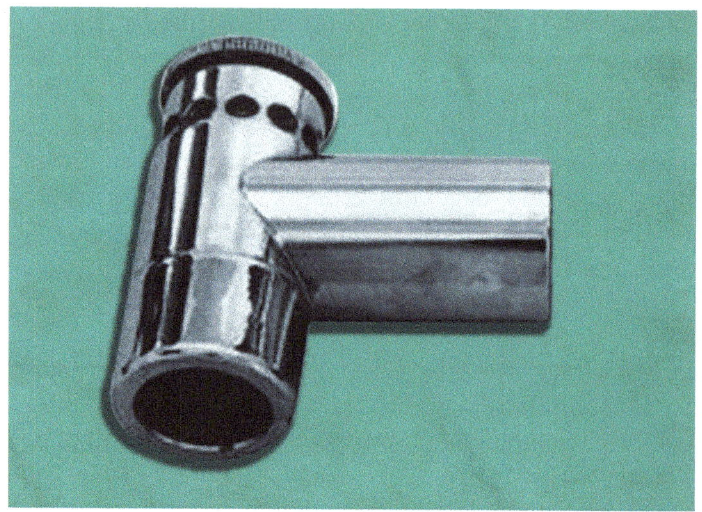

Fig. 4: Stephen Slater valve.

As the patient exhales, the increased pressure lifts the disk valve, so that the gas escapes to the atmosphere. When the chimney is rotated 90° counterclockwise, gas can then leak through the valve to atmosphere. This provides a safety factor by preventing pressure increases in the system.

The valve can be gas sterilized or via cold chemical sterilization technique.

Ruben (Danish) valve: Ruben resuscitation valve can be used only for controlled respiration, while Ruben mark 2 is a dual purpose valve. It has a clear plastic body with metal fittings. It is a multicolored valve in which blue color is inlet, gold color is outlet and red color end is patients end. Perforated end is for exhaled gases to escape to atmosphere. Ruben valve has a spring loaded bobbin within the valve housing. A disk type valve is near the exhalation port.

At rest, the spring holds the bobbin away from the expiratory port and against the inspiratory port allowing exhalation to occur. When the bag is squeezed, the bobbin is forced across the valve housing, so that the expiratory port is occluded and the inspiratory port is connected to the patient port and prevents gases leaking out through the expiratory port. In spontaneous respiration, the patient draws air from the inspiratory limb, forcing the bobbin to move and occlude the expiratory port. When the pressure at the inlet drops, the force of the spring pushes the piston against the inlet. During exhalation the pressure of the exhaled gases causes the disk valve to open. The gas then passes to the atmosphere.

When the valve is to be used with resuscitation equipment, the exhalation valve is not present. This allows the patient to inspire from the atmosphere. It has a dead space of 9 mL.

It is a very noisy valve. With the presence of backward leak, exhaled gases may go back to reservoir bag and rebreathing can occur. If it sticks in inspiration, high pressure may be formed leading to barotrauma. If exposed to heat it may deteriorate.

It is difficult to clean and can be done by flushing the channels with soap and water. It can also be gas sterilized.

Stephen Slater valve ***(Fig. 4)****:* It is used only for spontaneous ventilation. The valve body is made of metal. It has two rubber flaps each secured by shaft at its center.

Inspiratory flap valve is opened by patient's negative pressure. During exhalation, pressure in valve rises, inspiratory flap opens and gas flows to atmosphere.

The valve can be gas sterilized after disassembling and washing the parts.

IDEAL NONREBREATHING VALVE

It should have minimal dead space, minimal resistance, no forward or backward leak, light weight, transparent, easy to clean and sterilize, non-noisy, nonsticky, compact and inexpensive with minimal opening pressure.

Nonrebreathing valves prevent rebreathing. The inspired concentration of gases and vapors can be controlled as there is no mixing. It helps in dissipation of heat and water vapor. It can be used for spontaneous and controlled respiration. They are compact, lightweight and mobile with minimal dead space. However, as large flows are needed, there is wastage of gases and loss of heat and humidity from the patient. It also leads to theater pollution.

CONCLUSION

Although several valves are available, use of valve in anesthesia practise is reducing as circle absorber is preferred.

REFERENCES

1. Dorsch JA, Dorsch SE. Manual Resuscitators. In: Dorsch JA, Dorsch SE (Eds). Understanding Anaesthesia Equipments, 5th edition. Philadelphia: Wolters Kluwer Health/Lippincott Williams and Wilkins; 2008.
2. Forbat AF, Her C. Correction of gas compression in mechanical ventilators. Anesth Analg. 1980;59(7):488-93.

18

CHAPTER

Airways

Prerana N Shah

ABSTRACT

Airways are devices that can be passed orally or through nose to maintain the patency of air passages. They are available in different sizes and varieties depending on the utility. The oropharyngeal, initially they were made up of metal but were replaced by plastic one. The advantages of plastic have been highlighted. The airways were modified as per needs, such as for suction, as intubator was designed for blind orotracheal intubations and lateral suction channels, groove in the center of the lingual surface for fiberoptic scope and a slit in the distal end that allows manipulation in the anteroposterior direction.

The nasopharyngeal airway is useful in clinical situation, such as maintain the airway, patients who have limited mouth opening, or pathology of oral cavity that makes it difficult to insert oral airway.

INTRODUCTION

Airway is a device which helps maintain the patency of the air passage for unobstructed breathing. Unlike other maneuvers to maintain a patent airway, including chin lift, jaw thrust and tracheal intubation, insertion of an airway does not affect the stability of the cervical spine.[1]

TYPES

They can be of various types viz. oropharyngeal, nasopharyngeal, modified-laryngeal mask airway, cuffed oropharyngeal airway (COPA), etc.

USES

- It prevents obstruction of the upper air passage by lifting the tongue and epiglottis away from the posterior pharyngeal wall
- It prevents biting and occlusion of the orotracheal tube
- It protects the tongue during biting and seizure activity
- It facilitates oropharyngeal suctioning
- It provides a better mask fit for ventilation
- It helps insertion of tubular devices into pharynx or esophagus.

OROPHARYNGEAL AIRWAY

It is a curved apparatus made of metal, plastic or hard rubber. It has a flange at the proximal (buccal) end which limits the depth of insertion. It may also serve as a means to fix the airway in place. The flange may or may not rest on the patients lips depending on whether the particular airway being used is the correct size. The bite portion is straight and fits between the teeth or gums. It should be firm so that the patient cannot close the air channel by biting hard.

The pharyngeal end is the curved portion of the airway that extends upward and backward to correspond to the shape of the tongue and palate. It separates the tongue from posterior pharyngeal wall and by pressures along the base of the tongue pulls the epiglottis slightly forward. When inserted, the distal end should lie just above the epiglottis so as to not irritate the laryngeal inlet **(Figs. 1 and 2)**.

The oropharyngeal airways are oval or circular in cross section and are produced in varying lengths and diameters to suit different sizes of patients (from neonates to large adults). Oropharyngeal airway has a flange to prevent over insertion, a straight bite block portion and a curved section.

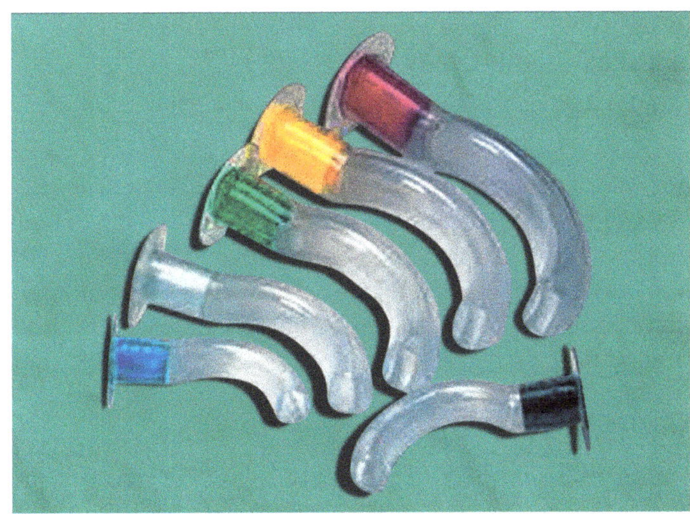

Fig. 1: Oropharyngeal airway.

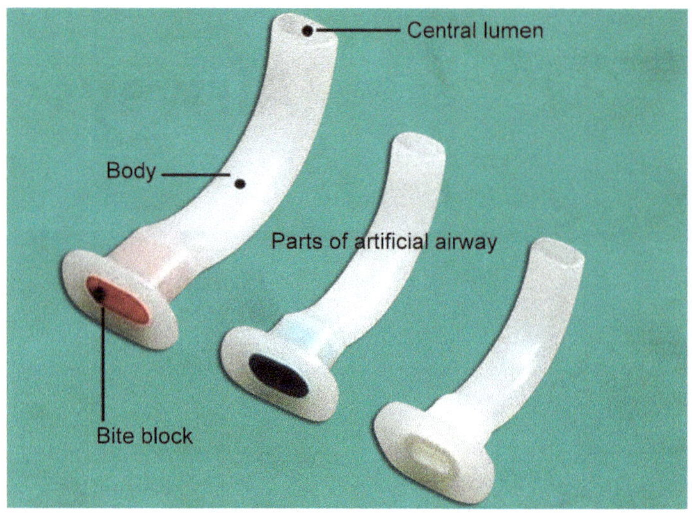

Fig. 2: Parts of oropharyngeal airway.

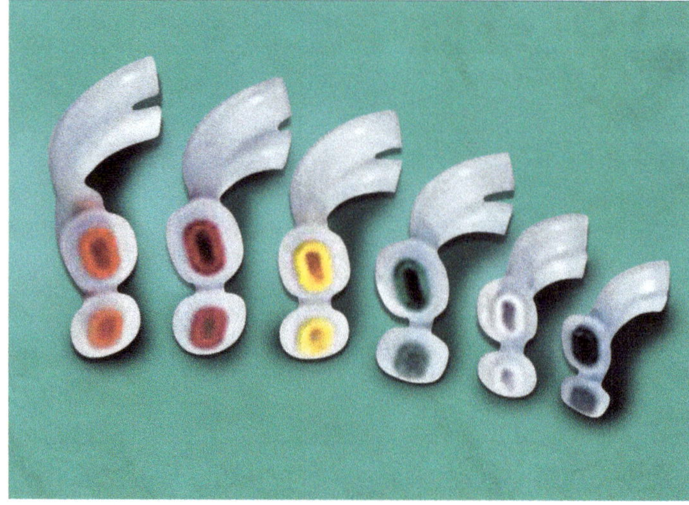

Fig. 3: Guedel airway.

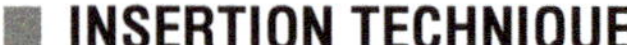

INSERTION TECHNIQUE

An estimate of the appropriate size is obtained by selecting it with the length corresponding to the vertical distance between the patient's incisor and the angle of the jaw. Too small an airway may cause kinking of the tongue and obstructing gas movement. Too large an airway may cause obstruction by displacing the epiglottis and may traumatize the larynx. The patient's mouth is opened and a well-lubricated airway is inserted into the oral cavity in the upside down position as far as the junction between the head and the soft palate and then rotated through 180°. It is then inserted further until it lies in the oropharynx. This rotation technique minimizes the chance of pushing the tongue backward and downward. Correct placement is shown by improvement in airway patency and by seating of the flattened reinforced section between the patient's teeth or alveolar margins if the patient is edentulous. Alternatively, a tongue blade may be used to depress the tongue. The airway is held horizontal as the tip is inserted into the mouth. As the airway is advanced it is rotated into a vertical position. This causes it to slide around behind the tongue.

TYPES OF ORAL AIRWAY

Guedel Airway[1]

It is most frequent airway that is used. The bite portions are color coded to provide easy identification of size. It is available in sizes 0-6. It is made up of rubber and is a hollow oropharyngeal airway with a large flange and a reinforced bite portion. It has a gentle curve that follows the contour of the tongue and has a tubular channel for air exchange and suction **(Fig. 3)**.

Waters Airway

It is named after Ralph Waters and is available in sizes 00, 0, 1-7. It is a metallic oropharyngeal airway with two holes at the pharyngeal end. It is hollow and has a nipple on the flange for oxygen and suction. It can be cleaned with soap and water **(Fig. 4)**.

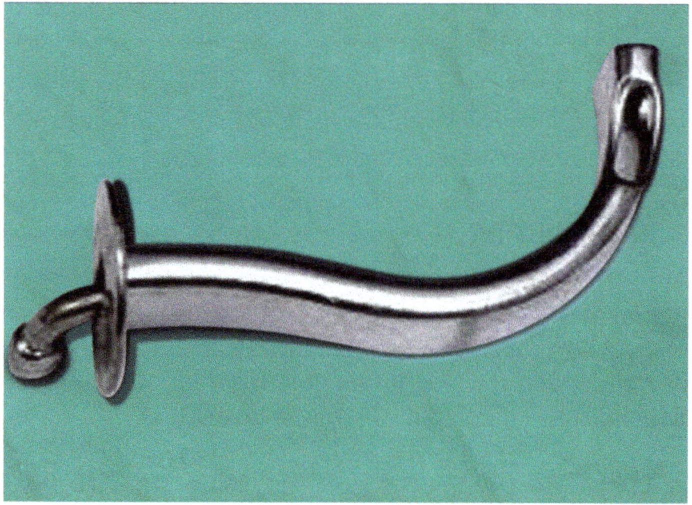

Fig. 4: Waters airway.

Safar's Airway

It is available in sizes for adult and pediatric. It is an "S" shaped airway that looks like two airways joined together. It is made of nontraumatic soft rubber. It is mainly used for artificial resuscitation **(Fig. 5)**.

Connell Airway

It is available in sizes 00, 0, 1-7. It is a metallic hollow oropharyngeal airway and is similar to waters airway but has no insufflation nipple. It can give problems to those who have latex allergy. It can be cleaned with soap and water. However, repeated sterilization may cause softening. Its design could have use in the management of a patient's airway during sedation **(Fig. 6)**.[2]

Berman Intubation Pharyngeal Airway

Sizes are available for infant, small child, child, medium adult, and large adult. It has no enclosed air channel.

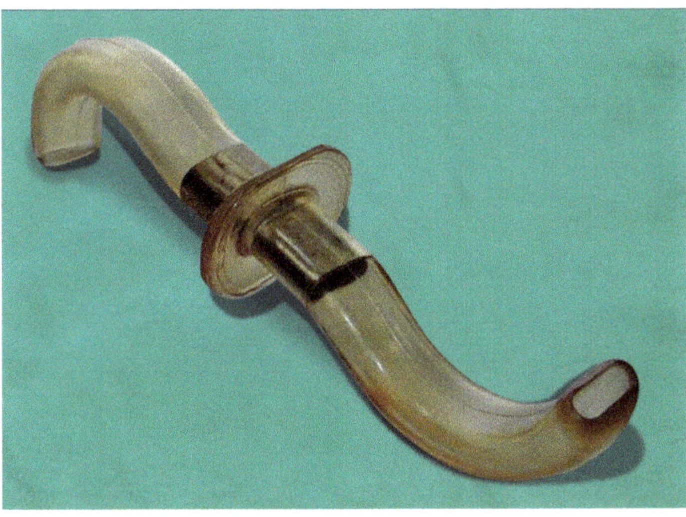

Fig. 5: Safar's airway.

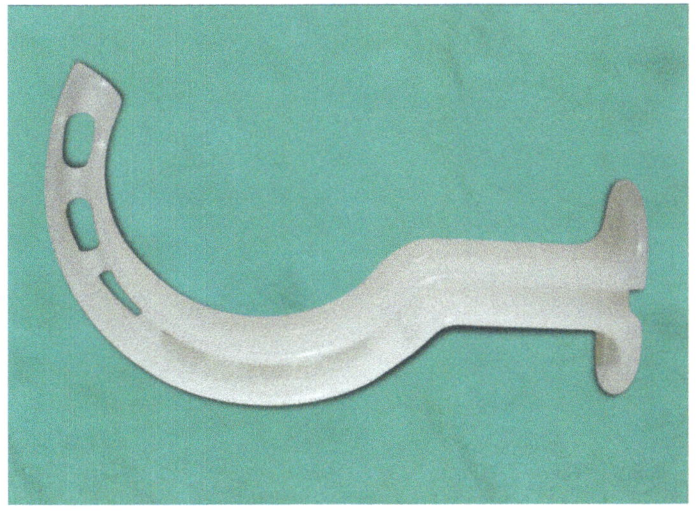

Fig. 7: Berman airway.

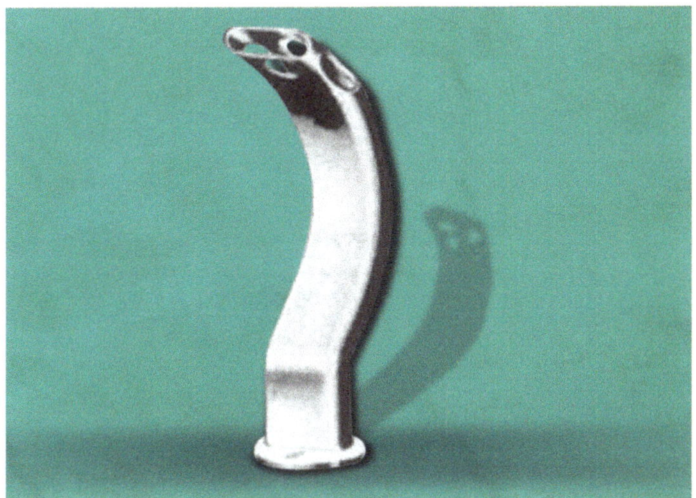

Fig. 6: Connell airway.

The sides are cut open and there is support through the center. The sides allow passage of suction catheters and provide air channels. The center may have openings in it to permit suction if the airway becomes lodged sideways. It has a flange at the buccal end. It is easier to clean and is less likely to become obstructed with foreign body or mucus. However, the anterior jaw lift was more effective than the Berman device for assisting fibreoptic orotracheal intubation.[3] Though the Williams Airway Intubator and the Berman Oropharyngeal Airway were superior to Ovassapian airway, further research is needed in this field to meet the requirements of endoscopists in situations when it is crucial that equipment reliably fulfills its function.[4] The Berman airway offers easier visualization of the vocal cords than the Ovassapian airway, provided that the Berman airway is of an adequate size and positioned in the midline. Upon impingement of the intubation tube, completing the tracheal intubation is more difficult with the Berman airway than the Ovassapian airway **(Fig. 7)**.[5]

Ovassapian Fiberoptic Intubating Airway

It is designed for use during fiberoptic intubation. The proximal end is tubular and narrow that gradually widens at the distal end. The distal part does not have any posterior wall. Hence, the distal end of the fiberscope can be maneuvered in this open space in the oropharynx. The lingual surface is flat. There are two side walls and two pairs of curved guide walls between the side walls. The guide walls curve toward each other, leaving a space for a tracheal tube up to size 9 and are flexible so that the airway can be removed from around the tracheal tube after intubation has been completed. It is not necessary to remove the tracheal tube connector when using this airway for fibreoptic intubation **(Fig. 8)**.

Patil-Syracuse Oral Airway or Patil Endoscopic Airway

It is made of aluminum and is useful for fiberoptic intubation. It has lateral suction channels, groove in the center of the lingual surface for fiberoptic scope and a slit in the distal end that allows manipulation in the anteroposterior direction **(Fig. 9)**.

Williams Airway Intubator

The Williams airway intubator was designed for blind orotracheal intubations. It can also be used to aid fiberoptic intubations or as an oral airway. It is made of plastic and available in two sizes, number 9 and number 10, which will admit up to an 8.0 or 8.5 internal diameter (ID) tracheal tube, respectively. The tracheal tube connector should be removed during intubation, because it will not pass through the airway unless the airway is modified. The proximal half is cylindrical, while the distal half is open on its lingual surface **(Fig. 10)**.

A comparison of the Williams airway intubator with the Ovassapian fiberoptic intubating airway found that the

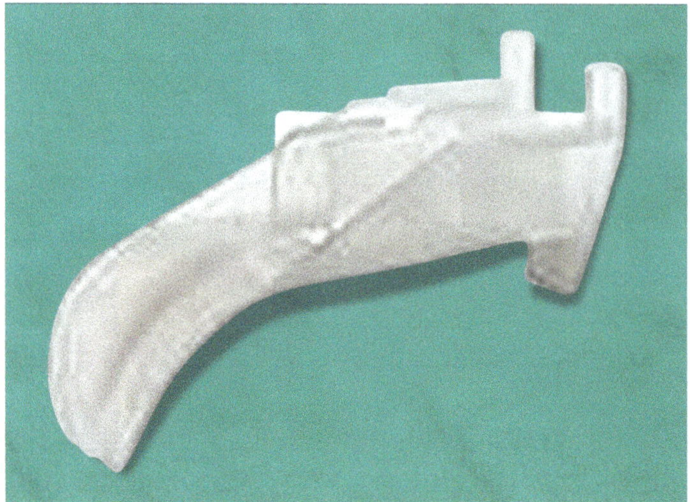

Fig. 8: Ovassapian fiberoptic intubating airway.

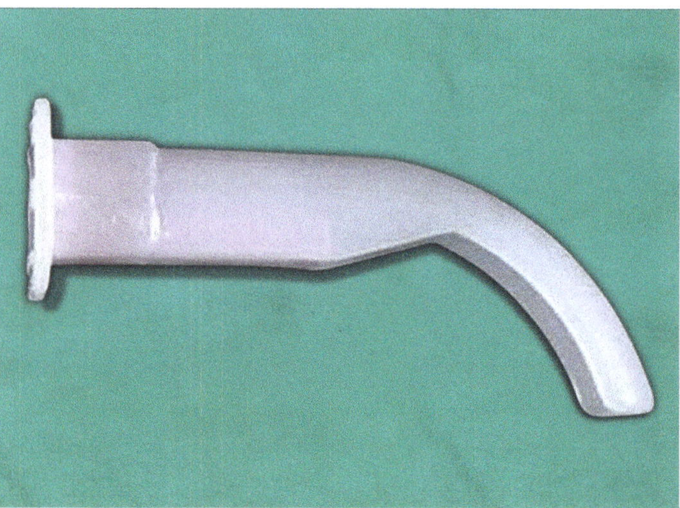

Fig. 10: Williams airway intubator.

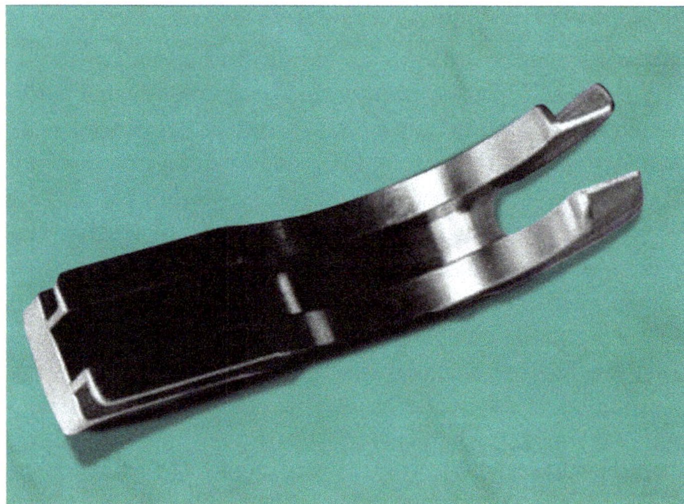

Fig. 9: Patil-Syracuse oral airway.

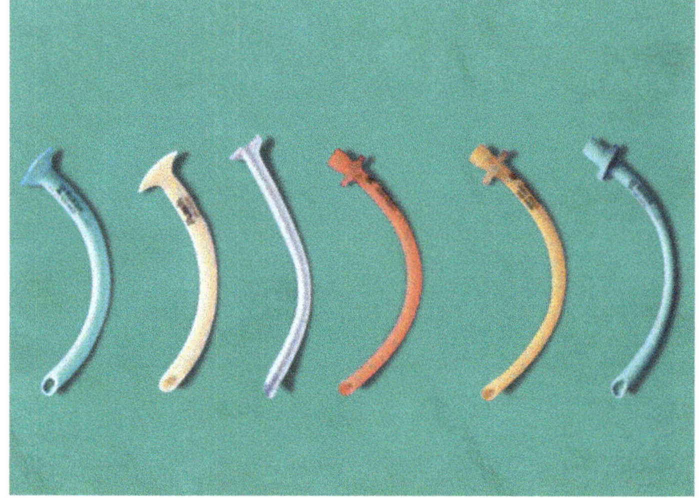

Fig. 11: Nasopharyngeal airways.

Williams airway intubator provided a better view of the glottis in a significant number of patients.[4]

Nasopharyngeal Airway

It is an alternative device that can be used to maintain the airway by inserting it through the nose. It is useful in patients who have limited mouth opening or pathology of oral cavity that makes it difficult to insert oral airway. Other uses of nasal airway are during pharyngeal surgery, fiberoptic bronchoscopy, to apply CPAP and facilitate suctioning. It is better tolerated in a semi-awake patient than an oral airway and is less likely to be accidentally displaced or removed **(Fig. 11)**.

Description

Nasopharyngeal airways are made of soft plastic, polyurethane or latex rubber and have either a fixed or adjustable flange at its proximal end and a beveled distal end. It curves to fit the curvature of the nasopharynx. It is available in a range of lengths and internal diameters.

Insertion Technique

The length of the airway needed for the patient is calculated as the distance from the tragus of the ear to the tip of the nose plus 1 inch or the distance from the tip of the nose to the meatus of the ear. After lubricating it along its entire length, it is held in the hand on the same side as it is to be inserted. It is inserted through the nares, bevel end first. It is passed vertically along the floor of the nose with slight twisting action and the curve of the airway should be directed toward the patient's feet. Do not proceed further if resistance is encountered. Either it should be redirected or passed through the other nostril or a smaller sized airway should be used. If placed appropriately, the pharyngeal end lies above the epiglottis and below the base of the tongue with the flange just outside the nostrils.

TYPES OF NASAL AIRWAY

Bardex Airway

It is made of rubber and has a large flange at the nasal end with bevel at pharyngeal end **(Fig. 12)**.

Binasal Airway

It consists of two nasal airways joined together by a connection that has a 15 mm adaptor for attachment to the breathing system. The distal tips are near the larynx just below the tip of epiglottis **(Fig. 13)**.

Cuffed Nasopharyngeal Airway

The cuffed nasopharyngeal (pharyngeal) airway is similar to a short cuffed tracheal tube. It is inserted through the nose into the pharynx. After inflating the cuff, it is pulled back until resistance is felt.

Epistaxis Airway

It is inserted into the nose and inflated. It is useful in epistaxis by providing local pressure and is available in several sizes **(Fig. 14)**.

Linder Nasopharyngeal Airway

It is a clear plastic airway with a large flange. The distal end is flat and not beveled. It is supplied with an introducer which has a balloon that can be inflated and deflated by attaching a Luer syringe to the one way valve at the other end of the introducer **(Fig. 15)**.

Rusch Airway

It is made of red rubber. It has an adjustable flange at the nasal end. The pharyngeal end has a short bevel **(Fig. 16)**.

Cuffed Oropharyngeal Airway

It was invented by Robert Greenberg at the John Hopkins Hospital, Baltimore, Maryland in 1990, and can be as an alternative to the face mask use during spontaneous ventilation anesthesia **(Fig. 17)**.

Description

It is color-coded according to sizes and is available in sizes 8–11. It is a modified Guedel type of oropharyngeal airway with an integral bite portion. The proximal end has a standard

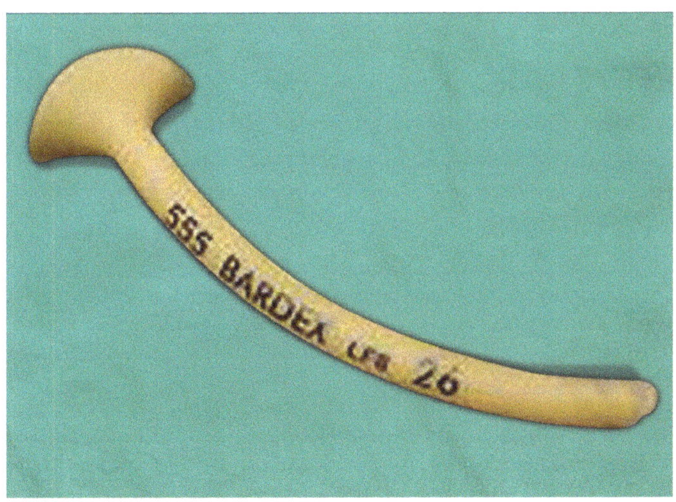

Fig. 12: Bardex nasopharyngeal airway.

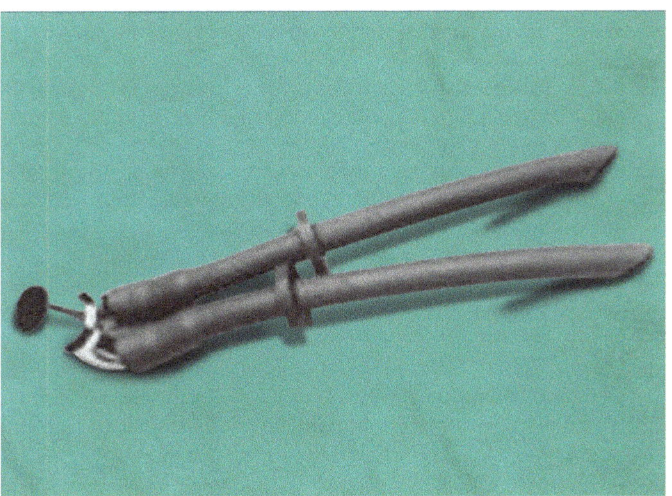
Fig. 13: Binasal airway.

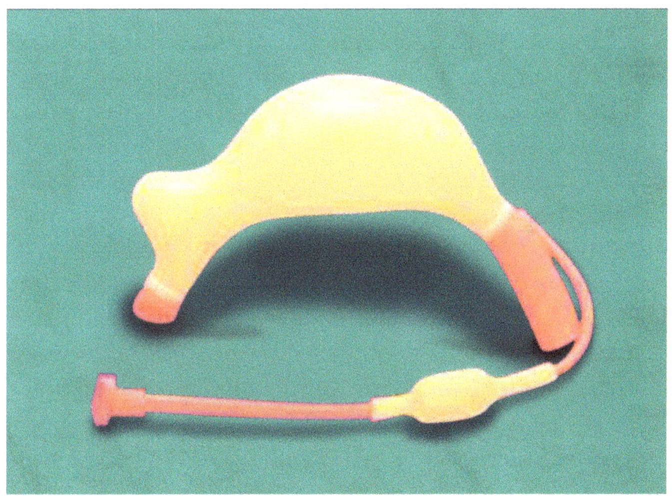
Fig. 14: Epistaxis airway.

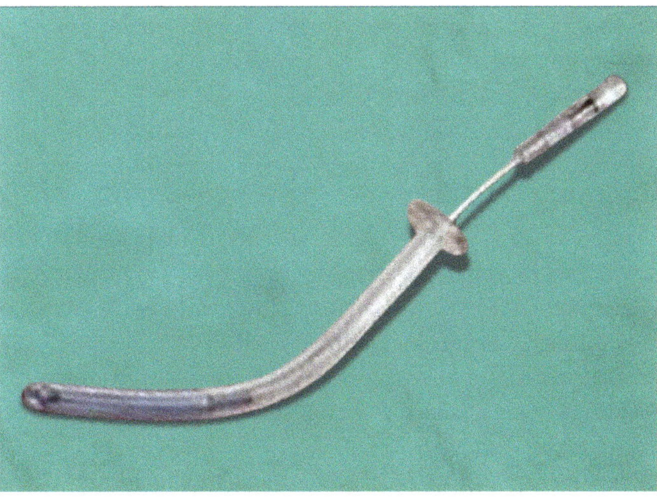
Fig. 15: Linder nasopharyngeal airway.

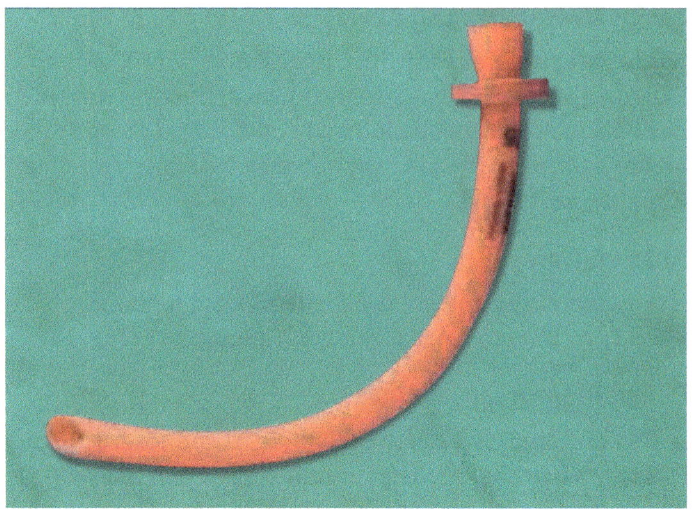

Fig. 16: Rusch airway.

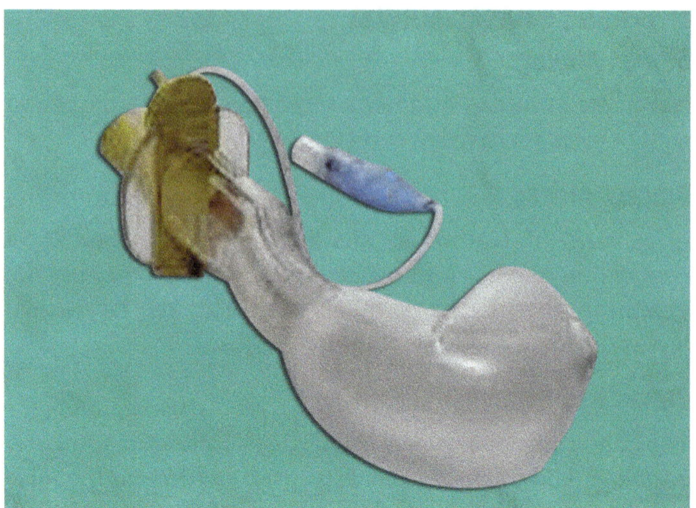

Fig. 17: Cuffed oropharyngeal airway.

15 mm connector for attachment to the breathing circuit. At its proximal end it has two posts for attaching a nonlatex elastic fixation strap which is used to stabilize the COPA device in the mouth. It is made of polyvinyl chloride. The inflatable cuff (capacity of 25–40 mL of air) at the distal end seals the oropharynx. It is inflated through a one way valve attached to a pilot balloon which emerges at the tooth lip guard. When inflated the cuff is broad and flattened posteriorly and shorter and more pointed anteriorly. On inflation, it displaces the base of the tongue, forms a low pressure seal with the pharynx and passively elevates the epiglottis from the posterior pharyngeal wall to provide a clear airway.[6] The cuffed oropharyngeal airway can be inserted easily by inexperienced users with a high first-attempt success rate (>90%); manipulations of the device may be required to maintain a patent airway.[7] Cuffed oropharyngeal airway is less reliable for "hands-free" ventilation than the laryngeal mask airway. However, the incidence of laryngopharyngeal discomfort and salivation is less with the COPA.[8]

Precautions to be Taken during Insertion of the Airway

- Pharyngeal and laryngeal reflex should be depressed to prevent coughing and laryngospasm
- Appropriate size must be used
- The airways must be inserted after lubrication.

Problems of the Airway

- *Airway obstruction:* If larger sized airway is used, it may act as a foreign body in the airway
- *Epistaxis:* Trauma to septal mucosa, nasal polyps or adenoidal tissue can cause epistaxis
- Trauma to the tongue, nose, uvula, pharynx, and teeth
- Long oropharyngeal or nasopharyngeal airway can cause laryngospasm
- Latex allergy
- Tissue edema
- Ulceration and necrosis
- Central nervous system trauma in a patient with basilar skull fracture
- Retention, aspiration, or swallowing.

CONCLUSION

Oral and nasopharyngeal airways constitute an important mandatory accessory in airway management.

REFERENCES

1. Dorsch JA, Dorsch SE. Understanding Anaesthesia Equipments, 5th edition. Wolters Kluwer Health/Lippincott Williams and Wilkins; 2008.
2. Capizzi F, Greenberg RS. The Connell airway: a feasibility study. AANA J. 2001;69(6):473-5.
3. Iqbal R, Gardner-Thorpe C, Thompson J, et al. A comparison of an anterior jaw lift manoeuvre with the Berman airway for assisting fibreoptic orotracheal intubation. Anaesthesia. 2006;61(11):1048-52.
4. Greenland KB, Irwin MG. The Williams Airway Intubator, the Ovassapian Airway and the Berman Airway as upper airway conduits for fibreoptic bronchoscopy in patients with difficult airways. Curr Opin Anaesthesiol. 2004;17(6): 505-10.
5. Randell T, Valli H, Hakala P. Comparison between the Ovassapian intubating airway and the Berman intubating airway in fibreoptic intubation. Eur J Anaesthesiol. 1997;14(4):380-4.
6. Greenberg RS, Kay NH. Cuffed oropharyngeal airway (COPA) helps in supporting the airway during fibreoptic tracheal intubation. Br J Anaesth. 1999;82(3):395-8.
7. van Vlymen JM, Fu W, White PF, et al. Use of the cuffed oropharyngeal airway as an alternative to the laryngeal mask airway with positive-pressure ventilation. Anesthesiology. 1999; 90(5):1306-10.
8. Heringlake M, Doerges V, Ocker H, et al. A comparison of the cuffed oropharyngeal airway (COPA) with the laryngeal mask airway (LMA) during manually controlled positive pressure ventilation. J Clin Anesth. 1999;11(7):590-5.

Ventilating Systems: Manual Resuscitators

Prerana N Shah

ABSTRACT

Manual resuscitators are more commonly called as "artificial manual breathing unit bag". Their use is mostly confined to emergency scenarios of resuscitation and failure of anesthesia machine.

INTRODUCTION

Nowadays, ventilating devices with nonrebreathing valves do have a role in current practice during resuscitation or during transport of patient.[1] Manual resuscitators are portable manual ventilating devices used for ventilating the patient during:

- Resuscitation
- Transport of the patient
- As a standby measure for nonfunctioning of anesthesia machine
- Administering anesthesia when anesthesia machine is not available, e.g., in field situation.

They are known by many names, the most common being "artificial manual breathing unit (AMBU) bag", i.e., artificial mandatory breathing unit or air mask bag unit. They are inflated at rest.

VARIOUS TYPES OF RESUSCITATORS

- Laerdal resuscitator bag: most commonly used
- AMBU bag resuscitator
- Air-viva resuscitator
- Samson Blease manual infant resuscitator.

The devices are available in three sizes:

1. *Adult:* It delivers tidal volume of 600 mL and has a capacity of 1,600 mL. It can be used in adults more than 30 kg weight.
2. *Child:* It has a capacity of 500 mL and can be used in patients weighing between 7 and 30 kg.
3. *Neonatal:* It is capable of delivering the tidal volume up to 20–50 mL and can be used in infants up to 7 kg.

The various components of any ventilating system are:

- Self-inflating bag
- Nonrebreathing valve
- Bag refill valve
- Attachment for oxygen enrichment
- Pressure limiting device for pediatric bags
- Attachment to the scavenging system if any.

Self-inflating Bag

It is usually oval, cylindrical or shaped like a base ball. It usually has a nonrebreathing valve at one end and a bag refill valve at the other end. On release after squeezing, the bag expands. If there is deficit in volume of oxygen to inflate the bag, it is compensated by intake of air. The rate at which the bag reinflates determines the maximum respiratory rate. Squeezing the bag requires considerable physical effort and during prolonged use the operator may become fatigued. Also, size of the operator's hands determines the actual tidal volume going to the patient and if the hands are small then it can cause hypoventilation. It can also be folded to a smaller size to facilitate storage. With prolonged exposure to cold conditions, the cycling rate of the bag may be reduced and the unit may become incapable of delivering satisfactory ventilation.

Nonrebreathing Valve

It ensures unidirectional flow of air from the bag to the patient and from the patient to the atmosphere. As the self-inflating bag is pressed, the valve directs the gas to the patient. Simultaneously, the expiration port gets blocked. When the squeezing of the bag is stopped and the bag is released, the expiration port opens and allows exhalation of the gases to the atmosphere.

Bag Refill Valve

This is the inlet valve which allows entry of oxygen and air in the bag. It is usually located on the opposite to the end of the nonrebreathing valve but can be at the same end also. It is a one-way valve that is opened by the negative pressure inside the bag. When the bag is squeezed, the valve closes automatically to prevent flow of the air back through the inlet.

Oxygen Enrichment Device

The manual resuscitator can deliver fraction of inspired oxygen (FiO_2) of at least 0.21. To increase the FiO_2 oxygen has to be mixed with the air that is drawn from the atmosphere. This can be achieved by delivering oxygen near the bag inlet valve or directly into the bag. A tubing from the oxygen flow meter can be connected to the inlet nozzle of the manual resuscitator. However, the oxygen enrichment is limited and can be enhanced by increasing the oxygen flow rate. This has limitations because most of the flow meters cannot deliver oxygen above 15 L. When delivered directly into the bag, delivery of higher concentration of oxygen can be achieved.

Reservoir

When the bag is not filling, the continuous flow of air and/or oxygen can be stored in a reservoir. Open reservoir can be corrugated tubing that is placed around the inlet valve and is open to atmosphere. Closed reservoir has an over flow and an air intake valve. The inflation of the reservoir bag gives a visual impression whether it is receiving sufficient oxygen. A deflated bag implies a defect in the bag or oxygen supply. The bag should be capable of delivering an inspired oxygen concentration of at least 40% at the oxygen flow rate of 15 L/min and at least 85% when an oxygen enrichment device is attached. A positive end expiratory pressure valve or a scavenging device can be attached to the expiratory port.

Pressure Limiting Devices

It is also called as pressure relief valve or pop-off valve. It opens at an opening pressure of 45 cm of water for infant and pediatric bags and thus prevents lung injury because of barotraumas and also the gastric inflation. In adults the opening pressure is kept at 60 cm of water.

The tidal volume delivered by a manual resuscitator to the patient depends on how the bag is pressed, the size of hands compressing, whether pressed with one or both hands and whether compressed against any solid surface. The ventilatory rate will depend on how rapidly the bag re-expands.

When the bag is pressed the air or enriched air in the bag is delivered to the patient via the nonrebreathing valve. Simultaneously, the inlet valve and the expiratory port of the nonrebreathing valve close. During this period, if oxygen is attached and available, it will get collected in the reservoir. When the bag is released, the negative pressure inside the bag will take in oxygen from the reservoir and from fresh gas flowing continuously in the inlet valve.

The delivered oxygen concentration is determined by minute volume, higher the minute volume lesser will be the oxygen concentration; the oxygen flow rate and the technique of bag squeeze.

Laerdal Silicone Manual Resuscitator

It has a Laerdal fish mouth type of valve, air inlet and optional reservoir bag. Delivered oxygen fraction depends on tidal volume, ventilator rate, oxygen flow rate, and type of reservoir and both the 250 mL and 500 mL corrugated tubes can be used as substitutes **(Fig. 1)**.[2]

AMBU Resuscitator

It is a black colored self-inflating double ended with foam rubber lining. It is available in two sizes. It has an AMBU E_2 nonrebreathing valve containing bobbin, disk, spring, steel ball; air inlet valve and oxygen inlet connection with or without attached oxygen reservoir **(Fig. 2)**.

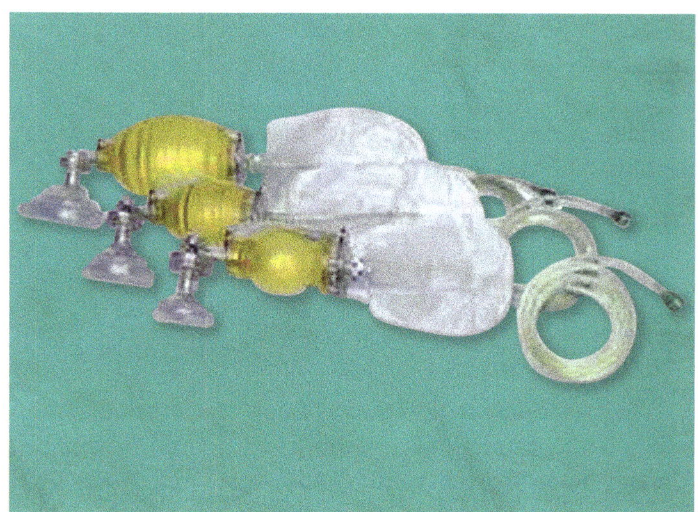

Fig. 1: Laerdal manual resuscitator.

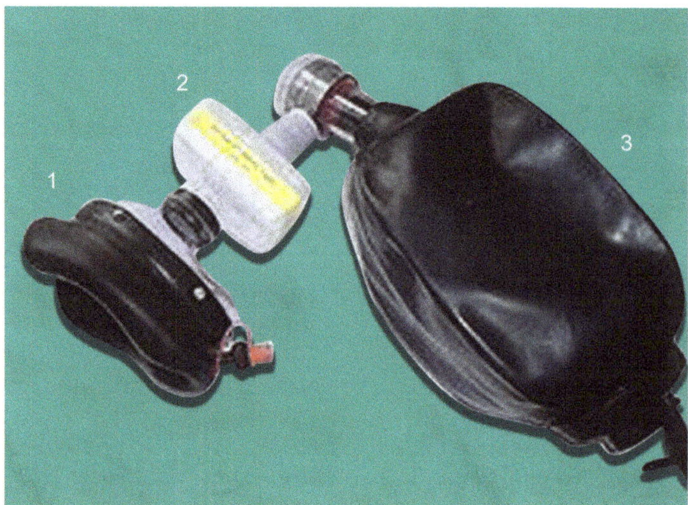

Fig. 2: Artificial mandatory breathing unit or air mask bag unit bag. Part 1 is the flexible mask to seal over the patients face. Part 2 has a filter and value to prevent pack flow into the bag itself. Part 3 is the soft bag element that is squeezed to expel air to the patient.

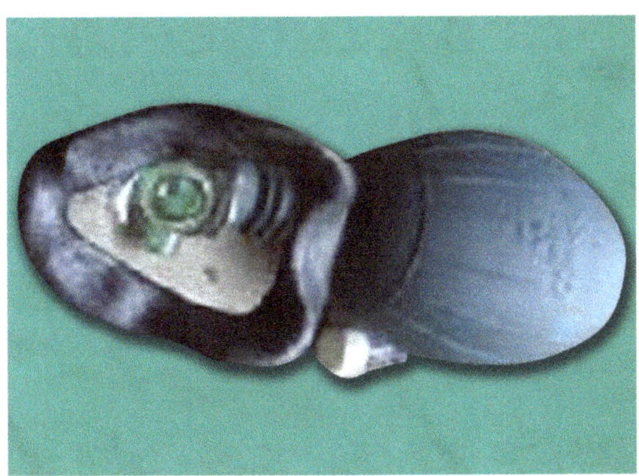

Fig. 3: Air-viva resuscitator.

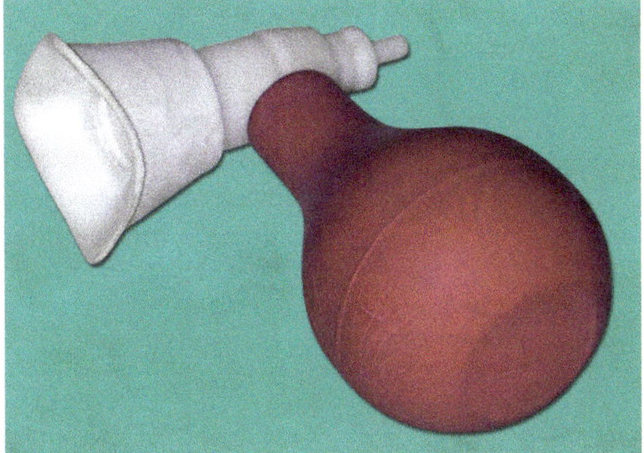

Fig. 4: Samson Blease manual infant resuscitator.

Air-viva Resuscitator

It is green colored, self-inflating single ended bag. It is closed distally and has an oxygen nipple and an expiratory valve at the opposite end. It causes partial rebreathing. It cannot be used to give anesthesia **(Fig. 3)**.

Samson Blease Manual Infant Resuscitator

It has a bulb, body, face piece, oxygen inlet tube, air inlet holes, valve, and pressure regulating holes **(Fig. 4)**.

CONCLUSION

Manual resuscitators continue to remain an essential component in the list of equipment mandatory in perioperative management.

REFERENCES

1. Dorsch JA, Dorsch SE. Manual resuscitators. In: Dorsch JA, Dorsch SE (Eds). Understanding Anesthesia Equipments, 5th edition. Philadelphia: Wolters Kluwer Health/Lippincott Williams & Wilkins; 2008.
2. Nam SH, Kim KJ, Nam YT, et al. The changes in delivered oxygen fractions using Laerdal resuscitator bag with different types of reservoir. Yonsei Med J. 2001;42(2):242-6.

Accessories, Connectors, Bite Block, Magill's Forceps, Stylet, and Laryngeal Sprays

Prerana N Shah

ABSTRACT

In addition to the standard anesthesia machine, there are several additional equipment that are needed during the conduct of anesthesia. Connector, dental block, Magill's forceps, stylet, and laryngeal spray are described below.

INTRODUCTION

Accessories that are often needed and used with anesthesia equipment include connectors, dental block, Magill's forceps, stylet, and laryngeal sprays. They should be available in the anesthesia cart.

CONNECTORS

A connector, as the name implies, is accessory equipment that joins together two or more parts.[1] However, one must distinguish it from an adaptor that is a special connector that joins functionally incompatible parts **(Figs. 1 to 8)**.

They can be differentiated by:

- Shape (straight, right angle or elbow, T or Y)
- Parts to which it is attached
- Added feature (with nipple or pop-off)
- Size and type of fitting at either end (15 mm male, 22 mm female).

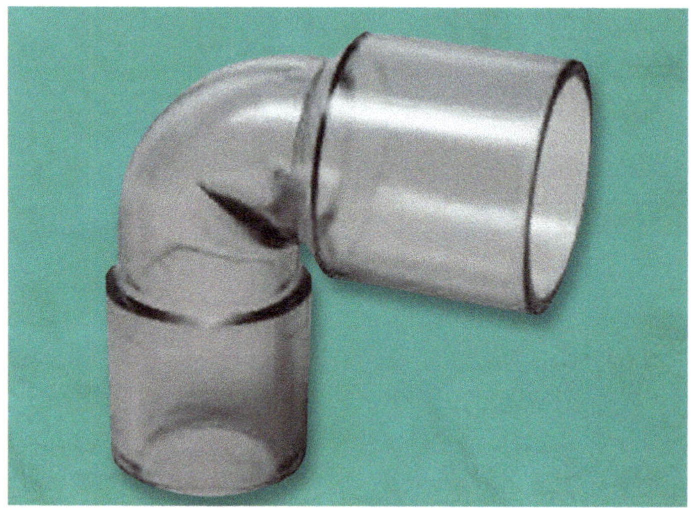

Fig. 1: Right angled (90°) connector—22 mm male and 15 mm female closed.

All anesthesia systems end at the patient end by connection to a mask, supraglottic device or endotracheal tube (ETT) adaptor. All face masks have a 22 mm female and a

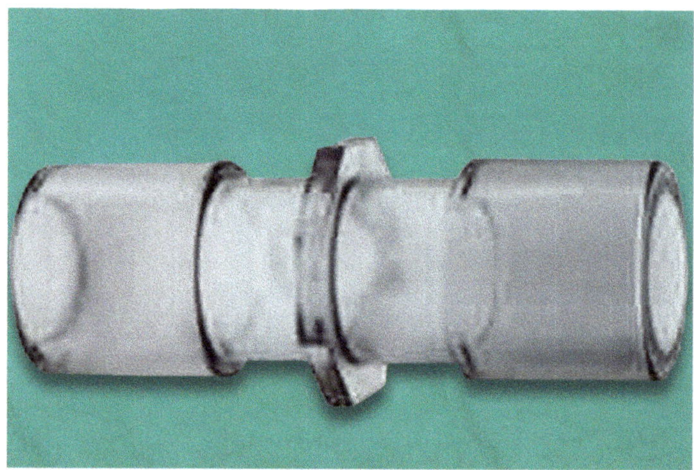

Fig. 2: Straight connector 15 mm female and 22 mm male connected to 15 mm female and 22 mm male.

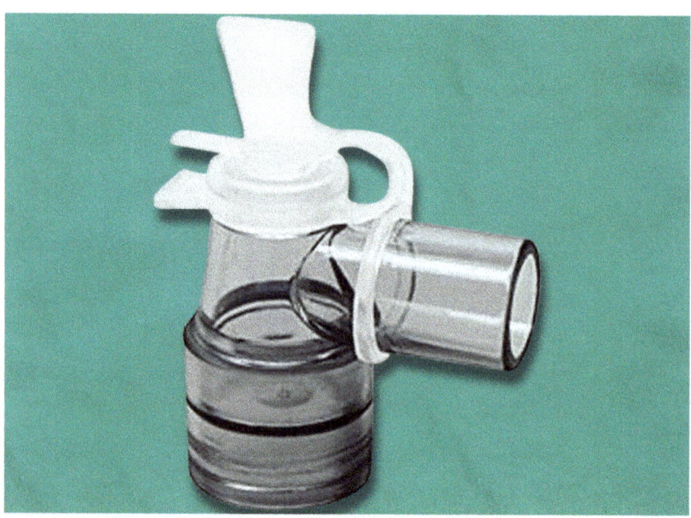

Fig. 3: Right-angled swivel connector 22 mm male and 15 mm female with clear silicone 5 mm cap.

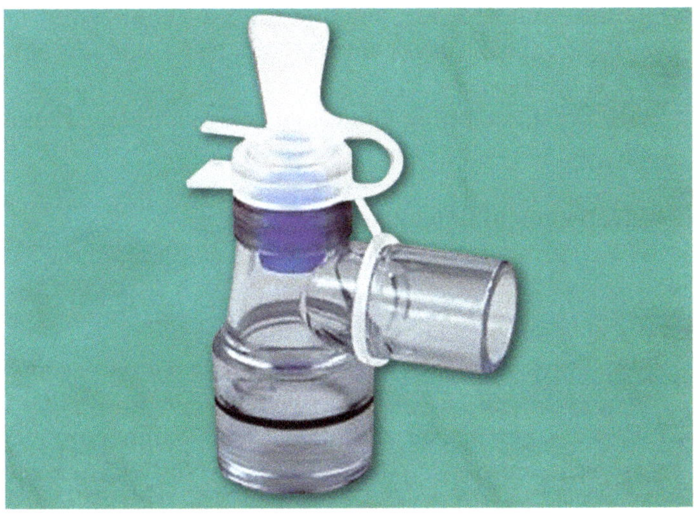

Fig. 4: Right-angled swivel bronchoscope connector 5 mm with suction cap.

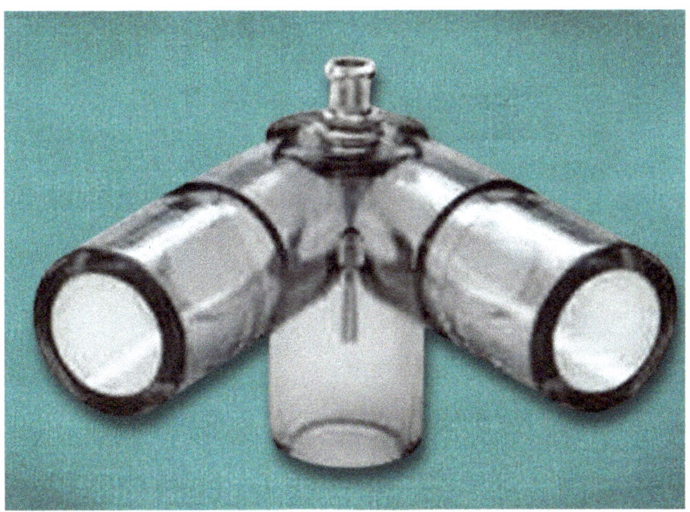

Fig. 7: Right-angled Y-connector 15 mm female 22 mm male metal female Luer lock.

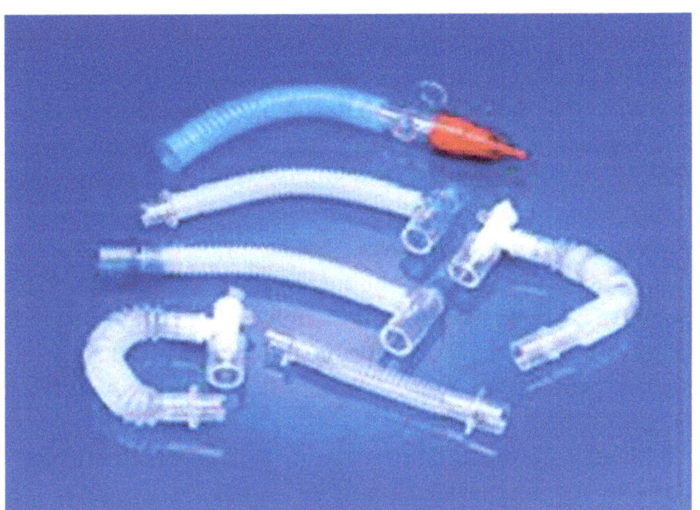

Fig. 5: Catheter mount.

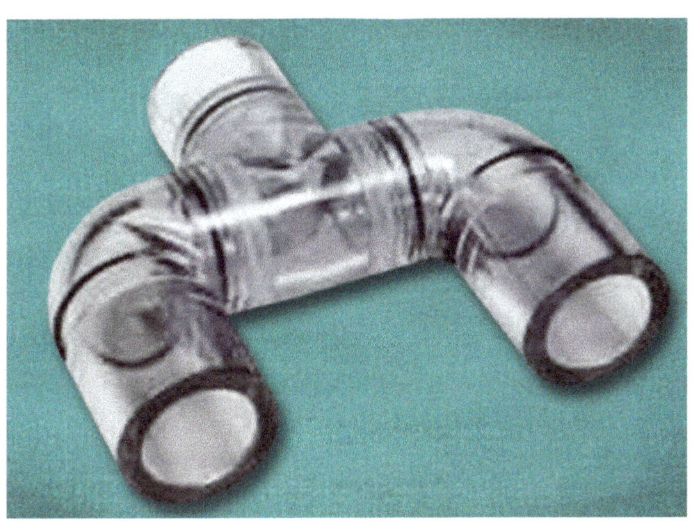

Fig. 8: Right-angled Y-connector 15 mm female 22 mm male with adjustable connectors.

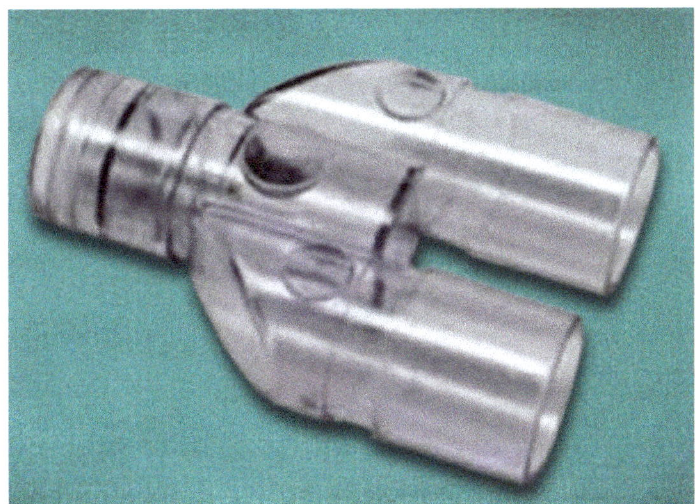

Fig. 6: Straight Y-connector 15 mm female 22 mm male with 22 mm tube connection.

15 mm male fitting. To facilitate the change from mask to tracheal tube or supraglottic device and vice versa, a component having a 22-mm male fitting with a concentric 15 mm female opening to fit either a mask or a connector is used at the patient end of most of the systems. It is usually right angled and may be called as elbow adaptor, elbow joint, elbow connector, face mask angle piece, mask adaptor or mask elbow.[1]

Bushings (Mounts)

A bushing changes the internal diameter of a part. It is usually cylindrical in shape and is inserted into and becomes part of, a pliable component such as a reservoir bag or a breathing tube **(Figs. 9 and 10)**.

Sleeves

In contrast to a bushing, a sleeve alters the external diameter of a component.

Functions of Connectors and Adaptors

- To increase the length of the circuit between the patient and the breathing system (head and neck surgery)
- To change the angle of connection between the tracheal tube or supraglottic device and the breathing system
- To allow flexibility between the tracheal tube or supraglottic device and the breathing system
- To increase the dead space, especially in cases of prolonged mechanical ventilation.[1]

Requirements of Connectors

- 15 mm male fitting at the machine end and either

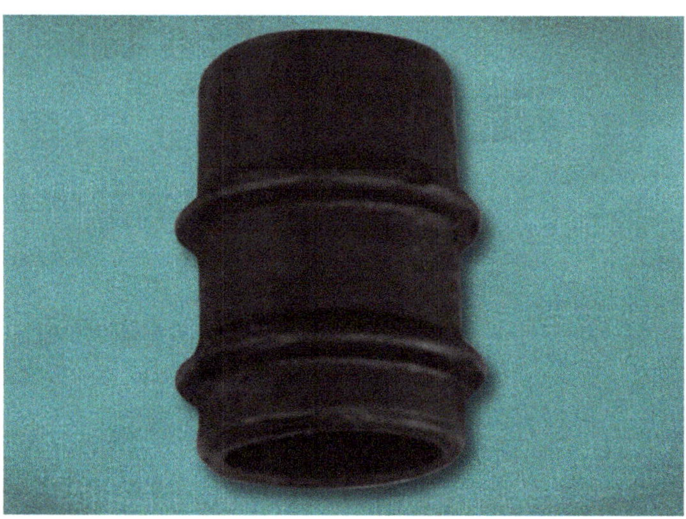

Fig. 9: Bag bushing reduces 7–8 inches bag or tube to 15 mm female.

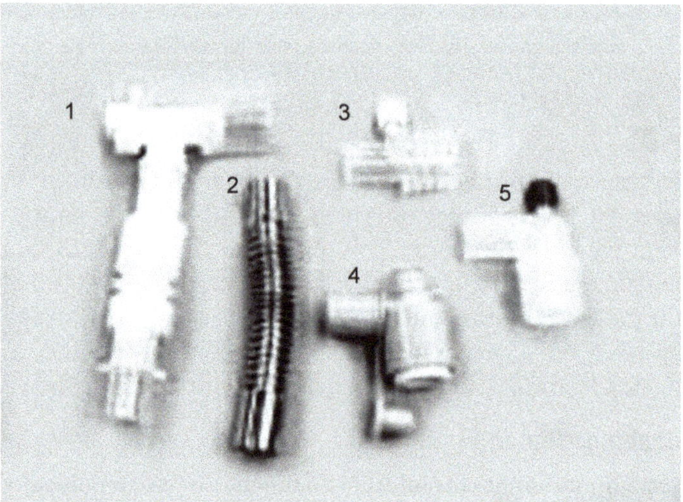

Fig. 10: Connectors[1]. 1. A swivel connector that can be used to insert a flexible fiberscope. It has a flexible accordion-type side arm, 2. A flexible metal connector that can be used between the tracheal tube and the breathing system. It cannot be used with a mask, 3. Straight connector with a side gas sampling port, 4. Right angle connector for insertion of a flexible fiberscope. It can accommodate different sized fiberscopes by changing the diaphragm. The large cap is used if no diaphragm is present, 5. Right angle connector with gas sampling port.

- 22 mm male/15 mm female fitting for connection to either tracheal tube or supraglottic device adaptor or a mask or
- 15 mm female fitting for connection to a tracheal tube adaptor.

Disadvantages of Connectors

- They increase dead space (important in infants)
- Any addition of a connector increases the chances of possible disconnections
- Resistance increases markedly with sharp curves and rough side walls, e.g., Cobb's suction union, Rowbotham adaptors, corrugated and pliable metal connector, etc. To minimize it, use adaptors that are straight or have gentle curves.

Tracheal Tube Connector

It is attached to the component of the breathing system. The size of the connector is designated by the internal diameter of the patient end in millimeters. The end that connects to the breathing system is called the machine end and has a 15 mm male fitting. It is fitted with a tapered cone and is pushed into the lumen of the ETT. It is slightly bigger than the tube so that the tube material has to be stretched to fit.

Various varieties include Magill's oral curved, Magill's nasal curved, Magill's suction union, Magill's Y-type pediatric, Cobb suction union, Rowbotham right angled **(Fig. 11)**, universal/nose worthy metallic or plastic, Carlen suction port, Robertshaw suction port, Swivel, Twin metallic **(Fig. 12)**, etc.

Magill's connectors are smoothly curved with corrugations at the tracheal end and an expanded flange at the wider machine end. The oral connectors are angled at slightly less than 90° while the nasal connectors have an acute angle curve.

Pediatric Endotracheal Tube Connector

Before standards were laid down, connectors were designed as per convenience (Magill's connectors, 13 mm; Worcester, 12 mm; Metal Cardiff, 12 mm; Knight, 9 mm; Bennett, 14 mm).

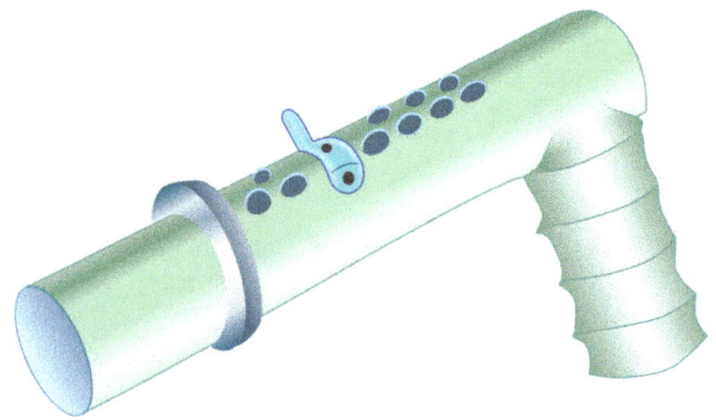

Fig. 11: Rowbotham connector.

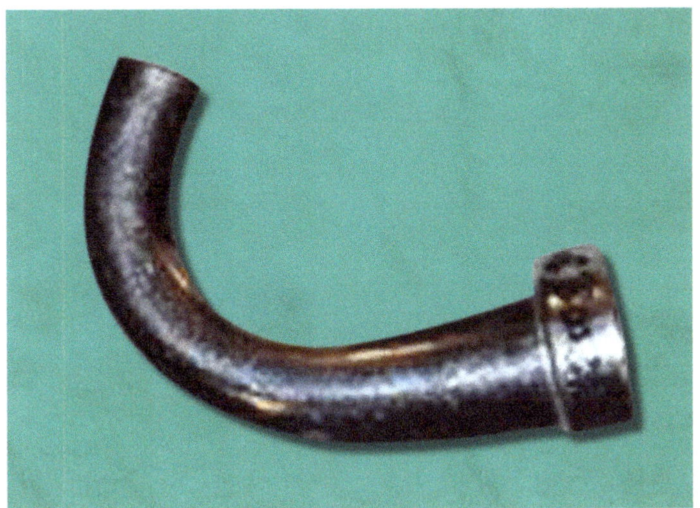

Fig. 12: Metal connector.

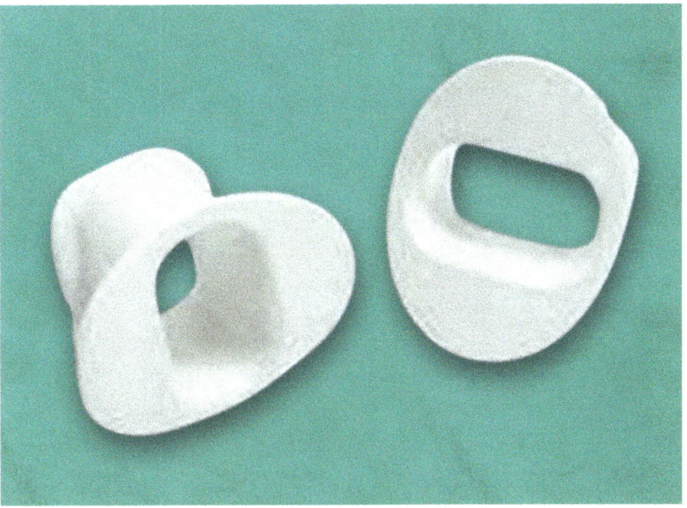

Fig. 13: Bite block.

Today, a standard 15 mm connection is supplied with most ETTs or supraglottic device. They have higher resistance to flow even though they do not have a bend in them because of the turbulence caused at the junction with the taper used for attachment to an ETT and is not the one with least resistance to gas flow.

Tapered Connection (Adaptors)

They are used to join rigid tubes or other components so that the joint will not leak. The joint is described as having a male half and a female half, which are pushed together with a slight twist to form a gas tight fit. The joint can be easily dismantled and reassembled.

Current standard recommendations are:
- 30 mm tapered connectors for scavenging hose
- 22 mm tapered connectors within the breathing system
- 15 mm connectors for ETT or supraglottic device.

Sterilization

Most connectors available today are of disposable variety. However, if they are not available, the nondisposable ones must be sterilized before every use.

Cleaning

After use, they should be rinsed under running water, then placed in a solution of detergent and water and soaked.

Disinfection

Rubber and plastic connectors may be sterilized with ethylene oxide or in a liquid, such, as gluteraldehyde. Metal connectors may be boiled, autoclaved, or pasteurized.

BITE BLOCK

A bite block is an accessory to protect the ETT, supraglottic device, fibreoptic scope, etc. from getting damaged by

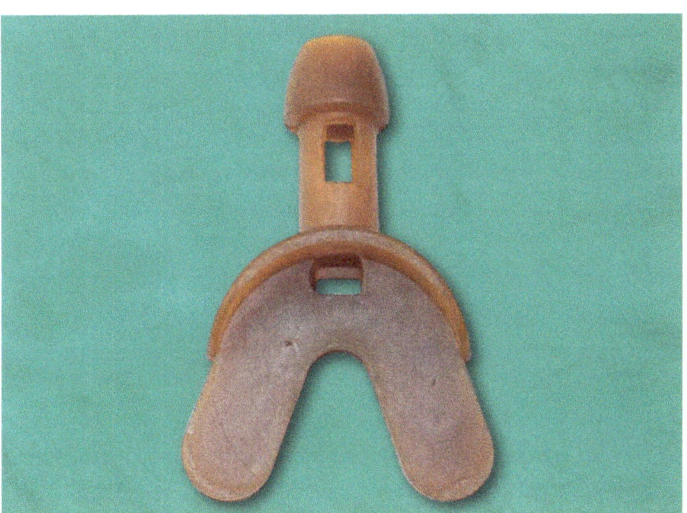

Fig. 14: Oberto mouth prop used for protecting the teeth during electroconvulsive therapy.

the teeth. It is also called as gag, mouth prop, bite protector **(Fig. 13)**.[2]

It is placed between the molar teeth or gums and not between the incisors. It is less irritable than the oral airway. It prevents the teeth from biting on a tracheal tube, supraglottic airway device, fiberscope, etc. It is also used during electroconvulsive therapy and in unconscious patients to prevent the teeth from biting the tongue and lips. It also helps keep the mouth open for suctioning **(Fig. 14)**. An oral airway may be harmful to the patient as all the power of the bite is concentrated on the incisors, which are not designed for this pressure and are liable to break or loosen.[2]

MAGILL'S FORCEPS

Magill's forceps is a common forceps that is essential constituent of intubation cart **(Fig. 15)**.

Description

It is a handheld, angled, nonlocking hinged in the middle type of forceps with flat grasping surface at the tip. It is used

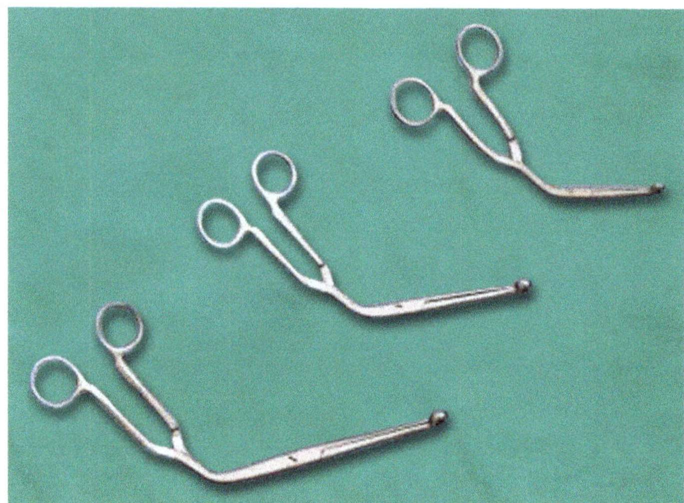

Fig. 15: Magill's forceps.

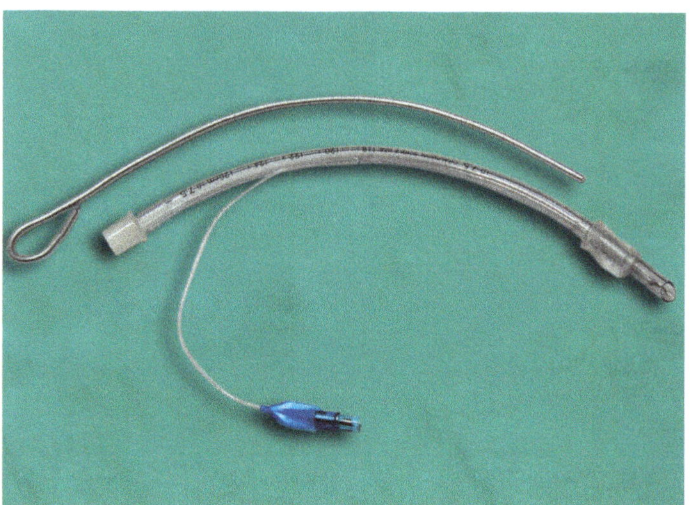

Fig. 16: Stylet.

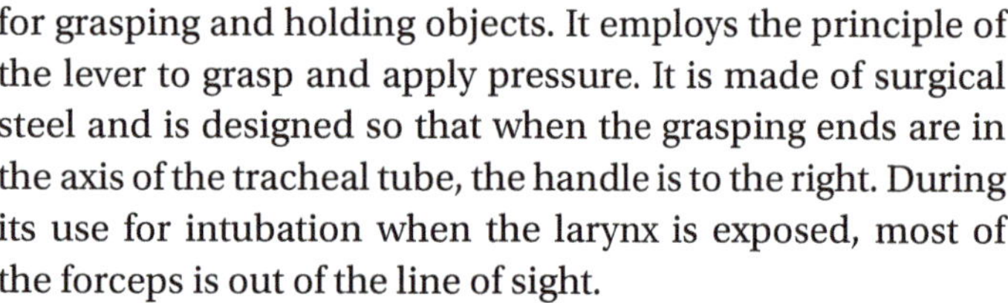

for grasping and holding objects. It employs the principle of the lever to grasp and apply pressure. It is made of surgical steel and is designed so that when the grasping ends are in the axis of the tracheal tube, the handle is to the right. During its use for intubation when the larynx is exposed, most of the forceps is out of the line of sight.

Uses

- It can be used to direct a tracheal tube into the larynx
- It can be used to direct a gastric tube or other device into the esophagus
- It can be used to insert or remove pharyngeal packing
- It can be used to remove foreign bodies from the upper airway or esophagus.

Problems

The tracheal tube cuff may become damaged or perforated especially when forceps are used with high volume, low pressure cuffs. Hence, the tube should never be grasped at the cuff. There is also a risk of damaging the mucosa.[3] The standard Magill's forceps has been modified by changing the jaws of the forceps to give curved atraumatic parts without any serrations or sharp edges.[3]

STYLET

Stylet is a slender, stiff, long instrument that is usually inserted in the ETT to facilitate intubation **(Fig. 16)**.

A stylet, also called as introducer when used fits inside and changes the shape of the tracheal tube to aid intubation. It is also an essential constituent of intubation cart. Many anesthesiologists routinely use it, while others use it for difficult intubation.

Description

A variety of stylets are available. Some have special nonstick surfaces. There is usually a guard to limit the depth of its insertion so that it does not protrude out of the stylet during intubation. It should be malleable so that its shape can be changed easily and rigid enough to maintain its shape during intubation. It should have a smooth surface devoid of sharp edges.

It is also useful to check the patency of a tracheal tube.

The stylet may have a light at the end to assist in visualization during and after placement.

Prior to its use, it must be lubricated over its entire length and then inserted into the tube until the distal end reaches the bevel. At this level, the guard must be fixed so that it cannot advance. It is desirable to remove the connector from the tube before inserting the stylet. The tube and stylet should then be bent to the desired shape, usually curved slightly for routine use and into a "J" or "hockey stick" shape for anterior larynx. Once the tracheal tube passes beyond the vocal cords, it is withdrawn from the tube.

Problems

It may be associated with trauma to the airway or esophagus especially if the tip protrudes from the patient end of the tube.

LARYNGEAL SPRAYS

Endotracheal intubation stimulates the sympathetic nervous system that causes a rise in arterial blood pressure. If this is associated with light plane of anesthesia, laryngeal spasm can occur. Local anesthetic applied to the vocal cords and trachea can limit this response. There are various types of sprays **(Fig. 17)**.

Macintosh® Spray

It has a flexible tip to anesthetize the oral cavity and larynx for application of topical anesthesia **(Fig. 18)**.

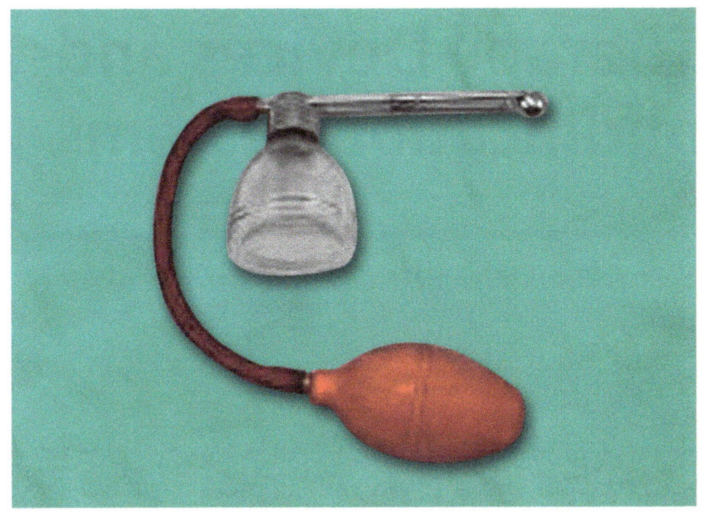

Fig. 17: Laryngeal spray.

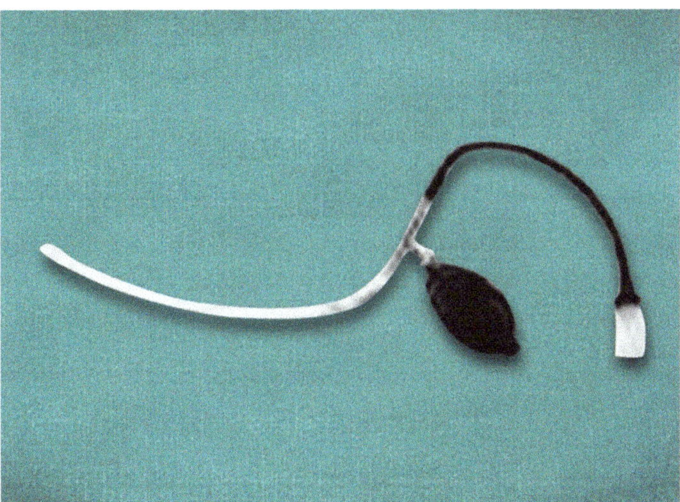

Fig. 19: Forrester laryngeal spray.

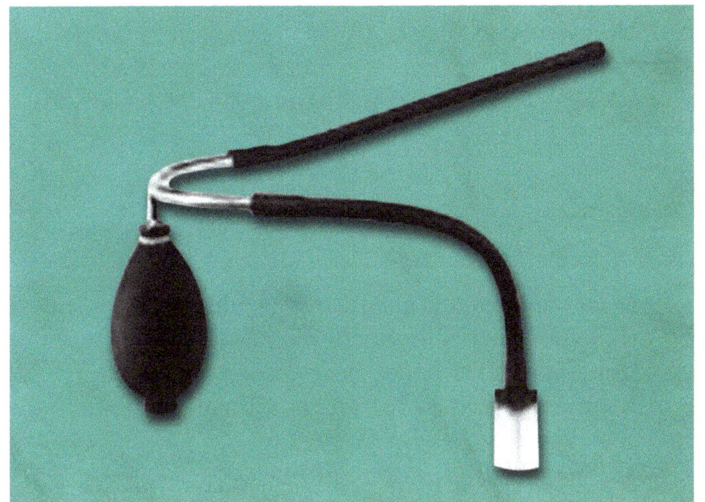

Fig. 18: Macintosh® laryngeal spray.

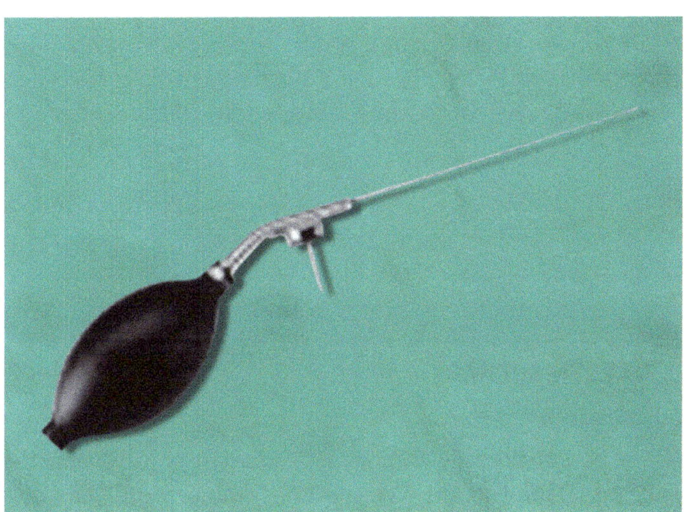

Fig. 20: Swerdlow laryngeal spray.

Forrester Spray

It has a rigid curved spray nozzle designed for application of topical anesthesia. The bottle is below the level of the nozzle so that risk of siphoning is minimized **(Fig. 19)**.

Swerdlow Spray

It has a rigid long nozzle designed for single handed application of topical anesthesia **(Fig. 20)**.

For each Macintosh® spray device tested, the dose delivered by a single maximal hand squeeze of the atomizer bulb was variable and was not dependent upon the user. A single, maximal hand squeeze of the Macintosh® laryngeal spray atomizer bulb can deliver a toxic dose of local anesthetic.[4]

After use, the spray must be washed with warm water otherwise crystals can get deposited in the nozzle and hamper its function. Hence, before every use, it must be tested for its functioning and patent nozzle.

CONCLUSION

The above mentioned accessories constitute essential equipment especially in anticipated difficult intubation.

REFERENCES

1. Dorsch JA, Dorsch SE. The breathing system: General principles, common components, and classifications. In: Dorsch JA, Dorsch SE (Eds). Understanding Anaesthesia Equipments, 5th edition. Philadelphia: Wolters Kluwer Health/Lippincott Williams & Wilkins; 2008.
2. Dorsch JA, Dorsch SE. Face masks and airways. In: Dorsch JA, Dorsch SE (Eds). Understanding Anaesthesia Equipments, 5th edition. Philadelphia: Wolters Kluwer Health/Lippincott Williams & Wilkins; 2008.
3. Ehrensperger C, Gross J, Hempel V, et al. The modified Magill forceps. Anaesthesist. 1992;41(4):218-20.
4. Ing RJ, Craig DM, Nowosad A, et al. Anaesthetic safety of the Macintosh® oral laryngeal spray device: original research. South Afr J Anaesth Analg. 2013;19(4):212-5.

Oxygen Therapy Devices and Humidification Systems

Raghbirsingh P Gehdoo, Azra Z Kakroo

ABSTRACT

Oxygen therapy devices (OTDs) are in use since long time; over the time, technology and efficiency of these devices improved and have been steadily focused on improving the facilities for continuous ambulatory oxygen therapy. The choice of delivery devices depends on the individual's oxygen requirement, efficacy of the devices, reliability, and patient acceptance. The main goal and aim of oxygen therapy is to treat alveolar and tissue hypoxia. Therefore, any medical or physical disorder causing hypoxia is a potential indication for oxygen administration. As the tissue oxygen delivery depends on a properly functioning of heart, lungs and hematological system. Therefore, only oxygen is not enough to treat and reverse tissue hypoxia—functioning of all the three organ systems also needs to be improved. At the same time, for a successful use of prolonged oxygenation particularly in postoperative period or mechanical ventilation, it always needs to be combined with humidification.

Keywords: Hypoxia, oxygenation, humidification devices.

PART I

OXYGEN THERAPY

Introduction

Being beneficial and without risk, oxygen is most commonly prescribed worldwide method in acutely ill patients. Although the primary indication of oxygen therapy is arterial hypoxemia, but most physicians and acute care practitioners use it very commonly in many conditions such as myocardial infarction or ischemia, shock, sepsis, chest pain, breathlessness, during childbirth, routine surgery, and anxiety regardless of the presence or absence of hypoxemia.[1-4]

Oxygen therapy is aimed to increase the fraction of inspired oxygen concentration (FiO_2) available to a patient. The rationale for oxygen therapy is prevention of cellular hypoxia, caused by hypoxemia [low partial pressure of O_2 (PaO_2)], and thus prevention of potentially irreversible damage to vital organs.

Main indications[5] of oxygen therapy are:

- *Acute hypoxemia:* Diminished blood oxygen levels [oxygen saturation (SpO_2) < 90%]
- Cardiac and respiratory arrest
- Low cardiac output along with metabolic acidosis (HCO_3 < 18 mmol/L)
- Respiratory distress [respiratory rate (RR) > 24 breaths/min), e.g., pneumonia, pulmonary embolus, and acute asthma
- Myocardial ischemia and infarction, but only if associated with hypoxemia (abnormally high levels may be harmful to patients with ischemic heart disease and stroke)
- Chronic type II respiratory failure (hypoxia and hypercapnia)
- Carbon monoxide poisoning
- *In postanesthesia care unit:* After major abdominal and thoracic surgery under general anesthesia, there is decrease in functional residual capacity (FRC) and resulting hypoxemia.

Less common indications are:

- *Pneumothorax:* There is increase in rate of resolution of small pneumothorax without intercostal drain, with oxygen.
- *Pneumocephalus:* It also increases the resolution of pneumocephalus in patients with a basal skull fracture.
- *Long-term oxygen therapy:*[6]
  - *During sleep:* PaO_2 < 55 mm Hg/SpO_2 < 88%) with associated complications
    - Pulmonary hypertension
    - Daytime somnolence, obstructive sleep apnea patient

Contraindications

No absolute contraindications of oxygen therapy exist.

Risk of Oxygen Therapy

In patients with chronic carbon dioxide retention (these patients have low PaO_2 as breathing stimulus), oxygen administration may depress respiratory drive. So careful monitoring for hypoventilation is mandatory during oxygen therapy. Cancer patients on bleomycin-based chemotherapy are at risk of pulmonary toxicity (pulmonary fibrosis and emphysema), if given high oxygen. Patients with paraquat poisoning and acid inhalation are also at risk of oxygen toxicity.

Side Effects of Oxygen Therapy

- Oxygen toxicity
- Retrolental fibroplasias (in premature neonates, if given 100% O_2 for long time)
- Absorption atelectasis
- Pulmonary fibrosis (in patient's on bleomycin chemotherapy)

Goals of Oxygen Therapy

The goal of oxygen therapy is to increase the alveolar oxygen tension thereby relieve hypoxemia, decrease myocardial work and work of breathing. Frequent arterial blood gas analysis is required in patients with acute respiratory failure, on supplemental oxygen therapy (goal is PaO_2 > 60 mm Hg).[5]

Oxygen Therapy Devices[7-9]

They are used to administer, regulate, and supplement oxygen to a patient in need, so as to increase the arterial oxygenation. To provide adequate oxygen, an appropriate oxygen delivery device must be chosen and is based on:

- Age and size (built) of the patient
- Oxygen requirements and therapeutic goals
- Acceptability of a particular method of oxygenation
- Humidification needs

OXYGEN DELIVERY SYSTEMS[10-13]

Classification of oxygen delivery systems are shown in **Flowchart 1**.

Classification of Oxygen Therapy Devices

Oxygen therapy devices are classified as low-flow or variable performance and high-flow or fixed performance, as shown in **Flowchart 2**.

Low Flow (Variable Performance)

Ideally, low-flow systems do not provide the patient's entire ventilator requirements through the delivery device. Some amount of air is entrained to meet the patient's ventilatory requirement. These are:

- Nasal prongs or cannula
- Nasal catheter
- Transtracheal catheter
- Simple face mask or Hudson's mask (without entrainment device)
- Partial rebreathing mask
- Nonrebreather face mask
- Tracheostomy mask (without entrainment device)
- Oxygen hood

High Flow (Fixed Performance)

The whole ventilatory requirement of the patient is provided by the delivery devices. Air entrainment devices

Flowchart 1: Classification of oxygen delivery systems.

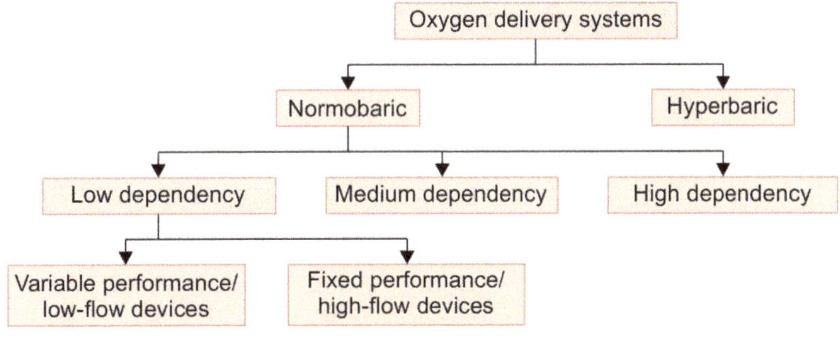

Flowchart 2: Classification of oxygen therapy devices.

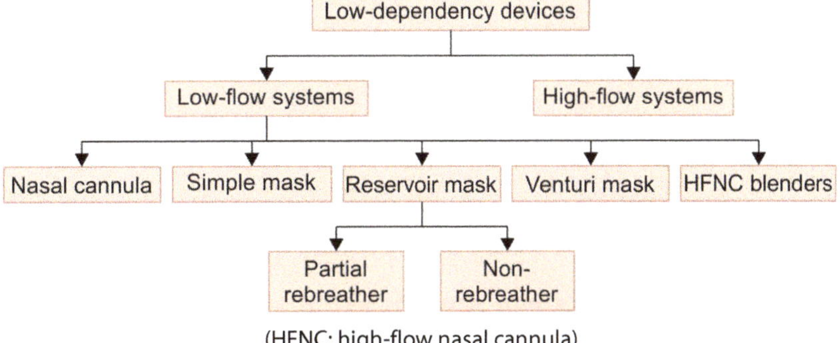

(HFNC: high-flow nasal cannula)

allow titration of inspired oxygen concentration (FiO_2%) by altering the amount of room air entrained through the device. These are:

- Venturi mask, multivent mask, and Aquapac
- Tracheostomy mask and face mask used in with an entrainment device
- Ventilators
- Continuous positive airway pressure (CPAP) and bilevel positive airway pressure (BiPAP)®

In such systems, oxygen-flow meters are available as high-flow and low-flow meters—low-flow range from 0 to 3 L/min and high-flow range from 0 to 15 L/min.

Apneic Oxygenation

- NO DESAT (nasal oxygen during efforts securing a tube)
- THRIVE (transnasal humidified rapid insufflation ventilatory exchange)
- Buccal oxygen therapy

Low-flow (Variable FiO_2) Devices

Nasal cannulae are the most commonly used devices for oxygen therapy as they are comfortable and well tolerated by most of the patients **(Fig. 1)**. Oxygen is provided at a certain flow rate in L/min. The patient's rate and depth of breathing determines the FiO_2 and is mostly not fixed at a fixed flow rate. Fast and deep breathing results into lower FiO_2 because it draws more room air into lungs and thus dilutes the inspiratory gas and oxygen concentration.

Nasal Cannula

It consists of two soft prongs attached to oxygen supply tubing. Nasopharynx acts as a reservoir. If patient breathes through mouth, air flow produces Venturi effect in the posterior pharynx entraining oxygen from the nose.

Amount of FiO_2 delivered as per the flow of O_2 per minute is shown in **Table 1**.

Advantages:

- It is available in different sizes and different prong shapes.
- Ideal for patient on long-term oxygen therapy.
- Low cost, light weight, and comfortable.
- More acceptable by patients because patients can communicate, eat, drink, and wear glasses to read without any difficulty.
- Mostly used for patients who do not tolerate a face mask.
- Humidification is not required.
- It can be easily used in home setting.

Disadvantages:

- It cannot provide high-flow oxygen, i.e., >6 L/min, as it makes patient uncomfortable.

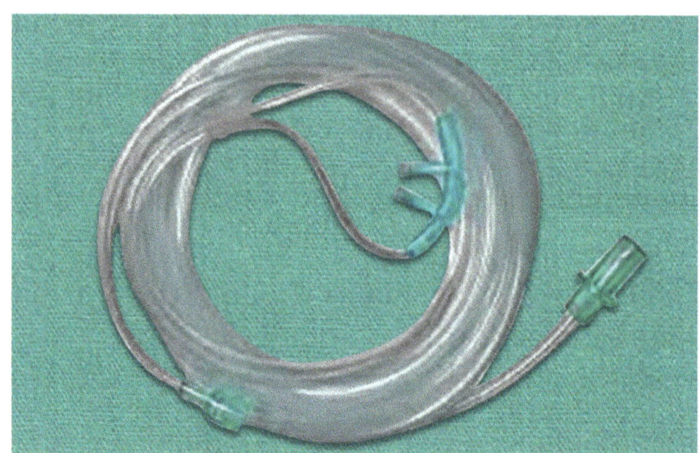

Fig. 1: Nasal cannula.

TABLE 1: Amount of FiO_2 delivered as per the flow of O_2/min.

Amount delivered (FiO_2)	*L/min (LPM)*
24%	1
28%	2
32%	3
36%	4
40%	5
44%	6

(FiO_2: fraction of inspired oxygen concentration)

- Above a flow rates of 4 L/min (without humidification), there is an increased chances of nasal irritation.
- Fraction of inspired oxygen concentration varies with respiratory efforts.
- In a patient with a blocked nose, FiO_2 may be much reduced.
- Never deliver >2–3 L/min to patient with chronic lung disease.

Nasal cannula can be used in pediatric patients (limiting flow rate to 3–4 L/min with humidifier) and in neonates and infants (flow rate 0.025–1.0 L/min). Nasal cannula can be considered a high-flow device for infants and neonates because inspiratory flow rate for infants and neonates is very low.

Nasal Catheter

It is a single lumen catheter **(Figs. 2A and B)**, which in lodged into the anterior nares by a foam collar and inserted just above the uvula. Oxygen flows of 2–3 L/min provide FiO_2 of 35–40%.

It needs to be repositioned after every 8 hours to prevent breakdown.

Contraindications:

- It should not be used if nasal mucosa tear is suspected as there is risk of surgical emphysema.
- Deep insertion can cause air swallowing and gastric distension.

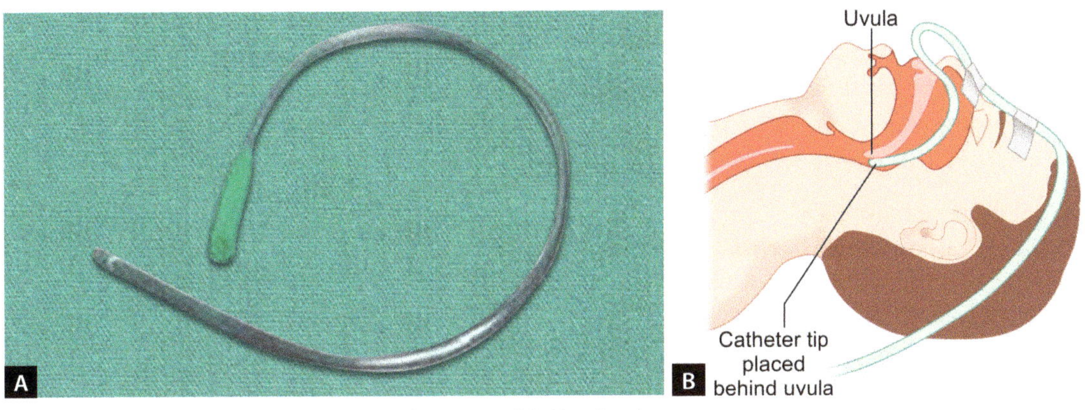

Figs. 2A and B: Nasal catheter.

Transtracheal Catheter

Most useful in a tracheostomized patients, as it is easy to insert and stays stable for a longer time as compared to the tracheostomy mask **(Fig. 3)**.

Advantages: It reduces total O_2 usage by 50–75%:

- Lack of nasal or facial irritation
- Lesser chances of catheter displacement during sleep

Disadvantages: Chances of infection:

- Mucous plug, leading to blockage
- Catheter breakage

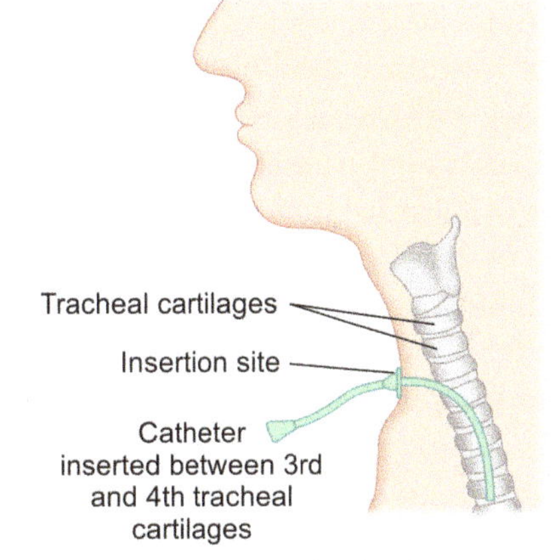

Fig. 3: Transtracheal catheter.

Simple Face Mask (Hudson Mask)

This is a simple plastic mask with several small vent holes on each side **(Fig. 4)**. Oxygen is delivered through a 7-mm diameter oxygen tubing from oxygen source. This is most commonly used in postanesthesia care units in patients recovering from anesthesia. This is always recommended for short-term use in patients with chronic lung disease for acute hypoxic breathlessness and prolonged use in patients with chronic lung disease may be problematic. It has a reservoir capacity of 100–250 mL. It uses a flow rate of 3–8 L/min and delivers 35–50% FiO_2 depending upon flow rate and respiratory drive of the patients. A flow rate of <3–4 L/min may cause rebreathing of expired gases. Flow rate of > 8 L/min does not increase FiO_2.

It should be better used with some humidification devices, if planned for prolonged use or used in pediatric or neonatal patients.

Advantages:

- Delivery of oxygen is more for a short period of time.
- It can also be used for mouth breathers.
- Less expensive

Disadvantages:

- Tight seal required to deliver higher concentrations
- Difficult to keep mask in position over nose and mouth for a long time
- Uncomfortable for patient while eating or talking

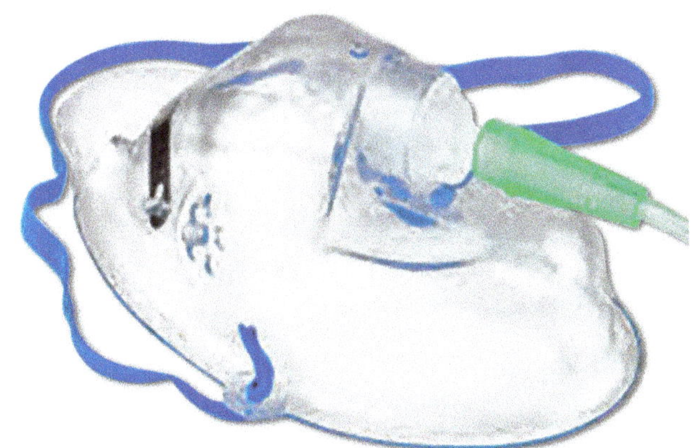
Fig. 4: Hudson mask.

- Chances of skin breakdown (due to pressure and moisture)
- Fraction of inspired oxygen concentration varies with breathing effects
- High chances of rebreathing.

Partial Rebreathing Mask

It needs a minimum of 8 L/min of oxygen flow to enter the mask to remove exhaled carbon dioxide and to refill oxygen reservoir. Flow rate must be sufficient to keep bag 1/3 to ½ inflated at all the times **(Fig. 5)**.

Advantages:
- Inspired gas is not mixed with room air.
- Patient can breathe room air through exhalation ports, if O_2 supply gets interrupted.

Disadvantages:
- More O_2 flow does not increase FiO_2.
- It interferes with eating and drinking.

Nonrebreathing Face Mask

It is modification of a simple face mask with attachment of an oxygen reservoir and a unidirectional valve system to prevent mixing of expired gases and fresh gas flow. The nonrebreathing mask system also has a valve on the side ports or vent holes of the mask which prevents mixing of room air with fresh gas flow into the mask. This nonrebreathing mask provides an FiO_2 of 60–80% with a flow rate of 10 L/min or more (in pediatric patients, it can be used with a flow rate of 5 L/min) **(Fig. 6)**.

In this type of mask, one needs high flow to prevent the rebreathing. Mainly used in patients who require urgent or emergent but for short-term, high FiO_2. A humidification system is never used with nonrebreathing system, because a condensation inside the reservoir bag may make bag stiff and resulting into inability to expand. So, long-term use of nonrebreathing mask may cause nasal and oral-mucosal irritation due to dry gas.

Tracheostomy Mask

These are same as simple face mask used at tracheostomy site in patients with permanent or temporary tracheostomy or stoma in patients who underwent total laryngectomy **(Fig. 7)**. The minimum flow rate required as in facemask is 3–4 L/min to prevent expired gas rebreathing, carbon dioxide accumulation, and subsequent drowsiness. The delivered FiO_2 is highly variable based on the patient's inspiratory flow, fitting of mask, and patient's RR and pattern.

Oxygen Hood

In this type of oxygenation, a plastic dome or box with warm and humidified oxygen inside is used for babies who can breathe on their own but still need extra oxygen. Here, the oxygen enters through a gas inlet port, and exhaled gases exit through the opening for the neck **(Fig. 8)**. Oxygen hood provides 80–90% oxygen, controlled temperature, and humidification.

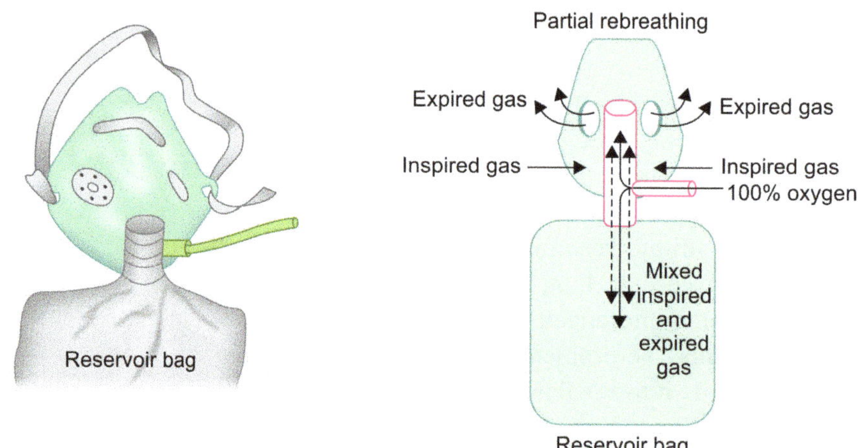

Fig. 5: Partial rebreathing mask.

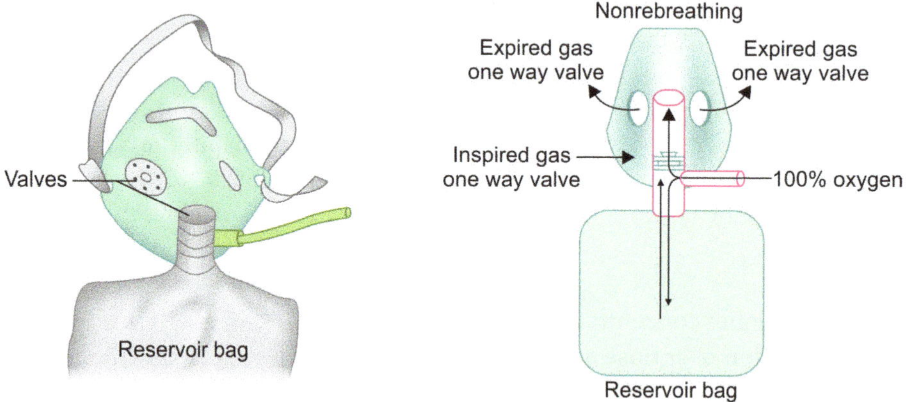

Fig. 6: Nonrebreathing mask.

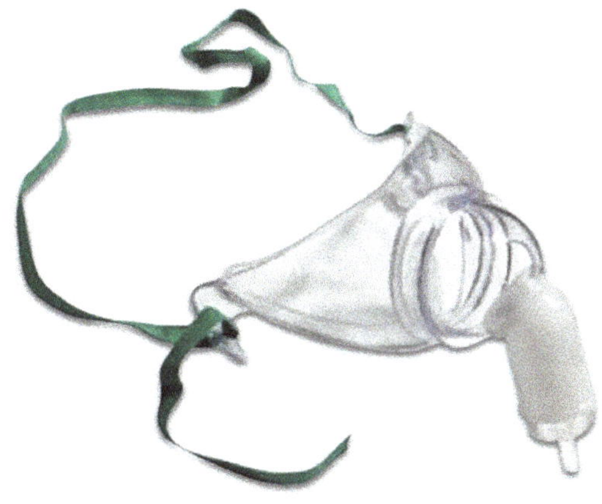

Fig. 7: Tracheostomy mask.

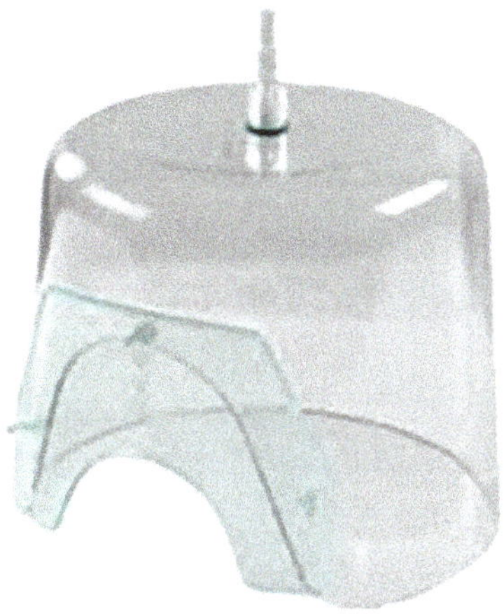

Fig. 8: Oxygen hood.

High-flow (Fixed FiO_2) Devices

High-flow or fixed performance OTDs provide oxygen at a certain concentration or FiO_2. They are based on Venturi modification of Bernoulli principle. With a properly functioning and setup of device, fixed or predetermined FiO_2 is always available to the patient, but it may provide false FiO_2 if the patient's inspiratory flow rate is unusually high. If patient's inspiratory demand exceeds the output of this device, it can no longer be classified as "high-flow" and FiO_2 will decrease.

The high-flow devices provide a total flow (mixture of oxygen and air) to fulfill the ventilatory requirement of patients regardless of RR or depth of breathing but if the patient's inspiratory demand is more than the maximum out of a particular device, other device has to be used to fulfill all the ventilatory requirements of the patient.

Air Entrainment Mask or Venturi Mask

A Venturi is a simple design of valve that uses high-flow oxygen supplied through a narrow port which allows room air to be drawn in from atmosphere **(Fig. 9)**.

The rate of flow generated by this Venturi principle and Venturi mask may be equal to peak inspiratory flow

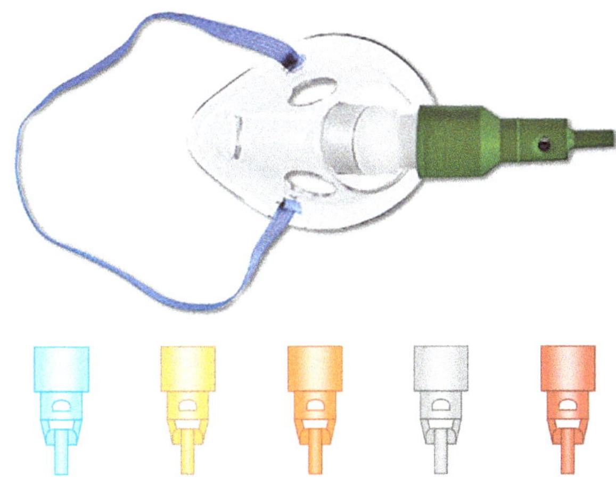

Fig. 9: Venturi mask.

TABLE 2: Venturi dilutor valve rating, color coding and O_2 flow rate.

Color coding	*O_2 concentration (%)*	*O_2 flow (L/min)*	*Air entrainment (L/min)*
Blue	24	2–4	50–100
White	28	4–6	40–60
Orange	32	6–8	56
Yellow	36	8–10	40
Red	40	8–12	24–36
Green	60	12	33

of patient. There are different colored dilutor jets which deliver a particular FiO_2 (24–50% depending upon the use of dilutor jet) at a particular flow rate set and marked or embossed onto bottom of the dilutor **(Table 2)**. As forward flow of inspired gas increases, the lateral pressure adjacent and perpendicular to the vector of flow decreases, resulting in entrainment of gas. Because of the high-flow rate, the exhaled gases are rapidly flushed from the mask, via its holes. Therefore, there is no rebreathing and no increase in dead space. These masks are recommended when fixed oxygen concentration is desired in patients whose ventilation is dependent on hypoxic drive. It is most commonly used for chronic obstructive pulmonary disease patients requiring a specific FiO_2 that will not fluctuate **(Table 2)** with changes in breathing pattern and also may be used in patient during weaning from long-term oxygen therapy to gradually lower the FiO_2. Long-term and high-flow dilutor mostly need humidification device to be used.

Advantages:

- It gives a fine control of FiO_2 at fixed rate.
- It gives a fine, reliable, and precise FiO_2.
- There is a high-flow entrainment of air, thereby saving oxygen cost.
- It can be used for low FiO_2 as well.
- It helps in deciding whether the O_2 requirement is increasing or decreasing.

Disadvantages:
- Uncomfortable
- Expensive
- It cannot deliver higher FiO_2
- It interferes with eating and drinking.

Multivent Masks

Multivent Venturi mask is an adjustable Venturi mask, in which, in same mask it is possible to use different flow rate and desired FiO_2 for changing oxygen requirement **(Figs. 10A and B)**. It has color-coded air-entrainment low concentrator dilutor (green colored) for 24%, 26%, 28%, and 30% FiO_2 and medium-concentration diluters (white colored) for 35%, 40%, and 50% FiO_2 with locking ring for securing flow setting. It also has an adapter for high humidity.

Aquapac Mask

This is a disposable adjustable Venturi mask, used with aerosol tubing and aerosol mask. It is suitable for patients who require low to moderate oxygen concentration. A water bottle is connected to the tubing at the bottom of the mask and it attaches to an oxygen flow meter to regulate the oxygen flow **(Fig. 11)**. If a heater is attached to the water bottle, it can be converted into a heated humidification system from a cold nebulization. FiO_2 delivered can be up to 98%.

Reservoir Bag Mask

Reservoir bag mask is designed for patients who require short-term high concentrations of oxygen **(Fig. 12)**. The FiO_2 depends on the flow rate, at 15 L/min of flow rate FiO_2 is about 90%; whereas at 10 L/min of flow rate, FiO_2 is almost 70%. Control over the flow rate and FiO_2 is rapid and can be useful in emergent and acute conditions. Although it provides high flow but performance is variable and should be used only for less time (preferably not more than 3 hours) to decrease complications related to dry gases.

High-flow Nasal Cannula

It delivers heated and humidified oxygen via special devices[14] **(Fig. 13)**.

There are three main proposed benefits of high-flow nasal cannula (HFNC):
1. Precise oxygen delivery
2. Functional residual capacity enhancement
3. Dead space washout

This system delivers greater and prescribed oxygen concentrations in the lungs with a lesser entrainment of room air, at a flow rates up to 8 L/min in infants and up to 40 L/min in children and adults. In patients with respiratory distress or failure, oxygen by humidified HFNC may be better tolerated than by face mask. Such high flow also helps to wash out carbon dioxide in anatomical dead space. FRC also increases by 25% with HFNC.

While the FiO_2 remains relatively constant. As gas is generally warmed to 37°C and completely humidified, so mucociliary function remains good and there is less discomfort.

High-flow High FiO_2 Nebulizer (Misty-Ox®)

The amount of FiO_2 provided by this is almost 100% (no oxygen dilution) and patients requiring this amount of oxygen are generally having critical oxygenation problems and they should be either in intensive care units or high dependency units **(Fig. 14)**.

High-flow Oxygen and Continuous Positive Airway Pressure

This device is mainly used in critical care units, pulmonary ward, coronary care units, and casualty department. This OTD provides high flow and supports to the spontaneous respiration of patients and provides sufficient oxygen for management in ward or transfers to a more suitable clinical area.

Bag-valve-mask or Manual Resuscitator or Ventilation Units

Bag-valve-mask (BMV) or manual resuscitator is mainly used for resuscitation purpose by positive pressure ventilation **(Fig. 15)**, but in emergency condition they can be used to provide 100% oxygen (if the patient is spontaneously breathing or ventilation is manual) for short period.

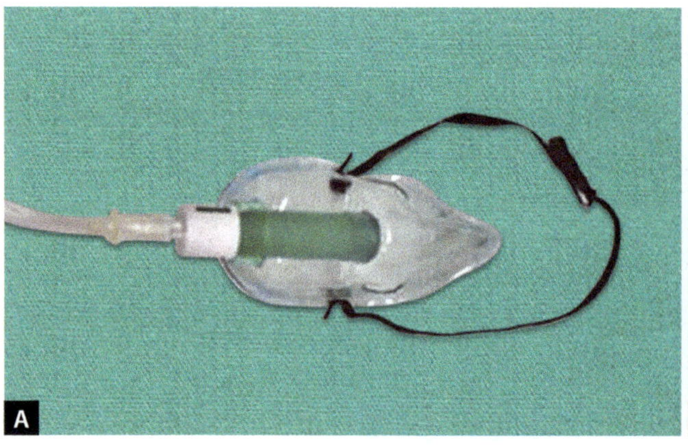

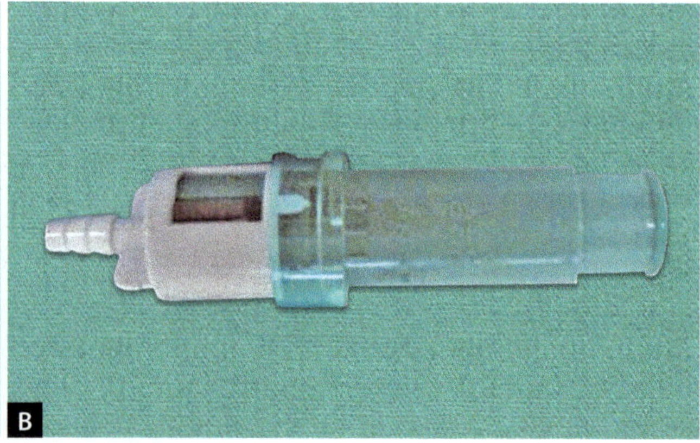

Figs. 10A and B: (A) Multivent mask; (B) Medium concentrator.

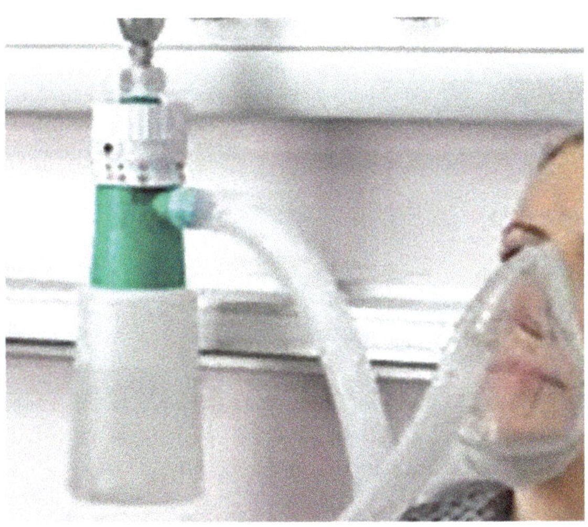

Fig. 11: Aquapac mask.

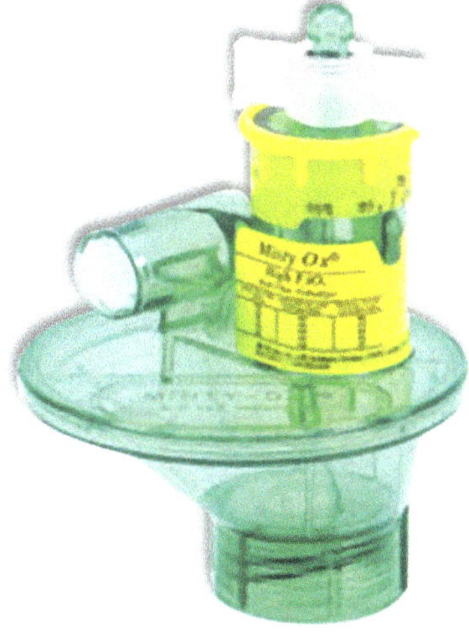

Fig. 14: Misty-Ox.

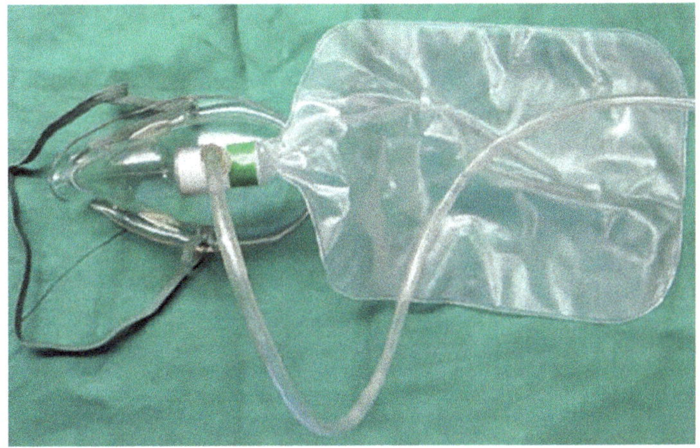

Fig. 12: Reservoir bag mask.

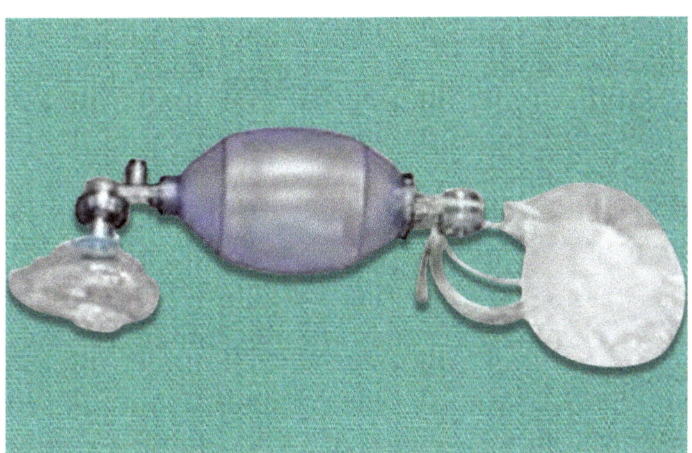

Fig. 15: Bag-valve-mask.

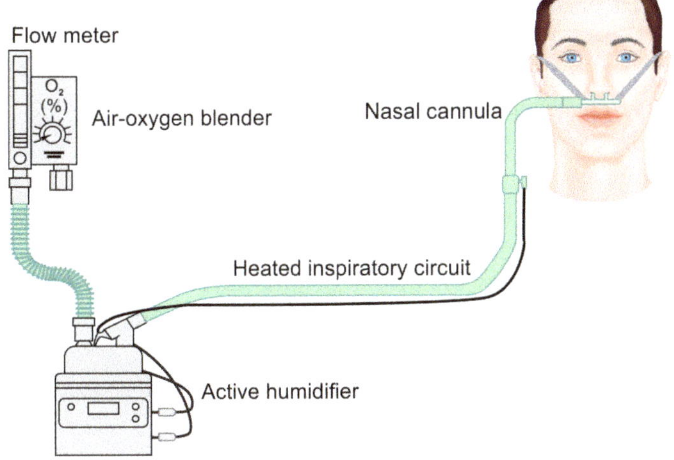

Fig. 13: High-flow nasal cannula.

There are various types of nonrebreathing valves that can be used with manual resuscitator for purpose of controlled and spontaneous respiration.

A comparison of different types of OTDs is given in **Table 3**.

TABLE 3: Comparison of various types of oxygen therapy devices.[15]

Delivery system	*Flow of oxygen (L/min)*	*Delivered FiO_2 (%)*
Nasal cannula	0.5–4	22–40
Hudson mask	5–10	40–60
Venturi mask	Variable (depend on required FiO_2)	24–50 (depend on flow selected)
Reservoir mask	10–15	60–90
CPAP or NIV	0.5–60	22–60

(CPAP: continuous positive airway pressure; FiO_2: fraction of inspired oxygen concentration; NIV: noninvasive ventilation)

PART II

APNEIC OXYGENATION[16]

Apneic oxygenation is the delivery of supplemental oxygen to the nasopharynx during apnea. Alveolar oxygen diffuses into the bloodstream and is consumed into carbon dioxide even during the period of apnea. At rest about 250 mL of oxygen is consumed per minute and about 5–20 mL of carbon dioxide is produced per minute and returned to alveoli. Because of carbon dioxide's high affinity for hemoglobin and effective buffering, the volume of carbon dioxide returned to the alveoli is less than the volume of oxygen removed. As a result, alveolar pressure decreases and gas is drawn down from the nasopharynx. This is called as aventilatory mass flow (AVMF). By increasing the fraction of oxygen in the gas moving from the nasopharynx to the lungs, apneic oxygenation aims to prevent arterial desaturation. For apneic oxygenation, 15 L/min of oxygen is given with advantages of no oxygen desaturation for a longer time.

The main advantage of this approach is that it is extremely simple and fast. Apneic oxygenation requires excellent preoxygenation and maintenance of a high concentration of oxygen extending from the nasal cannula to the alveoli.

Preoxygenation with nasal cannula may be performed *while* a patient is lying on their side and actively vomiting. This technique may be used in patients who cannot accept a mask due to facial surgery or trauma. The primary disadvantage is that the nasal cannula is uncomfortable at this flow rate without heating or humidification.

TECHNIQUES FOR APNEIC OXYGENATION

NO DESAT

Nasal oxygen during efforts securing a tube,[17] which uses a simple nasal cannula with standard low-flow cold dry oxygen at a rate up to 15 L/min. NO DESAT allows apneic oxygenation to continue while attempts at tracheal intubation are performed, and it increases apnea times by 2–5 minutes.

Apart from traditional oxygen therapy, noninvasive ventilation and invasive mechanical ventilation; recently patient with the respiratory failure can be treated with a high-flow nasal oxygenation. Nasal high flow (NHF) allows the delivery of up to 70 L/min of heated and humidified gas via a wide bore nasal cannula. It has got a blender which allows operator to choose the required FiO_2 and thus prevents oxygen toxicity.

THRIVE

Transnasal humidified rapid-insufflation ventilatory exchange[18] uses high-flow oxygen at a rate up to 70 L/min with warmed humidified nasal oxygen **(Fig. 16)**. It can either deliver varying fraction of oxygen from 21 to 100% (*Optiflow*™) or fixed 100% oxygen. THRIVE combines the benefits of apneic oxygenation with continuous positive airway pressure and gaseous exchange through flow-dependent dead space flushing. THRIVE increases apnea time by enhancing apneic oxygenation and provides apneic ventilation, reducing the rate of rise of CO_2 to approximately one-third of that expected. In patients with nonhypercapnic acute hypoxemic respiratory failure, treatment with high-flow oxygen has shown to reduce 90-day mortality.

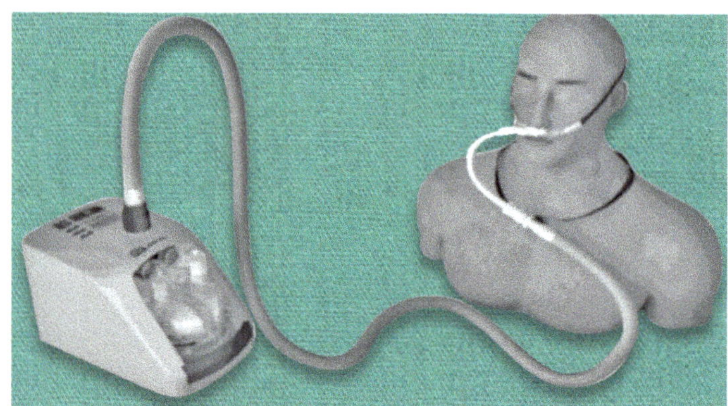

Fig. 16: Transnasal humidified rapid-insufflation ventilatory exchange (THRIVE).

Buccal Oxygen Delivery

Supplementary oxygen flow is delivered via the oral route using an adapted right angle endotracheal (RAE) tube secured in the left buccal space. This technique allows the benefits of apneic oxygenation during laryngoscopy and does not interfere with the ability to face mask ventilation. Theoretically, this technique is superior to NO DESAT and THRIVE because it offers additional protection from risk of pulmonary or gastric barotrauma, because oxygen source remains in the oral cavity and this ensures that any rise in pharyngeal pressure will be vented via the mouth.

PART III

HUMIDIFICATION

Humidification is like addition of heat and moisture to the inspired gas.

Rationale or the use of humidification is as follows:

- To liquefy and remove the retained thick secretions from the lower respiratory tract
- To reduce inflammatory and allergic responses in the upper respiratory tract
- To correct humidity deficit resulting from inspired air bypassing the airway during the use of mechanical ventilation in critically ill and postsurgical patients
- Cold and dry air increases heat and fluid loss
- Medical gases including air and oxygen have a drying effect on mucous membranes resulting in the airway damage
- In conditions such as asthma, hyperventilation of dry gases can worsen bronchoconstriction
- It may also help to manage hypothermia.

Indications

- Patients with copious secretions
- Noninvasive and invasive ventilation
- In children, nasal cannula and Hudson mask will need a flow rates of >2–4 L/min[16]
- Facial mask flow rates >5 L/min

- All high-flow systems require humidification
- Whenever oxygen is being delivered for longer time
- Patients with tracheostomy

Hazards and Complications from Humidification during Mechanical Ventilation

- High-flow rates during disconnect may aerosolize contaminated condense in the heated humidified circuit
- Increased work of breathing [heat-moisture exchanger (HME)]
- Elevated airway pressures caused by condensation of water
- Inadvertent overfilling resulting in unintended tracheal lavage in heated humidifiers
- Inadvertent tracheal lavage from pooled condensate in circuit in heated humidifiers

Methods of Humidification

Humidification systems are either active or passive:

- *Active humidification systems:* These include bubble through humidifiers such as Woulff bottle or improved version such as Aquinox heaters, humidification chambers, nebulization, and prefilled bags.
- *Passive humidification systems:* These include HMEs, which actually recycle the exhaled heat and humidity from the patient. It may be available with filters and can be hydrophobic or hygroscopic.[15]

The type of humidification device selected will depend on the oxygen delivery system in use, and the patient's requirements.

Active Humidifiers

It uses external sources of heat and water.

- *Low-flow humidifiers (unheated):*
  - *Passover humidifiers (Woulff bottle):* In this, O_2 and gas pass over the surface of water bath, picking up moisture. These are simple and easily available sources of humidification **(Fig. 17)**. But bubblers are water reservoir, hence can support the growth of *Pseudomonas aeruginosa* and may lead to nosocomial respiratory infection and also there are always chances of accidental spillage of hot water and risk of thermal burn.
- *High-flow humidifiers (heated):*
  - *Heated passover:* Directs gas over a reservoir of heated water. Problem with this type of humidification is accidental spillage of hot water and risk of burns **(Fig. 18)**.
  - *Diffuser cascade:* A more efficient design of the low-flow diffusion (bubbler) humidifier. Besides being heated, the area for gas-water interface is increased by use of large diffusion tower.
  - *Bubble humidifiers:* Usually, uses foam or mesh diffuser through which the mainstream flow must pass, producing smaller bubbles, thereby allowing greater surface area for gas/water interaction and aerosols at higher flow rates **(Fig. 19)**. Water levels of all humidifiers must be maintained as marked to ensure maximum humidity output. Inspired gas temperature should be monitored continuously

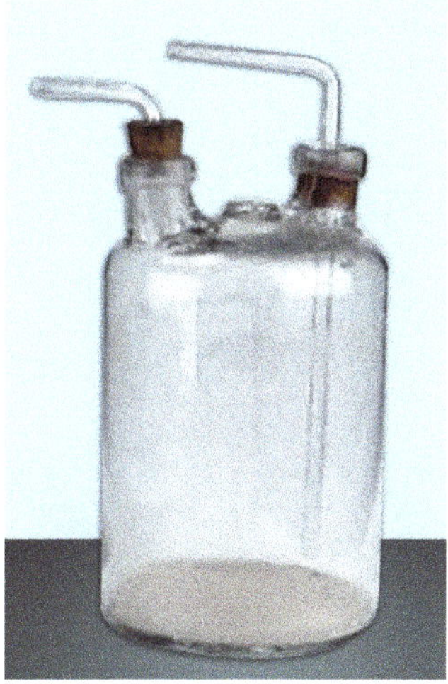

Fig. 17: Woulff bottle.

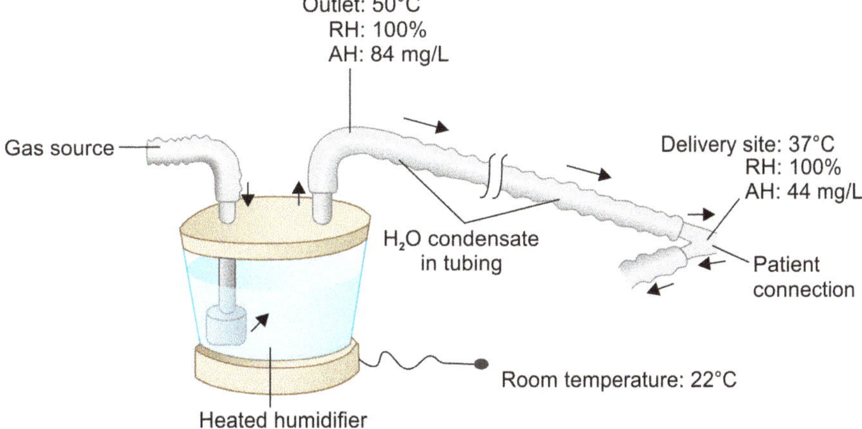

Fig. 18: Heated passover humidifier.

with an inline thermometer when using heated humidifiers. The thermometer should be as close to the patient as possible. One problem with this is that the warm and moist areas become the breeding grounds for microorganisms (especially *Pseudomonas*). The humidifier should be changed every 24 hours.

Passive Humidifiers

Heat-moisture exchangers (artificial nose): It mimics and functions like the nasal cavity and upper airways in gas humidification.

It is also called as condenser humidifier, Swedish nose, nose humidifier, regenerative humidifier, and vapor condenser. It traps the exhaled heat and moisture during the patients expiration and returns it to the patient during the next inspiration. These are the greatest source of contaminated moisture to the patient, hence ideally, should be changed every 12–24 hours **(Fig. 20)**.

Heated humidifiers are better in terms of preservation of relative humidity and temperature than HME,[17] however, most modern HMEs are cost effective and are able to maintain physiological air-conditioning even in long-term ventilated patients.[18] In spontaneously breathing patients and in tracheostomized patients, both HH and HMEs are equal in performance and in term of cost-effectiveness HMEs are preferred.[19]

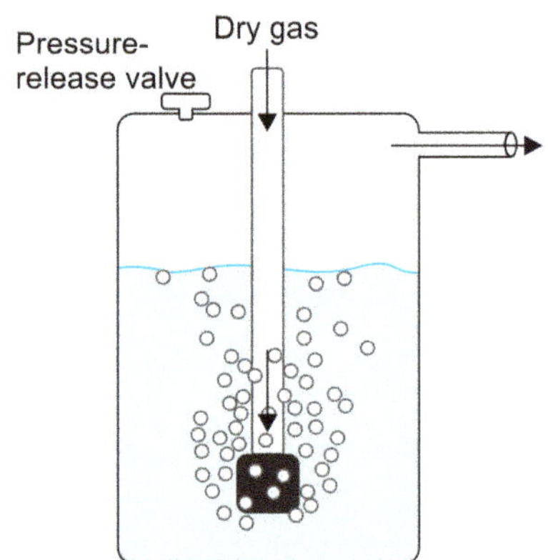

Fig. 19: Bubble humidifier.

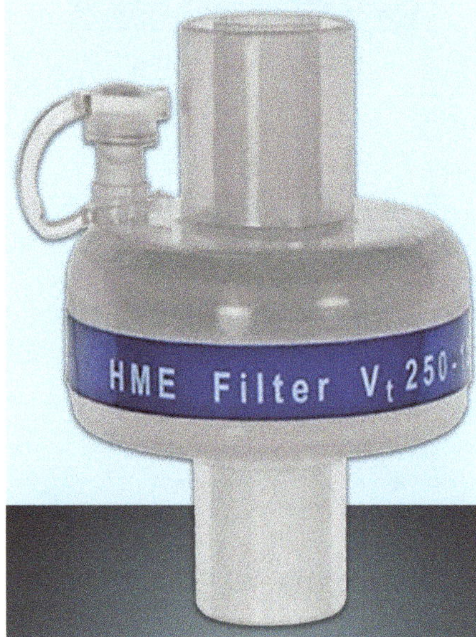

Fig. 20: Heat-moisture exchanger.

Indications of passive humidifiers:
- To increase heat and humidity during both short- and long-term ventilation.
- As transport ventilators do not have any source for humidification of inspired gases so it is used in transportation of intubated patients.
- For supplying supplemental oxygen to patients who are intubated or having supraglottic airway, by connecting oxygen tubing to gas sampling port.

Advantages of passive humidifiers:
- Inexpensive
- Easy-to-use small, light weight, and simple in design
- Silent in operation
- No requirement of external source energy, water, temperature monitor, and alarms
- No danger from hyperthermia, overhydration, electrical shock, and burns

Disadvantages:
- Delivery of limited humidity
- Insignificant contribution to temperature preservation
- Increased dead space, may lead to increase work of breathing
- Less effective than active humidifiers.

Contraindications for HME according to American Association for Respiratory Care (AARC) Clinical Practical Guidelines[20]

- Patients with thick or copious secretion
- When there is loss in expired tidal volume, (e.g., large bronchopleurocutaneous fistulas or presence of endotracheal tube cuff leak)
- In patients managed with low tidal volumes like those ARDS
- In difficult to wean patients and those with limited respiratory reserve
- Hypothermic patients with body temperature <32°C
- In patients with high minute ventilation volume (>10 L/min)

CONCLUSION

Long-term oxygen therapy is very important. The options in oxygen delivery sources, devices, and accessories should be fully understood in order to help attain the highest quality of life possible while using oxygen. Oxygen is a drug, and should be used only when required. Airway humidification also plays a vital role in the mechanically-ventilated patients along with oxygenation.

REFERENCES

1. Beasley R, Aldington S, Weatherall M, et al. Oxygen therapy in myocardial infarction: An historical perspective. JR Soc Med. 2007;100(3):130-3.
2. Cabello JB, Burls A, Emparanza JI, et al. Oxygen therapy for acute myocardial infarction. Cochrane Database Syst Rev. 2010;(6):CD007160.
3. Cranston JM, Crockett A, Currow D. Oxygen therapy for dyspnoea in adults. Cochrane Database Syst Rev. 2008;(3):CD004769.
4. Fawole B, Hofmeyr GJ. Maternal oxygen administration for fetal distress. Cochrane Database Syst Rev. 2003;(4):CD000136.
5. Singh CP, Singh N, Singh J, et al. Oxygen therapy. J Indian Acad Clin Med. 2001;2(3):178-84.
6. Grippi MA, Elias JA, Fishman JA, et al. Fishman's Book on Pulmonary Disease and Disorder, 5th edition. United States: McGraw-Hill Education/Medical; 2015.
7. Burton GG, Hodgkin JE, Ward JJ. Respiratory Care: A Guide to Clinical Practice, 4th edition. Philadelphia: Lippincott-Raven; 1997. pp. 381-95.
8. Kory RC, Bergmann JC, Sweet RD, et al. Comparative evaluation of oxygen therapy techniques. JAMA. 1962;179:123-8.
9. Leigh JM. Variation in performance of oxygen therapy devices. Anaesthesia.1970;25:210-22.
10. Davey A, Diba A. Ward's Textbook of Anaesthetic Equipment, 6th edition. Philadelphia: Saunders; 2012.
11. Dorsch JA, Dorsch SE. Understanding Anaesthesia Equipment, 5th edition. Philadelphia: Lippincott Williams and Wilkins; 2017.
12. Marino P. The ICU Book, 4th edition. Philadelphia: Lippincott Williams and Wilkins; 2013.
13. Wasnick J, Butterworth J, Mackey D. Morgan and Mikhail's Clinical Anaesthesiology, 5th edition. United States: McGraw Hill Education; 2013.
14. Nishimura. High-flow nasal cannula oxygen therapy in adults. J Intensive Care. 2015;3:15.
15. Swmantic Scholar. (2011). Guidelines for acute oxygen therapy for western australian hospitals. [online] Available from https://www.semanticscholar.org/paper/GUIDELINES-FOR-ACUTE-OXYGEN-THERAPY-FOR-WESTERN/32184604f8e8ebcf8df71591221def7e2a5db77b [Last accessed May, 2021].
16. Saraswat V. Inhalational therapy and humidification. Indian J Anaesth. 2008;52(Suppl 5):632-41.
17. Miyamoto K. Is it necessary to humidify inhaled low flow oxygen or low-concentration oxygen? Nihon Kokyuki Gakkai Zasshi. 2004;42:138-44.
18. Luchetti M, Stuani A, Castelli G, et al. Comparison of three different humidification systems during prolonged mechanical ventilation. Minerva Anestesiol. 1998;64:75-81.
19. Rathgeber J, Henze D, Züchner K. Air conditioning with a high-performance HME (heat and moisture exchanger)—an effective and economical alternative to active humidifiers in ventilated patients. A prospective and randomized clinical study. Anaesthesist. 1996;45:518-25.
20. American Association for Respiratory Care, Restrepo RD, Walsh BK. Humidification during invasive and noninvasive mechanical ventilation: 2012. Respiratory Care. 2012;57(5):782-8.

Video Laryngoscopy

Manoj R Shahane

ABSTRACT

Video laryngoscopy (VL) is a newer noninvasive method for endotracheal intubation. It has shown to improve the laryngeal view in difficult airway management. Video laryngoscopy is recently incorporated into the difficult airway algorithm. Detailed discussion of the history and evolution of the VL and its advantages over direct laryngoscopy are discussed in this chapter.

INTRODUCTION

Difficult airway management has been the foremost challenge faced by an anesthesia professional. A difficult airway can be defined as "the clinical situation in which a conventionally trained anesthesiologist experiences difficulty with facemask ventilation of the upper airway, difficulty with tracheal intubation or both."[1] This definition is very vague and depends on various factors including but not limited to patient factors, clinician factors and clinical settings.

In this chapter, we will review the video laryngoscopy (VL), a newer noninvasive method for endotracheal intubation. Video laryngoscopy has shown improved laryngeal views compared with direct laryngoscopy (DL) in patients with predicted and simulated difficult airways.[2]

HISTORY OF VIDEO LARYNGOSCOPY

Bullard laryngoscope was the first commercially available video device used for endotracheal intubation in 1980s. In late 1990s, many new indirect-optical laryngoscopes were developed. These laryngoscopes provided a non-line-of-sight view and the use of a dedicated monitor with an attached video camera, which laid down the foundation of VL. Weiss's modified Macintosh DL, had a fiberoptic bundle built in an angular blade,[3] and the Storz (Karl Storz Endoskope GmbH) DCI Video-Macintosh had a proprietary light source, video processor and a monitor with the Macintosh laryngoscope.[4] These devices functioned like a laryngoscope but did not need lot of force and distraction. In 2001, Canadian surgeon John A Pacey incorporated a miniature video chip into a modified Macintosh laryngoscope also known as a GlideScope (GVL, Verathon).[5] The original GlideScope had a 7 inch liquid-crystal display (LCD) black and white screen. Newer versions consist of color LCD screen and a bigger screen along with a lower profile blade (14 mm). Several similar products have been manufactured including the McGRATH® series 5 (Aircraft Medical), the C-MAC® (Storz), the AWS-100 (Pentax), and the disposable optical Airtraq® (Prodol, Spain).[6]

VIDEO LARYNGOSCOPY INDICATIONS AND POSSIBLE RECOMMENDED USE

- Elective oral intubation
- Elective nasal intubation
- Anticipated difficult intubation
- Awake intubation strategy
  - Rapid sequence intubation
- Unanticipated failed laryngoscopy
- Combined use of the GlideScope with fiberoptic bronchoscope in a very difficult airway
- Combined use of the GlideScope with various airway devices
- Diagnostic modality to document the recurrent laryngeal nerve status after the neck operations
- Placement of esophageal echoprobes under direct vision
- Placement of double lumen tubes for thoracic surgery
- Emergency room airway management for airway trauma, trismus and uncooperative patients
- Airway management for patients with inline neck stabilization
- Intensive care unit applications including endotracheal extubation backup support, endotracheal tube (ETT) exchange, placement of nasogastric tube to avoid lung feeding errors
- Air medical application like air transport and intubation
- Pediatric airway management
- Teaching airway anatomy to medical professionals and students.

EQUIPMENT

Video laryngoscopes consist of the following parts as shown in **Figures 1A and B**:

- LCD video monitor (color)
- Connecting cable with a fiberoptic bundle
- Laryngoscope blades of various sizes
- Intubating stylet
- Disposable laryngoscope blades.

The **Figures 1A and B** are representative figures of the VL, though multiple different models exist in different countries, which may look slightly different.

Video laryngoscope has an added advantage in lieu of their design compared to the DL:

- Video laryngoscopy has shorter interincisor distance compared to DL
- Video laryngoscopy blade has a relatively curved design compared to DL
- Video laryngoscopy has a non-line-of-sight view compared to DL.

TECHNIQUE

1. Review the VL's basic functioning and menu before use
2. Turn the VL on before its use. This helps to confirm its working condition and also heats the lens before its use to avoid fogging
3. Endotracheal tube is prepared in advance with the stylet, which is specifically designed for the VL
4. The rigid stylet is first lubricated to facilitate passing the ETT. The tube is at a 180° angle from its usual orientation on the stylet. The radiopaque stripe is on the concave side of the tube (convex side in a conventional stylet)
5. The plastic end of the VL stylet prevents it from spinning to its normal orientation
6. Blades of different sizes are available for VL; commonly used sizes are size 3 and 4
7. Load the VL blade on the video base unit if using the disposable blade and advance the scope like a DL into the midline of the oropharynx and gently advance the blade tip beyond posterior tongue
8. No lateral movement of the tongue is needed with VL
9. Once the vocal cords are visualized on the video screen, ETT is inserted
10. Video laryngoscopy blade should not be lifted once vocal cords are visualized as that can make the insertion of the tube more difficult **(Video 5)**.

VIDEO LARYNGOSCOPE BLADE SIZE

See **Table 1**.

COMMON CHALLENGES AND RESOLUTIONS

- Common cause of failure with VL is passing the scope too deep (esophageal view). It is necessary to look at the screen as the scope is passed to avoid this issue
- Insufficient space for tube insertion due to the midline approach with VL. The blade can be moved laterally to have adequate space to accommodate the tube
- Lifting the VL blade makes the vocal cords view more difficult. Minimal withdrawal with slight external pressure will make the view better
- Fogging of the video lens is common if the scope has not been turned on for at least 10 seconds. Prior 10 seconds warm up is needed to defog the lens.

TABLE 1: Video laryngoscope blade size.

Patient weight	<10 kg	10 kg adult	Adult (high body mass index)
Blade size	2	3	4

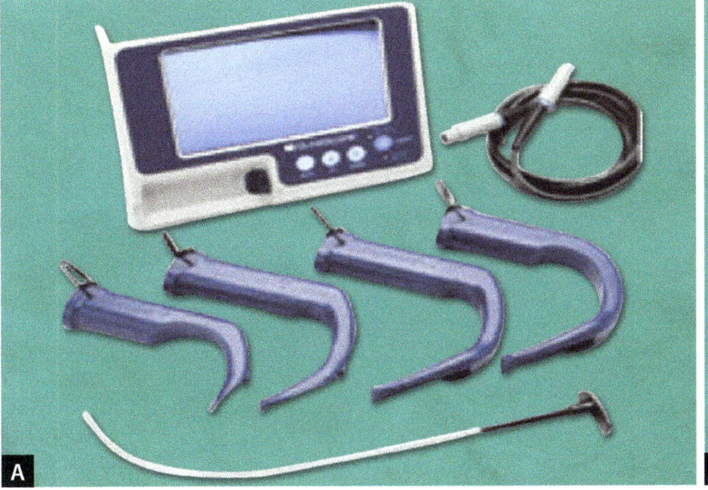
A

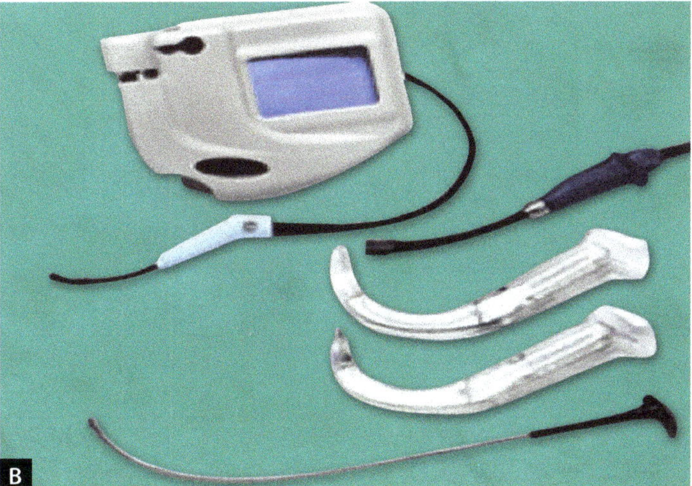
B

Figs. 1A and B: Video laryngoscope with disposable blades.

ROLE OF VIDEO LARYNGOSCOPY AND PROS AND CONS

- Video laryngoscopy has better efficacy in the patients with predicted difficult tracheal intubation[7,8]
- Video laryngoscopy has been shown to improve endotracheal intubation efficacy in infants[9]
- Video laryngoscope has been shown to improve success rate of intubation in adults[10]
- The time required to perform VL is significantly longer than the DL and thus can cause further increase in the heart rate, blood pressure and prolong apnea time[8,9]
- Proper training and preparation may reduce the time taken to use VL in future.

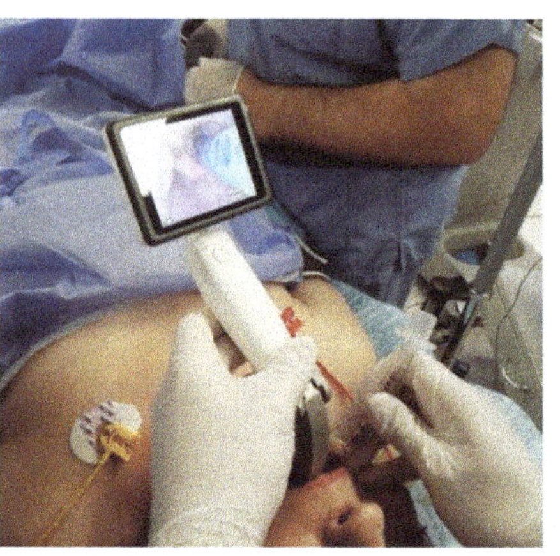

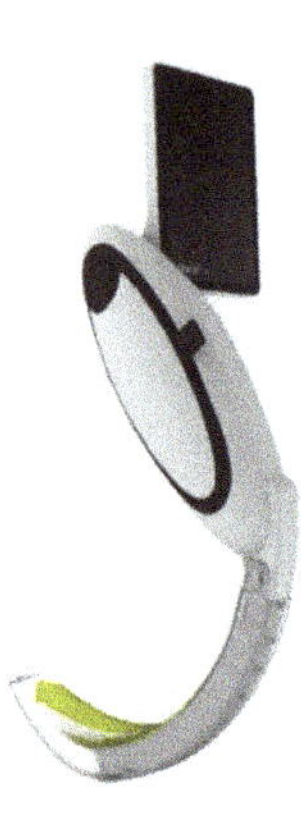

Fig. 2: McGrath video laryngoscope: Picture and demonstration.

We have seen new and improved versions of the video laryngoscope in last few years. I will mention two new and noteworthy video laryngoscopes at this time.

1. *McGrath video laryngoscope* is simple, easy to use, and not very expensive. It is as small as conventional laryngoscope with different sizes of McGrath disposable blades that click in place on a sturdy body with a small, swivel ready screen. I have used it on multiple occasions on patients with difficult airway with great result **(Fig. 2)**.
2. *GlideScope video laryngoscope core by Verathon* is a new and improved version of their original GlideScope model which has a picture-in-picture technology with two inputs. It enables us to use a conventional GlideScope handle along with a fiberoptic bronchoscope at the same time. An anesthesia provider can easily use this handle to insert double lumen tube and check with the attached fiberoptic scope with a single scope. Routinely, we do not need two channels, but it is a great addition specially for thoracic anesthesia. Anesthesia provider can also monitor heart rate and pulse oximetry measurements on the same screen. There is an option for recording a snapshot picture or a video for documentation or teaching perspective. I would consider this as a "Top of the line Video Laryngoscope" at current time **(Fig. 3)**.

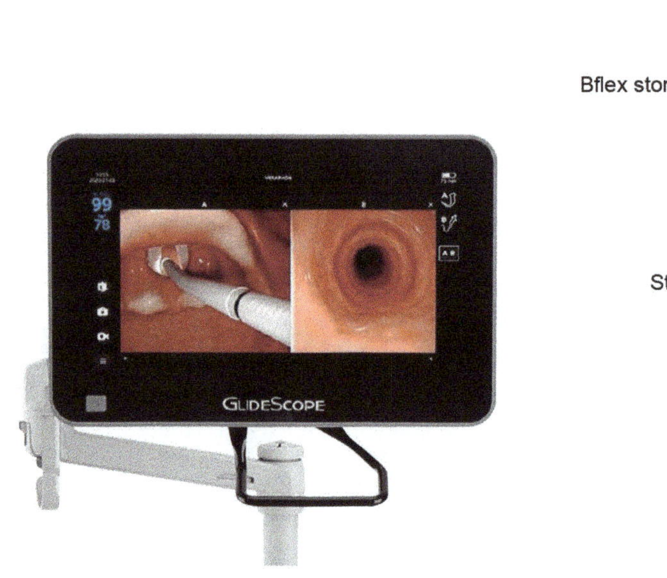

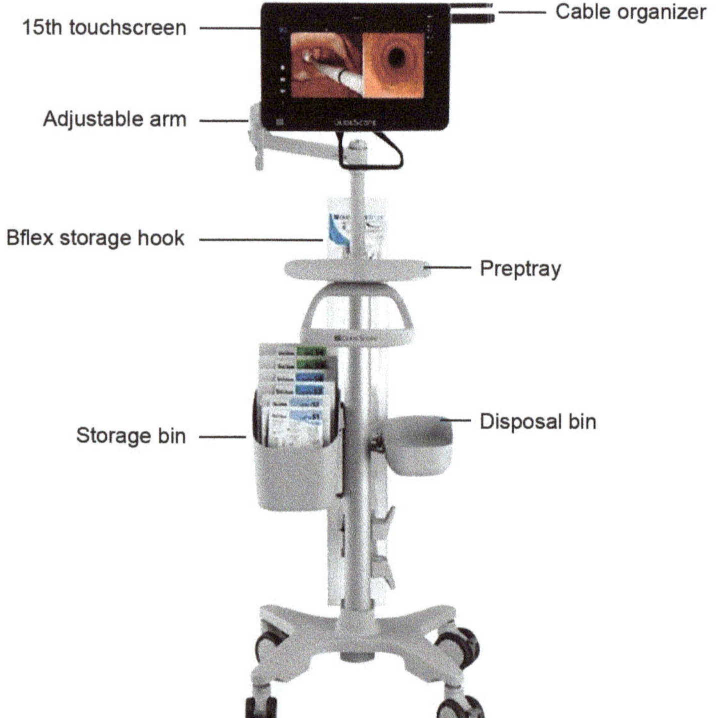

Fig. 3: GlideScope core by Verathon: Demonstration and picture.

CONCLUSION

Video laryngoscopy provides a better view of the glottis and a higher success rate of endotracheal intubation compared to the conventional laryngoscopy in adults and children. The time taken to perform the VL is improving as more experience is gained with this technique. The complication, which may occur due to increased time, is a concern and more evidence-based trials should be undertaken to review this further. The efficacy of VL is unequivocal and will enhance the scope of anesthesiology going forward.

REFERENCES

1. Apfelbaum JL, Hagberg CA, Caplan RA, et al. Practice guidelines for management of the difficult airway: An updated report by the American Society of Anesthesiologists Task Force on Management of the Difficult Airway. Anesthesiology. 2013; 118(2):251-70.
2. Jungbauer A, Schumann M, Brunkhorst V, et al. Expected difficult tracheal intubation: A prospective comparison of direct laryngoscopy and video laryngoscopy in 200 patients. Br J Anaesth. 2009;102(4):546-50.
3. Weiss M. Video-intuboscopy: a new aid to routine and difficult tracheal intubation. Br J Anaesth. 1998;80(4):525-7.
4. Kaplan MB, Ward DS, Berci G. A new video laryngoscope—an aid to intubation and teaching. J Clin Anesth. 2002;14(8):620-6.
5. Cooper RM, Pacey JA, Bishop MJ, et al. Early clinical experience with a new video laryngoscope (Glide Scope). Can J Anaesth. 2005;52(2):191-8.
6. Pott LM, Murray WB. Review of video laryngoscopy and rigid fiberoptic laryngoscopy. Curr Opin Anaesthesiol. 2008; 21(6):750-8.
7. Rosenblatt WH, Wagner PJ, Ovassapian A, et al. Practice patterns in managing difficult airway by anesthesiologists in the United States. Anesth Analg. 1998;87(1):153-7.
8. Aziz MF, Dillman D, Fu R, et al. Comparative effectiveness of the C-MAC video laryngoscope versus direct laryngoscopy in the setting of the predicted difficult airway. Anesthesiology. 2012; 116(3):629-36.
9. Fiadjoe JE, Gurnaney H, Dalesio N, et al. Prospective randomized equivalence trial of the GlideScope Cobalt® video laryngoscope to traditional direct laryngoscopy in neonates and infants. Anesthesiology. 2012;116(3):622-8.
10. Asai T, Liu EH, Matsumoto S, et al. Use of the Pentax-AWS in 293 patients with difficult airways. Anesthesiology. 2009; 110(4):898-904.

Fiberoptic Airway Management

Anil Parakh, Ameya Panchwagh

ABSTRACT

The field of airway management has undergone a vigorous revolution in the last 20 years. The array of devices, algorithms and pharmaceuticals in the modern airway armamentarium can be daunting. Supraglottic airways (SGAs) are firmly established in routine anesthetic care as well as airway rescue, but the advent of video laryngoscopy promises to remove many of the failings of a technique that has been in use for more than 100 years. Now, when faced with a difficult airway, the anesthesiologist has a plethora of devices to choose from. The fiberoptic bronchoscopy-guided intubation has however stood the test of time and is still considered the gold standard in airway management. Hence, it is prudent that every clinician dealing with difficult airways masters the art of fiberoptic bronchoscopic intubation. This chapter focuses on the equipment and technique of fiberoptic bronchoscopy and its use in combination with other airway devices as well as the intricacies involved in its troubleshooting.

INTRODUCTION AND HISTORY

The use of a fiberoptic bronchoscope (FOB) to assist in endotracheal intubation dates back to 1967, when a choledococoscope was first used to intubate a patient with Still's disease.[1] The first case series of the use of fiberscopes for intubation was published in 1972.[2] Initially clinicians used FOB for diagnostic purposes, ordinary intubation procedures and eventually for airway management in patients with very challenging airways and very soon became an instrument of the first choice in difficult intubation (DI) cases particularly after the publication of the American Society of Anesthesiologists (ASA) guidelines on difficult airway (DA) management.[3]

In the 1980s, the Asahi Pentax Company integrated FOB with the charge-coupled device (CCD) which allowed video monitor viewing of the airway and revolutionized its clinical benefits.[4] Later features like full color imaging, working suction or channel, light emitting diodes (LED) and micro-video complementary metal-oxide semiconductor (CMOS) chips were integrated. The "single use patients contact instruments" either as a reusable FOB with a disposable, sheath-like protective barrier or as an entirely disposable "nonfiberoptic" flexible bronchoscopes are recently tried and are available for use.

Current uses include nasal and oral intubations, evaluation of the airway, cervical risk scenarios, airway stenosis, obstructive sleep apnea, tracheomalacia, verification of accurate placement of single or double lumen endotracheal tubes, laryngeal mask airways (LMAs), endotracheal tube exchange, and placement of bronchial blocker devices. Recently the scope of this technique has widened due to its use in combination with other airway devices as a multimodal approach to DA management.

DESIGN AND PRINCIPLES

Fiberoptic bronchoscope and nonfiberoptic flexible bronchoscopes (Non-FOBs) are available from several manufacturers including Olympus, Pentax, Karl Storz, Ambu and Vision Sciences. Most of the FOBs are quite expensive and delicate, hence knowledge of their functionality and care is paramount to prevent damage and loss of clinical availability.

The Components of Fiberoptic Bronchoscope

Eyepiece

It contains lenses and adjustable focusing ring which can be fine-tuned to sharpen the image according to the visual acuity of the operator. The video camera can be attached on the eyepiece.

Control Section

The control section comprises of angulation lever, suction and working channel port. The suction port has a valve, which when pushed or pressed, activates suction. Angulation lever is used for flexing and deflexing the distal tip of the FOB. These movements along with the rotation of the FOB, allows nearly 360° visualization. The working channel port can be used for the instillation of the local anesthetic agents in "as we go technique" **(Fig. 1A)**.

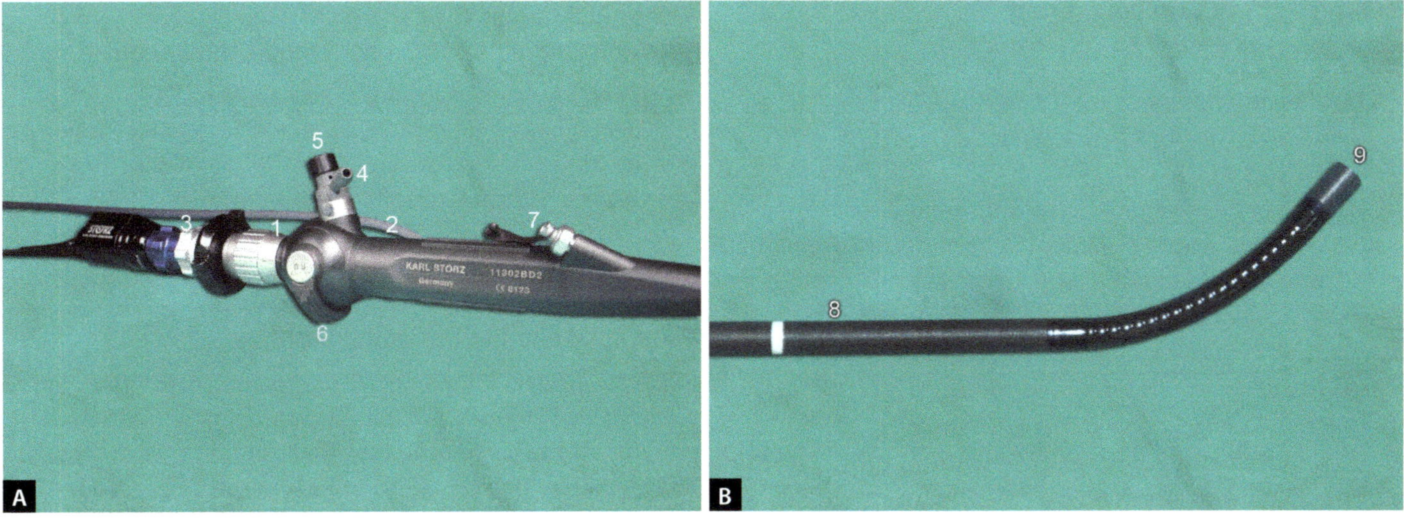

Figs. 1A and B: (A) Fiberoptic bronchoscope (FOB) handle (control section). 1. Focus adjusting ring; 2. Light source connection; 3. Video camera attachment; 4. Suction port; 5. Valve; 6. Lever; 7. Working channel; (B) Insertion cord and flexible tip. 8. Insertion cord; 9. Flexible tip.

Insertion Cord

The insertion cord consists of the following four components encased in a smooth plastic shell or sheath to provide airtight seal **(Fig. 1B)**:

1. Light guide bundles made up of noncoherent glass fiber, are one or two in number and allow the transmission of the light going towards the tip. Each bundle consists of 25,000–30,000 light fibers, which are of 25–30 µm in diameter
2. The fiberoptic bundle consists of 10,000–50,000 glass fibers, each 7–10 µm in diameter and arranged coherently to transmit the image to the visual section. The glass fibers are extremely sensitive to damage and black dots may become visible in the transmitted image, when damaged
3. Angulation wires are two in numbers and are controlled by angulation lever of the handle. Through an up and down movement of the angulation lever, the FOB tip moves in the opposite direction by as much as 240°–350°
4. The working channel is 1.2–2.8 mm in diameter and runs the length of the FOB from the suction or working port on the handle to the FOB tip. The FOB tip or the bending section is hinged and has an objective lens (2 mm in diameter) with fixed focal and short field of view (75°–120°).

Universal Cord

It transmits light from the light source and is attached at the level of control section of the FOB. The newer FOB have miniature battery operated light source at the control section.

Principle

The object is illuminated by the cold light, transmitted through two separate light transmission bundles.

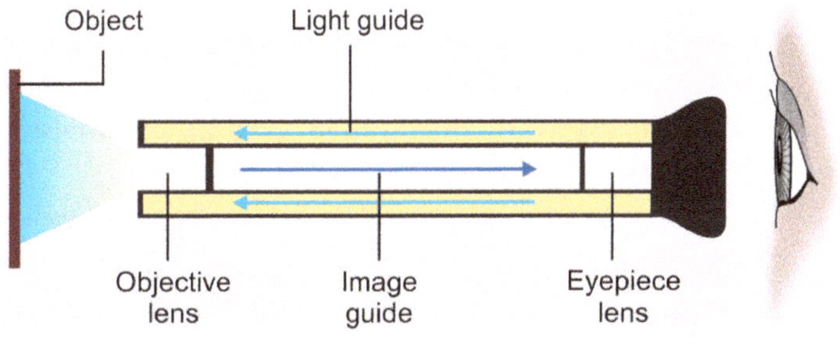

Fig. 2: Schematic drawing showing the transmission of light and images in an endoscope.

The reflected and back scattered light then enters the distal objective lens and is transmitted through the fiberoptic bundles to the eyepiece **(Fig. 2)**.

When the photons impact the tissue surface, some reflection occurs, depending on both the incident angle of the light and the refractive index of the tissue. The incident light beam is partially absorbed and partially scattered (changing direction) according to the optical properties of the tissue. Absorption and scattering substantially decrease the intensity of the light transmitted to the objective lens hence the output power of the light source must be high enough to cope with these conditions.

The image quality depends not only on the quality of the objective and eyepiece lenses, but also on the density and number of image or light fibers in the fiberoptic bundle.

INDICATIONS FOR FIBEROPTIC BRONCHOSCOPE INTUBATION

- Routine intubation
- Difficult intubations in following:
  - History of DI
  - History, physical examination and presence of congenital abnormalities (e.g., obesity, micrognathia, temporomandibular joint ankylosis)
  - Rescue of failed intubation attempt
- To prevent of cervical spine mobility in risky patients.
- To avoid trauma to a loose tooth, expensive dental prosthesis, nasal polyps
- To avoid aspiration of gastric contents
- For diagnostic purposes
  - Troubleshooting high airway pressures
  - Troubleshooting hypoxemia
  - Observation for airway pathology (e.g., stenosis, tracheomalacia, vocal cord paralysis)
  - Removal of airway pathology (e.g., secretions)
- For therapeutic purpose
  - Exchange of endotracheal tube
  - Assistance with airway placement (e.g., SGA devices, retrograde intubation, etc.)
  - Positioning of double lumen tubes or bronchial blockers
  - Correct positioning of the endotracheal tubes at specific depths
  - Intratracheal observation of tracheostomy instrument entry
- Awake intubation.

CONTRAINDICATIONS FOR AWAKE FIBEROPTIC BRONCHOSCOPIC INTUBATION

- Absolute contraindications
  - Uncooperative patient
  - Inexperienced endoscopic and assistant
  - Compromised equipment function
  - Significant upper airway obstruction except for diagnostic purposes
  - Massive trauma (but, if retrograde intubation is chosen, FOB may help)
- Moderate contraindications
  - Obstructing or obscuring blood, fluid, anatomy, or foreign body
- Relative contraindications
  - Concern for the vocal cord damage that might be caused by blind endotracheal tube (ETT) passage over the FOB
  - With some perilaryngeal masses or abscess, where blindly advancing the ETT can rupture the abscess or seed the tumor.

Contraindications for Asleep or Under Anesthesia Fiberoptic Bronchoscopic Intubation

- Inexperienced endoscopist and assistant
- Too high an aspiration risk or too difficult an airway
- Inability to tolerate even a short period of apnea
- Other contraindications are similar to those for awake FOB intubation.

EQUIPMENT

Fiberoptic and Nonfiberoptic Scopes

Various models of the FOB are available for use. Some FOBs have eyepiece or video attachments and others have varying degrees of portability. Sizes and ranges of view are also variable, from smallest infants to the largest adult size. Recently introduced FOB has lithium rechargeable battery operated FOB with a fixed, rotatable video screen by the handle and its CCD camera has a memory card.

Fiberoptic Bronchoscope Cart

Fiberoptic bronchoscope is an important part of a difficult intubation or difficult airway management algorithm hence it should be readily available to the users and all the members of the organization should be well aware about its availability and contents to increase the likelihood of success. Preferably, a mobile airway management cart equipped with the entire set of instruments, medications and consumables for fiberoptic intubation or advanced airway management should be available to all. The cart should have two widely separated tubular structures for hanging a clean FOB and, later a used one. The FOB cart should also have a light source, a video monitor, endoscopy masks, bronchoscope swivel adapters, oral intubating airways, bite blocks, atomizers, tongue blades, cotton-tipped swabs, gauzes, soft nasal airways, local anesthetics (e.g., 2 and 4% lidocaine) and suction catheters.

The entire FOB cart can be used as difficult airway cart and should contain a video laryngoscope and screen, SGA devices, intubating SGA devices, ETT introducer or exchangers[5,6] and percutaneous airway rescue sets.

Ancillary Equipment

Bronchoscopy Swivel Adapters and Endoscopy Masks

The bronchoscopy swivel adapters **(Fig. 3)** and the endoscopy masks **(Fig. 4)** are used in asleep or awake patients for the FOB examination, intubation, diagnosis or therapy. The bronchoscopy swivel adapter look like elbow adapters and can rotate and are placed between ventilating system and a mask, SGA or ETT and has a "flip-cap port", covering a diaphragm with a central opening. This allows passage of FOB without leakage during use of the continuous ventilation system on a patient. For intubation with swivel adapters the FOB is mounted through Aintree intubation catheter as mentioned later in the text. The endoscopy masks **(Fig. 4)**

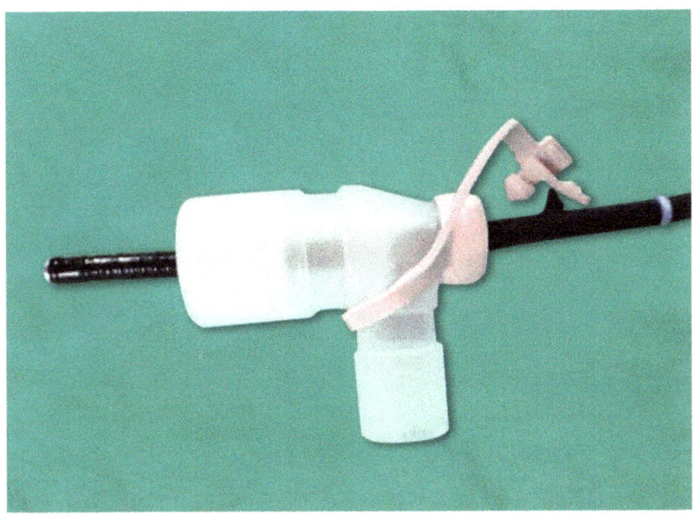

Fig. 3: Swivel adapter with fiberoptic bronchoscope.

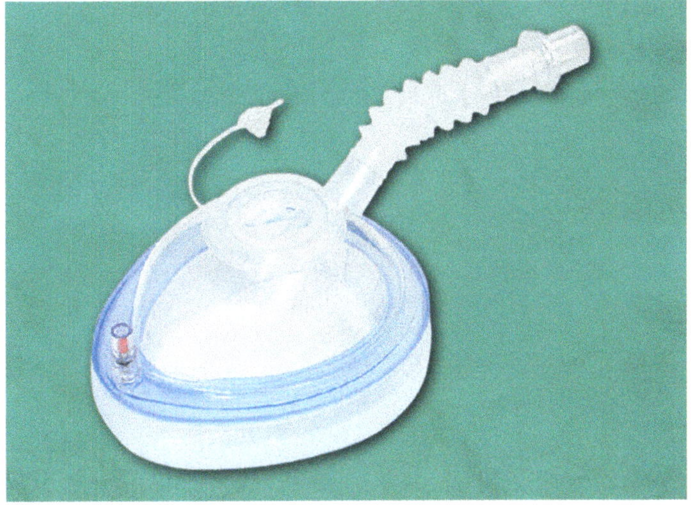

Fig. 4: Endoscopy mask.

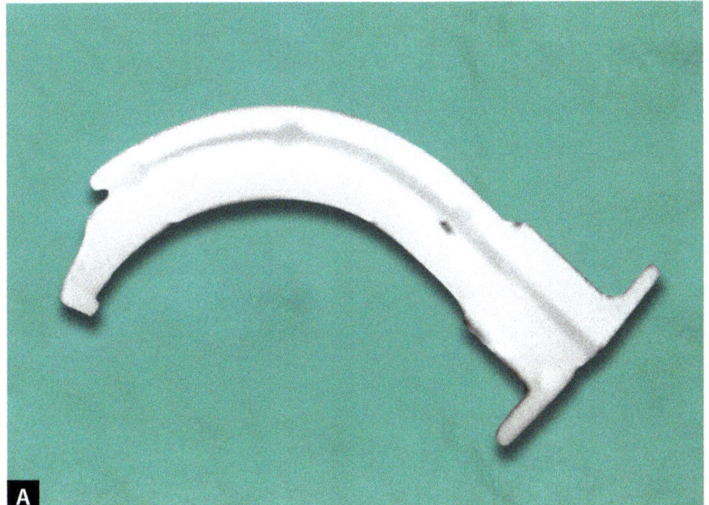

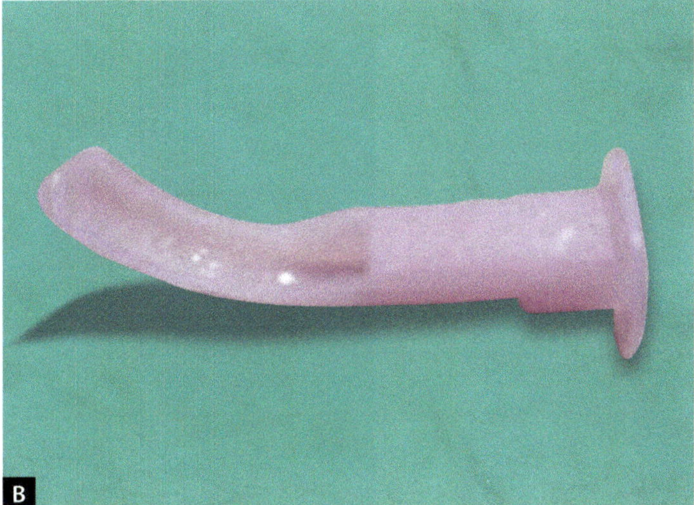

Figs. 5A and B: Intubating oral airways. (A) Berman's; (B) William's.

have at least one large additional opening through which FOB can be passed without any leakage. This opening allows the passage of ETT for intubation during continuous mask ventilation.

Intubating Oral Airways

Intubating oral airways (IOAs) are usually used in unconscious patients or in the totally anesthetized oropharynx of an awake patient, through which the FOB is inserted for the oral intubation. The commonly used IOAs are Berman's, William's **(Figs. 5A and B)** and Ovassapian **(Figs. 6A and B)**. These airways are useful in maintaining the midline while intubating the patient orally. Most of these IOAs has a channel that permits the passage of an ETT. The appropriate sizes IOAs should be selected for an individual patient for the smooth passage of ETT. Alternatively bite blocks **(Fig. 7)** can be used between the molars to prevent FOB damage.

Nasopharyngeal airways: There are two techniques of use of nasopharyngeal airways (NPAs) during FOB intubation.

1. Before inserting NPA make a lengthwise cut **(Fig. 8A)**, lubricate and gently insert into one nostril. Now guide lubricated FOB through NPA to lead tip of FOB towards the glottis. Once the FOB has entered just above the carina, the NPA is stripped away **(Fig. 8B)** and the ETT is railroaded over the FOB into the trachea

   In pediatric patients via NPA one can provide oxygenation and administer inhalational anesthesia administration
2. A lubricated NPA is inserted in one nostril and attached to a breathing circuit by an ETT adapter, and FOB intubation can be done either orally or nasally, through the opposite nostril.[7]

Endotracheal tubes: For FOB insertion, a regular polyvinyl chloride (PVC) ETTs are used. At times, the most distal ETT tip area can get caught on the arytenoids, especially the right, causing difficulty for the passage into the trachea. The centrally-curved soft tip ETTs have been reported to have greater success rate of passage.[8-10]

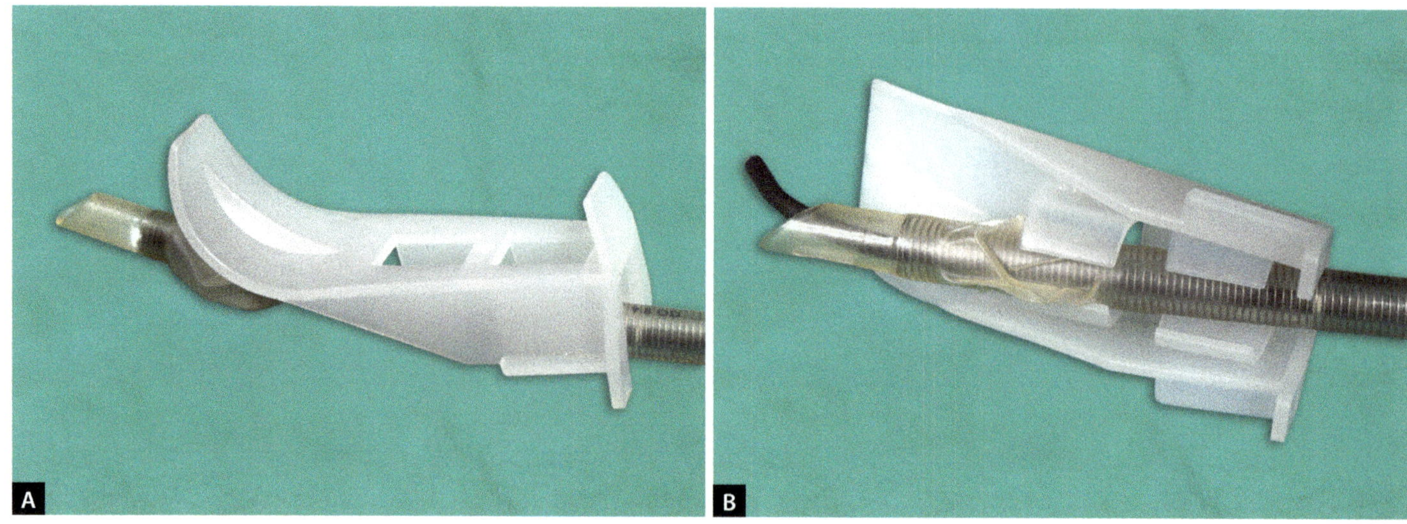

Figs. 6A and B: Ovassapian airway.

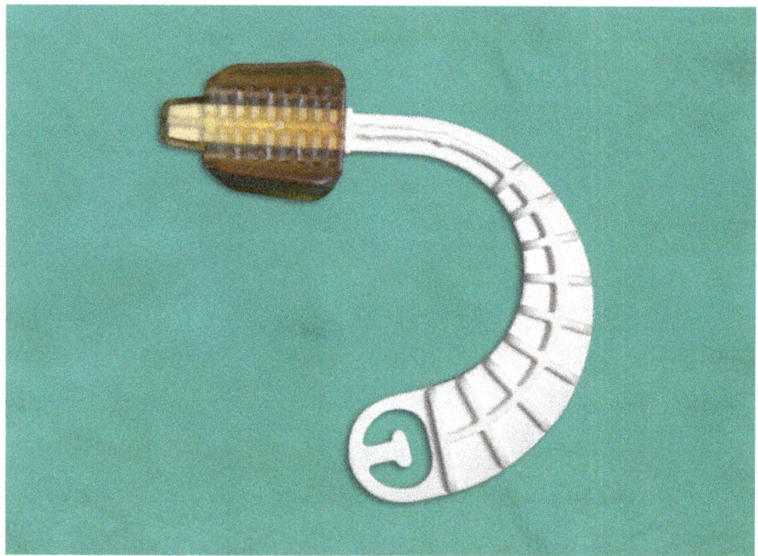

Fig. 7: Bite block.

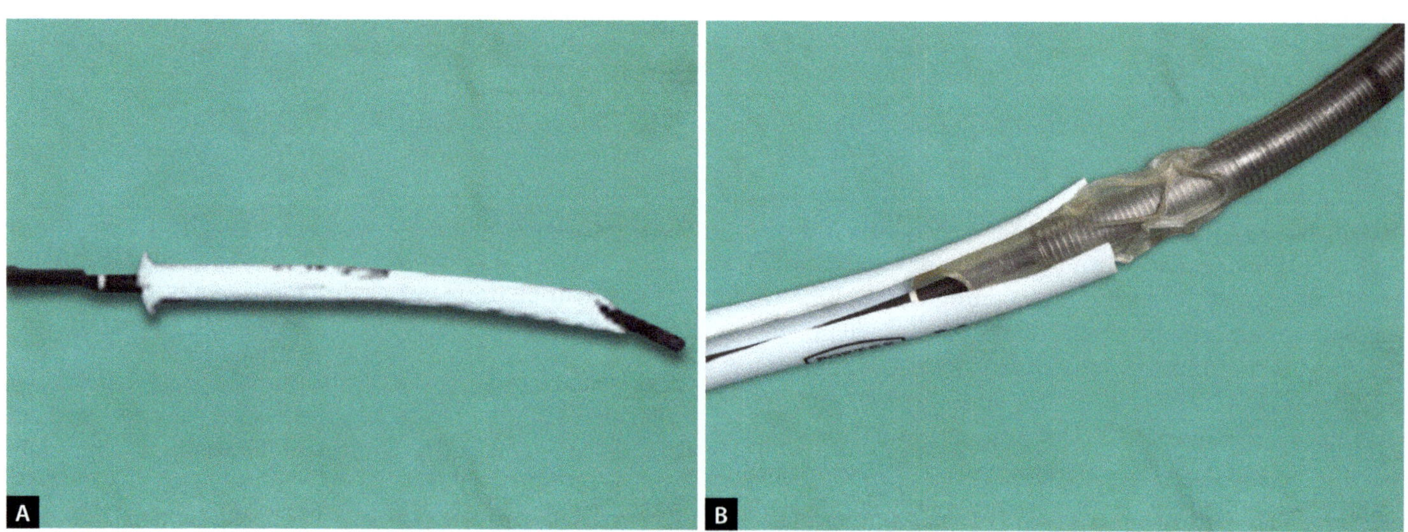

Figs. 8A and B: Nasopharyngeal airway. (A) Lengthwise split; (B) Stripping and removal.

CLINICAL CONSIDERATIONS

Once it is decided that the FOB intubation is the appropriate choice, one should decide whether to use a nasal or oral approach and whether to keep the patient awake until the control of airway is established or to perform the procedure in an anesthetized patient.

In general, the nasal route is easier for FOB intubation because the angle or curvature of the ETT naturally coincide that with the patient's upper airway hence it is easier to maintain a midline position and direct the scope into the trachea. When nasal route is used, the patient cannot bite or chew on the scope and also the gag reflex is less pronounced as compare to oral route. On the other hand, the risk of causing bleeding is higher and it is relatively contraindicated in patients with coagulation disorders.

The decision to perform the procedure in an awake versus anesthetized patient depends on the risk of losing the airway control. If there is any concern about the one's ability to manage the patient's airway, it is safest to have the patient maintain his or her own oxygenation and ventilation. One should not give up wakefulness easily.

TECHNIQUE OF FIBEROPTIC INTUBATION

Fiberoptic Bronchoscopic Intubation of the Conscious Patient

Awake FOB intubation is safe with a higher success rate due to following reasons:

- Preserved muscle tone avoids collapse of soft tissues and hence keeps the airway patent and avoids obstruction
- Spontaneous breathing dilates airway structures and deep breathing on command can open the obstructed airway passages
- Chances of desaturation of the patient is minimized in spontaneous breathing patients
- Proper local anesthesia (LA) of the airway will minimize the hemodynamic changes, severe coughing, laryngospasm, and failure of intubation.

General Preparation

A good intravenous access should be secured before the start of the procedure. Patient's monitoring equipment [like electrocardiography (ECG), blood pressure (BP), pulse oximetry], difficult airway cart with all the accessory devices, oxygen delivery systems, two suctions, drugs (like local anesthetics, vasoconstrictors, sedatives, narcotics, inhalation agents) and target controlled infusion devices should be kept ready.

Preparation of the Patient

The key of success for FOB intubation is adequate planning and patient's preparation, hence preparation should begin as soon as the decision has been made to use the technique.

- *Psychological preparation of the patient:* The psychological preparation of the patient is a basic step that is easily achieved with an explanatory, reassuring and professional discussion. The aim of the psychological preparation should be better patient's acceptance of the procedure and cooperation. During the preoperative visit, the degree of the difficulty should be assessed properly and justification for the use of awake FOB technique should be explained to the patient. Every step of the FOB intubation procedure should be explained in detail to the patient. LA should be described as sprays, as injections or as nebulization. Patient should be informed about any unpleasant taste of the local anesthetics, gargling, swallowing, taking deep breaths, if needed
- *Pharmacological preparation of the patient:*
  - *Antisialogogues:* Fiberoptic bronchoscope intubation requires a clear visual pathway. Blood and secretions prevents visualization, hence administration of an antisialogogue is essential. If any topical intraoral anesthetic is planned, the antisialogogue is given 15–20 minutes before hand, to allow sufficient onset time. These agents minimize the dilution of the local anesthetics, formation of a secretion barrier between LAs and the mucosa and washing away of topical agents down the esophagus. Glycopyrrolate (4 µg/kg) is preferred over atropine (10 µg/kg) except in children.
  - *Sedation:* The goal of sedation is to produce a cooperative patient, not an apneic patient. Sedation should be administered incrementally and titrated to drowsiness or slurring of the speech. Various drugs that may be used include midazolam (1–2 mg) for amnesia and sedation, fentanyl (0.7–1.5 µg/kg) for analgesia and antitussive effects, which reduce the discomfort and hemodynamic changes associated with topical anesthesia of the airway, nerve blocks and airway instrumentation. Other agents commonly used include ketamine (0.025–0.15 mg/kg) for sedation and analgesia, a combination of ketamine and Propofol, Propofol (25–75 µg/kg/min) for sedation, remifentanil (0.05–0.01 µg/kg bolus followed by 0.03–0.05 µg/kg/min infusion) for analgesia.

    Dexmedetomidine (0.2–0.7 µg/kg/h), a newer agent, started 20–30 minutes before the procedure provides hypnosis, amnesia, analgesia without respiratory depression. If titrated well, the patient remains responsive to verbal command. Target-controlled infusions are the most appropriate.
- *Local anesthesia:* Innervation of the upper airway—the ophthalmic (V1) and maxillary (V2) divisions of the trigeminal nerve provides innervation to the nasal mucosa as the anterior ethmoidal nerve, the nasopalatine nerve, and the sphenopalatine ganglion.[11,12]

  The anterior two-thirds of tongue rarely needs anesthesia. The sensory innervation to soft palate, posterior third of tongue, tonsils, and most of pharyngeal mucosa coms from Glossopharyngeal nerve (cranial nerve IX).[13,14] Some of its fibers supply lingual surface of epiglottis.[15] The gag reflex is controlled by afferent components of this nerve.

The motor function of soft palate and pharyngeal muscles is provided by vagus (cranial nerve X). The sensory supply to the laryngopharynx comes from superior and inferior laryngeal branches of vagus nerve.

The interior division of superior laryngeal nerve supplies sensory innervations to the base of the tongue, vallecula, epiglottis, pyriform recesses, epiglottis mucosa, and the laryngeal vestibule above the vocal cords. Its external division provides motor control to the adductor or tensors, the cricothyroid muscle and the cricopharyngeal part of the inferior constrictor of the pharynx.

The recurrent laryngeal nerve (RLN) is a branch of the vagus nerve (cranial nerve X). There are two recurrent laryngeal nerves, right and left, supplies all the intrinsic muscles of the larynx, except for the cricothyroid muscles.

Topical Orotracheal Anesthesia Technique

The LA of the airway should be performed without sedation but sedation can be given before any deep pharyngeal and laryngeal anesthesia.

The mouth can be anesthetized with lidocaine spray or viscous lidocaine. A commercial flavored preparation of 10% solution of lidocaine is available. This preparation is sold in pressurized bottles that deliver a metered spray. Alternatively, a 4% solution of the lidocaine can be sprayed in the mouth to the palate, tonsillar pillars, valleculae, epiglottis, and larynx during deep inspiration by bending the stylet-like applicator (atomizer) in whatever curve is needed **(Fig. 9)**.

Bilateral block of the glossopharyngeal nerve at the base of each anterior tonsillar pillar can be done by spraying LA **(Fig. 10)** or by placing swab or pledget soaked in local anesthetics in piriform fossa on each side for 5–10 minutes. 2 mL of Lidocaine can be injected at the base of anterior tonsillar pillar on each side to block this nerve but there are chances of hematoma formation and accidental vascular injection of the lidocaine.

Transtracheal Block

The transtracheal block provides rapid anesthesia of the entire trachea between the carina and the vocal cords. It is relatively simple to perform and requires no equipment other than a 10 cc syringe and 23 G needle. The complications of the trans tracheal block include bleeding, tracheal injury and the subcutaneous emphysema.

Technique

The transtracheal block should be performed approximately just prior to the start of FOB intubation. 2–4 mL of 4% lidocaine is taken into a 10 cc syringe with a 23 G needle. After applying antiseptic lotion, the cricothyroid membrane is identified **(Fig. 11A)**, and the syringe is directed posteriorly, perpendicular to the floor. When the needle is in trachea, a sudden loss of resistance is felt. The position of the needle is confirmed by aspirating air through the syringe. The lidocaine is then injected rapidly, and the needle is withdrawn quickly **(Fig. 11B)**. The patient will have a bout of cough, which would spread the local anesthetic down to the carina, trachea up to the vocal cords.

Superior Laryngeal Nerve Block

The superior laryngeal nerve (SLN), a branch of vagus nerve, provides sensory innervation to the epiglottis, arytenoids and vocal cords. The SLN blocks can be used in patient, who is not cooperative, and with limited mouth opening or as a rescue method when coughing or hemodynamic changes from the spray are undesirable.

The internal branch of the SLN is blocked by instilling LA, bilaterally, in the vicinity of the nerves, where they

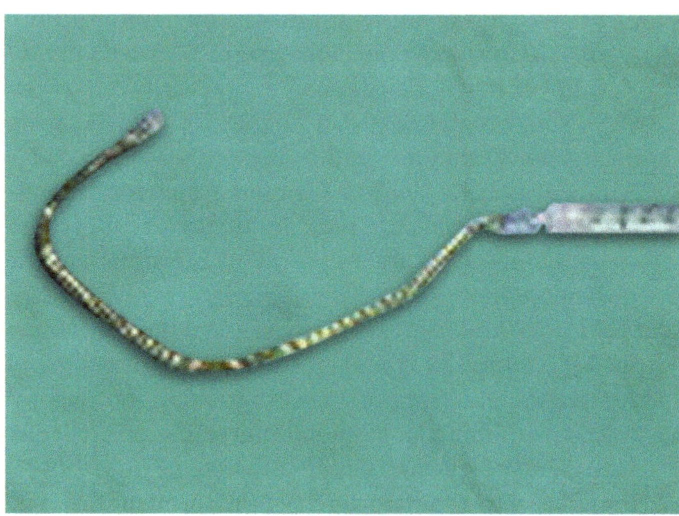

Fig. 9: Atomizer.

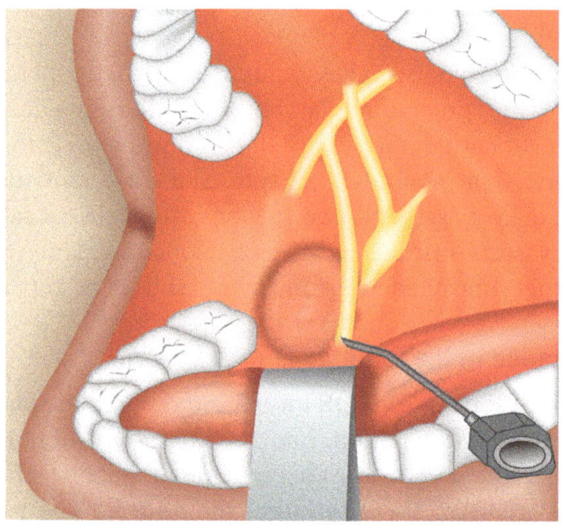

Fig. 10: Glossopharyngeal nerve block.

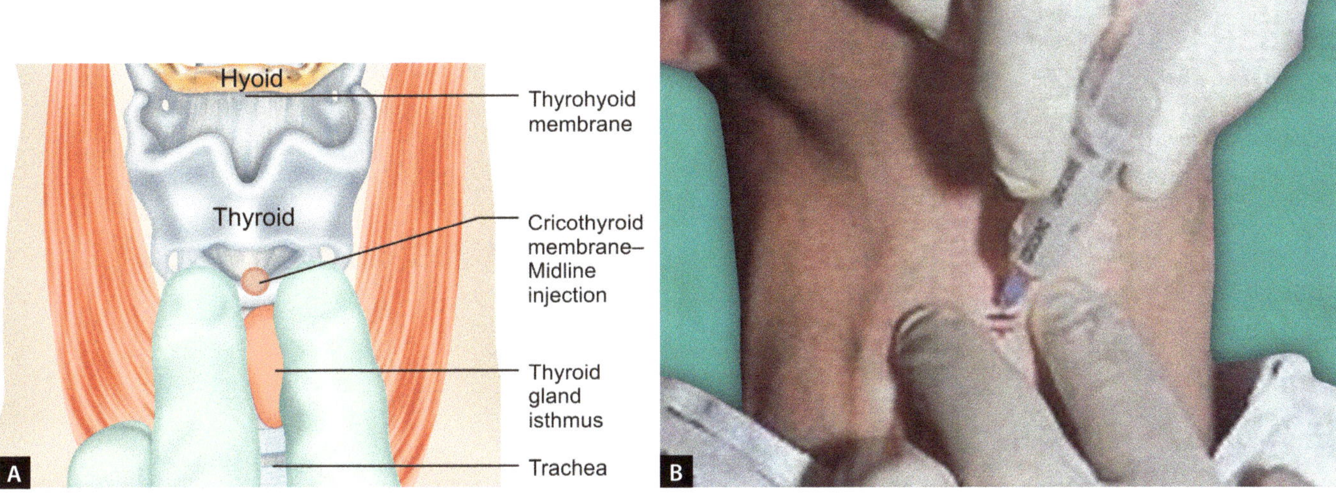

Figs. 11A and B: Transtracheal block. (A) Landmarks—cricothyroid membrane; (B) Injection.

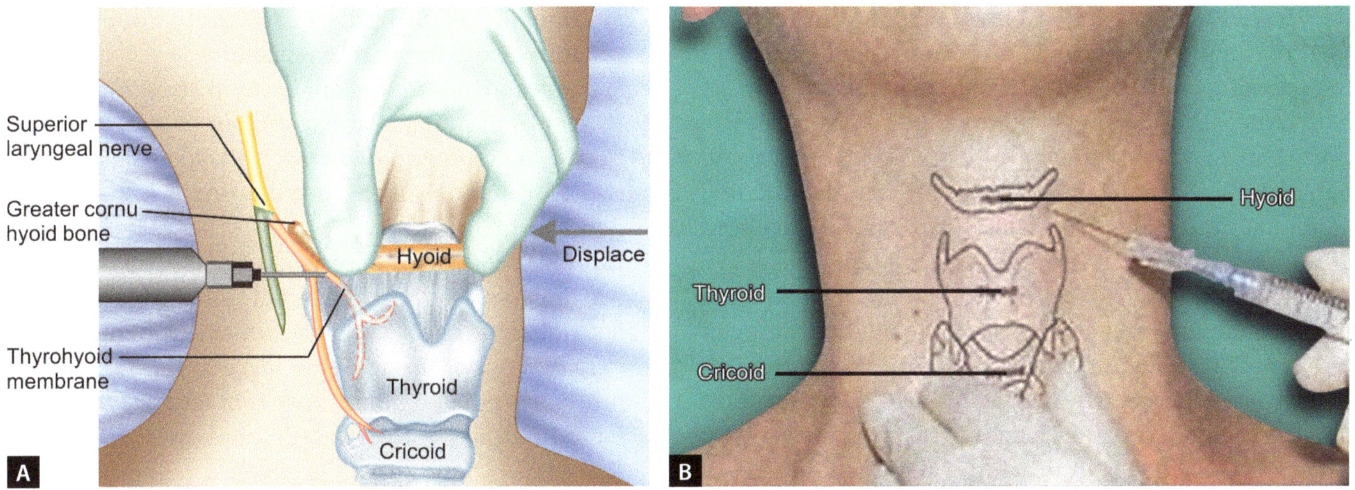

Figs. 12A and B: Superior laryngeal nerve block. (A) Landmarks; (B) Injection.

lie between the greater cornu of the hyoid bone and the superior cornu of the thyroid cartilage as they traverse the thyrohyoid membrane to the submucosa of the piriform sinus **(Fig. 12A)**. A 10 cc syringe containing 6 cc of 1% lidocaine, attached with a 23 G needle and inserted until it rests on the lateral most part of the hyoid bone and then it is withdrawn slightly and walked off the greater cornu, in the inferior direction. The needle is then advanced and passed through the thyrohyoid membrane, which should be felt as a slight resistance. The syringe is then aspirated, and the 2 cc of local anesthetic injected **(Fig. 12B)**. The procedure should be repeated on the opposite side.

Aerosol Method

The advantage of the aerosol method is that nebulized local anesthetic can be administered without needling and without much cooperation, if given by mask. Nebulized lidocaine (5 mL, 4%) can be given via a mouth piece **(Fig. 13)** for oral approach.

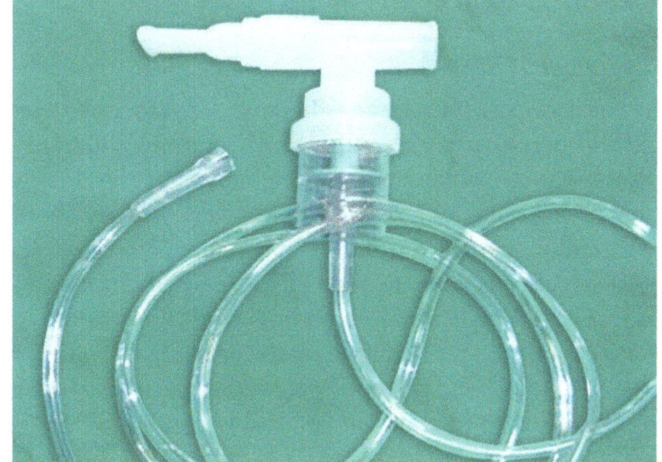

Fig. 13: Nebulizer.

"Spray As You Go" Technique

The "spray as you go" technique is used in patient who have partial or no pharyngeal, SLN or transtracheal anesthesia.

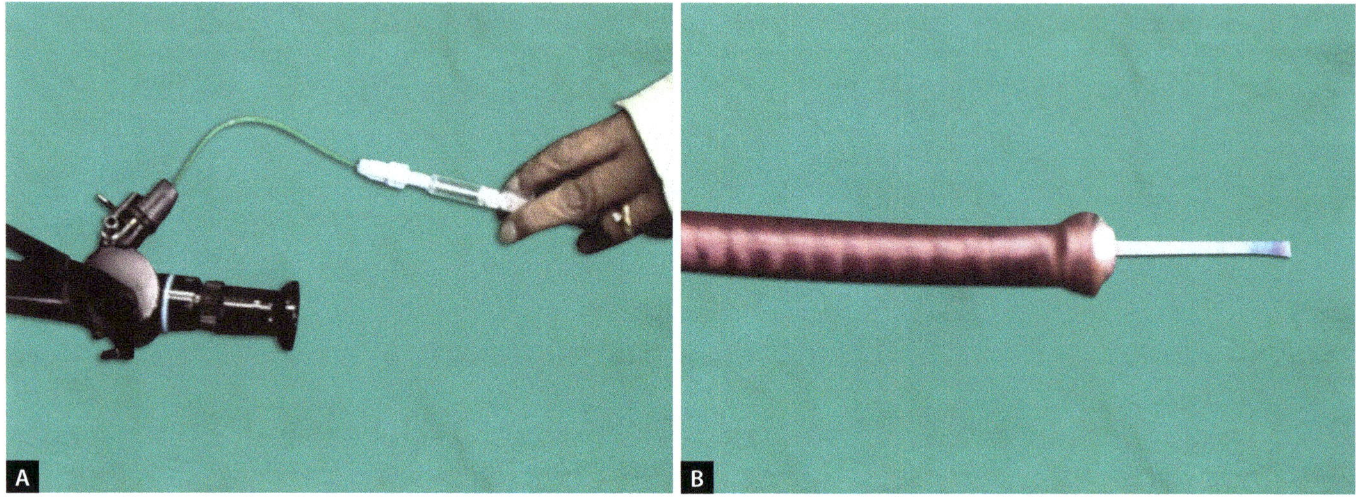

Figs. 14A and B: (A) Catheter through the working channel with a syringe; (B) Catheter tip beyond the fiberoptic bronchoscope tip.

The endoscopist uses an adult FOB with working channel and directs an assistant to give a quick pulse of 1 mL of 2–4% lidocaine (total 4 cc), when the tip of the scope reaches with areas of insufficient anesthesia. While injecting, make sure that the suction stopped; otherwise the local agent will be lost in the suction. Patients are more likely to react and cough after these sprays and the FOB view may be obscured for some seconds, after which the FOB can be advanced until another unanesthetized area is reached.[16]

A technique to avoid the obscured view is to attach a syringe containing local anesthetics to an epidural catheter (0.5–1.0 mm ID, single distant hole) and pass it through a three way stopcock attached at the FOB injection port through the working channel **(Fig. 14A)**. Extend the catheter tip 1 cm beyond the FOB tip **(Fig. 14B)** so that as LA is injected, the spray goes a further distance away, causing less visual disturbance to the FOB. The proximal epidural catheter at the working channel can be taped to keep its tip a fixed distance.

Preparation of Nasal Mucosa

The nasal mucosa must be anesthetized and vasoconstricted, typically performed with either a 4% cocaine solution or a combination of lidocaine and phenylephrine (1 cc of phenylephrine in 3 cc of lidocaine). These agents should be carefully used in parturient and patients with cardiac vascular diseases due to risk of decrease uteroplacental perfusion and myocardial infarction. Both the nostrils are packed and prepared with the swabs or pledgets soaked in these solutions.[17-26] The more patent or the larger passage side is used to avoid injury and bleeding.

Practical Application

Whichever method is chosen for FOB following sequence is advised:

- One must look in to patient concerns; equipment and patient preparation; medications such as antisialogogues, sedatives, narcotics, Las; monitoring and nasal cannula oxygen; the FOB; light source and proper working suctions before the start of procedure
- Set table lowest with patient in supine position
- To keep FOB straight use a step stool
- In case of dyspneic patient use FOB facing patient
- Use FOB handle in the nondominant hand, for easy directing of tip
- Hold FOB like pen in dominant hand's thumb and first two fingers to control progress of FOB during procedure
- For stabilization of FOB place 4th and 5th fingers on the patient's upper lip or cheek to keep the FOB straight, prevent bending damage, to lessen fatigue, and rest the hand holding the FOB handle high on that extremity's shoulder
- Use FOB as a unit to look left or right and lever to look up and down
- To look left, loosen the grip on the distal FOB insertion section between the thumb and two fingers while simultaneously rotating the handle section counter clockwise, to avoid torque
- To look right, turn the handle section clockwise in a similar fashion. Alternatively, rotate both hands equally in the same direction.

Awake Oral Fiberoptic Bronchoscopic Intubation

Once the airway is anesthetized, a lubricated ETT, which is at least 1.5 mm larger than the diameter of the FOB, is used. A bite block or an intraoral airway (IOA) may be introduced orally. Slowly the FOB is passed 6–8 cm in the mouth through the bite block or IOA, past the palate and then the uvula and the lever is used to look up, for the first landmark—the epiglottis **(Fig. 15A) (Video 6)**. If nothing is recognizable along the path, backup and try to look around with slow lever motion until structures are familiar, then proceed again. Once the epiglottis is identified, advance the FOB towards the laryngeal opening. If the topical anesthesia is not adequate, the first dose of local anesthetic, 2 mL lidocaine 2%, through the working channel should be instilled at this stage **(Fig. 15A)**. This may precipitate a bout of cough hence inform the patient beforehand. Wait for 1-2 minutes for the local anesthetics to act and then advance the FOB until it reaches the subglottic space.

Identify the second landmark—the trachea **(Fig. 15B)**. Clearly identify the tracheal rings. The second dose of the local anesthetic, 2 mL lidocaine 2% through the working channel should be instilled at this stage. Retract the FOB to just before the laryngeal opening to prevent mucosal irritation inside the trachea, wait for 1-2 minutes for the local anesthetic to act and then advance the FOB once again into the trachea.

Identify the third landmark—the bifurcation **(Fig. 15C)**. Do not go too close to the carina, which will be unlikely to be anesthetized hence will provoke the coughing. Local anesthetic is instilled at this stage for inadequate anesthesia and after waiting for 1-2 minutes and slide the ETT forward with Murphy eye oriented anteriorly if using a PVC-ETT to prevent it from getting hung up on the arytenoids. Most of the time, it gets caught on the right side.[27]

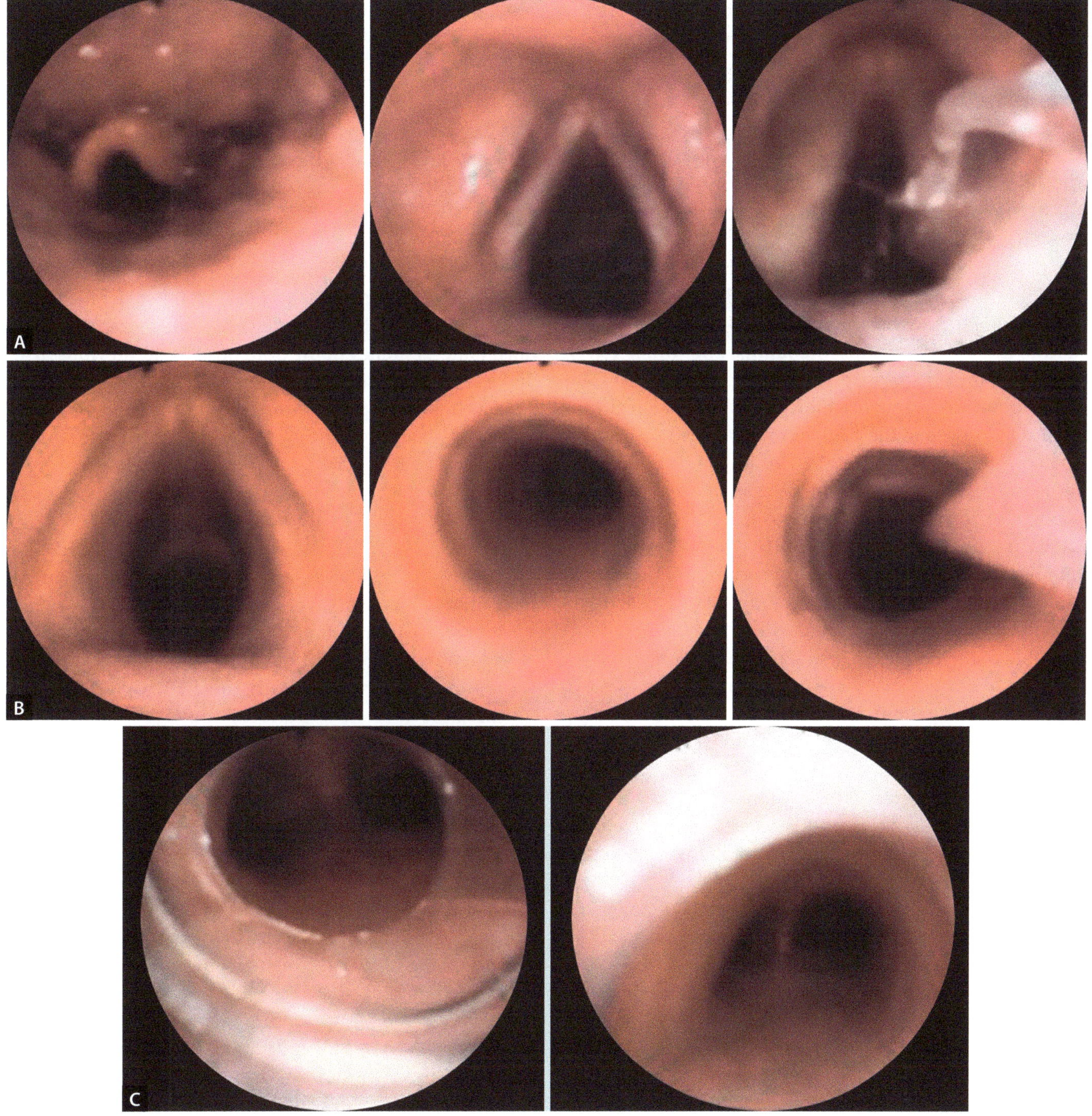

Figs. 15A to C: Landmarks. (A) Epiglottis; (B) Trachea; (C) Bifurcation.

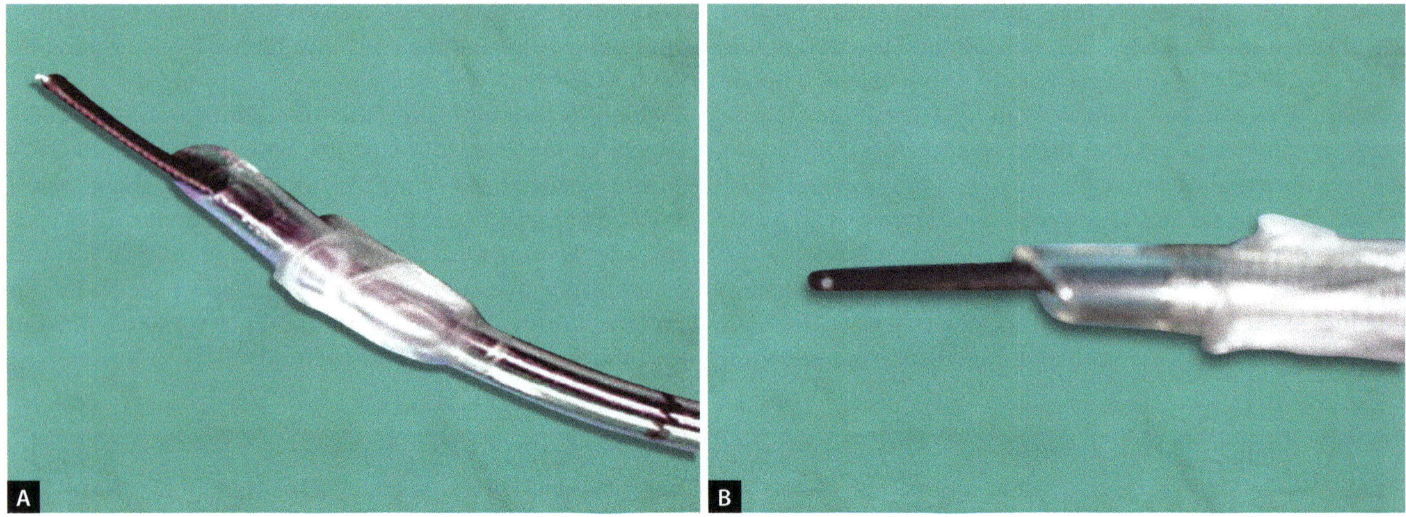

Figs. 16A and B: Endotracheal tube tip. (A) Usual position; (B) After 180° counter, clockwise rotation.

Do not let the FOB go forward as the ETT advances toward the back of the oropharynx. To prevent the dislocation of the FOB, the bifurcation must be kept in the field of vision all the time while advancing the ETT. At this point, look at the patient to judge when the ETT may be near the larynx by listening the breathing sounds. Ask the patient to take some deep breaths so that the vocal cords open more widely to admit the ETT. Time the breathing, and when ready, quickly push the ETT forward. After judging that the ETT has gone beyond the vocal cords, look at the FOB tracheal view again and gently slide the ETT until it reaches two to three rings above the carina, inflate the ETT cuff and stabilized it. Remove the FOB with its tip in the neutral position to prevent its damage. Attach the ventilating system while checking the end-tidal carbon dioxide pressure ($ETCO_2$), fixed the ETT and proceed for the anticipated next care.

If the patient has excessive oropharyngeal secretion or blood, and the visualization with the FOB is almost impossible then an assistant suctions the oropharynx, even continuously if necessary. FOB may be fogged due to warm exhaled air of the patient. For defogging, touch the FOB tip on the mucosa or otherwise remove the FOB, clean the tip and dip into warm saline.

If FOB cannot get under the epiglottis because it is stuck on the posterior pharynx, ask the assistant to pull the tongue out further and perform a jaw-thrust maneuver to lift the epiglottis.

If patient is gagging or coughing as the FOB advances, consider repeating the LA blocks or use the "spray as you go" technique.

In many situations the FOB is above the carina, but the ETT fails to enter the trachea. Withdraw the ETT 1-2 cm, turn it 180° counterclockwise, and advance it rapidly after asking patient for a deep breath and listening the expiratory gas noise at the connector of the ETT. By turning ETT by 180° counterclockwise, the tip of the ETT rests on the insertion cord of the FOB (**Figs. 16A and B**), hence when pushed in, it goes easily.

Nasal Fiberoptic Bronchoscopic Intubation of a Conscious Patient

Prior to attempting the nasal FOB intubation, detailed history of coagulation status or anticoagulation therapy, nasal abnormalities, patency of the both nostril and previous history of nasal surgery should be taken in detail.

Psychological preparation, monitoring and pharmacological preparation of the patient and concerns are similar to that of oral FOB intubation.

Nasal Fiberoptic Bronchoscopic Intubation Technique

There are several techniques for achieving nasal FOB intubation:

- Pass well-lubricated soft nasal airway with gradual dilatation of the nasal nostril to ascertain good patency. Replace this airway with the ETT, up to the same distance and now perform the fiberscopy through the ETT
- Load the ETT over the insertion cord up to the level of the control section, remove the nasal airway after gradual dilation of the patent nostril, and introduce the FOB directly through the nose
- As above, but introduce the FOB through a slit nasal airway to facilitate the fiberscopy and subsequently easy removal of the slit nasal airway via the split
- Access the airway through an anesthetic mask designed to accommodate FOB.

Whichever method is chosen, once the FOB reaches up to nasopharynx, identify the structures and direct the fiberoptic tip towards the larynx and identified the first landmark—the Epiglottis. The rest of the steps are similar to that for the orotracheal intubation.

Fiberoptic Bronchoscopic Intubation of the Anesthetized Patient

Fiberoptic bronchoscope intubation under general anesthesia (GA) should be considered only if the adequate oxygenation and ventilation can be maintained. Nasal or oral intubation is possible, and the technique can be performed with the patient breathing spontaneously or, while control ventilation.

In the anesthetized patient, the tongue and the soft tissues of the pharynx relax and close down the space of the hypopharynx and there is less space for manipulation of the tip of the FOB. A good jaw thrust and pulling the patient's tongue will help in opening the pharyngeal space.

To facilitate intubation under GA and minimize apnea time, the help of an assistant is important who can monitor the vital parameters and help in managing the jaw thrust, if required.

The FOB intubation under GA should only be attempted by trained personnel, who are well versed with the technique of the FOB intubation.

The elective FOB intubation after induction of general anesthesia is indicated in too young patient to understand the procedure, uncooperative patient

After checking the FOB equipment, setting up of monitoring and positioning now administer antisialogugue and premedication.

In case of nasotracheal intubation spray nostrils with a vasoconstrictor spray while patient is in awake and in sitting position.

A smaller size tube is preferred due to laxity of tissue which may obscure airway. After induction and muscle relaxant has acted, ask assistant to pull tongue and place or give a thrust as needed. Now insert FOB and intubate as described above. If unsuccessful, give additional dosage of induction agent and muscle relaxant and do mask ventilation and intubate.

Fiberoptic Bronchoscopic Intubation of Unconscious, Unanesthetized Patient

This is an emergency one needs to keep everything ready before FOB intubation. These patients may have full stomach so adequate precautions such as cricoid pressure must be employed and ask for an experienced FOB endoscopist to perform the procedure. If airway is already secured by some device, the FOB intubation can be performed by combination techniques.

Combination Techniques

Fiberoptic bronchoscopy can be combined with ancillary devices and laryngoscopy instrument to accomplish intubation in patients both in awake or under GA. FOB combination improves the airway control, rescues failed intubation, increases the rate of success and may be useful in unanticipated difficult mask ventilation and intubation.

Combination with endoscopy masks: Endoscopy masks are designed with a port that accommodate FOB through a diaphragm, which is air tight and does not allow air to leak while ventilating the patients. It allows for spontaneous or controlled ventilation while both nasal and oral FOB intubation can be performed.

The same preparation is required for FOB-endoscopy mask combination during GA as described above. To start with remove ETT connector and load the ETT over FOB and keep ready. After induction and muscle relaxant insert IOA and ventilate with 100% Oxygen. Instill LA spray if needed. Now introduce ETT loaded FOB. Once tip of FOB is at the level of bifurcation of trachea, push the tube in to trachea, remove FOB and mask and connect ETT to ventilator.

FOB and ETT both inserted simultaneously into endoscopy mask at beginning of planned orotracheal intubation and for nasotracheal intubation better not to insert initially to avoid limitation in FOB maneuvering while entering nasopharynx.

Combination with swivel adapters-for FOB examination or intubation connect bronchoscopy swivel adapter between ventilation circuit and an ordinary face mask, an SGA device or an ETT.

The FOB and swivel adapter in combination is used for GA or oxygen enrichment conditions such as FOB-endoscopy mask **(Fig. 17)**.

After induction insert pediatric FOB within Aintree intubation catheter through swivel adapter with spontaneous breathing. Now slide Aintree until two to three tracheal rings above bifurcation, secure Aintree and take out FOB. Now remove the Aintree connector to extract the mask, SGA, or old ETT and slide the lubricated ETT-loaded FOB through the Aintree. One needs to hold firmly the ETT and remove the FOB and the Aintree and reconnect the ETT to the ventilation circuit.

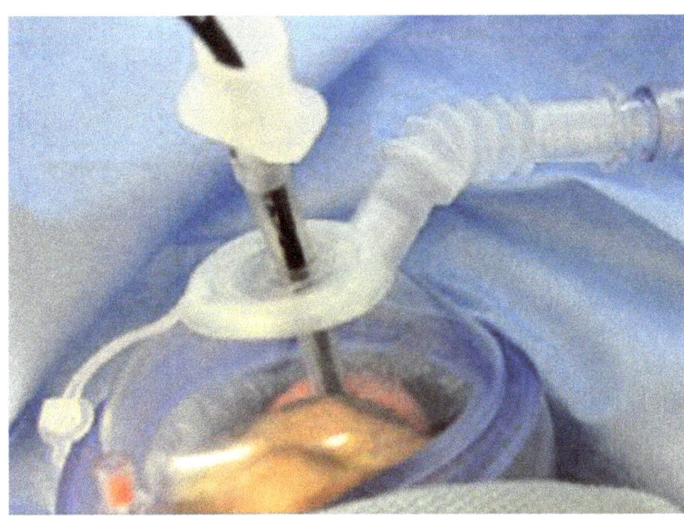

Fig. 17: Endoscopy mask and orotracheal intubation.

Combination using nasal airways: For awake nasotracheal intubation use of short and soft nasal airways are advised.

An intact soft nasal airway with a 15 mm ETT connector is inserted after proper lubrication in one of the nostril and connected to anesthesia circuit in a spontaneously breathing, anesthetized patient. Considerable amount of anesthetic gases are lost in the atmosphere but is a useful choice for the pediatric patients, who are prone for desaturation when intubation attempts are made during stoppages in the mask ventilation. If nasal intubation is planned, the other nostril is used for introduction of the FOB (Binasal technique).

Supraglottic Airways and Fiberoptic Bronchoscopic Intubation

The supraglottic airway devices have an important place in the ASA DA algorithm and can be used in unconscious, awake with LA, or under GA. The combination of FOB-SGA for the ETT intubation has been successfully tried with numerous SGA brands. To begin with induce GA and position the SGA while administrating 100% oxygen, in a spontaneously breathing, deeply anesthetized patient or a ventilated, muscle-relaxed patient, then disconnect the SGA from the circuit and slide the ETT-loaded FOB down the SGA until the glottis is visualized and secure the FOB tip at the bifurcation of the trachea and the ETT tube is railroaded on the FOB and confirm the ETT position by capnography.

Usually a smaller sized ETT traverses through the SGA **(Fig. 18)** hence proper sized ETT should be selected and it should be prechecked before the intubation (size 6 uncuffed ETT can be passed through size 4 LMA™). Once airway is secured, with the help of tube exchanger, smaller sized ETT can be changed to appropriate size ETT.

Combination with SGA and Aintree: Pass Aintree loaded FOB via SGA till carina, now fix Aintree and remove FOB and SGA. Finally intubate with ETT loaded FOB via Aintree.

Intubating Supraglottic Airways and Fiberoptic Bronchoscopic Intubation

For blind intubation, the intubating SGA act as conduit so larger ETT can be deployed for high success rate. The combination of FOB-SGA **(Fig. 18)** success rate is more than 98%.[28]

Combination with rigid laryngoscope: In case of upper airway edema which prevent entry in to glottis the lifting of mandible with rigid laryngoscope improves route for FOB. The FOB-RL technique requires two people, endoscopist inserts FOB and ETT while assistant makes RL immobile after optimal placement.[29] This combination is also used in intensive care patients also in patients with secretions.

Combination with video laryngoscope (VLs) or optical laryngoscope (OL): It has gained a place in DA algorithm. It has wide angle camera, clear optics. It has 60° angulation design with video to improve Cormack-Lehane view of larynx than RL[30-32] due to optical mirror capability. with improves optical mirror capability. The flexibility and ability to direct ETT mechanically of FOB are scoring points over VL.

Both techniques are good for airway management. The VL has greater range of vision and FOB-VL provides visualization and smooth passage even in soiled airway conditions as in FOB-RL technique.

At time failure of ETT occurs with Airtraq a channel loading type VL r OL even if it provides perfect visualization, in such cases VL may be used. In such case insert the FOB within an ETT, either in the channel **(Fig. 19)**, or next to the device and direct it towards the epiglottis.

Combination with high-flow nasal oxygen (HFNO): FOB can be combined with HFNO while performing awake or apneic oral fiberoptic bronchoscopy to maintain oxygenation. This may offer the benefit of greater patient and operator comfort and prolongs apnea time without desaturation.

Fig. 18: Fiberoptic bronchoscope with intubating supraglottic airways.

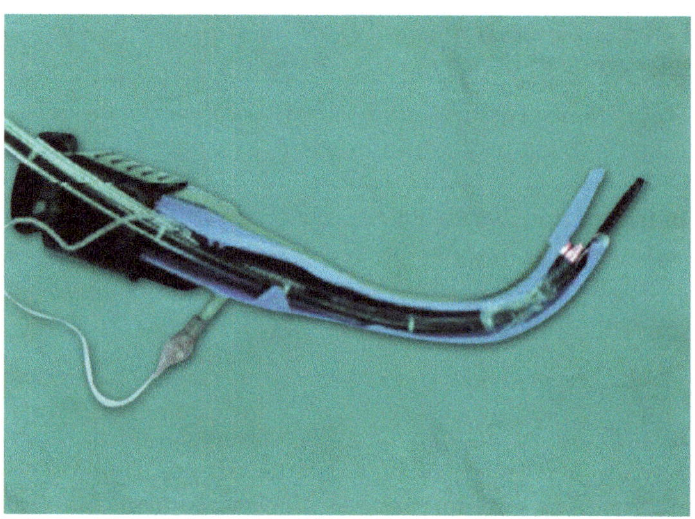

Fig. 19: Airtraq with fiberoptic bronchoscope.

Special Uses of Fiberoptic Bronchoscope

Endotracheal Tube Exchange

To exchange ETT in DA patient's fiberoptic bronchoscope is useful for chances of airway lost and reduce morbidity and mortality. Following techniques are used:

FOB-Aintree-Carry out exchange of ETT by passing FOB within an Aintree catheter in the old tube, remove FOB while securing Aintree. Now remove old ETT, and insert ETT-loaded FOB until just above carina, fix new ETT and remove FOB and Aintree.

Fiberoptic bronchoscope-wire-thread wire into a working channel of FOB, 2-3 cm beyond tip and slide in to old ETT, keep wire and remove FOB with tube. Now load new ETT over FOB and this assembly insert over the wire and advance into trachea and railroad ETT into the patient.

Fiberoptic bronchoscope-ETT or FOB-wire—In this by the side of existing ETT and new ETT loaded FOB is inserted under vision till it reaches old ETT, now deflate cuff of old ETT and advance new one.[33]

Fiberoptic Bronchoscope for Retrograde Intubation

The fiberoptic bronchoscope-retrograde intubation technique can be used when the FOB or other methods of intubation fails, particularly in patients who have anatomical difficult or soiled airway. A guidewire is passed through a cricothyroid needle or angiocath, directing cephalically. The wire exits the mouth or nose, is introduce through ETT loaded on FOB **(Fig. 20A)** or working channel of the FOB loaded ETT **(Fig. 20B)**, by holding the wire at its neck insertion site, until it exits near the handle. Slide the FOB along the tense wire by retrograde method into the trachea till it reaches up to its entry point. The wire is then removed and the ETT is secured after confirming its exact position.

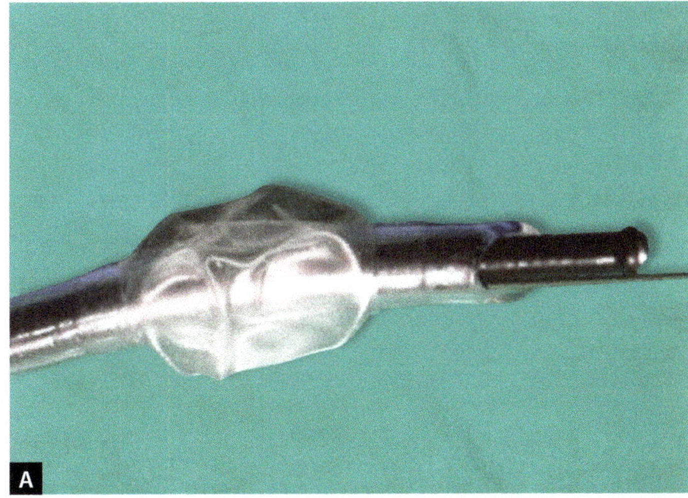

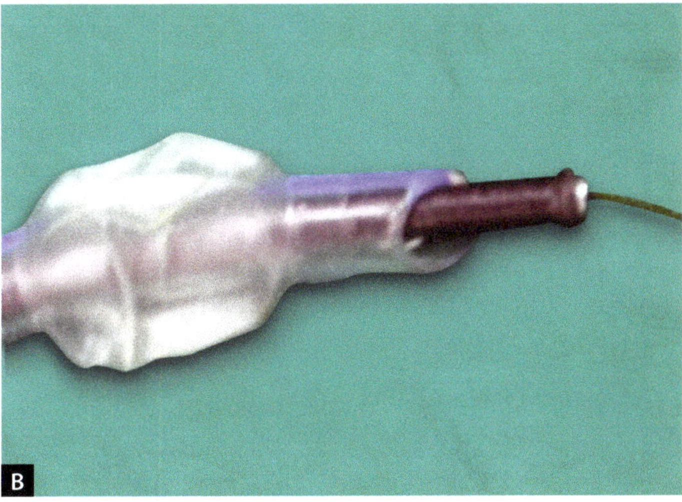

Figs. 20A and B: Fiberoptic bronchoscopic intubation with retrograde technique. (A) Wire through the endotracheal tube, outside the fiberoptic bronchoscope; (B) Wire through the working channel.

Fiberoptic Bronchoscopic Intubation in Infants and Children

Anatomical Characteristics of Pediatric Airways

The airways of adult, child and infants are anatomical different. In pediatric patient's presence of large tongue, cephalad larynx, and inclined vocal cords are there.[34,35] In new-borns larynx is relatively smaller, softer and more sensitive and in addition it is funnel shaped and narrow at cricoid cartilage. As infant grows larynx descends caudally.

The epiglottis is omega shaped, floppier, longer, and tubular in infants as compare to adults and is posterior. The FOB is indicated in congenital and hereditary conditions.

Equipment Monitoring and Drugs Availability

A standard monitoring, capnography or FOB cart, full airway equipment, oxygen, suctioning equipment, sedatives, opiates, local anesthetics, and vasoconstrictor is needed. The routes for medications can be intravenous, intramuscular, intranasal, oral, rectal, or inhalational.

Psychological Preparation

The psychological preparation and presence of guardians provides patient cooperation and understanding.

Pharmacological Preparation (Table 1)

The use of antisialagogues and in younger patient's short-acting sedatives or narcotics are preferred to avoid desaturation or respiration depression.

The preferred agent is Ketamine in infants, smaller children but transient apnea of less than 6 seconds duration has been reported.[36] However, with DA or respiratory compromise, ketamine may be useful due to less respiratory effects.[37]

Topical Orotracheal Anesthesia Technique

General anesthesia is useful for reducing hemodynamic responses and the reflexes that are prone to occur in pediatric patients. The technique for the local airway anesthesia is similar in the pediatric population and in adults with some exceptions, mostly involving younger patients.

TABLE 1: Pediatric drug dosage for fiberoptic bronchoscopic intubation.

Drugs	Dosage	Route
Atropine	0.01 mg/kg	IV or IM
Glycopyrrolate	0.004 mg/kg	IV or IM
Fentanyl	0.5 µg/kg	IV increments
Ketamine	0.5 mg/kg	IV increments
	4–5 mg/kg	IM
Ketamine	2 mg per mL Propofol infused as a Propofol drip at 50–200 µg/kg/min	–
Midazolam	10–20 µg/kg	IV increments
Propofol	0.5–2 mg/kg 50–200 µg/kg	IV bolus IV infusion
Remifentanil	0.05–0.1 µg/kg/min	IV infusion
Dexmedetomidine	0.2–0.7 µg/kg/h	IV infusion

(IV: intravenous; IM: intramuscular)

In infants younger than 6 months of age, the cricothyroid area is much smaller and difficult to palpate for the trans tracheal anesthesia. In addition, needling of very small tracheas should be avoided as any drop of blood within the trachea will compromise the airway to a larger extent than in larger patients. In cooperative children, intraoral and aerosolized techniques may work well.

Positioning of Infants and Smaller Children

Usually, the head and neck remain in neutral position. As the size of the head is larger in the infants, a towel under upper thorax can avoid excessive flexion of the neck and provide slight extension of the neck.

Endotracheal Tubes: Uncuffed versus Cuffed

The incidences of repeat laryngoscopy and trauma is 15 times lesser in cuffed ETT in comparison with the uncuffed ETT group due to repeated laryngoscopy but the incidences of stridor was almost identical.[38] The other advantages of use of cuffed ETT are better aspiration protection, better seal pressure for ventilation and less atmospheric contamination under GA.

Fiberoptic Bronchoscope Orotracheal Intubation Technique

Fiberoptic bronchoscope intubation of infants and children uses similar procedure technique and aiding maneuvers (e.g., tongue pulling) as in adults.

Antisialogogues should be administered before the instrumentation and an IOA can be used. Regular mask with a bronchoscopy swivel adapter is also useful. Supplement oxygen during the procedure to avoid desaturation of the patient. As the size of the ETT is smaller in pediatric patient, it is advisable to introduce the FOB before the ETT as the smaller size of the ETT may limit the maneuverability of the FOB.

Two-staged Fiberoptic Bronchoscopic Intubation

Fiberoptic bronchoscopic intubation can be carried out in two stages if the patient's airways are too small to FOB. First thread a guidewire from an airway exchange catheter set [Cook's pediatrics airway exchange catheter (PAEC)] through the working channel, about 1 cm beyond the FOB tip, as the scope is introduced into the oropharynx. When the glottis is visualized, advance the wire into the trachea till the carina. Remove the FOB, keeping the wire tip at the carina and in second stage, use the Cook's catheter set up and pass an appropriately sized ETT over the wire, in a manner similar to ETT exchanger technique.

Nasal Fiberoptic Bronchoscopic Intubation Technique

History and examination of nasal anomalies should always be kept in mind before doing nasal intubation. Softening of ETT by warming and pretreatment with Phenylephrine or Oxymetazoline is advocated to reduce the incidences of nasal bleeding. Anti-sialogogues, sedatives or narcotics, and LA dosage should be adjusted according to the patient's size.

Hypertrophied adenoids are common between 2 years and 6 years, and are susceptible to trauma of blind ETT entry. The technique is similar to that for adults in regards to preparation. Swivel adapters are useful.

Oral or Nasal Fiberoptic Bronchoscopic Intubation of the Anesthetized Pediatric Patient

Use antisialogogues agents and topical anesthesia of airway to limit reflexes if patient is cooperative enough. If difficult airway and difficult mask ventilation are not anticipated, induce GA and perform mask ventilation with 100% oxygen along with inhalation agent. With the patient under deep anesthesia with spontaneous respiration or lighter GA with muscle relaxant, remove the mask and execute the FOB intubation. Muscle relaxants help to avoid laryngospasm in patients who are uncooperative for LA of upper airway.

If spontaneous ventilation is more desirable, 2–4% xylocaine may be used on vocal cords in a "spray as you go" technique. Remember to promptly return to mask ventilation between brief periods of instrumentation to avoid rapid desaturation of the patient. Endoscopic mask or bronchoscopy swivel adapter useful in such circumstances. An FOB can also assist with proper SGA placement, and the FOB-SGA combination for successful insertion of the ETT.

General Anesthesia using Nasopharyngeal Airway

Insert a nasopharyngeal airway with a 15 mm adapter on it, into one of the nostril after LA and vasoconstrictor. Connect the anesthesia circuit to the adapter to supply the inhalation agents to the spontaneous breathing patient and proceed with FOB intubation, orally or nasally through the opposite nostril.

CAUSES OF FAILURE OF FIBEROPTIC BRONCHOSCOPE INTUBATION

Fiberoptic bronchoscope intubation is a complex technique. The failure may occur due to several reasons.

- Improper selection of the patient—choose the right patient after proper understanding of the proper indication and contraindication of the procedure
- Inexperienced endoscopist—must have proper training and practice in day-to-day cases so that DA can be handled
- Presence of secretions and blood—excessive secretions and blood obscure the vision—use proper anti-sialogogues, sedatives, narcotics and LA
- Lack of preparation—psychological preparation, equipment, antisialogogues, sedatives, narcotics and local anesthetics must be optimized and individualized for each patient. Improper preparation of the patients and equipment may pose difficulty or failure of FOB intubation
- Improper cleaning, focus and fogging of FOB—FOB should be properly cleaned after each use. Defoggers or warm water should be used on the tip of the scope
- Inadequate local anesthetics—blockage of GPN and SLN should be properly performed before starting the FOB intubation. If one of these is inadequate, the block can be repeated or the "spray as you go" technique can be used
- Larger diameter difference between the ETT and FOB—causes impingement problem hence the difference between the diameter of the ETT and the FOB should be minimum. If pediatric sized FOB is used for adult, Aintree catheter is used over the scope to minimize the space between ETT and FOB.

Complications of Fiberoptic Bronchoscope Intubation

The common complications of FOB intubation include nasal bleeding, sore throat, hoarseness of voice, tissue trauma, laryngospasm, bronchospasm, and aspiration but, the most frequent complication is damage to scope by biting, twisting, kinking and dropping hence proper care is advocated.

FIBEROPTIC BRONCHOSCOPE: CLEANING AND CARE

Fiberoptic bronchoscopes are delicate and expensive devices hence tender baby care must be taken when using and processing these instruments. When using the scope it must be placed such that it is not at risk of being crushed in anyway. Processing the endoscope after each use is important to avoid the transmission of the communicable diseases. All classes of microorganism, including bacteria, fungi and viruses have been implicated.[39-41] When an FOB is being used for patient management, involved clinical sites anatomically fall under the aegis of mandatory universal precautions. Constant care, vigilance in FOB care and high level disinfection are advocated. Once used, an FOB should be directly handed off to trained assistant and should be placed in a vertical holding tube. As soon as possible after using the FOB, all surfaces should be cleaned with enzymatic detergent followed by rinsing to remove organic material. The channel should be irrigated with the detergent solution and a specially designed brush used to remove particulate material.

Next, the FOB has to be diligently inspected for any damage, tear, indentation, or abnormalities along its entire length. A leak test to detect holes in the insertion tube sheath is essential at this point and failures necessitate sending FOB for the repair without any further sterilization. After successful leak testing, the scope is either liquid or gas sterilized. The disinfecting agent must be in contact with all the surfaces of the FOB for the recommended period of time. Agents for the high level disinfection include 2% alkaline or acid glutaraldehyde, 6% hydrogen peroxide, 0.85% phosphoric acid, and 1% peracetic acid.

After liquid processing, the external surfaces and channel should be then rinsed with disinfectant and water. The working channel should be then suctioned or air aspirated for 60 seconds and allowed to dry. Each manufacturer of FOBs has specific recommendations for processing their scopes and should be strictly followed.

Recent innovations in fiberoptic bronchoscopes: In situations such as the current pandemic of COVID-19, it is good to use single use devices so we can avoid cross infection.

Ambu A/S, a Denmark-based medical device company with expertise in single-use medical devices, launched first "fiberless-single use endoscope" called the "aScope" **(Figs. 21A and B)**.

The aScope™ 4 Broncho Slim endoscope is a single-use, flexible, ready-to-go bronchoscopy solution. aScope is available with an outer diameter of 3.8 mm, 5.0 mm, and 5.8 mm with the working channel of 1.2,2.2, and 2.8. The scope has been approved by regulators body (FDA and European CE) and extensively marketed across the globe.

The single-use scope is packed in a sterile jacket with sterilization credentials imparting to nullifying the chances of cross infection from the scope. It can do autofocus and white balancing automatically making it a "ready to use device."

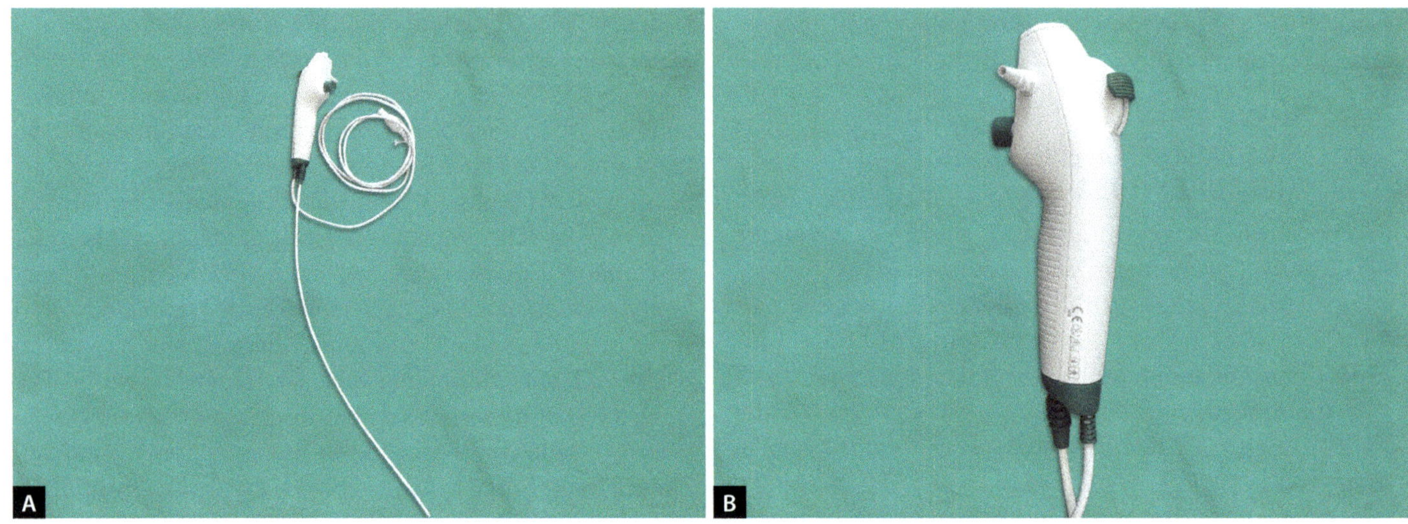

Figs. 21A and B: Disposable fiberoptic bronchoscope.

CONCLUSION

Fiberoptic bronchoscope intubation has an important place in difficult airway management and still a gold standard and safe mode of difficult intubation in spite of availability of many sophisticated techniques and gadgets for intubation; hence everyone should learn and practice the art of use of FOB technique. The FOBs are expensive but the cost of FOB purchase and maintenance should be balanced in relation to the cost of intubation failure and associated morbidity and mortality. The expense of airway failure and resulting complication may exceed the cost of one FOB system. The FOB intubation technique requires skill and has a place in the armamentarium of every professional airway management care provider like anesthesiologist, critical care and emergency medicine.

When a topical intraoral anesthesia is planned, anti-sialogogues like glycopyrrolate or atropine should be administered 15–20 minutes before the procedure. Supplementation of oxygen is advocated. Use of sedatives, narcotics and local anesthetics is dependent upon the patient's condition, respiratory status and urgency of the procedure. Proper topical anesthesia should prevent discomfort, psychological distress, hemodynamic changes and lack of patient cooperation.

The most common cause of FOB intubation failure is inexperience due to insufficient training, practice and patient's preparation; hence one should master the technique of FOB intubation solely or, in combination with other airway devices and intubation techniques to avoid any unwanted complication.

This technique takes time and should be entertained only if the anesthesia care provider is able to maintain adequate oxygenation and ventilation until the airway is secured.

REFERENCES

1. Murphy P. A fibreoptic endoscope used for nasal intubation. Anaesthesia. 1967;22:489-91.
2. Stiles CM, Stiles QR, Denson JS. A flexible fiberoptic laryngoscope. JAMA. 1972;221:1246-7.
3. American Society of Anesthesiology Task Force on the Difficult Airway. Practice guidelines for management of the difficult airway. Anesthesiology. 1993;78:597-602.
4. Miyazawa T. History of the flexible bronchoscope. In: Bolliger CT, Mathur PN (Eds). Progress in respiratory research. Basel: Karger; 2000. pp. 16-21.
5. Wong DM, Prabhu A, Chakraborty S, et al. Cervical spine motion during flexible bronchoscopy compared with the Lo-Pro Glidescope. Br J Anaesth. 2009;102:424-30.
6. El-Orbany MI, Salem MR, Joseph NJ. The Eschmann tracheal tube introducer is not gum, elastic, or a bougie. Anesthesiology. 2004;101:1240-4.
7. Beattie C. The modified nasal trumpet maneuver. Anesth Analg. 2002;94:467-9.
8. Sanuki T, Hirokane M, Matsuda Y, et al. The parker flex-tip tube for the nasotracheal intubation: the influence on nasal mucosal trauma. Anaesthesia. 2012;65:8-11.
9. Greer JR, Smith SP, Strang T. A comparison of the tracheal tube tip designs on the passage of an endotracheal tube during oral fiberoptic intubation. Anesthesiology. 2001;94:729-31.
10. Kristensen MS. The Parker flex-tip tube versus a standard tube for the fiberoptic orotracheal intubation: a randomized double-blind study. Anesthesiology. 2003;98:354-8.
11. Stackhouse R, Bainton CR. Difficult airway management. In: Hughes SC, Rosen M, Levinson G (Eds). Anesthesia for obstetrics, 4th edition. Baltimore: Williams and Wilkins; 2001, pp. 375-90.
12. Stackhouse R, Marks JD, Boynton CR. Performing fiberoptic endotracheal intubation: clinical aspects. Int Anesthesiol Clin. 1994;32:57-73.
13. Van de Water T, Staecker H. Otolaryngology: basic science and clinical review, 1st edition. New York: Thieme Medical Publishers; 2006. p. 562.
14. Becker W, Behrbohm H, Kaschke O, et al. Ear, Nose, and Throat Disease: With Head and Neck Surgery, 3rd edition. New York: Thieme Medical Publishers; 2009. p. 123.
15. Mu I, Sanders I. Sensory nerve supply of the human oro- and laryngopharynx: a preliminary study. Anat Rec. 2000;258:406-20.
16. Webb AR, Farnando S, Dalton H, et al. Local anesthesia for fiberoptic brochoscopy. Transcricoid and "spray as you go" technique. Thorax. 1990;45:474-7.
17. Barnett G, Hawks R, Resnick R. Cocaine pharmacokinetics in humans. J Ethnopharmacol. 1981;3:353-66.

18. Cone EJ. Pharmacokinetics and pharmacodynamics of cocaine. J Anal Toxicol. 1995;19:459-78.
19. Daniel WC, Mark PJ, Horton RP, et al. Electrophysiologic effects of intranasal cocaine. Am J Cardiol. 1995;76:398-400.
20. Greinwald JH, Holtel MR. Absorption of topical cocaine in rhinologic procedures. Laryngoscope. 1996;106:1223-5.
21. Hecker RB, Hays JV, Champ JD, et al. Myocardial ischemia and stunning induced by topical intranasal phenylephrine pledgets. Mil Med. 1997;162:832-5.
22. Jeffcoat A, Perex-Reyes M, Hill J, et al. Cocaine disposition in humans after intravenous injection, nasal insufflation (snorting), or smoking. Drug Metab Dispos. 1989;17:153-9.
23. Kalyanaraman M, Carpenter RL, McGlew MJ, et al. Cardiopulmonary compromise after use of topical and submucosal alpha-agonist: possible added complication by the use of beta-blocker therapy. Otolaryngol Head Neck Surg. 1997;117: 56-61.
24. Kumar V, Schoenwald R, Barcellos W, et al. Aqueous vs. viscous phenylephrine: systemic absorption and cardiovascular effects. Arch Ophthalmol. 1986;104:1189-91.
25. Lange RA, Hillis LD. Cardiovascular complications of cocaine use. N Engl J Med. 2001;345:351-8.
26. Vongpatanasin W, Lange RA, Hillis LD. Comparison of cocaine-induced vasoconstriction of left and right coronary arterial systems. Am J Cardiol. 1997;79(4):492-3.
27. Johnson DM, From A, Smith RB, et al. Endoscopic study of mechanism of failure of endotracheal tube advancement into the trachea during awake fiberoptic orotracheal intubation. Anesthesiology. 2005;102:910-4.
28. Erlacher W, Tiefenbrunner H, Kastenbauer T, et al. Cobra PLUS and Cooks air-Q versus Fastrach for blind endotracheal intubation: a randomized trial. Eur J Anaesthesiol. 2011;28: 181-6.
29. Kanaya N, Nakayama M, Seki S, et al. Two-person technique for fiberoptic-aided tracheal intubation in a patient with a long and narrow retropharyngeal air space. Anesth Analg. 2001;92: 1611-3.
30. Asai T, Enomoto Y, Shimizu K, et al. The pentax-AWS® video-laryngoscope: the first experience in one hundred patients. Anesth Analg. 2008;106:257-9.
31. Cooper RM, Pacey JA, Bishop MJ, et al. Early clinical experience with a new video laryngoscope (Glidoscope®) in 728 patients. Can J Anaesth. 2005;2:191-8.
32. Sasano N, Yamauchi H, Fujita Y. Failure of the airway Scope® to reach the larynx. Can J Anaesth. 2007;54:774-5.
33. Ovassapian A, Wheeler M. Fiberoptic endoscopy-aided techniques. In: Benumof JL (Ed). Airway Management: principles and practice, 1st edition. St. Louis: Mosby; 1996. pp. 282-319.
34. Eckenhoff JE. Some anatomical considerations of the infant larynx influencing endotracheal anesthesia. Anesthesiology. 1951;12:401-10.
35. Wheeler M, Ovassapian A. Fiberoptic endoscopy-aided technique. In: Hagberg C (Ed). Benumof's airway management, 2nd edition. Philadelphia, PA: Mosby Elsevier; 2007. pp. 399-438.
36. Green S, Rothrock S, Lynch E, et al. Intramuscular ketamine for the paediatric sedation in the emergency department: safety profile in 1,022 cases. Ann Emerg Med. 1998;31:688-97.
37. Hostetler MA, Barnard JA. Removal of esophageal foreign bodies in the pediatric ED: is ketamine an option? Am J Emerg Med. 2000;20:96-8.
38. Weiss M, Dullenkopf A, Fisher JE, et al. European Paediatric Endotracheal Intubation Study Group. Prospective randomized controlled multicentre trial of cuffed or uncuffed endotracheal tubes in smaller children. Br J Anaesth. 2009;103:867-73.
39. Agerton T, Valway S, Gore B, et al. Transmission of a highly drug resistance strain (strain W1) of Mycobacterium tuberculosis. Community outbreak and nosocomial transmission via a contaminated bronchoscope. JAMA. 1997;278:1073-7.
40. Bronowicki JP, Venard V, Botte C. Patient-to-patient transmission of hepatitis C virus during colonoscopy. N Engl J Med. 1997; 337:237-40.
41. Michele TM, Cronin WA, Graham NM. Transmission of Mycobacterium tuberculosis by a fiberoptic bronchoscope. JAMA. 1997;278:1093-5.

Monitoring Equipment

SECTION

Electrocardiogram Monitoring and Defibrillators

Samhita Kulkarni

ABSTRACT

The electrocardiogram (ECG) is a simple, cheap and readily available test to identify heart rate, rhythm, conduction pattern, myocardial ischemia, electrolyte abnormality, etc. Monitoring of the ECG is a very useful tool in the perioperative period. ECG monitoring helps to identify the cardiac status in patients with known heart disease or those with cardiac risk factors; it also helps to monitor the effects of anesthesia and importantly identify the electrolyte, metabolic, hypoxia and fluid shifts in the perioperative period. Identifying cardiac changes in the operative period at an early stage would facilitate taking appropriate remedial actions and these interventions can be life-saving. Defibrillators are very important to restore sinus rhythm in patients with ventricular flutter or fibrillation and to cardiovert various ventricular and supraventricular tachycardias.

ELECTROCARDIOGRAM MONITORING

The European Society of Cardiology (ESC), in its guidelines in perioperative risk assessment states that electrocardiogram (ECG) monitoring is recommended for all patients undergoing surgery.[1] Many believe ECG monitoring as very important, irrespective of the age, pre-existing cardiac disease or form of anesthesia, especially if sedation is used. Electrocardiogram monitoring, thus is a simple yet important parameter to be utilized in the perioperative period.

A 12-lead ECG is ideal to identify rhythm disturbances and myocardial ischemia.[2] However, during surgery one requires a continuous ECG monitoring, which is then limited to one to three or five ECG leads or some of the monitors are able to give a derived 12-lead ECG. The ECG monitoring during surgery and perioperatively is often done with multipara monitors which enable the simultaneous monitoring of various parameters like ECG, invasive and noninvasive blood pressure (BP) monitoring, oxygen saturation and end-tidal carbon dioxide ($ETCO_2$) concentration in the expired air **(Fig. 1)**.

Continuous ECG monitoring is essential intraoperatively to detect arrhythmias as well as myocardial ischemia. A single lead ECG monitoring at times will not allow accurate diagnosis of rhythm and ischemic changes. Lead II and V5 have been conventionally used to identify arrhythmias and ischemia respectively. However, a 12 lead ECG is often necessary for accurate rhythm diagnosis and similarly the sensitivity of identifying ischemia increases with addition of more leads, especially the inferior and adjacent V4 lead to V5. Thus, though it is practical to have a 3–5 ECG lead monitoring in most patients undergoing surgery, a 12-lead ECG is recommended in patients suspected to have ischemia or arrhythmia.

A continuous automated ST trending monitors is used in advanced operating room ECG monitors to facilitate ischemia detection. Such facility does increase the sensitivity of ECG ischemia detection. The secondary ST–T changes in patients with intraventricular conduction abnormalities and ventricular paced rhythms can limit the sensitivity of identifying ischemia, however the fluctuations of ST segment as identified in the ST trend monitoring helps to resolve the issue. It is very important that patients with baseline ECG changes should be evaluated preoperatively to rule out structural heart disease and functional capacity with additional tests like echocardiography, Holter and exercise stress test.

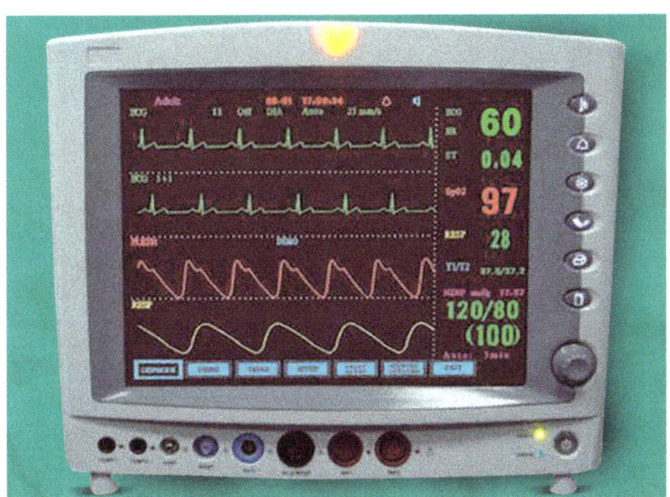

Fig. 1: Electrocardiogram monitoring in a multiple-parameter monitoring equipment.

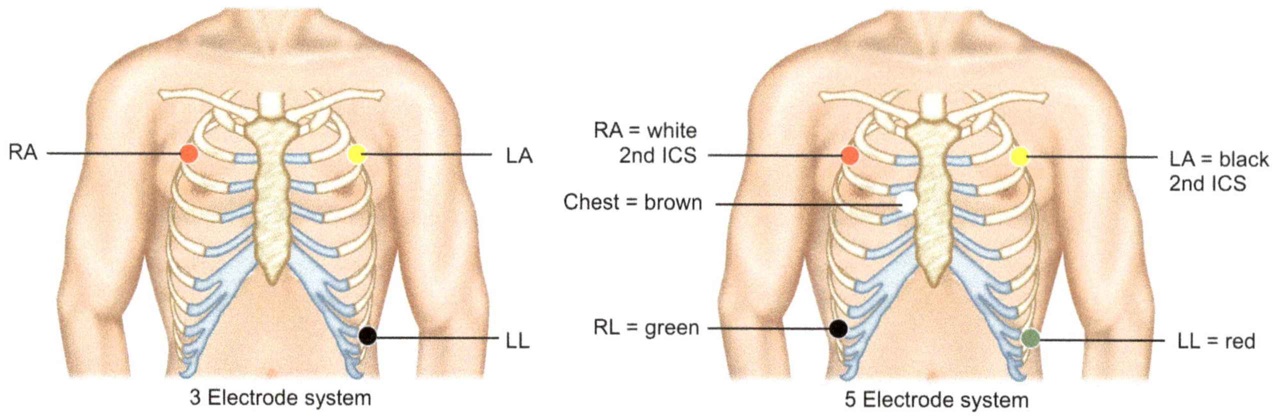

Fig. 2: Electrode placement in a 3 and 5 lead electrocardiogram monitoring system. (ICS: intercostal space; LA: left arm; RA: right arm; LL: left leg; RL: right leg)

Placing the Electrodes

The electrodes for ECG monitoring are placed in specific locations on the surface of the body. The electrodes of the arm are placed on the shoulders as close as possible to the point where the arm and the trunk are connected, whereas the lower limb electrodes are placed in the midaxillary line or above the hips. By convention the electrodes are color coded and across different companies same coding is used. For the right shoulder the electrode has red color, for the left shoulder is yellow, the left leg is encoded with green color, the right leg with black and for the precordial electrode, white color is used. **Figure 2** shows the location of the electrodes in a 3 and 5 lead ECG monitoring.

The five-electrode system incorporates four extremity and one precordial lead and can be used to monitor seven leads (I, II, III, aVF, aVL, aVR and a precordial lead). The precordial lead can be selected by placing the electrode at any position between V1 and V6. The right leg electrode is a ground placed anywhere often on the right side of chest or abdomen.

The three-lead system allows monitoring along one bipolar lead between two electrodes, third serves as ground. Although a five-lead system is the norm for ischemia monitoring during surgery, a modified three-lead system may be needed if a five-lead system is unavailable or cannot be used because of the site of surgery.

Modified three-lead system can be used to monitor for anterior ischemia, limb I is selected on the monitor.

1. *CS5:* Monitor lead I with left arm electrode placed on left fifth intercostal space on the anterior axillary line; right arm electrode is placed under right clavicle, left leg electrode is placed anywhere on the left side.
2. *CM5:* Monitor lead I with right arm electrode on sternal manubrium and left arm electrode on left fifth intercostal space on anterior axillary line. Left leg electrode is placed anywhere on left side.
3. *CB5:* Monitor lead I with right arm electrode over center of right scapula and left arm electrode on left fifth intercostal space on anterior axillary line.

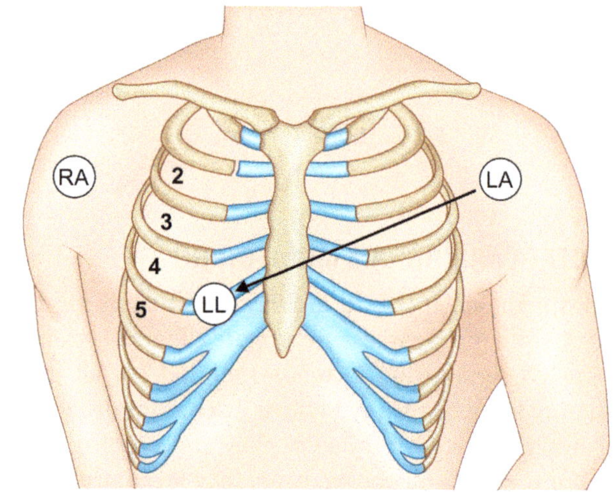

Fig. 3: MCL1 lead placement. (LA: left arm; RA: right arm; LL: left leg)

4. *CC5:* Monitor lead I with right arm electrode in mid chest at right anterior axillary line, left arm placed in V5 location, left leg electrode is placed anywhere on the left side.
5. *MCL1:* Monitor lead III with left leg electrode placed at V2R to V3R, left arm below left clavicle and right arm anywhere on right side. It can elicit p wave and QRS morphology adequate to detect some dysrhythmias **(Fig. 3)**.

Possible Fallacies

An improper electrode placement can result in inaccurate diagnosis of morphological ECG changes. A good contact between the electrodes and the body surface is to be assured by cleaning and scrubbing the skin with alcohol, so that the desquamated cells are removed, or by shaving if necessary, or by using an inductive cream. The electrodes are placed on bony surface and not in areas with loose skin, the surface should be dry and not moist, as the latter increases the resistance and prevents adequate adherence **(Box 1)**.

The most important tenet is that in case of any suspicion of ischemia or arrhythmia, instead of solely relying on the cardioscope monitoring, a thorough clinical examination by palpating the pulse, manually recording the BP and a 12-lead ECG should be obtained. **Figure 4** shows an example of how an inappropriate lead monitoring and cable artefact can result in wrong treatment, if one does not make a proper clinical assessment and solely relies on monitored information. Also, always keep the heart rate alarm on, such that not only a visual but an audible assessment of the heart rate is done intraoperatively.

Blood Pressure, Oxygen Saturation, and $ETCO_2$ Monitoring

Most multipara monitors include measurements of both invasive and noninvasive blood pressure recordings and O_2 saturation monitoring. Minor surgeries, in stable patients can be carried out with noninvasive BP monitoring, whereas major surgeries and in patients with compromised cardiac status require invasive arterial BP monitoring. Noninvasive monitoring can be done by attaching a standard BP cuff and recording BP at the brachial artery. The cuff can be programmed to inflate and deflate at fixed intervals. Noninvasive monitoring can sometimes give false readings due to wrong method or size of cuff application. A baseline manual recording should be taken and compared accordingly. O_2 saturation monitoring is essential for every surgical procedure. In case of mechanical ventilation, $ETCO_2$ monitoring is helpful. In case of hypotension or vasoconstriction, false low saturation can be recorded and therefore correlating with the pulse waveform and in doubtful cases an arterial blood gas analysis should be done.

BOX 1: Principles in electrode placement for perioperative electrocardiogram monitoring.

- Place the electrodes in appropriate location as per the color coding and wide apart
- Preferably use bony prominence to place the electrodes so as to ensure good contact
- Scrub the skin surface (avoid/shave hairy area) well with ether/spirit, dry the area and apply KY jelly
- Secure the electrodes with a nonallergic adhesive tape to ensure good contact through the surgery despite the use of betadine paint or soaking of the area
- Ensure that the monitor is attached to the power outlet with proper grounding

DEFIBRILLATORS

Defibrillators are equipment **(Figs. 5A to C)** which administer electric shocks to the heart. Defibrillation is the term used when asynchronous electric energy is delivered to terminate life-threatening ventricular flutter or fibrillation. Cardioversion is the term used when a synchronous direct current shock is used to restore sinus rhythm in various supraventricular and ventricular tachycardias. Synchronization of the delivery of electric shock to the R wave is chosen for all tachycardias with well-defined and identifiable QRS complex, e.g., all supraventricular and monomorphic ventricular tachycardias **(Box 2)**. This is essential so that defibrillation does not occur in the vulnerable period of cardiac repolarization when ventricular fibrillation (VF) can be induced. Asynchronous shock is used for polymorphic ventricular tachycardia or ventricular flutter and fibrillation where there is no well-defined QRS complex **(Fig. 6)**.

Transient delivery of electrical current causes a momentary depolarization of most cardiac cells allowing the sinus node to resume normal pacemaker activity. In the presence of reentrant-induced arrhythmia, such as paroxysmal supraventricular tachycardia (PSVT) and ventricular tachycardia (VT), electrical cardioversion interrupts the self-perpetuating circuit and restores sinus rhythm. Electrical cardioversion is less effective in treating arrhythmia caused

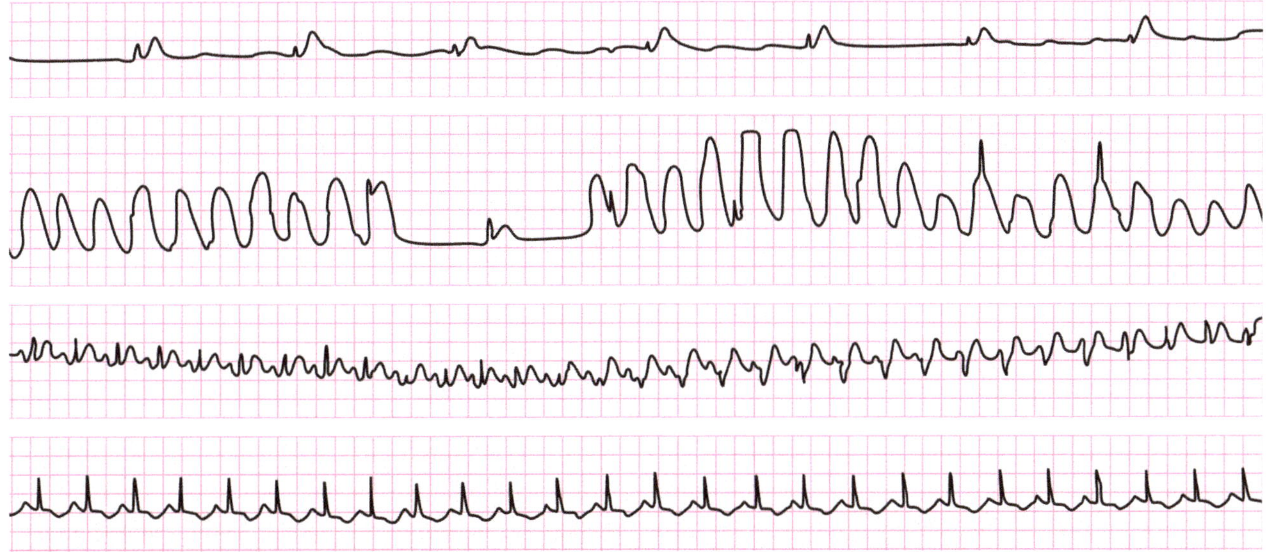

Fig. 4: Electrocardiogram (ECG) cable artefact. The first ECG monitoring lead shows a very small QRS complex and a larger T wave (inappropriate electrode placement). The second strip shows movement artefact of the cable; note the narrow, regular QRS complex within the bizarre looking wide rhythm. The bottom two strips show inappropriate treatment with atropine, digoxin, etc.

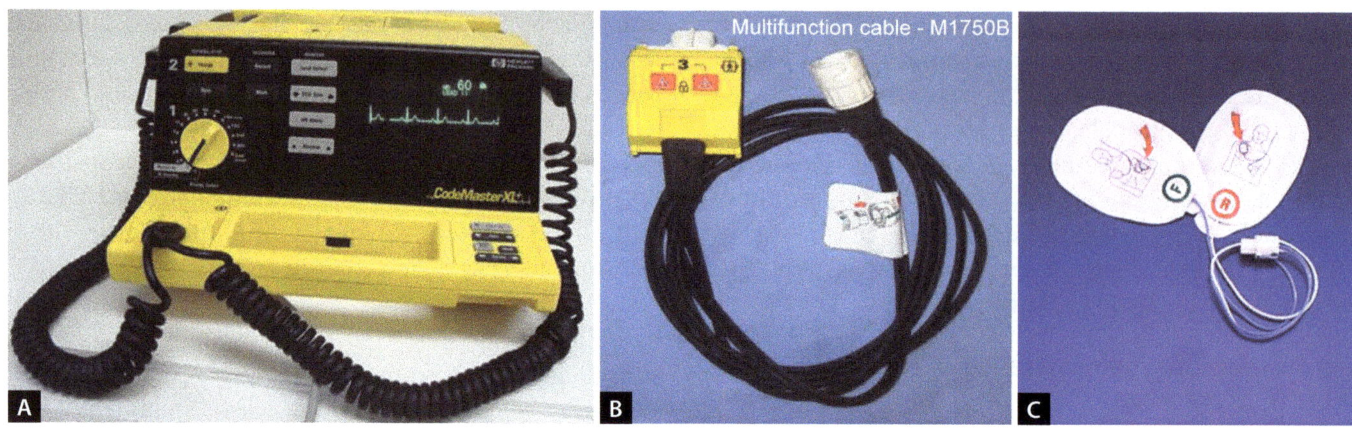

Figs. 5A to C: Defibrillator with R2 pads.

BOX 2: Indications for asynchronous versus synchronous shock.

- Asynchronous shock (defibrillation) is used in the following situations
  - Pulseless ventricular tachycardia
  - Ventricular fibrillation
  - Cardiac arrest due to or resulting in ventricular fibrillation
- Indications for synchronized electrical shock (cardioversion) include the following:
  - Monomorphic ventricular tachycardia
  - Atrial fibrillation
  - Atrial flutter
  - Paroxysmal supraventricular tachycardia

by increased automaticity (e.g., digitalis-induced tachycardia, catecholamine-induced arrhythmia) since the mechanism of the arrhythmia remains after the arrhythmia is terminated and therefore are likely to recur. These arrhythmias will require appropriate antiarrhythmic and antisympathetic drugs.

The first successful use of external defibrillation for human resuscitation for ventricular standstill was reported in 1952. Zoll in 1956 used alternating current for the resuscitation of patients with ventricular fibrillation. The current generation defibrillators use direct current (DC) energy which is more efficacious and safe.

The Lown waveform was the standard for defibrillation until the late 1980s when numerous studies showed that a biphasic truncated waveform (BTE) was equally efficacious while requiring the delivery of lower levels of energy to produce defibrillation. And the added advantage was a significant reduction in weight of the machine. The BTE waveform, combined with automatic measurement of transthoracic impedance is the basis for modern defibrillators. With a monophasic shock, the electrical charge does not change polarity, and this constant polarity necessitates the delivery of higher energy to achieve successful cardioversion. Biphasic defibrillation delivers a charge in one direction for half of the shock and in the electrically opposite direction for the second half. Biphasic waveforms thus defibrillate more effectively and at lower energies than monophasic waveforms.[3,4]

The defibrillator paddle placement on the chest wall has two conventional positions—anterolateral and anteroposterior. In the anterolateral position, a single paddle is placed on the left fourth or fifth intercostal space on the midaxillary line. The second paddle is placed just to the right of the sternal edge on the second or third intercostal space. In the anteroposterior position, a single paddle is placed to the right of the sternum, as above, and the other paddle is placed between the tip of the left scapula and the spine. An anteroposterior electrode position is more effective than the anterolateral position for external cardioversion of persistent atrial fibrillation (AF) and in obese individuals or dilated hearts. The anteroposterior approach is also preferred in patients with left infraclavicular implanted devices, to avoid shunting current to the implantable device and damaging its system.[5]

Because the skin can conduct away a significant portion of the current, it is common practice to employ conductive gel or pregelled pads so as to ensure good contact. Even in ideal circumstances, only 10–30% of the total current reaches the heart.

In patients with permanent pacemaker and intracardiac defibrillator implants, care should be taken such that the external defibrillator paddles should be at least 10 cm away from the implanted devices and the current vector of the external defibrillator should be perpendicular to the implanted device. The implanted device should be assessed for any malfunction after cardioversion.

Energy Selection

In case of life-threatening arrhythmias with cardiac arrest, highest energy shock (360 J monophasic or 200 J biphasic), asynchronous shock should be given. In the event of well defined QRS tachycardia, the defibrillator should be used in the synchronized mode. Atrial flutter and PSVT require less energy for correction: 50 J initially, then 100 J if needed. Cardioversion of VT requires shock of 50–100 J initially, then 200 J if the initial shock is unsuccessful. Energy requirements for correction of AF are higher at 100–200 J initially and

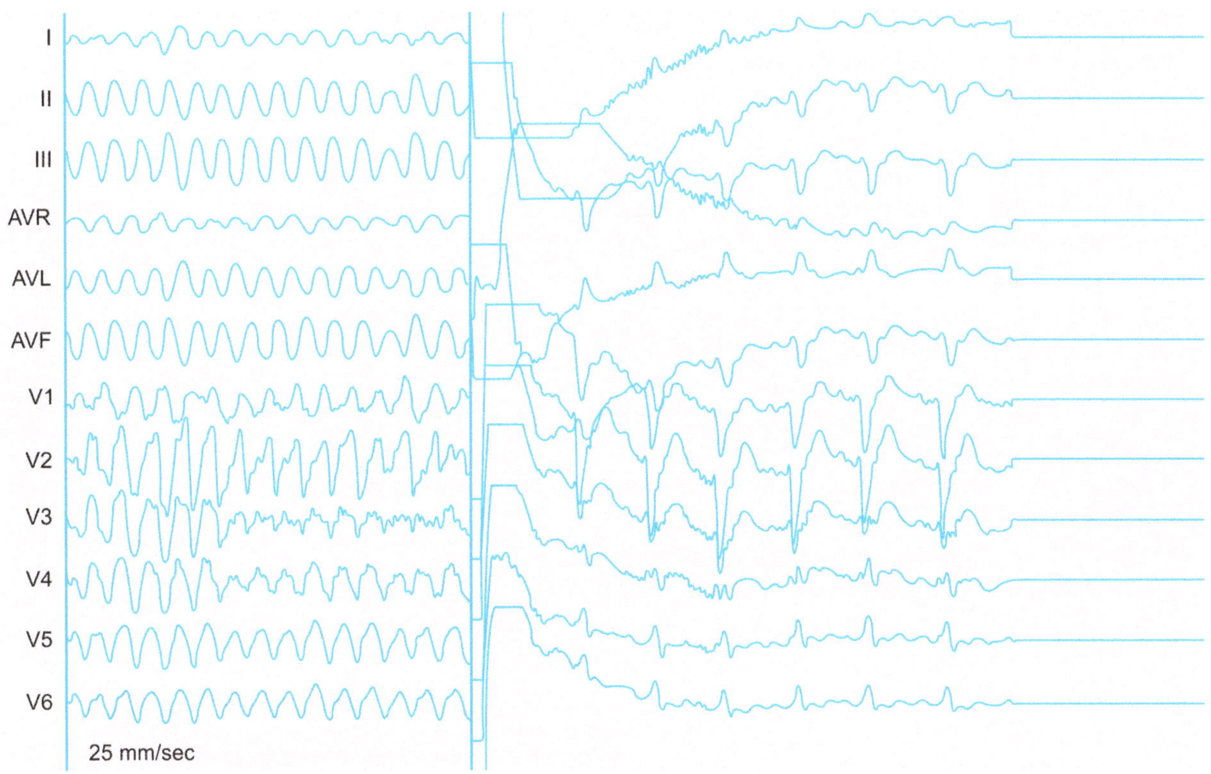

Fig. 6: Successful defibrillation using asynchronous, 200 J biphasic shock.

360 J for subsequent shocks **(Table 1)**. In children, smaller paddle size should be used (3 cm diameter) and also the energy selection is lower, i.e., 0.5–2 J/kg for cardioversion and 2–4 J/kg for defibrillation.

Complications resulting from the use of an external cardioverter defibrillator may include failure to shock, failure to sense or identify the rhythm, chest wall discomfort, and skin burns. Adequate sedation and amnesia is very essential to avoid any chest pain. Inadequate sedation can result in pain, resulting in increased sympathetic discharge perpetuating the tachycardia. Appropriate gelly application is also necessary to avoid any skin burns and reduce the transthoracic impedance allowing maximum delivery of energy to the myocardium. Importantly adequate and firm pressure should be applied while delivering the shock with complete contact of the defibrillator paddles to the body surface for effective defibrillation or cardioversion **(Box 3)**.

TABLE 1: Energy selection for defibrillation or cardioversion.

Arrhythmia	*Energy (biphasic/monophasic Joules)*
Pulseless ventricular tachycardia/ ventricular fibrillation	200/360
Atrial fibrillation	100–200/200–360
Atrial flutter	50–100/100–200
Paroxysmal supraventricular tachycardia	20–50/50–100

BOX 3: Principles of effective defibrillation or cardioversion.

- Adequate sedation or amnesia
- Proper mode of energy delivery—synchronous versus asynchronous
- Proper paddle location—anterolateral or anteroposterior
- Appropriate jelly application on the paddles
- Firm pressure and thorough skin contact of the paddles
- Identifying the tachyarrhythmia suitable for electrical shock
- Maintaining correct internal milieu (electrolyte or acid-base balance)
- Appropriate use of depth of anesthesia, antiarrhythmic drugs, and antisympathetic measures

R2 Pads

These are defibrillator pads which are flexible and firmly stick to the chest wall with the help of adhesive gel. These pads are then electrically connected to the defibrillator. The pads are imprinted to show proper placement. These self-adhesive electrode pads are used in situations where the sterile operative field covers the chest wall region; in patients likely to require repeated electric shocks; and in automated defibrillators used for out-of-hospital defibrillation. The apex pad covers the cardiac apex in the V5 and V6 electrode position, while the posterior pad is placed over the right infrascapular area, which reduces the risk of hazardous current concentration. The pads can be connected to a R2 cable adaptor compatible with the regular defibrillating system. The use of hand-held paddle electrodes may be more effective than self-adhesive patch electrodes. The success rates are slightly higher for patients assigned to paddled electrodes because these hand-held electrodes improve electrode-to-skin contact and reduce the transthoracic impedance. Some of the defibrillators also has transcutaneous pacing capability through these R2 pads.

However pacing is very rarely used as the ventricular capture is ineffective and often painful, hence used in the rare event of an emergency with severe, unexpected bradycardia.

CONCLUSION

Electrocardiogram cardioscopes and defibrillators form an integral and essential monitoring in operation theaters and recovery rooms. These equipment are mandatory for all patients undergoing surgery irrespective of the type of surgery, mode of anesthesia and the risk status of the patient. However, the most important caveat is to know and understand all the features of the equipment very well. A daily check-list should include proper charging and testing of the equipment along with noting the presence of all necessary accessories and cables. Finally using the information provided by the equipment judiciously, confirming and correlating with clinical assessment is the key to success.

REFERENCES

1. Poldermans D, Bax JJ, Boersma E, et al. Guidelines for pre-operative cardiac risk assessment and perioperative cardiac management in noncardiac surgery. Eur Heart J. 2009;30:2769-812.
2. Meek S, Morris F. ABC of clinical electrocardiography introduction. I-Leads, rate, rhythm, and cardiac axis. BMJ. 2002;324:415-8.
3. Kirchhof P, Eckardt L, Loh P, et al. Anterior-posterior versus anterior-lateral electrode positions for external cardioversion of atrial fibrillation: a randomised trial. Lancet. 2002;360(9342):1275-9.
4. Schneider T, Martens PR, Paschen H, et al. Multicenter, randomized, controlled trial of 150-J biphasic shocks compared with 200- to 360-J monophasic shocks in the resuscitation of out-of-hospital cardiac arrest victims. Optimized response to cardiac arrest (ORCA) investigators. Circulation. 2000;102(15):1780-7.
5. Niebauer MJ, Brewer JE, Chung MK, et al. Comparison of the rectilinear biphasic waveform with the monophasic damped sine waveform for external cardioversion of atrial fibrillation and flutter. Am J Cardiol. 2004;93(12):1495-9.

Pulse Oximeters

Anila D Malde

ABSTRACT

Pulse oximetry is a simple, noninvasive, reliable, reasonably accurate, cheap, continuous and risk-free method of measuring arterial oxygen saturation in all patient age groups. Pulse oximetry combines the technology of spectrophotometry and plethysmography. It is based on the Beer-Lambert's law. Oxyhemoglobin absorbs more infrared light (wavelength of 940 nm) than red light (wavelength of 660 nm) and deoxyhemoglobin absorbs more red light than infrared light. Conventional pulse oximetry measures the "functional" saturation. While interpreting results, one should keep in mind, sigmoid shape of oxygen dissociation curve. Finger, thumb, toe, pinna, the lobe of the ear in adults and palm or the sole for neonates and infants are the most common measuring sites. Monitoring oxygenation under anesthesia, in postanesthesia care unit, intensive care units and emergency department is the most common use. Perfusion index (PI) and pleth variability index (PVI) are the new features used for assessment of circulation. Motion artefacts, poor perfusion, skin pigmentation, nail polish, artificial nails, irregular rhythms, and electromagnetic interference can result in inaccuracy in the displayed oxygen saturation (SpO_2). However, here the cause is recognizable, and the observer is usually warned by the device (alarm) about the problem. Inability to detect hyperoxia, hypoventilation and delay in the detection of hypoxic events are some of the potentially unsafe limitations. Ambient light interference, abnormal hemoglobin molecules, venous pulsation and intravenous dyes can cause inaccuracy which is difficult to recognize. Error correction, multiwavelength and reflectance pulse oximetry are some of the recent advances in pulse oximetry.

INTRODUCTION

Hypoxemia is a dangerous and potentially avoidable cause of morbidity and mortality in emergency department, operating room, procedure suite and the intensive care unit (ICU). Human eye is a poor detector of cyanosis. Pulse oximetry is a simple, noninvasive, reliable, reasonably accurate, cheap, continuous and risk free method of measuring arterial oxygen saturation in all patient age groups. Pulse oximetry is now universally used and it has been called the "fifth vital sign".[1]

OPERATING PRINCIPLE

Pulse oximetry combines the technology of spectrophotometry and plethysmography.

Spectrophotometry

It is based on Beer-Lambert's law, a combination of two laws describing absorption of monochromatic light by a transparent substance through which it passes.

Beer's Law

The intensity of transmitted light decreases exponentially as the concentration of the substance increases. [August Beer, German Physicist (1825–1863)]

Lambert's Law

The intensity of transmitted light decreases exponentially as the distance traveled through the substance increases. [Johann Lambert, German Physicist (1728–1777)]

The Beer-Lambert's law is expressed as the following equation:

$$I_e = I_o \times e^{-DCa}$$

where I_e is the intensity of transmitted light, I_o is the intensity of the incident light, D is the distance that the light is transmitted through the medium, C is the concentration of the solute (hemoglobin), and the extinction coefficient a is a constant for a given solute at a specified wavelength; e = base of natural logarithms (approximately 2.7182818285) **(Fig. 1)**.

Oxyhemoglobin absorbs more infrared light (wavelength of 940 nm) than red light (wavelength of 660 nm) and deoxyhemoglobin absorbs more red light than infrared light **(Fig. 2)**. Isosbestic point is the point at which two substances absorb a certain wavelength of light to the same extent. This point may be used as reference points where light absorption is independent of the degree of saturation.

Pulse oximeters use a type of light source called "light emitting diodes (LEDs)" as they are cheap, very compact, emit light in accurate wavelengths, do not heat up much

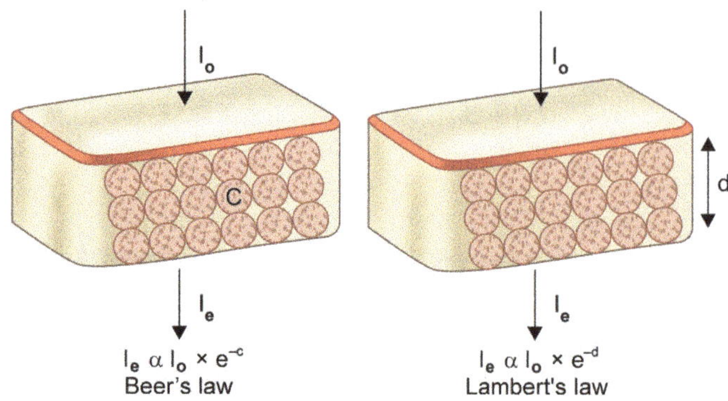

Fig. 1: Beer-Lambert's law. [I_e: intensity of transmitted light; I_o: intensity of the incident light; d: distance; c: concentration of the solute (hemoglobin)]

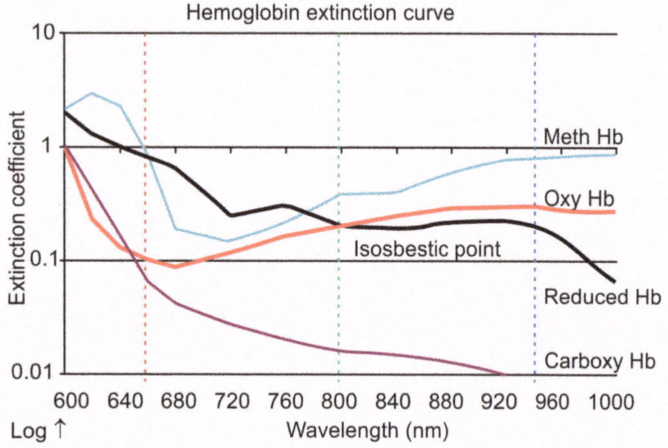

Fig. 2: Hemoglobin extinction curve. (Hb: hemoglobin)

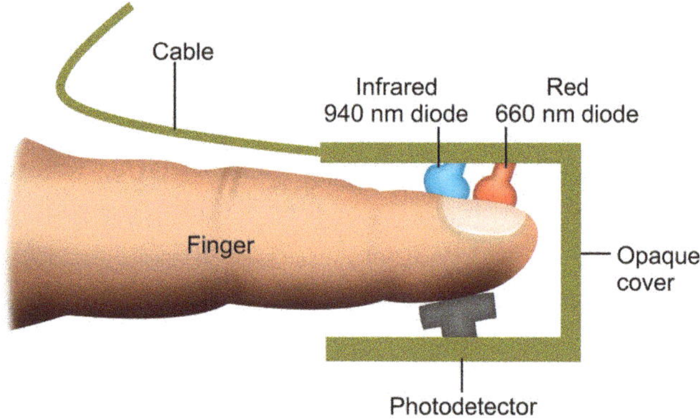

Fig. 3: Diagrammatic representation of a pulse oximeter probe.

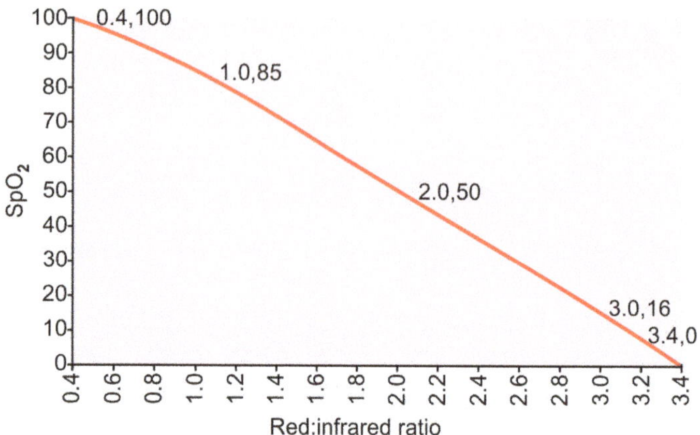

Fig. 4: Relation between oxygen saturation and red: infrared ratio.

during use and hence less likely to cause burns. Conventional pulse oximeters have two LEDs that emit light in the red light (660 nm) and infrared light (940 nm) wavelengths.[2] Emission of these two wavelengths alternates at frequencies of 0.6–1.0 kHz, and the nonabsorbed energy is detected by a photodetector **(Fig. 3)**.

Depending on the amounts of oxyhemoglobin and deoxyhemoglobin present, the ratio of the amount of red light absorbed compared to the amount of infrared light absorbed changes. Using this ratio, the pulse oximeter can then work out the oxygen saturation (SpO_2) **(Fig. 4)**.

The pulse oximeter needs to analyze only arterial blood, ignoring the other tissues around the blood. Principle of plethysmography is used for this.

Plethysmography

During each cardiac cycle, light absorption by tissue beds varies cyclically **(Fig. 5)**. During "diastole", absorption is caused by nonpulsatile arterial blood, venous blood, tissue, bone, and pigments [direct current (DC) component]. During "systole", the pulsatile expansion of the arteriolar bed produces an increase in path length thereby increasing the absorbance [alternating current (AC) component]. The microprocessor first determines the AC component of absorbance at each wavelength and divides this by the corresponding DC component. SpO_2 determines the red: infrared absorption ratio. Thus, the red: Infrared ratio of these pulsatile differences can be used to compute the pulse oximeter reading (SpO_2), which is an estimate of arterial oxygen saturation (SaO_2).[3]

$$SpO_2 = \frac{f(AC660/DC660)}{(AC940/DC940)}$$

The measured ratio is compared with stored ones in the microprocessor of the device and corresponding SpO_2 is displayed. These algorithms are derived through SaO_2 measurements in healthy volunteers breathing mixtures of decreasing oxygen concentrations and are usually unique for each manufacturer.[4-6]

The displayed SpO_2 represents the mean of the measurements obtained during the previous 3–6 seconds, whereas the data are updated every 0.5–1.0 second. The performance of each device is based on the reliability and complexity of the algorithms used in signal processing and to the speed and quality of the microprocessor.[4,5,7-10]

Accounting for Ambient (Room) Light[2]

Photodetector is exposed to three sources of light, namely red and infrared LED light, and ambient light. The room (ambient) light is unwanted "noise". To eliminate the effect of ambient light, pulse oximeter has following sequence **(Figs. 6A to D)**:

- Only red LED is on. Sensor measures red plus room light
- Only infrared LED is on. Sensor measures infrared plus room light
- Both LEDs off. Sensor measures only room light.

Thus, ultimately processor minuses out the effect of ambient light.

Conventional pulse oximetry measures the "functional" saturation, which is defined by the following equation:

$$\text{Functional } SaO_2 = \left[\frac{O_2\,Hb}{(O_2\,Hb + \text{reduced Hb})}\right] \times 100$$

where, Hb = hemoglobin

Laboratory co-oximeters use multiple wavelengths to distinguish other types of hemoglobin (Hb) by their characteristic absorption. Co-oximeters measure the "fractional" saturation, which is defined by the following equation:

$$\text{Fractional } SaO_2 = \left[\frac{O_2\,Hb}{(O_2\,Hb + \text{reduced Hb} + COHb + MetHb)}\right] \times 100$$

where, COHb is carboxyhemoglobin and MetHb is methemoglobin.

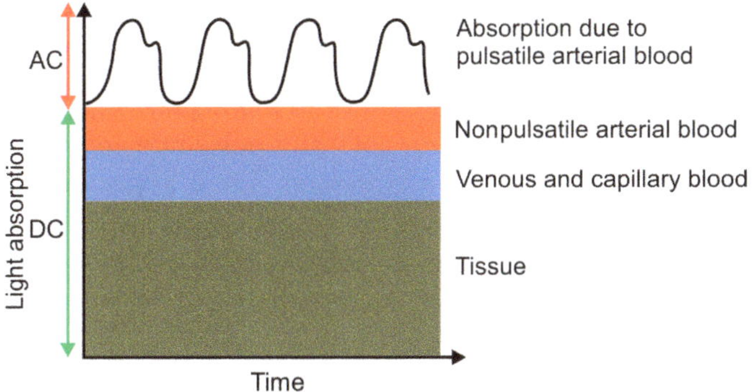

Fig. 5: Components of light absorption by a tissue bed.

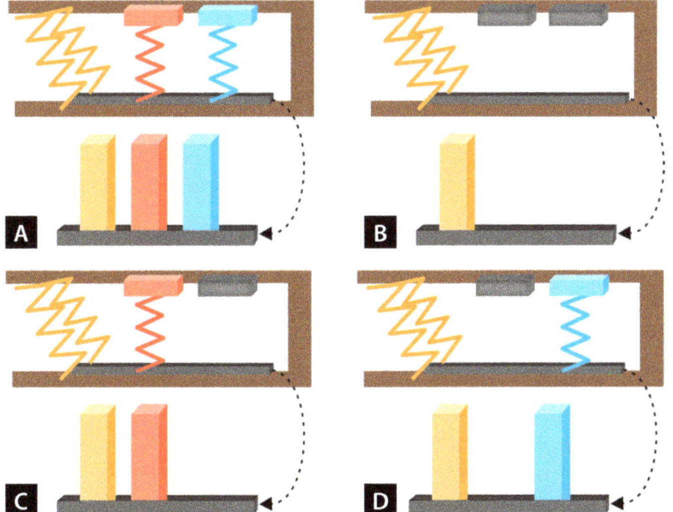

Figs. 6A to D: Diagrammatic representation of the mechanism by which pulse oximeter eliminates the effect of ambient light. (A) Red, Infrared light LEDs on; (B) Red, Infrared light LEDs off; (C) Red light LED on, Infrared light LEDs off; (D) Red light LED off, Infrared light LEDs on.

TYPES

Transmission Pulse Oximetry

Here the emitter and photodetector are placed opposite of each other. Measuring site is kept in-between the two. It is the most commonly used method.

Reflectance Pulse Oximetry

Here the emitter and photodetector are side-by-side on the measuring site. The light gets reflected from the emitter to the detector across the site. It was developed to overcome problems with signal transmission during hypoperfusion and nonavailability of transmission path. Forehead is the most commonly used probe site, where motion artifact and hypoperfusion are less problematic compared to other sites.[11] Forehead probes can detect hypoxemia earlier compared to ear or finger probes.[12] Three most common sources of inaccuracy with reflectance oximetry are (1) excessive edema, (2) poor skin contact, and (3) motion artifact. Probe placement directly over a pulsating superficial artery can lead to artifact.[13] Some of the recent advances in the use of reflectance pulse oximetry are discussed at the end of this chapter.

PHYSIOLOGY

While interpreting SpO_2, one should remember shape of the oxygen dissociation curve. On the middle steep part of the curve, a good correlation exists between SaO_2 and oxygen pressure (PaO_2). At a PaO_2 of more than 75 mm Hg, the SaO_2 plateaus and does not reflect changes in PaO_2. For example, when the fraction of inspired oxygen (FiO_2) is high, measured oxygen saturation may remain normal despite a significant deterioration in pulmonary gas exchange **(Fig. 7)**. However, since delivery of oxygen to the tissues is proportional to arterial oxygen saturation, pulse oximeters will detect changes in pulmonary gas exchange before tissue oxygenation is impaired.[3,14,15]

EQUIPMENT

Probes

Probes may be reusable or disposable. A disposable probe is usually attached using adhesive. Reusable probes are either clip on or are attached by using adhesive or Velcro®. Self-adhesive (band, wrap) probes are less susceptible to motion artefact and are less likely to come off if the patient moves compared to clip on probes. However, they are less well shielded from ambient light. Probes lined with soft material may be associated with fewer motion artefacts. Some probes are available in different sizes **(Figs. 8 to 10)**.

Cable

The probe is connected to the oximeter by an electrical cable. Cables from different manufacturers are not interchangeable.

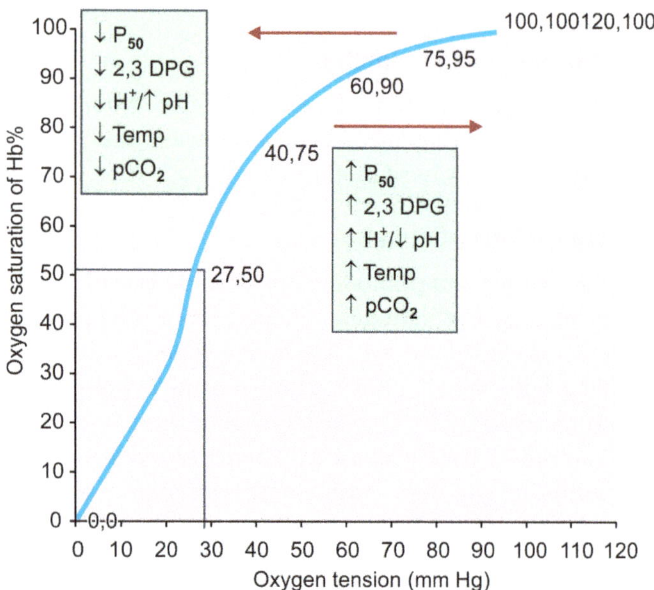

Fig. 7: Oxygen dissociation curve. (2,3 DPG: 2,3-diphosphoglycerate; pCO_2: partial pressure of carbon dioxide)

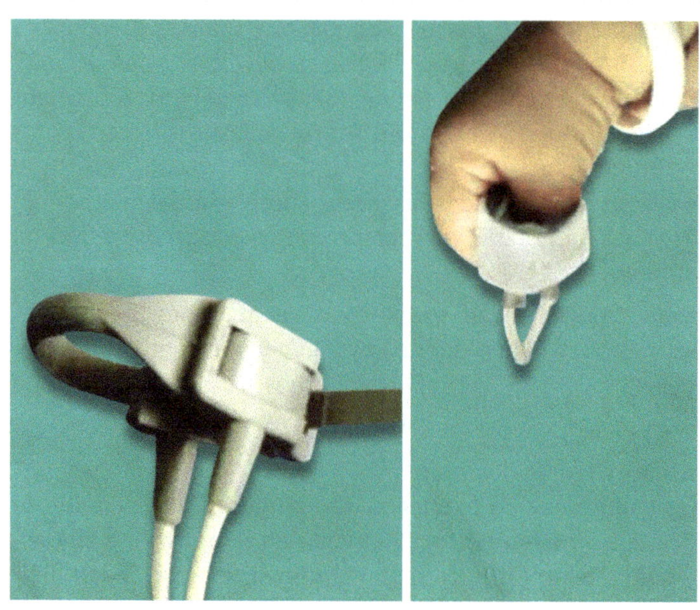

Fig. 10: Flexi probe.

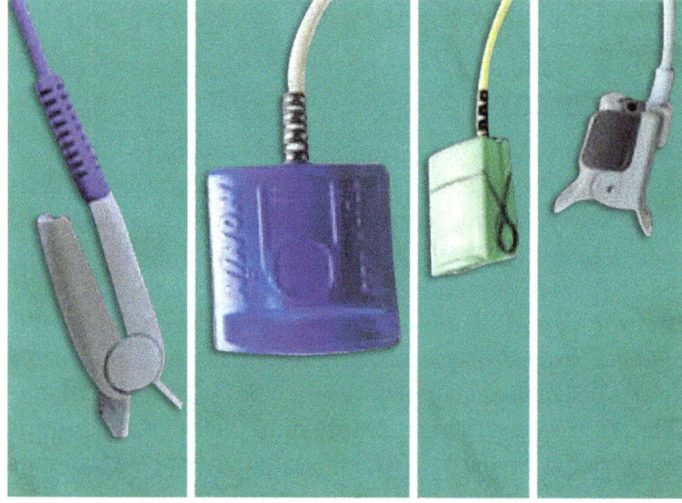

Fig. 8: Finger probes of various types and sizes.

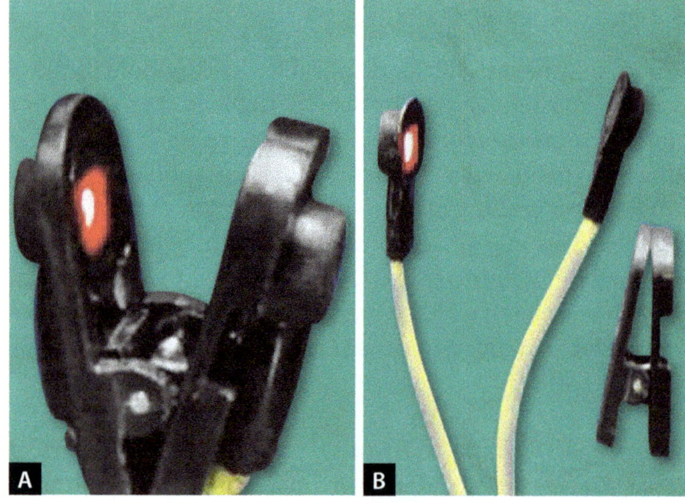

Figs. 9A and B: Ear clip probe. (A) Assembled; (B) Disassembled.

Console

It can be stand alone or a part of multiparameter monitor. Majority have battery backup.

The panel usually displays plethysmograph or pulse amplitude indicator, SpO_2, pulse rate, alarm limits and messages like improper application of probe or inadequate signal.

The displayed values for SpO_2 and pulse rate are usually weighted averages. Some oximeters allow adjustment of the averaging period. Longer averaging period is preferred if there is too much probe motion. Changes in pulse rate or saturation will be reflected more rapidly if the averaging is done over a shorter period of time.

Signal Strength

Some pulse oximeters like (Catalyst, Data scope, In vivo, Ohmeda) have indicator of the signal strength. Full strength signals suggest good perfusion. Low strength signals indicate vasoconstriction and low cardiac output. Thus, it can be of help in the diagnosis of intraoperative hypotension.

Pulse Beep

All pulse oximeters emit a beep after detecting a plethysmographic pulse. This coincides with each heartbeat. In better quality pulse oximeters, the pitch of this beep is proportional to SpO_2. Thus user can be alerted of changes in SpO_2, before alarm sounds, even if the digital value is away from visual sight.[3]

The application of oximeter probe on same side as blood pressure (BP) cuff is usually avoided as it can cause annoying false alarms. For majority of oximeters, the only way to prevent alarms during BP cuff inflation is the dangerous practice of disabling all alarms.[3] At times, patient position, site of operation or patient anatomy demands application of pulse oximeter probe on ipsilateral hand as the blood pressure cuff. Pulse oximeters with the ability to disable specific alarms are useful over here. For example, in Ohmeda oximeters one can turn off the low pulse rate alarm; this will prevent it from alarming when a BP cuff is inflated for up to 30 seconds. In Nellcor™ oximeter, electrocardiogram (ECG) synchronization allows the heart rate display to remain accurate despite BP cuff inflation; this prevents false "low heart rate" alarms during BP determination. Continuous display of alarm settings is another advantage.

TYPES OF PULSE OXIMETER MODELS

Fingertip Model

This light, handy simple model of pulse oximeter is attached to the finger of a patient and has a small computer and screen. It is stored in pocket or purse.

Wrist Model

It can be worn just like a watch and its sensor can be put into a finger. A short wire joins the two components. It is normally utilized for an uninterrupted monitoring during sleep studies. It has capacity to store 24 hours of data that can be downloaded in the computer afterward.

Handheld Model

It is most commonly used. It can be placed on the patient's earlobe, fingertip or on the toe of the patient.

Table-top Model

These are usually multiparameter monitors with multiple features.

SITES FOR MEASUREMENT

Most commonly used measuring sites include the finger, thumb, toe, pinna, and the lobe of the ear in adults and children. For neonates and infants measurements are commonly obtained from the palm or the sole by using specially designed probes. Less commonly used sites are the cheek and the tongue.[16-19]

Finger pulse oximeters can have delay of 30 seconds in detecting acute changes in arterial saturation. However, when placed on the ear, it responds within 5–10 seconds. Therefore, when acute changes in SaO_2 are expected, one should utilize earlobe oximetry.[3,20,21]

In addition to standard, slide-on finger probes, many manufacturers provide an option of tape-on probes. These may be disposable (Nellcor™) or reusable (Catalyst, Data scope, Ohmeda, Sensor Medics). They are designed to be fixed to the finger with double-stick tapes and wraps. They are taped to the palm or sole of neonate or infant. Tape-on probes are less susceptible to motion artifact compared to slide on probes. However, they are not as well shielded from ambient light sources as the slide-on design, increasing the risk of interference.

Clip-on probes, which are suitable for application to the earlobe or tongue are also available; these are especially useful in cases where the arms are inaccessible, peripheral perfusion is poor, or a rapid response to changes in oxygenation is critical. Rubbing the ear with alcohol or a small dab of nitroglycerin ointment can increase earlobe perfusion, and improve pulse oximeter signal.

Nellcor™ forehead SpO_2 sensor can provide earlier and better signal compared to finger sensors during poor perfusion conditions.[12,22-24] Other probes have been developed to monitor fetal oxygenation during labor. Esophageal probe has been used for monitoring SpO_2 when extremities are unavailable or have a pulse of insufficient amplitude.

APPLICATIONS OF PULSE OXIMETRY (BOX 1)

Monitoring Oxygenation under Anesthesia

Pulse oximetry is most useful as an early warning sign of hypoxemia. Hence, it has become a standard of care in anesthesia practice since 1986. Cullen, et al. demonstrated that the introduction of pulse oximetry to areas where anesthesia was administered decreased the overall rate of unanticipated admissions to the ICU.[25] In a trial in which 20,802 patients scheduled for surgery were randomly assigned to receive monitoring with pulse oximetry or not, hypoxemia was detected during anesthesia 20 times and hypoventilation three times as frequently in the pulse oximetry group. Myocardial ischemia was more common in the control group versus the oximetry group (26 and 12 patients, respectively).[26]

BOX 1: Different applications of pulse oximetry.

1. Monitoring oxygenation for adult and children in critical areas
   - A. Anesthesia
     - I. In operation room or general anesthesia
     - II. Monitored anesthesia care or during conscious sedation
   - B. Postanesthesia care unit
   - C. Intensive care units
   - D. Emergency department
2. Monitoring oxygenation in neonatal areas
   - A. Intensive care
   - B. Newborn nursery
   - C. Delivery suites
3. Transport
   - A. Internal (within the hospital)
   - B. External
     - I. Ambulance
     - II. Air transport
4. Diagnostic lab
   - A. Pulmonary function test lab
   - B. Exercise lab
   - C. Sleep lab
5. Subacute care centers
6. Home care patients
7. Controlling oxygen administration
8. Avoiding hyperoxemia
9. Monitoring peripheral circulation
10. Determining systolic blood pressure
11. Locating arteries
12. Monitoring vascular volume and sympathetic tone
13. Intrapartum fetal monitoring

Monitoring Oxygenation in Postanesthesia Care Unit

A few studies report detections of hypoxemia several days postoperatively with pulse oximetry.[27,28] The peak effects of analgesia may correlate with hypoxemia, so monitoring of patients receiving narcotics may be important to prevent adverse cardiac events.[29] After cardiac surgery, use of pulse oximetry has been shown to increase detection of hypoxemic episodes and decrease the number of arterial blood gases (ABGs) performed in the ICU.[30]

Monitoring Oxygenation for Critically Ill Adult and Children

Jubran and Tobin found that pulse oximeters accurately estimate SaO_2 in critically ill patients when SaO_2 is greater than 90% (bias, 1.7%; precision, ±1.2%) but are less accurate when SaO_2 falls below 90%.[31] SpO_2 of 92% was indicative of adequate oxygenation when titrating O_2 in white patients. However, significant hypoxemia was commonly present with SpO_2 of 92% in black patients, and SpO_2 of 95% was needed to ensure adequate oxygenation.

Monitoring Oxygenation in Emergency Department

In a study involving 12,000 adult patients in the triage area of an emergency department Mower, et al. showed a weak inverse relationship between SpO_2 and respiratory rate (correlation coefficients of 0.378 to –0.454 with a weighted mean of –0.160). Overall, only 33% of patients with SpO_2 below 90% exhibited an increase in respiratory rate, so SpO_2 should be considered as "pulmonary vital sign".[32]

Reduction in the number of unjustified ABGs (as determined by independent experts) over a 2-month period from 29% when pulse oximetry was unavailable to 12% when oximetry was available has been shown by Bourdelles et al. in an emergency department.[33]

Pulse oximetry has also been used for following:

- Diagnosing and managing a severe exacerbation of chronic obstructive pulmonary disease (COPD) in the community
- *Grading the severity of an asthma attack:* Attack is considered potentially life-threatening if saturations are <92% while breathing air
- Assessing severity and oxygen requirements for patients with community-acquired pneumonia
- Assessing severity and determining management in infants with bronchiolitis.

Monitoring of Oxygenation in COVID-19 Pandemic

Pulse oximetry is useful in evaluating the severity of the illness and, in conjunction with other criteria, determining whether to refer patients for further assessment and/or treatment. In low-resource settings where oxygen supplies and monitored beds are scarce, pulse oximetry is a crucial device for triaging patients and establishing the need for supplemental oxygen. Silent hypoxia (abnormally low oxygen saturation without symptoms of dyspnea) is common in patients with COVID-19. Prehospital pulse oximetry might be used as a red flag for early detection of "silent hypoxemia" in COVID-19 patients. Patients with COVID-19 who do not need immediate hospital attention but are at high risk of developing serious symptoms are given pulse oximeters to use at home to reduce the risk of serious deterioration. It may be useful to aid the monitoring of patients who have been discharged from hospital having been diagnosed with COVID-19 infection but now deemed well enough to return home.

Neonatal Applications

Neonatal Resuscitation

In immediate postnatal period, the skin color is not a reliable indicator of status of oxygenation.[34] In several studies during neonatal resuscitation the pulse oximetry is proved to be feasible and reliable.[35-38] It is now recommended in neonates that SpO_2 monitoring is recommended for persistent cyanosis and in neonates requiring assisted ventilation or supplementary oxygen or neonatal resuscitation is anticipated (high-risk deliveries).[34]

Neonatal Screening for Congenital Heart Disease

For early detection of asymptomatic newborns with critical congenital heart disease pulse oximetry can be a screening tool and single lower-extremity values after 24 postnatal hours is enough for large scale screening. At low altitudes SpO_2 threshold of less than 95% is considered appropriate.[39,40]

Prevention of Hyperoxia

A single best range has not been established yet. However, there is evidence that SpO_2 values between 85% and 93% are sufficient to maintain normoxemia and to decrease the incidence of retinopathy of prematurity in infants receiving supplemental oxygen.[41-45]

Monitoring Vascular Volume and Sympathetic Tone

Plethysmographic waveform analysis has been recommended for assessing volume status, fluid responsiveness, and few other clinical variables.[46,47] Respiratory variations in systolic pressure (dPs) and arterial pulse pressure (dPp) have been shown to be accurate indicators of volume status and fluid responsiveness in mechanically ventilated patients.[48] However, arterial cannulation for this purpose is not justified. Recently, variation in the pulse oximeter plethysmograph (dPOP) amplitude was shown to be a reliable noninvasive surrogate for dPp as both parameters are dependent on stroke volume.[49] Cannesson and colleagues found that baseline dPOP was correlated with percent change in cardiac index induced by volume expansion.[50] Feissel, et al. in study on critically ill septic patients concluded that dPOP can

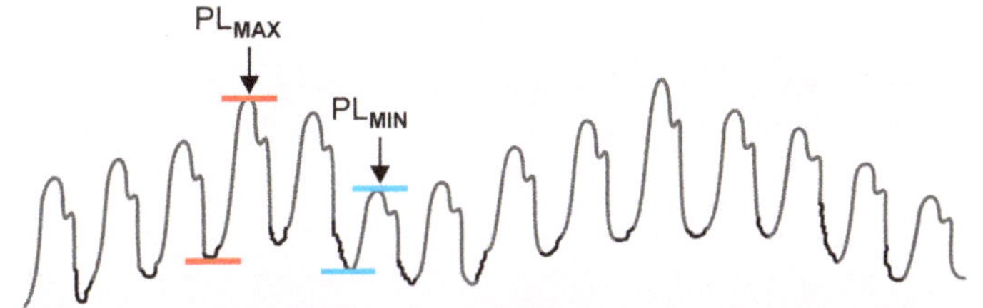

Fig. 11: Respiratory variations in pulse oximetry plethysmographic waveform amplitude in a patient with hypovolemia. (PL_{MAX}: maximum amplitude of plethysmograph wave; PL_{MIN}: minimum amplitude of plethysmograph wave)

predict response to fluid administration.[51] Shelley, et al. demonstrated that the ear and forehead may be better monitoring sites than the finger for detection of variation in respiratory waveform.[52] Error and artifact correction in most commercial pulse oximeters can obscure the subtle respiratory variations. Therefore, unaltered plethysmographic waveforms are needed for such analysis.

Perfusion index is the numerical value of the plethysmograph waveform amplitude. It is the ratio of pulsatile to nonpulsatile blood flow through the peripheral capillary bed. It indicates the vasomotor tone. Higher the vasomotor tone, i.e., vasoconstriction, lower is the PI. In case of vasodilatation, higher is the PI. Pleth variability index is an automatic measure of the dynamic change in PI that occurs during the respiratory cycle. The greater the PVI, the more likely the patient will respond to fluid administration **(Fig. 11)**.[53]

$$\text{Pleth variability index (PVI)} = (PL_{MAX} - PL_{MIN}) \times 100/PL_{MAX}$$

where, PL_{MAX}: Maximum amplitude of plethysmograph wave; PL_{MIN}: Minimum amplitude of plethysmograph wave.

Many other novel applications of pulse oximetry in anesthetic practice have been studied. Mowafi found that plethysmographic pulse wave amplitude (PPWA) may be a better indicator of intravascular test dose injection during epidural placement than traditional hemodynamic markers are (i.e., heart rate and systolic blood pressure). A 10% decrease in PPWA indicated intravascular injection with 100% sensitivity, specificity, positive predictive value, and negative predictive value. Sensitivities using heart rate and systolic blood pressure change as criteria were 85–95%.[54]

Many modern oximeters are programmed to measure perfusion index. Changes in perfusion index (defined as AC 940/DC 940) have been used as confirmation of epidural placement and as an indicator of painful stimulus under anesthesia.[55,56]

The plethysmographic waveform has been shown to be useful in the estimation of blood pressure when manometry fails.[57]

Intrapartum Fetal Monitoring

Intrapartum fetal pulse oximetry in the presence of a nonreassuring fetal heart rate is associated with a reduction in operative interventions.[58]

ADVANTAGES

- *Accuracy:* The accuracy of commercially available oximeters is quite variable, probably because of the different algorithms employed in signal processing.[59] These algorithms are limited, as volunteers cannot be made too hypoxic, i.e., SaO_2 less than 80%, and also the accuracy of the measurement standard (Co-oximeter) differs.[14] In healthy volunteers, oximeters commonly have a mean difference (bias) of less than 2% and a standard deviation (precision) of less than 3% when SaO_2 is 90% or above. Accuracy of pulse oximeters deteriorates when SaO_2 falls to 80% or less. In healthy volunteers under hypoxic conditions, bias of pulse oximetry varies from 15.0 to 13.1 while the precision ranges from 1.0 to 16.0.[20,60-63] In a study of 54 ventilator-dependent patients, the accuracy of oximetry deteriorated significantly at low SaO_2 values. Bias ± precision was 1.7 ± 1.2% for SaO_2 values more than 90%, and it increased to 5.1 ± 2.7% when SaO_2 was 90%.[31]
- Independence from gases and vapors
- Fast response time
- Noninvasive
- Continuous measurements
- Separate respiratory and circulatory variables
- Convenience
- Tone modulation
- User-friendliness
- Light weight and compactness
- Probe variety
- No heating required
- Battery operated
- Economy.

PRECAUTIONS TO BE TAKEN WHILE USING AN OXIMETER

- Do not use one manufacturer's sensor with another manufacturer's pulse oximeter unless compatibility has been verified
- Select appropriate size of probe for children and infants
- Select desired sensor site. Assess for arterial blood flow, warmth and capillary refill in the digit
- Avoid sites distal to indwelling arterial catheters, BP cuffs, military antishock trousers, or venous engorgement (e.g., arteriovenous fistula) to obtain accurate SpO_2 measurements
- Avoid placing the sensor on an extremity that has decreased or absent sensation because the patient may not be able to identify discomfort or the signs and symptoms of loss of circulation or tissue
- Ensure that the digit is inserted fully into the slide on probe
- Attach flexible probes correctly
- Emitters and detectors must oppose one another and light should not bypass the tissue reaching directly to the detector

- Resting readings should be taken for at least 5 minutes
- Check that the displayed heart rate correlates to a manually checked heart rate (within 5 beats/min). This generally rules out significant motion artifact
- Poor perfusion (due to cold or hypotension) is the main cause of an inadequate pulse wave. A sharp waveform with a dicrotic notch indicates good perfusion whilst a sine wave-like waveform suggests poor perfusion
- Set appropriate alarm limits according to the patient's condition (oxygen saturation limits should be 5% less than patient acceptable baseline)
- Periodic evaluation of sensor site for skin breakdown or loss of vascular flow is must (2–4 hourly for disposable sensor, 2 hourly for rigid encased nondisposable sensor)
- Frequent (4 hourly) change of the probe site is advisable
- Pulse oximeters are most unreliable in the newborn, as minor changes in skin temperature can affect the reading. Minor manipulation in contact can cause motion artefacts and a poor signal. It is advisable to use two pulse oximeters to improve accuracy.

LIMITATIONS AND DISADVANTAGES[64]

Safe Limitations (Table 1)

Motion Artefacts

Motion of the sensor relative to the skin can cause an artifact that the pulse oximeter is unable to differentiate from normal arterial pulsations. Motion may produce a prolongation in the detection time for hypoxemia without giving a warning.[65] Motion artifact continues to be a significant source of error and false alarms.[26,66,67]

Causes

- Shivering
- Movements during inhalation induction of small children
- Transport
- Evoked potential monitors and nerve stimulators can produce motion artifacts if the pulse oximeter sensor is on the same extremity
- Neonates and children with their tiny digits and poor contact with probes are most susceptible to motion artifact.

TABLE 1: Safe and potentially unsafe limitations.

Safe limitations	*Potentially unsafe limitations*
• Limitation where the inaccuracy in the displayed SpO_2 can be suspected and its cause is recognizable. The device alarms and alerts the observer about the problem	• Limitation where the inaccuracy is difficult to recognize; the displayed SpO_2 is incorrect, but there is no alarm and warning to the observer about the problem
• Motion artefacts	• Calibration assumptions
• Poor perfusion	• Delay in detection of hypoxia
• Skin pigmentation, nail polish, and artificial nails	• Probe positioning
• Irregular rhythms	• Ambient light interference
• Electromagnetic interference	• Abnormal hemoglobin molecules
	• Venous pulsation
	• Intravenous dyes

Mechanisms for Motion Interference[3]

- Depending upon the mass and shape of the oximeter probe, the orientation of the probe with respect to the finger tends to change during motion. For this reason, flexible, adhesive probes, which are taped in place, tend to be less susceptible to motion artifacts than clip-on probes
- Current is induced in the connecting cable when it moves with respect to the earth's magnetic field.

Recognition: The distorted plethysmographic waveforms and erratic display of pulse rate can be because of motion artefacts and increased pulse amplitude is an indicator of movement.

Measures for reduction of artifacts caused by motion are:
- Proper position of sensor on a different extremity from that being stimulated
- In restless patients probes for ear, cheek and nose are more useful than finger probes
- Motion artefacts can be reduced by tapping of flexible probes
- Avoid clip-on probe and use probe lined with soft material
- Lengthening the averaging mode will increase the likelihood that enough true pulses will be detected to reject motion artifacts
- Use R-wave of the patient's ECG to synchronize the optical measurement
- A new technology, termed Masimo signal extraction technology (SET™; Masimo Corporation, Mission Viejo, California, USA), was developed to extract the true signal from artifact due to noise and low perfusion.[68]
  It has new algorithms for processing the pulse oximeter's red and infrared light signals that enable the noise component, which is common to the two wavelengths, to be measured and subtracted. Masimo SET™ in healthy volunteers exhibited much lower error rates (defined as percentage of time that the oximeter error exceeded 5%, 7%, and 10%) and dropout rates (defined as the percentage of time that the oximeter provided no SpO_2 data) than did the Nellcor—N-200 and Nellcor™—N-3000 oximeters (Nellcor Puritan Bennett), during standardized motion for all test conditions.[69]

Poor Perfusion

To distinguish the light absorbed by arterial blood from that absorbed by venous blood and tissue, good quality arterial pulsations are necessary. In case of loss or diminution of peripheral pulse the reading may be unavailable or unreliable.

The causes of poor perfusion are:[70]
- Proximal blood pressure cuff inflation
- Leaning on an extremity

- Improper positioning
- Hypotension
- Hypothermia
- Cardiopulmonary bypass
- Low cardiac output
- Hypovolemia
- Peripheral vascular disease
- Infusion of vasoactive drugs.

Pulse oximeter may blank signal or display in above conditions[71] it may freeze the display at the previous reading in case pulse wave is inconsistent. Therefore, presence of a functioning pulse oximeter should not be construed as evidence of adequate tissue oxygenation or oxygen delivery to vital organs.

Methods to improve the signal include:

- Try an alternative probe site
- Try a different probe
- Try a different machine
- Application of vasodilating cream, e.g., glyceryl trinitrate (GTN) cream
- Digital nerve blocks[72]
- Administration of intra-arterial vasodilators
- Warm the extremity. This may increase the pulse amplitude, if cardiac output is normal
- Use pulse oximeters with signal extraction technology as they may perform better during low perfusion states.

Skin Pigmentation, Nail Polish, and Artificial Nails

Ideally, skin pigmentation results in constant level of absorption that is subtracted in the calculation of SpO_2 and, therefore, should not affect the reading. However, dark skin pigmentation has caused erroneous SpO_2 readings, especially at low SaO_2 values.[6,73,74] In critically ill patients, bias ± precision was greater in black patients, 3.3 ± 2.7%, than in white patients, 2.2 ± 1.8%; also, a bias >4% occurred more frequently in black patients (27%) than in white patients (11%).[31]

Nail Polish and Coverings

Polish of black, blue, or green color and synthetic nails might interfere with pulse oximetry and result in an underestimation of SaO_2.[75-79] It is recommended to apply the probe on the finger sideways.[80] Acrylic nails do not interfere with pulse oximetry readings.[81] Onychomycosis (a yellowish gray color caused by fungus) can cause falsely low SpO_2 readings. Dirt under the nail can lead to difficulty in obtaining reliable readings.

Irregular Rhythms

Irregular heart rhythms can cause erratic performance. During aortic balloon pulsation, because of augmentation of diastolic pressure more than systolic pressure, there is double or triple-peaked arterial pressure waveform. This confuses the pulse oximeter so that it may not provide a reading. Pulse oximetry is unreliable in the presence of rapid atrial fibrillation. Inaccurate oximetry readings can be observed during tachyarrhythmias. These artifacts can usually be recognized by observing the plethysmographic wave form. Many new devices possess signal-extraction technologies that can identify such events.[5,6,80]

Electromagnetic Interference

Electrical interference from an electrosurgical unit can cause the oximeter to give an incorrect pulse count (usually by counting extra beats) or to falsely register decrease in oxygen saturation. This problem may be increased in patients with weak pulse signals. The effect is transient and limited to the duration of the cauterization.

Measures to overcome this problem:[82]

- Manufacturers have made significant progress in reducing their instruments sensitivity to electrical interference. Special shielding and suppression circuitry enabled one oximeter (Data scope) to be totally immune to cautery interference
- Some monitors display a notice when significant interference is present
- Ohmeda oximeters give an error message and stops acquiring data whenever cautery interference exceeds a threshold which is independent of pulse signal strength. Because data acquisition is discontinued, the Ohmeda design avoids erroneous readings and false alarms during electrocautery in patients with weak pulse signals[3]
- Locate the electro surgery grounding plate as close to and the oximeter sensor as far from, the surgical field as possible
- Route the cable from the sensor to the oximeter away from the electrosurgery apparatus
- Keep the pulse oximeter sensor and console as far away as possible from the surgical site and the electrosurgery grounding plate
- Raise the high pulse rate alarm
- Operate the unit in a rapid response mode
- The electrosurgical apparatus and pulse oximeter should not be plugged in to the same power source.

Electromagnetic energy from cellular phones might interfere with pulse oximeters and lead to inaccurate SpO_2 readings.[83] During MRI, devices with fiberoptic technology should be used to avoid both interference with image quality and potentially dangerous heating of the sensor with subsequent thermal injury.[83,84] There are reports of interference with pulse oximeter readings, from a nerve stimulator.

Potentially Unsafe Limitations

Problem of not Detecting Hyperoxia

The pulse oximeter has a limited ability to distinguish high but safe levels of arterial oxygen from excess oxygenation.

This may be harmful, in premature newborns, and hypoxic drive-dependent COPD patients.[2]

Calibration Assumptions

Calibration algorithms are derived by correlating the absorption ratios with arterial SaO_2 measurements in volunteers over a range of saturation values. As it is unethical to desaturate volunteers below SaO_2 levels of <80%, lower SpO_2 values are derived by extrapolation and, therefore, are less accurate.[4,8,60,80,85] For calibration purposes healthy young adults are recruited, so the applicability of algorithms at the extremes of age is doubtful.[4,17,80,86,87]

Delay in the Detection of Hypoxia

While the response time of the pulse oximeter is generally fast, there may be a significant delay between a change in alveolar oxygen tension and a change in the oximeter reading. It is possible for arterial oxygen to reach dangerous levels before the pulse oximeter alarm is activated.

It depends on:

- Complexity of the algorithms used and might exceed 15 to 20 seconds[21,80,88,89]
- Location of sensor placement. Desaturation is detected earlier when the sensor is placed more centrally[6,21,86]
- Perfusion. Lag time will be increased with poor perfusion
- Motion artifacts delay detection of hypoxemia
- Increasing the time over which the pulse signals are averaged also increases the delay time.

Pulse oximetry should not be used as a substitute for cardiorespiratory monitoring in critically ill patients.[17,80]

Probe Positioning

The pulse oximeter operates best when all the light passes through arterial blood. However, if the probe is of the wrong size or has not being applied properly, some of the light, can be projected tangentially to the detector, sometimes without crossing an arterial bed. This is labeled as the "penumbra" or "optical shunting" effect.[90,91] Lower SpO_2 readings might occur when the probe is improperly placed, especially on the small fingers of neonates and infants. This problem can be avoided by positioning the emitter and the detector exactly opposite to each other and by using probes of appropriate size for neonates and infants.[16,86]

Ambient Light Interference

In addition to the light from the LEDs, ambient (room) light also reaches the detector. For good functioning of the pulse oximeter, the strength of the LED light falling on the detector should be superior compared that of ambient light falling on the detector. If the ambient light is too strong, the LED light signal gets "submerged" in the noise of the ambient light. This can lead to erroneous readings.

The pulsatile interference at physiological frequency depends upon relationship between sampling frequency of pulse oximeter and flicker frequency of light source. In such case oximeter reading is high or low. There are case reports of oximeter interference form overhead xenon-arc surgical lamps.[92-94]

Following are the ways to minimze the problems:

- The prevention of external light from reaching the photo-detector (Criticare, SARA) is achieved by good probe
- The covering of oximeter probe with opaque drape can rectify this problem.

Nellcor which lack both wave form and diagnostic message display gives high and low reading during such interference without indication of its presence.[95]

Those who handle neonates exposed to phototherapy, must be cautious of this potential limitation. It is important to minimize the amount of ambient light falling on the detector. Either move away the strong sources of room light or cover the pulse oximeter probe and finger with non-transparent material like cloth.[6,80,94,96]

Abnormal Hemoglobin Molecules

Carboxyhemoglobin

Carboxyhemoglobin (COHb) levels in nonsmokers are less than 2%, while they may be as high as 10–20% in heavy smokers. COHb absorbs very little light at 940 nm, while at 660 nm its extinction coefficient is very similar to oxyhemoglobin. Thus, the presence of significant COHb will resemble the curve of oxyhemoglobin in the red range, with no effect on the infrared, and "look like" oxyhemoglobin, causing the pulse oximeter to over read. For every 1% of circulating carboxyhemoglobin, the pulse oximeter over reads by 1%.[97-99] SpO_2 values should be verified by SaO_2 measurements using a co-oximetry method when the presence of COHb is suspected (e.g., carbon monoxide intoxication).[6,100-102]

Methemoglobin

There is absorption of equal amounts of red and near infrared light, when the normal ferrous (Fe^{+2}) state of the iron moiety in hemoglobin is oxidized to the ferric state (Fe^{+3}) the Methemoglobin (MetHb) occurs. The ratio of pulsatile and nonpulsatile absorbances in the two wavelengths is equal to 1 at a hemoglobin oxygen saturation of 85%. A high concentration of MetHb causes the saturation to approximate 85%. In hypoxic (saturation 40–50%) state, the MetHb artifactually increases the pulse oximeter reading to 85% and if the oxygen saturation is 100%, the MetHb spuriously decreases the pulse oximeter reading to 85%.[103] A multiwavelength co-oximeter will show decreasing oxygen saturations at increasing MetHb levels. It is necessary to check an arterial blood sample in a co-oximeter to measure the amount of oxyhemoglobin and methemoglobin if significant methemoglobinemia is suspected.

Fetal Hemoglobin and Hemoglobin S

Fetal hemoglobin and hemoglobin S have light-absorption property similar to that of adult hemoglobin and therefore, do not interfere with pulse oximetry.[104-107] However, abnormal hemoglobin molecules affect ODC and hence tissue oxygenation is low, particularly for children with sickle cell disease.

Venous Pulsation

Prominent venous pulsation, in case of severe tricuspid regurgitation, affect signal-to-noise ratio and result in wrong SpO_2 readings.[108,109]

Intravenous Dyes

Isosulfan blue (patent blue V) does not have significant effect at low dose; prolonged reduction in SpO_2 occurs at high dose. Methylene blue, and to a lesser extent indocyanine green have significant absorption bands at 660 nm. Oximeters interpret increased 660 nm absorption as resulting from decreased oxyhemoglobin. Therefore, low saturation is displayed. This effect is short-lived (5–10 minutes) because of redistribution to the nonpulsatile tissue compartment.[4,80,110-112]

Bilirubin

Bilirubin has no effect on pulse oximetry, because it presents a different spectrum of light absorption (at approximately 450 nm). It can be used for monitoring jaundiced patients, including neonates.[4,5,6,16,17,80,86,113]

Anemia

Anemia does not affect the accuracy of pulse oximetry.[80,114,115] However, in patients with sickle cell anemia presenting with acute vaso-occlusive crisis, mean bias of pulse oximetry was 4.5% (in some patients it was as high as 8%), which was significantly greater than in a control group of patients without sickle cell anemia.[116] Polycythemia does not affect pulse oximetry.[106]

Pressure on the Sensor

For accurate SpO_2 pressure there should be no pressure on the sensor to avoid in inaccurate SpO_2 readings without affecting pulse rate.

Hyperemia

The flow of capillary and venous blood becomes pulsatile in hyperemic limb. The absorption of light from these sources will be included in the saturation computations with resulting decrease in accuracy of the oxygen saturation measured by pulse oximetry.

A transient decrease in oxygen saturation is seen with rapid blood transfusion if pulse oximeter is placed closed to site of blood transfusion.[82]

Failure to Detect Absence of Circulation

The adequacy of tissue perfusion may not be indicated by normal oximeter signal or reading and at times pulse can be seen with inadequate tissue perfusion or absent pulse, as ambient light may produce a false signal.

Discrepancies between Readings from Different Monitors

In same patient at a same time reading discrepancies are seen in different brands of oximeters[117] and reason could be differences in methods of calibration and the variation in the time taken for detecting desaturation.

Failure to Detect Hypoventilation

In the patients receiving higher fractional concentration of oxygen hypoventilation and hypercarbia may occur without a decrease in hemoglobin oxygen saturation. For adequacy of ventilation or detect disconnections or esophageal intubation the pulse oximetry cannot be relied upon as it detects only the effects of such a mishap, namely hypoxia, and precious time is lost.[82]

Lack of User Knowledge

Many users have a limited understanding of how it functions and the implications of its measurements. Some clinicians also have a limited knowledge of the O_2 dissociation curve, and they do not recognize that SpO_2 values in the high 80s represent seriously low values of PaO_2.

Complications like corneal abrasions, pressure and ischemic injuries and burns have been reported with the use of pulse oximeter.

RECENT ADVANCES IN PULSE OXIMETRY

Error Correction

Two most common errors with pulse oximetry are motion artifacts and signal loss secondary to hypoperfusion. Recently quite a few manufacturers have incorporated new technologies of signal analysis reducing these inaccuracies. Several studies demonstrate that recent versions are better in detecting hypoxemia during motion and poor perfusion.[118,119] Accuracy in 92% of cases is shown in one study.[120]

Multiwavelength Pulse Oximeters

Eight-wavelength pulse oximeter capable of measuring several species of Hb has been developed. The Massimo Rad-57 (Massimo Corp, Irvine, CA) gained Food and Drug Administration (FDA) clearance in 2006. It claims capability to accurately measure MetHb and COHb. However, two large studies compared results from the unit with conventional co-oximetry in emergency department patients showing equivocal results, with one reporting a significant number of false-positive readings.[121,122] One smaller study in healthy volunteers reported good agreement between oximeter and laboratory measurements.[123] Still studies are ongoing to determine accuracy of the device.

Reflectance Pulse Oximetry

Reflectance oximetry has been used to monitor fetal oxygen saturation with scalp probes and has shown to decrease surgical intervention in the face of nonreassuring fetal status.[58] Esophageal probes have been designed and have shown success in measuring SpO_2 during cardiothoracic surgery when finger probes have failed.[124] The investigators reported minimal bias and narrow limits of agreement when compared with finger probes used in the study. Monitoring of gastric SpO_2 as an indicator of splanchnic perfusion has also shown promise.[125]

CONCLUSION

Pulse oximeter is a most vital monitor for early detection of hypoxia in perioperative settings. Lack of detection of hypoventilation and hyperoxia are two important limitations. Recent advances in technology have overcome errors due to motion artefacts and hypoperfusion. Novel uses are being developed.

REFERENCES

1. Neff TA. Routine oximetry. A fifth vital sign? Chest. 1988;94:227.
2. Pulse oximeter. [online] Available from www.howeqipments-works.com. [Last accessed May, 2014].
3. Alexander CM, Teller LE, and Gross JB. Principles of Pulse Oximetry: Theoretical and Practical Considerations. Anesth Analg. 1989;68:368-76.
4. Sinex JE. Pulse oximetry: principles and limitations. Am J Emerg Med. 1999;17(1):59-67.
5. Jubran A. Pulse oximetry. Intensive Care Med. 2004;30(11): 2017-20.
6. Callahan JM. Pulse oximetry in emergency medicine. Emerg Med Clin North Am. 2008;26(4):869-79.
7. Aoyagi T. Pulse oximetry: its invention, theory, and future. J Anesth. 2003;17(4):259-66.
8. Zonios G, Shankar U, Iyer VK. Pulse oximetry theory and calibration for low saturations. IEEE Trans Biomed Eng. 2004; 51(5):818-22.
9. Hanning CD, Alexander-Williams JM. Pulse oximetry: a practical review. BMJ. 1995;311(7001):367-70.
10. Hess DR, Branson RD. Noninvasive respiratory monitoring equipment. In: Branson RD, Hess DR, Chatburn RL (Eds). Respiratory Care Equipment Philadelphia, PA: J. P. Lippincott; 1995. p. 193.
11. Dassel ACM, Graaff R, Sikkema M, et al. Reflectance pulse oximetry at the forehead improves by pressure on the probe. J Clin Monit. 1995;11:237-44.
12. Bebout DE, Mannheimer PD, Wun CC. Site-dependent differences in the time to detect changes in saturation during low perfusion [abstract]. Crit Care Med. 2001;29:A115.
13. Nijland R, Jongsma HW, van den Berg PP, et al. The effects of pulsating arteries on reflectance pulse oximetry: Measurements in adults and neonates. J Clin Monit. 1995;11:118-22.
14. Ralston AC, Webb RK, Runciman WB. Potential errors in pulse oximetry. I. Pulse oximeter evaluation. Anaesthesia. 1991;46: 202-6.
15. Jubran A, Tobin MJ. Monitoring during mechanical ventilation. Clin Chest Med. 1996;17:453-73.
16. Salyer JW. Neonatal and pediatric pulse oximetry. Respir Care. 2003;48(4):386-96.
17. Marr J, Abramo TJ. Monitoring in critically ill children. In: Baren JM, Rothrock SG, Brennan JA, Brown L (Eds). Pediatric Emergency Medicine Philadelphia, PA: Saunders Elsevier; 2008. pp. 50-52.
18. Bell C, Luther MA, Nicholson JJ, et al. Effect of probe design on accuracy and reliability of pulse oximetry in pediatric patients. J Clin Anesth. 1999;11(4):323-7.
19. Sedaghat-Yazdi F, Torres A, Fortuna R, et al. Pulse oximeter accuracy and precision affected by sensor location in cyanotic children. Pediatr Crit Care Med. 2008;9(4):393-7.
20. Severing Haus JW, Naifeh KH. Accuracy of response of six pulse oximeters to profound hypoxia. Anesthesiology. 1987;67:551-8.
21. Young D, Jewkes C, Spittal M, et al. Response time of pulse oximeters assessed using acute decompression. Anesth Analg. 1992;74:189-95.
22. Branson R, Davis B, Davis K, et al. Comparison of forehead and finger oximetry in mechanically ventilated patients with poor perfusion. Respir Care. 2003;48:1086.
23. Schallom L, Sona C, McSweeney M, et al. Comparison of reflective and transmission oximetry in surgical/trauma patients with poor perfusion. Crit Care Med. 2005;32:S138.
24. MacLeod DB, Cortinez LI, Keifer JC, et al. The desaturation response time of finger pulse oximeters during mild hypothermia. Anaesthesia. 2005;60:65-71.
25. Cullen DJ, Nemeskal AR, Cooper JB, et al. Effect of pulse oximetry, age, ASA physical status on the frequency of patients admitted unexpectedly to a postoperative intensive care unit and the severity of their anesthesia-related complications. Anesth Analg. 1992;74:181-4.
26. Moller JT, Johannessen NW, Espersen K, et al. Randomized evaluation of pulse oximetry in 20,802 patients: II. Perioperative events and postoperative complications. Anesthesiology. 1993;78:445-53.
27. Wheatley RG, Shepherd D, Jackson IJ, et al. Hypoxaemia and pain relief after upper abdominal surgery: Comparison of im and patient-controlled analgesia. Br J Anaesth. 1992;69:558-61.
28. Rosenberg J, Oturai P, Erichsen CJ, et al. Effect of general anesthesia and major versus minor surgery on late postoperative episodic and constant hypoxemia. J Clin Anesth. 1994;6:212-6.
29. Gill NP, Wright B, Reilly CS. Relationship between hypoxaemic and cardiac ischaemic events in the perioperative period. Br J Anaesth. 1992;68:471-3.
30. Bierman MI, Stein KL, Snyder JV. Pulse oximetry in the postoperative care of cardiac surgical patients: A randomized controlled trial. Chest. 1992;102:1367-70.
31. Jubran A, Tobin MJ. Reliability of pulse oximetry in titrating supplemental oxygen therapy in ventilator dependent patients. Chest. 1990;97:1420-5.
32. Mower WR, Sachs C, Nicklin EL, et al. A comparison of pulse oximetry and respiratory rate in patient screening. Respir Med. 1996;90:593-9.
33. Bourdelles Le G, Estagnasie P, Lenoir F, et al. Use of a pulse oximeter in an adult emergency department: impact on the number of arterial blood gas analyses ordered. Chest. 1998; 113:1042-7.
34. Kattwinkel J, Perlman JM, Aziz K, et al. American Heart Association. Neonatal resuscitation: 2010 American Heart Association Guidelines for cardiopulmonary resuscitation and emergency cardiovascular care. Pediatrics. 2010;126(5). [online] Available from www.pediatrics.org/cgi/content/full/126/5/e1400. [Last accessed April, 2021].
35. Kamlin CO, O'Donnell CP, Davis PG, et al. Oxygen saturation in healthy infants immediately after birth. J Pediatr. 2006; 148(5):585-9.

36. Rabi Y, Yee W, Chen SY, et al. Oxygen saturation trends immediately after birth. J Pediatr. 2006;148(5):590-4.
37. Altuncu E, Ozek E, Bilgen H, et al. Percentiles of oxygen saturation in healthy term newborns in the first minutes of life. Eur J Pediatr. 2008;167(6):687-8.
38. Mariani G, Dik PB, Ezquer A, et al. Preductal and post-ductal O_2 saturation in healthy term neonates after birth. J Pediatr. 2007;150(4):418-21.
39. Hoffman JIE. It is time for routine neonatal screening by pulse oximetry. Neonatology. 2011;99(1):1-9.
40. Mahle WT, Newburger JW, Matherne GP, et al. American Heart Association, Congenital Heart Defects Committee of the Council on Cardiovascular Disease in the Young, Council on Cardiovascular Nursing, and Interdisciplinary Council on Quality of Care and Outcomes Research; American Academy of Pediatrics, Section on Cardiology and Cardiac Surgery, Committee on Fetus and Newborn. Role of pulse oximetry in examining newborns for congenital heart disease: a scientific statement from the AHA and AAP. Pediatrics. 2009;124(2):823-36.
41. Castillo A, Sola A, Baquero H, et al. Pulse oxygen saturation levels and arterial oxygen tension values in newborns receiving oxygen therapy in the neonatal intensive care unit: is 85% to 93% an acceptable range? Pediatrics. 2008;121(5):882-9.
42. Castillo A, Deulofeut R, Critz A, et al. Prevention of retinopathy of prematurity in preterm infants through changes in clinical practice and SpO_2 technology. Acta Pediatr. 2011;100(2): 188-92.
43. Deulofeut R, Critz A, Adams-Chapman I, et al. Avoiding hyperoxia in infants <1250 g is associated with improved short- and long-term outcomes. J Paerinatol. 2006;26(11):700-5.
44. Tokuhiro Y, Yoshida T, Nakabayashi Y, et al. Reduced oxygen protocol decreases the incidence of threshold retinopathy of prematurity in infants of <33 weeks gestation. Pediatr Int. 2009;51(6):804-6.
45. Askie LM, Henderson-Smart DJ, Ko H. Restricted versus liberal oxygen exposure for preventing morbidity and mortality in preterm or low birth weight infants. Cochrane Database Syst Rev. 2009;(1):CD001077.
46. Shamir M, Eidelman LA, Floman Y, et al. Pulse oximetry plethysmographic waveform during changes in blood volume. Br J Anaesth. 1999;82:178-81.
47. Monnet X, Lamia B, Teboul JL. Pulse oximeter as a sensor of fluid responsiveness: Do we have our finger on the best solution? Crit Care. 2005;9:429-30.
48. Michard F, Boussat S, Chemla D, et al. Relation between respiratory changes in arterial pulse pressure and fluid responsiveness in septic patients with acute circulatory failure. Am J Respir Crit Care Med. 2000;162:134-8.
49. Cannesson M, Besnard C, Durand PG, et al. Relation between respiratory variations in pulse oximetry plethysmographic waveform amplitude and arterial pulse pressure in ventilated patients. Crit Care. 2005;9: R562-8.
50. Cannesson M, Attof Y, Rosamel P, et al. Respiratory variations in pulse oximetry plethysmographic waveform amplitude to predict fluid responsiveness in the operating room. Anesthesiology. 2007;106:1105-11.
51. Feissel M, Teboul JL, Merlani P, et al. Plethysmographic dynamic indices predict fluid responsiveness in septic ventilated patients. Intensive Care Med. 2007;33:993-9.
52. Shelley KH, Jablonka DH, Awad AA, et al. What is the best site for measuring the effect of ventilation on the pulse oximeter waveform? Anesth Analg. 2006;103:372-7.
53. Cannesson M, Desebbe O, Rosamel P, et al. Pleth variability index to monitor the respiratory variations in the pulse oximeter plethysmographic waveform amplitude and predict fluid responsiveness in the operating theatre. Br J Anaesth. 2008;101(2):200-6.
54. Mowafi HA. The efficacy of plethysmographic pulse wave amplitude as an indicator for intravascular injection of epinephrine-containing epidural test dose in anesthetized adults. Anesth Analg. 2005;101:1506-11.
55. Uemura A, Yagihara M, Miyabe M. Pulse oximeter perfusion index as a predictor for the effect of pediatric epidural block. Anesthesiology. 2006;105: A1354.
56. Hager H, Church S, Mandadi G, et al. The perfusion index measured by a pulse oximeter indicates pain stimuli in anesthetized volunteers. Anesthesiology. 2004;101: A514.
57. Bendjelid K. The pulse oximetry plethysmographic curve revisited. Curr Opin Crit Care. 2008;14(3):348-53.
58. East CE, Brennecke SP, King JF, et al. The effect of intrapartum fetal pulse oximetry, in the presence of a non-reassuring fetal heart rate pattern, on operative delivery rates: A multicenter, randomized, controlled trial (the FOREMOST trial). Am J Obstet Gynecol. 2006;194:606.
59. Jubran A. Pulse oximetry. In: Tobin MJ (Ed). Principles and Practice of Intensive Care Monitoring. New York: McGraw Hill, Inc.; 1998. pp. 261-87.
60. Nickerson BG, Sarkisian C, Tremper KK. Bias and precision of pulse oximeters and arterial oximeters. Chest. 1988;93:515-7.
61. Morris RW, Nairn M, Torda TA. A comparison of fifteen pulse oximeters. Part I: a clinical comparison; Part II: a test of performance under conditions of poor perfusion. Anaesth Intensive Care. 1989;17:62-82.
62. Hannhart B, Haberer JP, Saunier C, et al. Accuracy and precision of fourteen pulse oximeters. Eur Respir J. 1991;4:115-9.
63. Severinghaus JW, Nafen KH, Koh SO. Errors in 14 pulse oximeters during profound hypoxemia. J Clin Monit. 1989;5:72-81.
64. Fouzas S, Priftis KN, Anthracopoulos MB. Pulse Oximetry in Pediatric Practice. Pediatrics. 2011;128:740.
65. Trivedi NS, Ghouri AF, Shah NK, et al. Effects of motion, ambient light, and hypoperfusion on pulse oximeter function. J Clin Anesth. 1997;3:179-83.
66. Reich DL, Timcenko A, Bodian CA, et al. Predictors of pulse oximetry data failure. Anesthesiology. 1996;84:859-64.
67. Runciman WB, Webb RK, Barker L, et al. The pulse oximeter: applications and limitations: an analysis of 2000 incident reports. Anaesth Intens Care. 1993;21:543-50.
68. Pollard V, Prough DS. Signal extraction technology: A better mousetrap? [Editorial]. Anesth Analg. 1996;83:213-4.
69. Barker SJ, Shah NK. Effects of motion on the performance of pulse oximeters in volunteers. Anesthesiology. 1997;86:101-8.
70. Severinghaus JW, Spellman MJ. Pulse oximeter failure thresholds in hypotension and vasoconstriction. Anesthesiology. 1990;73: 532-7.
71. Pologe JA. Pulse oximetry: Technical aspects of machine design. Int Anesthesiol Clinics. 1987;25:137-53.
72. Bourke DL, Grayson RF. Digital nerve blocks can restore pulse oximeter signal detection. Anesthesia and Analgesia. 1991;73: 815-7.
73. Feiner JR, Severinghaus JW, Bickler PE. Dark skin decreases the accuracy of pulse oximeters at low oxygen saturation: the effects of oximeter probe type and gender. Anesth Analg. 2007;105(6):S18-23.
74. Bickler PE, Feiner JR, Severinghaus JW. Effects of skin pigmentation on pulse oximeter accuracy at low saturation. Anesthesiology. 2005;102(4):715-9.
75. Coté CJ, Goldstein EA, Fuchsman WH, et al. The effect of nail polish on pulse oximetry. Anesth Analg. 1988;67(7):683-6.
76. Yamamoto LG, Yamamoto JA, Yamamoto JB, et al. Nail polish does not significantly affect pulse oximetry measurements in mildly hypoxic subjects. Respir Care. 2008;53(11):1470-4.
77. Hinkelbein J, Genzwuerker HV. Fingernail polish does not influence pulse oximetry to a clinically relevant dimension. Intensive Crit Care Nurs. 2008;24(1):4-5.

78. Brand TM, Brand ME, Jay GD. Enamel nail polish does not interfere with pulse oximetry among normoxic volunteers. J Clin Monit Comput. 2002;17(2):93-6.
79. Hinkelbein J, Koehler H, Genzwuerker HV, et al. Artificial acrylic finger nails may alter pulse oximetry measurement. Resuscitation. 2007;74(1):75-82.
80. Mechem CC. Pulse oximetry. [online] Available from www.uptodateonline.com/online/content/topic.do?topicKey_cc_medi/16589. [Last accessed January, 2011].
81. Edelist G. Acrylic nails and pulse oximetry [letter]. Anesth Analg. 1995;81:882-91.
82. Kamat V. Pulse Oximetry. Indian J Anaesth. 2002;46(4):261-8.
83. Rajkumar A, Karmarkar A, Knott J. Pulse oximetry: an overview. J Perioper Pract. 2006;16(10):502-4.
84. Dempsey MF, Condon B. Thermal injuries associated with MRI. Clin Radiol. 2001;56(6):457-65.
85. Severinghaus JW, Kelleher JF. Recent developments in pulse oximetry. Anesthesiology. 1992;76(6):1018-38.
86. Poets CF, Southall DP. Noninvasive monitoring of oxygenation in infants and children: practical considerations and areas of concern. Pediatrics. 1994;93(5):737-46.
87. Fanconi S. Reliability of pulse oximetry in hypoxic infants. J Pediatr. 1988;112(3):424-7.
88. Pinnamaneni R, Kieran EA, O'Donnell CPF. Speed of data display by pulse oximeters in newborns: A randomized crossover study. Arch Dis Child fetal Neonatal Ed. 2010;95(5):F384-5.
89. Stoneham MD. Uses and limitations of pulse oximetry. Br J Hosp Med. 1995;54(1):35-41.
90. Kelleher JF, Ruff RH. The penumbra effect: vasomotion-dependent pulse oximeter artifact due to probe malposition. Anesthesiology. 1989;71(5):787-91.
91. Guan Z, Baker K, Sandberg WS. Misalignment of disposable pulse oximeter probes results in false saturation readings that influence anesthetic management. Anesth Anal. 2009;109(5):1530-3.
92. Brooks TD, Paulus DA, Winkle WE. Infrared heat lamps interfere with pulse oximeters. Anesthesiology. 1984;61:630.
93. Amar D, Neidzwski J, Wald A, et al. Fluorescent light interferes with pulse oximetry. J Clin Monit. 1989;5:135-6.
94. Mannheimer PD. The light-tissue interaction of pulse oximetry. Anesth Analg. 2007;105(6): S10-7.
95. Norley I. Erroneous actuation of the pulse oximeter. Anaesthesia. 1987;42:11-6.
96. Fluck RR Jr, Schroeder C, Frani G, et al. Does ambient light affect the accuracy of pulse oximetry? Respir Care. 2003;48(7):677-80.
97. Barker SJ, Tremper KK. The effects of carbon monoxide inhalation on pulse oximetry and transcutaneous PO_2. Anesthesiology. 1987;66:677-9.
98. Hampson NB. Pulse oximetry in severe carbon monoxide poisoning. Chest. 1998;114(4):1036-41.
99. Barker SJ, Curry J, Redford D, et al. Measurement of carboxyhemoglobin and methemoglobin by pulse oximetry: a human volunteer study. Anesthesiology. 2006;105(5):892-7.
100. Verhovsek M, Henderson MP, Cox G, et al. Unexpectedly low pulse oximetry measurements associated with variant hemoglobins: a systematic review. Am J Hematol. 2010;85(11):882-5.
101. Lee WW, Mayberry K, Crapo R, et al. The accuracy of pulse oximetry in the emergency department. Am J Emerg Med. 2000;18(4):427-31.
102. Akhtar J, Johnston BD, Krenzelok. Mind the gap. J Emerg Med. 2007;33(2):131-2.
103. Eisenkraft JB. Pulse oximeter desaturation due to methemoglobulin. Anesthesiology. 1988;68:279-85.
104. Zijlstra WG, Buursma A, Meeuwsen-van der Roest WP. Absorption spectra of human fetal and adult oxyhemoglobin, deoxyhemoglobin, carboxyhemoglobin and methemoglobin. Clin Chem. 1991;37(9):1633-8.
105. Harris AP, Sendak MJ, Donham RT, et al. Absorption characteristics of human fetal hemoglobin at wavelengths used in pulse oximetry. J Clin Monit. 1988;4(3):175-7.
106. Dawson JA, Davis PG, O'Donnell CP, et al. Pulse oximetry for monitoring infants in the delivery room: a review. Arch Dis Child Fetal Neonatal Ed. 2007;92(1):F4-7.
107. Ortiz FO, Aldrich TK, Nagel RL, et al. Accuracy of pulse oximetry in sickle cell disease. Am J Resp Crit Care Med. 1999;159(2):447-51.
108. Bucher HU, Keel M, Wolf M, et al. Artifactual pulse oximetry estimation in neonates. Lancet. 1994;343(8906):1135-6.
109. Stewart KG, Rowbottom SJ. Inaccuracy of pulse oximetry in patients with severe tricuspid regurgitation. Anaesthesia. 1991;46(8):668-70.
110. Unger R, Scheller MS. More on dyes and pulse oximeters. Anesthesiology. 1987;67:148-9.
111. Saito S, Fukura H, Shimada H, et al. Prolonged interference of blue dye "patent blue" with pulse oximetry readings. Acta Anesthesiol Scand. 1995;39(2):268-9.
112. Momeni R, Ariyan S. Pulse oximetry declines due to intradermal isosulfan blue dye: a controlled prospective study. Ann Surg Oncol. 2004;11(4):434-7.
113. Poets CF, Southall DP. Noninvasive monitoring of oxygenation in infants and children: practical considerations and areas of concern. Pediatrics. 1994;93(5):737-46.
114. Jay GD, Hughes L, Renzi FP. Pulse oximetry is accurate in acute anemia from hemorrhage. Ann Emerg Med. 1994;24(1):32-5.
115. McEwen MP, Bull GP, Reynolds KJ. Vessel caliber and hemoglobin effects on pulse oximetry. Physiol Meas. 2009;30(9):869-83.
116. Comber JT, Lopez BL. Evaluation of pulse oximetry in sickle cell anemia patients presenting to the emergency department in acute vaso-occlusive crisis. Am J Emerg Med. 1996;14:16-8.
117. Wutemberger G, Muller S, Matthys H, et al. Accuracy of nine commercially available pulse oximeters in monitoring patients with chronic respiratory insufficiency. Monaldi Arch Chest Diseases. 1994;49:348.
118. Bohnhorst B, Poets CF. Major reduction in alarm frequency with a new pulse oximeter. Intensive Care Med. 1998;24:277-8.
119. Irita K, Kai Y, Akiyoshi K, et al. Performance evaluation of a new pulse oximeter during mild hypothermic cardiopulmonary bypass. Anesth Analg. 2003;96:11-4.
120. Durban CG, Rostow SK. Advantages of new technology pulse oximetry with adults in extremis. Anesth Analg. 2002;94: S81-3.
121. O'Malley GF. Non-invasive carbon monoxide measurement is not accurate. Ann Emerg Med. 2006;48:477-8.
122. Suner S, Partridge R, Sucov A, et al. Non-invasive screening for carbon monoxide toxicity in the emergency department is valuable. Ann Emerg Med. 2007;49:718-9.
123. Barker SJ, Curry J, Redford D, et al. Measurement of carboxyhemoglobin and methemoglobin by pulse oximetry: A human volunteer study. Anesthesiology. 2007;107:892-7.
124. Kyriacou PA, Powell SL, Jones DP, et al. Evaluation of oesophageal pulse oximetry in patients undergoing cardiothoracic surgery. Anaesthesia. 2003;58:422-7.
125. Fournell A, Schwarte LA, Scheeren TW, et al. Assessment of microvascular oxygen saturation in gastric mucosa in volunteers breathing continuous positive airway pressure. Crit Care Med. 2003;31:1705-10.

Noninvasive and Invasive Blood Pressure Monitoring

Nandini M Dave, Amit Padvi

ABSTRACT

The blood pressure is a fundamental cardiovascular vital sign and a critical part of monitoring anesthetized or ill patients. Indirect cuff devices and direct arterial cannulation with pressure transduction are the two techniques of measuring blood pressure.

Most automated noninvasive blood pressure measuring devices use an oscillometric measurement technique and rarely cause complications. Direct arterial pressure monitoring is used in operative patients with severe cardiovascular diseases or those undergoing major surgical procedures that involve significant blood loss or fluid shifts. The accuracy of a directly recorded arterial pressure waveform is determined by the natural frequency and damping coefficient of the pressure monitoring system.

INTRODUCTION

The blood pressure (BP) measurement is a fundamental aspect of monitoring the cardiovascular system during conduct of anesthesia and in intensive care. The monitoring standards mandate that the BP should be recorded at least every 5 minutes during anesthesia.[1]

NONINVASIVE BLOOD PRESSURE MEASUREMENT

Manual Intermittent Technique

The first description was the Riva-Rocci method (1896), which determined the systolic blood pressure (SBP) using an inflatable cuff and mercury manometer. The pressure at which the arterial pulse disappeared on palpation during cuff inflation was the systolic pressure. A variation of the Riva-Rocci method called the return-to-flow technique, measures the pressure during cuff deflation at which the pulse reappears.

The most widely used manual method is the auscultatory technique described by Korotkoff (1905). Using a sphygmomanometer, cuff and stethoscope, systolic and diastolic blood pressure (DBP) is measured by auscultation. The SBP is considered equivalent to the appearance of the first Korotkoff sound, and disappearance of the sounds or a muffled tone is considered equivalent to the DBP. This method is simple, uses low-level technology, and has a long history of use.

The auscultatory method has limitations. It does not correlate well with invasive blood pressure (IBP) measurement under all circumstances. The erroneous readings are obtained in decreased peripheral blood flow states, e.g., shock or with use of inappropriate cuff size and rapid deflation. The method overestimates at low pressure and underestimates at high pressure, and has large interobserver variation. Also, frequent and regular readings may be difficult to perform.

These limitations have been overcome by use of automated monitors. The initial automated devices were standalone monitors. Nowadays, multiparameter monitors are integrated with anesthesia workstations.

Automated Intermittent Technique

Basic Operating Principle

Most devices are based on oscillometry, a technique first described by Marey in 1876.[2] Arterial pulsations (oscillations) during cuff deflation are sensed by the monitor. The peak amplitude of arterial pulsations corresponds to mean arterial pressure (MAP). Systolic and diastolic pressure values are derived from increasing and decreasing magnitude of oscillations based on proprietary algorithms which vary from manufacturer to manufacturer.[3] Different devices, therefore, do not always yield the same pressures.[4] A variety of cuff sizes makes it possible to use oscillometry in patients of all ages.

Factors Affecting Blood Pressure Measurements

Cuff Size

The optimal cuff should have a bladder length that is 80% and a width at least 40% of arm circumference.[5] An inappropriately large cuff will underestimate BP, and a small cuff will overestimate BP.

Site

The forearm and wrist or the ankles are alternate sites when the upper arm is not accessible or the cuff does not fit. The systolic pressure increases and the diastolic decreases as the measurement site moves peripherally. The cuff should ideally be at the level of the heart, 7.5 mm Hg should be added or subtracted for cuff positioned 10 cm above or below the level of the heart.[6]

Cardiac Rhythm

Oscillometry can be erroneous in patients with dysrhythmias.[7]

Standards

The international standard limits the maximum cuff pressure obtainable during normal use to 300 mm Hg for equipment specified for adults and 150 mm Hg for equipment specified for neonates.[8] In addition, means must be present to prevent the cuff from remaining inflated for long periods of time.

Studies comparing pressures obtained with noninvasive blood pressure (NIBP) monitors with those obtained directly show that the correlation is best in normal healthy patients and least accurate at the extremes of BP.[9,10] Oscillometric devices tend to overestimate low pressures and underestimate high pressures.

Tips for Correct Use

- Noninvasive blood pressure cuff should preferably not be placed on the same limb as the intravenous (IV) infusion. This may stop or slow the infusion or cause back flow of blood into the infusion tubing
- The cuff should not be applied over a bony prominence, superficial nerve or joint
- Padding should be placed under the cuff to prevent skin bruising and nerve damage in susceptible patients
- Too tight application can cause discomfort and venous congestion. Too loose an application will lead to erroneous reading or the monitor will be unable to make a measurement
- The frequency of measurement should be only as clinically necessary. Very frequent measurements can increase complications while not necessarily adding to clinically relevant information[11]
- During prolonged application, periodic inspection and change of cuff site to another location is recommended.

Complications

Generally, automated BP measurement techniques are noninvasive and safe; however, complications have been reported.[12] These events occur more frequently after prolonged periods of excessively frequent cycles of cuff inflation or deflation and are due to trauma or impaired distal limb perfusion.

- *Damage to underlying structures:* Skin bruising, pain, erythema, petechiae, ecchymoses, limb edema, peripheral neuropathies
- Compartment syndrome
- *Erroneous readings and artifacts:* This can be due to cuff malposition, incorrect size, leaking cuff, hose, or connector. Motion artifacts can occur due to intrinsic factors, e.g., patient movement, shivering, convulsions and extrinsic factors, e.g., external pressure on the cuff.

Advantages

- Simple to use, inexpensive
- Few complications compared to direct arterial pressure measurements
- Compared to manual method
  - Regular and reliable measurements of BP possible
  - Eliminates error due to extraneous noise, personal bias
  - Standardizes BP readings from one operator to the next
  - Frees the clinician to do other tasks
  - Provides audible alarms, can transfer data to computer.

Limitations

- Rapid BP changes cannot be monitored
- Noninvasive blood pressure monitors function poorly at extremes of heart rate and BP
- Prolonged cycle times, e.g., hypertensive patients, poor peripheral circulation, leaking cuff or hose, artifacts, causes patient discomfort.

Continuous Noninvasive Blood Pressure Measurements

Continuous noninvasive blood pressure measurement using the Peñáz principle which states "a force exerted by a body can be determined by measuring an opposing force that prevents physical disruption" is an attractive option to direct arterial pressure measurement. Tonometric devices are clamped above the radial artery and measure the pressure transmitted to them through the overlying tissue. Volume clamp devices rely on the use of finger cuffs, photoplethysmographic signals from the fingers, and a rapid feedback loop that attempts to keep the photoplethysmographic signals flat by altering the pressure in the finger cuff.[13]

While reasonably accurate in vasodilated patients and those with normal circulation, these devices are less accurate in hypotensive patients, obese subjects, or those with vascular insufficiency. Small changes in positioning and tightness of the finger cuff can lead to variable readings. Both these technologies are relatively new, and their accuracy in comparison with oscillometry is not well described and they have not been widely incorporated into standard clinical practice.

The T-Line Tensymeter,[14] and Tensys TL-200[15] are devices that provide a calibrated arterial pressure waveform from which continuous BP measurements and heart rate are computed. These devices may enable physicians to circumvent arterial cannulation in certain circumstances (such as with low- or intermediate-risk procedures) on patients when beat-to-beat BP measurement is desirable.

INVASIVE BLOOD PRESSURE OR DIRECT ARTERIAL PRESSURE MEASUREMENT

The intra-arterial or direct BP provides a continuous display of the arterial waveform along with measurements of MAP, systolic and diastolic pressure. Arterial cannulation with continuous pressure transduction and waveform display remains the accepted standard for BP monitoring.[12,16]

Indications[17]

- Continuous real-time BP monitoring
- Arterial blood sampling
- Intentional pharmacological or mechanical cardiovascular manipulation, e.g., cardiopulmonary bypass, infusion of vasoactive drugs
- Failure of indirect BP measurement, e.g., burns, obese patient
- For additional information from the arterial waveform.

Components of Invasive Blood Pressure Monitoring[17,18]

- The measuring apparatus
- The transducer
- The monitor.

Measuring Apparatus

This consists of an arterial cannula connected to tubing containing a continuous column of saline which conducts the pressure wave to the transducer. The arterial line is also connected to a flushing system consisting of saline. The flush system provides continual flushing of the system at a slow rate of approximately 1–3 mL/h. A rapid flush can be delivered by manually opening the flush valve.

Transducer

The transducer consists of a flexible diaphragm with an electric current applied across it.

As pressure is applied to the diaphragm, it stretches and its resistance changes, altering the electrical output from the system.

Transducer setup: Before initiating patient monitoring, the pressure transducer must be zeroed, calibrated, and leveled to the appropriate position on the patient. The initial step in this process is to expose the transducer to atmospheric pressure by opening the adjacent stopcock to air, pressing the zero-pressure button on the monitor, and thereby establishing the zero-pressure reference value. The transducer now has a reference—ambient atmospheric pressure—against which all intravascular pressures are measured.[19] Whenever the level of the pressure transducer is adjusted, there is no need to re-zero the transducer because atmospheric pressure changes little over the few inches of height adjustment. However, calibration is no longer necessary because of accurate disposable transducers.

Leveling implies reference to a specific position on the patient's body. In the supine patient, it is common practice to align pressure transducers at mid chest position in the midaxillary line. However, more accurate readings are obtained when arterial pressure transducers are placed at a level that will best estimate aortic root pressure position; approximately 5 cm posterior to the sternal border.[20]

Common errors in BP measurement occur when pressure transducers are fixed to an IV pole and the height of the patient's bed is adjusted. Raising the height of the bed relative to the transducer will cause overestimation of BP, whereas lowering the patient below the transducer will cause underestimation of BP. Any air bubble in the tubing will cause underdamping of the system, leading to lower SBP and higher DBP.[18]

Monitor

Modern monitors amplify the input signal. They also filter the "noise" from the signal and display the arterial waveform in "real time" on a screen. They also give a digital display of systolic, diastolic and mean BP and most of the monitors incorporate safety features such as high and low BP alarms and tachycardia and bradycardia alerts.

Accuracy of Invasive Blood Pressure Monitoring

The accuracy of intra-arterial monitoring is affected by the oscillation, damping, natural frequency, and resonance of the system.[17]

Oscillation

The tendency of a system to move either side of set point is referred to as its tendency to oscillate.

Damping

How freely a system oscillates following an input of energy depends on the degree of damping in the system. A "well damped" system tends not to oscillate freely whereas a "poorly damped" system may oscillate wildly. The amount of damping inherent in a system is described by the damping coefficient (D) which usually lies between 0 and 1. The oscillations are undesirable in physiological measuring systems as these require accurate measurement of a maximum amplitude (e.g., that caused by the arterial pulsation), with a rapid response time and rapid return to the set point, ready for the next measurement.

A system with a D value close to 1 is overdamped, will not oscillate freely, but will take a long time to initially move away from and to return to its resting point. A system with a D value approaching 0 is underdamped, will oscillate freely and move rapidly away from its resting point and back again, but tends to overshoot and then oscillate around the resting point.

The ideal level of damping applied to a measuring system is a compromise between achieving a rapid response

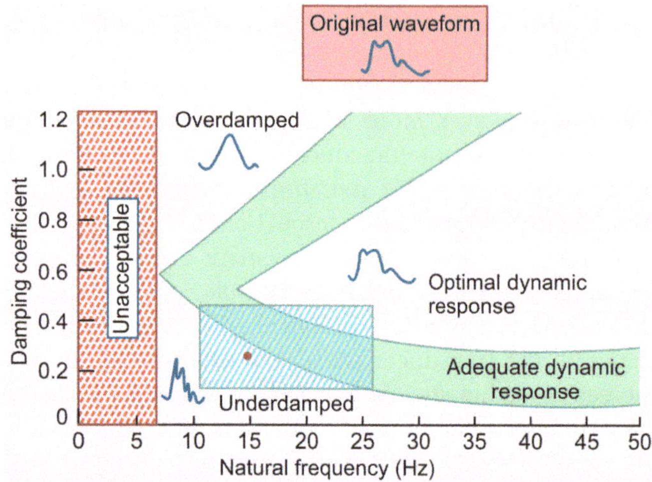

Fig. 1: Interaction between damping coefficient and natural frequency. Overdamped and underdamped systems introduce monitoring artifacts. Systems with a natural frequency less than 7 Hz are considered unacceptable.

Source: Mark JB. Technical requirements for direct blood pressure measurement. In: Mark JB (Ed). Atlas of Cardiovascular Monitoring. New York: Churchill Livingstone; 1998.

time and accurate reflection of maximum amplitude by designing a system with D close to 0, and needing a system that returns to the resting point without excess oscillation (D around 1). The optimal damping value of D for IBP monitoring equipment lies between 0.6 and 0.7.

An overdamped arterial pressure waveform is recognized by its slurred upstroke, absent dicrotic notch, and loss of fine detail. Underdamped pressure waveforms display systolic pressure overshoot and contain additional artifacts produced by the measurement system that are not part of the original intravascular pressure wave **(Fig. 1)**.

Natural Frequency and Resonance[21]

The frequency at which the system "naturally" oscillates is known as the natural frequency. If the input of energy into the system occurs at or close to the same frequency, a phenomenon called resonance occurs and the output amplitude of the oscillations is greatly magnified. This could lead to over-reading of the SBP. Arterial pulsation is a complex sine wave composed of many individual sine waves. It is important that the natural frequency of the measuring equipment does not correspond to any of the component frequencies of the arterial pulsation input. This is achieved by making sure that the natural frequency of the measuring system is raised above any of the component frequencies of the arterial sine waveform.[20]

To ensure that the natural frequency of the system is higher than that of the arterial pulsation:

- Arterial catheter must be short and with the maximum gauge possible
- Column of saline must be short
- The catheter and tubing must be stiff
- The transducer diaphragm must be rigid
- The number of stopcocks and other monitoring system appliances must be kept to a minimum.

DIFFERENCE BETWEEN NONINVASIVE AND INVASIVE BLOOD PRESSURE MEASUREMENT WITH LATERAL DECUBITUS POSITION[18]

When a patient is in the lateral decubitus position, one arm is higher than the heart (and aortic root) and the other arm is lower. If the pressure transducer remains fixed at the level of the heart, the location of the arms has no influence on the measured arterial pressure. However, NIBP measurements will be different in the two arms, higher in the dependent arm and lower in the nondependent arm. However, if the arterial pressure transducers were attached to the arms rather than fixed at the level of the heart, pressures recorded from the right and left radial artery catheters would equal those recorded by the ipsilateral noninvasive cuffs.

SITES FOR ARTERIAL CANNULATION

The radial artery is the most common site for IBP monitoring because it is technically easy to cannulate and complications are uncommon.[22] Arterial catheterization can be performed with a standard IV catheter or an integrated guidewire catheter assembly designed for this purpose. Ultrasound imaging can be used to facilitate catheter insertion.[23]

The alternative cannulation sites are the ulnar, femoral, axillary, brachial and occasionally other peripheral arteries including the dorsalis pedis, posterior tibial, and superficial temporal arteries.[24]

COMPLICATIONS[25]

- Distal ischemia
- Pseudoaneurysm
- Arteriovenous fistula
- Hemorrhage
- Arterial embolization
- Infection
- Peripheral neuropathy.

CONCLUSION

The standards for basic anesthetic monitoring mandate measurement of arterial BP at least every 5 minutes in all anesthetized patients. The techniques for measuring BP include indirect cuff devices and direct arterial cannulation and pressure transduction. These methods differ primarily in their degree of invasiveness. Although IBP is considered the gold standard, this technique can also record erroneous readings. Direct arterial pressure monitoring should be preferred in operative patients with severe cardiovascular diseases or those undergoing major surgical procedures that involve significant blood loss or fluid shifts. The anesthesiologist should be aware of the physics of BP monitoring, common errors and possible complications.

REFERENCES

1. American Society of Anesthesiologists. Standards for basic anesthetic monitoring. [online] Available from http: //www.asahq.org/For-Members/Standards-Guidelines-and-Statements.aspx. [Last accessed November, 2017].
2. Pickering TG, Hall JE, Appel LJ, et al. Recommendations for blood pressure measurement in humans and experimental animals. Part 1: blood pressure measurement in humans: a statement for professionals from the Subcommittee of Professional and Public Education of the American Heart Association Council on High Blood Pressure Research. Hypertension. 2005;45(5):142-61.
3. Yelderman M, Ream AK. Indirect measurement of mean blood pressure in the anesthetized patient. Anesthesiology. 1979;50: 253-6.
4. Kaufmann MA, Pargger H, Drop LJ. Oscillometric blood pressure measurements by different devices are not interchangeable. Anesth Analg. 1996;82:377-81.
5. Pickering TG, Hall JE, Appel LJ, et al. Recommendations for blood pressure measurement in humans and experimental animals: Part 1: blood pressure measurement in humans: a statement for professionals from the Subcommittee of Professional and Public Education of the American Heart Association Council on high blood pressure research. Circulation. 2005;111:697-716.
6. Quill TJ. Blood pressure monitoring. In: Ehrenwerth J, Eisenkraft JB (Eds). Anesthesia Equipment: Principles and Applications. St. Louis: Mosby; 1993. pp. 274-83.
7. Cleland M, Pham B, Miller D. Influence of arrhythmias on accuracy of non-invasive blood pressure monitors. Can J Anaesth. 1998;45:699-705.
8. Dorsch JA, Dorsch SE. Noninvasive blood pressure monitors. In: Dorsch JA, Dorsch SE (Eds). Understanding Anesthesia Equipment, 5th edition. Philadelphia: Lippincott Williams & Wilkins; 2008. pp. 838-44.
9. Loubser PG. Comparing direct and indirect arterial blood pressures. Anesthesiology. 1985;63:566-7.
10. Gourdeau M, Martin R, Lamarche Y, et al. Oscillometry and direct blood pressure: a comparative clinical study during deliberate hypotension. Can Anaesth Soc J. 1986;33:300-7.
11. Kennedy R. The effect of the interval between blood pressure determinations on the delay in the detection of changes—a computer simulation. Anaesth Intens Care. 1999;27:84.
12. Cockings JG, Webb RK, Klepper ID, et al. The Australian Incident Monitoring Study. Blood pressure monitoring—applications and limitations: an analysis of 2000 incident reports. Anaesth Intensive Care. 1993;21:565-9.
13. Roach JK, Thiele RH. Perioperative blood pressure monitoring. Best Pract Res Clin Anaesthesiol. 2019;33:127-38.
14. Janelle GM, Gravenstein N. An accuracy evaluation of the T-Line Tensymeter (continuous noninvasive blood pressure management device) versus conventional invasive radial artery monitoring in surgical patients. Anesth Analg. 2006;102(2):484-90.
15. Dueck R, Goedje O, Clopton P. Noninvasive continuous beat-to-beat radial artery pressure via TL-200 applanation tonometry. J Clin Monit Comput. 2012;26(2):75-83.
16. Gardner RM. Direct arterial pressure monitoring. Curr Anaesth Crit Care. 1990;1(4):239-46.
17. Gupta B. Invasive blood pressure monitoring. [online] Available from http://update.anaesthesiologists.org/wp-content/uploads/2009/09/Invasive-Blood-Pressure-Monitoring.pdf. [Last accessed November, 2017].
18. Schroeder RA, Barbeito A, Bar-Yosef S, et al. Cardiovascular monitoring. In: Miller RD (Ed). Anesthesia, 7th edition. London: Churchill Livingstone Elsevier; 2010. pp. 1267-328.
19. Courtois M, Fattal PG, Kovacs SJ, et al. Anatomically and physiologically based reference level for measurement of intracardiac pressures. Circulation. 1995;92:1994-2000.
20. Mark JB. Technical requirements for direct blood pressure measurement. In: Mark JB (Ed). Atlas of Cardiovascular Monitoring. New York: Churchill Livingstone; 1998. pp. 99-126.
21. Kleinman B. Understanding natural frequency and damping and how they relate to the measurement of blood pressure. J Clin Monit. 1989;5:137-47.
22. Slogoff S, Keats AS, Arlund C. On the safety of radial artery cannulation. Anesthesiology. 1983;59:42-7.
23. Levin PD, Sheinin O, Gozal Y. Use of ultrasound guidance in the insertion of radial artery catheters. Crit Care Med. 2003;31:481-4.
24. Scheer B, Perel A, Pfeiffer UJ. Clinical review: complications and risk factors of peripheral arterial catheters used for haemodynamic monitoring in anaesthesia and intensive care medicine. Crit Care. 2002;6:199-204.
25. Singleton RJ, Webb RK, Ludbrook GL, et al. The Australian Incident Monitoring Study. Problems associated with vascular access: an analysis of 2000 incident reports. Anaesth Intensive Care. 1993;21:664-9.

Capnography

Dinesh K Jagannathan, Bhavani S Kodali

ABSTRACT

The capnography is a valuable tool that helps to monitor carbon dioxide (CO_2) production in the tissues and organs, transportation to lungs via the cardiovascular system, and final elimination of CO_2 by the pulmonary system. It is an indirect monitor unlike pulse oximetry. It serves as an adjuvant in the differential diagnosis of hypoxia in determining the etiology so that corrective measures can be implemented before irreversible brain damage. The value of capnography in the operating room is unquestionable, and therefore many societies around the world have included capnography as a standard of monitoring during anesthesia to enhance patient safety and prevent avoidable morbidity and mortality associated with anesthesia.

In recent years, the value of capnography has been recognized outside of the operating rooms resulting in the change in the standards of monitoring in these locations. Although the value of capnography has been well recognized by anesthesiologists in many developed countries, its value is under recognized by many in developing countries. Blaming the scarcity of resources does not seem to be a factor in many areas, but lack of diligent understanding of the value of capnography may be responsible for underutilization. It is only a question of time when capnography will be accepted universally as the standard of monitoring during anesthesia, sedation, and in intensive care units.

INTRODUCTION

The capnography is the continuous monitoring of instantaneous CO_2 concentration in respired gases during the respiratory cycle. The graphic display of this concentration as a function of time or volume produces a waveform, and it is called capnogram.

The measurement of CO_2 in expired gases directly indicates elimination of CO_2 from the lungs (pulmonary processes). Indirectly, it indicates the production of CO_2 at the tissue level (metabolic processes) and delivery of CO_2 to the lungs (circulatory processes). For patients on mechanical ventilation, be it in operating rooms (ORs) or in intensive care units (ICUs), exhaled CO_2 monitoring ensures the integrity and patency of the airway, helps to guide ventilator settings and enhances patient safety. Capnography has significant clinical applications not just in respiratory monitoring but also in monitoring of cardiac function like assessment of adequacy of cardiopulmonary resuscitation (CPR) and aid in diagnosis of special situations like pulmonary embolism.

The purpose of this chapter is to go over briefly the basic principles involved in CO_2 measurement, history of its development, normal capnogram, interpretation of abnormal capnograms, clinical correlations, current practice standards in place and its future role.

TECHNOLOGY

A number of technologies are available for measurement of CO_2. These include mass spectrometry, Raman spectroscopy, photoacoustic measurement and infrared (IR) spectrometry.[1] IR-based monitors are currently the most economical and popular in clinical use.

The infrared technology is because CO_2, being a polyatomic gas, absorbs light at a specific wavelength (4.3 μm, **Fig. 1**) in the far IR light spectrum and the absorption is proportional to the concentration of CO_2 in the analyzing chamber.[2] The measured CO_2 is displayed as either volume

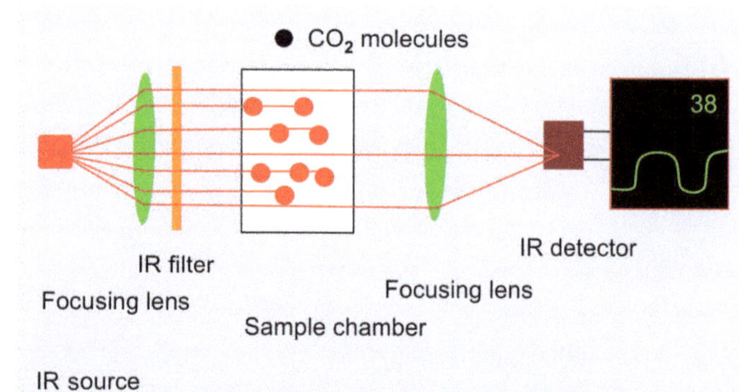

Fig. 1: Infrared (IR) beam from the detector travels through the analyzing chamber to the detector. An infrared filter selectively allows 4.3 μm wavelength to pass through to the chamber.

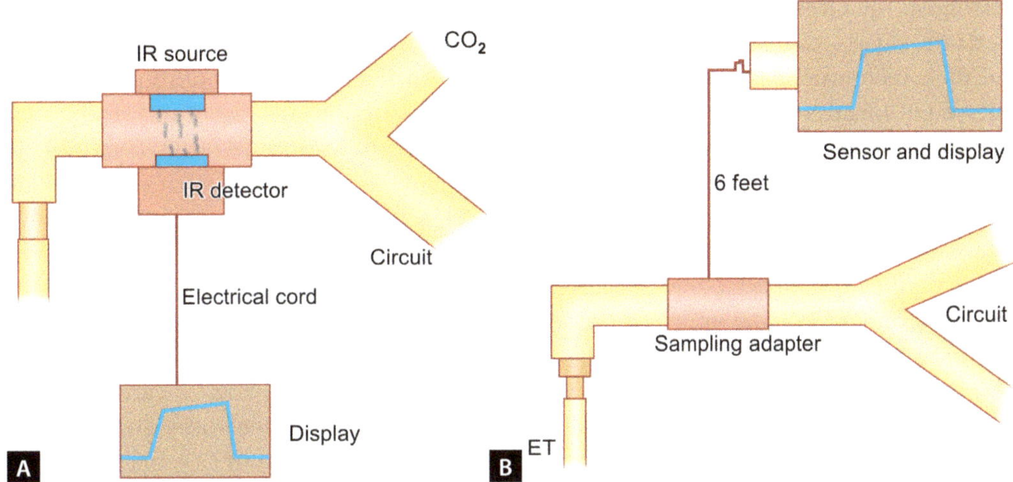

Figs. 2A and B: Mainstream capnography has a sensor located across the airway. In sidestream capnograph, the respiratory gases are aspirated into the device by a pump via a 6 feet sampling tube into the device. (IR: infrared; ET: endotracheal tube)

TABLE 1: Differences between mainstream and sidestream technology.

Mainstream	*Sidestream*
CO_2 sensor is inserted between the breathing circuit and endotracheal tube	CO_2 sensor is housed external to the breathing circuit
No gas removed from circuit	Gas is constantly aspirated from circuit via a 6 feet sampling tube into the unit containing CO_2 sensor
Increase in mechanical dead space	Minimal dead space
Earlier sensors were heavy and might have caused kinking or disconnection of circuit. Modern sensors are light weight and small	Light-weight adapter
Sensor may be damaged or lost	Sampling line may clog
Waveform in real time	Waveform is delayed (1–4 seconds) due to transportation of gases from the patient's airway to the unit containing the sensor
Difficult to adapt to nonintubated patients. Modifications are made to this type to enable connection to the oxygen mask or mimic side stream sensors by aspirating the sample via sampling line to the mainstream sensor plugged to the side of the display unit	Easily adapted to nonintubated patients

percent or as partial pressure (mm Hg). Based on the location of the IR sensor, there are two types of capnographs, (i) side stream and (ii) mainstream **(Figs. 2A and B)**. The characteristics of these two varieties are presented in **Table 1**.

The modern capnographs are fairly accurate within the clinical range of measurements (0–70 mm Hg) and usually utilize a self-calibration process. However, periodic calibration of the units is necessary with 5% CO_2 calibrating gas to maintain accuracy of capnographs to measure CO_2 in the clinical range of measurement. Variations in atmospheric pressure, humidity and the presence of nitrous oxide can affect the CO_2 measurements. However, their affect is minimal in clinical practice. There is an automatic compensation system to account for the nitrous oxide in most of the capnographs in clinical practice.

HISTORICAL NOTES

The modern IR-based technology for measurement of CO_2 was first developed by Karl Friedrich Luft in 1937.[3] However, its clinical application took several decades to be appreciated, even though papers were published as early as 1960s showing the utility of CO_2 monitoring for respiratory and circulatory changes.[4]

One of the earliest studies that showed the importance of continuous monitoring of expired CO_2 was done by Cote et al. in 331 children.[5] The study showed that 31 intraoperative events were detected by use of end-tidal CO_2 ($EtCO_2$) monitoring including life-threatening conditions like malignant hyperthermia as against 2 detected clinically. The earliest uses of CO_2 analysis were in early detecting of esophageal intubation.[6] Furthermore, an American Society of Anesthesiologists (ASA) closed claim analysis study[7] showed that the application of capnography and pulse oximetry together could have helped in the prevention of 93% of avoidable anesthesia mishaps. These studies helped the ASA and many other professional anesthesia societies to adopt capnography as a standard of monitoring during anesthesia care. The ASA mandates the use of a quantitative method of continual $EtCO_2$ analysis whenever general anesthesia is performed, especially with endotracheal or laryngeal mask airway use (ASA Standards for Basic Anesthesia Monitoring 3.1.11). In the last 2 years, the ASA,

Association of Anesthetists of Great Britain and Ireland (AAGBI), and American Heart Association (AHA) have revised and updated their recommendations on the use of capnography outside of OR locations. Recent studies have also highlighted the morbidity and mortality related to the underuse of capnography in ICUs. With these recommendations, the use of capnography to monitor ventilation during sedation has increased in areas outside of the ORs.[8] However, in developing countries like India, due to scarcity of resources, capnography is not mandated except in certain procedures like laparoscopy.[9] Hopefully, better standards of monitoring will be imposed in future that will entail the use of capnography during anesthesia as well as sedation for all surgical and other procedures.

TIME CAPNOGRAM

The graphical display of CO_2 concentration versus time produces a time capnogram and is most commonly used in clinical settings. The recording of the time capnogram can be of two speeds (sweep speed)—slow speed (0.7 mm/sec) that produces a trend capnogram or overall change in the CO_2, or a high speed (7 mm/sec) that produces a characteristic waveform with detailed information of each breath. A normal high-speed time capnogram consists of two segments: (i) an inspiratory and (ii) an expiratory segment as shown in **Figure 3**.[10,11] The expiratory segment consists of phase I, II, III, and occasionally IV (representing terminal rise of CO_2 due to emptying of alveoli with long-time constants having higher CO_2 concentration). Phase I represents the initial stage of expiration where there is no rise in CO_2 due to expiration of gases from the anatomic and apparatus dead space. This is followed by phase II which is characterized by a sharp rise in CO_2 concentration as mixing of alveolar gas and dead space gas occur. Phase III is the alveolar plateau phase representing CO_2 evolution from the alveoli. The maximum concentration at the end of the alveolar plateau (phase III) is referred to as end-tidal CO_2 ($PetCO_2$). $PetCO_2$ is the best reflection of alveolar CO_2 ($PaCO_2$). Normal lungs have high a CO_2 diffusion coefficient (i.e., CO_2 equilibrates across the alveolar membrane rapidly) and hence alveolar CO_2 [$PaCO_2$] closely reflects the arterial CO_2 [$PaCO_2$] concentration. The difference between $PetCO_2$ and $PaCO_2$ ($PaCO_2$-$PetCO_2$) is usually 3–5 mm Hg, and this is an indirect measure of physiological dead space. Towards the end of phase III, the CO_2 concentration decreases abruptly to the baseline and represents inhalation of CO_2 free gases. This is the inspiratory segment, otherwise called phase 0, and continues until the start of expiration.

There are two angles, alpha and beta angles **(Fig. 3)**. Alpha angle is the angle between phase II and III and is usually 100–110°. It increases as the slope of phase III increases as is seen in chronic obstructive pulmonary disease. The slope also indirectly represents the ventilation/perfusion (V/Q) status of the lung. Other factors that influence this angle include respiratory rate, response time of the capnograph and the sweep speed. The angle between phase III and phase 0 is called the beta angle and is usually 90°. This angle increases during rebreathing.

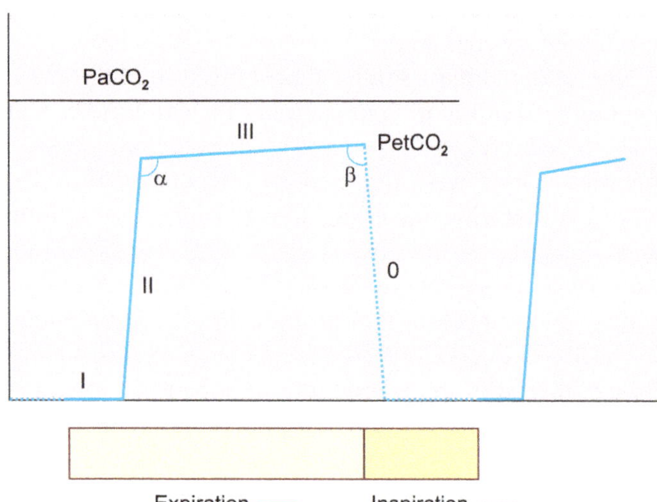

Fig. 3: Time capnogram and its components. Time capnogram showing segments, phases and angles. Inspiratory segment is phase 0, and expiratory segment is divided into three phases: I, II, and III. Maximum value of CO_2 at the end of the breath is designated as end-tidal pCO_2. It is lower than arterial CO_2 by about 5 mm Hg.
Source: Kodali BS. Capnography outside the operating rooms. Anesthesiology. 2013;118:192-201.

VOLUME CAPNOGRAM

In volume capnogram **(Fig. 4)**, the CO_2 concentration is plotted against the expired volume and it has similar characteristics. However, there is no inspiratory component in volume capnogram. The slope of the phase III is a better reflection of the V/Q status of the lung compared to time capnogram. This is because in a time capnogram, most of the exhalation is predominantly completed in the proximal one-third of the phase III and remaining portion of the plateau represents expiratory pause with continuous CO_2 sampling from the airways. A volume capnogram can be divided into various components of tidal volume **(Fig. 4)** so that the capnogram analysis offers a mode estimating physiological dead space.

ANALYSIS OF SHAPE OF CAPNOGRAMS

In analyzing capnograms, several characteristics should be assessed including the height of the capnogram indicating $PetCO_2$ concentration, baseline and shape of the curve. **Boxes 1 and 2** show causes of increased or decreased $PetCO_2$ values. Normal $PetCO_2$ is 35–40 mm Hg.

The shapes of capnograms offer diagnostic clues towards specific clinical conditions and are very useful both in ORs and out of OR locations. **Figures 5A to O** illustrate various shapes of capnograms that are encountered in clinical practice.

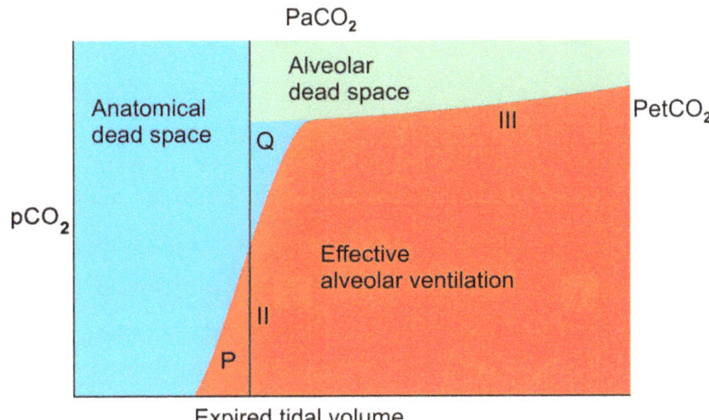

Fig. 4: A volume capnogram and its components. Volume capnogram (pCO_2 versus expired volume): Volume capnogram showing subdivisions of tidal volume. Area under the CO_2 curve is effective alveolar ventilation. Area above the CO_2 curve and the arterial $PaCO_2$ line indicates physiological dead space. A vertical line is drawn across phase II such that the two triangles P and Q are equal in area. This divides physiological dead space into anatomical and alveolar dead space.
Source: Kodali BS. Capnography outside the operating rooms. Anesthesiology. 2013;118:192-201.

BOX 1: Causes of increase of partial pressure of end-tidal carbon dioxide.

- Due to increase in CO_2 production
  - Malignant hyperthermia
  - Thyroid storm or hyperthyroidism
  - Malignant neuroleptic syndrome
  - Sepsis
  - Any other cause of increased metabolic rate like fever, shivering
  - Extraneous CO_2—laparoscopic procedures
- Due to decrease in CO_2 elimination
  - Hypoventilation due to any cause
  - Rebreathing
  - CO_2 absorber exhaustion
- Due to technical failure
  - Improper calibration
  - Malfunction or contamination of measuring system

BOX 2: Some causes of decrease of partial pressure of end-tidal carbon dioxide.

- Due to decrease in CO_2 production
  - Hypothermia
  - Hypothyroidism
  - Any other cause of decreased metabolic rate like general anesthesia
- Due to increase CO_2 elimination
  - Hyperventilation
- Due to decrease in alveolar delivery of CO_2
  - Decrease cardiac output states or hypoperfusion
  - Pulmonary embolism
  - Pulmonary edema
  - Intrapulmonary or intracardiac shunts
- Due to technical failure
  - Sampling tube leak or block
  - Disconnection of breathing system

SPECIFIC SITUATIONS

Cardiopulmonary Resuscitation

The usefulness of capnography and continuous monitoring of $EtCO_2$ during resuscitation has been demonstrated in multiple studies.[12-14] However, it has taken nearly two decades before its role in CPR has been widely accepted. Use of waveform capnography during cardiac arrest was recommended in the 2010 International Consensus on Cardiopulmonary Resuscitation Science with Treatment Recommendations.[15] These changes are based on the fact that capnography not only confirms tracheal intubation but also indirectly gives information regarding adequacy of chest compressions. Furthermore, it has been shown that return of spontaneous circulation is heralded by sudden increase in $EtCO_2$ values, even when other signs like recordable blood pressure or pulse are absent **(Fig. 6)**. Based on the current guidelines, a stand equipped with capnograph and video laryngoscope is taken to all codes at our institution **(Fig. 7)**.

Postoperative Monitoring of Patients Requiring Narcotic Pain Medications

Narcotic pain medications have the potential to cause respiratory depression and hypoventilation.[16] There is some evidence the capnography along with pulse oximetry can detect significant respiratory depression in patients receiving patient controlled opioids analgesics.[17] Although the routine use of capnography is limited to some extent by technological challenges, it should be considered in select high-risk populations like in patients with elevated body mass index.

Ventilation in Intensive Care Units

Use of capnography for ventilated patients in ICUs has been growing, but its incidence varies.[18-20] A 1-year nationwide audit undertaken in the UK involving ORs, emergency departments, and ICUs showed that there is a 66 times greater risk of airway complications in ICU ventilated patients when capnography is not routinely used as compared to ORs where capnography is the standard of care.[21] The audit recommends the use of capnography in all patients undergoing mechanical ventilation and for confirmation of tracheal intubation. Additional costs and availability of equipment may impede implementation of these recommendations, but there is growing consensus that widespread use of capnography will improve safety of critically ill patients. Additionally, volume capnograph can also aid in management of ventilator settings and in weaning patients.[22,23]

Procedural Sedation

Many procedures are being performed in out of OR locations under procedural sedation by nonanesthesiologists including nurses under the supervision of physicians. These include interventional radiology, endoscopy, cardiac catheterization, and electrophysiological (EP) procedures. Studies indicate a significant percentage of patients have evidence of respiratory depression and/or hypoxia during the sedation.[24,25] Furthermore, it has been shown that use of capnography can decrease the incidence of hypoxic events by early detection of hypoventilation.[26-28]

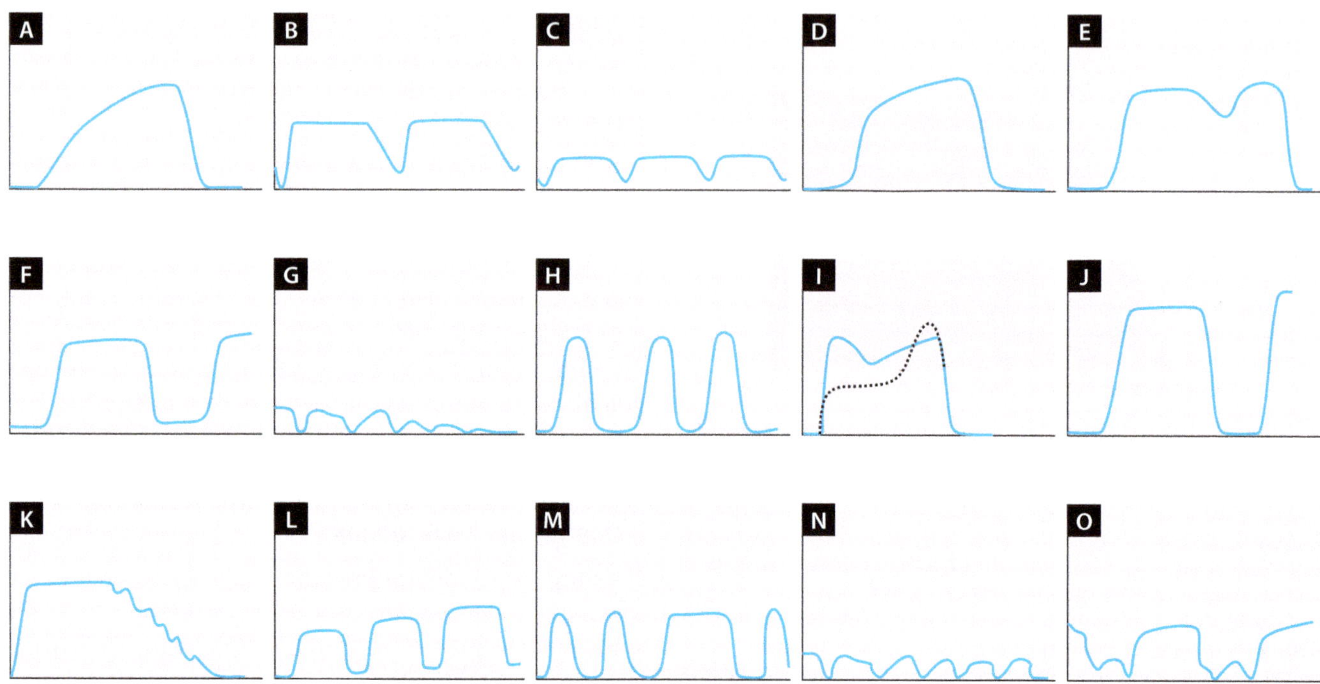

Figs. 5A to O: (A) Prolonged phase II and steeper phase III suggestive of bronchospasm, or airway obstruction; (B) Expiratory valve malfunction resulting in elevation of the baseline and obtuse down stroke of inspiratory down stroke. This is due to rebreathing of expiratory gases from the expiratory limb during inspiration; (C) Inspiratory valve malfunction resulting in rebreathing of expired gases from inspiratory limb during inspiration; (D) Capnogram with normal phase II but with increased slope of phase III. Observed in pregnant subjects under general anesthesia. (Normal physiological variant[9]); (E) Curare cleft: Patient is attempting to breathe during partial muscle paralysis. Surgical movements on the chest and abdomen can also result in the curare cleft; (F) Baseline is elevated as a result of CO_2 rebreathing; (G) Esophageal intubation resulting in the gastric washout of residual CO_2 and subsequent CO_2 will be zero; (H) Spontaneously breathing capnograms where phase III is not well delineated; (I) Dual capnogram in one lung transplantation patient. The first of peak of phase III is from the transplanted normal lung, whereas the second peak is from the native disease lung. A leak around the sidestream sensor port at the monitor can also result in a dual peaked capnogram. This is because of the dilution of expired pCO_2 with atmospheric; (J) Malignant hyperpyrexia where CO_2 is raising gradually with zero baseline suggesting increased CO_2 production with CO_2 absorption by the soda lime; (K) Ripple effect during the expiratory pause showing cardiogenic oscillations. These occur as a result of to and fro movement of expired gases at the sensor due to motion of the heartbeat; (L) Sudden raise of baseline and the partial pressure of end-tidal carbon dioxide ($PetCO_2$) due to contamination of the sensor with secretions or water vapor; (M) Intermittent mechanical ventilation breaths in the midst of spontaneously breathing patient. A comparison of the height of spontaneous breaths compared to the mechanical breaths is useful to assess spontaneous ventilation during the weaning process; (N) Cardiopulmonary resuscitation: Capnogram showing positive waveforms during each compression suggesting effective cardiac compression generating pulmonary blood; (O) Capnogram showing rebreathing during inspiration. This is normal in rebreathing circuits such as Mapelson D or Bain circuit.
Source: Anesthesiology. 2013;118:192-201.

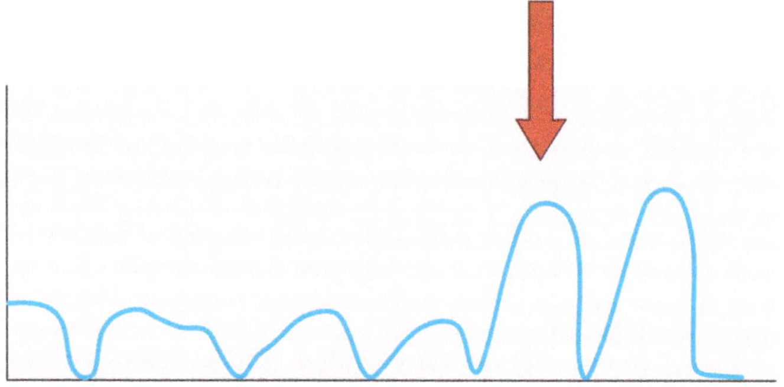

Fig. 6: Graph showing abrupt increase in partial pressure of end-tidal carbon dioxide values suggest spontaneous return of circulation during cardiopulmonary resuscitation.

In 2011, the ASA and the AAGBI issued revised standards to monitor ventilation by capnography to enhance safety of patients undergoing sedation, irrespective of the location of procedural sedation. There is a hope that other professional societies including physicians supervising nurse-administered conscious sedation employ these guidelines

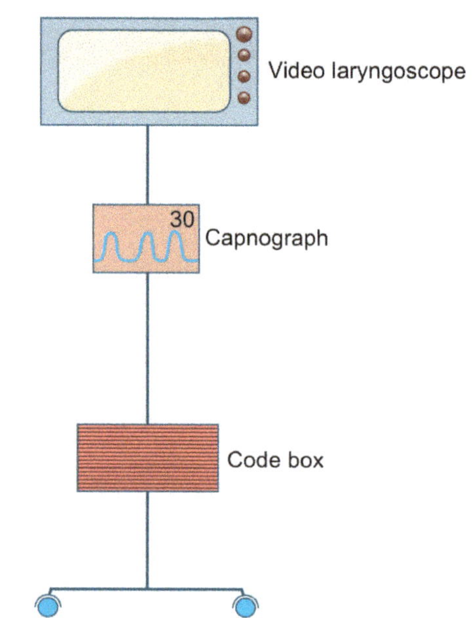

Fig. 7: A stand equipped with capnograph and video laryngoscope is taken to all locations of cardiac arrest at our institution.

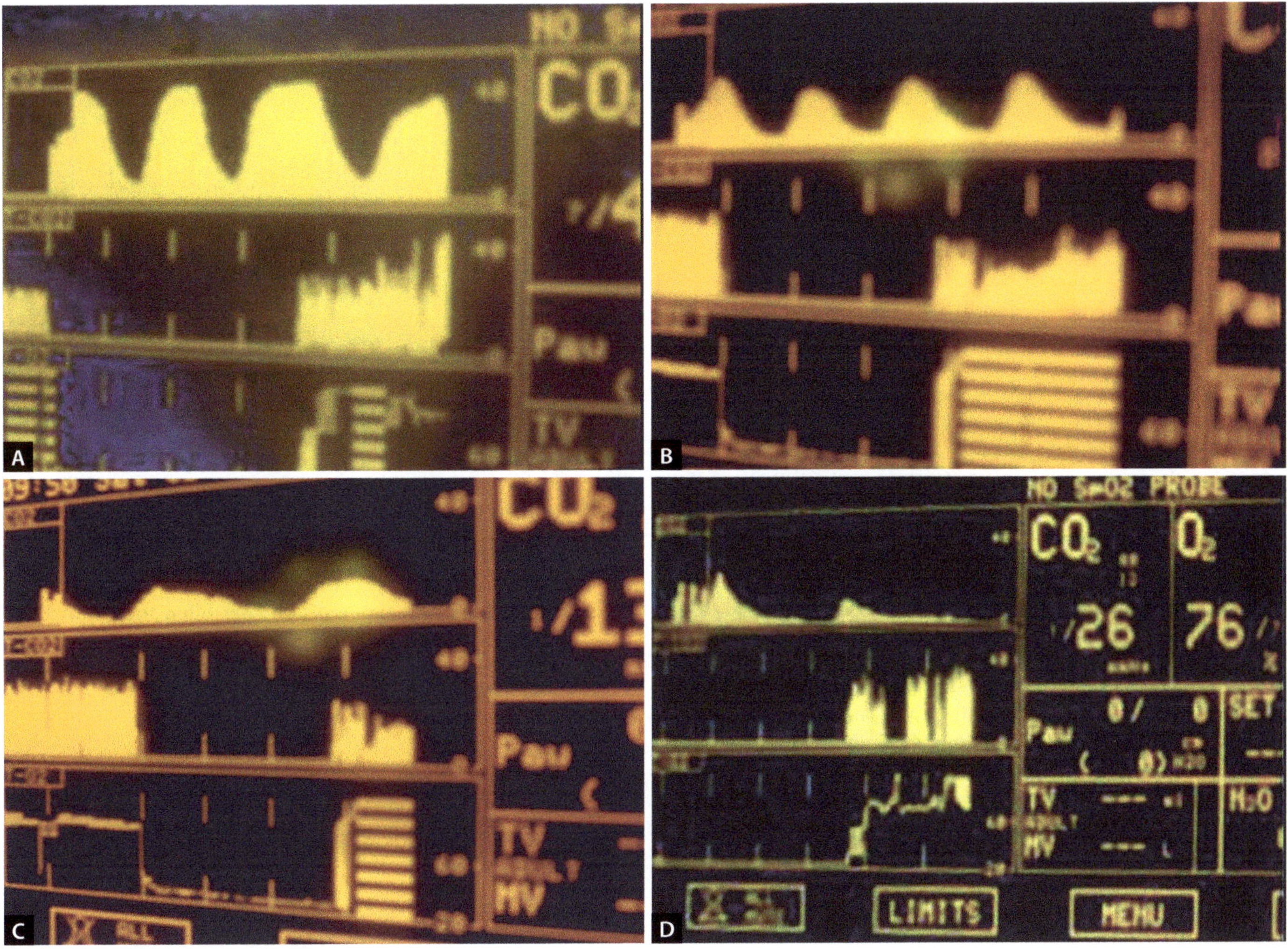

Figs. 8A to D: Capnograms before and during sedation. Changes from baseline are the important factor to note.

to monitor respiratory status and enhance patient safety. **Figures 8A to D** show capnograms during sedation. It is important to realize that changes from baseline capnograms are more important than the absolute values because of dilution of $PetCO_2$ by the oxygen flow, or atmospheric air.

CONCLUSION

Capnography or continual monitoring of expired CO_2 concentration has grown from its humble beginnings in the early half of the 20th century to become an integral part of anesthesia monitoring. Its usefulness beyond the confines of the operating room in promoting patient safety, including procedural sedation and postoperative respiratory monitoring, is being understood. There is an expanded role for capnography in other areas of patient care like CPR and ICU management. Understanding the basic physiology of capnograms will facilitate the ability to interpret the cause of abnormal $PetCO_2$ values and shapes of capnogram so that corrective measures can be initiated before the patient experiences significant harm.

REFERENCES

1. Bhavani-Shankar K, Kumar AY, Moseley H, et al. Capnometry and Anesthesia. Can J Anesth. 1992;39(6):617-32.
2. Jaffe MB. Infrared measurement of carbon dioxide in the human breath: "breathe-through" devices from Tyndall to the present day. Anesthesiology. 2008;107(3):890-904.
3. Westhorpe RN, Ball C. The history of capnography. Anaesth Intensive Care. 2010;38(4):611.
4. Leigh MD, Jones JC, Motley HL. The expired carbon dioxide as a continuous guide of the pulmonary and circulatory systems during anesthesia and surgery. J Thorac Cardiovasc Surg. 1961; 41:597-610.
5. Coté CJ, Liu LM, Szyfelbein SK, et al. Intraoperative events diagnosed by expired carbon dioxide monitoring in children. Can Anaesth Soc J. 1986;33:315-20.
6. Guggenberger H, Lenz G, Federle R. Early detection of inadvertent oesophageal intubation: pulse oximetry vs. capnography. Acta Anaesthesiol Scand. 1989;33(2):112-5.
7. Tinker JH, Dull DL, Caplan RA, et al. Role of monitoring devices in prevention of anesthetic mishaps: a closed claims analysis. Anesthesiology. 1989;71:541-6.
8. Kodali BS. Capnography outside the operating rooms. Anesthesiology. 2013;118(1):192-201.
9. Capnography is mandatory for laparoscopic surgeries for reimbursement. India, Government of Andhra Pradesh Order, AST/775/F25/September; 2011.

10. Bhavani-Shankar K, Philp JH. Defining segments and phases of a time capnogram. Anesth Analg. 2000;91:973-7.
11. Bhavani-Shankar K, Kumar AY, Moseley HS, et al. Terminology and the current limitations of time capnography: a brief review. J Clin Monit. 1995;11:175-82.
12. Kalenda Z. The capnogram as a guide to the efficacy of cardiac massage. Resuscitation. 1978;6(4):259-63.
13. Falk JL, Rackow EC, Weil MH. End-tidal carbon dioxide concentration during cardiopulmonary resuscitation. N Engl J Med. 1988;318:607-11.
14. Sanders AB, Kern KB, Otto CW, et al. End-tidal carbon dioxide monitoring during cardiopulmonary resuscitation. A prognostic indicator for survival. JAMA. 1989;262:1347-51.
15. Deakin CD, Morrison LJ, Morley PT. 2010 International Consensus on Cardiopulmonary Resuscitation and Emergency Cardiovascular Care Science with Treatment Recommendations part 8: advanced life support. Resuscitation. 2010;81:e93-174.
16. Weigner MB, Lee LA. No patient shall be harmed by opioid-induced respiratory depression (for the Anesthesia Patient Safety Foundation). APSF Newsletter. 2011;26:21-40.
17. Overdyk FJ, Carter R, Maddox RR, et al. Continuous oximetry/capnometry monitoring reveals frequent desaturation and bradypnea during patient controlled analgesia. Anesth Analg. 2007;105:412-8.
18. Kannan S, Manji M. Survey of use of end-tidal carbon dioxide for confirming tracheal tube placement in intensive care units in the UK. Anaesthesia. 2003;58:476-9.
19. Georgiou AP, Gouldson S, Amphlett AM. The use of capnography and the availability of airway equipment on intensive care units in the UK and the Republic of Ireland. Anaesthesia. 2010;65:462-7.
20. Husain T, Gatward JJ, Hambidge OR, et al. Strategies to prevent airway complications: a survey of adult intensive care units in Australia and New Zealand. Br J Anaesth. 2012;108:800-6.
21. Cook TM, Woodall N, Harper J, et al. Major complications of airway management in the UK: results of the Fourth National Audit Project of the Royal College of Anesthetists and the Difficult Airway Society. Part 2: intensive care and emergency departments. Br J Anaesth. 2011;106:632-42.
22. Tusman G, Sipmann FS, Bohm SH. Rationale of dead space measurement by volumetric capnography. Anesth Analg. 2012;114:866-74.
23. Thompson JE, Jaffe MB. Capnographic waveforms in the mechanically ventilated patient. Resp Care. 2005;50(1):100-9.
24. Chudnofsky CR, Weber JE, Stoyanoff PJ, et al. A combination of midazolam and ketamine for procedural sedation and analgesia in adult emergency department patients. Acad Emerg Med. 2000;7:228-35.
25. Sacchetti A, Senula G, Strickland J, et al. Procedural sedation in the community emergency department: Initial results of the ProSCED registry. Acid Emerg Med. 2007;14:41-6.
26. Deitch K, Miner J, Chudnofsky CR, et al. Does end-tidal CO_2 monitoring during emergency department procedural sedation and analgesia with Propofol decrease the incidence of hypoxic events? A randomized, controlled trial. Ann Emerg Med. 2010;55:258-64.
27. Waugh JB, Epps CA, Khodneva YA. Capnography enhances surveillance of respiratory events during procedural sedation: a meta-analysis. J Clin Anesth. 2011;23:189-96.
28. Beitz A, Riphaus A, Meining A, et al. Capnographic monitoring reduces the incidence of arterial oxygen desaturation and hypoxemia during Propofol sedation for colonoscopy: a randomized, controlled study (ColoCap Study). Am J Gastroenterol. 2012;107:1205-12.

Respiratory Gas Monitoring and Minimum Alveolar Concentration

Sheila N Myatra, Sohan L Solanki

ABSTRACT

The concern for patient safety during anesthesia has given rise to the development of several technologies like respiratory gas monitoring. The early gas monitoring systems were large stand-alone units that were usually placed on a shelf on the anesthesia machine. Anesthesia monitors in use now a days, mostly incorporates the major anesthetic gas monitoring systems. The ongoing advancements in the field of respiratory gas monitoring of inhaled anesthetic agents, N_2O, CO_2 and O_2, the valuable clinical information they provide to the anesthesiologist and the decrease in the size and cost of these sensors and monitors, has led to their widespread use in the modern operating rooms.

Monitoring of respiratory gases can alert the anesthesiologist of a number of potentially adverse, preventable and correctable conditions, such as vapor overdose, wrong agent in vaporizer, CO_2 retreating, excessive end-tidal CO_2 ($PetCO_2$), timing to reach minimum alveolar concentration awake, monitoring of uptake and distribution, and during low-flow anesthesia it can assure that the desired agent concentration is being delivered. The aim of this chapter is to provide a framework for the understanding of the methods whereby respiratory gases are analyzed, as well as their clinical applications and limitations.

RESPIRATORY GAS MONITORING

INTRODUCTION

Respiratory gas monitoring is now an essential part of all patients with an artificial respiration especially operating room, and also in critical care unit, for transport of ventilated patients. The Association of Anesthetist of Great Britain and Ireland (AAGBI), recommended respiratory gas monitoring an essential component during anesthesia and included, an oxygen analyzer with an audible alarm and a CO_2 analyzer; a vapor analyzer whenever a volatile anesthetic is delivered.[1]

Respiratory gas monitoring is today a part of most of the modern anesthesia room as they provide valuable information to the anesthesiologist, also they are available and included with most modern multiparameter monitors or they are also part of anesthesia workstation monitor **(Figs. 1A and B)**.

Monitoring of respiratory gases can alert the anesthesiologist of a number of potentially adverse, preventable and correctable conditions such as vapor overdose, wrong agent in vaporizer, CO_2 rebreathing and excessive ($PetCO_2$), timing to reach minimum alveolar concentration (MAC) awake, monitoring of uptake and distribution, and in the setting of

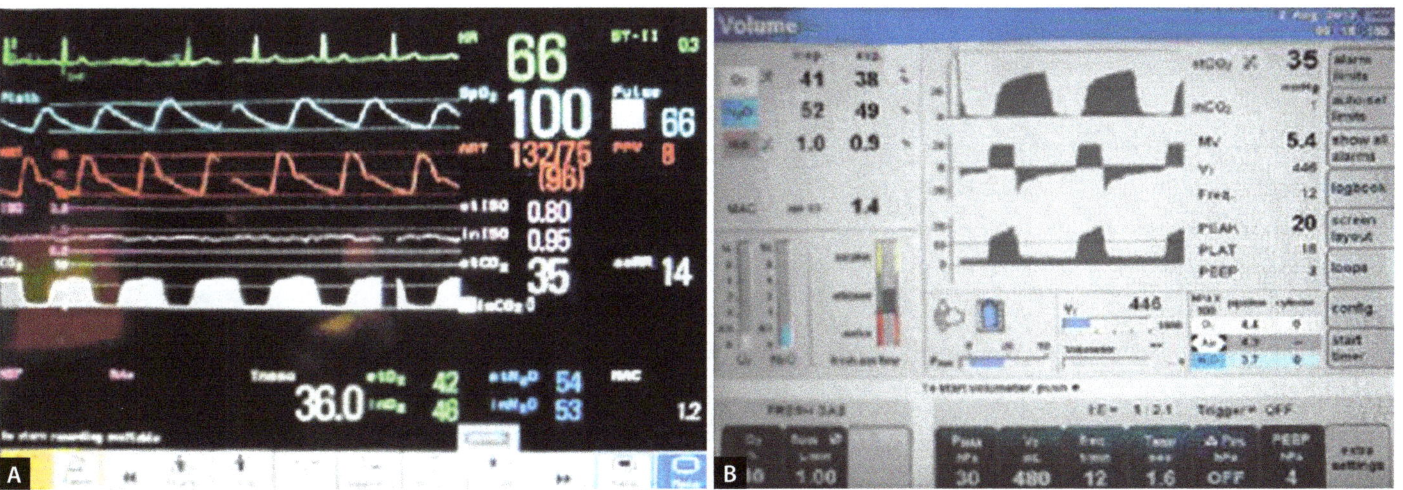

Figs. 1A and B: Multiparameter monitor: Respiratory gas monitoring is today included with: (A) Multipurpose monitor that include ECG, blood pressure, invasive monitoring, pulse oximetry, temperature, etc.; (B) Part of the anesthesia workstation monitor.

low-flow anesthesia it can assure that the desired agent concentration is being delivered.

American Society of Anesthesiologists (ASA) Closed Claims study published in 1997[2] regarding the role of equipment related problems to malpractice litigations in the US, observed that 72 (2%) claims out of 3,791 claims were related to gas delivery system. Of the 72 claims, 21% were related to vaporizers that lead to excessive airway pressure and anesthetic agent overdose. They also reported two cases where vaporizer failures were associated with intraoperative awareness due to lower inhalational agent concentrations.

TYPES OF MONITOR

Two types of monitor are in clinical use for respiratory gas monitoring: mainstream or nondiverting and sidestream or diverting based on the site of measurement of gases.[3,4]

Mainstream or Nondiverting

Mainstream gas monitor is used for monitoring of oxygen and CO_2 only. In this type of gas monitor, sensor is placed and measurement is done directly in the main gas stream. Mainstream gas monitor can be used both for intubated and nonintubated patients and it is attached to nasal or oral mask in case of nonintubated patients **(Table 1)**.

Technology

Mainstream monitor for CO_2 monitoring use infrared technology and the sensor is placed between circuit and patient and monitor for O_2 monitoring use electrochemical technology and the sensor is placed in the inspiratory limb of the breathing system for only inspiratory O_2 monitoring and between the patient and the breathing system if used for both inspiratory and end-tidal O_2 concentration **(Figs. 2A and B)**.

Sidestream or Diverting

In sidestream monitor, gas from the breathing circuits is aspirated by a pump through the sampling tubing into the sensor in to the main unit near or into the main monitor **(Figs. 3A and B)**.

TABLE 1: Advantages and disadvantages of mainstream gas monitor.

Advantages	*Disadvantages*
Fast response time (no delay time)	Only used for CO_2 and O_2
Better CO_2 waveform than that generated by sidestream monitor	Bulky sensor is placed near the patient and there is increased dead space
No sampling tube and no problem of blockage by expiratory water vapor and secretions	In CO_2 monitor, the sensor may become dislodged from the cuvette and waveform may lost or incorrect
No effect due to pressure drop	Leak, disconnection and obstruction may occur
No pollution	Risk of infection with cross-contamination

Technology

This type of respiratory monitor also uses same technology as used in main stream monitor.

Advantages over the mainstream monitor is that there is no bulky assembly near the patient, no risk of cross-contamination between the patients and it can be used for volatile anesthetic agents as well as for N_2O apart from CO_2 and O_2. But, there is always a delay time because gases have to be aspirated to the main sensor and analyzed, also risk of sampling tube blockage by expiratory water vapor and secretion or sometimes with some foreign body.[5] Time delay can be shortened by using a short sample tube. Sometimes a mainstream monitor with diverting capability can be used.

GAS MEASUREMENT

Oxygen Analysis and Monitoring

Electrochemical Oxygen Analysis

An electrochemical oxygen analyzer consists of a sensor (containing cathode, anode and surrounding electrolytes), and an analyzer (containing electronic circuit, display of partial pressure or percentage of O_2 and alarm). The sensor is placed in the inspiratory limb of the breathing system **(Figs. 4A and B)**. They have a lag time, so mostly respond slowly to change in O_2 pressure and in most of the cases used for measuring inspiratory O_2 only.[6,7] Two types of electrochemical sensor are in use for O_2 analysis.

Galvanic Cell, Hersch or Fuel Sensor

This is made of an anode (made up of Pb) and two cathodes (made up of Au or Ag) surrounded by electrolytes

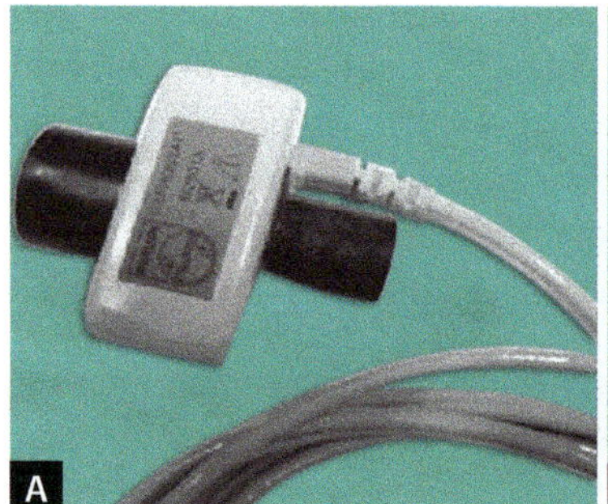

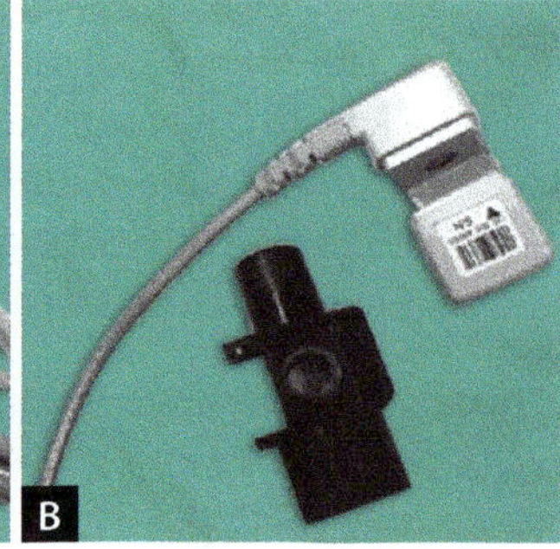

Figs. 2A and B: Main stream gas analyzer, it is directly connected to the breathing circuits and sense gas at the source.

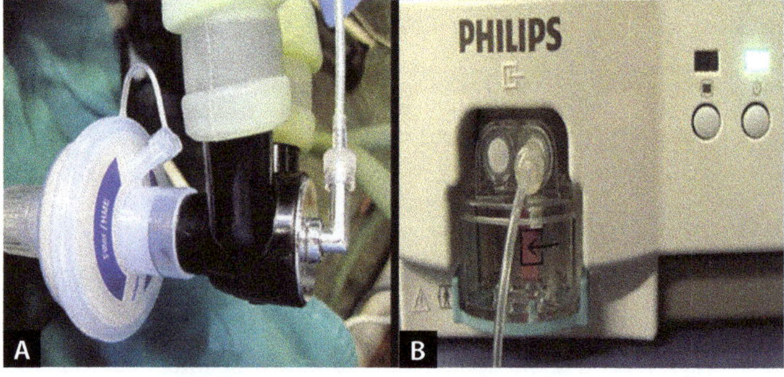

Figs. 3A and B: Sidestream gas analyzer with a sampling tube.

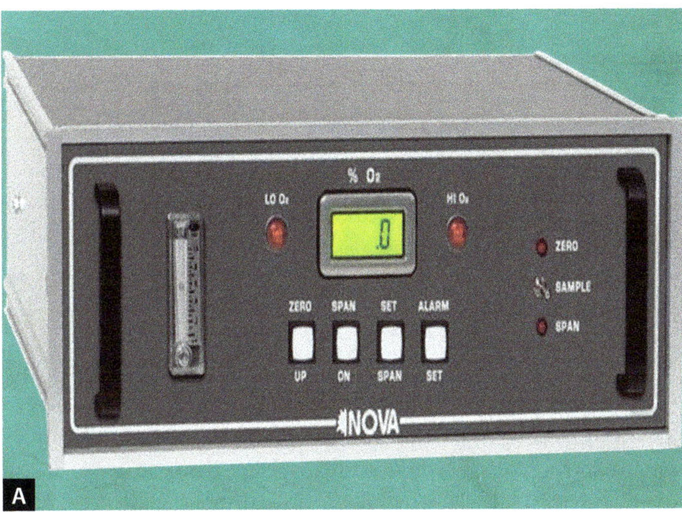

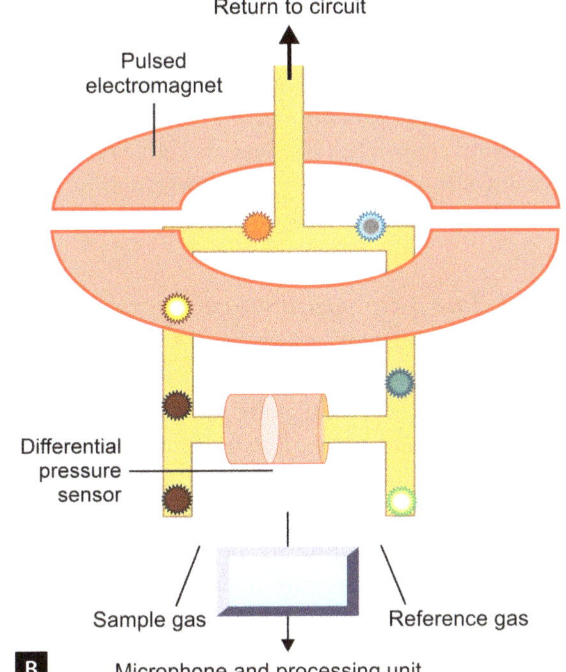

Figs. 4A and B: Paramagnetic O_2 analyzer and its working principle.

(mostly KOH). Only O_2 can diffuses through the electrochemical sensor membrane and electrolyte to the cathode, where it is reduced, causing a current to flow.[8,9]

The partial pressure of O_2 is proportional to the rate of O_2 entering into the cell and generating the current. This partial pressure of O_2 is displayed as percentage of O_2 on monitor. Reactions at cathodes and anode are as follows:

Cathode reaction:

$$O_2 + 2H_2O + 4e^- \rightarrow 4OH^-$$

Anode reaction:

$$4OH^- + 2Pb \rightarrow 2PbO + 2H_2O + 4e^-$$

Life of the galvanic sensor is decreased when it is exposed to a high O_2 concentration. Sensor life can be prolonged by removing it from the breathing system and exposing it to air when not in use **(Figs. 5A to C)**.

Polarographic (Clark) Sensor

Polarographic or Clark sensor consists of an anode (Ag or AgCl), a cathode (Au or Pt), an electrolyte (KCl or KBr) and a gas-permeable membrane. An external current source is required to drive the cathode reaction (hence named polarographic) **(Fig. 6)**. Oxygen diffuses through the membrane and external current is applied to the cathode, cathode reaction take place:

$$O_2 + 2H_2O + 4e^- \rightarrow 4OH^-$$

And at the anode, following reductive reaction is generated:

$$4Ag^+ + 4Cl^- + 4e^- \rightarrow 4AgCl$$

Polarographic sensor over reads O_2 when used in presence of N_2O because contamination with silver reduces the N_2O at cathode, so falsely high percentage of O_2 is measured.

International and US standards on respiratory gas monitors analyzers[10,11] recommended O_2 readings within ±2.5% of the actual level and this accuracy shall be maintained

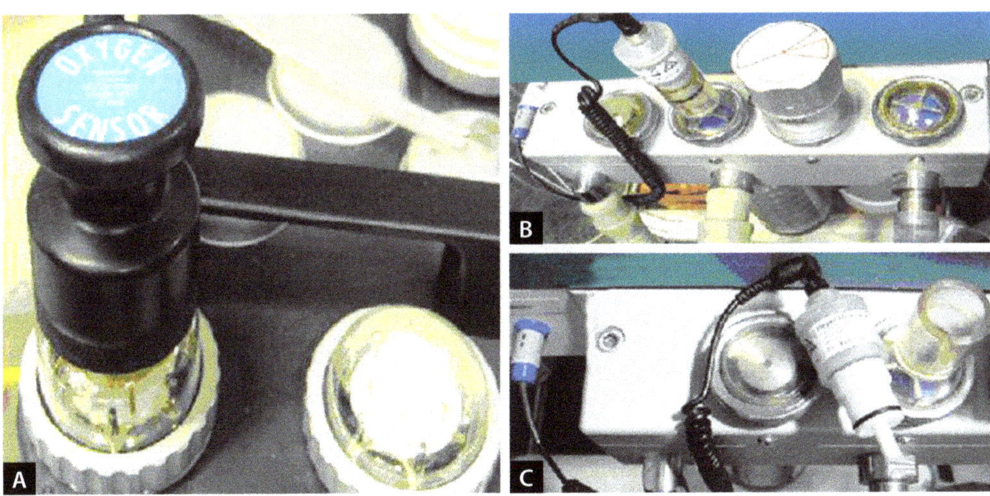

Figs. 5A to C: (A and B) Galvanic or fuel cell oxygen sensor in place (in inspiratory limb); (C) When not in use, it should be kept open to air to increase its self-life.

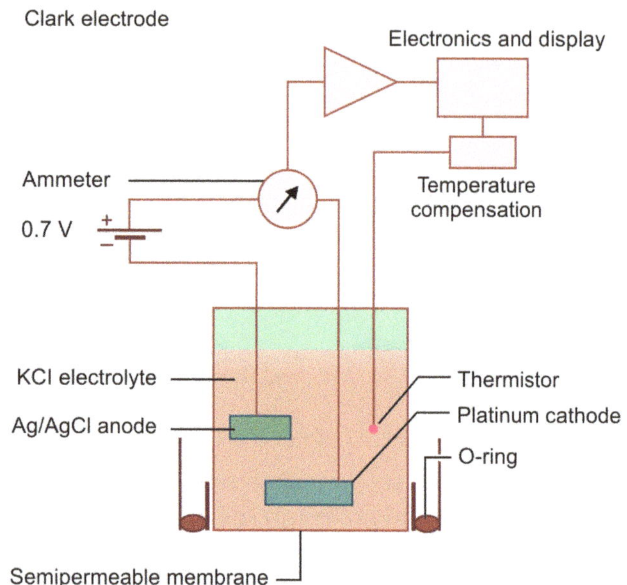

Fig. 6: Polarographic or Clark's oxygen sensor.

for at least 6 hours of continuous use and high and low O_2 level alarms must be at least medium priority with a high-priority alarm for an inspiratory O_2 concentration below 18%.

Carbon Dioxide Analysis

Basis for CO_2 monitoring is assessment of metabolism, circulation and ventilation while patient is under anesthesia. CO_2 monitoring is included in basic anesthetic monitoring by ASA and AAGBI. American Heart Association also recommends using CO_2 monitoring to judge the effectiveness of chest compression during cardiopulmonary cerebral resuscitation (CPCR). Partial pressure of end-tidal CO_2 ($PetCO_2$) is recommended for confirming the correct positioning of tracheal tube or supraglottic airway device. $PetCO_2$ monitoring is also recommended throughout during the general anesthesia and an audible alarm is also included for any deviation from normal.

A closed claims analysis and many other studies found that end-tidal monitoring of CO_2 can prevent or detect many general anesthesia related hazard and guides the anesthesiologist for timely management of preventable anesthesia complications.[12-14]

Capnometry is the measurement of CO_2 in a gas mixture and capnography is the graphical recording of CO_2 concentration with time. A capnometer is available both as a portable single monitor device as well as included in multi-parameter monitor.

Physical Principles of Capnography

There are five physical principles of capnography:

1. Infrared spectrography
2. Molecular correlation spectrography
3. Mass spectrography
4. Raman spectrography
5. Photoacoustic spectrography.

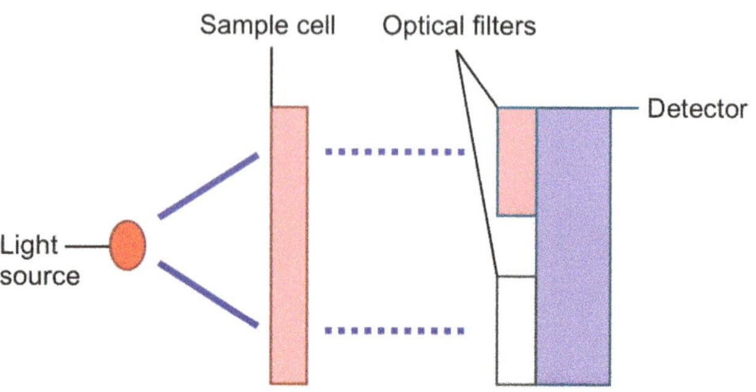

Fig. 7: Infrared CO_2 analyzer.

Infrared spectrography: This technique of CO_2 monitoring is most commonly used and more compact and economical too. Infrared rays (wavelength more than 1.0 mμ) are used and they are absorbed by polyatomic gases like CO_2, N_2O and water vapor. Absorption is according to the Beer-Lambert law, which states that there is a logarithmic dependence between the transmission of light through a substance and the concentration of that substance. CO_2 selectively absorb 4.3 mμ wavelength of infrared light. The concentration of CO_2 can be determined by measured absorbance and it is displayed as mm Hg on monitor **(Fig. 7)**.[15]

Factors affecting CO_2 measurement by infrared spectrography: Several factors can affect the infrared spectrography like atmospheric pressure, N_2O, O_2, inhalational agents (although insignificant), and water vapor.

If the atmospheric pressure is high, $PetCO_2$ percentage will be high by increasing number of infrared light absorbing molecules and increasing intermolecular forces; whereas, at low atmospheric pressure (high altitude), $PetCO_2$ percentage will be low. This effect on atmospheric pressure can be minimized by measuring the $PetCO_2$ as partial pressure, calibrating the equipment with known CO_2 concentration at the place of measurement and keeping the sampling flow rate of capnometer constant.

Use of N_2O can also affect CO_2 measurement and can give falsely high value of CO_2, because N_2O also absorb infrared light (wavelength 4.5 mμ). This interference can be decreased by using a very narrow band of infrared light (4.3 mμ, used by CO_2).[16]

Oxygen can also affect the CO_2 measurement and results in falsely low CO_2. Although it does not absorb infrared light, it affects the absorption of infrared light by CO_2 by collision with CO_2 molecules and broadens its absorption peak.

Inhalational agents at low doses do not affect CO_2 measurement by infrared light because they absorb infrared light at different wavelength (3.3 mμ).

Water vapor can affect CO_2 measurement by condensing on infrared cell and also by condensing and blocking the sampling tube in sidestream sensors.

Molecular correlation spectrography: This is a laser-based technology used to generate infrared light that correlates with absorption spectrum of CO_2. This is high accuracy method of CO_2 analysis with rapid response and can be useful in extreme low flow (150 mL/min).

Mass spectrography: This technology is rarely used in clinical practice as it is very expensive and bulky apparatus. The mass spectrography separates molecules on the basis of mass to charge ratio.[15]

Raman spectrography: This is based on "Raman scattering" (unstable vibrational or rotational energy) principle of CO_2 monitoring. The CO_2 mixed gas is aspirated into a chamber and is illuminated by a high intensity monochromatic argon laser beam. The Raman scattering light is of low intensity light and is measured at right angle to laser beam. This technology is used now in many newer anesthetic monitors (RASCAL monitors) for CO_2 and anesthetic agent monitoring.[17]

Photoacoustic spectrography: This use same principle as used by infrared spectrography, only difference is that infrared spectrography uses optical methods whereas photoacoustic spectrography uses acoustic methods. It is more accurate, reliable and requires less maintenance.

An international and a US standard on capnometers[10,11] recommends the CO_2 reading within ±12% of the actual value or ±4 mm Hg, whichever is greater and the manufacturer must disclose any interference caused by ethanol, acetone, methane, helium, tetrafluoroethane and dichlorodifluoromethane as well as commonly used halogenated anesthetic agents. An alarm for high CO_2 for both inspired and exhaled CO_2 should be there and there should also be an alarm for low exhaled CO_2.

Most of the capnometers are included in a multiparameter monitoring system but portable, battery-operated CO_2 monitors are also available for use in emergency medicine and patient transport. Magnetic resonance imaging (MRI)-compatible infrared CO_2 monitors are also available.

Physiologic Basis of CO_2 Monitoring

Metabolism

End-tidal CO_2 monitoring indicates patient's metabolic rate.[18] In a patient with controlled ventilation, $PetCO_2$ monitoring is a reliable indicator of metabolism but not in spontaneously breathing patients because of compensatory mechanisms.

Conditions with increased metabolism and therefore increased $PetCO_2$ include fever (increased body temperature), shivering, seizures, high catecholamine production, and parenteral hyperalimentation. Increased $PetCO_2$ may be because of CO_2 used for endoscopic and laparoscopic surgeries. One of the most dreaded intraoperative complications, malignant hyperthermia, may be because of extreme CO_2 production and capnography is very useful in early detection of this.[13,14]

Circulation

End-tidal CO_2 increase or decrease with increase or decrease in cardiac output if ventilation remains constant.[19,20] Compression of major blood vessels during surgery may also decrease pulmonary blood flow and subsequent decrease in $PetCO_2$. Any form of pulmonary embolism dramatically reduce $PetCO_2$ (sudden fall), but in case of CO_2 embolism, there is initial rise in $PetCO_2$ followed by fall.

American Heart Association[21] recommends the use of capnography not only for confirmation of tracheal tube placement, but also to monitor the effectiveness of chest compressions during CPCR. The $PetCO_2$ values should be maintained between 10 and 20 mm Hg during chest compression. This serves to give feedback to optimize chest compression for effective CPR and monitor effectiveness. A $PetCO_2$ value less than 10 mm Hg measured after initiation of CPR is associated with poor outcome **(Table 2)**.

Respiration

Carbon dioxide is better monitor for the frequency and depth of respiration. Capnography is best mean for assuring correct positioning of an endotracheal tube (single lumen as well as double lumen) or supraglottic airway device and can diagnose esophageal intubation, circuit disconnection, endotracheal tube cuff leak, airway obstruction, change in compliance and ventilator malfunction.

There is some transient and small CO_2 waveform with esophageal intubation, these CO_2 waveform is due to CO_2 that has entered the stomach during mask ventilation.

Capnography can also be used to diagnose tracheobronchial injury during thoracoscopic procedures.[22]

TABLE 2: Differential diagnosis to be considered during increase or decrease in $PetCO_2$.

Causes of abnormal $PetCO_2$	***$PetCO_2$ increase***	***$PetCO_2$ decrease***
Metabolic	• Shivering during recovery from anesthesia • Thyroid storm • Severe sepsis • Malignant hyperthermia • Neuroleptic malignant syndrome	• Hypothermia • Metabolic acidosis
Circulatory	• Tourniquet release • CO_2 insufflations • Laparoscopic surgery • Treatment of acidosis	• Induction of anesthesia • Pulmonary embolism • Profound hypovolemia • Cardiogenic shock • Hemorrhagic shock • Intracardiac shunt
Respiratory	• Hypoventilation • COPD • Asthma	• Hyperventilation • Pulmonary edema • Intrapulmonary shunts
Technical	• Exhausted soda lime • Contamination of the monitor	• Disconnection or blockage in circuit

($PetCO_2$: partial pressure of end-tidal CO_2; COPD: chronic obstructive pulmonary disease)

Capnogram

Physiology of Normal Capnogram

Carbon dioxide is produced in the body tissues, carried by the blood to the lungs, excreted by the lungs by exchange with fresh O_2, and removed by the breathing system. Therefore, any changes in respiratory CO_2 may reflect alterations in metabolism, circulation, respiration or the breathing system.

In a normal healthy patient, at the end of normal tidal inspiration, if there is no rebreathing, the airway and alveoli are filled with fresh air (containing almost zero CO_2). The CO_2 present in alveoli (depending on the ventilation/perfusion ratio of those alveoli) is exchanged by O_2 in fresh air. In the proximal airway (trachea and left and right main bronchi) there is almost no exchange between CO_2 and O_2 and air filled in these airways are devoid of CO_2 (respiratory dead space). During expiration, as the initial gas from respiratory dead space have no CO_2, the CO_2 sensor detects no CO_2 but as the expiration continue, CO_2 concentration increases and reaches at a plateau level when gas from CO_2 rich alveoli come to the CO_2 sensor. At the end of expiration, CO_2 concentration falls abruptly to baseline because next inspiration is started.[15]

Normal Capnogram

The shape of the normal capnogram is shown in **Figure 8**. It has four phases:

1. Phase I (inspiratory baseline) begins at start of expiration and is normally zero, reflecting expired gases from respiratory dead space, which is normally devoid of CO_2
2. Phase II (expiratory upstroke) is rapid S-shaped upswing represents the transition from gas from the respiratory dead space (zero CO_2) and alveolar gas that contains CO_2
3. Phase III is plateau phase because gas is coming entirely from alveoli. If a plateau is not seen, the maximum value (peak) obtained, may not be equivalent to the end-tidal level. The last portion of phase III is referred to as the end-tidal point. The CO_2 level here is normally at its maximum.
   The angle between phases II and III is called a angle.[23] Normally, it is between 100° and 110°.
   The angle between the end of phase III and the descending limb of the capnogram is called the a angle. Normally, it is approximately 90°
4. In phase IV, the patient inhales. Normally, CO_2 falls abruptly to zero and remains at zero until the next exhalation.

Common Conditions with Deviation from Normal Capnogram

- *Curare notch:* Patient on control ventilation who is showing some spontaneous respiratory activities during respiratory cycle of controlled ventilation **(Fig. 9)**. It is usually present on later third part of waveform[24]
- A biphasic capnogram (two peaks) is generally caused by unilateral hypoventilation or unilateral high airway pressure, single lung transplantation, endobronchial intubation, or severe kyphoscoliosis **(Fig. 10)**[25,26]
- A capnogram not touching to baseline **(Fig. 11)** is normally caused by breathing of expired CO_2 and may be because of exhausted CO_2 absorber, malfunctioning expiratory valve or extremely low flow of fresh gas
- A capnogram with increased α angle **(Fig. 12)** is normally caused by airway obstruction, either mechanical (tracheal tube kinking or blockade by secretions or foreign body) or pathological (bronchial asthma, chronic obstructive pulmonary disease)
- A capnogram with increased β angle may be caused by rebreathing or an inefficient inspiratory valve **(Fig. 13)**.

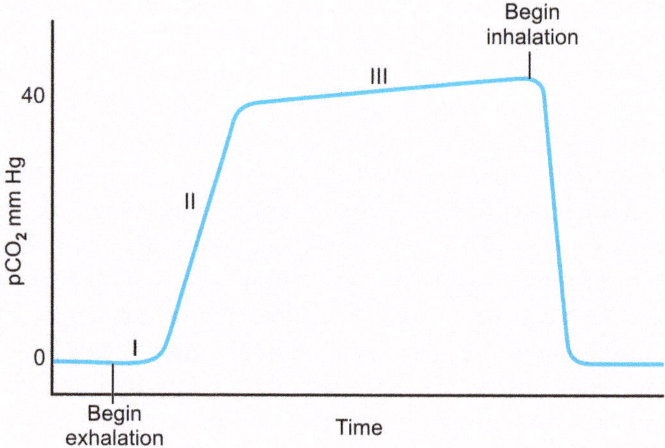

Fig. 8: A normal capnogram.

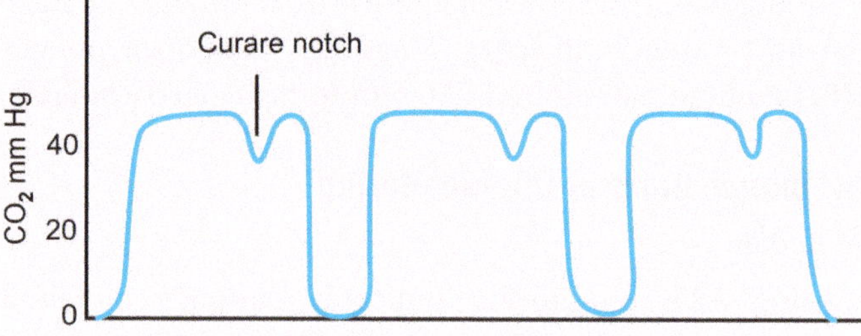

Fig. 9: Capnograph showing "curare notch" indicating spontaneous respiratory efforts.

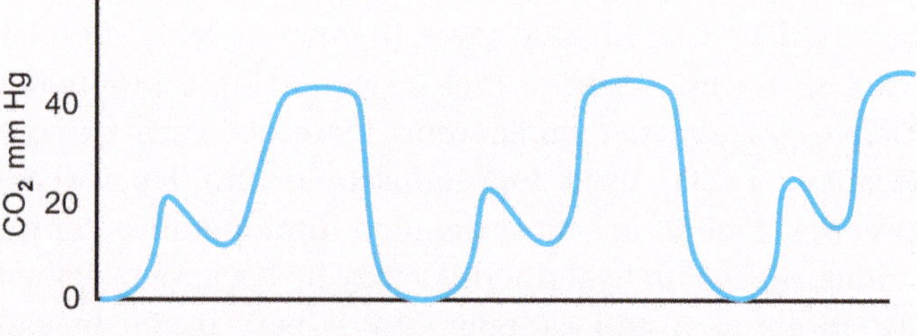

Fig. 10: Biphasic capnograph.

Uncommon Conditions with Capnogram Waveform Variations

Positive end expiratory pressure (PEEP) valve malfunctioning can cause distorted capnogram waveform and shows alternate normal and abnormal waveform. The accumulation of moisture in PEEP valve leads to increased adhesion of the diaphragm of PEEP valve to the metal rim and thus the pressure needed to open the valve may be more than set PEEP. This results into failure of expiration of every alternate breath and monitor may show double expired tidal volume and half respiratory rate than those of ventilatory settings **(Fig. 14)**.[27]

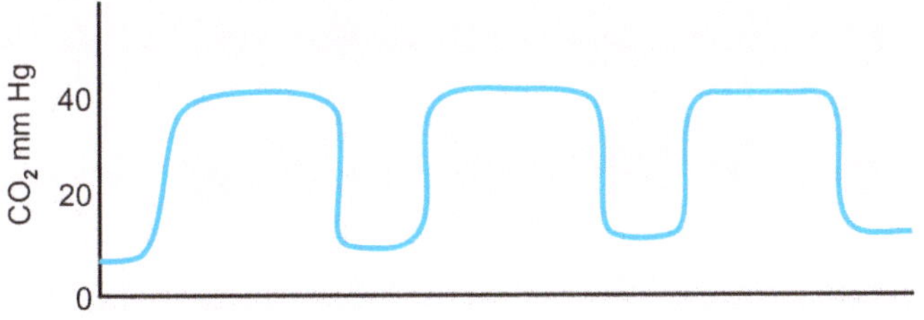

Fig. 11: Capnograph not touching the baseline.

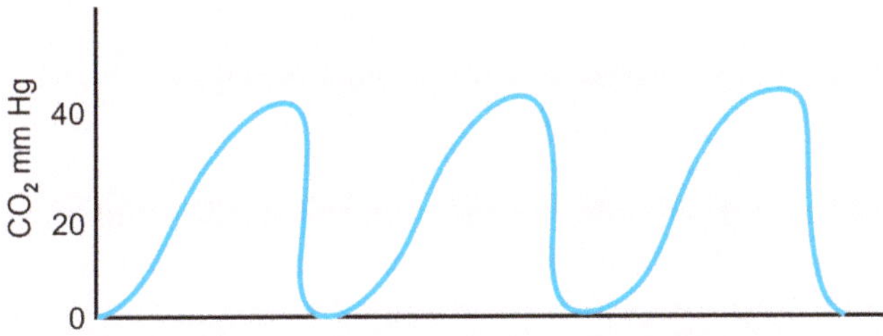

Fig. 12: Capnograph with increased alpha angle.

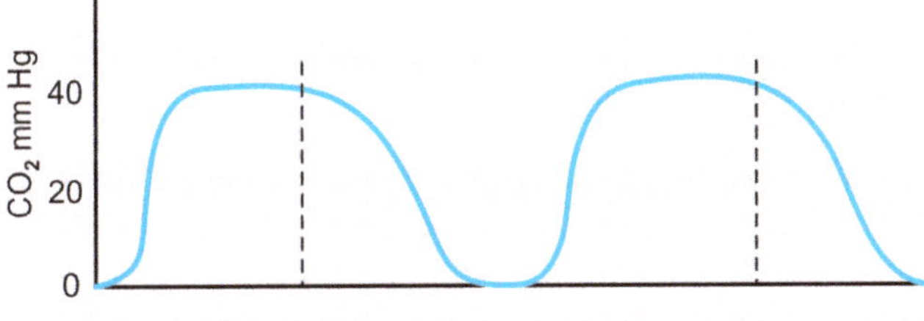

Fig. 13: Capnograph with increased beta angle.

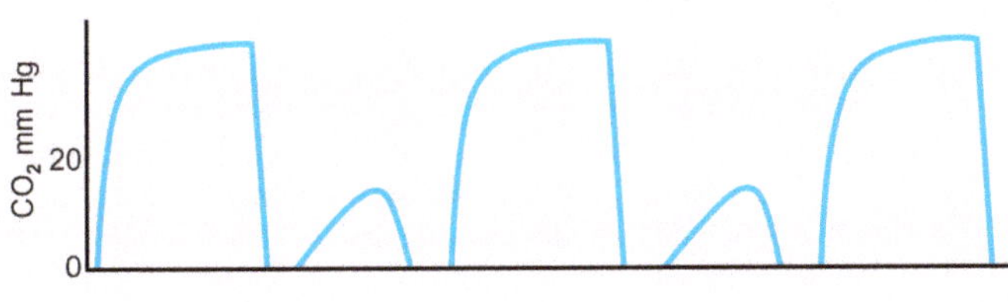

Fig. 14: Capnograph showing alternate normal and abnormal waveforms.

Other Uses of Capnography

Guide for blind tracheal intubation, to confirm the correct placement of cricothyrotomy needle or percutaneous tracheostomy and to localize the site of leak in CO_2 insufflation equipment.

Capnometer-related Problem and Drawbacks

Leak or break in sampling tube of sidestream sensor may add air in the sample and falsely low CO_2 will be detected. If sampling tube is obstructed by water vapor or some foreign body, the capnogram will get damp or may fall to zero[5] and cause falsely high inspired and falsely low end-expired CO_2 values.[28]

VOLATILE ANESTHETIC AGENTS

Monitoring of volatile anesthetic agent is now included as standard of care during general anesthesia in many countries. Both end-tidal and inspiratory concentrations of anesthetic agents are monitored and provide valuable information regarding depth of anesthesia.

Now a days, most anesthetic agent monitoring systems are included as part of multi-parameter monitor.

According to international and US standard for anesthetic gas monitors[10,11] for halogenated anesthetic gases, the difference between the mean anesthetic gas reading and the anesthetic gas level shall be within ±0.2% vol% + 15% of the anesthetic gas level and a high concentration alarm is mandatory.

Technology

Anesthetic agents can be monitored by:

- Infrared light
- Refractrometry
- Piezoelectric analysis.

Clinical Applications and Advantages

- Anesthetic agent gas monitoring can effectively assess the ability of a vaporizer, its accuracy and agent contained in it. Now a days, agent specific vaporizers are more commonly used and agent gas monitoring can detect the incorrect agent filling. It also detects the mixing of volatile agent when one agent is turned "off" and other agent is turn "on"
- Anesthetic agent gas monitoring provides information about depth of anesthesia in a paralyzed patient and helps the clinician administer adequate (neither low nor high) anesthetic agent. It helps the anesthesiologist for faster awakening of patient at end of surgical procedure as well as avoiding anesthetic awareness. High agent concentration may also cause hemodynamic instability especially in pediatric patients due to excessive myocardial depression

- Anesthetic agent gas monitoring alerts the anesthesiologist when a vaporizer has become empty, inadvertently turned "off" or turned "on"
- The difference between the dial setting and inspiratory concentration is usually high at the beginning and becomes equal as equilibrium is achieved
- Agent gas monitoring give valuable information on uptake and elimination of particular volatile agent.

NITROUS OXIDE MONITORING

Nitrous oxide can be measured directly only by infrared technology (N_2O absorb infrared light at 4.5 mμ). Both inspiratory and end-tidal concentration of N_2O is displayed on monitor.

MINIMAL ALVEOLAR CONCENTRATION

First devised by Edmund Eger and colleagues in 1965; MAC is used for assessment of the anesthetic potency of a volatile anesthetic agent. By definition, MAC is "the minimum concentration of volatile anesthetic agent that prevents movement in 50% of the patients in response to an incision". In reality it is the median alveolar concentration. Minimum alveolar concentration helps to predict the amount of volatile anesthetic required to immobilize the patient during surgery. Minimum alveolar concentration is a useful measure because it mirrors brain partial pressure, and allows comparisons of potency between agents. Meyer-Overton hypothesis was put forward in 1899–1901 by Hans Horst Meyer and Charles Ernest Overton. This states that the MAC of a volatile substance is inversely proportional to its lipid solubility (oil:gas coefficient), in most cases. Minimum alveolar concentration is inversely related to potency. A lower MAC value represents a more potent volatile anesthetic. This hypothesis relates the lipid solubility of an anesthetic agent **(Table 3)** with its potency (1/MAC). It suggests that onset of anesthesia occurs, when sufficient number of molecules of the anesthetic agent have dissolved in the cell's lipid membranes. Factors affecting the MAC values are shown in **Table 4**.

Minimum alveolar concentration values are additive. For example, when using 0.3 MAC of agent A and 1 MAC of agent B, the total MAC achieved is 1.3 MAC. In a similar way N_2O is used as a "carrier" gas to reduce the anesthetic requirement of other agents.

Minimum alveolar concentration-awake is the MAC at which an anesthetized patient responds appropriately to verbal commands like "open your eyes" or "show your tongue". MAC-awake helps to predict the minimum anesthetic required to prevent anesthesia awareness in paralyzed patients. For volatile anesthetics, MAC-awake is generally about one-third of MAC, but for N_2O, MAC-awake is about two-third of MAC.

The MAC_{95} is the MAC that prevents movement in roughly 95% of patients and it is equal to 1.3 times of MAC.

TABLE 3: Anesthetic volatile agents and their minimum alveolar concentration values.

Anesthetic agent	*Minimum alveolar concentration value*
Chloroform	0.5
Halothane	0.75
Isoflurane	1.15
Enflurane	1.70
Diethyl ether	1.9
Sevoflurane	2.00
Desflurane	6.00
Xenon	71
Nitrous oxide	104

TABLE 4: Factors affecting the minimum alveolar concentration values.

Factors increasing MAC	*Factors decreasing MAC*
Hyperthermia	Hypothermia
Hypercapnia	Hypothyroidism
Hypernatremia	Increasing age
Chronic alcohol abuse	Acute alcohol intoxication
Thyrotoxicosis	Opioid analgesics
Sympathoadrenal stimulation	• Pregnancy • Nitrous oxide • Alpha-2 adrenergic agonist • Hypotension • Hyponatremia

(MAC: minimum alveolar concentration)

Minimum alveolar concentration-blockade of adrenergic responses (MAC-BAR) is the potency of volatile agent for ablating tachycardia and hypertension in response to noxious stimuli during anesthesia.

Strong analgesics reduce MAC-immobility and MAC-BAR. Analgesics also reduce MAC-awake if noxious stimulation is occurring simultaneously with spoken commands to test for awareness.

CONCLUSION

The ability to monitor anesthetic gas concentrations being respired by a patient under general anesthesia has made an immeasurable contribution to patient safety. These devices have changed the practice of anesthesia for the better and effective control over delivered and required concentration of expensive anesthetic gases.

REFERENCES

1. The Association of Anaesthetists of Great Britain and Ireland. Recommendations for standards of monitoring during anaesthesia and recovery, 4th edition. (2007). [online] Available from http://www.aagbi.org/publications/guidelines/docs/standardsofmonitoring07.pdf [Last accessed February, 2014].
2. Caplan RA, Vistica MF, Posner KL, et al. Adverse anesthetic outcomes arising from gas delivery equipment: a closed claims analysis. Anesthesiology. 1997;87(4):741-8.
3. Block FE, McDonald JS. Sidestream versus mainstream carbon dioxide analyzers. J Clin Monit. 1992;8(2):139-41.

4. Jaffe MB. Carbon dioxide measurement. In: Gravenstein JS, Jaffe MB, Paulus DA (Eds). Capnography: Clinical Aspects. Cambridge: Cambridge University Press; 2004. pp. 399-412.
5. Bansal S, Solanki SL, Yadav R. An unsual foreign body in breathing circuit detected by capnography. Anesth Essays Res. 2011;5(2):245-6.
6. Meriläinen PT. A fast differential paramagnetic O_2-sensor. Int J Clin Monit Comput. 1988;5(3):187-95.
7. Meriläinen PT. A differential paramagnetic sensor for breath-by-breath oximetry. J Clin Monit. 1990;6(1):65-73.
8. Gas monitoring and the standard of care in the OR. Health Devices. 1990;19(7):207-35.
9. Overview of oxygen monitors. Technol Anesth. 2004;24:1-2.
10. American Society for Testing and Materials. Medical electrical equipment—particular requirements for the basic safety and essential performances of respiratory gas monitors (ASTM/ISO 21647). West Conshohocken, PA; 2005.
11. International Standards Organization. Medical electrical equipment: Particular requirements for basic safety and essential performance of respiratory gas monitors. Geneva, Switzerland. (2004). [online] Available from http://webstore.iec.ch/preview/info_iso80601-2-55%7Bed1.0%7Den.pdf [Last accessed February, 2014].
12. Tinker JH, Dull DL, Caplan RA, et al. Role of monitoring devices in prevention of anesthetic mishaps: a closed claims analysis. Anesthesiology. 1989;71(4):541-6.
13. Cote CJ, Liu LM, Szyfelbein SK, et al. Intraoperative events diagnosed by expired carbon dioxide monitoring in children. Can Anaesth Soc J. 1986;33(3 Pt 1):315-20.
14. Brown ML. End-tidal carbon dioxide monitoring in the detection of anesthesia-related critical incidents. AANA J. 1992;60(1): 33-40.
15. Kalenda Z. Mastering Infrared Capnography. The Netherlands: Kerckebosch-Zeist; 1989.
16. Kennell EM, Andrews RW, Wollman H. Correction factors for nitrous oxide in the infrared analysis of carbon dioxide. Anesthesiology. 1973;39(4):441-3.
17. Tremper KK, Barker SJ. Fundamental principles of monitoring instrumentation. In: Miller RD (Ed). Anesthesia, 3rd edition. New York: Churchill Livingstone; 1990. pp. 957-99.
18. Wilner D, Weissman C. Carbon dioxide production and anesthesia. In: Gravenstein JS, Jaffe MB, Paulus DA (Eds). Capnography: Clinical Aspects. Cambridge: Cambridge University Press; 2004. pp. 231-40.
19. Wahba RW, Tessler MJ, Beique F, et al. Changes in pCO_2 with acute changes in cardiac index. Can J Anaesth. 1996;43(3): 243-5.
20. Nakagawa Y, Weil MH, Jin X, et al. $ETCO_2$ as non-invasive indicator of cardiac output during hemorrhagic shock. Crit Care Med. 1997;25:A132.
21. Sayre MR, O'Connor RE, Atkins DL, et al. 2010 American Heart Association Guidelines for Cardiopulmonary Resuscitation and Emergency Cardiovascular Care Science. Circulation. 2010;122:S657-64.
22. Goode JG, Gumnit RY, Carel WD, et al. Hypercapnia during laser arthroscopy of the knee. Anesthesiology. 1990;73(3): 551-3.
23. Krauss B, Deykin A, Lam A, et al. Capnogram shape in obstructive lung disease. Anesth Analg. 2005;100(3):884-8.
24. Bissinger U, Lenz G. Capnographic detection of diaphragm movements ("curare clefts") during complete vecuronium neuromuscular block of the adductor pollicis muscle. Anesth Analg. 1993;77(6):1303-4.
25. Srinivasa V, Kodali BS, Hartigan PM. Evolving capnograms after single lung transplant. Anesth Analg. 2004;98(5):1504.
26. Williams EL, Jellish WS, Modica PA, et al. Capnography in a patient after single lung transplantation. Anesthesiology. 1991;74(3):621-2.
27. Solanki SL, Doctor JR, Patil VP, Rana M. Positive end-expiratory pressure valve malfunctioning detected by capnography and airway pressure waveform. Ann Card Anaesth. 2014;17:255-7.
28. Gravenstein JS, Paulus DA. Clinical perspectives. In: Gravenstein JS, Jaffe MB, Paulus DA (Eds). Capnography: Clinical Aspects. Cambridge: Cambridge University Press; 2004. pp. 3-12.

Bispectral Index

Ajit C Pillai

ABSTRACT

The bispectral index (BIS) is used for monitoring depth of anesthesia using a proprietary algorithm derived from complex electroencephalogram (EEG) parameters. Various studies over the years have suggested its clinical use in preventing intraoperative awareness and guiding the anesthetist to administer hypnotic drugs especially in high-risk patients. It also decreases the requirement of intraoperative anesthetic drug besides facilitating early extubation and postoperatively decreasing the recovery time and the incidence of postoperative nausea and vomiting, delirium and cognitive dysfunction. Though recent studies have questioned these benefits, its use as a valuable tool to preventing intraoperative awareness and recall is finding widespread acceptance all over the world and its scope is gradually increasing beyond the operating room to critical care units and others locations where anesthesia services are provided like the endoscopy suite, radiology, dental offices and emergency units.

Bispectral index algorithm is undergoing constant modifications but may be affected by certain factors such as electrical and mechanical interference, limitations of the equipment, certain clinical states and may not accurately reflect the hypnotic state when used with certain agents (nitrous oxide, ketamine, opioids) and should be interpreted with caution and interpreted taking into account other clinical factors and data. Large scale prospective randomized control trials are required to validate the various clinical correlations, both in and outside the operating room, and appropriate guidelines drawn up to help anesthetists apply and interpret this information.

INTRODUCTION

The bispectral monitoring system was introduced for clinical use in October 1996 (Aspect Medical Systems Inc., later acquired by Covidien in 2009), as a technique of measuring the depth of anesthesia induced by hypnotics and sedatives.

In 2004, bispectral index (BIS) was approved by the United States Food and Drug Administration (FDA) as a technique for monitoring the depth of anesthesia and reducing the incidence of intraoperative awareness during general anesthesia.

HISTORY AND DEVELOPMENT

Since the late 1930s, studies have suggested a link between the measured electrical activity of the brain and the electroencephalogram (EEG) and the changes produced by anesthetic agents.[1]

Bispectral analysis is the statistical study of phenomena made at two wavelengths of nonlinear character. The BIS index derives data from a complex EEG parameter combining several variables from the frequency domain (power spectrum, bispectrum, beta ratio, SyncFastSlow) and time domain (burst suppression) analyzed in real time. This data is processed using a proprietary algorithm, with advanced artifact detection, developed using data from normal EEG from individuals correlating to corresponding states of hypnosis and anesthetic drug levels. The BIS index is a continuous processed multifactorial EEG parameter denoted by a dimensionless number with a range from 0 to 100. Nonanesthetized awake patients have a BIS reading between 90 and 100 and total brain cortical activity suppression (isoelectric) results in a 0 reading. Readings over 70 are suggestive of patients most likely to be conscious and probably able to follow verbal commands and the ability to recall events during the procedure. The optimal suggested BIS value for general anesthesia with low probability of explicit recall and nonresponsive to verbal stimulus is between 40 and 60. A BIS value below 40 corresponds to deep sedation with increasing burst suppression on the EEG signal till cortical silence (isoelectric EEG) at 0 BIS value **(Fig. 1)**.[2]

EQUIPMENT

The BIS monitoring system consists of the following components **(Fig. 2)**:

- BIS Sensor
- BISx (Digital Signal Converter and Processing Unit) with the Monitor Interface Cable and the Patient Interface Cable (PIC)
- BIS Monitor.

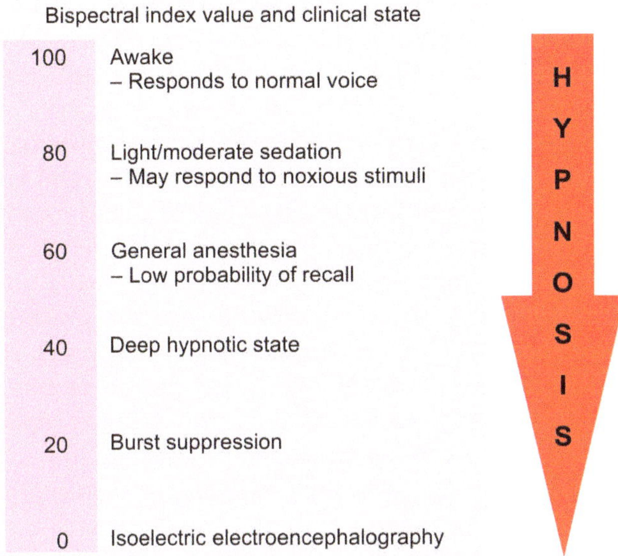

Fig. 1: Bispectral index scale of 0–100 with recommended score of 40–60 for general anesthesia and between 65 and 85 for sedation.

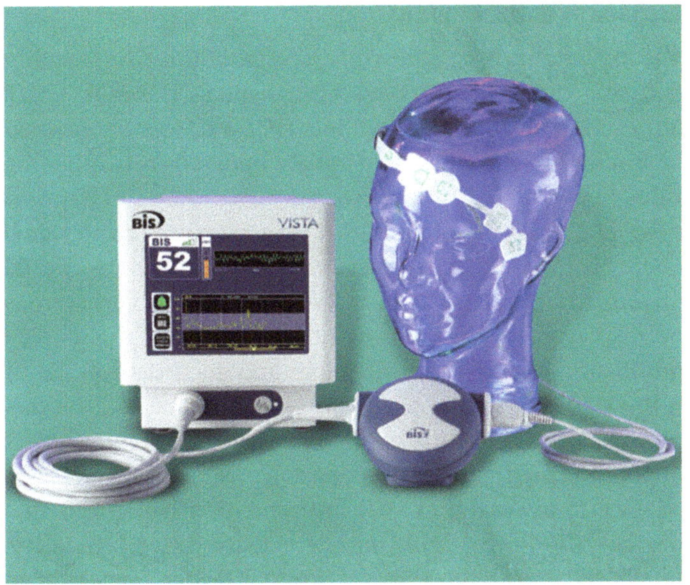

Fig. 2: Bispectral index monitor and various components.

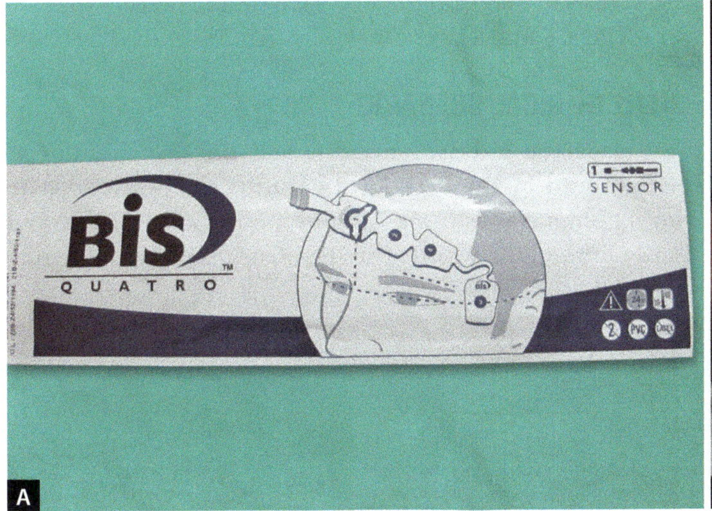

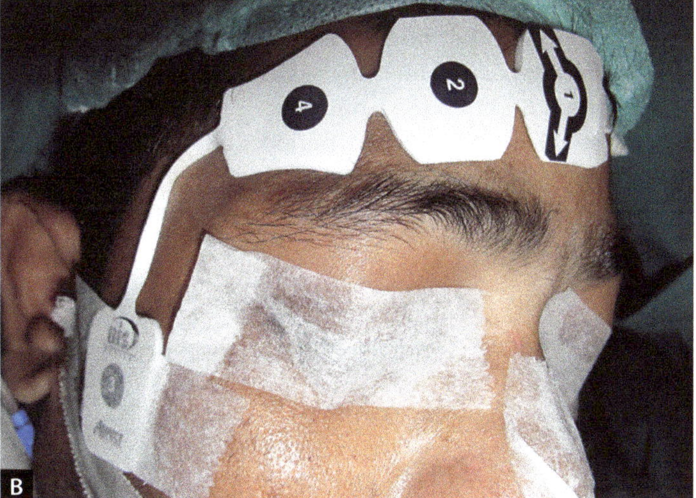

Figs. 3A and B: (A) Bispectral index sensor; (B) Sensor applied to forehead (note the position of the electrodes).

Bispectral Index Sensor

The BIS sensor is a replaceable single-use self-prepped multielectrode component. After wiping the patient's forehead with an alcohol swab and letting it dry to ensure a signal of reasonable good quality, the four electrodes are applied to the patient's forehead **(Figs. 3A and B)**. The leads correspond to the international standardized 10-20 system for location of EEG scalp electrodes as follows: lead 1—Fz (Fpz or Apz), lead 2—F3 (AF3) and lead 3—F7 (FT9 or F9). Lead 4 measures the electromyography (EMG) signal of the Frontalis muscle. The BIS Sensor connects to the BIS device through the PIC.

Bispectral Index-X Device

The BISx device consists of the digital signal converter and is the component that continuously receives and processes the patient's EEG signals. It computes the data based on the BIS algorithm while at the same time filtering detected artifacts to calculate the BIS. It also calculates other parameters such as signal quality indicator (SQI), EMG, burst count and suppression ratio (discussed in BIS monitor). These are transferred and displayed on the BIS monitor through the monitor interface cable which connects to the front of the monitor.

The BISx stores EEG parameters, including the BIS value along with the time and date of acquisition for approximately 1,200 hours and the data may be acquired to view the BISx history for a specific case.

The BISx device is placed close to the patients head to prevent interference of the EEG signal from other medical equipment.

Bispectral Index Monitor

The BIS monitor is a touch screen monitor, which, other than the numeric BIS value also displays the SQI, EMG, burst count and suppression ratio **(Fig. 4)**. Most parameters including the BIS are continuously updated to display the value in real time.

Signal quality indicator (SQI) is a measure of the signal quality for the EEG channel source and is calculated based on impedance data, artifact, and other variables. It may be displayed in bar form or numerically and higher SQI numbers indicate a more reliable and accurate BIS value. If the signal quality is poor, the BIS value may not be displayed along with the other trend variables and parameters depending on the cause or artifact.

Electromyograph (EMG) indicator is a bar graph that displays the power from muscle activity (i.e., EMG in the frequency range 70–110 Hz) and indicates presence of muscle activity or other high-frequency artifacts (oscillating ventilator modes, convective warming blanket, fluid warmer, oscillating air mattress). BIS monitoring conditions are optimal when the bar is empty. A high EMG may occur as a result of pain or other noxious stimuli, lightening sedation, and/or neuromuscular blocking agent (NMB) wearing off.

Suppression ratio (SR) number is the percentage of time over the last 63 second period that the EEG signal is considered to be in suppressed state. It is a calculated parameter designed to indicate when an isoelectric (flat line) condition may exist.

Burst count (burst per minute) is another method of quantifying suppression and measured as number of EEG bursts per minute and displayed when the BIS extend sensor is used.

Depending on the monitor and the type of sensor a single or multichannel EEG maybe displayed. A BIS trend graph may also be obtained which plots the BIS values over time with a target range indicator. A unique case identification number is assigned when a new sensor is attached to the PIC and displayed for each individual case after passing the sensor check. Three ports on the back of the system allow for data transfer to an USB drive or a patient monitoring or recordkeeping system, printing and software updates as approved by the manufacturer. The monitor stores recorded trend data with time and date of acquisition for approximately 72 hours.

The newer BIS Vista™ bilateral monitoring system allows advanced monitoring capabilities with detection of hemispheric differences in the brain. It provides for four channel EEG monitoring, asymmetry indicator for differences in hemispheric EEG activity and density spectral array **(Figs. 5 and 6)**.

THE CLINICAL SCENARIO

The bispectral index monitoring was the first monitor to be approved by the FDA for measuring the hypnotic state during general anesthesia. Various models are available and in use around the world. The BIS algorithm has undergone

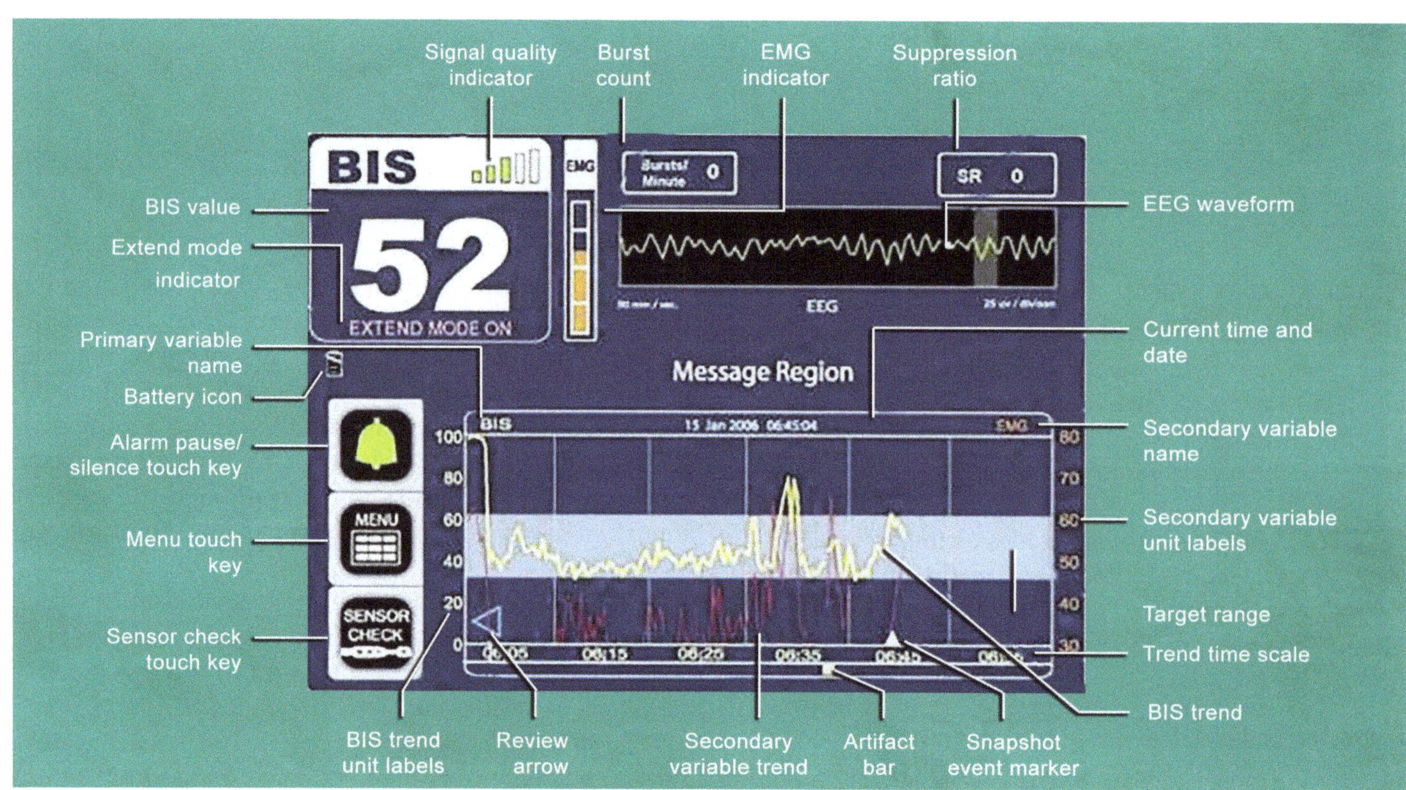

Fig. 4: Bispectral index monitor display.

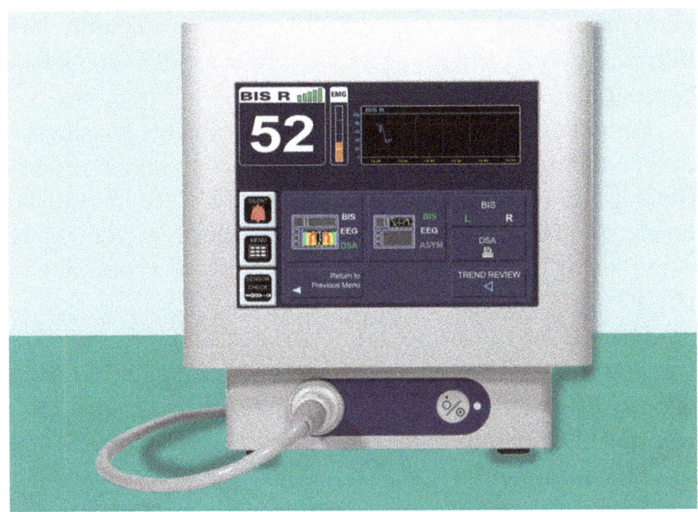

Fig. 5: Bispectral index bilateral monitoring system showing the right hemispheric electroencephalography and density spectral array.

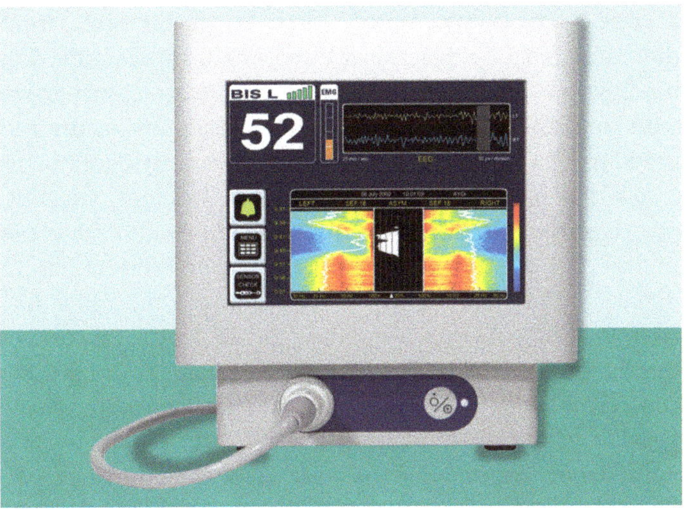

Fig. 6: Bispectral index bilateral monitoring system showing the left hemispheric electroencephalography and density spectral array.

various modifications for better performance and artefact detection.

Numerous studies over the years have suggested that BIS-guided general anesthesia (within the ranges 40–60) reduced the requirement of propofol or volatile agents, reduced the recovery time, time to extubation, early response to verbal command, duration of postanesthesia care unit (PACU) recovery and stay, postoperative delirium and cognitive dysfunction, decreased incidence of postoperative nausea and vomiting.[3-10] The cognitive dysfunction after anaesthesia (CODA) trial by Chan and colleagues concluded that BIS-guided anesthesia for major surgery reduced anesthesia requirements and decreased the risk of postoperative cognitive dysfunction (POCD) incidence by 31% and reduced postoperative delirium by 35%.[10] Radtke et al. in their study determined that intraoperative neuromonitoring is associated with a lower incidence of postoperative delirium in elderly high risk patients more than 60 years of age undergoing elective surgery, probably by avoiding extremely low (<20) BIS values but showed no significant reduction in POCD, which can probably be attributed to the similar overall average BIS levels in the study and control groups.[11] The above mentioned proof-of-concept trials and various studies[12-14] meta-analytical reviews[15] have demonstrated that optimal intraoperative management and neuromonitoring may avoid possible neurotoxic effects in vulnerable elderly patients undergoing major surgery and reduce the incidence of postoperative delirium and POCD and result in favorable postoperative outcome. A review by Klopman, et al. examined the cost-effectiveness and justified the beneficial use in every general anesthetic.[16]

However, there have also been a few conflicting studies like the "B-UNAWARE" trial, and the "BAG-RECALL" trial which found no significant difference between BIS-guided and end-tidal anesthetic concentrations (ETAC)-guided groups of patients at high risk of intraoperative awareness.[17,18] In a recent large randomized controlled trial (n = 21,601) there was no significant difference between the BIS and anesthetic concentration protocol groups with respect to intraoperative awareness to explicit recall and in terms with postoperative recovery criteria of early discharge or postoperative nausea and vomiting, or decreased anesthetic agent use. By "posthoc" analysis the study concluded that BIS monitoring may decrease intraoperative awareness compared with no intervention.[19]

FACTORS AFFECTING THE BISPECTRAL INDEX VALUE

While most studies have proven the clinical reliability of the BIS monitoring system, there are still certain circumstances that may affect its accuracy leading to BIS values inconsistent with the patient's hypnotic state.

Equipment-related Factors

Erroneous placement of the BIS sensor or lesser adherence can cause difference in the BIS values (usually false high due to elevated electrode impedance).[20]

Newer versions of BIS (BIS-XP version 4.0) gave lower readings compared to the older versions when used concomitantly in patients in two recent studies.[20-23] This could be as a result of the difference and modifications made in the BIS algorithm in the newer versions to reduce the interferences, reduce the level of noise and EMG activity. Also the concomitant use of two BIS-XP monitors gave 10% variability in the readings in the same patient.[24] This suggests a lack of consistent intrapatient reproducibility. There is also a time lag range of 14–155 seconds to update the BIS levels and this could limit the efficiency of the monitor in the period of transition from an awake state to the unconsciousness and vice versa.[25]

The electromyographic activity (especially from the patients facial or forehead muscles) can affect the BIS readings and often low frequency EMG signals may interfere with the EEG signals, causing a false elevation in the BIS reading.[22,26] This increase in the muscle activity could be as a result of pain, other noxious stimuli, twitches, seizures, or eye movement. The recent modifications and advances in the BIS algorithm have taken into consideration to decrease these factors from interfering with the BIS value. Also, the EMG bar on the monitor gives a good indication of the muscle activity. Higher the EMG, greater is the muscle activity and greater the chances of the BIS value being falsely elevated. Clinically this may indicate that the patient may be more deeply sedated than what is reflected on the displayed BIS value. The anesthetist may be required to take into account other factors such as SQI, the BIS trend, and other clinical parameters to make a decision and subsequent administration or top up of neuromuscular blocking drugs (NMBD) may reduce the EMG activity (and the BIS) without changing the patient's level of sedation. Kim et al. in their study on effects of neuromuscular blockade reversal agents noted an increase in both BIS and EMG values, irrespective of the reversal agent used and inferred it is difficult to determine if the BIS value is true reflection of the arousal state or correlating to the raised EMG.[27] The interpretation of BIS value needs to be applied carefully to measure depth of monitoring after administration of neuromuscular blockade reversal drugs.

Anesthetic or Clinical Factors

Certain drugs routinely used in anesthesia may affect the BIS values. Drugs such as Ketamine, Nitrous Oxide (N_2O), Etomidate may result in either no alteration or an elevation in the BIS values.

Nitrous oxide has weak cortical action and at concentrations ranging from 50 to 70% does not change the BIS value.[28] In volunteers receiving target controlled infusions (TCI) of propofol[20,29] and patients receiving propofol and remifentanil,[20,30] the addition of N_2O decreased the response to laryngoscopy and tracheal intubation without affecting the BIS value. Rampil et al. in their study confirmed the unchanged BIS level with N_2O but noted in some individuals a paradoxical decrease in the BIS after N_2O was withdrawn.[28] This was attributed to a unique suppression phenomenon after the sudden withdrawal of N_2O characterized by low frequency EEG activity.

Ketamine in doses ranging from 0.25 to 0.5 mg/kg, a rapid bolus shows a rise in the BIS value in anesthetized patients receiving propofol or sevoflurane, with deepening of the hypnotic state.[31,32] Ketamine causes an increase in high frequency EEG activity reflecting the high BIS value.

Etomidate, when used for induction of anesthesia, frequently causes myoclonus and hence raised EMG activity and can display a falsely high BIS value. Significantly, the decrease in BIS values reflected hypnotic levels better when compared to spectral entropy.[33]

Equipotent concentrations of different volatile anesthetics reflect different BIS values at equipotent concentrations (halothane > sevoflurane > isoflurane).[34] Care should be taken to prevent an inadvertent overdose of halothane when using a BIS monitor in such cases, especially in children and infants.[34,35]

There is also a case report of paradoxical increase in BIS values on increasing the concentration of isoflurane from 0.79 to 1.26% due to the increase in high frequency EEG waveform, and return to baseline levels after decreasing the concentration.[36]

Opioid receptors are mainly concentrated in the subcortical structures. The hypnotic effects of Propofol is increased by the addition of opioids, resulting in decreased Propofol requirement but the reflected BIS value is higher and may lead to an inadvertent anesthetic overdose.[20,37,38] BIS values monitored during a balanced Propofol-opioid regimen can be used to detect an elevation in BIS values to noxious stimuli thus, indicating a need for higher dose of analgesics.[22]

Case reports of an increase in the BIS values (>70) after administration of Isoproterenol in response to beta adrenergic stimulation (notably without intraoperative recall) and the sudden decrease in BIS values after successive doses of Methylene Blue followed by a recovery to the pre-drug levels have been reported.[39,40]

Electrical or Mechanical Interference

Use of different electrical equipment in the operating room during surgery can affect the BIS values. Electrical interference has been reported in literature from the use of atrial pacemaker during cardiac surgeries[41] and theoretically other equipment such as electric scalpel can also cause similar interference. Recent modifications in the BIS algorithm have decreased the probability interference and clinically monitoring the SQI bar can help detect these.

There are reports of instances where the monitor did not identify the interference, creating a clinical scenario for potential anesthetic overdose. Fine vibrations of the plastic face cover of a forced air warming device against the BIS sensor causing elevated BIS values with no change in SQI or visible artifact have been reported.[42] Bose, et al. also reported a similar case with an elevated EMG value on the monitor with a negative "train of four" test.[43] BIS values decreased on placing a barrier between the plastic flap and the BIS sensor or on shutting off the device. Similar changes were noted from oscillations of the endoscopic shaver during shoulder arthroscopy[44] and from an electromagnetic field created by an ear, nose, and throat (ENT) positioning system around the head.[45] In these cases the BIS values returned to their actual reading on switching off the devices.

CLINICAL CONDITIONS AFFECTING THE BISPECTRAL INDEX VALUE

The BIS algorithm is derived empirically from statistical data processed and calculated from normal healthy individuals. In children, the nervous system is characterized by rapid development till the age of 12 years and typically reflects age dependant variability in the EEG patterns. Wang et al. suggested age as an important factor affecting BIS in children above the age of 1 year.[46] BIS values under single dose Propofol administered for induction of anesthesia showed a more rapid change in the >5 - <12-year group than in the >1 - <5-year group.

Any pathophysiological state resulting in an abnormal EEG waveform can be misinterpreted by the BIS monitoring system and the displayed BIS value may not accurately represent the clinical state of sedation.

Approximately 5–10% of the population exhibit a normal low voltage genetically determined EEG variant not associated with any cerebral dysfunction and is not recognized by the monitor.[47] It is thus important that the BIS monitor be applied before anesthetic induction.

After electroconvulsive therapy (ECT), in the post-ECT state, after eye opening is characterized by an EEG pattern similar to deep planes of anesthesia.[48] The BIS values in between 45 and 57 reflect this state of brain activity irrespective of the anesthetic agent used during emergence from anesthesia.

Other studies have shown a reduced BIS value in patients with dementia related to Alzheimer's (mean BIS 89) compared to a control population of elderly individuals (mean BIS 95) and in children with cerebral palsy compared to normal children both during anesthesia and during emergence from the anesthetic.[49,50] BIS signals are also highly vulnerable to the electrical interference or artifacts when the EEG signals are isoelectric (BIS 0 as in brain death or severe hypothermia), as demonstrated in two confirmed brain dead patients, in whom the BIS values were elevated from the misinterpretation of synchronized electrocardiogram (ECG) signals.[22,51]

BIS monitoring during two reported cases of hypovolemic cardiac arrest showed a corresponding decrease in the BIS values to 0 (isoelectric EEG).[52,53] Fluid resuscitation and restoration of arterial blood pressure returned the BIS values to prearrest status. This variation in the BIS value is related to the cerebral and brain perfusion and reflected in the hemodynamic changes occurring during asystole following cardiac arrest and also in focal ischemia, following carotid artery clamping, which resulted in decrease in the BIS value and its return to normal on restoration of blood circulation.[54,55] Hypothermia may affect BIS monitoring and values were seen to decrease by an average of 1.12 units for every degree Celsius drop in body temperature, in a study ($n = 100$), during hypothermic cardiopulmonary bypass (CPB) with isoflurane.[56] This is attributed to the pharmacokinetics of the inhalational agent (greater lipid solubility and cellular level concentration at decreasing temperature) and the linear reduction in the drug requirement and a reduction in the brain function.

Hypoglycemia causes a gradual increase in low frequency waves as the blood glucose levels decrease from 72 to 54 mg/dL. On further reduction in blood glucose levels to 32 mg/ dL, the waveform is similar to one during general anesthesia and reflected correspondingly by decreased BIS values.[57,58] In two reported cases of hypoglycemic coma, correction and return to normoglycemic levels with return of conscious state increased the BIS values to 80.[59,60] Xi et al. reported two cases under general anesthesia for diabetic retinopathy surgery with severe perioperative hypoglycemia associated with abnormally low BIS values which increased with the correction of hypoglycemia.[61]

BISPECTRAL INDEX BEYOND THE OPERATING ROOM

BIS was designed for intraoperative use to prevent awareness and improve patient outcome. It is gradually finding a wide area of practical application in some critical care units and locations outside the operating room where anesthesia services are provided like the Dental Suite, Endoscopy Suite, in Radiology and the Accident and Emergency Department to administer sedation and improve patient safety.[7] In Critical Care Units besides monitoring sedation for bedside procedures it is also used to monitor patients receiving neuromuscular blocking drugs, certain coma states (e.g., drug-induced coma), and as an adjunct to neurological examination to confirm brain activity. BIS serves as an valuable tool for monitoring patients during procedural sedation and analgesia however further trials and modifications are required to identify and prove its usefulness in various clinical situations and its effect on the patient outcome as various reports are available debating the exact nature and limitations of BIS in these settings.[7,62-66]

CONCLUSION

The BIS monitor is a valuable intraoperative tool to monitor the hypnotic state and used as guide for the administration of various drugs. Its use in clinical practice is gradually increasing all over the world with respect to preventing intraoperative awareness during anesthesia and its scope is also being widely recognized beyond the operating room—to critical care units, accident and emergency units and to office based anesthesia suites for monitoring sedation and improving patient care. Despite certain limitations in its use, it is still an valuable addendum to clinical monitoring along with other monitors and clinical data and the clinical experience of the anesthetist. Some recent studies have questioned the reliability of the use of BIS but at the same time conclude by "posthoc" analysis that BIS monitoring may decrease incidence of intraoperative awareness compared with routine care without a protocol. However, large prospective randomized clinical trials and studies are required to definitively validate its clinical usefulness with respect to BIS value and intraoperative recall and also with intermediate outcomes related to perioperative anesthetic drug administration and postoperative extubation time, nausea and vomiting, and recovery room discharge time and its use outside the operating room to provide safe anesthesia.

ACKNOWLEDGMENT

The author would like to thank "Medtronic India Pvt. Ltd." for providing technical data and contributing to the photographs **(Figs. 4 to 6)** in the article.

REFERENCES

1. Rampil IJ. A primer for EEG signals processing in anesthesia. Anesthesiology. 1998;89:980-1002.
2. BIS VISTA™ operating system manual. Aspect medical systems, Newton, Massachusetts, USA; 2008.
3. Gan TJ, Glass PS, Windsor A, et al. Bispectral index monitoring allows faster emergence and improved recovery from propofol, alfentanil, and nitrous oxide anesthesia. BIS Utility Study Group. Anesthesiology. 1997;87:808-15.
4. Guignard B, Coste C, Menigaux C, et al. Reduced isoflurane consumption with bispectral index monitoring. Acta Anaesthesiologica Scandinavica. 2001;45:308-14.
5. Lehmann A, Boldt J, Thaler E, et al. Bispectral index in patients with target-controlled or manually controlled infusion of propofol. Anesth Analg. 2002;95:639-44.
6. Liu SS. Effects of bispectral index monitoring on ambulatory anesthesia: a meta-analysis of randomized controlled trials and a cost analysis. Anesthesiology. 2004;101:311-5.
7. Johansen J. Update on BIS. Best Prac Res Clin Anaesthesiol. 2006;20:81-99.
8. Oliveira CR, Bernardo WM, Nunes VM. Benefit of general anesthesia monitored by bispectral index compared with monitoring guided only by clinical parameters. Systematic review and meta-analysis. Rev Bras Anestesiol. 2017;67(1):72-84.
9. Chiang MH, Wu SC, Hsu SW, Chin JC. Bispectral Index and non-Bispectral Index anesthetic protocols on postoperative recovery outcomes. Minerva Anestesiol. 2018;84(2):216-28.
10. Chan MT, Cheng BC, Lee TM, Gin T. BIS-guided anesthesia decreases postoperative delirium and cognitive decline. J Neurosurg Anesthesiol. 2013;25:33-42.
11. Radtke FM, Franck M, Lendner J, Kruger S, Wernecke KD, Spies CD. Monitoring depth of anaesthesia in a randomized trial decreases the rate of postoperative delirium but not postoperative cognitive dysfunction. Br J Anaesth. 2013;110(Suppl. 1):i98-105.
12. Ballard C, Jones E, Gauge N, et al. Optimised anaesthesia to reduce postoperative cognitive decline (POCD) in older patients undergoing elective surgery, a randomised controlled trial. PLoS One. 2012;7:e37410.
13. Fedorow C, Grocott HP. Cerebral monitoring to optimize outcomes after cardiac surgery. Curr Opin Anaesthesiol. 2010;23: 89-94.
14. Rundshagen I, Hardt T, Cortina K, et al. Narcotrend-assisted propofol/remifentanil anaesthesia vs clinical practice: does it make a difference? Br J Anaesth. 2007;99:686-93.
15. Bocskai T, Kovács M, Szakács Z, et al. Is the bispectral index monitoring protective against postoperative cognitive decline? A systematic review with metaanalysis. PLoS ONE. 2020;15(2): e0229018.
16. Klopman MA, Sebel PS. Cost-effectiveness of bispectral index monitoring. Curr Opin Anaesthesiol. 2011;24(2):177-81.
17. Avidan MS, Zhang L, Burnside B, et al. Anesthesia awareness and the bispectral index. New Engl J Med. 2008;358:1097-108.
18. Avidan MS, Jacobsohn E, Glick D, et al. Prevention of intraoperative awareness in a high-risk surgical population. New Engl J Med. 2011;365:591-600.
19. Mashour GA, Shanks A, Tremper KK, et al. Prevention of intraoperative awareness with explicit recall in an unselected surgical population. Anesthesiology. 2012;117:717-25.
20. Duarte LT, Saraiva RA. When the bispectral index can give false results. Rev Bras Anesthesiol. 2009;59(1):99-101.
21. Dahaba AA, Mattweber M, Fuchs A, et al. Effects of different stages of neuromuscular block on the bispectral index and the bispectral index-XP under remifentanil propofol anaesthesia. Anesth Analg. 2004;99:781-7.
22. Dahaba AA. Different conditions that could result in the bispectral index indicating an incorrect hypnotic state. Anesth Analg. 2005;101:765-73.
23. Tonner PH, Wei C, Bein B, et al. Comparison of two bispectral index algorithms in monitoring sedation in postoperative intensive care patients. Crit Care Med. 2005;33:580-4.
24. Niedhart D, Kaiser H, Jacobsohn E, et al. Intrapatient reproducibility of the BISxp monitor. Anesthesiology. 2006;104:242-8.
25. Pilge S, Zanner R, Schneider G, et al. Time delay of index calculation: analysis of cerebral state, bispectral and narcotrend indices. Anesthesiology. 2006;104:488-94.
26. Baldesi O, Bruder N, Velly L, et al. Spurious bispectral index values due to electromyographic activity. Eur J Anaesthesiol. 2004;21:324-5.
27. Kim D, Ahn JH, Jung H, et al. Effects of neuromuscular blockade reversal on bispectral index and frontal electromyogram during steady-state desflurane anesthesia: a randomized trial. Sci Rep. 2019;9:10486.
28. Rampil IJ, Kim JS, Lenhardt R, et al. Bispectral EEG index during nitrous oxide administration. Anesthesiology. 1998;89:671-7.
29. Kearse LA, Rosow C, Zaslavsky A, et al. Bispectral analysis of the electroencephalogram predicts conscious processing of information during propofol sedation and hypnosis. Anesthesiology. 1998;88:25-34.
30. Coste C, Guignard B, Menigaux C, et al. Nitrous oxide prevents movement during orotracheal intubation without affecting BIS value. Anesth Analg. 2000;91:130-5.
31. Hans P, Dewandre PY, Brichant JF, et al. Comparative effects of ketamine on bispectral index and spectral entropy of the electroencephalogram under sevoflurane anaesthesia. Br J Anaesth. 2005;94:336-40.
32. Vereecke HE, Struys MM, Mortier EP. A comparison of bispectral index and ARX-derived auditory evoked potential index in measuring the clinical interaction between ketamine and propofol anaesthesia. Anaesthesia. 2003;58:957-61.
33. Kim HM, Shin SW, Yoon JY, et al. Effects of etomidate on bispectral index scale and spectral entropy during induction of anesthesia by means of the raw electroencephalographic and electromyographic characteristics. Korean J Anesthesiol. 2012;62(3):230-3.
34. Edwards JJ, Soto RG, Thrush DM, et al. Bispectral index scale is higher for halothane than sevoflurane during intraoperative anesthesia. Anesthesiology. 2003;99:1453-5.
35. Davidson AJ, Czarnecki C. The bispectral index in children: comparing isoflurane and halothane. Br J Anaesth. 2004;92:14-7.
36. Detsch O, Schneider G, Kochs E, et al. Increasing isoflurane concentration may cause paradoxical increases in the EEG bispectral index in surgical patients. Br J Anaesth. 2000;84:33-7.
37. Struys MM, Vereecke H, Moerman A, et al. Ability of the bispectral index, autoregressive modelling with exogenous input

derived auditory evoked potentials, and predicted propofol concentrations to measure patient responsiveness during anesthesia with propofol and remifentanil. Anesthesiology. 2003;99:802-12.

38. Lysakowski C, Dumont L, Pellegrini M, et al. Effects of fentanyl, alfentanil, remifentanil and sufentanil on loss of consciousness and bispectral index during propofol induction of anaesthesia. Br J Anaesth. 2001;86:523-7.
39. Matthews R. Isoproterenol-induced elevated bispectral indexes while undergoing radiofrequency ablation: a case report. AANA J. 2006;74:193-5.
40. Matisoff AJ, Panni MK. Methylene blue treatment for methemoglobinemia and subsequent dramatic bispectral index reduction. Anesthesiology. 2006;105:228.
41. Gallagher JD. Pacer-induced artefact in the bispectral index during cardiac surgery. Anesthesiology. 1999;90:636.
42. Hemmerling TM, Fortier JD. Falsely increased bispectral index values in a series of patients undergoing cardiac surgery using forced-air-warming therapy of the head. Anesth Analg. 2002;95:322-3.
43. Bose S, Lewis B, Farag E. Interference with BIS™ values from a forced-air warming device. Br J Anaesth. 2012;108(1):168.
44. Hemmerling TM, Migneault B. Falsely increased bispectral index during endoscopic shoulder surgery attributed to interferences with the endoscopic shaver device. Anesth Analg. 2002;95: 1678-9.
45. Hemmerling TM, Desrosiers M. Interference of electromagnetic operating systems in otorhinolaryngology surgery with bispectral index monitoring. Anesth Analg. 2003;96:1698-9.
46. Wang F, Zhang J, Yu J, et al. Variation of bispectral index in children aged 1-12 years under propofol anesthesia: an observational study. BMC Anesthesiol. 2019;19:145.
47. Schnider TW, Luginbuehl M, Petersen-Felix S, et al. Unreasonably low bispectral index values in a volunteer with genetically determined low-voltage electroencephalographic signal. Anesthesiology. 1998;89:1607-8.
48. Gunawardane PO, Murphy PA, Sleigh JW. Bispectral index monitoring during electroconvulsive therapy. Anesth Analg. 2002;88:184-7.
49. Renna M, Handy J, Shah A. Low baseline bispectral index of the electroencephalogram in patients with dementia. Anesth Analg. 2003;96:1380-5.
50. Choudhry DK, Brenn BR. Bispectral index monitoring: a normal children and children with quadriplegic cerebral palsy. Anesth Analg. 2002;95:1582-5.
51. Myles PS, Cairo S. Artifact in the bispectral index in a patient with severe ischemic brain injury. Anesth Analg. 2004;98:706-7.
52. Engl MR. The changes in bispectral index during a hypovolemic cardiac arrest. Anesthesiology. 1999;91:1947-9.
53. Azim N, Wang CY. The use of bispectral index during a cardio pulmonary arrest: a potential predictor of cerebral perfusion. Anaesthesia. 2004;59:610-2.
54. Merat S, Levecque JP, Le Gulluche Y, et al. BIS monitoring may allow the detection of severe cerebral ischemia. Can J Anaesth. 2001;48:1066-9.
55. Billard V. Brain injury under anesthesia: is monitoring of the EEG helpful? Can J Anaesth. 2001;48:1055-60.
56. Mathew JP, Weatherwax KJ, East CJ, et al. Bispectral analysis during cardiopulmonary bypass: the effect of hypothermia on the hypnotic state. J Clin Anaesth. 2001;13:301-5.
57. Bjorgaas M, Sand T, Vik T, et al. Quantitative EEG during controlled hypoglycemia in diabetic and non-diabetic children. Diabet Med. 1998;15:30-7.
58. Tribl G, Howorka K, Heger G, et al. EEG topography during insulin-induced hypoglycemia in patients with insulin dependent diabetes mellitus. Eur Neurol. 1996;36:303-9.
59. Wu CC, Lin CS, Mok MS. Bispectral index monitoring during hypoglycemic coma. J Clin Anesth. 2002;14:305-6.
60. Vivien B, Langeron O, Riou B. Increase in bispectral index (BIS) while correcting a severe hypoglycemia. Anesth Analg. 2002;95:1824-5.
61. Xi C, Pan C, Li T. Abnormally low bispectral index and severe hypoglycemia during maintenance of and recovery from general anesthesia in diabetic retinopathy surgery: Two case reports. BMC Anesthesiology. 2018;18:45.
62. Bigham C, Bigham S, Jones C. Does the bispectral index monitor have a role in intensive care? JICS. 2012;13(4):314-9.
63. Haenggi M, Ypparila-Wolters H, Hauser K, et al. Intra- and inter individual variation of BIS-index® and Entropy® during controlled sedation with midazolam/remifentanil and dexmedetomidine/ remifentanil in healthy volunteers: an interventional study. Crit Care. 2009;13:R20. Also available online from http://ccforum.com/content/13/1/R20.
64. Vivien B, Di Maria S, Ouattara A, et al. Overestimation of bispectral index in sedated intensive care unit patients revealed by administration of muscle relaxant. Anesthesiology. 2003;99: 9-17.
65. Frenzel D, Greim CA, Sommer C, et al. Is the bispectral index appropriate for monitoring the sedation level of mechanically ventilated surgical ICU patients? Intensive Care Med. 2002; 28:178-83.
66. Tonner PH, Wei C, Bein B, et al. Comparison of two bispectral index algorithms in monitoring sedation in postoperative intensive care patients. Crit Care Med. 2005;33:580-4.

Temperature Regulation and Patient Warming Devices

Satish K Kulkarni, Aaliya Mehmood

ABSTRACT

Mild hypothermia is common during general as well as regional anesthesia and has been associated with perioperative complications and poor outcomes. It is important and reasonable to monitor and maintain normothermia in the perioperative period and improve the quality of care and outcomes. Principles of monitoring equipment, sites and devices available in our practice for maintenance of temperature are discussed.

INTRODUCTION

Human body core temperature, i.e., temperature of the deep tissues of the body is maintained within a very narrow limit, i.e., 36.5–37.5°C under various physiological and environmental variations by a central servomechanism in the posterior hypothalamus of the brain.[1] In contrast the peripheral or skin temperature can vary as per the environmental temperature and surrounding conditions. Temperature measurement is one of the vital parameters monitored on the wards in all patients and changes in temperature and the pattern of change can be useful in diagnosis and management of the patients. Fever is a very common symptom for which medical help is sought for and is associated with infective as well as various inflammatory conditions.

Temperature regulation is one of the most finely tuned controlled mechanisms with afferent receptors and pathways, central thermostat control, i.e., temperature regulation center and the efferent pathways and mechanisms. It is a very important to maintain core temperature within a very narrow limit for optimal functioning of the sensitive enzyme systems in the core organs. The afferent pathways consist of various sensory inputs from the warm and cold receptors from the skin, spinal cord, brain and the various deep tissues of the human body. The sensory input is integrated in the hypothalamus and when a threshold is reached for a particular stimulus or change in the sensory input, the effecter responses are initiated.

The most important early effect or responses are the behavioral changes (e.g., moving away from an adverse environmental surrounding or dressing appropriately). The physiological effector responses are mainly by the autonomic nervous system. In response to the detection of cold, there is generalized vasoconstriction to prevent loss of heat from periphery and shivering to generate heat. Piloerection is important in animals.

The endocrine system and the hormone thyroxine are important in chronic exposure in cold environments. Nonshivering thermogenesis by metabolism of brown adipose tissue is an important mechanism to maintain temperature in neonates and infants. In response to the increase in temperature, vasodilatation and sweating are important autonomic responses to lose heat and reduce body temperature.

In the perioperative period especially intraoperative, unintentional and inadvertent hypothermia is common and to an extent preventable. Intraoperatively core temperature decrease has been associated with poor surgical outcomes.[2] The problems of increase in cardiac morbidity[3] in the postoperative period, increase in bleeding and transfusion requirements,[4] increase in surgical site skin infections[5] and delayed recovery[6] with cost implications have been well documented. Patients remember the discomfort and shivering when awake in the recovery area and is one of the reasons, apart from pain, nausea and vomiting, associated with dissatisfaction of the overall surgical experience. Shivering also interferes with monitoring in the recovery ward.

The decrease in the core temperature intraoperatively follows a typical pattern[7] and in the first 20–30 minutes, there is rapid fall in the core temperature by 1–2°C. This is mainly because of peripheral vasodilatation induced by anesthetic drugs and redistribution of core body heat to periphery. The abolition of behavioral responses and shivering under anesthesia, the effects of anesthetic drugs on central regulatory control by changes in response thresholds, exposure to cold in the operating room environment, cold intravenous and antiseptic fluids, and evaporative losses from surgical site contributes to the decrease in core temperature. The laminar airflow in the modern operating theaters contributes to convection losses. The initial drop is followed by linear decrease in the core temperature as heat loss exceeds heat production. Later core temperature stabilizes and decreases very slowly or starts to increase gradually if measures are being taken to maintain temperature or warm the patient.

Monitoring of core temperature is not common during regional anesthesia. Regional anesthesia is also associated with decrease of core temperature especially spinal and epidural anesthesia and is because of peripheral and central impairment of thermoregulatory control.[8] However, regional anesthesia alters perception of cold and patients feel warm. The thermoregulatory central control misinterprets skin temperature as increased in the blocked area. Concomitant addition of sedative drugs contributes as well to impair central regulatory mechanisms.[8]

TEMPERATURE MEASUREMENT PRINCIPLES[9]

- *Mercury thermometer:* Mercury glass thermometers are slow and cumbersome and have been replaced by electronic systems in clinical practice. Spilled mercury is also a biohazard. However, they are still used for laboratory calibration of other systems.[10]
- *Thermistor, e.g., pulmonary artery catheter tip:* A small bead of semiconductor which can be covered by plastic or stainless steel and can be sterilized chemically. The electrical resistance changes in the bead nonlinearly with temperature and the signal is made linear electronically. The response time is rapid. However, the resistance can change over time and needs recalibration.
- *Infrared thermometer, e.g., tympanic membrane thermometer:* A small probe with a disposable transparent cover receives infrared radiation from the tympanic membrane. The signal is converted into an electrical signal. Such probes are accurate but provide intermittent readings. Wax in the ear can affect the accuracy. Also, they must be accurately aimed at the tympanic membrane. These infrared technology-based screening devices are extensively being used during the COVID-19 pandemic.
- *Thermocouples, e.g., skin temperature sensors:* They are based on the Seeback effect. They are two strips of dissimilar metals of different specific heats and in contact at both ends. The metals expand and contract to different degrees with change in temperature and the electrical potential generated is compared to a reference junction. The current produced is directly proportional to the temperature difference between the two junctions and it is measured and amplified. Response time is rapid, stable and measurement is accurate to 0.1°C.
- *Zero heat flux (ZHF) thermometry:* In well-perfused parts of the body, tissue temperature slightly below the skin surface reasonably approximates core temperature; based on this principle, ZHF thermometry's specially designed sensor which consists of two thermometers, separated by an insulator and covered by a heater which is based on servo-controlled mechanism creates an isothermic tunnel between the skin surface and the subcutaneous tissue where the temperature correlates well with the core temperature **(Figs. 1 and 2)**.[11]

TEMPERATURE MONITORING SITES[9-13]

Ideally temperature measurements perioperatively should be from the same sites in the pre-, intra- and postoperative period. However, no single site can be used accurately and constantly during the perioperative period.

- *Skin (surface) temperature:* Axilla is the preferred site for skin and muscle temperature making it suitable for detecting malignant hyperthermia and validity of peripheral neuromuscular monitors.
- *Core temperature*
  - *Temporal artery thermometer:* Temporal temperature scanner gives a quick, noninvasive and easy method of core temperature measurement. These are based on infrared radiation detection. Measurements are intermittent and unreliable and various studies do not support their use in the perioperative period.
  - *Tympanic membrane:* It correlates well with core esophageal and brain temperatures. May not be always accurate. The auditory canal needs to be free from wax. The readings are intermittent and may be useful in the recovery rooms.
  - *Nasopharynx:* The temperature probe should be positioned just behind the soft palate. Gives a good estimate of the core temperature. These are prone to inaccurate results if positioning is incorrect because of ambient temperature or expired tracheal gases if there is leak around the endotracheal tube.
  - *Esophageal:* Accurately reflects the core temperature when positioned in the lower third of the esophagus. May not be accurate during a thoracotomy.
  - *Rectal:* The detected temperature can be higher than the core temperature by 0.5–1.0°C and the response time is slow. In an anesthetized patient does not reflect core temperature accurately where temperature changes can be rapid.
  - *Blood:* Measured by the pulmonary artery catheter tip positioned in the pulmonary circulation. It is the best estimate of core temperature. Pulmonary artery catheterization is an invasive procedure.
  - *Bladder:* Foley's catheters with a temperature sensor are available in various sizes to monitor urine flow and temperature. High urine flow is necessary for accurate reflection of core temperature.
  - *Forehead:* A single use, ZHF technology based specially designed sensor is applied on the forehead (above left eyebrow). It reliably and accurately estimates core temperature as per published studies. It is a noninvasive, easy-to-use temperature monitoring site that continuously measures patient's core body temperature throughout the perioperative journey.[11]

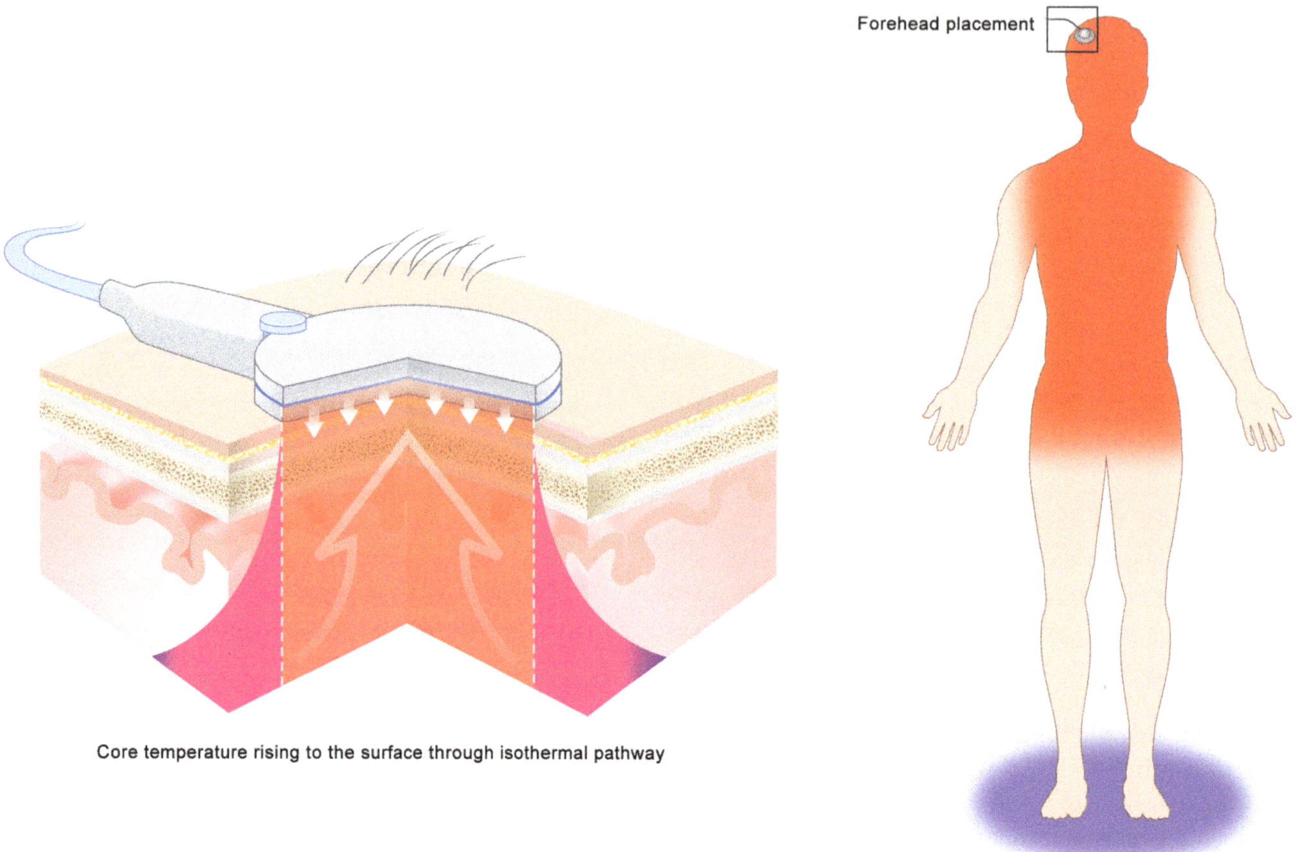

Fig. 1: Principle of zero heat flux thermometry (3M™ Bair Hugger™).

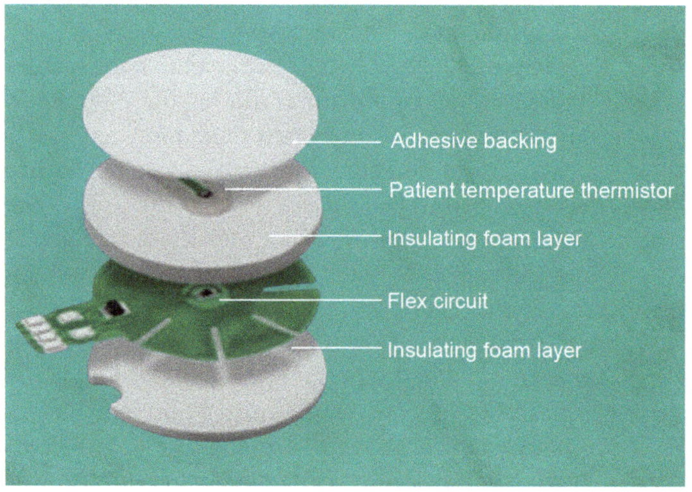

Fig. 2: Parts of zero heat flux sensor (3M™ Bair Hugger™).

TEMPERATURE MONITORING GUIDELINES

Various societies have suggested guidelines based on available data for temperature management perioperatively.

The American Society of Anesthesiologists (ASA) recommends that, "every patient receiving anesthesia shall have temperature monitored when clinically significant changes in body temperature are intended, anticipated or suspected." The body temperature of pediatric patient shall be measured continuously.

Generally, core temperature should be monitored in most patients requiring general anesthesia for longer than 30 minutes. Efforts should be made to maintain core temperature above 36°C. Patients may be discharged from recovery rooms once normothermia is established.

WARMING DEVICES

Various devices are available for fluid warming and to monitor and maintain patient temperature in the perioperative period. Different sensors to monitor skin and esophageal or rectal temperatures and temperature monitoring modules are inbuilt or available separately with monitors **(Figs. 3 to 5)**.

Forced air warming devices are most commonly used **(Fig. 6)**. They are cost-effective and used as standard to compare other devices or technology. They are used for prewarming in the preoperative areas, intraoperatively are being used to cover the nonoperative body surface area as much as possible and are used in the recovery areas as well **(Fig. 7)**. Injuries with the use are rare and mainly because of inappropriate or incorrect use.[12] Electric heating mattresses and pads may be as effective as forced air devices.[14] Fluids should be warmed. Various inline fluid warming devices

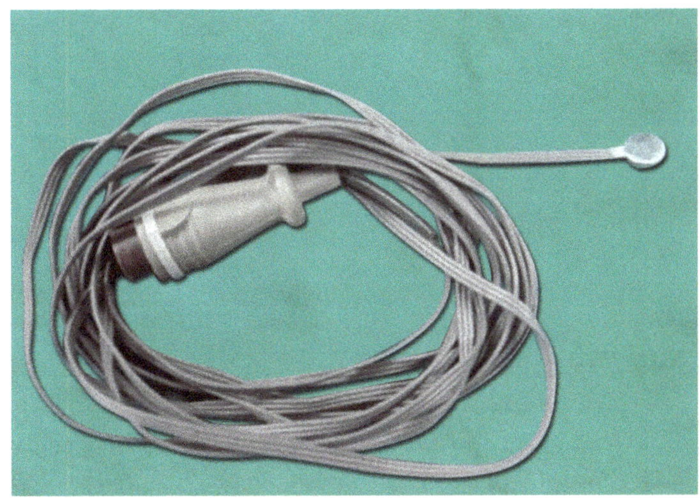

Fig. 3: Skin temperature monitoring probe.

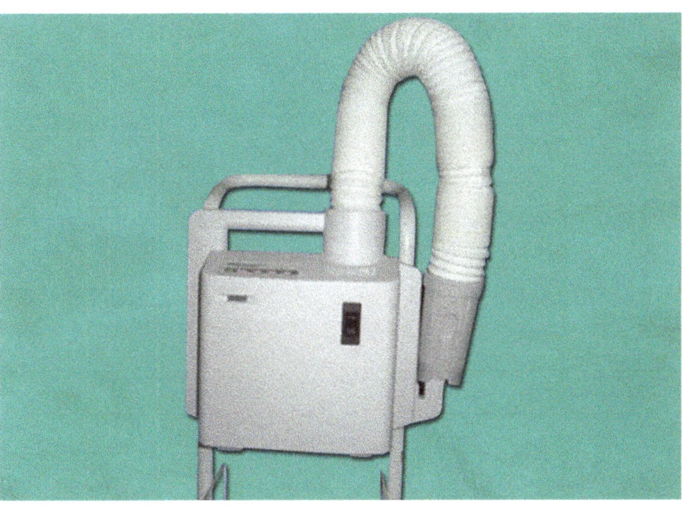

Fig. 6: Forced air warming device. It consists of an electrically operated heater blower and a disposable paper or fabric patient cover.

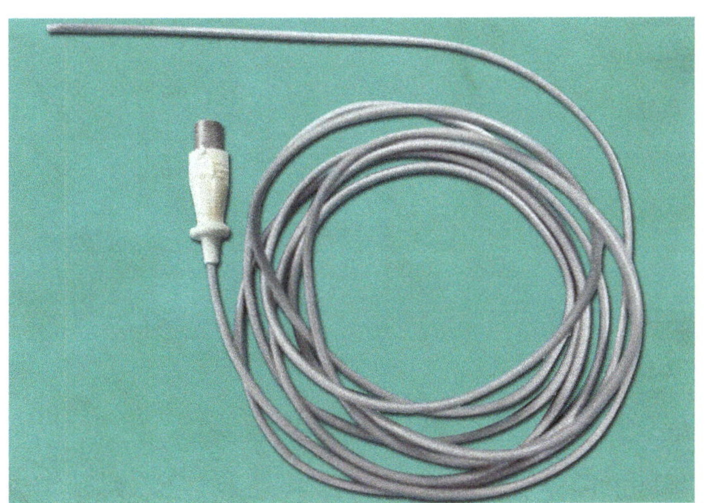

Fig. 4: Esophageal/rectal temperature monitoring probe.

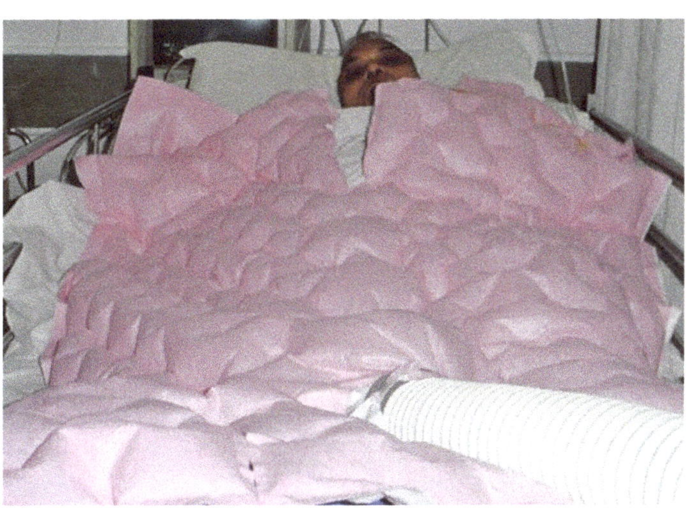

Fig. 7: Forced air device being used in recovery areas.

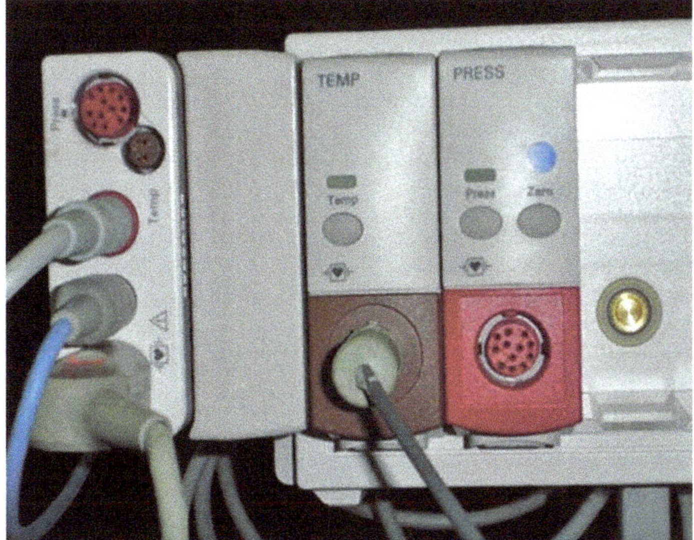

Fig. 5: Temperature monitoring module.

are available to be used according to the rate of fluid administration **(Figs. 8 to 10)**. Radiant warmers are used mainly on neonatology wards and neonatal intensive care units.

CONCLUSION

Inadvertent intraoperative hypothermia has been associated with adverse outcomes and it is reasonable to monitor temperature and maintain normothermia in surgical patients. External forced air warming devices are effective and along with fluid warming devices should be used whenever possible. Every effort should be made to improve patient comfort and reduce perioperative morbidity.

ACKNOWLEDGMENT

Figures 1 and 2 Courtesy of 3M. © 2021 3M. All rights reserved. 3M and the other marks shown are marks and/or registered marks. Unauthorized use prohibited.

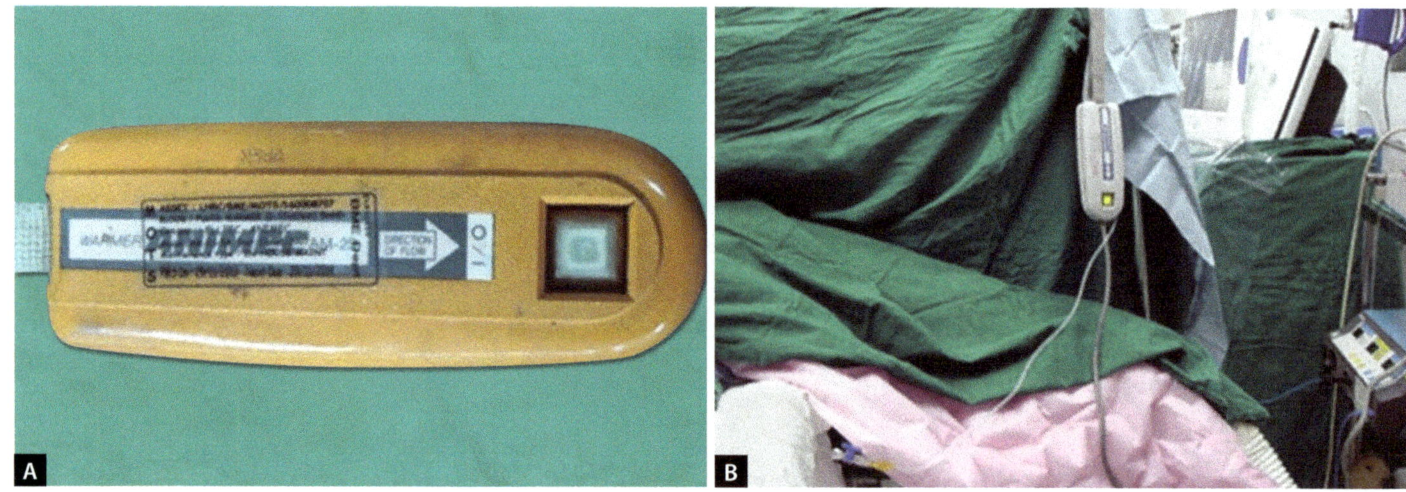

Figs. 8A and B: (A) Inline fluid warmer. The intravenous fluid infusion or blood transfusion sets passes through the warmer and is effective for slow infusion rates. The device should be placed as near to patient as possible and is particularly useful for slow blood transfusions in theaters, recovery rooms and wards; (B) Inline fluid warmer in use along with forced air warming intraoperatively.

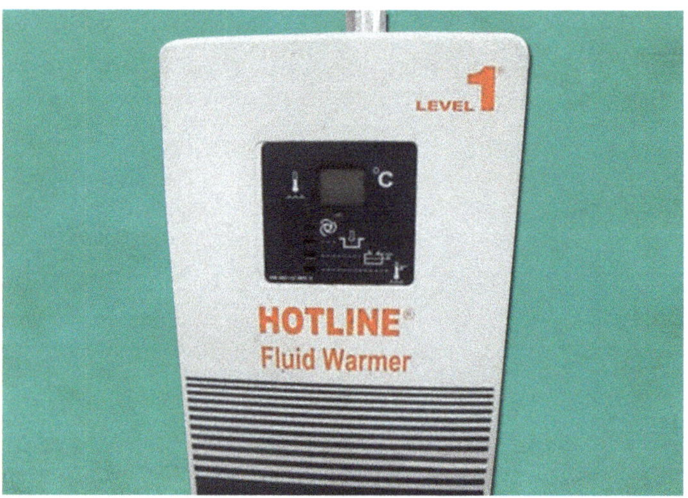

Fig. 9: Inline fluid warmer. This system does involve an additional cost of the required disposable tubing and is useful and effective for high fluid or blood transfusion rates and for major surgeries.

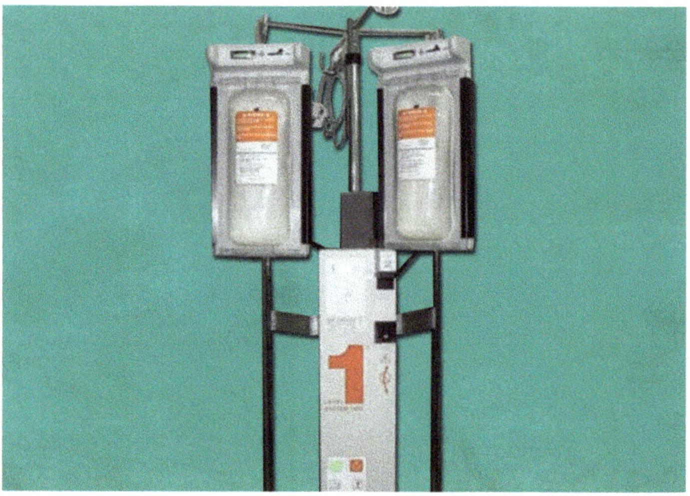

Fig. 10: Rapid infusion system. Useful for thermoregulation during major trauma and liver transplants.

REFERENCES

1. Buggy DJ, Crossley WA. Thermoregulation, mild perioperative hypothermia and postanaesthetic shivering. Br J Anaesth. 2000; 84(5):615-28.
2. Sessler DI. Complications and treatment of mild hypothermia. Anesthesiology. 2001;95:531-43.
3. Frank SM, Fleisher LA, Breslow MJ, et al. Perioperative maintenance of normothermia reduces the incidence of morbid cardiac events. A randomized clinical trial. J Am Med Assoc. 1997; 277:1127-34.
4. Rajagopalan S, Mascha E, Na J, et al. The effects of mild perioperative hypothermia on blood loss and transfusion requirement. Anesthesiology. 2008;108:71-7.
5. Kurz A, Sessler DI, Lenhardt R. Perioperative normothermia to reduce the incidence of surgical wound infection and shorten hospitalization. N Engl J Med. 1996;334:1209-15.
6. Lenhardt R, Marker E, Goll V, et al. Mild intraoperative hypothermia prolongs postanaesthetic recovery. Anesthesiology. 1997;87:1318-23.
7. Sessler DI. Temperature Monitoring and Regulation. Miller's Anesthesia, 7th edition; 2010.
8. Pestel GJ, Kurz A. Hypothermia-it's more than a toy. Curr Opin Anaesthesiol. 2005;18:151-6.
9. Al-Shaikh B, Stacey S. Essentials of Anaesthetic Equipment, 3rd edition; 2007.
10. Sessler DI. Temperature monitoring and perioperative thermoregulation. Anesthesiology. 2008;109:318-38.
11. Eshraghi Y, Nasr V, Parra-Sanchez I, et al. An evaluation of a zero-heat-flux cutaneous thermometer in cardiac surgical patients. Anesth Analg. 2014;119(3):543-9.
12. Abreu MM. New concepts in perioperative normothermia. Anesthesiol News; 2011.
13. Anaesthesia UK. Temperature measurement sites. [online] Available from http://www.frca.co.uk/. [Last accessed April, 2021].
14. The Management of inadvertent perioperative hypothermia. NICE Clinical Guideline 65. National Collaborating Centre for Nursing and Supportive Care (UK). London: Royal College of Nursing (UK); 2008.

Neuromuscular Block and its Monitoring with Peripheral Nerve Stimulator

Falguni R Shah, Preeti A Padwal

ABSTRACT

Muscle relaxants are employed in anesthesia to provide muscle relaxation and/or abolish movements. There exists enormous variation in patient's response to muscle relaxants. The disease states and perioperative medication can also modify the responses to these medications. It is difficult and often impossible to exclude with certainty, clinically significant residual curarization by clinical evaluation of neuromuscular (NM) function alone. The depth of neuromuscular blockade (NMB) should be monitored when muscle relaxants are used to avoid drug over dosage or under dosage and residual NMB during recovery.

There are several different varieties of stimulators and stimulating patterns available, which can be used in clinical practice during various stages of anesthesia. This aids in optimizing dosage and effects of NM blocking drugs and ensures complete recovery from muscle relaxants in postoperative period.

INTRODUCTION

The modern anesthesia is based on concept of balanced anesthesia, which is nothing but a fine tuning of equilibrium between hypnosis, analgesia, and neuromuscular blockade (NMB).[1]

The use of muscle relaxants in clinical practice dates back to 1942 when Griffith and Johnson used d-tubocurarine safely for clinical anesthesia. However, it was found to increase morbidity and mortality in subsequent years due to reasons well-known now, hence its use went out of practice. Succinylcholine was introduced in 1952, and it changed the anesthesia practice drastically. It was in late 1960s and early 1970s that significance of monitoring with peripheral nerve stimulator (PNS) to decrease the risk of residual muscle weakness in recovery room was realized.[2]

The residual postoperative NMB causes decrease in chemoreceptor sensitivity to hypoxia, functional impairment of pharyngeal and upper esophageal muscles, impaired ability to maintain the airway, and increase the risk of post-operative pulmonary complications and aspiration.[2]

The latest monitoring guidelines published all over the world (American Society of Anesthesiologists, Society of Great Britain and Ireland, Canadian Anesthesiologists' Society, etc.) mentions that NMB monitoring with PNS should always be available if NMB drugs are in use. Though it is not one of the mandatory monitoring devices, its use is highly recommended.[3]

This chapter will discuss basic physiology and pharmacology of NMB and use of neuromuscular (NM) monitoring with different stimulation patterns or modes available for clinical use during various phases of anesthesia and recovery to have perfect intubating conditions, optimal surgical relaxation, and complete recovery.[4]

MORPHOLOGY OF THE NEUROMUSCULAR JUNCTION

Each motor neuron runs from the ventral horn of the spinal cord or medulla to the NM junction as a large myelinated axon. It runs without interruption.[2] It approaches the muscles, branches repeatedly and along with many muscle cells forms a functional motor unit. The NM junction consists of prejunctional motor nerve ending separated from a highly folded postjunctional membrane.[5]

The nerve is separated from the surface of the muscle by synaptic cleft that is separated by a gap which is approximately 20–30 nm wide. The muscle surface is heavily corrugated with deep invaginations making the total surface area very large. The shoulders of the folds are densely populated with acetylcholine receptors about 5 million of them in each junction. With the, exception of the extraocular muscles, which have multiple innervations, all other muscles have only one NM junction per cell **(Fig. 1)**.

NEUROMUSCULAR TRANSMISSION

The components needed by the nerve ending for the synthesis, storage, and release of the neurotransmitter acetylcholine are made in the nerve cell body itself. This is then transmitted to the nerve ending by axonal transport.[2] The choline and acetate obtained from the environment of the nerve ending in the presence of choline acetyltransferase forms acetylcholine, which is stored in the form of vesicles. The nerve stimulation causes these vesicles to rupture and

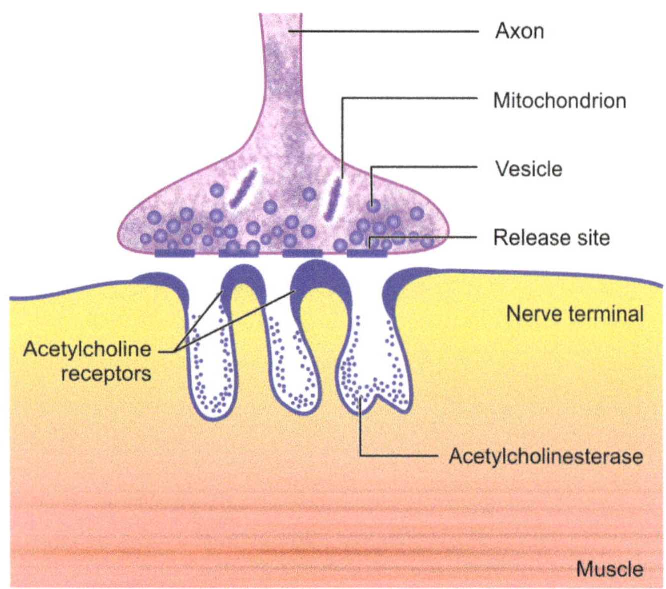

Fig. 1: Neuromuscular junction.

release acetylcholine into the synaptic cleft. There are two pools of vesicles releasing acetylcholine VP_1 which is the reserve pool and VP_2 which is the readily releasable pool.

During the nerve action potential, sodium from outside flows across the membrane causing depolarization, thus, opening the calcium channels which in turn results in release of acetylcholine. The ionized calcium concentration determines the quanta of acetylcholine released. The calcium channels are of two types, the P channels and the slower L channels. Along with the calcium channels, the potassium channels are present whose function is to limit the entry of calcium and hence depolarization.[2]

Under normal circumstances, a molecule of acetylcholine reacts with only one receptor before it is hydrolyzed by acetylcholinesterase. The action of acetylcholine is very short-lived, and it is destroyed in less than a millisecond after it is released.[5]

PHARMACOLOGY OF MUSCLE RELAXANTS

The principal pharmacologic effect of NM blocking drugs is to interrupt the transmission of nerve impulses at the NM junction.

They are classified as follows **(Table 1)**.

Based on Their Mode of Action

Depolarizing and Nondepolarizing Drugs

The depolarizing muscle relaxants (DMR) mimic the action of acetylcholine (ACh), while nondepolarizing muscle relaxants (NDMR) interfere with action of ACh. As we know, DMR have a biphasic action on muscle—an initial contraction giving rise to fasciculations, followed by relaxation. NDMR blocks the NM transmission by competitively preventing the binding of ACh to its receptors. Acetylcholinesterase (AChE) inhibitors like neostigmine acts by inhibiting enzyme AChE, thus concentration of ACh in the synaptic cleft remains high, resulting in displacement of NDMR molecules from receptors on the muscle end plate.[5]

TABLE 1: Classification of muscle relaxants.

Clinical classification	***Chemical classification***
Depolarizers	
Succinylcholine (less than 10–12 minutes duration)	
Nondepolarizers	
Long acting (>50 minutes)	
Pancuronium	Amino steroid
Doxacurium	Amino steroid
Pipecuronium	Amino steroid
Intermediate acting (20–50 minutes)	
Atracurium	Benzylisoquinoline
Vecuronium	Amino steroid
Rocuronium	Amino steroid
Cisatracurium	Benzylisoquinoline
Short-acting (15–20 minutes)	
Mivacurium	Benzylisoquinoline
Ultrashort-acting (<10–12 minutes)	
Gantacurium	Asymmetric mixed-onium chlorofumarates

Based on Their Chemical Classification

Benzylisoquinoline compounds and aminosteroid compounds.

Based on Their Duration of Action

- Long-acting
- Intermediate acting
- Short-acting
- Ultrashort-acting.

METHODS TO QUANTIFY THE DEGREE OF NEUROMUSCULAR BLOCKADE

Subjective

Visual Assessment

The observer should be at an angle of 90° to the motion.[6] It is the simplest method. The number of responses with train-of-four (TOF), post-tetanic count (PTC), or double-burst stimulation (DBS) can be counted.

Tactile Assessment

It can be evaluated by placing the fingertips lightly over the muscle to be stimulated and feeling the strength of contraction.[6] It can also be used to determine the presence or absence of the response with TOF, PTC, or DBS like visual assessment; however, it is more sensitive.

Objective

Mechanomyography

This technique measures thumb movement after application of preload of around 200–300 g. When the ulnar nerve is stimulated, the thumb acts on a force displacement transducer. The force of contraction is then converted into an electrical signal which is amplified, displayed and recorded.

It is important to avoid overloading the transducer and aligning the thumb in its direction. This method is very cumbersome and impractical in operating rooms.

Acceleromyography

It is based on the Newton's second law, i.e., force is equal mass times acceleration.

It is useful in the operating room and the intensive care unit (ICU) setting also. This technique applies the piezoelectric transducer with electrodes fixed on both side of the moving part. As the part moves, voltage which is proportional to the acceleration of the moving part is generated.[6] Extra-movements at the thumb should be avoided.

This is a nonisometric measurement, and there are less stringent requirements for immobilization of the arm, fingers, and thumb, and no preload is necessary.[7]

Kinemyography[6]

It utilizes a bending sensor that is placed between the thumb and forefinger. The core of the sensor is a piezoelectric material.

The movement is determined by the change in shape of the material when it is bent by adductor pollicis muscle contraction. When the piezoelectric material changes shape, the electric charge in the material is redistributed, and this leads to an electron flow to balance the charges. This flow is measured as a potential change that is proportional to the amount of distortion. The hand need not be immobilized. The device can be included in a multipara monitor. It lags mechanomyography (MMG) in determining recovery from NMB.

Electromyography[6]

It records the muscle action potential by five electrodes, two stimulating electrodes are placed over the nerve to be stimulated; three electrodes, two receiving and one ground are used for recording.

The ulnar and the median nerves are commonly used; two new sites include the larynx and the diaphragm. The electromyography (EMG) machine determines the supramaximal stimulus, determines the control, stimulates at the selected interval, measures response, and compares with the control. Less immobilization is required as compared to MMG; however, it is sensitive to electrical interference and temperature.

Phonomyography

It is based on the principle that contraction of muscles generates low frequency sound, which can be recorded with a piezoelectric microphone. The phonomyogram is easy to use and can be used on several different muscles.

Piezoelectric Film

It uses a disposable piezoelectric film that spans a movable joint. Muscle movement from evoked stimulation bends the film and generates a voltage that is proportional to the amount of bending. It can be used with the patient's thumb, fifth digit and great toe.[6] It is not as accurate as MMG.

Peripheral nerve stimulator can be a part of multiparameter monitor or a separate unit by itself. The stimulation can be accomplished by proper placement of the electrodes along the nerve course and then passing a current through them. The electrodes can be surface (most commonly used in clinical practice), metal or needle electrodes. The positive electrode is generally placed proximally along the course of the nerve. Most of the time, positive electrode is red and negative is black.

PROPERTIES OF AN IDEAL PERIPHERAL NERVE STIMULATOR[2]

- It must produce both monophasic and rectangular waveforms
- The length of the pulse should not exceed 0.2–0.3 ms
- Capability to stimulate the nerve at a constant current as compared to a constant voltage because current is the determinant of the nerve stimulation.
- Preferably, battery operated with an indicator for battery status. Low battery can result in generation of only three pulses during TOF stimulation giving rise to faulty interpretation of NMB
- Indicator for polarity of the electrodes
- It should deliver TOF stimulation, single twitch stimulation at 0.1 and 1 Hz, tetanic stimulation at 50 Hz, DBS, PTC, etc.
- Desirable to have an alarm system to warn if selected current is not delivered
- It should be reproducible
- Compact, lightweight, and simple to operate
- Temperature sensor/thermistor incorporated
- Optical interface with software for PC.

SITES FOR MONITORING NEUROMUSCULAR BLOCKADE

There are various sites described in literature for monitoring of NMB. However, the electrodes should not be applied in areas where inflammation, edema, or injury is evident.

Selection of site depends on following factors:

- Should be away from surgical site
- Easily accessible to anesthesiologist for intraoperative monitoring
- Preferably pulse oximeter probe and blood pressure cuff should not be applied on the same extremity as the PNS
- Peripheral nerve stimulator should not be applied on the paretic extremity as it may misinterpret resistance to NDMRs.

Various Sites[6]

Ulnar Nerve

Stimulation of ulnar nerve leading to contraction of adductor pollicis muscle (thumb) is most commonly monitored site. As this muscle is on the side of the arm opposite to that of the nerve, there is remote chance of direct muscle stimulation.

Ulnar nerve can be stimulated at the wrist, elbow, or hand.

Wrist: At the wrist, the two electrodes should be placed along the medial aspect of the distal forearm approximate 2 cm proximal to the proximal skin crease with the negative electrode distal **(Fig. 2)**. Stimulation will cause thumb adduction and finger flexion.

Elbow: At the elbow, the electrodes should be placed over the sulcus of the medial epicondyle of the humerus. Caution should be exercised to ensure that the electrodes do not cause ulnar nerve compression **(Fig. 3)**. Stimulation will cause thumb adduction, finger flexion along with hand adduction.

Hand: The electrodes may also be placed on the hand with the negative electrode on the palm between the base of the thumb and the second finger and the positive electrode in the same position on the dorsal side of the hand.

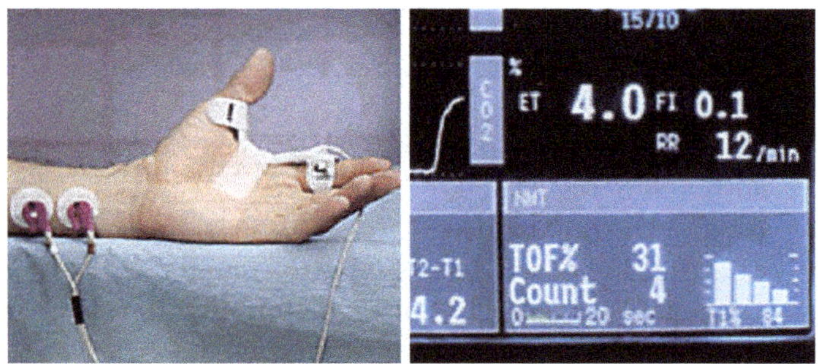

Fig. 2: Ulnar nerve stimulation at the wrist.

Median Nerve

It can be stimulated at the wrist. The electrodes are to be placed medial to where the electrodes would be placed while stimulating the ulnar nerve. The response is that of thumb adduction.

Tibial Nerve

Two electrodes are placed along the lateral side of the popliteal fossa. Gastrocnemius muscle is stimulated.

Posterior Tibial Nerve

The electrodes are applied behind the medial malleolus and anterior to the Achilles tendon at the ankle. Response is seen in the form of plantar flexion of the foot and big toe **(Fig. 4)**.

Peroneal Nerve (Lateral Popliteal)

The electrodes are placed on the lateral aspect of the knee. Response is elicited in the form of dorsiflexion of the foot **(Fig. 5)**.

Muscular Branch of the Femoral Nerve

It can be stimulated in vastus medialis muscle. It is useful in monitoring NM function, especially in the prone patient.

Facial Nerve

It is the best in detecting the onset of relaxation in the muscles of the jaw, larynx, and diaphragm. The negative electrode is placed anterior to the inferior part of the ear lobe, and the other electrode is placed just posterior or inferior to the lobe **(Fig. 6)**.

Other method includes, one electrode placed lateral to and below the lateral canthus of the eye and the other electrode is placed anterior to the ear lobe.

The facial muscles are relatively resistant to NMB drugs. Thus, the facial nerve should not be used to assess the recovery from NMB drugs.

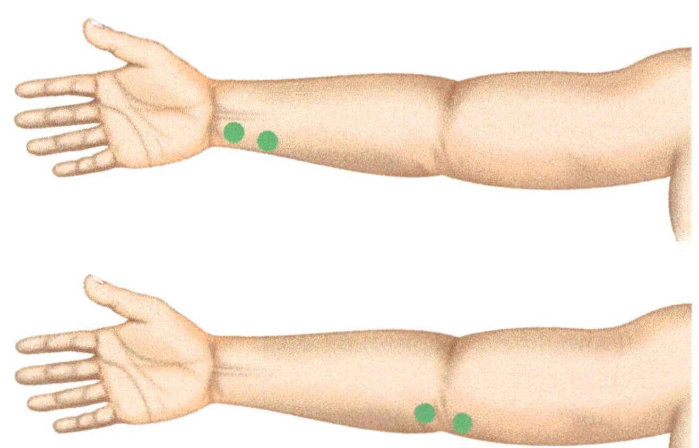

Fig. 3: Ulnar nerve stimulation at the elbow and wrist.

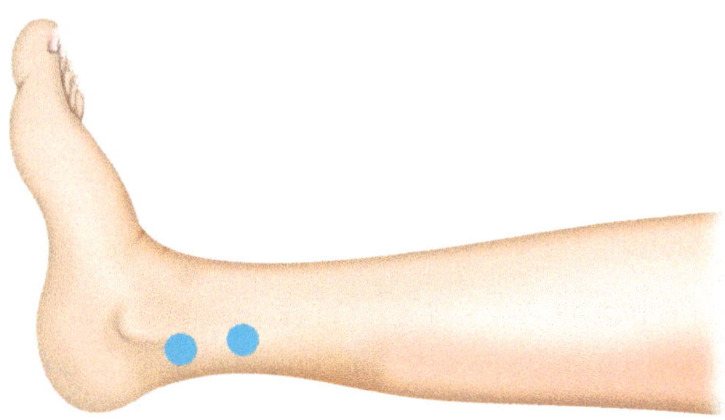

Fig. 4: Posterior tibial nerve stimulation.

Mandibular Nerve

The negative electrode is placed anterior and inferior to the zygomatic arch, and the positive electrode is placed over the forehead. The stimulation of this nerve causes the jaw to close.

Spinal Accessory Nerve

The electrodes are placed over the depression between the ramus of the mandible and the mastoid process/sternocleidomastoid (SCM) muscle. Stimulation is seen in the form of contraction of the SCM and the trapezius muscle.

Recurrent Laryngeal Nerve

Percutaneous stimulation can be done by placing the two electrodes between the notch, between the thyroid and cricoid cartilages. Response can be measured by placing the tracheal tube cuff between the vocal cords and measuring pressure changes within the cuff or by phonomyography.

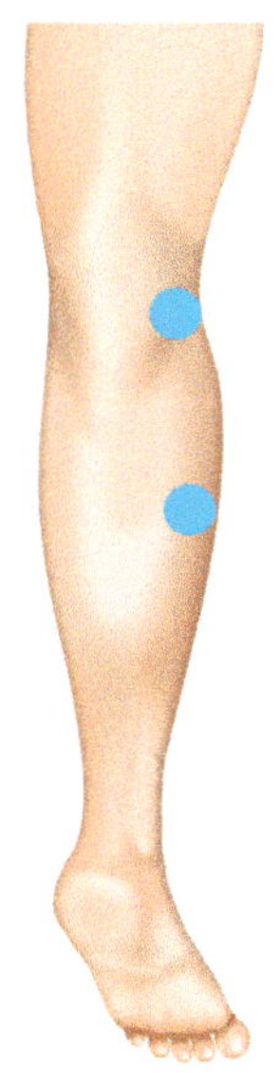

Fig. 5: Peroneal nerve stimulation.

Various muscle groups have different sensitivity to neuromuscular blocking drugs (NMBD). Fine muscles like those of eyes and digits are affected earlier as compared to trunk and abdomen. Ultimately, intercostal muscles and diaphragm are the last to be paralyzed. Recovery occurs in reverse order of paralysis.[5]

PATTERNS OF STIMULATION

Various modes or patterns of stimulation are described, and each one has its own indication during different stages of anesthesia **(Figs. 7 and 8, Table 2, and Video 14)**.

Single Twitch Stimulation

Single supramaximal electrical stimulus (current which is 10–20% higher than the current required to depolarize all the fibers nerve bundle, i.e., to elicit maximal contraction) is applied to a peripheral motor nerve from 0.1 to 1 Hz.[2] It is the simplest form of neurostimulation. The height of the evoked muscle potential depends on the number of unblocked junctions.[7] It requires a pre-relaxant control value for comparison. The strengths of subsequent twitches are then compared with the control and expressed as a percentage of the control. In both depolarizing and nondepolarizing agents, there is a progressive decrease in the twitch height as the block develops **(Fig. 9)**. A decrease in the temperature will also cause a reduced response.[6]

Advantages

Using 1 Hz stimulation shortens the time required for supramaximal stimulation, so it is preferable during induction of anesthesia.[2]

Disadvantages

- Requirement of a control value
- It cannot distinguish between depolarizing and nondepolarizing block.

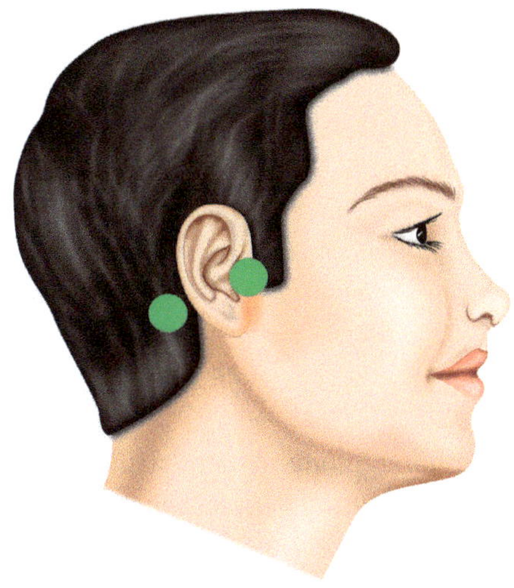

Fig. 6: Facial nerve stimulation.

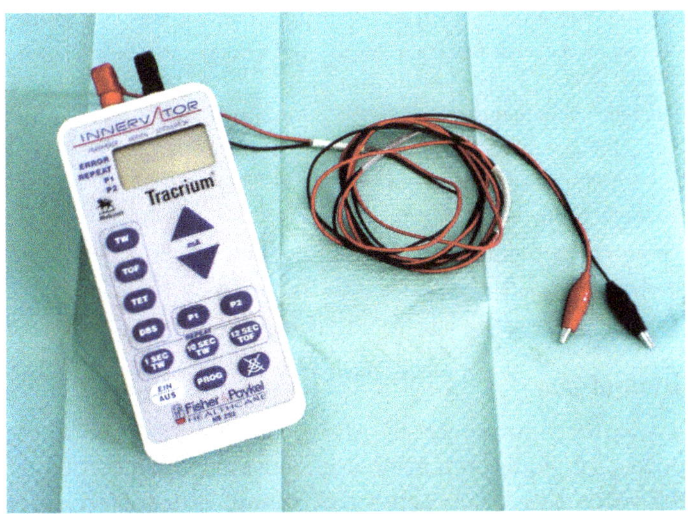

Fig. 7: Peripheral nerve stimulator with different modes for stimulation.

Pulse patterns

Twitch
- Single twitch
- Used with depolarizing blockade
- Degree of twitch depression used to calculate level of blockade

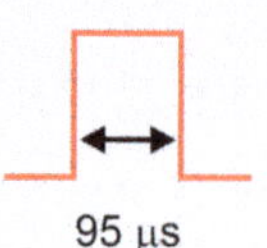

Double burst stimulation
- Two bursts 0.5 s apart
- Either 3 pulses followed by 2 pulses (3:2) or 3 followed by 3 (3:3)
- Used under light paralysis where train-of-four ratio is difficult to distinguish

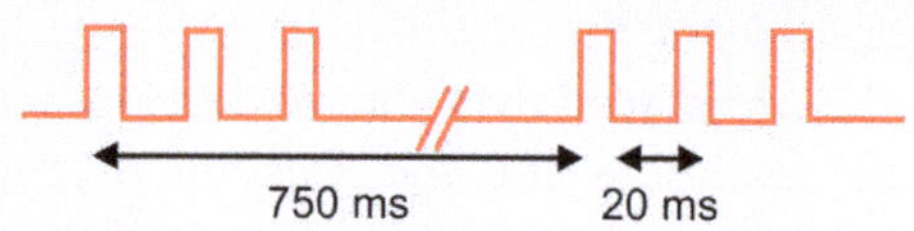

Train-of-four
- Four single pulses at 2 Hz
- Shows fade
- Ratio of first to fourth twitch used to calculate level of blockade

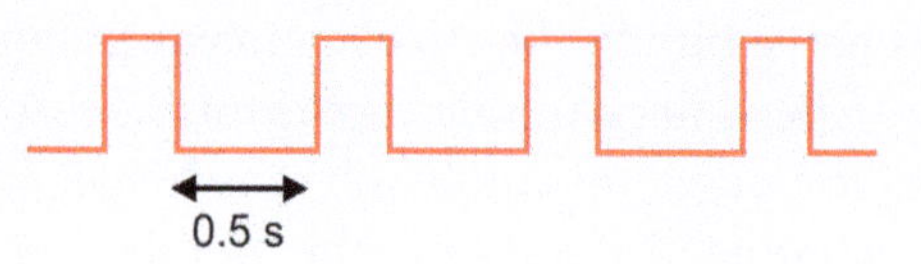

Post-tetanic count
- 5 s tetanus followed by 20 pulses at 2 Hz
- Shows fade response earlier than train-of-four
- Used under deep paralysis to estimate time to recovery

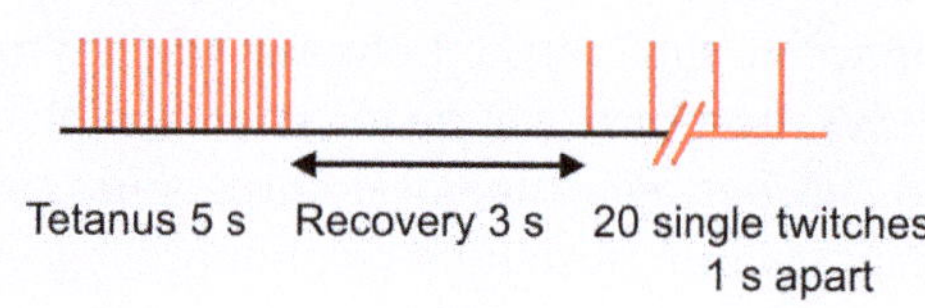

Tetanus
- Sustained burst of pulses at 50 or 100 Hz
- Usually held for around 5 s
- Used to 'kick start' the nerve under deep paralysis

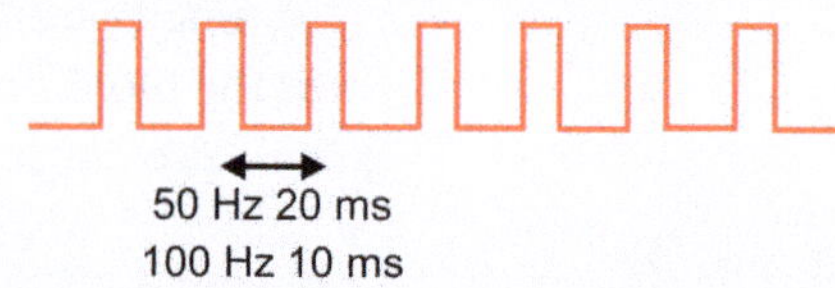

Fig. 8: Summary of patterns neuromuscular stimulation.

TABLE 2: Summary of patterns of neuromuscular stimulation.[7]

Feature	*ST*	*TOF*	*Tetanus*	*DBS*	*PTC*
Current strength	Supra-maximal	Supra- or submaximal	Supra- or sub-maximal	Supra- or submaximal	Supra- or submaximal
Frequency	0.1–1 Hz	2 Hz four stimuli	30–50 Hz for 5 seconds	Three impulses at 50 Hz repeated after 750 ms	50 Hz for 5 seconds, 3 seconds later ST at 1 Hz
Pre-relaxant control	Needed	Not needed	Not needed	Not needed	Not needed
Pain on stimulation	–	–/+	++	++	++
Sensitivity of manual detection (visual and tactile)	Not sensitive	Not sensitive at TOFR of 0.4 or more	Sensitive	Highly sensitive	Sensitive
Alteration of subsequent responses	Not altered	Not altered	Altered (post-tetanic facilitation)	Not altered	Altered
Interval between successive stimuli	5 seconds	12 seconds	2 minutes	12–15 seconds	6 minutes
Receptor occupancy detection	75–90%	70–90%	70–90%	70–90%	>90%
Sensitivity for detection of subtle block	Not sensitive	Sensitive	Sensitive	Sensitive	Not applicable
Monitoring of profound block	Not useful	Not useful	Not useful	Not useful	Useful

(ST: single twitch; TOF: train-of-four; PTC: post-tetanic count; DBS: double-burst stimulation)

Train-of-four

It was first introduced by Ali and associates. Four single pulses of equal intensity are delivered at intervals of 0.5 second (2 Hz).[6] Each set of stimuli is repeated every 10–20 seconds.[2]

It forms the differentiating point with DMR and NDMR **(Fig. 10)**. In case of a partial depolarizing block, there is equal depression of all four twitches and with a nondepolarizing block there is a progressive depression of height with each twitch called as fade.[6] Fade seen in the TOF response

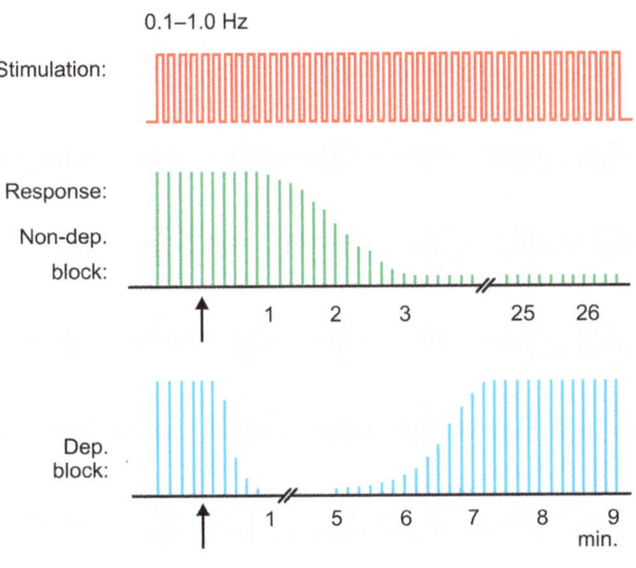

Fig. 9: Single twitch stimulation.

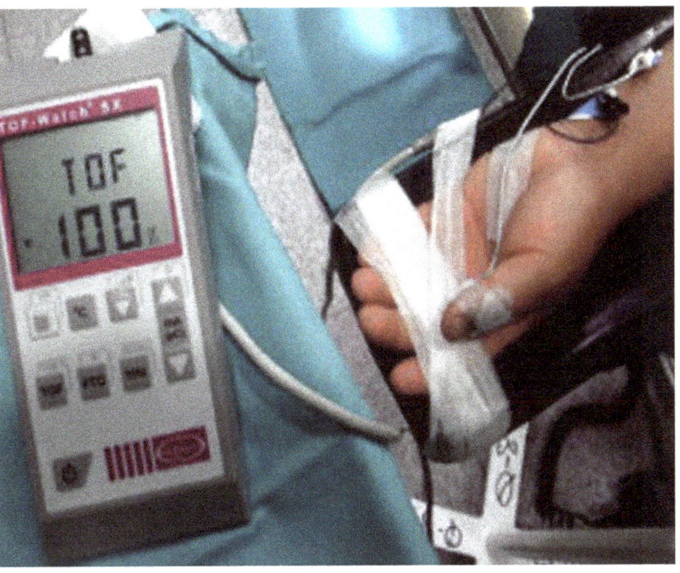

Fig. 11: Train-of-four ratio—1 (100%).

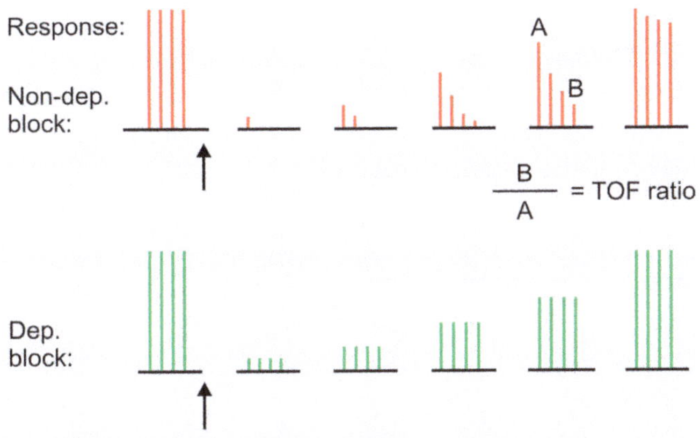

Fig. 10: Train-of-four stimulation.

after the succinylcholine injection signifies development of phase II block.[2]

The amplitude of the fourth response is divided by the amplitude of the first response and provides the TOF ratio (TOFR) **(Fig. 11)**.[2]

Advantages[4]

- A control value is not necessary
- It is more sensitive than single twitch stimulation. Train-of-four ratio is only 70% when single twitch has completely recovered
- It can differentiate between DMR and NDMR blockade
- Good correlation between fade and degree of NMB
- It is less painful
- It is repeatable after 10–12 seconds. TOF is in fact a very small tetanic stimulation, which produces virtually no facilitation. Hence, it can be repeated every 10–12 seconds and is less painful
- Unlike tetanic stimulation, TOF does not affect the degree of NM blockade
- It is relatively simple to use.

Disadvantage

It does not guarantee a reliable value at profound NMB and near complete recovery.

Tetanic Stimulation

It consists of rapid delivery of electrical stimuli. Most commonly, 50 Hz stimulation is given for 5 seconds. 50 Hz frequency is considered physiological as it is the same generated during maximal voluntary effort.[7] However, 50, 100, and 200 Hz stimulation is also used for 1 second.[2] The tetanic stimulation should not be repeated more often than every 2 minutes.[6] In case of a pure depolarizing block, the muscle response to 50 Hz for 5 seconds is sustained. In case of a nondepolarizing block and a phase II block after succinylcholine, the fade response occurs. The degree of fade depends on the degree of NM blockade, frequency and length of stimulation, and on how often tetanic stimuli are applied.[2]

Post-tetanic Facilitation

Post-tetanic facilitation is enhanced transmission after tetanus.[4] Mobilization and enhanced synthesis of ACh continued during and after cessation of tetanic stimulation is responsible for post-tetanic facilitation.[7]

Post-tetanic stimulation is useful when during intense NM blockade, there is no response to single twitch, tetanic, or TOF stimulation. It can be useful in surgeries where sudden movements can be dangerous, e.g., ophthalmic surgeries.

A tetanic stimulus of 50 Hz is applied for 5 seconds. After a 3-second pause, single twitch stimuli are applied at 1 Hz and the number of post-tetanic responses are counted. The number of twitches elicited increases as the depth of NMB decreases.[6]

Disadvantage

It is very painful so to be avoided in un anesthetized patients.

Double-burst Stimulation

It consists of two short bursts of 50 Hz tetanic stimulation separated by 750 ms. The duration of each square wave impulse in the burst is 0.2 seconds **(Fig. 12)**.[2] The clinician detects whether the second burst is weaker than the first, i.e., whether DBS fade exists.[4] The commonly used DBS are $DBS_{3,3}$ with three impulses in each of the two tetanic bursts. Other types include $DBS_{3,2}$ and $DBS_{3,3}$ 80–40 Hz and modified DBS consisting of first two stimuli of 0.3 ms duration at 50 Hz and then two stimuli of 0.2 ms duration at 50 Hz. It should not be repeated at intervals of less than 12 seconds.[6]

It is mainly used to detect residual NMB.

Advantages

- Fade is detected better with DBS than TOF **(Fig. 13)**; however, there is a close relationship between the two.[6] Studies have shown that DBS fade is detected at TOFR of 0.5–0.6, which is considerable improvement over the TOF mode where fade is detected only in the range of TOFR 0.3 or less[4]
- Better in assessing deep blocks as compared to TOF.[6]

Disadvantage

It is painful to the patient.

USES

Peripheral nerve stimulator is useful during various stages of anesthesia, e.g., during induction, maintenance, recovery, and postoperative period **(Fig. 14 and Table 3)**. It also can be used for electroconvulsive therapies (ECTs) and in ICU patients.

Before Induction

The stimulator should be connected to the electrodes, which are positioned over the selected nerve. The skin where the electrodes are applied should be properly cleansed with alcohol, thoroughly dried and then rubbed with a gauze piece. Care should be taken to avoid spreading the gel while placing the electrodes. A tape should be applied over the electrodes to hold them in position and prevent any movement.

At Induction[6]

During induction, the stimulator can be used to determine the onset of NMB and the extent of relaxation achieved for intubating the patient **(Video 14)**.

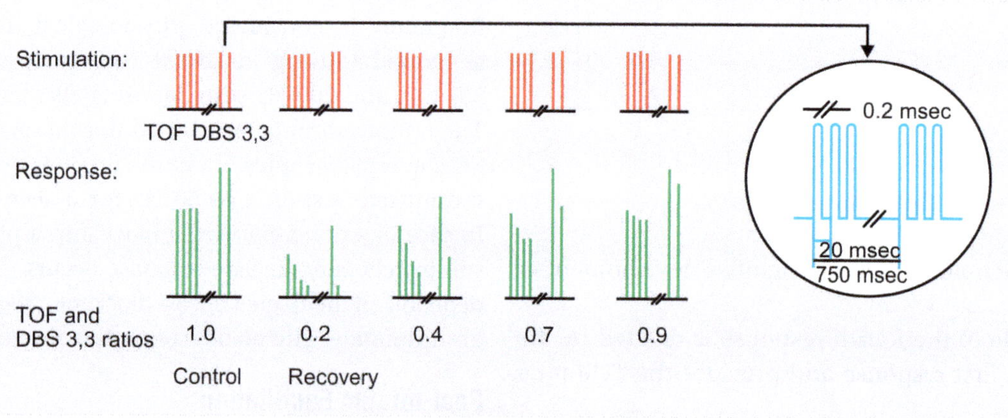

Fig. 12: Double-burst stimulation.

No drug	Nondepolarizing block	Depolarizing block	
		Phase I	Phase II
Train-of-four TOF–R = 1.0	Fade TOF–R = 0.4	Constant but diminished TOF–R = 1.0	Fade TOF–R = 0.4
Double burst	Fade	No fade	Fade

Fig. 13: Double-burst stimulation and train-of-four fade.

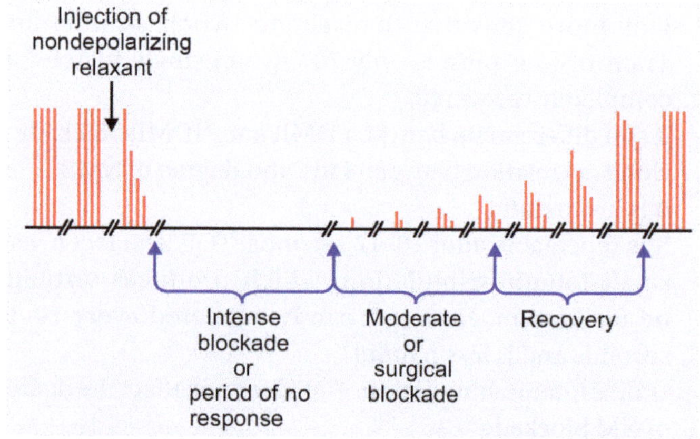

Fig. 14: Train-of-four during various phases of anesthesia.

TABLE 3: Uses of various patterns and sites of stimulation.[4]

Test	*Onset*	*Maintenance of deep block*	*Maintenance of shallow block*	*Prerecovery (before reversal)*	*Recovery*
TOF–AP	+	0	+++	+++	+
DBS–AP	0	0	++	++	++
TOF–OO	++	+++	+	0	0
PTC–AP	0	+++	0	0	0
Tetanus–AP	0	0	+	0	+
Accelerography–AP	+	0	+++	+++	++

(AP: adductor pollicis; OO: orbicularis oculi)

Note: +++: Reliable; ++: Not always reliable, but useful; +: Poor reliability, but sometimes useful; 0: Unreliable, useless and occasionally misleading.

Once the patient is induced, the stimulator should be set to deliver single twitch stimuli at 0.1 Hz. The output of the stimulator should be gradually increased. With increasing current strength, the response will also increase till a point when no further increase is noted even with rise in current strength. This point is point of maximal stimulation. The current is further increased by 10–20% to achieve supramaximal stimulation.

Inability to achieve maximal stimulation even at a current of 50–70 mA, warrants rechecking of the electrode placement. Even after doing this if maximal stimulation is not achieved, needle electrodes should be used.

The needle electrodes should be inserted subcutaneously with the angle of insertion parallel to the nerve to prevent direct nerve injury and should be secured with tapes.

During Intubation

Neuromuscular blockade and adequate depth of anesthesia are essential features during intubation **(Video 14)**.

The central muscles like the diaphragm and the larynx have a faster onset and offset of the block as compared to the peripheral muscles like adductor pollicis. The diaphragm is most resistant to both depolarizing and nondepolarizing agents. The diaphragm and the muscles of the jaw and larynx should be completely paralyzed during intubation.

Monitoring the response of the eye muscles particularly orbicularis oculi will be more precise in estimating the time of onset of NMB at the laryngeal muscles and diaphragm as compared to the peripheral muscles.

The anesthesiologist must wait before laryngoscopy and intubation until there is no response to single twitch at 0.1 Hz.

During Maintenance Phase

Use of the PNS during maintenance phase avoids under dosing and overdosing of relaxant **(Video 14)**. There are multiple factors responsible in determining the degree of NMB during surgery. These include the type of surgery, the anesthetic technique and the depth of anesthesia. The assessment is also dependent on factors like the temperature of the patient and skin resistance.

Correlation of patient's reaction to nerve stimulation and clinical condition is vital, as there may be discrepancy between the degree of relaxation of the monitored muscles and that of the muscles at the surgical site.

Train-of-four ratio is commonly used in operation theaters for NM monitoring during maintenance. A supramaximal stimulus at the ulnar nerve is generally used. Twitch depression of at least 90% is confirmatory of adequate muscle relaxation in most of the surgeries.[2] The paralysis of the diaphragm can be ensured only when the post-tetanic stimulation is zero in the thumb.[2] For adequate abdominal muscle relaxation, there should be not more than one response to TOF stimulation. If no response is present, further muscle relaxation is not required. If two responses are present, abdominal relaxation would be adequate only with balanced anesthesia. Presence of three twitches is usually associated with adequate relaxation if a volatile agent is used, but may need top-up of muscle relaxant.

Recovery and Reversal

The stimulator is helpful at the end of the surgery to assess the reversibility of the block and adjust the dose of the reversal agent accordingly **(Video 14)**. The reversal drug should not be administered till at least two responses to TOF stimulation are present or till clinically NM recovery is demonstrable.[2] It is now recommended by most researchers that a TOFR at the adductor pollicis should be at least 90% measured by MMG before extubation. Manual evaluation of the response to TOF is not confirmatory in excluding residual NMB so DBS is preferred along with correlation of the clinical signs and symptoms (e.g., sustained head lift for 5 seconds, sustained leg lift and hand grip for 5 seconds, maximum inspiratory pressure 40–50 cmH_2O or more, etc.) to rule out residual NMB.[2]

Monitoring of TOF ratio helps in titrating Neostigmine dosages. Various studies have shown that limiting the dose of Neostigmine to less than 60 μg/kg decreases the incidence of postoperative pulmonary complications.[8] The TOF count and the post tetanic count also helps in deciding the dosages of Sugammadex as shown in some studies.[9] Sugammadex has a better potential to offer fast, complete, and predictable reversal of both moderate and deep NM blockade. Current recommendations state in case of profound NM block, acetylcholinesterase inhibitors to be avoided and sugammadex to be used (4–16 mg/kg). In case of a moderate block, both sugammadex (2 mg/kg) and acetylcholinesterase inhibitors (0.07 mg/kg) neostigmine can be used. For reversibility of superficial block 0.02–0.03 mg/kg of neostigmine is sufficient.[10]

A third category of NM block antagonists, namely Calabadion is under various animal trials. This molecule is broad spectrum agent having action on both steroidal and benzylquinolone molecules with much faster action as compared to sugammadex.[10]

Postoperative Period

Currents less than the supramaximal stimulation are used if nerve stimulator is used in the postoperative period, as it is less painful to the patient if residual weakness is suspected.

Prolonged Muscle Relaxant Infusions

Long-term muscle relaxant infusions are used in ICU set up. Monitoring in this setting prevents over dosage as many of these patients may have hepatic and renal impairment, leading to deranged metabolism. Cautious interpretation is required in presence of severe edema and diabetic neuropathy.

Nerve Location

Nerve stimulators can also serve the function of a nerve locator.

Electroconvulsive Therapy

Premature delivery of the current is a common problem in ECT, so a single stimulus of 1 Hz is applied to the posterior tibial nerve. The ECT can be started after abolition of the response.[6]

Cleaning/Maintenance of Peripheral Nerve Stimulator

The simplest and safest way to clean the PNS is by using damp cloth. Preferred cleaning agents are 70% ethanol, methanol, a chlorhexidine solution or 0.5% hypochlorite. Use of other chemical cleaning agents may cause damage to the case finish and hence to be avoided. Care should be taken to prevent liquid from entering the case while cleaning.

RECENT ADVANCES IN NEUROMUSCULAR MONITORING: I-TOF[11]

Neuromuscular monitoring is here to stay and has a fundamental role in general anesthesia. To make it less cumbersome, practical and to incorporate it as a part of the daily usage by anesthesiologists, i-TOF comes to the rescue. i-TOF is a new wireless, neuromuscular monitoring device that associates Bluetooth technology combined with application downloadable on a smartphone. It is a portable device, consists of a triaxial accelerometer, two poles for nerve stimulation and wireless connection on a smartphone by application. Data memory is an additional advantage. Measured data can thus be saved and even attached to patient's medical records or used for clinical study purpose **(Fig. 15)**.

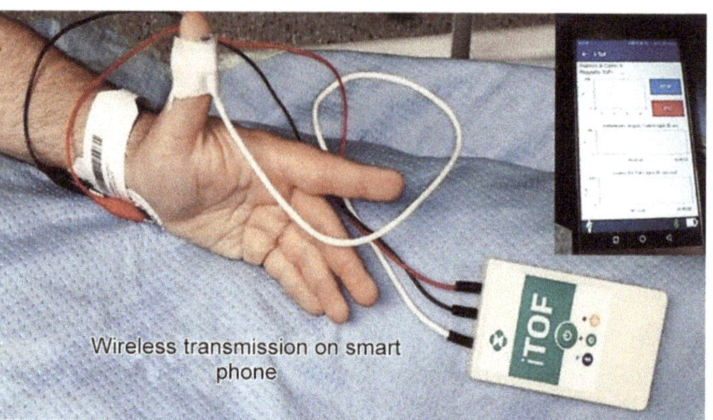

Fig. 15: i-TOF.
Source: Schiavoni L, Pascarella G, Grande S, et al. Neuromuscular block monitoring by smartphone application (i- TOF system): an observational pilot study. NPJ Digital Medicine. 2020;3:137.[11]

COMPLICATIONS AND PITFALLS[6]

Although relatively safe, inappropriate use of PNS can result in the following:

- *Burns:* It is commonly found with metal ball electrodes. Injuries can range from minor local tissue burns to permanent loss of hand function. Burns occur because electrodes provide good contact with minimal resistance for exit of high frequency current over a small area of skin
- *Nerve damage:* Nerve damage can occur due to pressure of the electrodes (e.g., ulnar nerve in elbow) or due to intraneural placement of the needle electrodes. It can vary from local paranesthesia to nerve palsy
- *Pain:* Incidence of pain is greater with use of higher current strengths, DBS and tetany, stimulation in awake or partially anesthetized patient and use of needle electrodes
- Needle electrodes can also be associated with complications like bleeding and infection
- *Electrical interference:* Peripheral nerve stimulator can interfere with ECG monitoring. It can also result in malfunctioning of implanted pacemakers and automated implantable cardioverter defibrillators (AICD)
- Patients with nerve damage, Bell's palsy, myasthenia gravis, diabetic neuropathy or other NM problems may 'not respond predictably' to stimulation.

CONCLUSION

The safe use of NM relaxants is dependent upon the accurate titration of the relaxants and their antagonists with the help of NM monitoring.[12]

The data obtained from NM monitoring should be interpreted in the light of patient factors, pharmacology of drugs used, site of monitoring, mode of stimulation and time during the surgical procedure (i.e., onset, maintenance, or recovery).[4]

Postoperative residual curarization (PORC) is not an unusual problem even in modern postanesthesia care units despite shorter and intermediate acting drugs available which are least dependent on renal and hepatic function. Postoperative residual curarization is a potentially preventable problem and therefore it is important to know and learn the ways to minimize its incidence. Hence quantitative neuromuscular monitoring is absolutely necessary. Chemical reversal with drugs like sugammadex will probably eliminate dangers of PORC soon.[13]

Valuable strategies to achieve appropriate muscle relaxation and blockade include avoidance of long-acting muscle relaxants, use of intermittent injections rather than continuous infusions, prevention of hypothermia, use of objective NM monitoring during procedure and use of reversal agents at the end of the case.[1]

REFERENCES

1. Plaud B. Neuromuscular monitoring, residual blockade, and reversal: time for re-evaluation of our clinical practice. Can J Anaesth. 2013;60(7):634-40.
2. Miller R, Eriksson LI, Fleisher LA. Miller's Anesthesia, 7th edition. Churchill Livingstone Elsevier; 2010.
3. Martin R, Bourdua I, Theriault S, et al. Neuromuscular monitoring: does it make a difference? Can J Anaesth. 1996;43(6):585-8.
4. Donati F. Neuromuscular monitoring: useless, optional or mandatory? Can J Anaesth. 1998;45(5 Pt 2):R106-16.
5. Stoelting RK, Hillier SC. Pharmacology & Physiology in Anesthetic Practice, 4th edition. Philadelphia: Lippincott Williams & Wilkins; 2006.
6. Dorsch JA, Dorsch SE. Understanding Anesthesia Equipment, 5th edition. Philadelphia: Wolters Kluwer-Lippincott Williams and Wilkins; 2008.
7. Padmaja D, Mantha S. Monitoring of neuromuscular junction. Indian J Anaesth. 2002;46(4):279-88.
8. Duncan J. McLean, M.B.Ch. B, Daniel Diaz- Gil, Hassan N Farhan, et al. Dose-dependent association between intermediate-acting neuromuscular-blocking agents and post-operative respiratory complications Anesthesiology. 2015;122:1201-13.
9. Shigeaki Otomo, Hajime Iwasaki, Kenichi Takahoko, Yoshiko Onodera, et al. Prediction of optimal reversal dose of Sugammadex after Rocuronium administration in adult surgical patients Anaesthesiology Research and Practice. 2014;848051:5.
10. Dutu M, Ivascu R, Tudorache O, et al. Neuromuscular monitoring: an update. Rom J Anaesth Intensive Care. 2018;25(1):55-60.
11. Schiavoni L, Pascarella G, Grande S, et al. Neuromuscular block monitoring by smartphone application (i-TOF system): an observational pilot study. npj Digital Medicine. 2020;3:137.
12. Bevan DR. Monitoring, new drugs, and reversal of neuromuscular blocking drugs. Can J Anaesth. 1991;38(4 Pt 2):R89-93.
13. Naguib M, Kopman AF, Ensor JE. Neuromuscular monitoring and postoperative residual curarisation: a meta-analysis. Br J Anaesth. 2007;98(3):302-16.

Pulmonary Function Tests

Charulata M Deshpande, Sarika Ingle

ABSTRACT

Pulmonary function tests are an important group of investigations for the comprehensive and complete assessment of all the components of the respiratory system. They also form an integral part of preanesthetic evaluation in a subset of patients who are at high risk of postoperative pulmonary complications, and patients undergoing thoracic or upper abdominal surgery. Although these tests are often conducted by a pulmonary technician, it is important for the anesthesiologist to understand the physiology, physics, and the working principle behind these tests to diagnose the nature, progress, and severity of an underlying pulmonary disease as well as to assess the effectiveness of treatment.

INTRODUCTION

Pulmonary function tests are a group of maneuvers carried out using standardized equipment to diagnose, determine the nature, progress, and severity of an underlying pulmonary disease as well as to assess the effectiveness of treatment. Pulmonary function tests assess the function of all four lung components, i.e., (i) the airways, (ii) lung parenchyma, (iii) pulmonary vasculature, and (iv) the bellows-pump mechanism of respiratory muscles.

For the anesthesiologist, these tests form an important part of preanesthetic evaluation to identify patients who are at high risk of postoperative pulmonary complications,[1] to formulate plan of anesthesia, and also to wean patients off ventilator.

Pulmonary function tests can be broadly classified as:

- *Static function tests:* These measure volumes and capacities, e.g., body plethysmography
- *Dynamic function tests:* These measure flow and airway resistance, e.g., spirometry
- *Diffusion capacity:* These assess the alveolar-capillary membrane
- Respiratory muscle strength
- *Cardiopulmonary exercise test:* It is a comprehensive test of cardiorespiratory system
- Metabolic measurements.

Alternatively, the pulmonary function tests (PFTs) can also be classified as:

- Tests for assessment of mechanical ventilatory function of respiratory system, e.g., static lung volumes, dynamic lung volumes, and respiratory muscle strength
- Tests for assessment of gas diffusion or exchange, e.g., diffusion capacity of lungs for carbon monoxide (CO) and arterial blood gas analysis
- Tests for assessment of cardiopulmonary interaction, e.g., 6-minute-walk test, ergospirometry (cardiopulmonary exercise test).

Out of all the PFTs, spirometry is the most commonly performed and the most basic test for assessing pulmonary function. The forced vital capacity (FVC) maneuver and flow-volume loops form an integral part of spirometry and provide vital information about the pulmonary system. The instrument used for spirometry is called a spirometer. The results of the test are presented in graph form, called the spirogram.

SPIROMETER

The spirometers are of the following two basic types: those which measure volume directly and those which derive volume from flow rate.

The direct volume measuring spirometers are bellows, rolling seal **(Figs. 1A and B)**, water seal **(Fig. 2)**, or dry type. These measure the volume of displaced air to derive lung volumes and capacities.

The flow measuring spirometers have a flow sensor (pneumotachometer)[2] of different types: Fleisch, screen (Lily), diaphragm, hot wire, or turbine. These calculate volume from the measured flow rate.

The core element of all modern spirometers is the flow sensor. These modern spirometers are computerized microprocessor driven machines, which measure lung volumes and flow rates as the patient breathes to and from

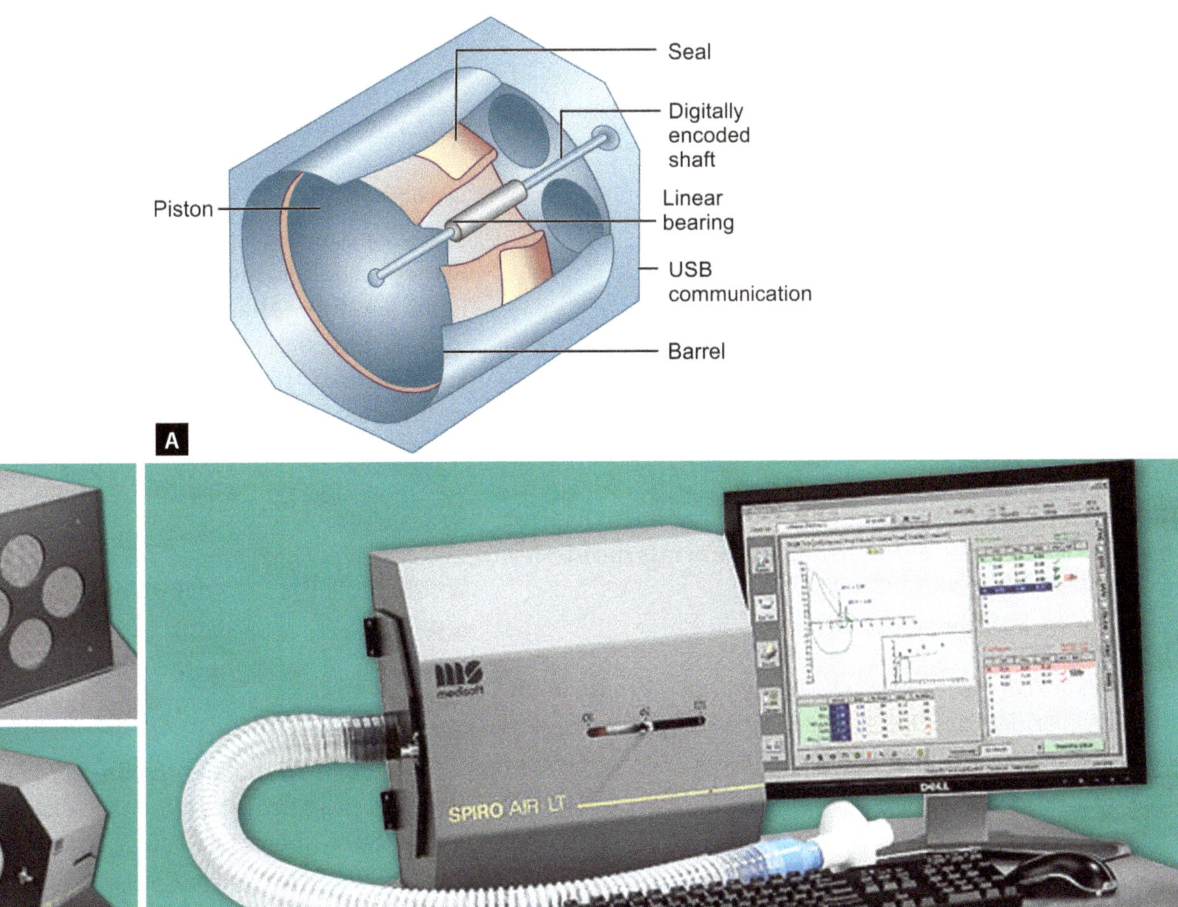

Figs. 1A and B: Rolling seal spirometer.

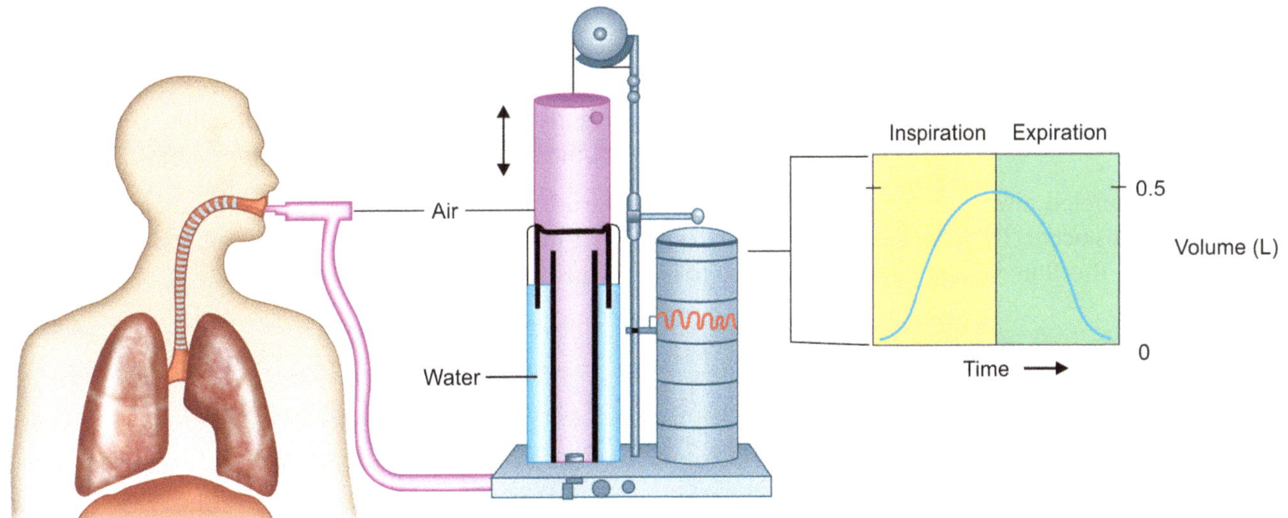

Fig. 2: Water seal spirometer.

the ambient air through a mouthpiece connected to the flow sensor. The sensor measures the flow and the integrated microprocessor or computer calculates volume, and other derived parameters.

The flow sensor measures the flow rate by detecting pressure difference caused by a resistive element placed in the breathing tube or flow tube.[2] The flow sensor (and hence the spirometer) gets its name depending on the type of resistor inserted. As only a laminar flow provides a pressure drop proportional to the flow rate, a flow rectifier (a breathing filter or a short tube) is inserted between the mouthpiece and flow sensor to laminarize the air flow.

TYPES OF SPIROMETERS

Pneumotachometer[2]

These measure flow rate from pressure difference across a resistive element and derive volume from the flow rate.

Fleisch

This flow sensor has a fixed resistive element in the form of an array capillaries (a roll of z-folded sheet metal) arranged in parallel with the direction of flow **(Fig. 3)**. The turbulent flow of air exhaled from trachea is converted into small threads of laminar flow by the capillaries. The pressure difference along the capillary is used to derive flow rate.

Lilly

The flow sensor has a close-mesh screen, single or in a series, as a resistive element. Pressure difference across the mesh is used to derive flow rate.

Hot Wire

This sensor has a Venturi tube with two hot wires linked in an electric bridge circuit. One wire, made up of two types of platinum, senses gas temperature and the other measures the heat flux into the passing gas. Temperature-corrected heat flux is proportional to gas flow.

Turbine

This sensor has a turbine or propeller built into the flow tube. The passing gas flow results in rotation of the turbine and these rotating elements interrupt or reflect the light from a light-emitting diode (LED). Photodiodes register the rotations, returning an electrical impulse frequency proportional to flow, while the total count of rotation is proportional to volume.

Vortex

The air flow is channeled toward a resistive element (bluff body), where vortices occur. The type and extent of vortices formed depend on the flow velocity and their number is evaluated by piezoelectric elements, thermistors or optodes. It can detect unidirectional flow only and an independent sensor, such as a pressure sensor is required for detection of flow; limiting its use in practice.

Ultrasound

The sensor technology has two built in ultrasound elements in the sensor housing and are placed oblique to the airstream in the flow tube. Alternating ultrasound impulses are emitted in both directions, and their transit times across the tube are measured. The difference in transit time is proportional to the flow velocity and independent of gas temperature, viscosity, or humidity. Advantages of ultrasound technology are freedom from calibration, high accuracy, and total hygiene.

Whole Body Plethysmography

It is used to measure lung-volume subdivisions and airway resistance. It works on the Boyle's law that states that the volume of gas at a constant temperature varies inversely with the pressure applied to it.

A body plethysmograph consists of an airtight chamber **(Fig. 4)**. The patient sits in the chamber and breathes through a flowmeter and a fast-acting shutter valve. The thoracic movements of the patient's breathing result in changes in the volume and proportional pressure change inside the lung and thoracic cavity of the patient. This is reflected by an identical volume and pressure swings inside the chamber, which are measured and evaluated.

An airway resistance loop is also graphed when the box pressure is measured against flow at the mouth during tidal breathing. Shape analysis of resistance loops allows diagnosis of homogeneous obstruction (bronchitis) from inhomogeneous obstruction (emphysema).

The advantages of using body plethysmography are:

- It measures intrathoracic volume and airway resistance in a single test.

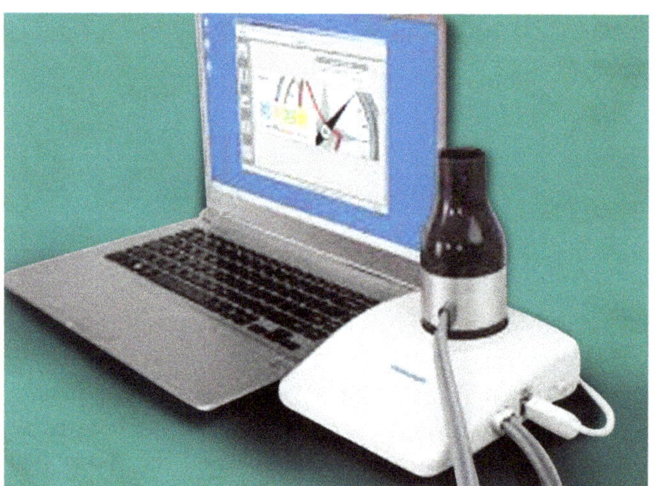

Fig. 3: Fleisch pneumotachograph.

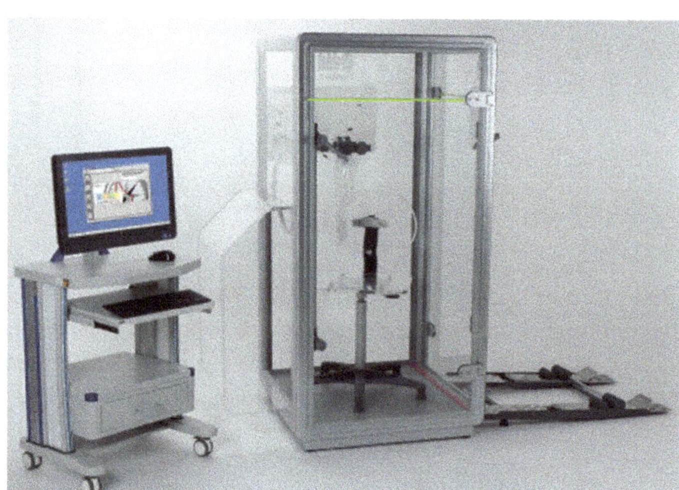

Fig. 4: Body plethysmography.

- It can be repeated multiple times, does not require much cooperation from the patient, and can measure not only the total volume of air in the chest but gas trapped in bullae also.
- When combined with forced spirometry and flow-volume loops (which can be performed with the chamber open), it gives valuable information about the entire pulmonary system.

Spirometry

The spirometry is the cornerstone of pulmonary system evaluation. It is a simple test and does not differ significantly with different spirometers used.

Procedure[3]

The test is conducted by a pulmonary function technician. The technician prepares the spirometer, conducts spirometer verification and/or calibration, and inserts a new mouthpiece or breathing filter in the flow tube to prevent contamination. The test procedure is explained to the patient as well as demonstrated. The patient is asked to sit comfortably in a chair. Soft nose clip is applied to prevent exhaled air escaping from nose and airtight lip seal around the mouthpiece is confirmed. The patient is encouraged to practice before recording the test results.

Forced Vital Capacity Maneuver

The most common and internationally standardized maneuver in spirometry is the "FVC maneuver". There are three distinct phases to the FVC maneuver: (i) maximal inspiration, (ii) a "blast" of exhalation, and (iii) continued complete exhalation to the end of test.

The patient is asked to breath normally through the mouthpiece for a few breaths. Then the patient is asked to take a maximally deep breath and then exhale through the mouthpiece as hard, as fast and as long as possible, followed by another rapid deep inhalation. The test is repeated, at least three times to ensure accurate and repeatable results. The test may be repeated after inhalation of bronchodilator to assess reversibility of airway obstruction. The normal value of FVC is 80–120% of predicted value.

A slow vital capacity (SVC) maneuver is also carried out **(Fig. 5)**. Breathing at resting baseline, patient is asked to take a slow, continuous, maximum inspiration followed by a slow, maximum expiration, followed again by a complete inspiration. The FVC and SVC are similar in normal healthy person. In patients with obstructive lung disease, forceful expiration causes dynamic collapse of the airways and leads to a much lower value of FVC than SVC.

The spirometry provides two types of graphs: flow volume loop and volume time curve **(Figs. 6A and B)**. In the second graph the test results are plotted as volume against time while in the flow-volume loop, the test results are plotted as volume against flow. A slow spirometry [tidal volume (TV) breathing] is also recorded.

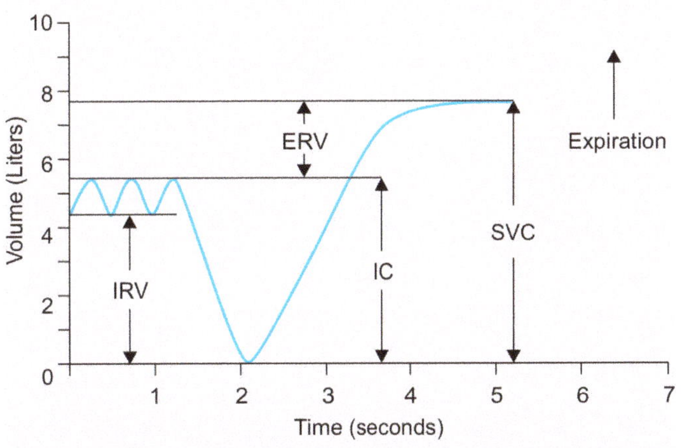

Fig. 5: Slow spirometry.

The performance of the test relies on comprehension and cooperation of the patient and can only be used on adults and children old enough to comprehend and follow the instructions. This test is not possible in unconscious, heavily sedated patients, and patients having limitations that interfere with vigorous respiratory efforts. Other types of PFTs are available for infants and unconscious persons.

Spirometry gives values of a vast number of lung parameters. The most important are the FVC, forced expiratory volume in 1 second (FEV1) and FEV1 as a percentage of forced vital capacity (VC) (FEV1%). The other parameters include peak expiratory flow (PEF), forced expiratory flow (FEF) when 25% of the FVC has been expired (FEF25), FEF when 50% of the FVC has been expired (FEF50), FEF when 75% of the FVC has been expired (FEF75) and peak inspiratory flow.

Results of spirometry are usually given in both actual data (liters, L/s) and percent predicted, i.e., the test result as a percent of the "predicted values" for the patients of similar height, weight, age, sex, and ethnicity. Results nearest to 100% predicted are the most normal, and results over 80% are considered normal.

Forced Vital Capacity

It is volume of air that can be forcefully expired after a maximum inspiratory effort. Normal value is 80–120% of predicted.

Interpretation of percentage predicted:
- *80–120%:* Normal
- *70–79%:* Mild reduction
- *50–69%:* Moderate reduction
- *Less than 50%:* Severe reduction.

The majority of FVC can be exhaled in less than 3 seconds in normal people, but is much more prolonged in obstructive diseases. FVC is critically important for diagnosis of obstructive and restrictive lung disease. FVC is reduced

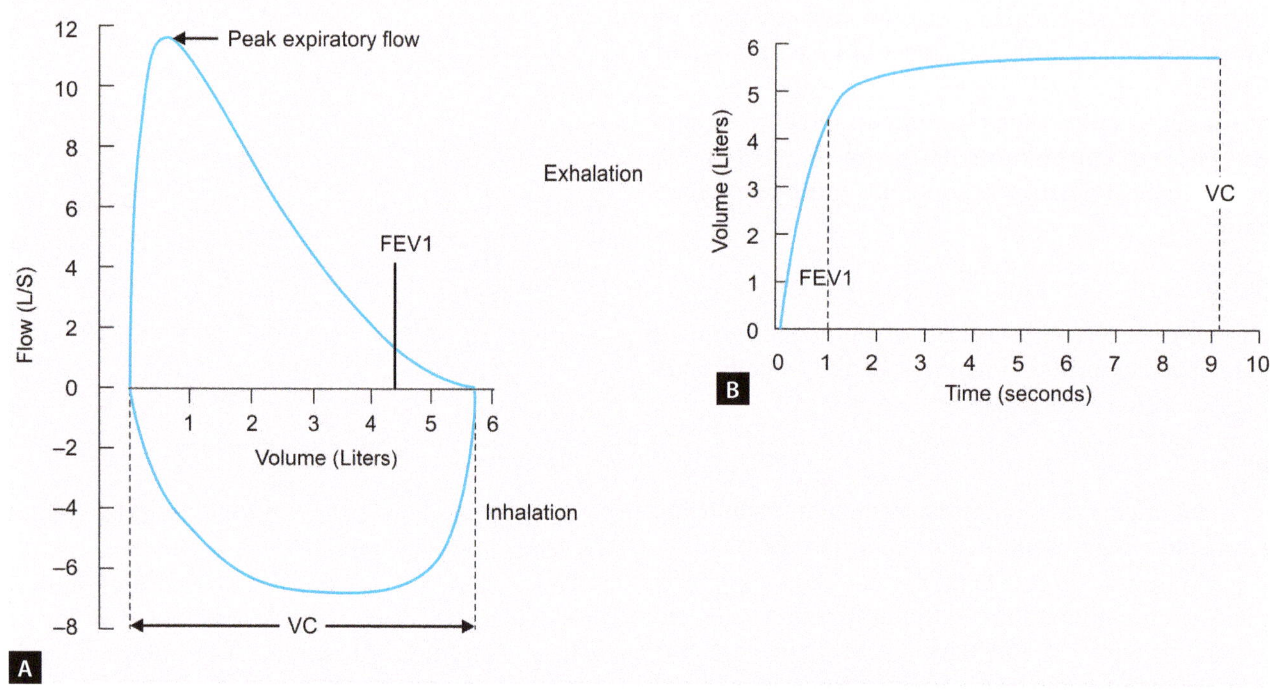

Figs. 6A and B: (A) Flow-volume loop; (B) Flow-time curve.

in restrictive lung diseases as well as in obstructive lung diseases and lung collapse.

Forced Expiratory Volume in 1 Second

This is most widely used parameter that reflects mechanical properties of both the large airways and medium-sized airways. It is the volume of air forcefully expired from maximal inspiration [total lung capacity (TLC)] in the first second. Normal people can exhale more than 75–80% of their FVC in the first second; thus, the FEV1/FVC can be utilized to characterize lung disease. Reduction in the ratio is specific for obstruction, and the ratio is normal in restriction.

Forced Expiratory Flow 25–75%

This is the mean FEF during middle half of FVC measured in L/s. It reflects effort independent expiration and the status of the small airways (<2 mm diameter). It is an indicator of obstruction and depends on FVC.

Interpretation of percentage predicted:

- *Greater than 60%:* Normal
- *40–60%:* Mild obstruction
- *20–40%:* Moderate obstruction
- *Less than 10%:* Severe obstruction.

Peak Expiratory Flow Rate

It gives the maximum flow rate achieved during FVC maneuver. This is a sensitive test for obstructive lung disease, useful to assess effectiveness of treatment. Normal value is 4–5 L/s.

Maximum Voluntary Ventilation

It is the maximum amount of air that the patient breathe in 1 minute. It is determined by breathing in and out as deeply and rapidly as possible for 12–15 seconds then extrapolated to 60 seconds. It reflects status of muscle bellows, lung compliance and airway resistance. This test is effort dependent; therefore, it may be a poor predictor of muscle strength and compliance. Normal value is 160–180 L/min. It can also be derived from FEV1 as maximum voluntary ventilation (MVV) = FEV1 × 40. A value of less than 50% is associated with high risk of postoperative complications. MVV is low in pulmonary, cardiovascular, and neuromuscular diseases.

Uses of Spirometry

Data from a spirometry help distinguish between obstructive pulmonary disorders that reduce airflow from restrictive disorders that reduce the total lung volumes.

A reduced FVC and FEV1 with normal or high FEV1/FVC ratio suggest a restrictive disorder. A reduced FEV1 and reduced FEV1/FVC ratio suggest obstructive disorder. The severity of reductions in the FVC and/or the FEV1 can be classified as:

- *Mild:* 70–79% of predicted
- *Moderate:* 60–69% of predicted
- *Moderately severe:* 50–59%
- *Severe:* 35–49% of predicted
- *Very severe:* Less than 35% of predicted.

The FVC, FEV1, and FEV1/FVC% can be normal in the presence of small airways obstruction and reduced mid expiratory flow rate.

The American Thoracic Society Standardization Guidelines for Acceptability and Reproducibility Criteria for Spirometry[3]

The acceptability criteria are a satisfactory start of test and a satisfactory end of test, i.e., a plateau in the volume-time curve. In addition, the technician should make sure that the subject understood the instructions and performed the test with a good start, maximum inspiration, a smooth continuous exhalation and maximal effort. It should also be observed that the test is free of any artifacts, such as cough or glottis closure during first second, hesitation to start, leak or obstructed mouthpiece, early termination of expiration, and extrabreath during test.

The repeatability criteria are that after three acceptable FVC maneuvers two largest FVC and FEV1 should be within 0.150 L of each other.

The American Thoracic Society (ATS) has recommended that the threshold for significant response is demonstration of an at least 12% increase and 0.2 L increase in either FVC or FEV1 and 20% increase in FEF 25–75% on a spirogram performed 10–15 minutes after inhalation of a therapeutic dose of a bronchodilating agent.

Flow-volume Loops

A flow-volume loop and a time-based spirogram are recorded in addition to the FVC maneuver during spirometry. The time-based spirogram gives important information about the expiratory time. The normal expiratory time is 3 seconds (most of the FVC is exhaled in about 3 seconds) in a healthy subject, but can be as prolonged as 10–20 seconds in a patient with obstructed airways.

In many laboratories, flow-volume loop is the primary maneuver for spirometry. Flow-volume loops are a graphical illustration of a patient's spirometric efforts **(Figs. 7A and B)**. During the procedure, the patient makes a full expiratory and inspiratory loop as a single maneuver and flow is plotted against volume. The overall shape of the flow-volume loop is important in identifying anatomical location of airway obstruction. The loop illustrates maximum expiratory and inspiratory flow and in normal person MIF50% greater than MEF50%.

Chronic obstructive pulmonary disease (COPD) results in characteristically concave descending limb of the expiratory loop. There is decreased FEV1, FEF25–75, FEV1/FVC ratio (<0.8). In obstructive lung disease, the volume-time curve shows slow rise in upstroke and failure to reach plateau. Obstruction of the large airways produce a variety of patterns of truncation or flattening of either one (inspiratory/expiratory) limb of the loop (variable upper airway obstruction) **(Fig. 7B-5 and 6)** or both limbs of the loop (fixed upper airway obstruction) **(Fig. 7B-4)**.

Restrictive lung disease is associated with diminished lung volume and normal or increased FEV1/FVC ratio. The volume-time curve shows a normal rapid upstroke but low plateau volume **(Fig. 8)**.

Volumes and Capacities

Spirometry measures four volumes and four capacities which are sum of two or more lung volumes.

- *Tidal volume:* It is the volume of air inspired and expired during normal quiet breathing. Normal value is 7–10 mL/kg
- *Inspiratory reserve volume (IRV):* The maximum amount of air that can be inhaled after a normal TV inspiration. Normal value is 2.5–3 L
- *Expiratory reserve volume (ERV):* Maximum amount of air that can be exhaled from the resting expiratory level. Normal value is 1–1.5 L
- *Residual volume (RV):* Volume of air remaining in the lungs at the end of maximum expiration. Normal value is 1.5–2 L
- *Inspiratory capacity (IC):* Maximum amount of air that can be inhaled from the end of a TV: IC = TV + IRV. Normal value is 3–3.5 L
- *Vital capacity:* Volume of air that can be exhaled from the lungs after a maximum inspiration. FVC: when VC exhaled forcefully and SVC: when VC is exhaled slowly. VC = IRV + TV + ERV. Normal value is 4–4.5 L
- *Functional residual capacity (FRC):* Volume of air remaining in the lungs at the end of a TV expiration. The elastic force of the chest wall is exactly balanced by the elastic force of the lungs. FRC = ERV + RV. Normal value is 3 L
- *Total lung capacity:* Volume of air in the lungs after a maximum inspiration. Total lung capacity = IRV + TV + ERV + RV. Normal value is 6–6.5 L. Total lung capacity is a very good indicator of restrictive lung disease.
  - TLC less than 80%, but greater than 70% of predicted: Mild restriction
  - TLC less than 70%, but greater than 60% of predicted: Moderate restriction
  - TLC less than 60% of predicted: Severe restriction.

Spirometry cannot measure residual volume (RV), FRC, and TLC. Whole-body plethysmography, N_2 washout test and inert gas (He) dilution method can measure these. The whole body plethysmography is the least invasive and accurate.

TESTS FOR TOTAL LUNG CAPACITY, RESIDUAL VOLUME, AND FUNCTIONAL RESIDUAL CAPACITY

The least invasive method for the assessment of TLC, RV, and FRC is body plethysmography, which has already been discussed. The other methods are described below.

Helium Dilution Method

Patient breathes in and out of a spirometer of known volume filled with 10% He (which is insoluble in blood) and 90% O_2, till equilibrium is reached between the lungs and spirometer. FRC can be calculated by the equation:

$$C1V1 = C2V2, V2 = (V1 + FRC)$$

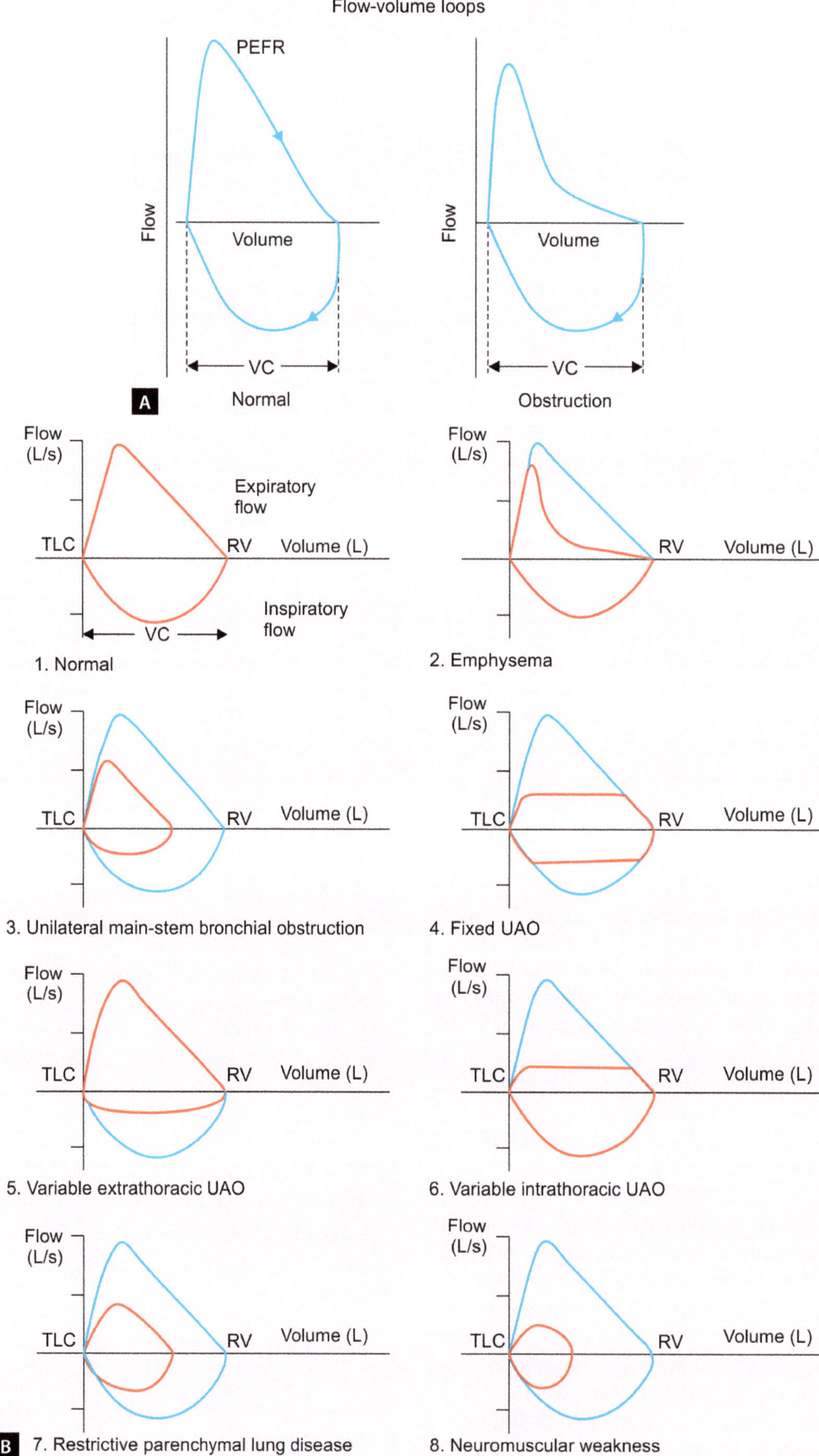

Figs. 7A and B: (A) Flow-volume loop in obstruction; (B) Flow-volume loops in different conditions. (PEFR: peak expiratory flow rate; TLC: total lung capacity; RV: residual volume; UAO: upper airway obstruction)

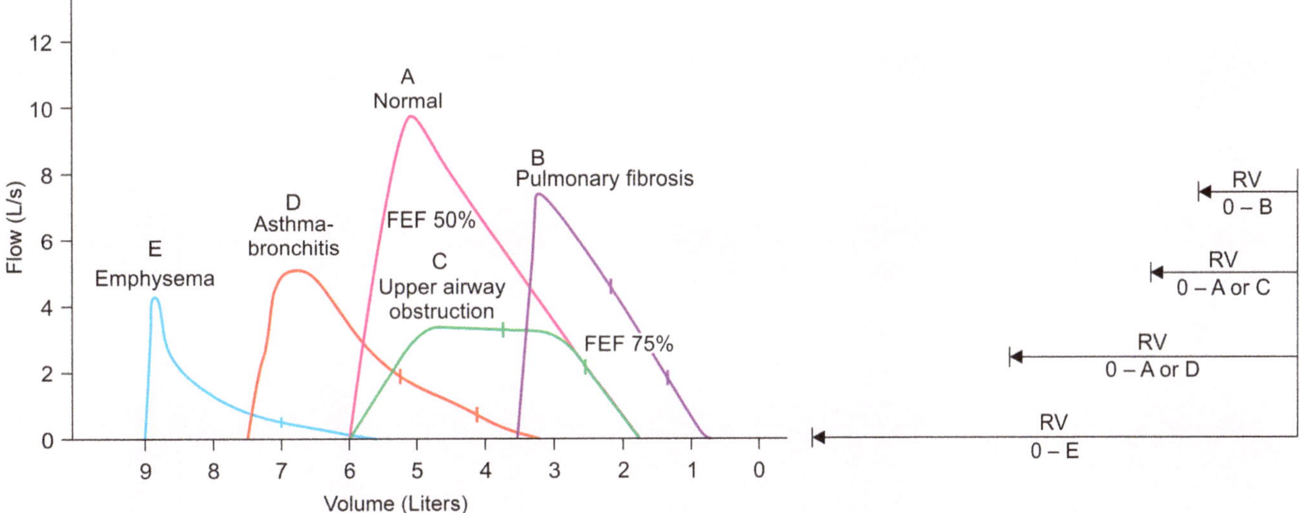

Fig. 8: Flow-volume curve in different conditions.

where, V1 = volume of spirometer, V2 = FRC, C1 = concentration of He in the spirometer before equilibrium, C2 = concentration of He in the spirometer after equilibrium. Unlike whole-body plethysmography, this test can only measure the communicating gas volume. Gas trapped behind closed airways, pneumothorax or bullae is not measured.

Nitrogen Washout Method

Following a maximal expiration (from RV) or normal expiration (from FRC), patient inspires 100% O_2 and then expires it into N_2 free spirometer till all the N_2 is washed out of the lungs, which usually takes about 6–7 minutes. Nitrogen concentration of spirometer as well as total volume of exhaled air is calculated. Normal air has 80% N_2, so actual FRC/RV is calculated.

The complications of this test may include atelectasis due to washout of N_2 from poorly ventilated lung zones (obstructed areas), elimination of hypoxic drive in COPD patients, and underestimation of FRC due to trapped gas in nonventilated regions, pneumothorax, and bullae.

DIFFUSING CAPACITY[4]

Diffusion capacity of lungs for carbon monoxide (DLCO) is a test that measures the rate of gas transfer (diffusion) across alveolar-capillary membrane.

The most widely used and standardized technique is the single breath technique which is relatively simple and recommended by ATS and European Respiratory Society (ERS) for routine use.

In this test, patient inspires a test gas mixture of 0.3% CO, a tracer gas which is usually 10% He, 21% O_2 and rest of N_2, starting from residual volume to maximal inspiratory capacity. At full inspiration, the patient is asked to hold his breath for a period of 10 seconds (9-11 seconds), allowing the gas mixture to distribute in the alveolar space. After 10 seconds, the patient exhales the gas sample, which is passed through a gas analyzer. Gas concentrations in exhaled air are displayed graphically on the monitor. The purpose of tracer gas is for estimation of alveolar CO concentration at the end of inhalation and for estimation of alveolar volume **(Figs. 9A to C)**.

The DLCO machine contains compressed gas cylinder of test gas, flow meter and gas analyzer **(Figs. 9A to C)**. The flow meter is equipped with an optoelectronic reader and a flow sensor (turbine or pneumotachometer) for gas flow and volume measurements. The flow meter of newer machines have demand valves that automatically connect the patient to room air, the test gas or portal to exhaled gas analyzer during the procedure.

Modern machines have infrared analyzers for determination of gas concentration. These rapidly analyze the exhaled gas and facilitate real-time graphical display of CO and tracer gas concentrations on the monitor **(Fig. 9A)**. The graphical display also helps to accurately locate the alveolar gas without contamination from anatomical dead space gas.

Normal value of DLCO is 17-25 mL/min/mm Hg. A DLCO result at least 80% of the predicted value is considered to be within normal limits. The degree of severity of reduction in the diffusing capacity is graded as follows: Less than the lower limit of normal (LLN) but greater than 60% of predicted is mild, between 40 and 60% of predicted is moderate, and less than 40% is severe. When DLCO is corrected for simultaneously measured TLC (VA) and hematocrit, it is Ht adjusted DLCO/VA.

Diffusion capacity of lungs for CO is reduced in interstitial lung disease due to increased alveolar membrane thickness, e.g., pulmonary fibrosis, sarcoidosis, allergic alveolitis, pulmonary edema, as well as in obstructive lung disease, such as emphysema and cystic fibrosis. It may also be reduced with pneumonectomy because of reduced alveolar surface area. DLCO is increased in left to right shunt

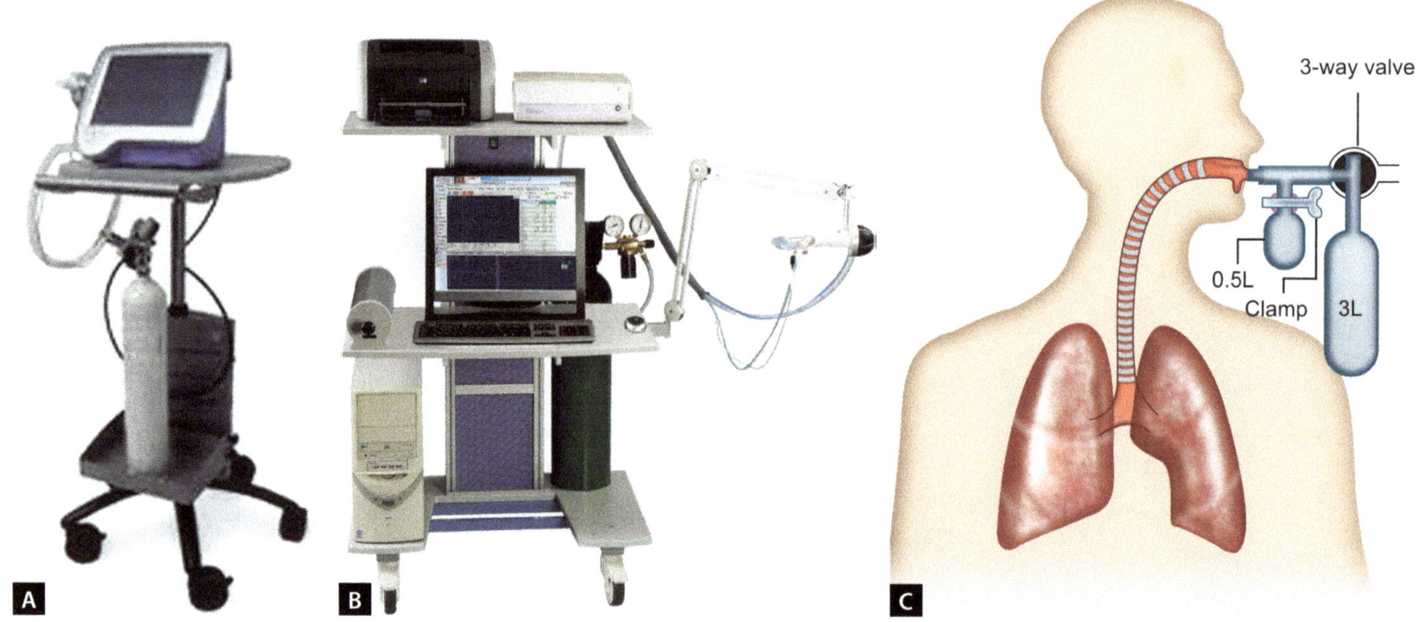

Figs. 9A to C: (A and B) DLCO monitor; (C) DLCO test.

and intrapulmonary bleeding. Low hemoglobin results under estimate DLCO and vice versa. If DLCO is decreased with associated airway obstruction or ↑TLC—indicates emphysema. If DLCO is decreased along with ↓TLC—indicates parenchymal disease, e.g., pulmonary fibrosis. If DLCO is decreased along with normal lung mechanics: indicates pulmonary vascular disease.

RESPIRATORY MUSCLE STRENGTH[5]

Respiratory muscle strength can be assessed by various tests.

Volitional Tests

- Measuring static maximal inspiratory and expiratory pressures PI_{max} and PE_{max}
- *Esophageal studies:*
    - Transdiaphragmatic pressures PI, di, max
    - Maximum sniff pressures
    - Cough pressures Pga, co.

The maximal static inspiratory and expiratory pressures are measured by body plethysmography. Inspiratory pressures are measured at FRC and expiratory pressures at TLC. These are volitional tests. Although simple to perform, these are not very reliable as maximal effort of the patient cannot be ascertained.

Esophageal studies involve insertion of double balloon esophageal catheter under local anesthesia. A pressure transducer and microprocessor compute the data. Maximum static transdiaphragmatic pressure provides specific information on diaphragm strength.

Maximum sniff pressures can be achieved by patients with practice. Sniff pressures are reproducible and have a narrower normal range than static mouth pressures or PI, di, max. Sniff nasal pressure provides a useful noninvasive measure of inspiratory muscle strength and has been validated in patients with neuromuscular disease **(Fig. 10)**.

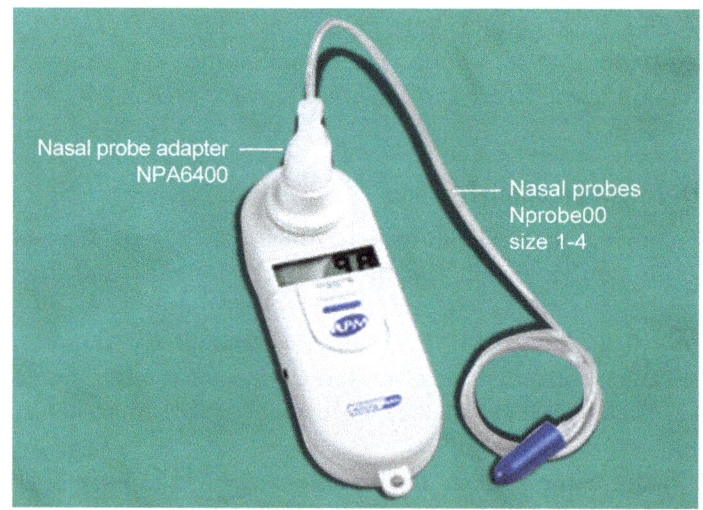

Fig. 10: Sniff nasal inspiratory pressure.

Cough gastric pressure is measured as an index of abdominal muscle strength. Pga, co is a useful test to supplement PE_{max}, particularly in patients unable to perform the PE_{max} maneuver reliably.

Nonvolitional Tests

- *Phrenic nerve stimulation:* Specific for the diaphragm and is not influenced by the central nervous system. It can be either electrical phrenic nerve stimulation (ES) or magnetic phrenic nerve stimulation (MS)
- *Abdominal muscle stimulation:* Magnetic stimulation over the eighth to 10th thoracic vertebrae posteriorly, and the recording of twitch gastric pressure, provide a clinically applicable nonvolitional test of abdominal muscle strength.

- Normal PI_{max} is -80 cmH_2O and PE_{max} is +80 cmH_2O. Both are reduced in neuromuscular disorders. A PE_{max} of less than 50 cmH_2O is indicative of ineffective cough and difficulty in clearing out secretions.

TESTS FOR CARDIOPULMONARY INTERACTION

- *Stair climbing test:* If a patient is able to climb three flights of stairs without stopping/dyspnea at his/her own pace indicates reduced morbidity and mortality. If not able to climb two flights indicates high risk
- *Six-minute walk test:* It is considered gold standard. If patient is able to walk more than 2,000 feet/6 min, VO_2 max greater than 15 mL/kg/min.

BEDSIDE PULMONARY FUNCTION TESTS

De Bono's Whistle Test[6]

The De Bono's whistle is a simple and easy to carry device introduced by EF De Bono in 1963. It is used to measure peak expiratory flow rate (PEFR) **(Fig. 11)**.

The whistle is made up of an outer disposable cardboard tube, which acts as a mouthpiece and slides over an inner wide bore plastic tube. The inner plastic tube has a slot on the side and a double orifice type whistle at the end. The slot on the plastic tube works as a leak hole. The outer cardboard tube can be slided over the inner plastic tube to adjust the size of the leak hole (slot) on the plastic tube. The plastic tube has a scale on it in the increments of 100 L/min.

The principle of the device is that for a given size of leak hole a minimum rate of airflow is required to sound the whistle. The patient blows forcibly into the cardboard mouthpiece initially with the smallest leak hole and then with gradually increasing size till the whistle cannot be sounded. The last size of the leak hole at which a whistle can be obtained is the patient's PEFR which can be read from the scale.

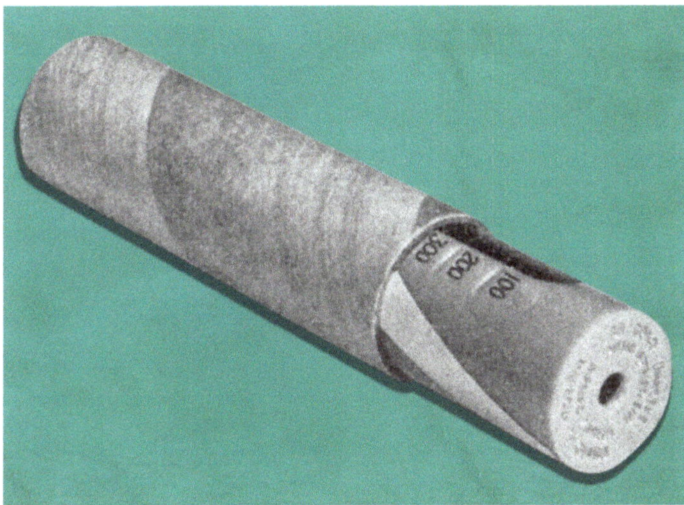

Fig. 11: De Bono whistle.

When compared with Wright's peak expiratory flow meter, the whistle gives satisfactory results for PEFR up to 300 L/min. It underestimates value at rates more than 300 L/min.

Snider's Match Test

The test was described by Thomas H Snider in 1959. It is a very simple test for objective assessment of pulmonary function. The only equipment needed is "match sticks or paper matches".

Method

The patient sits comfortably with head held erect and chin supported or rested. The physician holds a lighted match in front of the patient at a distance of 6 inches. The head and match should be at the same level. Once the initial match flare dies down the patient is asked to take a deep breath and exhale forcibly with the mouth wide open to blow out the match. Care is taken to prevent the patient from pursing his lips. The ability to blow out the match at 6 inches corresponds with the maximum breathing capacity (MBC) of greater than 60 L/min and FEV1 of greater than 1.6 L/min.

In the modified Snider's test, if the patient is unable to blow match at 6 inches, then the test is repeated with match at a distance of 3 inches. If the patient is able to blow the match indicates MBC of greater than 40 L/min but less than 60 L/min. The ability of a patient to blow a match held at the distance of 9 inches indicates MBC of greater than 150 L/min.

Sebrasez's Breath-holding Time

This test indicates overall cardiorespiratory reserve of the patient. No equipment is needed. The patient is asked to take a full breath and hold it for as long as possible. The breath-holding time of more than 25 seconds is normal and indicates normal cardiorespiratory reserve while less than 15 seconds indicates poor cardiorespiratory reserve.

Sebrasez's Single Breath Count

This test indicates VC. No equipment is needed. The patient is asked to take a deep breath and then exhale counting from 1, 2, 3,..., n till the time that patient cannot hold breath. Normal count is greater than 40 and indicates normal VC.

Cough Test

This test indicates VC and respiratory muscle strength. No instruments are required. The patient is asked to take a deep breath and then cough forcefully. An effective cough indicates good VC and respiratory muscle strength.

Weak or ineffective cough is an indicator of FVC less than 20 mL/kg, FEV1 less than 15 mL/kg and PEFR less than 200 mL/min. At the same time, cough with expectoration or continuous paroxysms of cough indicate high risk of post-operative pulmonary complications.

Forced Expiratory Time

For this test, only a simple stethoscope is needed. This test can be used to determine the nature of underlying pulmonary disease. The patient is asked to take a deep breath and then exhale forcefully and maximally while auscultating over the trachea.

Normal FET is 3–5 seconds. In obstructive lung disease, the FET is prolonged, i.e., greater than 5 seconds while in restrictive lung disease; the FET is shortened, i.e., less than 3 seconds.

Wright's Spirometer[7]

This is a simple, easy to use and portable instrument that measures the volume of air inspired and expired by the patient. Dr BM Wright developed the instrument in 1955. Later, he also developed Wright's peak flow meter in 1959.

It works on the principle of mechanical movement (rotation of a vane) caused by the kinetic energy of the gas flowing during inspiration or expiration. This rotation of the vane causes movement of a needle against a dial calibrated in liters and allows direct reading of the volume from it **(Fig. 12)**.

The Wright's spirometer can be used in a spontaneously breathing patient as well as in an intubated patient or patient using a face mask. With the patient in sitting or propped up position breaths through the spirometer for 1 minute and the minute volume is read directly from the dial. The TV can be derived by dividing the minute volume by respiratory rate. It gives accurate measurement in the range of 3.7–20 (± 10%) L/min.

The disadvantage of Wright's spirometer is that it under-reads at low flows and over-reads at high flows. The first because of friction and the latter, because of momentum. Wright's spirometer is very helpful for weaning patients off ventilator and for bed side PFTs.

Wright's Peak Flow Meter[8]

This instrument was designed and described in detail by Dr BM Wright and CB Mckerrow in 1959. It is specially designed to measure the peak flow rate during single forceful expiration. This instrument also works on the principle of rotation of vane. The design is modified from the Wright's spirometer in such a way that movement of the vane by expired gas causes gradual increase in the size of the gas outlet. The rotation of the vane also moves a needle across a scale calibrated in L/min **(Fig. 13)**.

The patient takes a VC breath and blows into the instrument through the mouthpiece forcefully. Usually, an average of three attempts is taken as the PEFR. The normal values are in male: 450–700 L/min and in female: 350–500 L/min. Value less than 200 L/min indicates poor cough and increased risk of postoperative pulmonary complications.

Even though the original Wright's peak flow meter is compact, it is still bulky and cumbersome to use. Newer versions of Wright's peak flow meter are now available specially designed for patients of asthma and other obstructive diseases. These are made of a light plastic tube with a mouthpiece and a scale located inside the device which measures the force of air expelled from the lungs into the tube. This force is measured in L/min from the scale. Examples of peak flow meters include Miniwright, ASSESS®, AsthmaCheck®, PocketPeak®, and MicroPeak®. Using these newer peak flow meters, the asthma patients can record the personal best reading and later self-assess the control of their disease status with the use of three zones (green, yellow, and red) marked on the scale. Most of these are still not available in Indian market.

Microspirometers

Many new models of the original Wright's spirometer are now available in market. Most of these monitor FVC, FEV1, PEF, and flow volume curves **(Fig. 14)**.

Fig. 12: Wright spirometer.

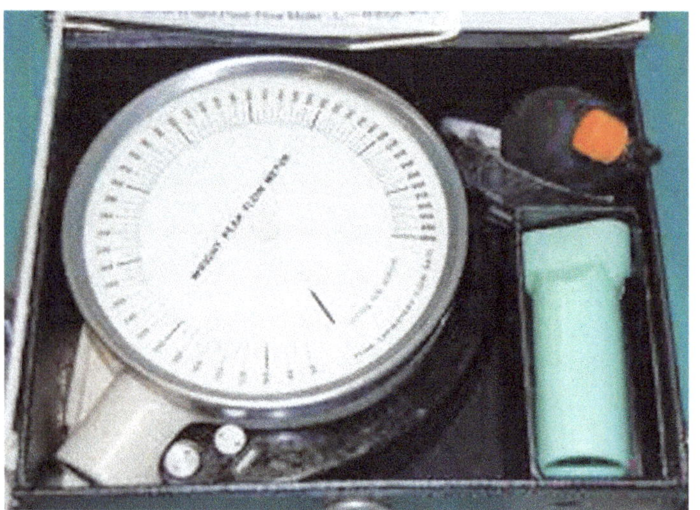

Fig. 13: Wright peak flow meter.

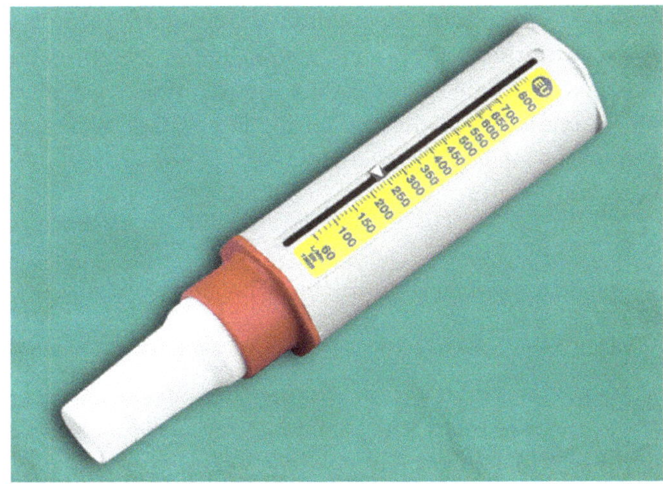

Fig. 14: Microspirometer.

These have been designed to be compact and user-friendly. They are designed using different principles of gas laws such as flow through variable orifice (mini Wright digital), fixed orifice or Ventury principle (Piko-1), stator or rotor device (Pulmo Life), pneumotachograph (Vitalograph Micro), Ultrasonic (EasyOne). These work well at ambient weather conditions.

Vitalograph

It is an instrument to record a single VC breath. It consists of a bellows which inflates when the patient expires into it after taking a VC breath. A recording pin is attached to the bellows which moves on a paper that moves at a constant speed by a motor. Volume is displayed on the Y-axis and time on the X-axis.

Bedside Pulse Oximetry and Arterial Blood Gas Analysis[9]

These are also important in comprehensive evaluation of cardiopulmonary system.

INTERPRETATION OF PULMONARY FUNCTION TESTS[10]

Step 1: Technical Quality

Verify "acceptability" and "reproducibility" criteria suggested by the ATS.

Step 2: Normal, Obstructive, or Restrictive Pattern?

- *Look for FEV1/FVC ratio:*
  - *If less than normal value:* Obstructive pattern
  - *If greater than or equal to normal value:* Normal or restrictive pattern
- *Restrictive pattern:* Look for FVC—If less than normal: Restrictive pattern → Confirm with TLC which will be reduced
- *Obstructive pattern:* Is obstruction reversible? Compare pre- and postbronchodilator values of FVC and FEV1—at least 12% or 200 mL increase with FEF 25-75%—an increase of greater than or equal to 20%. If yes: bronchial asthma; if no—chronic bronchitis or emphysema.

Step 3: How Severe is the Disease?

- *For obstruction:* Look at FEV1; and for restriction: Look at TLC
- *For obstruction:*
  - FEV1 greater than 100% of predicted: Normal variant
  - FEV1 less than 100% greater than 70% of predicted: Mild obstruction
  - FEV1 less than 70% greater than 60% of predicted: Moderate obstruction
  - FEV1 less than 60% greater than 50% of predicted: Moderately severe obstruction
  - FEV1 less than 50% greater than 34% of predicted: Severe obstruction
  - FEV1 less than 34% of predicted: Very severe obstruction.
- *For restriction:*
  - TLC less than 80%, but greater than 70% of predicted: Mild restriction
  - TLC less than 70%, but greater than 60% of predicted: Moderate restriction TLC less than 60% of predicted: Severe restriction.

Step 4: Differential Diagnosis?

Look at DLCO and lung volumes:

- *Obstruction:* DLCO less than 80% with ↑RV and FRC indicates "emphysema," DLCO greater than 80% and less affected RV and TLC indicates "asthma and chronic bronchitis"
- *Restriction:* DLCO less than 80% with ↓RV and FRC indicates "intrapulmonary restriction," DLCO greater than 80% and less affected RV and TLC indicates "extrapulmonary restriction".

PULMONARY FUNCTION TEST IN THE TIMES OF COVID-19

Coronavirus Disease 2019 (COVID-19) infection is associated with impairment of lung function in the form of restrictive pattern and which may extend from months to years.

In early convalescence phase, there is impaired diffusing capacity, decrease in respiratory muscle strength and lungs imaging abnormalities.

Performing pulmonary function test (PFT) in COVID-19 patient is known to increase risk of transmitting COVID-19 to people and healthcare personal present in PFT clinic, by producing aerosol droplets.

Practical considerations to be taken are:

- Avoiding PFT until absolutely necessary
- Postponing the PFTs till 30 days
- Performing PFTs at a safe distance of 2 meters

- Performing PFTs inside negative pressure room or leaving windows or door open
- Use of inline filters (bacterial as well as viral), disposable nose clips, and mouthpiece
- Cleaning the floor with 1% sodium hypochlorite and using PPEs and hand sanitizers.

The alternative methods like moving PFTs to point of care using hand held spirometers at home and personal peak flow meters should be adapted. Diagnostics questionnaire should be used instead of PFT in laboratories for diagnosis. In long term, point of care PFTs will help in early screening of COPD and asthmatic patients who are at risk of contracting COVID-19 infection by frequent visits to clinic.

CONCLUSION

Monitoring of pulmonary function is done by conducting PFTs. Pulmonary function tests are comprehensive tests, which assess and diagnose pulmonary problems of a patient. Pulmonary function tests should be an integral part of the preanesthetic evaluation of the patient with pulmonary problems, geriatric patients, and patients undergoing thoracic and upper abdominal surgeries. Performance of many of the PFTs is patient dependent and a single test may not always be adequate for diagnosis of underlying pulmonary problem. Although PFTs are conducted by a pulmonary technician, understanding the instruments used for these tests as well as the method of conducting these tests help in better interpretation of results. Better interpretation helps in adequate preoperative preparation of patient, determination of anesthesia plan and targeted postoperative pulmonary care for early recovery.

REFERENCES

1. Gass GD, Olsen GN. Preoperative pulmonary function testing to predict postoperative morbidity and mortality. Chest. 1986; 89(1):127-35.
2. Kwong Fah Koh. Gas, Tubes and Flows. Anaesth Intensive Care Med. 3(6):214-5.
3. Miller MR, Crapo R, Hankinson J, et al. General considerations for lung function testing. Eur Respir J. 2005;26(1):153-61.
4. Kumari Indira KS. Diffusion capacity of Lungs (DLCO) Part II–Technical standards and interpretative issues. Pulmonary. 2012;14(1):22-30.
5. Polkey MI, Green M, Moxham J. Measurement of respiratory muscle strength. Thorax. 1995;50:1131-5.
6. De Bono EF. Measurement of peak expiratory flow rate with a whistle. Br Med J. 1965;2(5469):1040-1.
7. Wright BM, Mckerrow CB. Maximum forced expiratory flow rate as a measure of ventilator capacity with a description of a new portable instrument for measuring it. British Med J. 1959; 2(5159):1041-6.
8. Moyle JT, Davey A. Ward's Anaesthetic Equipment, 4th edition. London: Saunders; 1998.
9. Miller RD, Eriksson LI, Lee A, et al. Miller's Anaesthesia, 7th edition. New York: Churchill Livingstone; 2010.
10. Pellegrino R, Viegi G, Brusasco V, et al. Interpretative strategies for lung function tests. Eur Respir J. 2005;26(5):948-68.

Peripheral Venous Cannulation

Anil Agarwal, Sujeet KS Gautam, Dwarkadas K Baheti

ABSTRACT

The intravenous (IV) cannulation is a common bedside medical procedure. It provides venous access for administration of IV fluid, drug administration, and transfusion of blood products. The procedure may be part of a planned intervention or investigation, or it might have to be carried out in an emergency. In this chapter, we have discussed the indications; technique; common problems encountered and methods of reducing pain on IV cannulation.

In the IV cannulation a needle is used to gain access to the target vein so that a cannula can be placed. When the cannula is stable the needle is removed and the cannula is fixed in place so that it cannot slide out. Although it looks like a very easy procedure, still adequate technical experience is required to minimize the common problems encountered such as difficulty in finding vein; difficulty in advancing IV cannula or venous valves.

The options available to reduce pain of IV cannulation are local anesthetic infiltration; applying of eutectic mixture of local anesthetic cream application and distraction techniques. We recommend the use of Valsalva procedure in adults and inflation of balloon in pediatric patients for attenuating venipuncture pain.

INTRODUCTION

The intravenous (IV) cannulation is a common bedside medical procedure and is first interventional encounter between doctor and patient. It provides venous access for administration of IV fluid, drug administration, and transfusion of blood products. The procedure may be part of a planned intervention or investigation, or it might have to be carried out in an emergency. It can act as lifeline to many patients.

Although it seems a small procedure and is a routine event for healthcare provider, many patients and their families associate it with dramatic events and serious illness. Hence, this can be both traumatic and painful for the patients and stressful so the patients and their families require support and encouragement to deal with the procedure.

In this procedure, a needle is used to gain access to the target vein so that a cannula can be placed. Once the cannula is stable, needle is removed and the cannula is fixed in place so that it cannot slide or come out. Usually, an upper extremity like dorsum of hand or forearm is chosen. The size of the IV cannula depends on the size of patient; condition of veins, and purpose and type of surgery. The larger the cannula size, the faster will be the rate at which fluids can be delivered.

The implications of IV cannulation should not be underestimated as introduction of a foreign body (i.e., IV cannula) inside any peripheral vein is an invasive intervention and carries infection risks. Hence, an aseptic nontouch technique should be employed throughout the procedure.

INDICATIONS

- Intravenous fluid therapy
- Intravenous drug administration
- Transfusion of blood products
- Blood sampling
- Intravenous administration of contrast agents for radiological interventions.

INTRAVENOUS CANNULA: SELECTION OF APPROPRIATE SIZE

The intravenous cannulas are available in various sizes mentioned as gauge (16–24 G; **Fig. 1**); lengths (25–44 mm); compositions and designs.

The flow rate of an IV cannula **(Table 1)** is directly proportional to its radius and inversely proportional to its length. In general, the smallest gauge of IV cannula should be selected for any prescribed therapy; in adult patients IV cannula of 18 G or 20 G is the usual choice, while in pediatric patients the usual choice is 22 G or 24 G. However, in emergency situations requiring large fluid volumes to be infused quickly, the largest gauge cannula (14 G or 16 G) is used.

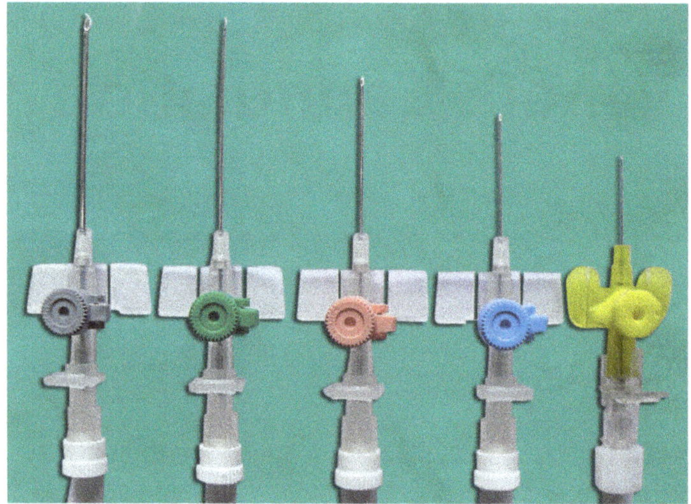

Fig. 1: Color-coding intravenous cannula of different gauge.

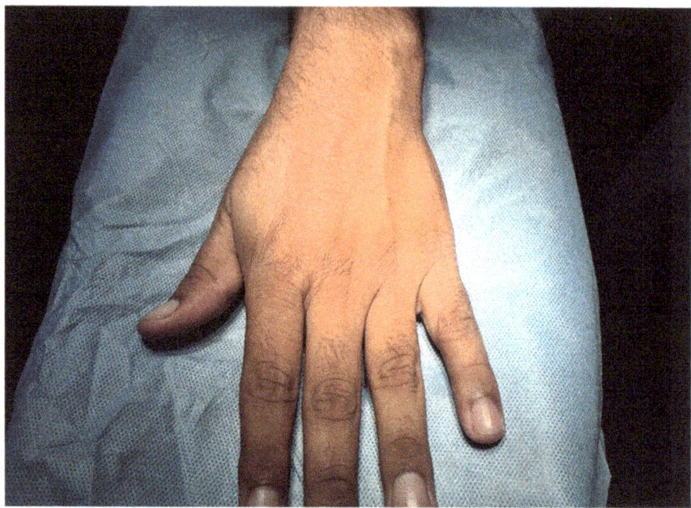

Fig. 2: Select site of venous cannulation.

TABLE 1: Maximal flow rate through different gauge cannula.

Gauge	*Color-code of cannula*	*Maximal flow rate (mL/min)*
24 G	Yellow	13
22 G	Blue	31
20 G	Pink	67
18 G	Green	103
16 G	Gray	236
14 G	Orange	270

TECHNIQUE OF INTRAVENOUS CANNULATION[1] (VIDEO 2)

Steps for intravenous cannulation are:

- *Prepare the patient:* Explain the procedure to the patient and take informed consent. Consider using local anesthesia
- *Select site of venous cannulation:* Commonly used positions for venous cannulation are the dorsal hand **(Fig. 2)**, forearm, or antecubital fossa. Apply a tourniquet proximally and encourage fist clenching to engorge the veins. Look for a straight, wide, "spongy" vein, with no evidence of valves. It is advised to use gloves or clean your hands with spirit or antiseptic solution
- Clean the site of venous cannulation with alcohol antiseptic and allow it to dry before cannulation **(Fig. 3)**. In case of children application of local or topical anesthetic gel is advised
- Before starting the procedure, warn the patient that there would be "sharp sting"
- Stretch the skin overlying the vein **(Fig. 4)** with non-dominant hand and insert cannula with your dominant hand as follows:
  - With the bevel facing up, slide the cannula through the skin and into the vein until flashback of blood is seen; this indicates that the needle tip has penetrated the vein **(Fig. 5)**

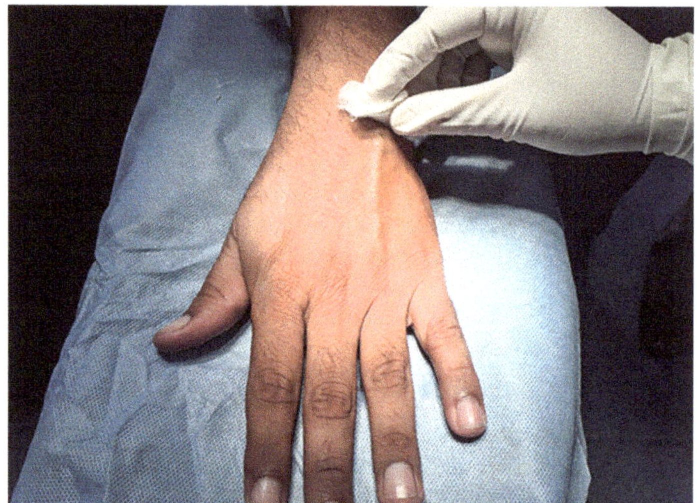

Fig. 3: Clean the site of venous cannulation with alcohol.

  - Advance the cannula a few millimeters further to ensure the catheter as well as needle tip enters the vein; withdraw the needle and advance the cannula inside the vein
  - Apply digital pressure of left thumb over the catheter tip **(Fig. 6)**, remove the needle, and put stylet into the cover of cannula held in nondominant hand, fix 10 cm extension line at the end of cannula
  - Pull the cannula 1–2 mm backward or downwards and apply sterile and transparent dressing (such as Tegaderm™) over the cannula with and write down date of cannulation over the dressing **(Fig. 7)**
  - Flush the cannula with 0.9% saline to confirm placement, watching for extravasations of fluid.

How to Reduce Incidence of Infection?

- Wipe your hands with antiseptic solution such as spirit, alcohol
- Pull cannula backward or downward to prevent tugging of cannula against wall of vein as it will cause pain while passing of fluid or injecting drug

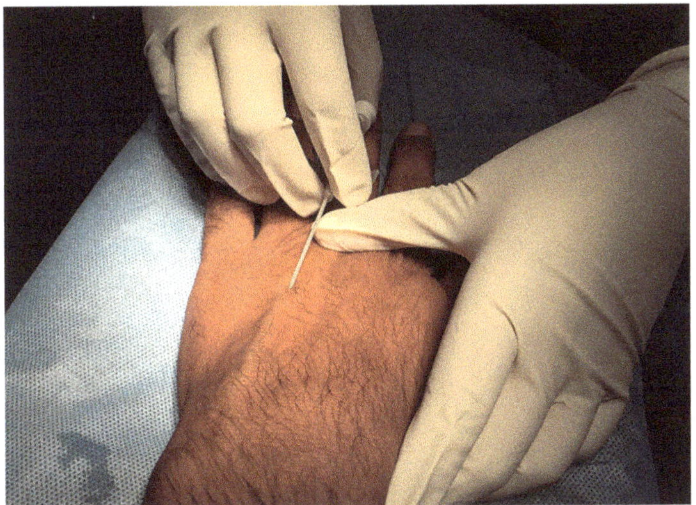

Fig. 4: Stretch the skin overlying the vein with nondominant hand.

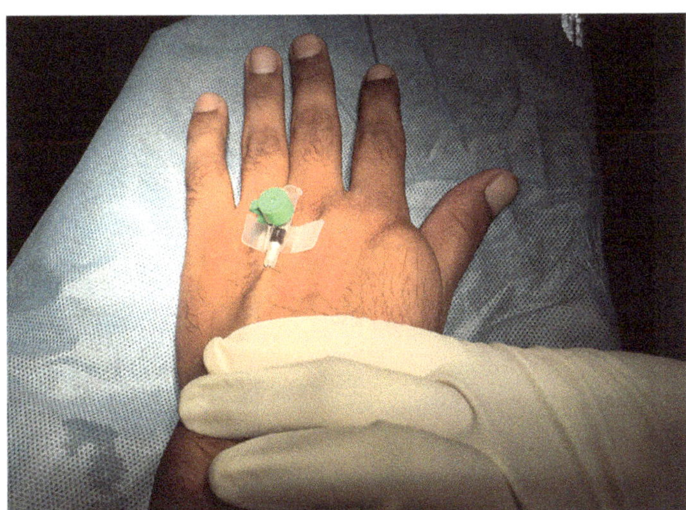

Fig. 6: Advance the cannula a few millimeters further to ensure the catheter as well as needle tip enters the vein; withdraw the needle and advance the cannula inside the vein.

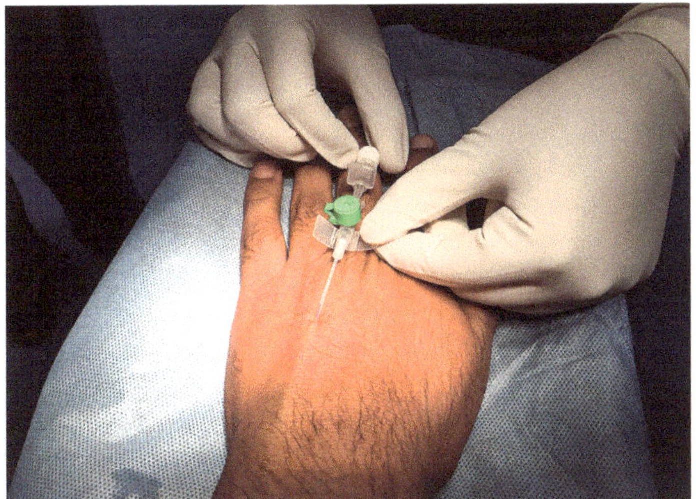

Fig. 5: With the bevel facing up, slide the cannula through the skin.

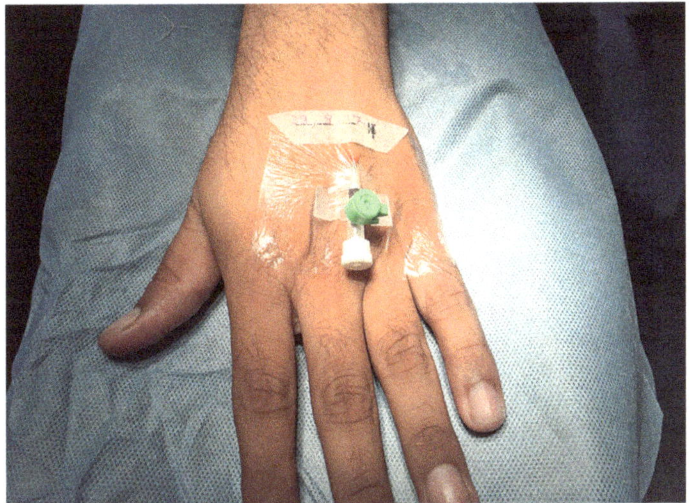

Fig. 7: Apply sterile and transparent dressing over the cannula and write down date of cannulation over the dressing.

- Use Tegaderam (sterile, transparent dressing) to fix cannula. Do not fix the cannula with sticking plaster, Elastoplast®, or any unsterile dressing **(Figs. 8A to C)**
- Use extension line instead of bivalve as movements while handling does cause pain during handling or injecting.

METHODS OF REDUCING PAIN ON INTRAVENOUS CANNULATION

A clinical study revealed that discomfort from IV catheter insertion ranked 5th among the 33 low morbidity clinical outcomes by expert anesthesiologists when both clinical importance and frequency were considered.[2] The pain experienced during venous cannulation has both somatic and psychological components. The pharmacological measures, such as the application of local anesthetics, treat only the somatic component of pain, whereas, attention diverting measures (e.g., cough trick) address only the psychological component of pain.[3,4]

There are two widely acceptable approaches to minimize this pain include application of local anesthetic cream and second is direct intradermal injection of local anesthetic at the site of venous cannulation. A comparison of intradermal injection and local anesthetic cream found them to be equally effective in relieving venipuncture pain.[5] The other methods have been tried to minimize venous cannulation pain with variable success ethyl chloride spray, nitrous oxide inhalation, distraction techniques, and "cough trick".

The pain relief prior to venous cannulation using topical analgesics is a growing practice as healthcare providers strive for a pain-free and pleasant hospital stay for patients. The eutectic mixture of local anesthetic (EMLA) cream is widely used topical analgesic since the early 1980s. The 1 g of EMLA contains 25 mg of lignocaine and 25 mg of prilocaine. It is formulated as an oil-in-water emulsion, yielding an 80% concentration in the oil droplets, which facilitates its skin penetration. However, EMLA has disadvantages like

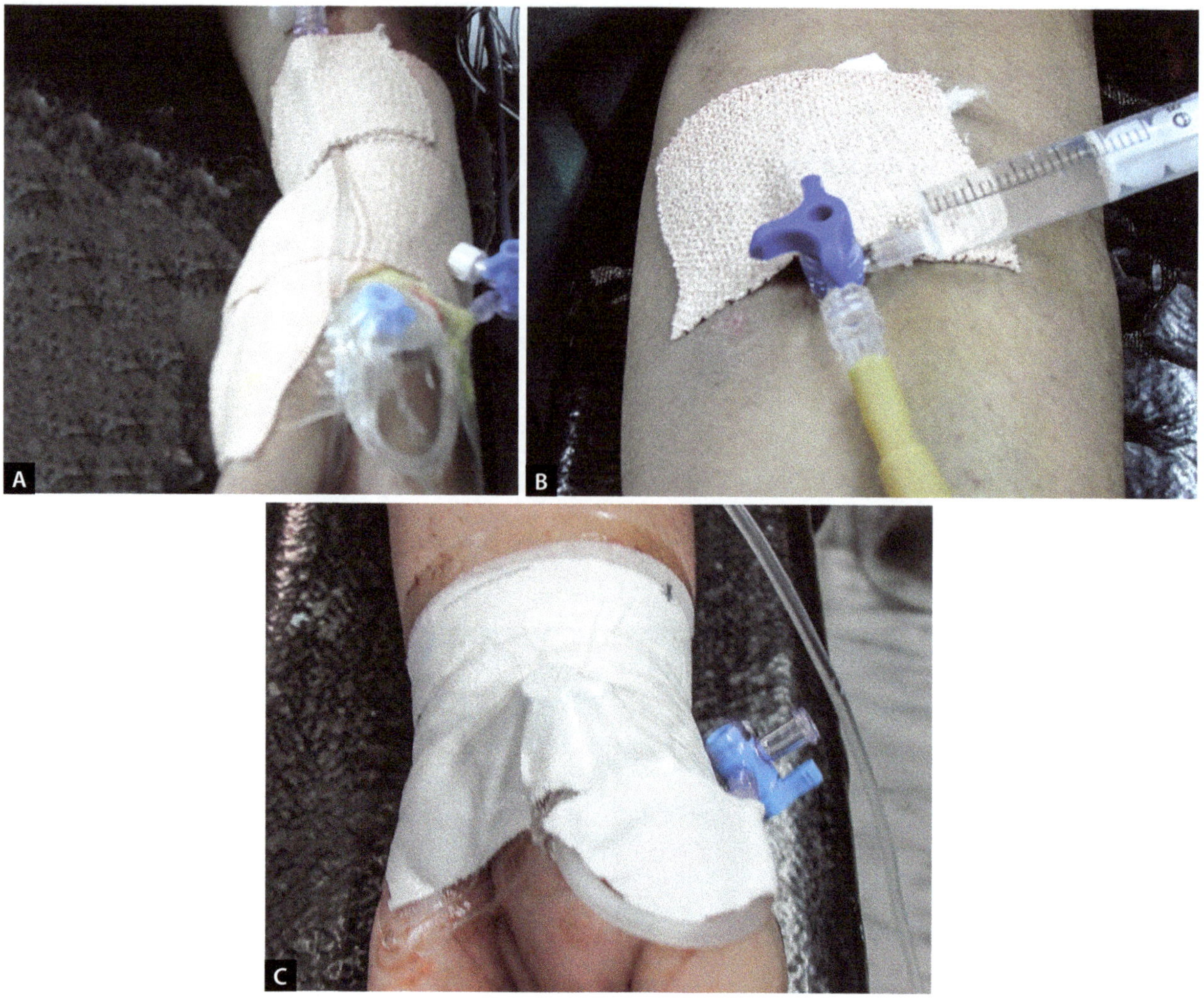

Figs. 8A to C: Do not fix the cannula with (A) Sticking plaster; (B) Elastoplast®; (C) Any unsterile dressing.

delayed onset of action, i.e., 60 minutes, a potential for complicated venous cannulation due to blanching of the skin, short duration of action, i.e., 30–60 minutes, and risk of methemoglobinemia in children below 1 year of age.

The Amethocaine is an ester local anesthetic that is more lipophilic than either lignocaine or prilocaine, facilitating its passage across the stratum corneum. In a 4% preparation, it has a more rapid onset of action of 30 minutes after application with occlusive dressing, lasts 4–6 hours, causes slight erythema, which may aid cannulation, and can be used in infants from 1 month of age with a seemingly better tolerability profile.[6]

We recommend performance of Valsalva procedure in adults by blowing into sphygmomanometer tubing as an effective method to reduce the incidence and severity of venipuncture pain with the added advantage that the number of patients in whom one needed to make the vein prominent before cannulation and the time taken for the same is also reduced.[7] We also recommend that inflation of a balloon during venipuncture in pediatric patients reduces both the incidence and severity of venipuncture pain. The observed reduction in the pain is secondary to distraction along with physiological effect of Valsalva on pain and increase in the intrathoracic pressure resulting in decrease in venous return and thus making the veins more prominent and easier to cannulate.[8]

A flash of light prior to venous cannulation (by stimulation of somatosensory thalamic has been reported to modulate nociceptive information) and is thus effective, simple and inexpensive method, which is devoid of any associated pain and side effects.[9]

The Diclofenac patch applied at the venipuncture site 1 hour prior to venous cannulation reduces both the incidence and severity of venipuncture pain.[10] Agarwal et al. further evaluated the efficacy of transdermal diclofenac patch (TDP) and compared it with EMLA for decreasing venous cannulation pain and peripheral venous thrombophlebitis and observed that both treatments were equally efficacious in reducing venous cannulation pain; however, TDP was associated with a lower incidence of thrombophlebitis.[11]

The topical application of miloxacin ointment (oleoresin capsicum equivalent to capsicum 0.075% w/w) has similar efficacy to EMLA but is a cheaper option and thus may be a suitable alternative for reducing the incidence and severity of venous cannulation pain.[12]

Recently, it has been reported that topical application of combination of capsaicin and EMLA have been found to be equally effective in minimizing the pain of venipuncture with the advantage that lower concentrations of individual drugs in this mixture may also be associated with reduced side effects.[13]

The search for an ideal option is still ongoing. However, till the time consensus is reached we suggest that one should try to minimize this intravenous cannulation pain with use of minimal or no medication and with minimal possible intervention. We therefore recommend the use of Valsalva procedure in adults and inflation of balloon in pediatric patients for attenuating venipuncture pain.

COMMON PROBLEMS ENCOUNTERED IN INTRAVENOUS CANNULATION

Common problems encountered in intravenous cannulation are mentioned as follows:

- *Difficulty in finding vein:* A common problem especially in patients after multiple cannulation during prolonged hospitalization; few solutions of this problem are to opt for any of the following alternative sites:
  - *Ventral forearm:* This site is often overlooked and usually has some wide flat veins
  - *Feet:* This site is useful in patients who have undergone axillary clearance surgeries
  - *Long saphenous vein:* This vein is located just anterior to the medial malleolus. Sometimes it is difficult to palpate this vein; a blind puncture at this site may be successful to identify this vein many times. Cannulation of this vein is especially useful in those cases in which fluid administration is desirable via inferior vena cava
  - *Neck:* External jugular vein is prominently seen most of the times traversing over the sternocleidomastoid muscle; this could serve as an important cannulation site, in case of inability to find veins at other conventional sites. Cannulation of this vein requires patient to lie in a supine position with head slightly lowered to facilitate engorgement; a finger could also be placed along the upper border of clavicle to compress the lower end of vein to facilitate its engorgement. Cannulation is performed keeping the cannula flat, almost parallel to the skin. This site serves as an important area in emergency situations for rapid fluid infusion
  - *Intraosseous fluid administration:* This serves as important alternative in pediatric patients if venous cannulation could not be performed; it is commonly done in the anterolateral tibial surface 2 cm below the tibial tuberosity
- *Enhancement of venous engorgement:* Many times veins seen in different body parts are of small caliber; in such cases, certain maneuvers could be done to enhance venous engorgement to facilitate cannulation:
  - *Warm the cannulation site:* This encourages venodilation and hence engorgement
  - *Fist clenching and unclenching with limb movement:* This enhances venous return
  - *Tapping of veins:* Veins dilate upon tapping along the length of vein
- *Difficulty in advancing IV cannula inside the vein:* This is because the cannula is not inside the vein; it could be because of the following reasons:
  - The cannula has passed through the vein outside the other side; in this case, withdraw the needle outside by 0.5–1 cm and then the cannula till flashback of blood followed by advancing the cannula inside the vein
  - Only the needle tip has entered the vein and cannula is superficial to the vein
- *Hematoma or bruise is forming at the site of cannulation:* This means that the needle has gone outside through the vein with extravasation of blood into the surrounding tissues
- *Highly mobile vein:* Seen in elderly population due to degradation of subcutaneous connective tissue; skin has be fixed tightly in these patients, to immobilize the vein, during cannulation
- *Venous valve prevents cannula advancement:* Valve in the lumen of vein may stop the cannula; cannula can be advanced by flushing the saline through cannula and simultaneously advancing the cannula. The hydrostatic pressure opens the valve and helps the cannula in crossing the valve.

Removal of Intravenous Cannula[14]

- Intravenous cannula should be removed or changed after 72–96 hours of insertion, or if there are any signs of phlebitis or infiltration or extravasation
- Intravenous cannula with port should be removed after 72 hours of use
- Intravenous cannula removal could serve as a source of infection, so asepsis must be ensured during this procedure.

Person removing the cannula should wash hands with antiseptic, remove the protective dressing and apply gentle pressure above the cannula tip while withdrawing the cannula. After removal of cannula apply firm pressure to the site, for approximately 2–3 minutes or more depending on the individual patient on anticoagulation. Once the bleeding has stopped apply a sterile plaster or dressing and document the removal in the notes and advise him or her to leave the dressing in place for 24 hours.

Complications of Intravenous Cannulation

- Pain, induration, and erythema
- Thrombophlebitis
- Infection
- Extravasation of fluids or drugs leads to swelling at the site of cannulation. It also depends upon type of fluid extravasated. The hypertonic solutions can be the irritant to the tissues so injection of saline with hyaluronidase may facilitate subcutaneous absorption
- Hematoma at the site of cannulation
- Skin and soft tissue necrosis around the site of cannulation
- Arterial puncture (rare).

CONCLUSION

In this chapter the indications, technique, tips for prevention of infection, common problems encountered and methods of reducing pain on venous cannulation are discussed. The peripheral venous cannulation is a common procedure required in most of the patients hence, it is mandatory to take maximum precautions. The choice of right size IV cannula; use of aseptic technique for cannulation with minimum pain is key.

REFERENCES

1. Harty E. Inserting peripheral intravenous cannulae—tips and tricks. Update in Anaesthesia. 2011;27:22-6.
2. Patterson P, Hussa AA, Fedele KA, et al. Comparison of four analgesic agents for venipuncture. AANA J. 2000;68:43-51.
3. Usichenko TI, Pavlovic D, Foellner S, et al. Reducing venipuncture pain by a cough trick: a randomized crossover volunteer study. Anesth Analg. 2004;98:343-5.
4. Macario A, Weinger M, Truong P, et al. Which clinical anesthesia outcomes are both common and important to avoid? The perspective of a panel of expert anesthesiologists. Anesth Analg. 1999;88:1085-91.
5. Soliman IE, Broadman LM, Hannallah RS, et al. Comparison of the analgesic effects of EMLA (eutectic mixture of local anesthetics) to intradermal lidocaine infiltration prior to venous cannulation in unpremeditated children. Anesthesiology. 1988;68:804-6.
6. Choy L, Collier J, Watson AR. Comparison of lignocaine-prilocaine cream and amethocaine gel for local analgesia before venipuncture in children. Acta Paediatr. 1999;88:961-4.
7. Agarwal A, Sinha PK, Tandon M, et al. Evaluation of efficacy of Valsalva on venous cannulation pain: a prospective, randomized study. Anesth Analg. 2005;101:1230-2.
8. Gupta D, Agarwal A, Dhiraaj S, et al. An evaluation of efficacy of the balloon inflation on venous cannulation pain in children: a prospective, randomized study. Anesth Analg. 2006;102:1372-5.
9. Agarwal A, Yadav G, Gupta D, et al. Role of flash of light for attenuation of venous cannulation pain: a prospective, randomized and placebo controlled study. Anesth Analg. 2008;106:814-6.
10. Agarwal A, Dhiraaj S, Kumar A, et al. Evaluation of a diclofenac transdermal patch for the attenuation of venous cannulation pain: a prospective, randomized, double-blind, placebo-controlled study. Anaesthesia. 2006;61:360-2.
11. Agarwal A, Gautam SKS, Gupta D, et al. Transdermal diclofenac patch vs. eutectic mixture of local anesthetics for venous cannulation pain. Can J Anesthesia. 2007;54:196-200.
12. Agarwal A, Yadav G, Gupta D, et al. Comparative evaluation of efficacy of miloxacin ointment and EMLA for attenuation of venipuncture pain: a prospective, randomized, double blind, placebo-controlled study. Anaesth Intensive Care. 2007;35:726-9.
13. Gupta D, Kishore K, Rastogi S, et al. A comparative evaluation of local application of the combination of eutectic mixture of local anesthetics and capsaicin for attenuation of venipuncture pain. Anesth Analg. 2013;116:568-71.
14. Ingram P, Lavery I. Peripheral intravenous cannulation: safe insertion and removal technique. Nurs Stand. 2007;22:44-8.

Central Venous and Arterial Cannulation

Lipika A Baliarsing, Anjana D Sahu

ABSTRACT

The anesthetist's role as a perioperative physician necessitates thorough knowledge of hemodynamic monitoring. Noninvasive monitoring suffices in most patients. However, the critically ill and surgeries involving large fluid shifts with hemodynamic instability require intensive monitoring. This is generally achieved by a combination of central venous, systemic arterial, and pulmonary artery catheter.

Central venous cannulation provides central venous pressure measurement and serves as a port for temporary hemodialysis, administration of vasoactive drugs, transvenous cardiac pacing, etc.

Arterial cannulation provides real-time continuous blood pressure monitoring and can be used for repeated blood sampling. Invasive (intra-arterial) blood pressure monitoring is a useful technique for blood pressure monitoring in the intensive care unit as well as in the operation theater. It provides beat-to-beat monitoring and its waveform morphology gives us idea about the hemodynamic status of the patient. Either central or peripheral artery can be cannulated depending upon the site of preference.

The pulmonary artery catheter measures right heart pressures, pulmonary arterial, and pulmonary capillary wedge pressures, estimates the left atrial and left ventricular end-diastolic pressures, measures mixed venous oxygen saturation, cardiac output by thermodilution technique, etc. It is discussed in Chapter 35: Pulmonary Artery Catheter.

Central cannulation provides vast data whose interpretation depends on the knowledge and experience of the anesthetist. These procedures are not without complications and the risk–benefit ratio must be considered. This chapter describes in detail the central venous and arterial pressure monitoring equipment and technique. It also provides valuable information about the pressure measurement system.

In our second edition we have highlighted the role of ultrasound in vascular cannulation. The recent updates on relationship of central venous pressure and Starling's curve have been added. We have also incorporated the recent guidelines for the prevention of central line-associated bloodstream infections.

CENTRAL VENOUS CANNULATION

INTRODUCTION

The central venous pressure (CVP) measurement is the mainstay of hemodynamic monitoring. This measures right atrial pressure (RAP) and indicates circulating blood volume, venous tone, and right ventricular (RV) function. Vasoactive drugs, fluids, chemotherapeutic agents are administered through central line. Transvenous pacing and pulmonary artery catheter placement are done through this route. Commonly right internal jugular vein (IJV) is preferred for venous cannulation and Seldinger technique is used for cannulating the vein. Complications like hematoma, arrhythmias can happen, but they are preventable. The CVP waveform can be analyzed for RV function and left ventricular (LV) filling pressure. Abnormal waves can be observed in atrioventricular (AV) dissociation, cardiac tamponade, valvular dysfunction, etc.

Central venous pressure monitoring is a useful monitor to assess the cardiovascular system. CVP is also known as RAP. It reflects the pressure of blood in thoracic vena cava, near right atrium (RA) of the heart and is an estimate of the amount of blood returning to the heart. Many factors influence the CVP, i.e., patient's blood volume, venous tone, and right ventricle (RV) performance. It is a good determinant of right ventricular end-diastolic volume (RVEDV). Although controversial, CVP is still being used as a surrogate for preload and a predictor of volume responsiveness.

MEASUREMENT OF CENTRAL VENOUS PRESSURE

The very basic aspect of cardiovascular assessment is assessment of CVP through physical examination of neck veins. There are two reference points from where CVP can be measured, i.e., (i) from the sternum (0–14 cmH_2O) and (ii) from the mid-axillary line (8–15 cmH_2O). When central venous catheter (CVC) is connected to a properly calibrated water column, the height of the column indicates the CVP. Water manometers were used in the past to measure CVP by observing the height of mercury column. Phlebostatic axis is a reference point used to estimate the level of *in situ* catheter. It is identified as the point midway between the anteroposterior chest wall at the level of fourth intercostal space. This is the precise anatomical point of origin of the hemodynamic pressures being measured. It is the cavo-atrial junction which lies approximately below superior vena cava (SVC). A normal CVP measurement in a spontaneously breathing patient is 5–10 cm of water, rising 3–5 cm during mechanical ventilation. The CVP measurement may still be in the normal range even with hypovolemia due to venoconstriction.

CENTRAL VENOUS CANNULATION METHOD

As a standard clinical method cannulation of a central large vein is performed, such as right-sided IJV, subclavian vein, femoral vein, and antecubital vein for measuring the CVP. Central venous catheters are available in various ranges of lengths, gauges, lumens, composition of catheter material for both adults and children. Most commonly 7-French, 20 cm multilumen catheter is used with one port of 16 gauge (G) and other two ports of 18 G allowing monitoring of CVP and infusion of drugs simultaneously. Catheters can be used for short-term (less than 6 weeks) as in the postoperative period and intensive care unit (ICU) or long term (more than 6 weeks) as in patients on dialysis or receiving chemotherapy. Catheter can be placed via internal jugular (most common) **(Video 16)**, subclavian, femoral, or antecubital vein approach. Multilumen lines are inserted using Seldinger technique. Single lumen lines may be sited using Seldinger technique or catheter-over-needle method. National Institute for Health and Care Excellence (NICE) in the United Kingdom guidelines (2002) recommend use of two-dimensional (2D) ultrasound to guide catheter placement particularly via IJV.[1] Otherwise, landmark method is used **(Video 16)**.

DESCRIPTION OF THE CATHETER AND THE DESIGN

Central venous catheters range from simple single lumen catheter to complex combination of introducer sheaths and multilumen catheters. Most catheters are supplied as self-contained catheters for percutaneous insertion using Seldinger technique or catheter-over-needle sets. Most single and multilumen catheters have a fixed length. The most important factor is to keep the tip of the catheter rightly placed. The US Food and Drug Administration prohibits the placement of the catheter tip in the RA. Introducer sheaths are available from 9- to 11-French. It aids in introducing the pulmonary artery catheter into the circulation and can function as a large bore CVC for resuscitation. There are lots of manufacturers in the market.[2] Depending on duration of use the catheters can be divided into (i) short-term or temporary catheters and (ii) long-term catheter.[2] Temporary catheters are placed for less than 1 week for perioperative use or for some acute event. Short-term catheters can be placed from 1 to 6 weeks before either exchanging or replacing it. The portion of the catheter near the skin can have silver incorporated collagen cuff, which can make the life of the catheter to be extended to 6 weeks by preventing infection. Long-term catheters are placed for more than 6 weeks usually for total parenteral nutrition, antibiotics administration for osteomyelitis, endocarditis, intravascular device-related infection, etc. The risk of infection increases with short-term catheters if they are kept for longer period, as they have no barriers to infection by design. ARROWgard Blue® available from Arrow International Inc. manufactures the catheters coated with antimicrobicidal molecules. The coating is chlorhexidine-silver sulfadiazine molecularly bonded to the external part of the intravascular portion of the CVC. Temporary catheters are usually made up of polyurethane, making the duration of cannulation limited. As this material is rigid at room temperature for ease of insertion, it can cause vessel erosion if left inside vein for longer time, in spite of becoming flexible when exposed to body temperature. It has the advantages of maintaining low thrombogenicity. It has good structural stability when exposed to variety of infusates. Long-term catheters are usually made of silicone elastomer or Silastic. These catheters are used in patients undergoing dialysis, requiring chemotherapy so need to be placed in the body for really long time. This molecule is more flexible and soft than the polyurethane as well as less thrombogenic. As it is soft, the insertion becomes difficult thus the use of peel away sheath is required to manipulate the catheter into the central veins. The lumen is of the double configuration type with both temporary and long-term catheters. The proximal lumen is used as arterial lumen and through the more distal lumen venous return occurs when long-term catheters are used for dialysis. The dual lumen format can be of three types like (i) side-by-side, (ii) coaxial, and (iii) recently introduced individual lumen. Side-by-side configuration is the most commonly used design (Hickman hemodialysis catheter by Bard Access System). In the triple lumen catheter system, the distal 18 G brown port is most proximal to RA, it is used for general access, CVP monitoring and administration of blood products. The middle port of blue color is of 18 G and used for general access and medication. The proximal white port is 18 G and used for general access, drawing blood samples and total parenteral nutrition. It has to be ensured that there are no leaks, loose connections or stopcocks in the wrong position and forward flow is maintained always. Thrombus formation is prevented by flushing the device with heparinized solution.[3]

INDICATIONS

The CVP monitoring is a good indicator of intravascular volume status. This reflects LV filling pressure in patients

BOX 1: Indications for placing the central venous cannula in the perioperative period.

- *Central venous pressure monitoring in:*
  - All cardiac surgical cases
  - Surgery involving large fluid shifts or blood loss in patients with reasonable cardiac function
- *Administering drugs and medications—hyperalimentation for critically ill patients:*
  - Vasoactive drugs
  - Chemotherapy
  - Antibiotic therapy for prolonged period
  - Irritant drugs to the peripheral veins
- Aspiration of air in case of air embolism in neurosurgical patients especially in sitting position, pelvic surgeries
- For fast fluid administration
- Peripheral veins unavailable
- Pulmonary artery catheterization and monitoring of pulmonary artery pressure
- Sampling site for repeated blood testing
- Temporary hemodialysis
- Transvenous cardiac pacing
- Major trauma

with good ventricular function. It does not reflect the left heart filling pressure in elderly patients, as they have associated coronary artery disease. The CVP placement is mandatory in all cardiac surgical patients during cardiopulmonary bypass (CPB). Sometimes SVC cannula can get kinked during CPB, showing high CVP and may cause alarming decrease in cerebral venous pressure in patients undergoing CPB. The tip of the catheter in the SVC indicates RAP and cerebral venous pressure. The indications for placing the central venous cannula in the perioperative period are given in **Box 1**.[4]

CONTRAINDICATIONS

The CVP catheter placement is absolutely contraindicated in patients having SVC syndrome.[1] The venous pressure is very high in the head and upper part of the body. If fluid is administered through the obstructed venous circulation, it will increase the edema and exacerbate the high venous pressure. The medications given through this might not reach the central circulation as it goes through the collateral circulation in slow fashion. In these cases, femoral vein should be cannulated. Duplex scanning or venography for patency of selected venous site should be done if cannulation has to done in the upper extremities. The contraindications for central venous cannulation are given in **Box 2**.

SITES

Internal Jugular Vein Cannulation[3]

The selection of the most suitable site for carrying out an effective and safe cannulation needs the judgment of indication for placement of CVP catheter, the clinical scenario, the medical condition of the patient and the level of expertise of the clinician performing the cannulation. In an emphysematous patient, internal jugular is safer approach than

BOX 2: Contraindications for central venous cannulation.

- *Absolute contraindications:*
  - The superior vena cava syndrome
  - Pneumothorax or hemothorax on the contralateral site
- *Relative contraindications:*
  - Coagulopathies
  - In presence of newly inserted pacemaker wire (4–6 weeks)
  - Presence of carotid disease
  - Diaphragmatic dysfunction
  - Thyromegaly
  - Previous neck surgery
  - Burns scar on the neck
  - Recent cannulation of the internal jugular vein
  - Skin infection over puncture site
  - Uncooperative patient
  - No consent for the procedure
  - Application of high positive end-expiratory pressure
  - Only one functioning lung

subclavian. Trauma patients with associated cervical spine injury are resuscitated effectively through a subclavian or femoral approach. Right IJV is the most suited vein for transvenous pacing, as it is the most direct and predictably accessible route to RV. In a patient with bleeding diathesis, IJV or external jugular vein (EJV) will be a preferable route than the subclavian route as compression can be applied readily. The length of the catheter inserted to position the catheter tip in the SVC varies according to puncture site; it is 3–5 cm more when the left IJV or EJV is chosen versus the right IJV. The percutaneous puncture of the right IJV is the most preferred method for central venous cannulation for the anesthesiologists since 1960s.[1,4] It is readily identifiable and approachable, the landmarks on the surface anatomy are palpable most of the time **(Table 1)**.[4] The rate of successful placement is 90–99% and the straight course to the SVC is a huge advantage.[4]

The steps for right IJV cannulation along with the rationale and possible problem in each step and the solution are discussed in **Table 2**[3] **(Figs. 1 to 3)**.

OTHER SITES FOR PLACEMENT OF CENTRAL VENOUS CATHETER

Internal Jugular Vein on the Left Side

The technique of IJV cannulation on the left side is more or less similar to right side IJV but other anatomical differences are like the higher dome of pleura increasing the risk of pneumothorax. The thoracic duct is close by the junction of IJV and subclavian vein so the risk of duct injury is higher. The vein itself is smaller in caliber than right side IJV. The carotid artery overlaps more on the vein when head is rotated more than 40° for cannulation. The catheter enters through left brachiocephalic and may rest against the lateral wall of SVC thus increasing the risk of vessel injury. So, the confirmation of the position of the tip of the catheter placement is a must through fluoroscopy, X-ray, ultrasonography. As this approach is not always used, it might give rise to more adverse events and morbidity.

TABLE 1: Comparison of different approaches to the internal jugular vein cannulation.

Approach to the IJV	*Anatomical landmarks*	*Complications*
Central approach	From the apex of the triangle formed by clavicular and sternal head of sternocleidomastoid the needle has to be aimed caudally and laterally toward same side nipple	• Pneumothorax (low incidence) • Hemothorax (low incidence)
Anterior approach	From the medial border of medial head of SCM approximately 5 cm above the clavicle. The needle direction toward same side nipple	• Carotid puncture (risk higher) • Risk reduces if carotid artery retracted medially • Hemothorax (high incidence)
Posterior approach	At the point of intersection of a line drawn from cricoid ring on the lateral border of clavicular head of SCM	• Carotid artery puncture (risk higher) • Pneumothorax and hemothorax (low risk)
Supraclavicular approach	At the interscalene groove 2 cm above the clavicle, the needle directs medially and caudally	• Pneumothorax (high incidence) • Subclavian artery puncture risk • Hemothorax

(IJV: internal jugular vein; SCM: sternocleidomastoid muscle)

TABLE 2: Steps for right internal jugular vein cannulation along with the rationale and possible problems.

Steps of IJV cannulation	*Rationale and possible problems*
1. Functioning cardioscope and pulse oximeter to be applied on the patient. Oxygen to be administered via polymask	1. Essential for monitoring arrhythmias, hypoxemia
2. Remove head pillow and rotate head to left. Patient's head to be lifted to note the position of both heads of SCM and mark the surface	2. Aids in visualization
3. Patient positioned in 15° Trendelenburg position. A wedge of 6–8 inches is kept below the shoulder and the head ring can be removed to make the anatomical landmark prominent	3. Distends IJV and decreases risk of air embolism. May increase the congestive heart failure symptoms
4. Under due asepsis, preparation and draping of the cannulation site to be done carefully	4. Mandatory sterile gown and full gloves for prevention of infection
5. Landmarks rechecked and skin weal raised if patient is awake, 1% infiltration with lignocaine in the deeper planes to be done	5. Sometimes IJV can be superficial and may be found while infiltrating, withdraw syringe before injecting LA
6. Finder needle of 22 gauge (G) 3.75 cm or 11/2 inch length attached to a Luer-lock 5 cc syringe	6. Use of finder needle reduces the risk of causing bigger hematoma in case the carotid artery is punctured
7. Surface anatomy reconfirmed and placing the syringe-needle assembly negative aspiration is applied in the appropriate direction as per the approach chosen	7. Constant aspiration as unit advanced is required to see flashback
8. Once the vein is located with free dark venous blood aspiration in the aspirating syringe a. Finder needle can be left in place or b. Remembering the direction finder needle can be removed keeping the skin and surface anatomy fixed by the left hand	8. Needle left in place serves as reminder of location and if finder needle interferes with cannulation can be removed
9. The vein is then punctured with an 18 G, 2 1/2 inch (6.4 cm) thin-walled needle attached to a 5-mL syringe along the same track when flashback of dark venous blood comes advance the unit by 1 mm	9. Once IJV is located end of needle is capped with finger or syringe to avoid air embolism
10. If blood is not aspirated freely a. Needle is to be removed b. Syringe to replaced and aspirate c. Withdraw needle till free flow of blood comes d. Advance the needle slowly into vein	10. The needle might have pierced the posterior wall or the patient might be hypovolemic and IV fluid bolus might increase success. Increased head down position might help
11. Confirm IV placement by a. Checking for lack of pulsatile flow b. Compare IJV and arterial samples, visually or by oximetry c. Compare the waveforms by attaching the transducer	11. If arterial cannulation is diagnosed, needle syringe assembly is removed and applies firm pressure for at least 5 minutes to avoid hematoma in the carotid artery
12. Now place the dilator on the needle length	12. While passing the guidewire through the needle arrhythmias can happen
13. Place the CVC over wire after removing the dilator	13. Skin nick might be needed to accommodate the introducer
14. Sterile dressing is applied after suturing the CVC firmly in place on the neck	14. Firm sterile dressing over the sutured CVC prevents the dislodgment and infection

(IJV: internal jugular vein; SCM: sternocleidomastoid muscle; LA: local anesthetic; CVC: central venous catheter)

Subclavian Vein

This route is a popular route in trauma patients where cervical spine is immobilized for collars, for long-term use in patients undergoing dialysis, for chemotherapy, total parenteral nutrition, for emergency resuscitation, long-term intravenous therapy. The advantages are many as (i) patient is comfortable as neck is free, and (ii) risk of infection is comparatively less than IJV and femoral route.[4]

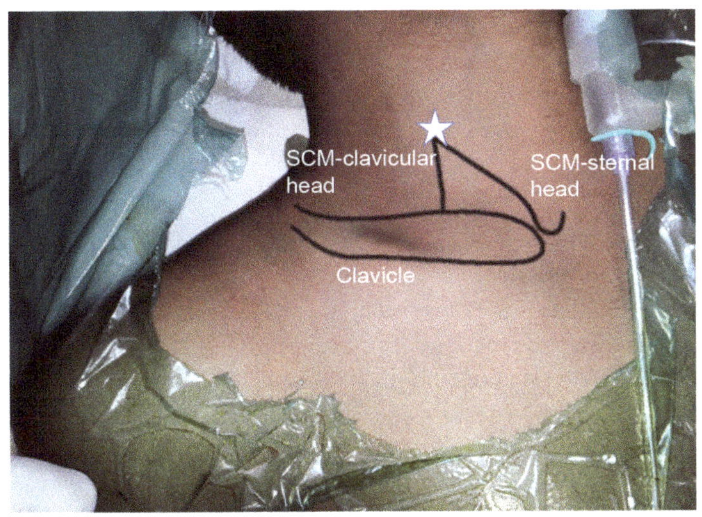

Fig. 1: Surface landmark for internal jugular vein cannulation.

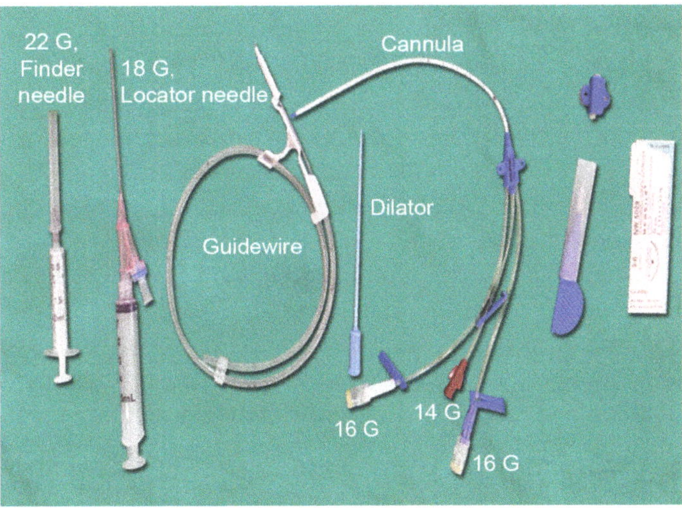

Fig. 2: Central venous pressure set.

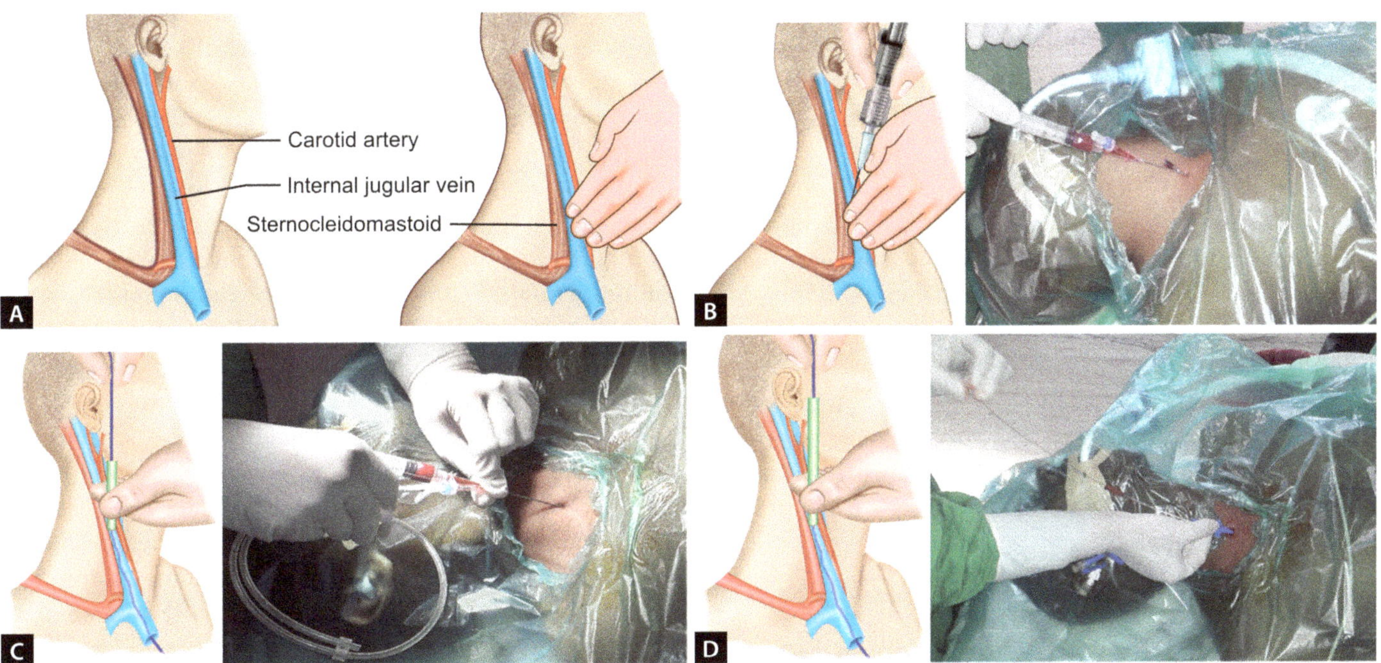

Figs. 3A to D: Steps of internal jugular vein cannulation (IJV). (A) Landmarks and palpation of internal carotid artery; (B) Cannulation of IJV; (C) Introduction of guidewire; (D) Advancement of central venous cannula.

Technique

The patient is placed in a head low position, the arms kept adducted fully and a roll is placed between the shoulder blades so that the infraclavicular area gets exposed properly, after thorough asepsis the skin is punctured 2–3 cm below the midpoint of clavicle with the needle directed toward the suprasternal notch, which should be identified by keeping the fingers of the other hand of the operator. The needle is advanced gently with a constant negative pressure aspiration on the plunger of the syringe. If in the first attempt, the subclavian vein is not entered the needle can be withdrawn a little bit and again in the next attempt the needle can be moved in more rostral direction keeping it close to the undersurface of clavicle and not increase the downward angle while advancing the needle. After the subclavian vein is punctured, the rest of the procedure is same as in IJV cannulation.

Complications

The incidence of pneumothorax is less than 2% and subclavian artery puncture is 5%. The incidence of complication is less in more experienced hands. The risk of hematoma and pneumothorax rise along with multiple attempts to cannulate. Bilateral attempts for this approach should not be attempted at all. If subclavian vein is not punctured in the second or third attempt, more attempts are discouraged at this point. The vein is usually punctured with the needle over which guidewire is to be threaded as the finder needle of a 6.8 cm length does not suffice to reach up to the thin-walled vein.

External Jugular Vein

This vein courses superficially across the sternocleidomastoid muscle to join the subclavian vein close to the junction of the IJV and subclavian vein. The course of this vein is tortuous in the neck and presence of valves makes it difficult to thread the guidewire and access the central line through this route.

External jugular vein under ultrasound guidance can be a choice of central vein cannulation in ICU during pandemic scenario of corona virus disease (COVID-19) or such, where large number of critical patients requiring central vein cannulation and there is unavailability of the skilled persons.[4A]

Technique

After the head down position once the vein is distended, applying traction to the vein an 18 G catheter instead of the needle is introduced into the vein and a J-tipped flexible guidewire is used to negotiate the tortuous course of the vein. Central passage of the catheter is usually and surprisingly easy from the left EJV. The remainder of the insertion technique is same as in IJV cannulation.

Advantage and Disadvantage

It is a safe and ready venous access via angiocatheter. The risk of vessel avulsion is higher in this route.

Femoral Vein

Femoral vein cannulation is a good site when jugular and subclavian veins are not accessible. This situation is encountered in patients with burns, trauma, surgical procedures involving the head, neck, upper thorax or during cardiopulmonary resuscitation.

Technique

The femoral artery is palpated as the femoral vein lies medial to the femoral artery. Below the inguinal ligament the femoral vein is punctured. A long catheter (40–70 cm) is positioned under electrocardiogram (ECG) or fluoroscopic guidance in the inferior vena cava (IVC) close to cavoatrial junction. A catheter of shorter length 15–20 cm can be inserted from the femoral vein into the common iliac vein. Intra-abdominal venous pressure measurement is obtained from both techniques which correlate well with SVC pressure, in mechanically-ventilated patients. This correlation might not be valid in spontaneously breathing patients, in patients who are not in supine position, and in patients with raised intrathoracic or intra-abdominal pressure.

Advantage and Disadvantage

The complications of central vein cannulation like pneumothorax, neck hematoma are avoided. But injury to femoral artery and nerve can happen. Risk of infection, thromboembolic complications, vascular injury can happen which may lead to intra-abdominal, retroperitoneal hemorrhage. In children below 6 months, avascular necrosis of femur, bladder injury, and gangrenous changes in the leg due to extravasation can happen.

Peripherally Inserted Central Cannula

Peripherally inserted central cannulas (PICCs) are a reliable alternative to short-term CVCs with a lower risk of complications. For venous access devices to be termed PICC, it must be inserted into the peripheral vasculature and the distal tip must terminate in the SVC, IVC, or proximal RA. For infants, the catheter must be inserted in the saphenous vein with the tip terminating in the IVC above the level of the diaphragm. Generally, PICCs are inserted into the basilic and cephalic veins of the antecubital space or brachial veins. Basilic vein is preferred as it offers the largest diameter (8 mm) of the upper extremity vessels and has a nontortuous entry into the subclavian vein. Cephalic vein (6 mm) is smaller and angles 90° to enter the terminal portion of the axillary vein, sometimes making catheter advancement difficult. Brachial veins lie in the center of the mid to upper arm and cannot be outwardly visualized or palpated; ultrasound guidance is required for access. Peripherally inserted central cannulas are not advisable in patients with renal failure and impending need for dialysis, in whom preservation of upper extremity veins is needed for fistula formation. Use the smallest gauge of PICC to reduce the risk of phlebitis. Polyurethane is a tougher material enabling thinner lumen valves and larger internal diameters of the lumina, this significantly increases flow rates and reduces the potential for breakage and rupture of the catheter. Polyurethane PICCs have higher risk of thrombosis compared to silicone. PICCs need to be regularly flushed; volume of the flush or lock should be equal to at least twice the volume of the catheter plus add-on devices. The volume of the lumen is generally less than 1 mL and an access device 0.1 mL, so a minimum volume of 2–3 mL of solution should be sufficient. Use a 10-mL or larger syringe to avoid excessive pressure and catheter rupture. Syringe smaller than 10 mL can produce high pressure in the lumen and risk of catheter rupture. Two methods of PICC insertion are, the peel-away technique and modified Seldinger technique.

- *Peel-away cannula technique:* Intravenous access is established like a regular intravenous cannula. The stylet is removed and the catheter inserted through the cannula. The cannula is then pulled back and peeled away from the catheter
- *Modified Seldinger technique:* The vein is accessed through a regular hypodermic needle, a guidewire is threaded several centimeters and the needle removed leaving the guidewire in place. The guidewire is not advanced past the shoulder. A nick is made in the skin beside the guidewire and an introducer sheath with

dilator is inserted over the guidewire. The guidewire and dilator are removed, the catheter is advanced through the introducer sheath which is then pulled back and peeled away.

- Infraclavicular SCV catheterization is associated with a significantly higher rate of pneumothorax during mechanical ventilation. To prevent this, if a short phase of apnea is justifiable in the patient, mechanical ventilation should be discontinued during the central vein cannulation.[4B] Inadvertent pulmonary artery cannulation can be a complication while performing subclavian artery cannulation.[4C] This emphasizes more of using ultrasound guidance for central venous cannulation.

Complications

These are phlebitis, thrombus formation, infection, and malposition. The catheter tip of the standard long venous catheter inserted from the antecubital vein may advance into the heart as the arm is abducted increasing the risk of cardiac perforation or arrhythmias. Be cautious while placing any CVCs while PICC line is in place due to the risk of shearing the PICC line within the central venous circulation.

Indications

These indications are parenteral nutrition, chemotherapy, CVP monitoring, and short-term infusion of vasoactive drugs.

The EJV runs from the angle of the mandible inferolaterally to the clavicle, crossing the sternocleidomastoid obliquely about 5 cm above the clavicle and terminates behind the middle of the clavicle, where it joins the subclavian vein. Being superficial in course the chances of pneumothorax or unintended arterial puncture are practically nil. It is best accessed at a 10–25° angle at a site about the midpoint of the vein. The head is turned to opposite side in Trendelenburg position, slight pressure above the clavicle and Valsalva maneuver help in making the EJV more prominent. A give-way sensation is perceived and blood appears in the chamber of the venous access device. The angle should be reduced to prevent puncture of the posterior wall of the vein and the catheter is gently advanced 2–3 mm into the vein.

It is possible to cannulate the IJV through the EJV. A guidewire should be introduced through the catheter rather than the thin-walled needle. The curved J-tip of the guidewire helps negotiate the tortuous course between the EJV and SCV. The ipsilateral shoulder may be abducted beyond 90° before advancing the wire to prevent it from moving peripherally into the subclavian vein. Applying mild caudal traction on the shoulder with the ipsilateral arm placed at the side helps to straighten the course of EJV as the wire is advanced.

Ultrasound-guided Central Venous Cannulation

The 2D ultrasound guidance of IJV cannulation in defining the anatomical variations of IJV, locating the vein and decreasing the incidence of arterial puncture has made it a popular technology in this procedure in the operating theater or ICU. Updates will be discussed at the end of the chapter.

Technique

Internal jugular vein cannulation is performed with a real time, 2D 7.5–10 MHz protected by a sterile sheath. The view of the target vessel is obtained by holding the ultrasound probe in the nondominant hand. The ultrasound images of the vein and artery appear as two circular black images. The compressibility, vein wall appearance and the anatomic location make the vein identified. The artery appears pulsatile. Either transverse (short axis) or longitudinal (long axis) views are adequate. By the transverse axis view both artery and vein can be visualized. By the longitudinal view the needle tip is visualized all the time. After the positioning of the vein in the center of ultrasound screen, the vein is punctured with the 18 G needle. Then after the confirmation of the intravenous location of the guidewire in the longitudinal view the dilator is applied and then the technique progresses as the landmark technique.

CATHETER POSITION CONFIRMATION

Central venous catheter placed in the operating room is used commonly for the duration of the surgery and the postoperative period. Inside the operation theater, the radiological confirmation of the tip of the catheter usually does not take place. Aspiration of the dark venous blood from each lumen of the multilumen catheter confirms the placement and makes it feasible to remove the air from the tubing. By placing an extension tubing and keeping it at the level of junction of SVC and RA and looking for movement of fluid column with intermittent positive-pressure ventilation (IPPV) or spontaneous respiration is another method to check the placement. Correct thoracic placement should be confirmed with a chest X-ray, after surgery, showing the catheter within the SVC and the tip at the level of the tracheal carina. Waveform and blood gas analysis (although acceptable for femoral cannulation) will only confirm venous intrathoracic placement and not position. If the catheter tip is located below the pericardial reflection of SVC, it increases risk of fatal cardiac tamponade, and atrial, ventricular perforation. The catheter tip should remain parallel to the vessel walls, within the SVC. The tip should be positioned above the level of third rib, the tracheal carina, T4–T5 interspace, division of the right main bronchus and the azygos vein. The tracheal carina is always above the pericardial reflection of SVC, so the catheter tip should always be above this important landmark.

COMPLICATIONS OF CENTRAL VENOUS CATHETERIZATION

Before performing the procedure, the procedure should be explained in detail to the patient and his relative in the language they understand. The risks, benefits, and alternatives should be explained. The complications due to the CVC placement are being recognized as a source of morbidity and mortality. Almost in 15% of patients some kind of untoward movement is witnessed. Complications can be due to the CVC placement or mechanical, due to thromboembolic phenomenon, and due to infection. The incidences of complication depend on the site chosen to cannulate and the medical condition of the patient. It is deciphered from large retrospective and observational studies that arterial puncture, which is unintentional is the most common acute complication, the incidence varying from 1.9 to 15%. Localized hematoma formation is the usual sequela. If arterial puncture occurs with small needle, then immediately needle has to be removed and firm compression at the hematoma site for some minutes makes itself-limiting. When the carotid artery gets cannulated with the catheter inadvertently, it can be managed conservatively by removing catheter and applying local compression to the arterial puncture site while monitoring patient's airway and neurological status. Injury to venous valves can occur. Aortic perforation and facial vein avulsion have been reported in literature but thankfully rarely. The delayed vascular complications can be aortoatrial fistula, venobronchial fistula, carotid artery-IJV fistula, and pseudoaneurysm formation in the carotid artery. The most catastrophic vascular complication is cardiac tamponade as a consequence to perforation of intrapericardial SVC, RA, RV, or unintentional pericardial instillation of intravenous fluid. In a closed claim study cited by American Society of Anesthesiologists in 2004, cardiac tamponade resulted in death in 81% of cases had a presentation after 1–5 days of cannulation. Alarmingly, it is the second most common complication happening as the evidences are emerging. It has more to do with the catheter maintenance and use other than the procedure itself. It is completely avoidable as it happens due to the catheter tip malposition inside within the heart chambers or getting against the wall of SVC. This complication is observed with peripheral site cannulation. The incidence is quite high and attributable mechanism is cited to be the shoulder abduction causing the catheter tip to advance into dangerous position. The symptom starts appearing suddenly so high index of suspicion has to be maintained all the time. The precise location of the catheter tip can be attained by anteroposterior and lateral chest X-ray and injection of radiopaque contrast material. Pneumothorax is the other most adverse complication reported though it is reportedly less frequent in the IJV route (0.5%) than in subclavian. If the cardiac surgery has taken place then the magnitude of pneumothorax can increase. Small pneumothorax can be managed conservatively. But if it is a large air collection, major surgery has to be done, patient requiring positive-pressure ventilation then it is safer to put thoracostomy tube.

Thrombosis, thromboembolism, infection, sepsis, endocarditis, arrhythmias and hydrothorax can be the complications. Transient atrial, and ventricular arrhythmias occur when the guidewire is passed into the RA or RV using the Seldinger technique. This kind of response is seen when a relatively inflexible guidewire touches the endocardium. There is 70% reduction in the incidence of arrhythmias when the guidewire is inserted to 22 cm. There are incidences of complete heart block due to guidewire insertion. This can be managed using a temporary transvenous or external pacemaker. Resuscitative drugs and equipment should be available to treat this complication. Decreasing angle of incidence less than 40°, single orifice catheters, polyurethane catheter, and silicone rubber catheter can all decrease the risk of perforation of the heart or vessel.

INTERPRETATION OF CENTRAL VENOUS PRESSURE WAVEFORMS

Attaching the transducer to the catheter port and checking the typical CVP waveform on the monitor screen is the best confirmatory sign of the catheter placement. Then the drugs and blood, fluid therapy can be given through the line. The line can be attached to the transducer of the monitor to get a CVP waveform. As the pressure keeps on changing inside the RA due to the cardiac cycle activity, the waveform goes up and down depending on the pressure characteristics of the event. The pressures are as depicted in **Table 3**. The normal CVP waveform has five waves, three upward waves namely "a", "c" and "v" waves and two downward descents ("x" and "y" descents). The right atrial contraction generates an average pressure of 6 mm Hg and the upward "a" wave happens just after the P wave on the ECG. The "c" wave happens due to the bulging of tricuspid valve into the RA during isovolumic ventricular contraction. Once the RV starts ejecting the tricuspid valve is pulled away from the RA and the "x" descent happens. Then the RA starts filling up and the pressure rises to 5 mm Hg leading to the upright "v" wave. The "y" descent happens as soon as the RA empties into the RV **(Fig. 4)**. Correlations of all the parameters of hemodynamic monitoring are shown in **Figure 5**.

TABLE 3: Pressure values in the right atrium.

Pressure	Average (mm Hg)	Range (mm Hg)
	Right atrium	
"a" wave	6	2–7
"v" wave	5	2–7
Mean	3	1–5

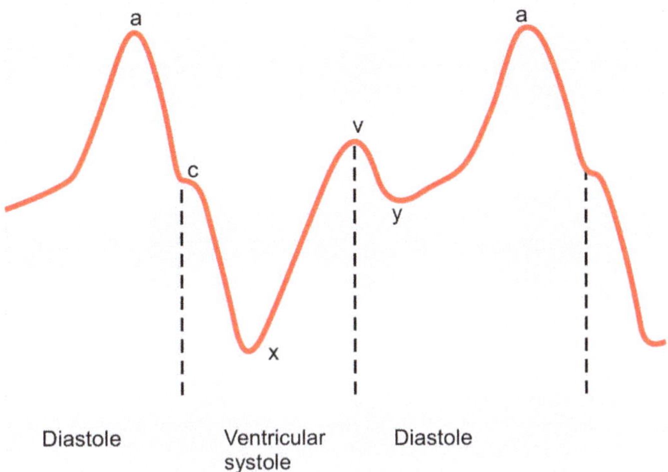

Fig. 4: Normal central venous pressure waveform showing upstroke waves a, c, v, and descendant waves x and y.

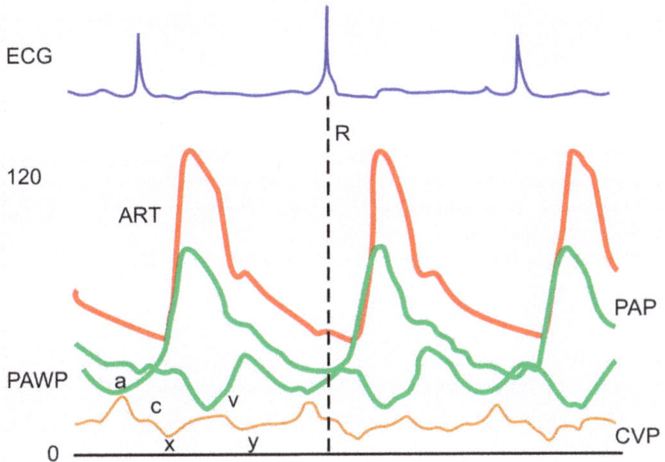

Fig. 5: Relationship between normal systemic arterial pressure, pulmonary artery pressure, central venous pressure, and pulmonary artery wedge pressure.

Interpretation of the Central Venous Pressure Waves

Normal waves of CVP as shown in **Figure 4** (normal range 6–12 mm Hg). Static measurement less helpful in guiding fluid resuscitation since compliance of right heart will affect reading for any given RVEDV. Dynamic measurements with response to fluid challenges are more informative. In the context of LV failure, higher values are more reliable since they reflect poorly compliant ventricle and "offloading" (diuresis/venodilatation) may be appropriate. Preload assessed by dynamic changes in response to a fluid challenge (discussed below).

- *Fluid challenge-assessing response to fast 250 mL fluid bolus:* If CVP rises then falls over 10 minutes with overall increase less than 3 mm Hg—under filled. CVP rises then equilibrates at a value between 3 and 5 mm Hg above baseline—optimal. CVP rises and equilibrates 5 mm Hg above baseline—fluid overload, further fluid may result in pulmonary edema. Trends in CVP can be useful in giving clue to estimate blood loss or fluid loss and help in guiding the replacement therapy. A significant alteration in circulating blood volume and RV preload gives rise to only a small change in CVP. This becomes a predictable indicator of fluid status when correlated well with blood pressure and urine output.
- Abnormal wave in different medical conditions as shown in **Table 4 and Figure 6**
- *RV function:* CVP actually offers direct measurement of RV filling pressure
- LV filling pressures can be measured using CVP as a guideline. Measurements represent RAP and hence right

TABLE 4: Abnormal wave in different medical conditions.

Condition	***Characteristics changes in the CVP waves***
Atrial fibrillation	Loss of a wave, prominent c wave
Atrioventricular dissociation	Cannon a wave
Tricuspid regurgitation	Tall systolic c-v wave, loss of x descent
Tricuspid stenosis	Tall a wave, attenuation of y descent
Right ventricular ischemia	Tall a and v waves, steep x and y descents, M or W configuration
Pericardial constriction	Tall a waves, steep x and y descents, M or Y configuration
Cardiac tamponade	y descent attenuation, x descent dominant
Respiratory variation during spontaneous ventilation or positive-pressure ventilation	Pressure to be measured at end of expiration

(CVP: central venous pressure)

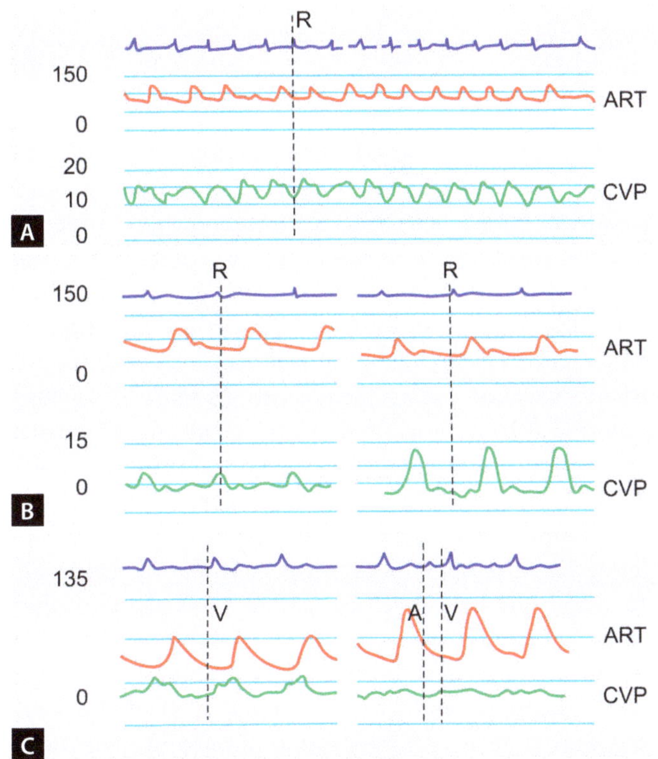

Figs. 6A to C: Abnormal central venous pressure waveform. (A) Atrial fibrillation; (B) Isorhythmic atrioventricular dissociation; (C) Ventricular pacing.

ventricular end-diastolic pressure (RVEDP). Commonly (and mistakenly) taken to represent preload, however preload is a function of RVEDV not RVEDP, which will be dependent on compliance of ventricle. Assuming normal anatomy and structure of heart and lungs, this will also represent left heart pressure

- Right IJV is the most preferred site for central venous cannulation. It was found by Troianos et al. that more than 75% of the IJV overlies carotid artery in 54% of patients.[5] The IJV overlaps the carotid artery more when the head is rotated to 80° rather than 40° or no rotation at all.[6,7] Maximum right IJV diameter is achievable with placement of patient in 15° Trendelenburg position, keeping the head close to midline, slightly elevating the head with a small head elevation and releasing the pressure applied to palpate the carotid artery before IJV cannulation.[7,8]

ARTERIAL CANNULATION

INTRODUCTION

In modern anesthesia, arterial cannulation is becoming the standard procedure for beat-to-beat real-time blood pressure monitoring. Major surgical procedures where excessive blood loss and major fluid shifts are expected, beat-to-beat blood pressure monitoring is needed to take measures against the untoward events intraoperatively. High-risk patients with severely compromised cardiac condition and those in shock are some of the indications for invasive blood pressure (IBP) monitoring. It is also useful during critical care, as meticulous blood pressure monitoring is needed in ICU. It also provides an access to withdraw frequent blood sample for analysis without pricking needle to the patient. The pressure monitoring has been started since 1733 when Stephen Hales measured the height of blood in a tube inserted into the artery of a horse. After that different methods have been adapted to monitor pressure. In 1947, Lambert and Wood introduced electrical strain gauge, and increase accuracy and durability of transducers. In 1953, Miller perfected catheter-tipped transducers by using unbound semiconductor half bridges.

INDICATIONS

The indications for invasive arterial blood pressure monitoring are shown in **Box 3**.

CONTRAINDICATIONS

Local infection at the site can lead to catheter induce sepsis. In case of bleeding disorders, artery bleeds profusely and forms hematoma; however, it is a relative contraindication. Raynaud's syndrome, Buerger's disease, and severe atherosclerosis may complicate the cannulation. Hypothermia of the hand can precipitate the Raynaud's vasospastic episode.[9] Therefore, axillary or femoral artery should be cannulated in these cases. Surgical procedure, such as radial artery harvesting or in case of brachial artery cut down for cardiac catheterization, these sites are not appropriate for IBP monitoring. The contraindications for invasive arterial blood pressure monitoring are shown in **Box 4**.

BOX 3: Indications and uses of arterial cannulation.

- *Indications:*
  - Invasive blood pressure monitoring
  - Major abdominal surgery (pheochromocytoma, Whipple's, large retroperitoneal masses, splenectomy, Wertheim's hysterectomy)
  - Neurosurgery—posterior fossa surgeries, meningioma, aneurysm, spinal surgeries
  - Cardiac procedures requiring cardiopulmonary bypass
  - Surgery on aorta, other vascular surgery
  - Orthopedic procedure
  - Oncosurgery
  - Organ transplants
  - Surgery with large fluid shift
  - Patient with recent history of myocardial infarction, unstable angina, low ejection fraction
  - Patient with right heart failure, chronic obstructive pulmonary disease, pulmonary hypertension, pulmonary embolism
  - Patient in cardiogenic shock, hypovolemic shock, septic shock
  - Patient requiring inotropes or intra-aortic balloon counterpulsation
  - Patients with electrolyte or metabolic disturbances
  - Massive trauma
  - Noninvasive blood pressure sites unavailable (severe burn, infection, morbid obesity)
- *Uses:*
  - Repeated blood sampling
  - Arterial blood gas analysis

BOX 4: Contraindications of invasive arterial blood pressure monitoring.

- Inadequate circulation to the extremity
- Raynaud's syndrome
- Thromboangiitis obliterans (Buerger's disease)
- Full-thickness burn over insertion site
- Skin infection over insertion site
- Uncontrolled coagulopathy
- Systemic anticoagulation
- Inadequate collateral flow from ulnar artery on Allen test
- Atherosclerosis

COMPONENTS OF THE PRESSURE MEASUREMENT SYSTEM

Invasive arterial blood pressure is measured by the pressure measurement system, which comprises of intravascular cannula, pressure transducer, flushing device, and analyzer display system **(Figs. 7 and 8; Box 5)**.

Intravascular Cannula

This provides access to the pressure wave which is electronically analyzed and displayed on the monitor. Nowadays various arterial kits are available depending on the site. These cannulas are made up of polyurethane or Teflon™ material as it decreases the risk of thrombus formation. The risk of arterial thrombus formation is increased with larger diameter of cannula; therefore, appropriate sized cannula should be used. Nonported cannula prevents inadvertent injection into artery.

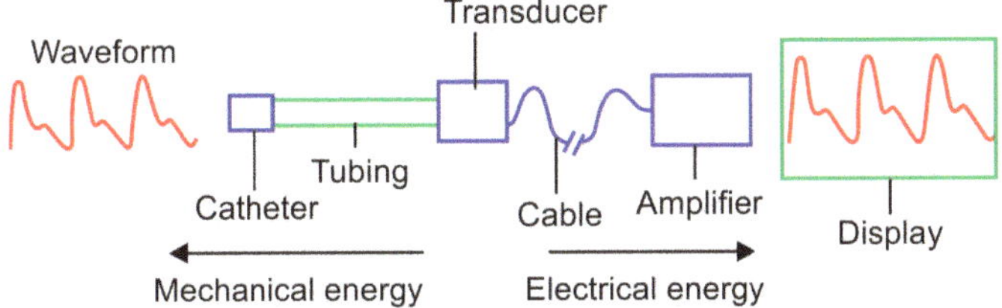

Fig. 7: Schematic diagram of simple and basic knowledge of pressure measurement system. Transducer converts the mechanical energy into electrical energy. This is then modified and analyzed by the amplifier and displayed on the monitor.

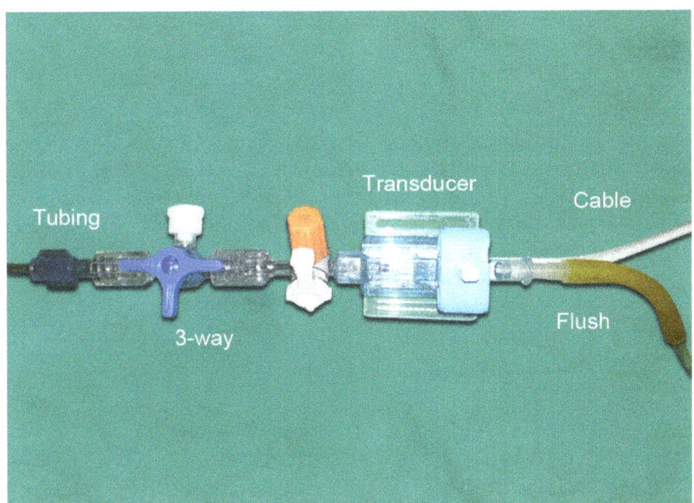

Fig. 8: Components of pressure measurement system: fluid-filled tubing, 3-way tap, transducer with flush system and cable (white color).

BOX 5: Components of pressure measurement system.

• Intravascular cannula 20 G or less • Coupling system • Transducer	• Analysis and display system • Flush system

Coupling System

The pressure measurement system requires a fluid-filled column for hydraulic coupling. Arterial extension tubing connects the cannula with the pressure transducer. Also a 3-way connecter is placed before transducer for the purpose of zeroing and withdrawing of blood sample. Tubing should be short in length, larger in diameter as far as possible, color-coded and noncompliant (stiff). These characteristics reduce the potential of amplification of actual arterial blood pressure by increasing the natural frequency of the system.[10] The fluid-coupling system adds compressibility, which is responsible for degrading the pressure signal input across the transducer membrane by increasing volume displacement. Low-density fluid eliminates this problem and water is a good example.

Transducer

The pressure measurement system is based on the physics that the transducer converts mechanical force into electric current or voltage. Nowadays, most transducers are of

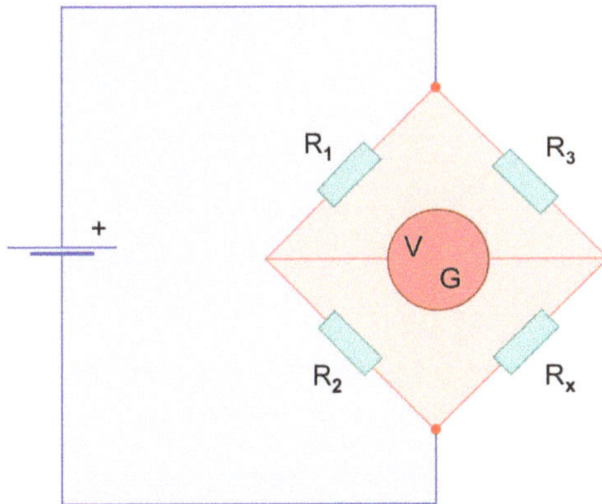

Fig. 9: Wheatstone bridge: There are two fixed resistors (R_1 and R_3) and third is adjustable standard resistor (R_2) while the fourth one is unknown resistor (R_X).

resistance type. In the Wheatstone bridge of electric circuit, two pairs of resistors are incorporated, one of them is a variable resistor known as Strain gauge. The disposable transducer has a silicone diaphragm into which resistive elements have been incorporated. The diaphragm of the transducer channelizes the fluid wave as electrical input. Any change in the pressure produces voltage alteration across the pair of resistors, incorporated in the Wheatstone bridge, reflecting as change in current. This is electronically modified and displayed on the monitor **(Fig. 9)**.

Analysis and Display System

Microprocessor unit in the system analyzes the electrical signal from the transducer. These signals are amplified and displayed on the screen as pressure waveform.

Flush System

Flush system helps in maintaining the patency of the cannula. It provides continuous flush of plain or heparinized 0.9% normal saline at 1–3 mL/h through a bag pressurized at 300 mm Hg. It reduces the risk of thrombus formation and prolongs the effectiveness of the cannula.[11] Some practice avoid use of heparin in the flush system as it can cause heparin-induced thrombocytopenia. Intermittent flushing with large volume should be avoided as it may result into central arterial embolization.[12] If required, small aliquots 2–4 mL can be used. Flush system also allows to do pop test for calculating natural frequency and damping.

PROPERTIES OF PRESSURE MEASUREMENT SYSTEM

The arterial pressure waveform is a complex periodic sine wave. Fundamental frequency is the first harmonic frequency which is equal to the heart rate. For example, if heart rate is 60 beats per minute (bpm) then fundamental frequency will be 1 Hz. Summation of such first ten harmonic will contribute to produce actual arterial pressure waveform **(Figs. 10A and B)**. Pressure waves are measured by transduction of force per unit area into an electric voltage which can easily be measured and displayed as a function of time.[10]

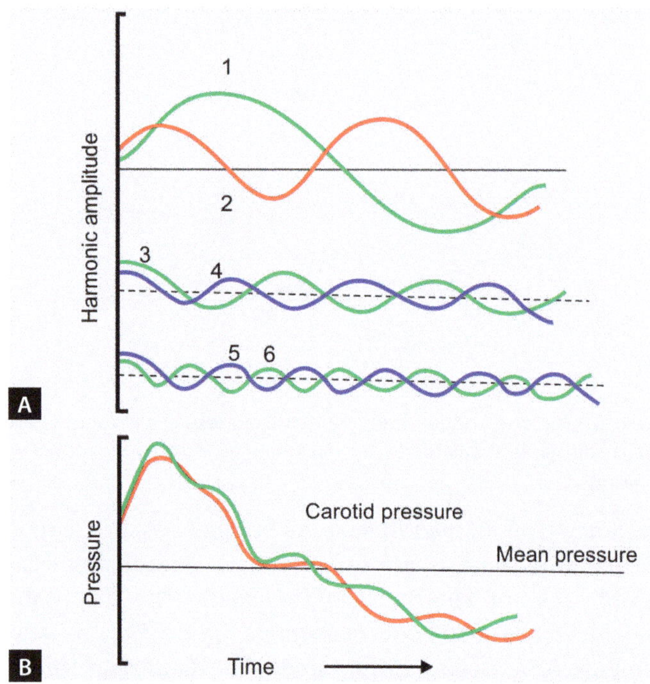

Figs. 10A and B: (A and B) Summation of first six harmonics of fundamental frequency will produce significant waveform.

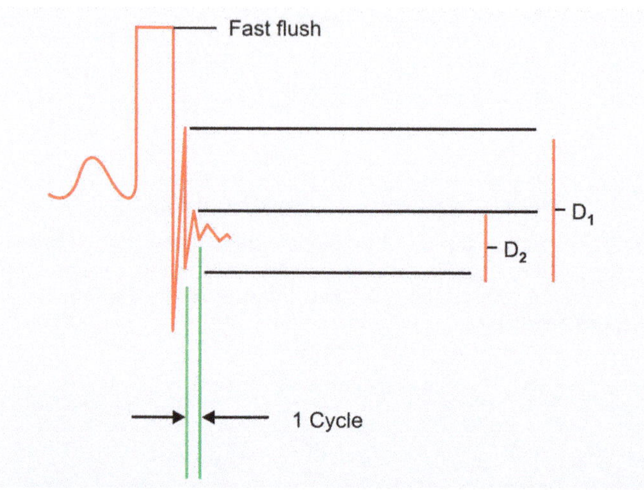

Fig. 11: Fast flush test allows bedside measurement of natural frequency and damping coefficient. Natural frequency can be derived by dividing the paper speed (mm/sec) with period of 1 cycle (mm). Damping coefficient by measuring the ratio of the amplitude of one induced resonant wave to next, D_2/D_1.

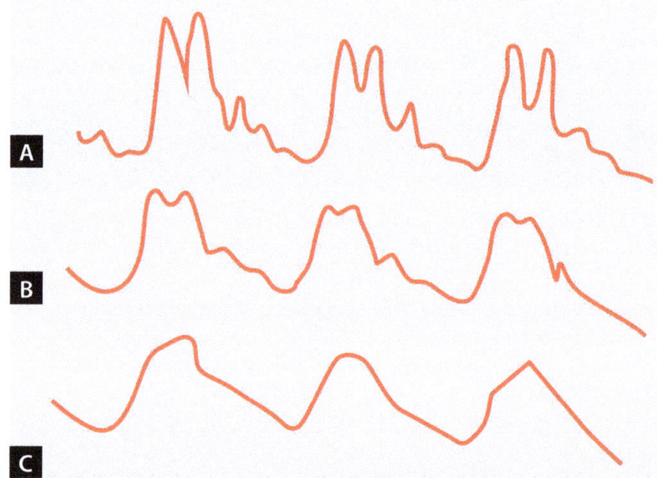

Figs. 12A to C: (A) An under-damped waveform (D <1); (B) A critically-damped waveform (D = 0.7); (C) An over-damped waveform (D >1).

Natural Frequency and Damping

Dynamic response of a pressure measurement system includes natural frequency and damping.[2] Rapid oscillation above and below the baseline of the pressure waveform is known as natural frequency, which is soon shifted to baseline due to friction known as damping effect. Normally 10–20 Hz of natural frequency is present in the arterial blood pressure signal which is the maximal signal frequency. The natural frequency is calculated by the formula:

$$\text{fn} = \frac{1}{2\pi}\sqrt{\frac{\pi D^2}{4\,\delta L}\,\frac{\Delta P}{\Delta V}} = \frac{\text{Paper speed (mm/sec)}}{\text{Length in 1 cycle (mm)}}$$

where, D is diameter of the tubing, L is length of the tubing, ($\Delta P/\Delta V$) is system compliance, and δ is the density of the fluid.

Damping arises due to friction, compliance of transducer tubing and air bubble in the system. This results into decrease in amplitude of peaks and troughs in the pressure tracing due to absorption of energy. The pressure measurement system can be underdamped, critically damped or over-damped. This can be assessed with high-pressure flush assembly. On flushing the pressure line, an under-damped system shows multiple oscillations for a prolonged period before shifting to baseline. An over-damped system shows no oscillation and takes long time to shift to baseline. A critically-damped system shows one or two oscillations and shifts to baseline. To minimize distortion in the system, some amount of damping is required. Nowadays, most transducers are under-damped system with low natural frequency.

Clinically, both the natural frequency and damping coefficient can be calculated by pop test or fast flush test[13] which is done by using high-pressure flush technique. The natural frequency is measured by calculating the time period of one oscillation as it shifts to baseline. The damping coefficient is calculated by measuring the amplitude ratio of two consecutive peaks. Ideally the damping coefficient should be 1, but optimal damping happens at 0.7 which gives an accurate estimation of blood pressure even at higher heart rate **(Figs. 11 and 12)**.

Volume Displacement

To produce more accurate pressure waveform, smaller amount of volume displacement is required across the transducer membrane. An elastic property of the transducer membrane plays an important role. To produce accurate pressure waveform, some amount of stiffness is required so that small volume displacement occurs across the membrane.

Zeroing and Leveling

Transducer should be at zero or electrically balanced. Zeroing means zero current at zero pressure. This is done by turning the 3-way so that transducer is exposed to the atmosphere pressure and calibrated the pressure at zero. For better accuracy, the transducer should be at the level of RA in the mid-axillary line. Zeroing will not be affected by leveling; however, change in room temperature may cause drifting of zero from baseline. Therefore, during the procedure, transducer needs to be zeroed periodically.

Errors

- Any condition which decreases the natural frequency should be avoided. Air or blood clot at the catheter tip in the system will result into damping of arterial pressure waveform
- Error may occur due to catheter whip that is the motion of the catheter tip in the arterial lumen causes distortion in the pressure waveform.

EQUIPMENT

- Arterial catheter kit (appropriate to the patient size and site)
    - Radial (20 G)/Femoral (18 G)/Angiocatheter **(Figs. 13A to C)**
    - 20 G for adult and large children
    - 22 G or 24 G for small children, infant or neonate
- Syringe, 2 cc 1% plain lignocaine with 25 G or 27 G needle
- Syringe, 5 cc with heparinized flush
- Adhesive tape
- Stopcock, 3-way
- Pressure tubing
- Pressure transducer kit with a flushing system.

SITES

Radial artery is preferred over other sites for cannulation, because it is superficial and is associated with less complication. Before proceeding for radial arterial cannulation, one should perform modified Allen's test to access the collateral circulation of the hand. The original Allen's test is a bedside test to assess arterial stenosis in the patient with thrombophlebitis obliterans of hands. It was described by EV Allen in 1929.[14] In modified Allen's test, ask the patient to clench his fist and simultaneously occlude both radial and ulnar artery to obstruct the blood flow to the hand then ask the patient to open his hand, palm turns pale. Release the pressure over ulnar artery first if color of the palm turns pink within 5–10 seconds. It indicates that the collateral through ulnar artery is good and there is no obstruction in the blood flow. This is called negative modified Allen's test. Pulse oximetry or plethysmography is other method to check collateral circulation.[15] Doppler probe is also a good technique to check collateral flow.

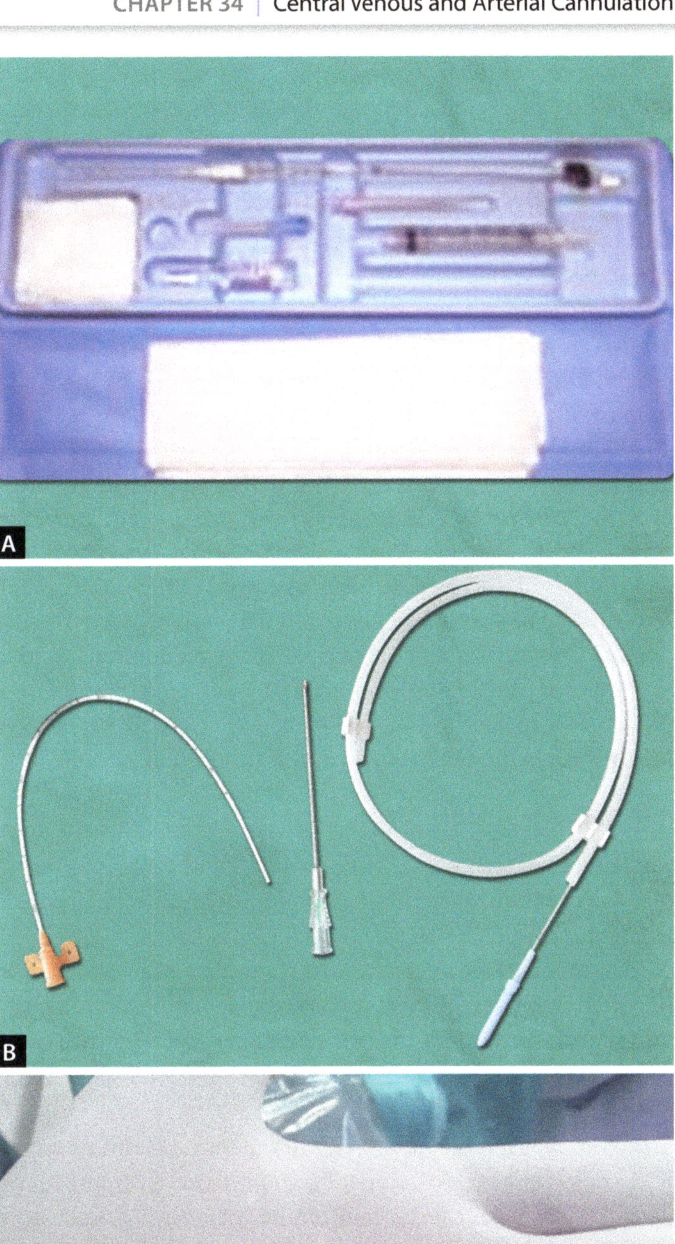

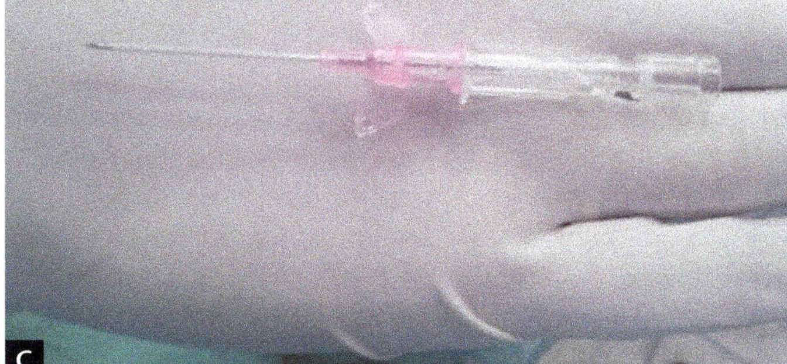

Figs. 13A to C: Arterial cannulation kit. (A) Radial set; (B) Femoral set; (C) Angiocath.

Radial and Ulnar Artery

Radial artery is the most common artery for cannulation as its course is superficial and straight over the wrist. It is easily accessible and easy to cannulate. But it should not be attempted in case of obstructed collateral circulation. About 90% of hand circulation is dependent on ulnar artery.

Ulnar artery is also a good option for cannulation when the hand circulation depends on radial artery or in case unavailability of radial artery. Complications include hematoma, thrombosis and in extreme case ischemic complication leads to gangrene of the hand. In case of brachial artery cut down for cardiac catheterization, radial or ulnar artery cannulation should not be performed as it may give false low pressure value.[16] More than three attempts are not feasible for cannulation of same artery as it causes vasospasm of the artery. Repeated attempts may cause ischemia of the hand in extreme case. Sometime on CPB the radial artery shows 10–20 mm Hg lesser value than the palpable central aortic pressure, an extra arterial tubing with a needle attached is inserted into the ascending aorta by the surgeon to know the accurate pressure. Right radial artery should be preferred in case of patent ductus arteriosus as clamp is applied over the left subclavian artery and perfusion may hampered to the left upper extremity for a short period. Right radial artery is also preferred in case of coronary artery bypass graft as retractors (Favaloro's retractor) used during left internal mammary artery harvesting may compress left subclavian artery.

Brachial Artery

The brachial artery lies in the antecubital fossa medial to bicipital tendon. Brachial artery cannulation can be done but better to avoid as there is no collateral flow to the hand in case of brachial artery occlusion. Therefore, other site should be preferred over it. Pressure tracing is like femoral artery and shows more proximity with central aortic pressure.

Axillary Artery

The axillary artery is the preferable site for cannulation in the ICU for long-term catheterization and in case of peripheral vascular diseases. It is cannulated near the junction of deltoid and pectoral muscle, best felt below the belly of bicep muscle. Artery is palpated and fixed against the humerus. It is the second largest artery next to femoral; therefore, risks of thrombus formation and ischemia of distal area are less. If it gets occluded then there are collateral vessels which maintain the distal perfusion. Axillary artery pressure measurement shows close proximity to central artery pressure, and there is decrease risk of contamination and blood loss. It is prone to kink in case of adduction of the arm in lateral decubitus position.[1] It is closely situated to cerebral circulation therefore increase risk of cerebral embolization on flushing.[1,4]

Femoral Artery

The femoral artery has a large diameter and it is the main artery of lower limb. The specific indication is descending thoracic aortic aneurysm for distal arterial pressure monitoring. It also provides access for placement of intra-aortic balloon pump. Cannulation of femoral artery is done by Seldinger technique and it shows more proximity to central aortic pressure. Though the risk of atherosclerotic plaque embolization is there during guidewire and catheter placement but being larger lumen, blood supply of the lower limb is not affected.

Dorsalis Pedis and Posterior Tibial Artery

The dorsalis pedis and posterior tibial arteries both are situated over the foot. Generally these arteries are preserved for pediatric patient.[4] Modified Allen's test can be performed on foot to know the efficacy of collateral blood supply. These arteries are far from central artery therefore prone to have distortion in pressure waveform and overestimation of systolic blood pressure.

Superficial Temporal Artery

It is present in front of tragus over the face. It has a tortuous course therefore difficult to cannulate. It is more close to the cerebral circulation, so the risk of cerebral embolization is high. It should not be cannulated in case of cerebrovascular or carotid occlusive disease.

POSITION

Here we discuss radial artery cannulation as it is most frequently attempted; however, the techniques are same in all cannulation. Dorsiflexion of wrist over rolled up towel in supination **(Fig. 14)**. Paint the area with 4% chlorhexidine gluconate or povidone-iodine and after draping local anesthetic agent 1% lignocaine (without adrenaline) is infiltrated at the site. After completion of the procedure, one should never forget to keep back the hand in anatomical neutral position as prolong hyperextension can lead to neuropathy of the hand.

In case of femoral artery cannulation, keep folded towel under the buttocks and upper one-third of the thigh, this makes the site flat especially in pediatric patient. In morbidly obese patient, assistant helps in pulling up the abdomen as it obstruct the plane of puncture site.

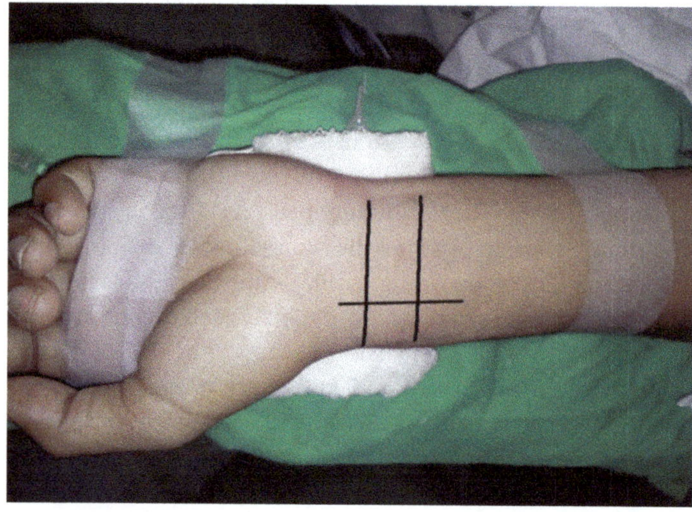

Fig. 14: Position and marking for radial artery cannulation.

TECHNIQUE

Direct Cannulation

Palpate the radial artery with three fingers. Introduce the intravenous cannula at an angle of 30–45° while feeling the pulse under the pulp of finger, simultaneously look at the hub of cannula, there will be flash of blood as it enters the artery. Depress the cannula about 10–15° and withdraw the needle a little, continuous flow of blood will be seen at the hub. Stabilize the needle and advance the catheter over it. Remove the needle and attach the 3-way with a syringe-filled with heparinized flush to the hub. Attach the pressure transducer tubing to it. Secure the catheter with suture or adhesive tape **(Fig. 15 and Video 16)**.

Transfixation

The steps of position, preparation and draping are same as mentioned above. Introduce the catheter-over-needle assembly at an angle of 30–45° toward the artery. When flow of blood occurs at the hub, advance the whole assembly further until the flow stops. This is called transfixing the artery **(Video 16)**. Now withdraw the needle completely off the catheter and slowly withdraw the catheter till good pulsatile flow occurs at the end. Advance the catheter slowly into the artery. Alternatively, the whole assembly can be withdrawn at one time until flow of blood seen at the hub. Depress the angle by 10–15° and thread the catheter over the needle into the artery.

Over-the-wire Technique (Seldinger)

Palpate the radial artery with three fingers. Introduce needle or catheter-over-needle unit at an angle of 30–45° where maximal pulsation is felt. Advance unit till flash of blood appears at the clear hub. Stabilize the introducer needle and thread the guidewire gently as far as into the lumen. Do not use force while threading, it might pierce the wall of the artery. If resistance is encountered, do not retract the guidewire, as this may damage the guidewire. Instead, withdraw the entire unit and attempt a new puncture. Advance catheter assembly 1–2 mm more into the vessel. Hold the introducer needle steady in place and advance the catheter forward over the guidewire. Hold the catheter in place and remove the needle, guidewire and feeding tube assembly **(Fig. 16 and Video 16)**.

Doppler Flow-guided

The Doppler-assisted technique is useful where artery localization is difficult like in case of obese patient, small children, and infants.

Ultrasonography-guided

Ultrasound can be used for arterial cannulation. It is high-frequency ultrasonic transducer (9 MHz), which helps in visualizing small structures. Doppler flow technique is often combined with ultrasonic method in case of difficult cannulation. Updates will be discussed at the end of the chapter.

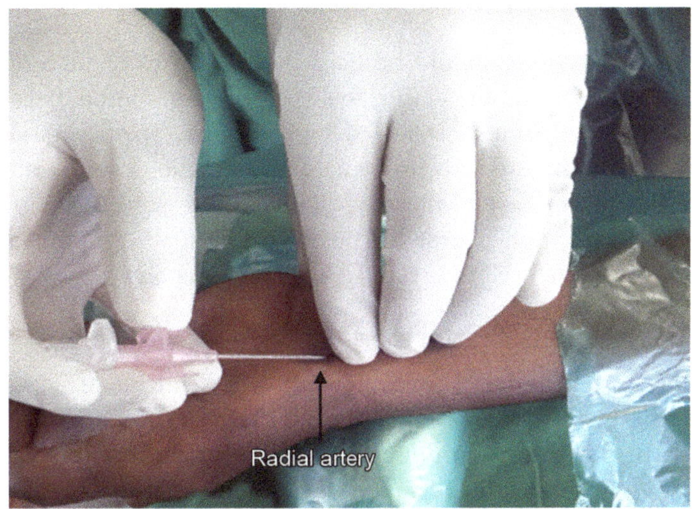

Fig. 15: Radial artery cannulation.

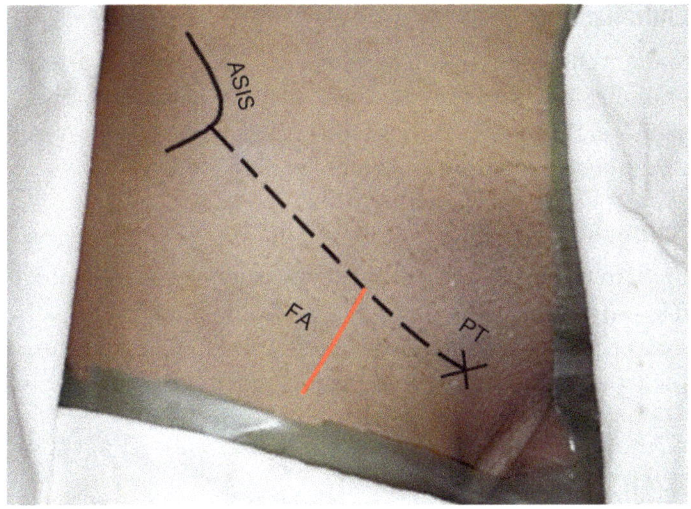

Fig. 16: Surface marking for femoral arterial (FA) cannulation. Imaginary line between, anterior superior iliac spine (ASIS) and pubic tubercle (PT) is the inguinal ligament.

Cut Down

If above measures fail then surgical cut down can be done. The target artery is cannulated under direct vision. A small incision is made over the skin and subcutaneous dissection is done to locate the artery. Two suture ligatures without tying are applied over the artery. Under direct vision the catheter-over-needle assembly is introduced.

COMPLICATIONS

Infection

Indwelling catheter infections occur due to poor aseptic technique, infection at the site, poor maintenance on prolong duration in ICU.[17] Catheter-induced sepsis and cellulitis require immediate removal of the cannula, wound cleaning and systemic antibiotic therapy.[18]

Bleeding

All connections should be tight fit so that no chance of exsanguination. Preferably the connections should have Luer-lock system instead of tapered one. Unsuccessful arterial puncture leads to hematoma formation. Condition is worsen in case of bleeding diathesis. Pressure bandage should be applied over the puncture site for 5–7 minutes (approximately clotting time) in case of hematoma.

Thrombosis and Distal Ischemia

Inadvertent arterial injection of drugs might lead to thrombosis. Radial artery occlusion due to thrombosis may occur therefore continuous flushing is needed. In case of lack of collateral blood supply, distal ischemia leads to skin necrosis.

Embolization

Sudden flushing may cause central or cerebral arterial embolization. Continuous flush with heparinized normal saline at 1–3 mL/h through the pressurized bag prevents thrombosis formation and embolization.

Neuropathy

Median nerve lies close to brachial artery in the antecubital fossa so the risk of injuring nerve more. Peripheral neuropathy may occur in case of large hematoma and hyperextension of the wrist. Axillary plexus and nerve injury can occur in case of axillary artery cannulation.

ARTERIAL LINE IN NEONATE

Arterial line in neonates is commonly used in intensive care unit for the management of critically ill infants and in operation theater for major surgeries. It can be achieved through central (umbilical) and peripheral arteries and known as umbilical arterial catheters (UACs) and peripheral arterial catheters (PALs) respectively. In critical care setting these arterial catheters are mainly used for invasive blood pressure monitoring and arterial blood sampling.

Selection of Site

Radial and posterior tibial arteries are preferred sites while ulnar and dorsalis pedis are acceptable sites. Temporal artery cannulation is usually avoided as it is an end artery. Brachial artery cannulation is rare and is used only in condition when other accesses are failed or in critical condition.

Femoral artery cannulation can be used inside the operation theater for major surgeries like cardiac, neurology, hepatic, organ transplants, etc.

Special Note

- Flush system should include 50 mL syringe of 0.45% heparinized saline (50 units heparin in 50 mL 0.45% sodium chloride) (most preferred). 5% dextrose can be used to decrease the sodium chloride load
- 0.45% sodium chloride flushes should be used in babies less than or equal to 28 weeks gestation
- 0.9% sodium chloride flushes can be used for babies more than 28 weeks gestation.

Complications

Apart from infection, bleeding, thrombosis, arteriospasm, air embolism, the specific complications in case of UACs are erosion of vessel wall, necrotizing enterocolitis, and poor perfusion of buttocks and lower limb need to be noted. However, these UACs complication are rare. Necrotizing enterocolitis is due to poor perfusion of gut and may be associated with early start of feed though there are not high quality literature available to support this; the commencement of feeding should be discussed with the concerned unit doctor when UAC is *in situ*.

CLINICAL INTERPRETATIONS

Normal arterial blood pressure waveform actually represents the ejection of blood from the left ventricle into the aorta during systole, followed by peripheral runoff during diastole. It shows systolic upstroke, systolic peak and then decline during diastole with a dicrotic notch, which is formed due to closure of aortic valve. This decline continues till end-diastole **(Fig. 17)**. Central aortic pressure waveform shows rounded contour with well-defined dicrotic notch termed as incisura while peripheral waveform shows steep upstroke, high systolic pressure with delayed appearance of dicrotic notch, prominent diastolic wave, and lower end-diastolic pressure. Therefore, peripheral waveform shows high systolic pressure, low diastolic pressure, wide pulse

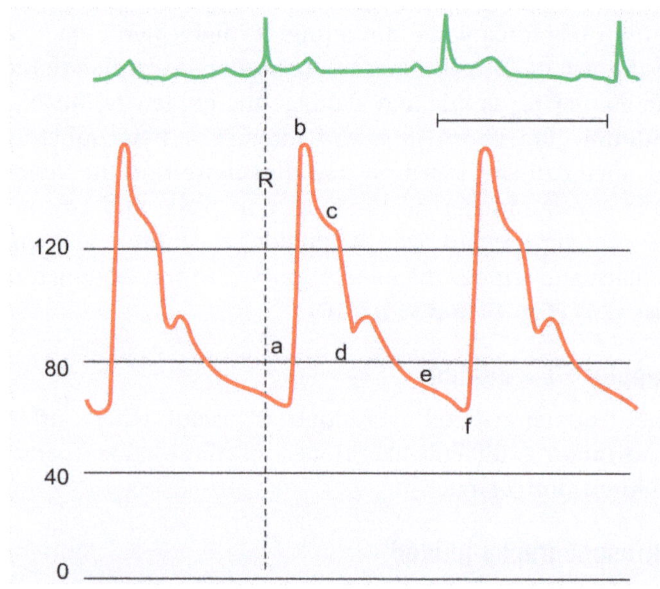

Fig. 17: Normal arterial pressure waveform: a, systolic upstroke; b, systolic peak pressure; c, systolic decline; d, dicrotic notch; e, diastolic runoff; f, end-diastolic pressure.

pressure and minimally low mean pressure. Upper extremity maintains dicrotic notch well while lower extremity shows slurring (femoral) and loss (dorsalis pedis) of dicrotic notch **(Fig. 18)**.

One can interpret the qualitative information by observing the morphology of the waveform, such as contractility, stroke volume, and vascular resistance. The contractility can be roughly estimated by the rate of pressure rise during systole. Stroke volume can be represented by the area under the arterial pressure waveform from the beginning of systole to the dicrotic notch. The heart rate, rhythm, pulse pressure can be assessed. Decrease in systolic pressure during the positive-pressure ventilation is suggestive of hypovolemia. Pulse pressure is estimated by subtracting diastolic pressure from systolic pressure, low pulse pressure (pulsus parvus) is seen in aortic stenosis while high in aortic regurgitation and sepsis **(Table 5)**.

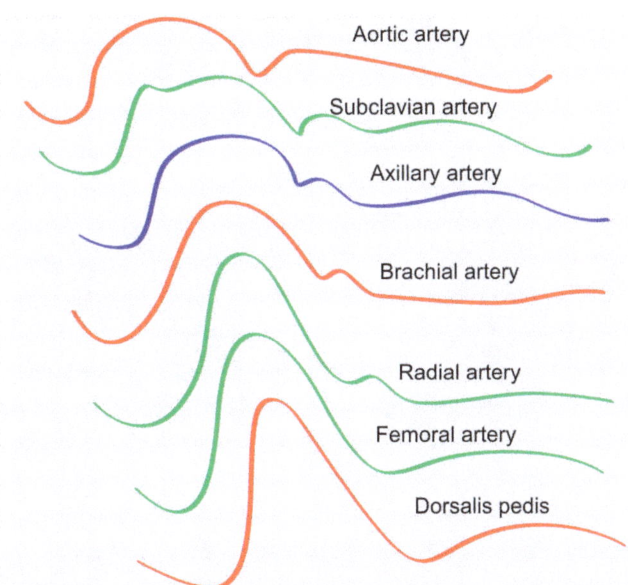

Fig. 18: Waveforms: as pressure wave travels from central to periphery, i.e., from aortic to dorsalis pedis, its morphology changes. The central tracing shows more rounded systolic contour and defined dicrotic notch while periphery shows high peak systolic pressure with delayed and smooth dicrotic notch. High systolic pressure, low diastolic pressure, and wide pulse pressure are observed in peripheral tracing because of high peripheral vascular resistance.

TABLE 5: Conditions with abnormal arterial waveform.

Condition	*Waveform characteristics*
Aortic stenosis	• Narrow pulse pressure (pulsus parvus) • Delayed systolic upstroke (pulsus tardus)
Aortic regurgitation	• Double systolic peak (pulsus bisferiens) • Wide pulse pressure
Hypertrophic cardiomyopathy	Spike and dome pattern
Systolic left ventricular failure	Alternating pulse pressure amplitude (pulsus alternans)
Cardiac tamponade	Exaggerated decrease in systolic blood pressure during spontaneous inspiration (pulsus paradoxus)

RECENT UPDATES

Central Venous Pressure and Starling Curve

In 2015, marking 100th anniversary of the Starling curve, Starling curve in relation to CVP reflecting is revisited again. On the x-axis or abscissa lies the CVP, making clinicians presume that patients having low CVP would benefit in terms of stroke volume and cardiac output when fluid resuscitated. Even many clinical guidelines practice fluid resuscitation of hypovolemic patients till CVP goes high. Later on numerous investigations have challenged this data. Actually in this review of Starling curves and central venous pressure by David A Berlin and Jan Bakker,[19] it is discussed in detail and observed that the model had excluded the effects of the pressure adjacent to the heart, which is an important factor in critically sick patients while considering the CVP as a dependent variable of venous return and cardiac function.

Dynamic hyperinflation state under anesthesia in mechanically-ventilated patients, like unnoticed autopositive end expiratory pressure (Auto-PEEP) can give rise to raised CVP, this state may lead to shock and death.[20] Other important causes of juxtacardiac pressures are excessive positive pressure ventilation, tension pneumothorax, cardiac tamponade. The venous return getting obstructed due to high juxtacardiac pressures, IV fluids, venoconstrictors are considered to return the venous gradient.[21]

Elevated CVP, as per the Starling's curve shows that venous return had exceeded beyond the limit of cardiac accommodation. In left ventricular heart failure, CVP might be normal, in right ventricular dysfunction and right ventricular outflow obstruction it is elevated. Rather than reduced cardiac index, elevated CVP correlates best with hepatic dysfunction and renal failure in congestive heart failure state. It is a marker for hepatic, renal congestion in heart failure and also development of renal failure in severe sepsis.[22,23]

If there is no tricuspid valve disease or juxtacardiac pressure rise, elevated CVP is an important marker of right heart failure due to elevated pulmonary vascular resistance. It is commonly due to acute respiratory distress syndrome or acute pulmonary embolism.[24] A rise in CVP in these situations indicates the severity of illness. Pulmonary vascular resistance increases beyond the limits of right ventricular compensation and as the cardiac output falls, pulmonary artery pressure falls. So CVP rises into double digits due to distended right-sided chambers. This coincides with a rapid rise in right ventricular systolic and diastolic pressure, this can end up in decreased coronary perfusion gradient in right ventricular myocardium. So this raised CVP with hypoperfusion alert us to take care of coronary circulation. Ultrasound measurements of IVC can predict CVP during spontaneous ventilation. Along with other functional hemodynamics and echogradiography CVP measurements can guide us clinically as a hemodynamics parameter in relation to venous return and Law of heart as per Starling's curve.[25]

Ultrasound-guided Vascular Cannulation

Ultrasound is unique and safe technique for vascular cannulation. It has become the gold standard method for the vascular cannulation. It not only gives the anesthesiologist and intensivists a real time snap shot of the target area but it also provides information about the surrounding anatomical structures dynamically. This real time dynamic information leads to better clinical correlation and safe approach.

Using ultrasound guidance for the central venous cannulation throughout the procedure is known as "direct" technique and using it only to identify and mark the vein before starting the puncture is known as "indirect" technique.

Points to be Remembered

- On ultrasound the view for both artery and vein is similar and both have an anechoic (black) lumen. However, arterial walls are little hyperechoic (brighter) then veins. It is generally in practice to say that the arteries are noncompressible but actually both artery and vein are compressible with varied amount of pressure. Their differentiation depends upon the amount of pressure exerted on the vessel which could help us to identify the vessels. Veins are compressible with relatively less amount of pressure. Presence of a thrombus in the vein can make it noncompressible. Doppler imaging (color or spectral) can be used for identification and differentiation of the vessel **(Figs. 19A and B)**. In past Doppler ultrasound (only sound no image) was used for identification of vessels but later it was proved that it does not provide a great help as compare to 2D (B-mode) ultrasound imaging.
- Static ultrasound provides the information about the location and patency of the vessel and dynamic ultrasound guidance provides real time performance of the procedure about the needle position and its tip placement.
- The needle surely enters the target vessel, if it is inserted at an angle of 45° towards the target vessel when it is kept at the same distance from the probe to the depth measured by the US scan. (Pythagorean law of isosceles right triangle). The entry of the needle may vary with the convenience of the operator. It may be inserted as close as to the probe or at variable distance from the probe, but in these conditions the angle of needle also vary as per the depth of target vessel for successful cannulation.
- Short-axis (out of plane image) and long-axis (in plane image) views are used for effective cannulation **(Figs. 20 to 22)**. In short-axis view the probe is placed transversely over the vessel and needle tip is seen as bright dot along the traversed path. In short-axis view the needle tip should lie directly over the vessel and if it has seen lateral or medial, it should be redirected and target vessel should be centralized on the screen. Once needle is seen entering the vessel, it is appreciated as a bright dot inside the vessel, known as "*target sign*" **(Figs. 20A and B)**. It is wiser to use *fanning* of the plane of the probe so that the plane of ultrasound beam intersecting the needle near its tip rather than its shaft to estimate the correct depth. In dehydrated or hypovolemic patient sometimes

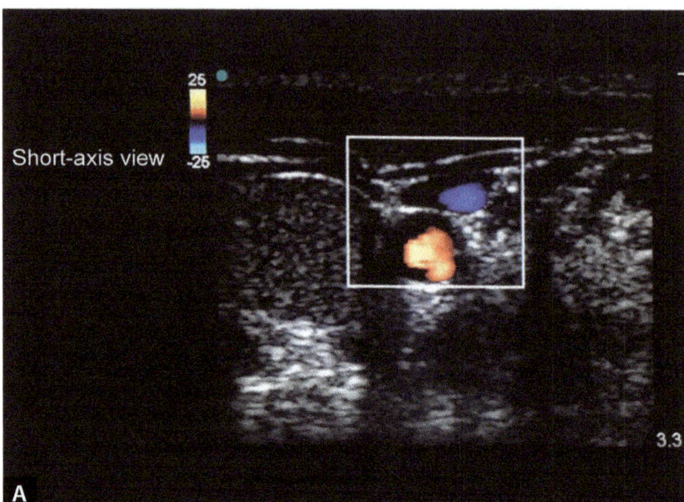

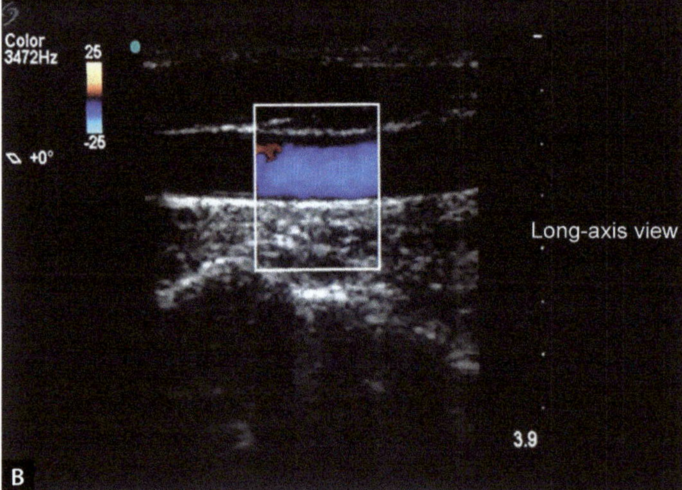

Figs. 19A and B: Color Doppler imaging of internal jugular vein and internal carotid artery.

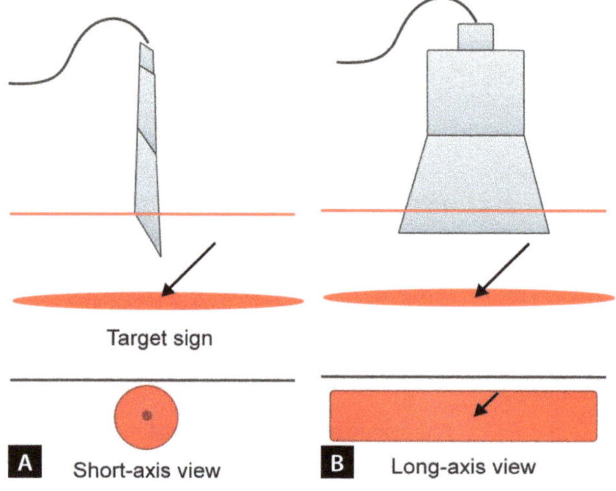

Figs. 20A and B: Probe position in short- and long-axis plane with target sign.

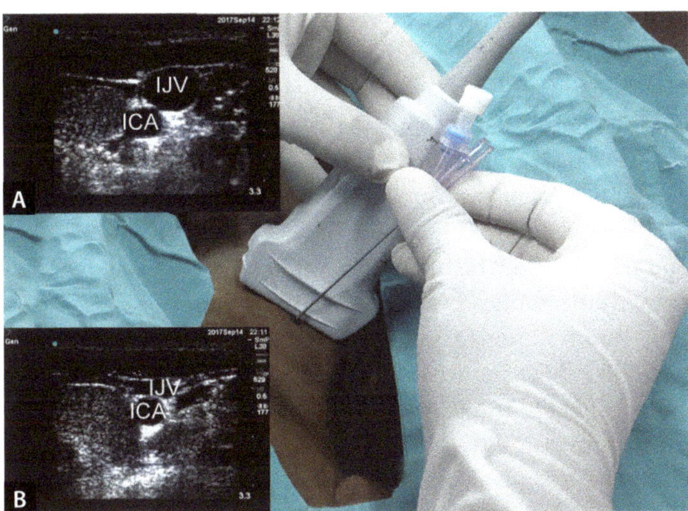

Figs. 21A and B: Short-axis view: Probe is placed transversely over the great vessels. (A) Internal carotid artery (ICA) and internal jugular vein (IJV), both show anechoic (black) lumen; (B) IJV is compressible while ICA has maintained its rounded shape.

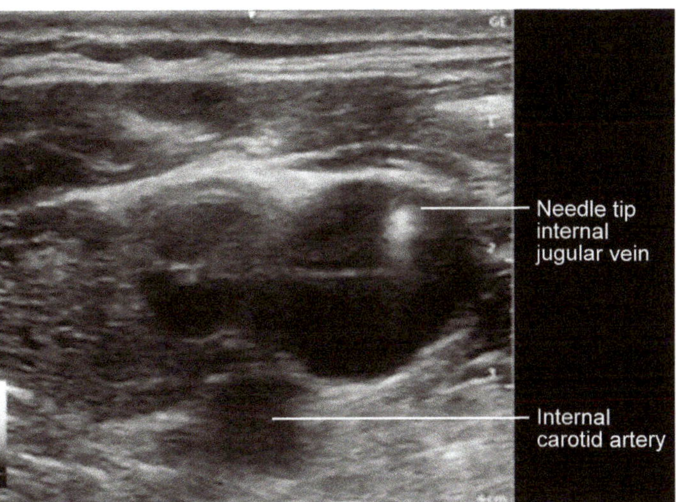

Fig. 23: Needle tip (target sign) inside the internal jugular vein.

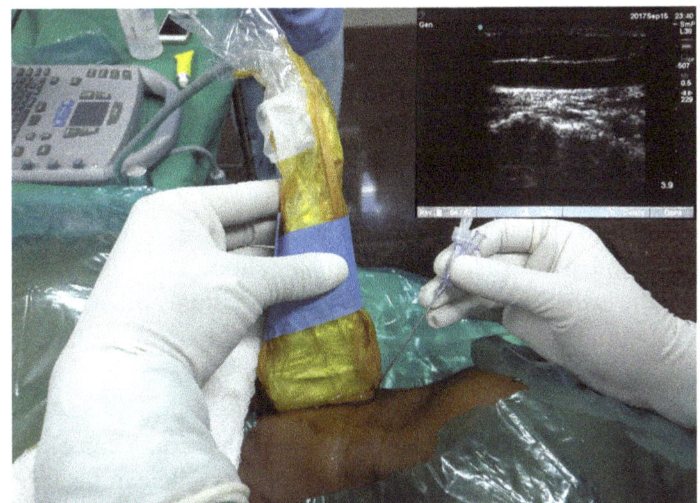
Fig. 22: Long-axis view: Probe is placed parallel to the course of great vessels.

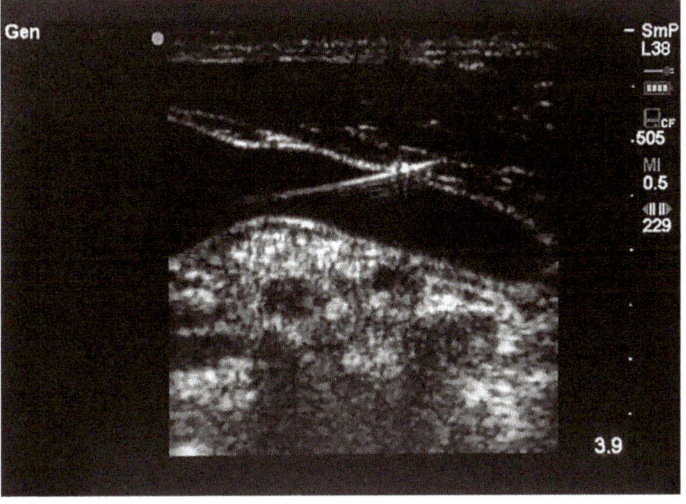

Fig. 24: Guidewire entering internal jugular vein.

needle may pierce the posterior wall of the vessel, which can be negotiated back by withdrawing the needle tip until the target sign appears on the screen, this confirms its intraluminal position. In long-axis view the probe is placed parallel to the vessel and traversing needle is seen with its shaft on the screen with the real time dynamic. Needle path and its tip should be observed continuously while performing the procedure irrespective of view taken **(Fig. 23)**. Once needle placement is confirmed, guidewire is advanced through the needle using Seldinger's technique **(Fig. 24)**. It is always better to begin with short-axis view with target sign and then shift to long-axis view as needle is advanced inside the vessel. It is advisable to re-confirm the correct intravascular position of guidewire, dilator and catheter placement on the ultrasound screen in the target vessel and not into the adjacent vessel.

- A preliminary scan should be done before starting the aseptic preparation to look for any thrombi, occlusion, and disfigured anatomy **(Fig. 25)**.

P Brass et al. analyzed the effectiveness and safety of 2D ultrasound (US)- or Doppler ultrasound (USD)-guided puncture techniques for subclavian vein, axillary vein, and femoral vein puncture during central venous catheter insertion using Cochrane database systemic review.[25A] Their primary objective was comparing US and USD with the landmark technique for complications. Their secondary objectives were mainly overall success rate, number of attempts until success, number of participants in arterial puncture and hematoma formation and time taken to cannulate. On the basis of available data, they concluded that 2D ultrasound offers small gains in safety and quality when compared with an anatomical landmark technique for subclavian (arterial puncture, hematoma formation) or

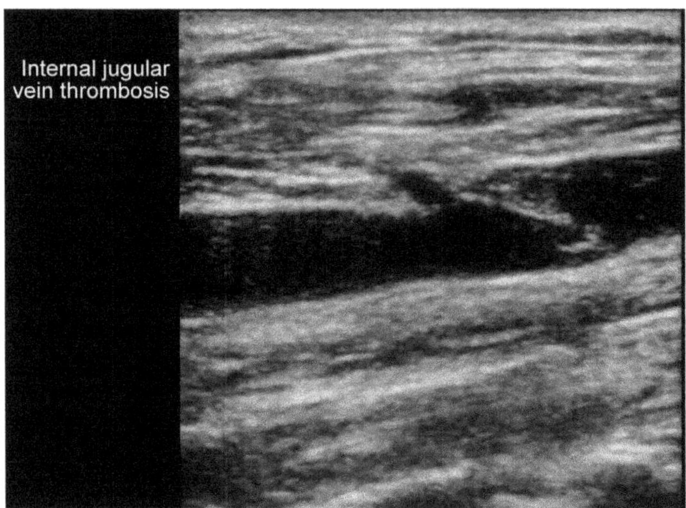

Fig. 25: Thrombus in internal jugular vein.

femoral vein (success on the first attempt) cannulation for central vein catheterization. Data on insertion by inexperienced or experienced users, or on patients at high risk for complications, are lacking. The results for Doppler ultrasound techniques versus anatomical landmark techniques are uncertain.

Central Venous Cannulation

Central venous cannulation includes—internal jugular, subclavian, and femoral veins. Internal jugular vein cannulation as described earlier in this chapter with the landmark is an easy and direct approach to get central venous access. It is easy to cannulate with ultrasound guidance with the same landmark technique. In subclavian vein cannulation clavicle obscure the view but it can be easily cannulated through axillary vein and supraclavicular approach. Subclavian venous cannulation is required for long-term monitoring, pharmacological support (inotropic/vasopressor/venodilator/inodilator/sedation, etc.), and total parenteral nutrition in intensive care unit. Femoral vein cannulation is performed when above two are contraindicated or fail to cannulate or have limitations to cannulate. It lies in the infection prone zone, therefore risk to catch an infection and its systemic transmission is always a concern. As described in upper section with ultrasound-guided vascular cannulation we can cannulate the central veins with great ease and with experience the time for the performance of the procedure is reduced effectively. Ultrasound-guided central venous cannulation pose a great help in obese patients and smaller children, it also helps in patients with burn to identifying the correct position of the vessels.

Ultrasound-guided Internal Jugular Cannulation

A portable ultrasound scanner in bi-dimensional (2D) mode with a linear transducer probe of 5–10 MHz is most commonly used. The transducer is covered with ultrasound gel and should be wrapped in a sterile sleeve. Patient's skin area should be covered with normal saline solution to remove the air interface between the skin and the sleeve. The transducer is placed in a transverse position (short axis out of plane) to the patient's neck axis, leveled with the separation of the sternal and clavicle head of the sternocleidomastoid muscle, or, if nonpalpable, lateral to the cricoid cartilage at the middle point between the lower jaw angle and the clavicle. The internal carotid artery (ICA) is identified as a well circular, pulsatile, and noncompressible vessel. The internal jugular vein is identified as compressible, nonpulsatile structure and is located in front and outwards with respect to the ICA. Cannulation is done after checking for compressibility. Noncompressible nature of the vein could be a sign of intraluminal thrombus with decreased luminal size or irregular lumen therefore cannulation should be done through the contralateral side. Once inside the vein, the central venous cannulation is placed using Seldinger's technique.

Lal J et al. (2020) did a prospective randomized comparative study to evaluate long axis, short axis, and medial oblique axis (M-OAX) approach for USG-guided IJV cannulation in which they found the medial oblique axis is safe and effective technique when compared with other two.[25B] In M-OAX technique, the linear transducer has been placed in SAX view first means parallel and superior to clavicle for IJV cannulation then rotated 30° counterclockwise in a medial cephalad to the lateral-caudad direction. The introducer needle is then inserted directly at the proximal end of the US probe and advanced in a plane laterally toward ipsilateral nipple. The advantage of M-OAX is, the IJV and carotid artery can be seen beside each other and the needle shaft and tip are clearly visualized in real-time cannulation. The risk of carotid artery puncture is less as entire needle can be seen while cannulating the IJV and direction is from medial to lateral which is away from the carotid artery.

Ultrasound-guided Arterial Line (Fig. 26)

Ultrasound-guided arterial catheterization is especially helpful in patient with obesity, disfigured anatomy, reduced perfusion pressure or nonpulsatile blood flow. It is also useful in patients, where multiple attempts of palpatory method of arterial cannulation have been failed. Ultrasound guidance provides high first pass success rate, decreased number of unsuccessful puncture, decreased procedural time, and decreased the risk of complication. Ultrasound-guided arterial cannulation is same as described in arterial section. Jijeh AM et al.[26] (2014) found 93% success rate in radial artery cannulation in pediatric cardiac critical care patients (6 days-11 years) with no complication. Aouad-Maroun et al.[27] (2017) did a review study through Cochrane database and identified moderate-quality evidence suggesting that ultrasound guidance for radial artery cannulation improves first and second attempt success rates and decreases the

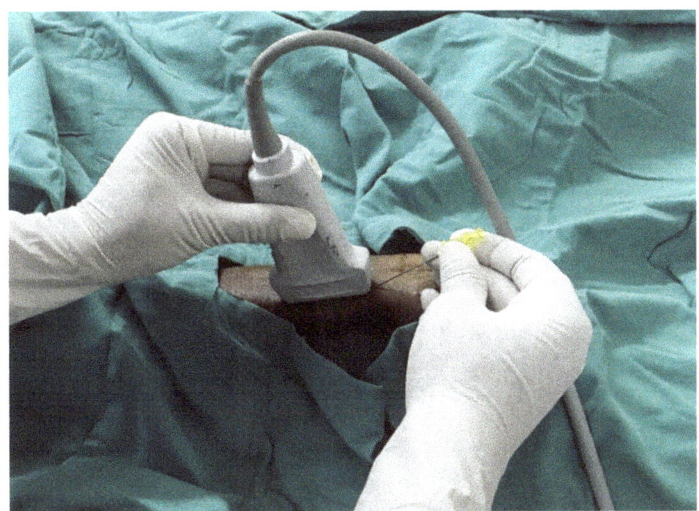

Fig. 26: Ultrasound-guided radial artery cannulation.

rate of complications as compared with palpation or Doppler auditory assistance. They said that the first attempt success rate is more pronounced in infants and small children, in whom arterial line cannulation is more challenging than in older children.

Guideline to Prevent Central Line–associated Bloodstream Infections

Central line-associated bloodstream infections, or CLABSIs, are associated with increased morbidity, mortality, and healthcare costs. As per recent article on prevention of CLABSI by Ling et al.[28] (2016) published in Antimicrobial Resistance and Infection Control (2016), the guidelines are:

- Catheter type and site should be selected as per the requirement. Femoral vein should be avoided as far as possible
- Ultrasound guidance should be used to minimize the complications
- Hand hygiene should be maintained as per the protocol for every invasive procedure. Wear sterile hand gloves before cannulation. Use new sterile gloves before handling the new catheter when guidewire exchanges are performed (II)
- Site should be cleaned with an alcoholic chlorhexidine solution containing 0.5–2% chlorhexidine and 70% alcohol before central venous cannulation and also during change of dressing. If there is a contraindication to chlorhexidine (e.g., hypersensitivity), tincture of iodine, an iodophor, or 70% alcohol can be used as alternatives (IA)
- Allow the skin antiseptic being used to dry completely before catheter insertion (IB)
- Disinfect catheter hubs, needleless connectors, taps and injection ports before accessing the catheter using an alcoholic chlorhexidine preparation or 70% alcohol (IIB)
- Promptly remove any central venous catheter that is no longer required (IA)
- Do not use guidewire exchanges to replace a nontunneled catheter suspected of infection (IB)
- Minimize contamination risk by scrubbing the access port with an appropriate antiseptic (alcohol-based chlorhexidine, povidone iodine, an alcohol-based iodophor, or 70% alcohol) and accessing the port only with sterile devices (IA)
- Minocycline-rifampin or chlorhexidine-silver sulfadiazine impregnated catheters should be considered in adult patients whose catheter dwell time is expected to be more than 7 days and in units where the CLABSI infection rate is not meeting the set goal (IA)
- Use either sterile gauze or sterile, transparent, semipermeable dressing to cover the catheter site (IA)
- If the patient is diaphoretic or if the site is bleeding or oozing, use a gauze dressing until this is resolved (II)
- Replace catheter site dressing if the dressing becomes damp, loosened, or visibly soiled (IB)
- Do not use topical antibiotic ointment or creams on insertion sites, except for dialysis catheters, because of their potential to promote fungal infections and antimicrobial resistance (IB)
- Replace transparent dressings used on CVC sites at least every 7 days, except in those pediatric patients in which the risk of dislodging the catheter may outweigh the benefit of changing the dressing (IB)
- Use a chlorhexidine-impregnated sponge dressing for central venous catheters in patients older than 2 months of age if the CLABSI infection rate high and not decreasing despite adherence to maintenance bundle prevention measures, including education and training (IB)
- In patients not receiving blood, blood products or fat emulsions, replace administration sets that are continuously used, including secondary sets and add-on devices, no more frequently than at 96-hour intervals, but at least every 7 days (IA)
- Replace tubing used to administer blood, blood products, or fat emulsions (those combined with amino acids and glucose in a 3-in-1 admixture or infused separately) within 24 hours, of initiating the infusion (IB)
- Replace tubing used to administer propofol infusions every 6 or 12 hours, when the vial is changed, refer to the manufacturer's recommendation (IA).

The current Centers for Disease Control and Prevention (CDC) guidelines suggest the use of sterile US cover shields in order to reduce the risk of CLABSI.

CURRENT CONCEPT OF CENTRAL VENOUS CANNULATION DURING COVID-19 PANDEMIC FOR ICU PATIENTS

COVID-19 patients may require endotracheal intubation and prone position management in severe acute respiratory distress syndrome to maintain adequate oxygenation.

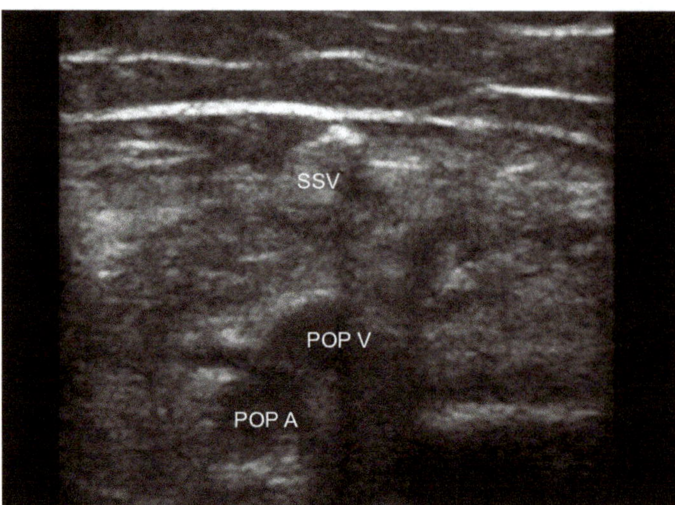

Fig. 27: Popliteal vein USG view in short axis. (SSV: small saphenous vein; POP V: popliteal vein, POP A: popliteal artery)

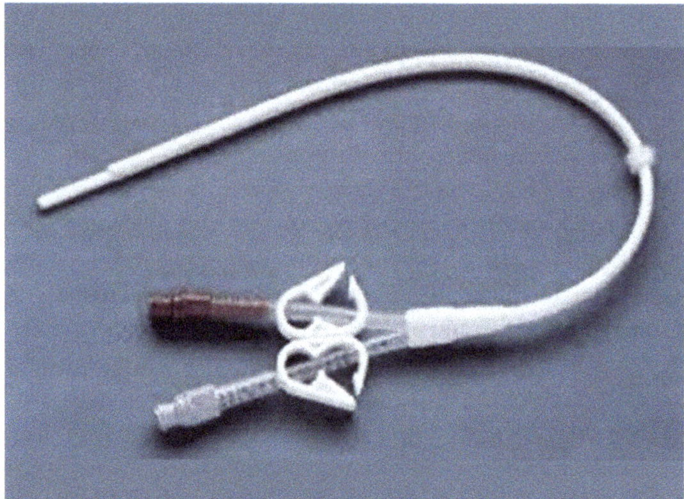

Fig. 28: Permcath 50.

These patients may also require central venous cannulation for vasopressor drug administration, fluid resuscitation and blood sampling along with an emergent continuous renal replacement therapy. Popliteal venous cannulation can easily be accessed in pronated patients under USG guidance **(Fig. 27)**.[29] Permcath (50 cm) can be used for such cannulation in ICU for emergent dialysis **(Fig. 28)**.

In this COVID-19 pandemic GAVeCeLT (Group Accessi Venosi Centrali a Lungo Termine), an Italian expert association has put forth few recommendations for the venous (central) access site, insertion and maintenance of the venous access devices. These devices are designed to protect the intensivist along with increase in success rate of catheter placement and to decrease complications and risks.[30]

- Peripherally inserted central cannula, FICC (femorally inserted central catheter) or CICC (centrally inserted central catheter) can be used for central line.
- Peripherally inserted central cannula decreases the risk of exposure of intensivist while putting central line in patients on CPAP/NIV and/or in tracheostomized patients.
- Peripherally inserted central cannula provides easy management of exit site in pronated patients.
- Femorally inserted central catheter also minimizes the exposure of intensivist to infected oral, nasal, and tracheal secretions of patients.
- Centrally inserted central catheter, infraclavicular approach should be preferred than supraclavicular (USG-guided axillary vein cannulation) for greater protection and stability of catheter.

CONCLUSION

There are many distinct advantages of CVP monitoring. But along with it comes many potential risks associated with invasive hemodynamic monitoring. The clinician is responsible for using appropriate techniques to prevent complications as well as continuously monitoring for the development of adverse consequences. Invasive blood pressure offers beat-to-beat blood pressure monitoring for patients undergoing major surgery and critically ill. It is a useful technique where a pressure measurement system is used for close blood pressure monitoring; however, common sources of error such as natural frequency, damping, zeroing, and leveling should be detected and corrected early to produce an accurate pressure waveform.

REFERENCES

1. Reich DL, Mittnacht AJ, London MJ, et al. Monitoring of the heart and vascular system. In: Kaplan JA, Reich DL, Lake CL, Konstadt SN (Eds). Kaplan's Cardiac Anesthesia, 5th edition. Philadelphia: Saunders Elsevier; 2006. pp. 385-436.
2. Fox K, Roach DJ, Berman SS. Central venous catheter: selection and placement techniques. In: Berman SS (Ed). Vascular Access in Clinical Practice; 2002.
3. Gerhardt MA, Skeehan TM. Monitoring the cardiac surgical patient. In: Hensley FA, Martin DE, Gravlee GP (Eds). A Practical Approach to Cardiac Anesthesia, 4th edition. Philadelphia: Lippincott Williams and Wilkins; 2008. pp. 104-41.
4. Schroeder RA, Barbeito A, Bar-Yosef S, et al. Cardiovascular monitoring. In: Miller RD, Eriksson LI, Fleisher LA, Wiener-Kronish JP, Young WL (Eds). Miller's Anesthesia, 7th edition. Philadelphia: Churchill Livingstone Elsevier; 2010. pp. 1267-328.

4A. Mitre C, Adela G, Acalovschi I, et al. Ultrasound-guided external jugular vein cannulation for central venous access by inexperienced trainees. Eur J Anaesthesiol. 2009;27(3):300-3.

4B. Palmaers T, Frank P, Eismann H, et al. Vena-subclavia-Katheter und Pneumothoraxrisiko: Maschinelle Beatmung erhöht das Pneumothoraxrisiko während infraklavikulärer landmarkengestützter V.-subclavia-Punktion: eine prospektive randomisierte Studie [Catheterization of the subclavian vein and the risk of pneumothorax: Mechanical ventilation increases the risk of pneumothorax during infraclavicular landmark-guided subclavian vein puncture: a prospective randomized study]. Anaesthesist. 2019;68(5):309-16.

4C. Papamichalis P, Alexiou E, Zafeiridis T, et al. Inadvertent direct pulmonary artery catheterization complicating the effort for subclavian venous cannulation and central venous catheter placement: A case report and review of the literature. Int J Crit Illn Inj Sci. 2020;10(3):143-7.

5. Troianos CA, Kuwik RJ, Pasqual JR, et al. Internal jugular vein and carotid artery anatomic relation as determined by ultrasonography. Anesthesiology. 1996;85(1):43-8.
6. Sulek CA, Gravenstein N, Blackshear RH, et al. Head rotation during internal jugular vein cannulation and the risk of carotid artery puncture. Anesth Analg. 1996;82(1):125-8.
7. Mallory DL, Shawker T, Evans RG, et al. Effects of clinical maneuvers on sonographically determined internal jugular vein size during venous cannulation. Crit Care Med. 1990;18(11): 1269-73.
8. Parry G. Trendelenburg position, head elevation and a midline position optimize right internal jugular vein diameter. Can J Anaesth. 2004;51(4):379-81.
9. Porter JM. Raynaud's syndrome. In: Sabiston DC (Ed). Textbook of Surgery. Philadelphia: WB Saunders Company; 1985. pp. 1925-32.
10. Kozak M, Robertson BJ, Chambers CE. Cardiac catheterization laboratory: diagnostic and therapeutic procedures in the adult patient. In: Kaplan JA, Reich DL, Lake CL, Konstadt SN (Eds). Kaplan's Cardiac Anesthesia, 5th edition. Philadelphia: Saunders Elsevier; 2006. pp. 299-354.
11. Tuncali BE, Kuvaki B, Tuncali B, et al. A comparison of the efficacy of heparinized and nonheparinized solutions for maintenance of perioperative radial arterial catheter patency and subsequent occlusion. Anesth Analg. 2005;100(4):1117-21.
12. Lowenstein E, Little JW, Lo HH. Prevention of cerebral embolization from flushing radial artery cannulas. N Engl J Med. 1971;285(25):1414-5.
13. Kleinman B, Powell S, Kumar P, et al. The fast flush test measures the dynamic response of the entire blood pressure monitoring system. Anesthesiology. 1992;77(6):1215-20.
14. Allen EV. Thromboangiitis obliterans: methods of diagnosis of chronic occlusive arterial lesions distal to the wrist with illustrated cases. Am J Med Sci. 1929;178:237.
15. Barbeau GR, Arsenault F, Dugas L, et al. Evaluation of the ulnopalmar arterial arches with pulse oximetry and plethysmography: comparison with the Allen's test in 1010 patients. Am Heart J. 2004;147(3):489-93.
16. Ryan JF, Raines J, Dalton BC, et al. Arterial dynamics of radial artery cannulation. Anesth Analg. 1973;52:1017-25.
17. Scheer B, Perel A, Pfeiffer UJ. Clinical review: complications and risk factors of peripheral arterial catheters used for haemodynamic monitoring in anaesthesia and intensive care medicine. Crit Care. 2002;6(3):199-204.
18. Lorente L, Santacreu R, Martín MM, et al. Arterial catheter-related infection of 2,949 catheters. Crit Care. 2006;10(3):R83.
19. Berlin DA, Bakker J. Review of Starling curves and central venous pressure. Critical Care. 2015;19(1):55.
20. Berlin D. Hemodynamic consequences of auto-PEEP. J Intensive Care Med. 2014;29(2):81-6.
21. Forrester JS, Diamond G, McHugh TJ, et al. Filling pressures in the right and left sides of the heart in acute myocardial infarction. N. England J Med.1971;285(4):190-3.
22. Boyd JH, Forbes J, Nakada TA, et al. Fluid resuscitation in septic shock: A positive fluid balance and elevated central venous pressure are associated with increased mortality. Crit care med. 2011;39(2):259-65.
23. Legrand M, Dupuis C, Simon C, et al. Association between systemic hemodynamics and septic acute kidney injury in critically ill patients: a retrospective observational study. Crit care. 2013;17(6):R278.
24. Jardin F, Vieillard- Baron A. A ultrasonographic examination of the venae cavae. Intensive Care Medicine. 2006;32:203-6
25. Guyton AC, Hall JE. Textbook of Medical Physiology, 11th edition, Philadelphia, Elsevier Saunders; 2006.
25A. Brass P, Hellmich M, Kolodziej L, et al. Ultrasound guidance versus anatomical landmarks for subclavian or femoral vein catheterization. Cochrane Database Syst Rev. 2015;1(1):CD011447.
25B. Lal J, Bhardwaj M, Verma M, et al. A prospective, randomised, comparative study to evaluate long axis, short axis and medial oblique axis approach for ultrasound-guided internal jugular vein cannulation. Indian J Anaesth. 2020;64(3):193-8.
26. Jijeh AM, Shaath G, Kabbani MS, et al. Ultrasound-guided vascular access in pediatric cardiac critical care. J Saudi Heart Assoc. 2014;26(4):199-203.
27. Aouad-Maroun M, Raphael CK, Sayyid SK, et al. Ultrasound-guided arterial cannulation for paediatrics. Cochrane Database Syst Rev. 2016;14;9:CD011364.
28. Ling ML, Apisarnthanarak A, Jaggi N, et al. APSIC guide for prevention of Central Line Associated Bloodstream Infections (CLABSI). Antimicrob Resist Infect Control. 2016;5:16.
29. Adams E, Mousa AY. Achieving a popliteal venous access for renal replacement therapy in critically ill COVID-19 patient in prone position. J Vasc Surg Cases Innov Tech. 2020;6(2):266-8.
30. Pittiruti M, Pinelli F, on behalf of the GAVeCeLT Working Group for Vascular Access in COVID-19. Recommendations for the use of vascular access in the COVID-19 patients: an Italian perspective. Crit Care. 2020;24:269.

Pulmonary Artery Catheterization

Sarita Fernandes

ABSTRACT

The pulmonary artery catheter (PAC) was introduced in the 1970s and has provided invaluable diagnostic information which has immensely helped the clinician. One of the main reasons for insertion of PAC is to measure the pulmonary capillary wedge pressure and pulmonary artery diastolic pressure, both of which are estimates of left atrial pressure, left ventricular end-diastolic pressure, and volume. Special purpose PACs for pacing, cardiac output monitoring, mixed venous oximetry, etc., are now available. An understanding of the potential benefits and pitfalls of pulmonary artery catheterization is essential for the anesthesiologist.

INTRODUCTION

The pulmonary artery catheter (PAC) was developed and used in humans by the US physicians Harold James Swan and William Ganz in the 1970s. A large number of hemodynamic measurements are possible with the use of the PAC. Special purpose PACs for continuous cardiac output (CO) monitoring, pacing, right ventricular (RV) ejection fraction monitoring, and continuous mixed venous oximetry are available. Clinical trials however have failed to demonstrate improved patient outcomes with its use. The PAC has fallen into disrepute in recent times due to complications involved and the availability of newer, lesser invasive methods of hemodynamic monitoring. Its usefulness depends on the experience of the user and his knowledge and interpretation of the information provided by the PAC.

CATHETER DESIGN (FIGS. 1 AND 2)

The PAC is a flexible, flow directed, balloon tipped catheter available in adult and pediatric sizes ranging from 60 to 110 cm in length, 4–7.5 Fr in caliber and balloon inflation volumes ranging from 0.5 to 1.5 mL. The material used is polyvinyl chloride, which softens at body temperature.[1] The standard catheter is 110 cm long, marked every 10 cm by thin and thick black lines to estimate the catheter tip location during insertion and mostly has 5 lumens or interior channels. The number of lumens may vary according to manufacturer design and the purpose of insertion. A percutaneous sheath introducer and contamination shield is provided along with the PAC.

Distal Lumen

It terminates at the distal tip. When connected to the pressure monitoring system, it measures pulmonary artery pressures (PAP), pulmonary capillary wedge pressure (PCWP), and can be used for withdrawal of samples to measure mixed venous oxygen saturation; it is not to be used for continuous fluid or drug administration.

Proximal Infusion Lumen

It terminates 30 cm proximal to the catheter tip and is positioned in the right atrium (RA) in most adults when the PAC is in the wedged position. This port allows for infusion of solutions, central venous pressure (CVP) monitoring, and blood sampling.

Proximal Injectate Lumen

It terminates at a port located 26 cm from the distal tip. When the distal tip is located in the pulmonary artery, this port will reside in the RA or vena cava, allowing for bolus

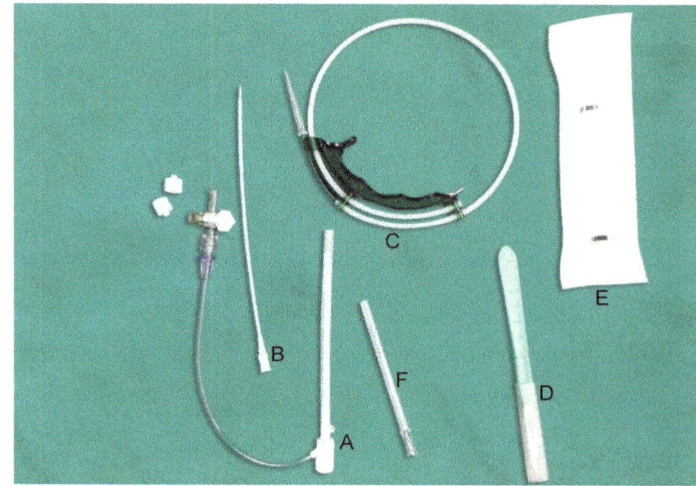

Fig. 1: Pulmonary artery catheter kit. A, introducer sheath with venous extension; B, dilator; C, guidewire; D, blade; E, syringe; F, introducer needle.

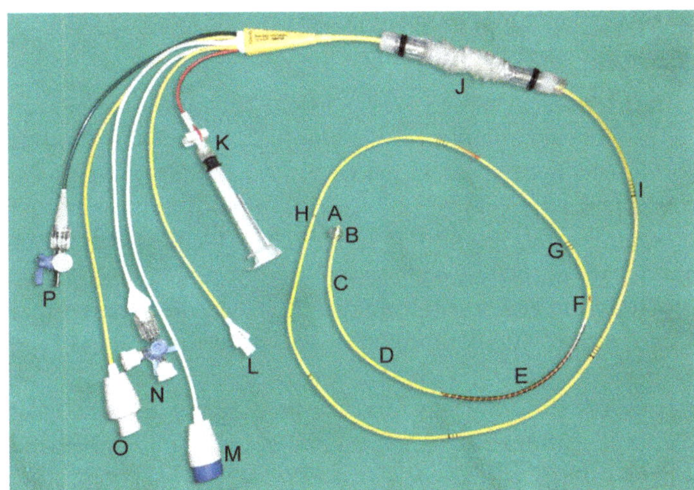

Fig. 2: Parts of pulmonary artery catheter. A, pulmonary artery distal lumen; B, balloon; C, thermistor at 4 cm; D, 10 cm mark; E, thermal filament; F, proximal injectate port at 26 cm; G, proximal infusion port at 30 cm; H, 50 cm mark; I, 90 cm mark; J, protective contamination shield; K, balloon inflation valve with syringe; L, pulmonary artery distal lumen hub; M, thermistor connector for cardiac output monitoring; N, proximal injectate lumen hub; O, thermal filament connector for cardiac output monitoring; P, proximal infusion lumen hub.

CO injections, RA pressure monitoring, blood sampling, or infusion of solutions.

Balloon Inflation Lumen

It terminates within the balloon located just proximal to the catheter tip.

Thermistor Connector Lumen

It is connected by wires to a small thermistor located 3.5-4 cm proximal to the catheter tip and is used to measure the CO using the thermodilution method.

Additional Venous Infusion Lumen

It provides separate access to the RA and can be used for continuous infusion of fluids even during CO measurement.

Oximetry Lumen

It terminates at the distal tip and contains fiber optic bundles through which light is transmitted to the pulmonary artery and reflected to the photodetector by the hemoglobin in the blood.

The specialized PACs with permanently implanted electrodes allow atrial, ventricular or atrioventricular pacing and intracardiac electrocardiogram recording. The standard PACs are equipped with a rapid response thermistor can measure right ventricular ejection fraction and right ventricular end-diastolic volume. PACs with incorporated fiberoptic bundles can continuously measure mixed venous hemoglobin saturation via a special computer attached to it. PACs treated with antimicrobial heparin coating are also available.

TECHNIQUE OF INSERTION (VIDEO 18)

The preferred site of cannulation is the internal jugular vein (IJV) although subclavian or femoral vein can also be used. With the subclavian route, there is a possibility of the introducer kinking during sternal retraction. The sterile sheath that covers the PAC must be secured at both ends to prevent contamination of the outer portion of the catheter. All the lumens are flushed with heparinized saline and the distal port hub is attached to the transducer. The IJV is punctured with an 18 G needle, a flexible guidewire is passed and the needle removed. The nick on the neck has to be larger to accommodate a large bore introducer sheath which has a hemostasis valve at its outer end and a sidearm extension for intravenous (IV) access. A stopcock can be attached to the extension to prevent spillage of blood during cannulation. An 8 Fr sheath with vein dilator is passed over the guide wire. The sheath remains in the IJV after the dilator and guidewire are removed. The patency and symmetry of the balloon is tested by inflating it with 1.5 mL of air from a volume limited syringe.

Typical waveforms are observed during the PAC transit. At a depth of 15-20 cm, when the PAC lies in the SVC or right atrium, a CVP waveform with a, c, v waves, and low mean pressure is observed. The balloon is now inflated. Orienting the PAC curve leftward to the sagittal plane and positioning the patient head down facilitates passage through the tricuspid valve. As the catheter tip enters the right ventricle (RV), there is a rise in systolic pressure to 15-30 mm Hg with minimal change in diastolic pressure to 0-8 mm Hg. Tilting the patient onto the right side and placing the head up supposedly minimizes arrhythmias and encourages floatation out of the RV.[2] As the catheter crosses the pulmonic valve a dicrotic notch appears on the pressure waveform with a sudden increase in diastolic pressure. During diastole, the pulmonary artery pressure will fall because of interruption of flow during pulmonic valve closure whereas the pressure in the RV will increase because of filling from the right atrium. The PAP waveform is similar to the systemic arterial waveform but is smaller and precedes it slightly. The normal PAPs are 15-20 mm Hg systolic and 5-12 mm Hg diastolic. When the catheter is advanced further by 3-5 cm the pulmonary artery occlusion pressure (PAOP) or the pulmonary artery wedge pressure (PAWP) tracing is obtained with morphology that resembles the CVP tracing. The PAWP is considered normal between 5 and 12 mm Hg. Deflate the balloon and confirm that the PAP waveform reappears. If it does not, withdraw the catheter till the PAP tracing is obtained. At, the time of catheter placement, the difference between pulmonary artery (PA) end-diastolic and mean PCWP should be determined. If the difference does not exceed 5 mm Hg, PA end-diastolic pressure can be used in place of PAOP. During normal catheter use, the inflation syringe is kept attached to the gate valve to prevent inadvertent injection of liquid into the balloon inflation lumen. Repeated cardiac manipulation and temperature changes that occur during cardiopulmonary bypass (CPB) can alter the stiffness of the catheter and cause the PAC to migrate distally even without balloon inflation.[3] The PAC may be withdrawn 3-5 cm before institution of CPB.[4] The pressure monitoring lumens should be kept patent by intermittent flush or continuous flow infusion with heparinized saline solution. Viscous solutions flow slowly and may occlude the catheter lumen. The catheter should never be flushed when the balloon is wedged in the pulmonary artery.

When the PAC is inserted from the right IJV, the RA should be reached at 20-25 cm, the RV at 30-35 cm, the PA at 40-45 cm, and the wedge position at 45-55 cm. If the RV waveform is not observed after inserting the catheter 40 cm, coiling in the RA is likely. If a PA waveform is not observed after inserting the catheter 50 cm, it has probably coiled in the RV. The balloon should be deflated, catheter withdrawn to 20 cm and the PAC floating sequence repeated. Additional distance of 5-10 cm from the left IJV, right and left external jugular veins, 15 cm from the femoral veins and 30-35 cm from the antecubital veins is needed. The tip of the PAC must lie in west zone III of the lung where the pulmonary arterial and venous pressures exceed the alveolar pressure. The supine position of the patient favors zone III conditions.[5] Benumof et al. found that most catheters pass into the right middle or lower lobes.[6] Pulmonary artery occlusion pressure should be measured at end expiration when the effect of intrathoracic pressure is minimal. The tip of the PAC should be within 2 cm of the cardiac silhouette on a standard anteroposterior (AP) chest film.[7]

INTERPRETATION OF PULMONARY ARTERY WEDGE PRESSURE

In the wedged position, a continuous static column of blood connects the PAC tip to the junction of the pulmonary veins and the left atrium. Ideally the PAWP and pulmonary artery diastolic pressure (PADP) are estimates of left atrial pressure (LAP), which reflects left ventricular end diastolic pressure (LVEDP) and left ventricular (LV) preload. These values, however, should be interpreted keeping in mind the patient's clinical condition. The PAWP will be greater than the LVEDP in cases of mitral stenosis and regurgitation, left atrial myxomas, increased intrathoracic pressure, COPD, etc. The PAWP will be less than the LVEDP in conditions where the LV is noncompliant (e.g., ischemia and hypertrophy) and when the LVEDP is greater than 25 mm Hg. The PAWP should be determined at end expiration in both spontaneously breathing and mechanically ventilated patients. A properly wedged catheter with balloon inflated does not allow mixing of shunted venous blood with the post capillary blood, so the oxygen saturation of a properly wedged catheter is around 20% higher than the one recorded with the balloon deflated.[8]

PULMONARY ARTERY CATHETER WAVEFORMS (FIGS. 3 TO 5)

Either before or after PAC insertion, the system is zeroed to ambient air pressure using the midpoint of the LA, i.e., the fourth intercostal space in the midaxillary line as the reference point. Most monitors perform an automated electronic calibration after zeroing. The PAP waveform has systolic phase, diastolic phase and dicrotic notch. The dicrotic notch on the PAP waveform reflects closure of the semilunar valves at the end of contraction and prior to refilling of the ventricles. The slight elevation seen at the dicrotic notch represents the transient increase in PAP due to backup of blood flow immediately after closure of the semilunar valves.[8]

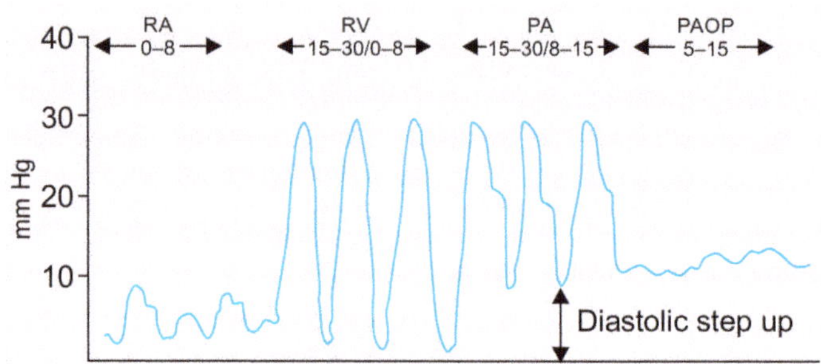

Fig. 3: The waveforms observed during flotation of a pulmonary artery catheter from the venous circulation to the pulmonary capillary wedge position. There is sudden increase in systolic pressure as the catheter enters the right ventricle and sudden increase in diastolic pressure as the catheter enters the pulmonary artery, followed by a decrease in mean pressure as the catheter reaches the wedge position. (RA: right atrium; RV: right ventricle; PA: pulmonary artery; PAOP: pulmonary artery occlusion pressure)

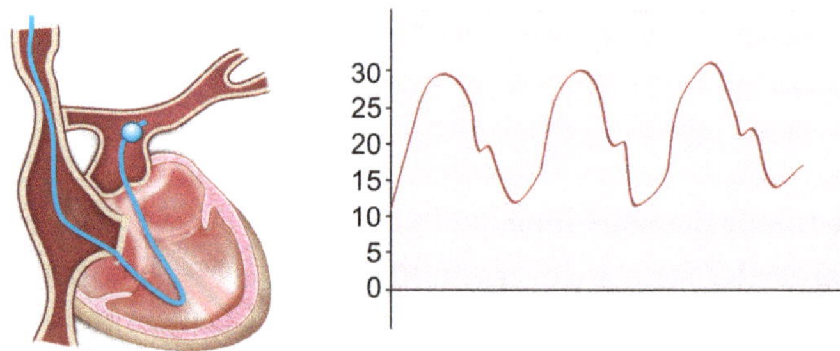

Fig. 4: The pulmonary artery catheter in the pulmonary artery with the balloon inflated. The characteristic pulmonary artery waveform with the dicrotic notch.

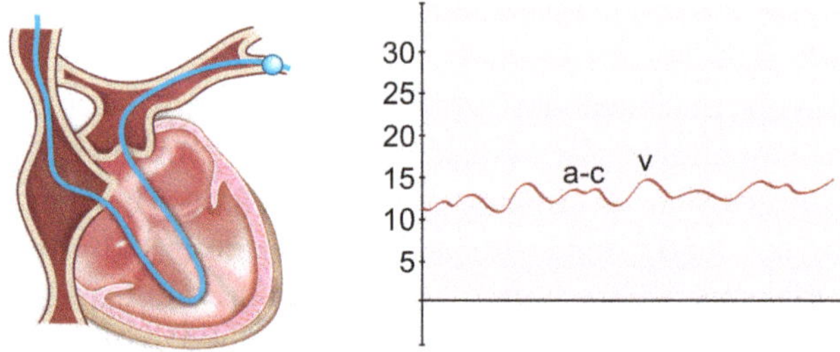

Fig. 5: The pulmonary artery catheter in the wedge position with the balloon inflated. This is obtained by passing the catheter 3-5 cm further from where the pulmonary artery waveform was observed. The pulmonary artery wedge pressure has a similar morphology to the right atrial pressure with a-c and v waves.

PCWP waveform resembles that of CVP with *a, c,* and *v* waves and x and y descents. The *a* wave of PAWP waveform may be increased in cases of higher resistance to LV filling, e.g., mitral stenosis, LV failure and decreased LV compliance. Large *v* waves are seen in myocardial infarction due to decrease in LV diastolic compliance or mitral regurgitation as a result of ischemic papillary muscle dysfunction.

Dampened Waveform

It is commonly the result of transducer malfunction, loose connection in the tubing, catheter impinging the vessel wall, air bubbles etc. A dampened system does not overshoot or oscillate and there is a delay in returning to the PAC waveform. The system is checked using the rapid flush test where an initial horizontal straight line with a high pressure reading is recorded when flushed. When the flushing is terminated, the pressure drops immediately, which is represented by a vertical line that plunges below the baseline. A brief and well-defined oscillation occurs, followed by return of the pulmonary artery (PA) waveform.

An artificially low pressure or a pressure peak that occurs simultaneous with the CVP *c* wave: This common PAC trace artifact occurs at the onset of systole due to excessive catheter movement.

Over Wedging

The over wedged pressure is devoid of pulsatality, is higher than expected and rises continuously to flush pressure. A continuous wedge trace with the balloon deflated or with minimal balloon inflation should arouse suspicion of distal catheter migration. Gently, withdrawing the catheter to a more proximal location in the pulmonary artery usually solves this problem.

INDICATIONS OF PULMONARY ARTERY CATHETER INSERTION

The American Society of Anesthesiologists Practice Guidelines state that the patient, surgery, and practice setting need to be considered prior to use of a PAC. It is mainly indicated in high risk patients undergoing high risk surgical procedures during which large fluid shifts and major hemodynamic fluctuations are anticipated. They can be used to guide treatment of patients after evaluating the risk-benefit ratio in patients with complicated myocardial infarction, cardiogenic shock, noncardiogenic pulmonary edema, septic shock, multi trauma necessitating massive transfusion, adult respiratory distress syndrome, perioperative cardiac surgical patients, critically ill patients on inotropes, vasopressors or vasodilators and surgeries like heart or liver transplant.

CONTRAINDICATIONS

Tricuspid or pulmonic stenosis, RA, RV or PA masses, tetralogy of Fallot (the right ventricular outflow tract being hypersensitive, the PAC may induce infundibular spasm), arrhythmias, coagulopathy, complete left bundle branch block (risk of complete heart block is increased), Wolff-Parkinson-White syndrome, Ebstein's malformation (risk of tachyarrhythmias), newly inserted pacemaker wires, cardiac resynchronization therapy or automatic implantable cardioverter-defibrillator.

COMPLICATIONS OF PULMONARY ARTERY CATHETER

Arrhythmias

The self-limited atrial and ventricular arrhythmias are common during PAC insertion and transient right bundle branch block can occur as the PAC strikes the interventricular septum. It is imperative to have an external pacemaker available or to use a pacing PAC in patients with left bundle branch block.[9]

Mechanical Problems

Pulmonary artery catheter may kink as it exits the introducer sheath,[10] may dislodge temporary transvenous pacing wires or form knots within the heart.[7] Insertion of a guidewire under fluoroscopic guidance may aid in unknotting the catheter. Ensure free movement of the PAC before chest closure as it may become entrapped in sutures or bypass cannulas. Damped appearance of the monitored pressure trace or difficulty infusing fluids or withdrawing blood through one of the catheter lumens should alert one to this problem. Failure of the PAC to enter the RV may occur in patients with an enlarged RA or ventricle particularly if the CO is low or in the presence of tricuspid or pulmonary incompetence or pulmonary hypertension. Deep inspiration by the patient during advancement may facilitate passage. This may also be overcome by filling the balloon with sterile saline instead of air and positioning the patient with left side down. When the RV is entered, the saline should be removed and replaced with air.[11] Stiffening the catheter by injecting 10–20 mL of ice cold solution through the distal lumen may help in proper placement. Balloon rupture causing air embolus is a possibility and should be suspected if no resistance is felt during injection of air and if there is failure to obtain the wedge waveform. In such cases, the balloon port may be left unused and the PADP monitored as an estimate of PCWP.[1] Air should never be used for balloon inflation in any situation where it may enter the arterial circulation, e.g., in all pediatric patients and in adults with suspected right to left intracardiac or intrapulmonary shunts. Bacteria-filtered carbon dioxide can be used for balloon inflation in patients with right to left shunts.[4]

Thrombus Formation

Heparin bonding to the external surface has reduced the thrombogenicity of PACs; however high dose aprotinin and epsilon-aminocaproic acid can increase the risk of thrombus formation on the PAC.[12]

Thrombocytopenia

Although rare can be triggered by heparin coated PACs.[7]

Pulmonary Artery Injury and Rupture

The risk factors include advanced age, hypothermia, pulmonary hypertension, coagulopathy, excessive depth of insertion, hyperinflation or improper inflation with liquid rather than air, pulmonary artery hypertension.[13] The measures to prevent this complication include avoiding over inflation and prolonged inflation of the balloon in the wedged position and avoiding insertion too far peripherally into a branch of the pulmonary artery. Transesophageal echocardiography[14] and videofluoroscopy[15] have been used to guide placement when floatation is predicted to be difficult, e.g., low cardiac output states, severe tricuspid regurgitation, septal defects, etc. Transthoracic echocardiography[16] has also been used to provide visualization of a mobile to and fro PAC balloon in the main or right pulmonary artery.

During hypothermic CPB there is a risk of distal migration of the catheter tip with movement of the heart and hardening of the PAC. The withdrawing of the PAC about 3-5 cm when CPB is instituted may help prevent this complication.

Pulmonary Infarction

The continuous monitoring the pulmonary artery waveform and keeping the balloon deflated when the PCWP is not being measured can prevent this complication. It could also result from embolization of a thrombus formed on the PAC.

Valvular Damage

The withdrawal of the catheter with the balloon inflated may result in injury to the tricuspid or pulmonic valves. There exists a risk of passing the catheter between the chordae tendineae if the PAC is advanced with the balloon deflated.[17]

HEMODYNAMIC VARIABLES MEASURED

The PAC directly measures RA and RV pressures, pulmonary artery systolic and diastolic pressures, PCWP estimates, left atrial and LV end-diastolic pressures and core body temperature. The cardiac output is measured by continuous or intermittent thermodilution methods. The current computers with the help of standard formulae can derive hemodynamic parameters, such as the cardiac index, systemic and pulmonary vascular resistance, LV and RV stroke work index, arterial oxygen content, mixed venous oxygen content, arteriovenous oxygen content difference, pulmonary capillary oxygen content, pulmonary shunt fraction, oxygen delivery and consumption, oxygen extraction ratio, etc.

CARDIAC OUTPUT MEASUREMENT

Intermittent Thermodilution Technique

Although the newer methods of measuring CO are less invasive, the PAC remains a valuable tool for CO monitoring. The thermodilution is an indicator-dilution method of measuring blood flow and is based on the principle that when an indicator substance is added to circulating blood, the rate of blood flow is inversely proportional to the change in concentration of the indicator over time.

The equipment required is the CO computer, a thermodilution PAC, catheter connecting cables, injectate solution and an injectate temperature probe. Prior to injection, confirm that the balloon is deflated and the thermistor hub connected to the cardiac output monitor. 10 mL of 0.9% saline or 5% D ice cold solution or solution at room temperature is injected as a bolus within 4 seconds into the RA. The resulting temperature change is detected by the thermistor in the pulmonary artery. The CO computer displays the temperature-time curve. The area under the curve is inversely proportional to the rate of blood flow in the pulmonary artery. In the absence of intracardiac shunts, this flow rate is equivalent to the average cardiac output. The modified Stewart-Hamilton equation is used to calculate the cardiac output.[4]

$$\frac{V(T_B - T_I)\times K_1 \times K_2}{\int_0^{\infty} \Delta T_B(t)dt}$$

Where CO (cardiac output in L/min), V (volume of injectate in mL), T_B (initial blood temperature in °C), T_I (initial injectate temperature in °C), K_1 (density factor), K_2 (computation constant) and $\int_0^{\infty} \Delta T_B(t)dt$ is the integral of blood temperature change over time. The injection should be timed during end expiration and the average value of three measurements is taken as the CO provided they do not differ from each other by more than 15%. The faster the rate of change in blood temperature, the greater will be the flow rate, and higher will be the cardiac output. There may be a discrepancy in the cardiac output measured by the thermodilution technique in cases of intracardiac shunts and severe TR due to prolonged transit time and recycling of the indicator.

Continuous Thermodilution Cardiac Output Monitoring

This method uses a specialized PA catheter with a 10 cm thermal filament incorporated into the RV portion of the PAC approximately 15-25 cm from the catheter tip. The filament generates low energy heat pulses that are transmitted to the surrounding blood and the resulting temperature change is measured by the thermistor at the PAC tip. The thermodilution temperature curve is plotted and the displayed value of CO updated every 30-60 seconds. It represents the average CO measured over the previous 3-6 minute.[7] Since it is an average over several minutes, beat to beat variations in stroke volume that occur during a single respiratory cycle are all equally represented.

REMOVAL OF THE PULMONARY ARTERY CATHETER

The possible causes of resistance while removing the PAC are catheter knotting, deformation and suture entrapment.[18] It is wise to check the recent X-ray film prior to PAC removal. The acute angulation of the PAC on chest radiograph suggests suture entrapment.[19] The transesophageal echocardiogram in this situation will show deformity of the heart contour wall when traction is applied on the PAC.[20]

The coagulation status must be checked prior to removal of the introducer. The patient is positioned head down to prevent air embolism and ensure that the balloon is deflated prior to catheter removal. The introducer sheath with side arm may be left in situ for IV access. Now unclip the hub of the protective catheter sheath and remove the catheter gently and steadily.

CONCLUSION

It is not the insertion of the PAC rather the correct interpretation of the data obtained and selecting the right treatment plan that makes a difference to patient outcome. The newer methods like esophageal Doppler and pulse contour analysis allow beat-to-beat estimation of LV stroke volume and are less invasive. Nevertheless, the PAC is a useful tool, which can guide the physician in making therapeutic decisions in critical care.

REFERENCES

1. Sunavala JD. Cardiac monitoring in adults. In: Udwadia FE (Ed). Principles of Critical Care, 2nd edition. New Delhi: Oxford University Press; 2007. pp. 59-76.
2. Keusch DJ, Winters S, Thys DM. The patient's position influences the incidence of dysrhythmias during pulmonary artery catheterization. Anesthesiology. 1989;70(4):582-4.
3. Johnston WE, Royster RL, Choplin RH, et al. Pulmonary artery catheter migration during cardiac surgery. Anesthesiology. 1986; 64(2):258-62.
4. Reich DL, Mittnacht AJ, London MJ, et al. Monitoring of the heart and Vascular System. In: Kaplan JA, Reich DL, Lake CL, Konstadt SN (Eds). Kaplan's Cardiac Anesthesia, 5th edition. Philadelphia: Saunders Elsevier, Churchill Livingstone Elsevier; 2010. pp. 399-436.
5. Kronberg GM, Quan SF, Schlobohm RM, et al. Anatomic locations of the tips of pulmonary artery catheters in supine patients. Anesthesiology. 1979;51(5):467-9.
6. Benumof JL, Saidman IJ, Arkin DB, et al. Where pulmonary artery catheters go: intrathoracic distribution. Anesthesiology. 1977;46(5):336-8.
7. Schroeder RA, Barbeito A, Yosef SB, et al. Cardiovascular monitoring. In: Miller RD, Erikson LI, Fleisher LA, Weiner Kronish JP, Young WL (Eds). Miller's Anesthesia, 7th edition. Philadelphia: Churchill Livingstone Elsevier; 2010. pp. 1267-328.
8. Chang DW, Hamelin G. Hemodynamic monitoring. In: Chang DW (Ed). Clinical Application of Mechanical Ventilation, 4th edition. New York: Thomson Delmar Learning; 2010. pp. 276-306.
9. Sprung CL, Elser CL, Schein RM, et al. Risk of right bundle branch block and complete heart block during pulmonary artery catheterization. Crit Care Med. 1989;17(1):1-3.
10. Bromley JL, Moorthy SS. Acute angulation of a pulmonary artery catheter. Anesthesiology. 1983;59(4):367-8.
11. Macartney F. The pulmonary artery catheter. In: Marino PL, Sutin KM (Eds). The ICU Book, 3rd edition. Philadelphia: Lippincott Williams & Wilkins; 2001.
12. Dentz ME, Slaughter TF, Mark JB. Early thrombus formation on heparin bonded pulmonary artery catheters in patients receiving epsilon aminocaproic acid. Anesthesiology. 1995; 82(2):583-6.
13. Hardy JF, Morissette M, Taillefer J, et al. Pathophysiology of rupture of the pulmonary artery by pulmonary artery balloon tipped catheters. Anesth Analg. 1983;62(10):925-30.
14. Cronin B, Robbins R, Maus T. Pulmonary artery catheter placement using TEE. J Cardiothoracic Vasc Anesth. 2017;31:178-83.
15. Weinberg L, Miles L, Suaf M, et al. Video fluoroscopy for positioning of PAC in patients undergoing cardiac surgery. J Cardiothorac Vasc Anaesth. 2015;29:1511-6.
16. Tan C, Weinberg L, Stoey D, et al. TTE assists appropriate pulmonary artery catheter placement: An observational study. World J Anesthesiol. 2015;4(2):30-8.
17. Kainuma M, Yamada M, Miyake T. Pulmonary artery catheter passing between the chordae tendineae of the tricuspid valve (correspondence). Anesthesiology. 1995;83(5):1130.
18. Bhatti WA, Sinha S, Rowlands P. Percutaneous untying of a knot in a retained Swan-Ganz catheter. Cardiovasc Intervent Radiol 2000;23(3):224-5.
19. Wholey MH, Zikria EA, Bolyle B. Inadvertent atrial fixation of a Swan-Ganz catheter by suture and a method for its percutaneous removal. Cardiovasc Intervent Radiol. 1987;10(3):171-4.
20. Dubois PE, Collard E, Xenitos P, Louagie YA. Early recognition of pulmonary artery catheter entrapment with TEE. J Cardiothoracic Vas Anesth 2003;17(1):142-3.

Cardiac Output Monitors

Vasundhra R Atre, Naina P Dalvi

ABSTRACT

The importance of "optimization" of fluid therapy in the critically ill and injured patients as well as those undergoing major surgery cannot be emphasized enough. Fluid loading is generally the first step used to resuscitate these groups of unstable patients where the clinical determination of the intravascular volume can be extremely difficult. Studies have shown that only about 50% of hemodynamically unstable patients in the intensive care unit (ICU) and operating room show response to a fluid challenge. In fact, in the setting of major surgery overzealous fluid resuscitation has been shown to increase not only complications, the length of ICU stay and hospital days but also mortality; while optimization of fluid therapy has been shown to reduce both postoperative complications and the length of hospital stay.

Traditionally, fluid management has been guided by measurement of cardiac filling pressures, including the central venous pressure (CVP) and pulmonary artery occlusion pressure. That cardiac filling pressures are not good predictors of fluid responsiveness has been demonstrated by various studies over the last three decades. It has also been shown that the pulmonary artery catheter (PAC) thermodilution (TD) technique considered as the "gold standard" for the measurement of cardiac output (CO) is invasive and is not without its "imperfections". The last decade has seen the search for and introduction of alternative methods of both invasive and minimally invasive methods for the measurement of CO.

All monitors in use today draw on one or a combination of different methods/principles to measure CO. The basic principles on which the monitors work are described, followed by a comparison of the various types of monitors in current use and a detailing of the possible parameters that the monitors could measure, calculate, and display.

INTRODUCTION

The need for fluid optimization in the management of the critically ill patients and those undergoing major surgery cannot be stressed enough. The study of Rivers et al. using a protocol of early goal directed therapy in patients with severe sepsis and septic shock showed reduced organ failure and improved patient survival.[1] In the setting of major surgery excessive fluid resuscitation has been shown to increase not only complications, the length of intensive care unit (ICU) stay and hospital days but also mortality; while optimization of fluid therapy has been shown to reduce both postoperative complications and the length of hospital stay.[2-5]

The traditionally measured parameters of blood pressure, pulse rate, CVP, and O_2 saturation have been shown to have limitations as adequate indicators of fluid resuscitation. Although fluid loading has been considered as the first step to resuscitating a hemodynamically unstable patient[6] and cardiac filling pressures and CVP, have been used universally to guide fluid therapy, only about 50% of hemodynamically unstable patients in the ICU and operating room respond to a fluid challenge.[7] During the past decade attention has shifted to tests that dynamically test volume responsiveness; assess cardiac function and tissue oxygen delivery.

In the critically ill or patient undergoing major surgery, cardiac output (CO) monitoring is standard practice. It is a hemodynamic parameter, which acts as a guide to appropriate fluid resuscitation and estimates whole body perfusion delivery. CO is the amount of blood pumped by the heart in L/min, being the product of the stroke volume (SV) measured in mL and heart rate (HR) measured as beats per minute.

$$CO = SV \times HR$$

Stroke volume is the amount of blood ejected by the ventricles with each ventricular contraction and is dependent on three factors: (i) preload, (ii) contractility, and (iii) afterload. Preload is the amount of blood in the ventricle before it contracts. Contractility is the force with which the ventricles contract. The afterload is the resistance against which the ventricles are contracting to push the blood into circulation.

Over the last three decades, the pulmonary artery catheter (PAC) TD technique has been the "gold standard" for the measurement of CO. It is, however, invasive and not without its "imperfections". Some suggesting that its use might not only be unnecessary, but also potentially harmful.[8]

This has led to the introduction of alternative methods of both invasive and minimally invasive methods for the measurement of CO.

The less invasive devices track SV continuously and provide dynamic indices of fluid responsiveness; others allow assessment of volumetric preload variables, while some also provide continuous measurement of central venous saturation through proprietary catheters attached to the same monitor.[9] Together these variables along with the CO could improve hemodynamic assessment of the critically ill patient.

The techniques used to measure CO are diagnostic and not therapeutic tools; clinical acumen remains most important in the decision making process.

METHODS/PRINCIPLES USED TO MEASURE CARDIAC OUTPUT

All monitors in use today draw on one or a combination of the following methods/principles to measure CO. Each has its inherent advantages and limitations. The basic principles on which the monitors work are described, followed by a comparative chart of the various types of monitors in current use.

Fick's Principle

In the 19th century, Adolf Fick,[10] a German physiologist (1829–1901) first described utilized O_2 concentrations in arterial and venous blood samples to compute an animal's CO. The principle described measures the blood flow through any organ that adds or removes substances from the blood.

The CO thus equals the pulmonary blood flow, while the lungs add O_2 to the blood and remove CO_2 from it.

The relationship described was:

$$Q = \frac{M}{(V\text{-}A)}$$

where, Q = the volume of blood that flows through an organ in a minute

M = the number of moles of a substance the organ adds to the blood in a minute

V = venous concentration of the substance

A = arterial concentration of the substance.

In 1886, Grehant and Quinquaud were the first to perform pulmonary artery catheterization in dogs,[11] although it took, another five decades before it was offered to humans.

Dilution Techniques

The "indicator-dilution" technique was next developed. Stewart pioneered animal experiments where sodium chloride was injected into the central circulation and its subsequent concentration was measured in the femoral artery.[12] The principle was modified for humans by Hamilton to account for the changing concentrations of the diluted injectate over time.

A known quantity of the dye is first injected into the pulmonary artery and its concentration in a peripheral artery is measured. To correct for recirculation of the dye the achieved curve is semilogarithmically replotted. The Stewart-Hamilton equation is used to calculate the CO.[13]

In 1954, Fegler introduced the TD technique, which is based on the same principle. Instead of a dye, he used a cold solution as an injectate and measured the blood temperature distally.[14] The CO is calculated using the Stewart-Hamilton equation.

The PAC developed in 1970 by Swan et al. a multilumen flow directed balloon tipped catheter,[15] made bedside and intraoperative CO monitoring, still considered the "gold standard" possible (Refer Chapter 35: Pulmonary Artery Catheter).

Using the same thermodilution principle, newer technologies applied to the PAC allow for continuous pulmonary artery TD.[16] An electric filament incorporated into the right ventricular bulb, about 15–25 cm proximal to the PAC tip, intermittently heats the blood, as it flows through the right ventricle. The thermistor at the catheter tip measures the resultant temperature. The continuous TD method was shown to correlate well with intermittent bolus measurement.[17] Although a continuous cardiac output (CCO) trend is provided and updated values displayed every 30–60 seconds, it is in fact the average CO value for the last 5–15 minutes that is reflected.[16]

Doppler Monitoring

In recent days, Doppler techniques that are noninvasive are finding favor as a way to assess blood flow. An ultrasonic vibration is transmitted into the body by these machines; the change in frequency in the signal caused by their reflection off the red blood cells is recorded. This measures the velocity, not the flows.

It works on the principle that there is an increase in the observed frequency of a signal when the signal source approaches the observer and decreases when the source moves away.

The CO is measured based on either, the measured or estimated, diameter of the aorta, the distribution of the CO to the descending aorta, and the measured flow velocity of blood in the aorta.[18]

Transesophageal Doppler Monitoring

Initially, suprasternal transthoracic ultrasound/Doppler probes were used to determine CO. Their use was limited by instability of the probe position for repeated measurements over extended time periods.

The esophageal probes, described in the 1970s,[19] gained better acceptance; the esophageal smooth muscle tone naturally maintains the probe in place for extended time intervals and the proximity of the esophagus to the aorta reduces signal interference improving measurement.

Pulse Contour Analysis

The pulse contour analysis model is based on the relationship between blood pressure, SV, the arterial compliance and systemic vascular resistance (SVR). If the arterial compliance and SVR are known, based on the arterial pressure waveform the SV or CO can be calculated. The SV is the area under the systolic portion of the arterial pulse wave divided by the aortic impedance. The CO is calculated by multiplying the calculated SV by the HR.

The commercially available pulse contour systems used to measure the CO draw on either[1] an indicator dilution CO measurement,[2] patient demographics and physical characteristics to estimate the arterial impedance or[3] a system that needs neither preloaded data nor calibration.[18]

Thoracic Impedance

The thoracic bioimpedance technology, developed by Kubicek et al. in the 1960s, is the least invasive of the CO monitors. It suggests that the thorax is a cylinder that is perfused with fluid (blood) with a high resistivity.[20]

Bioimpedance measurement detects the electrical changes that occur with altering fluid levels in the thorax. The levels change as the left ventricle contracts and blood flows into the thoracic aorta. This results in a corresponding change in resistance within the thorax because the fluid level in the aorta increases. This change in impedance is measured as a change in voltage passing between typically the six surface electrodes—two on either side of the neck and four in the lower thorax placed on the patient.

The current transmitted from the outermost set is sensed by the innermost set of electrodes. The rate of change of impedance, Zo is believed to be related to the instantaneous blood flow in the aorta and is used to measure and calculate hemodynamic parameters. Thus, bioimpedance measures the amplitude of the voltage change across the thorax.

Thoracic Bioreactance

Bioreactance is a newer way of processing the impedance signal. It is based on the principle that pulsatile changes in aortic fluid volumes induce changes in phase (phase shifts) of the thoracic impedance. Phase shifts can only occur because of pulsatile flow. Underlying tissue fluids and changes in them do not induce phase shifts and do not affect the flow information.

Thoracic bioreactance tracks the phase of the electrical currents traversing the chest and derives the flow information from the phase component of the thoracic bioimpedance.

Echocardiography

The movement of the anterior and posterior ventricular walls and the ejection fraction can be measured by two-dimensional echocardiography.

Magnetic Resonance

Resonance properties of protons in the nucleus do change with respect to velocity. Thus, magnetic resonance can be used as an accurate way to measure the flow in aorta (CO). The method is expensive; it is only used in research.

CARDIAC OUTPUT MONITORS

Choosing the Right Monitor

The purpose of hemodynamic monitoring being "optimization" of therapy to achieve set hemodynamic goals, it is necessary to choose a monitor that subserves the necessary function and is "tailor-made" for the patient. Given the number of monitors available today and having got an insight on the principles on which they work, the requirements, the different parameters that can be measured using them, their advantages and disadvantages, the choices are manifold and increasing.

Ideally, the hemodynamic monitoring system would be simple to use, safe, relatively adaptable and consistently applicable and of course it should be affordable and cost-effective.

The monitor choice would be dictated by how easily the monitoring systems, as well as the disposable components, are available. A tried and tested system with available expertise, training and literature will help gain confidence in use of the system and help in problem solving and troubleshooting. Given that an institution would more open to accepting technology that does not incur huge expenses, systems that can be integrated into the existing monitors and are uniformly acceptable would be easier to adapt. Systems chosen should be easy to operate and interpret, and preferably be independent of the operator. Depending on the area of patient care and the requirements and resources of the given area, a choice can be made between using a more noninvasive or invasive system and intermittent or continuous monitoring. The degree of accuracy and reproducibility of parameters and the required response time to intervention and, accurate and reliable trending would also be influencing factors.

Given that all the hemodynamic systems discussed are not without limitations, some limiting factors being patient dependent, certain patient-related considerations may also influence the choice of hemodynamic monitoring tool being adopted. The most common being the cardiac function and rhythm, and/or the presence of any preexisting valvular conditions, mechanical ventilation, vascular access and other anatomic considerations, the severity, stage and type of disease condition for which the monitoring is being planned as also the circulatory support measures that are to be planned and instituted and of course, patient tolerance.

All influencing factors need to be balanced when deciding on the hemodynamic tool that should be adopted by the institution and for a given work area.

WHAT DO WE MEASURE; WHAT DOES IT MEAN?

Cardiac output (normal values 4–8 L/min) is the volume of blood that is ejected from the heart with each contraction per minute;

$$CO = SV \times HR$$

Cardiac index (CI) (normal value 2.5–4 L/min/m^2) takes into account body size and CO.

Stroke volume (normal value 60–100 mL/min) is the amount of blood ejected by the ventricles with each contraction. It considers ventricular performance or ejection without HR influence.

Stroke volume index (SVI) (normal value 33–47 mL/beat/m^2) is the quantity of blood ejected from the heart, indexed to take into account body size.

Ejection fraction (normal is approximately 65%) is SV expressed as a percentage of end diastolic volume.

Systemic vascular resistance (normal value 800–1,000 dynes/cm^{-5}) is an indicator of the left ventricular after load being the force that is impeding the ejection of blood from the left ventricle.

Systemic vascular resistance index (SVRI) (normal value is approximately 1,800–2,400 dynes.sec/cm^5/m^2) is the (MAP-RAP) × 79.9/CI (dynes.sec/cm^5/m^2).

Stroke volume variation (SVV) is a naturally occurring phenomenon. During inspiration the arterial pulse pressure falls and rises during expiration. This is the result of changes in the intrathoracic pressure secondary to negative pressure ventilation in the spontaneously breathing and vice versa in a mechanically ventilated patient. Stroke volume variation and its comparable measurement, pulse pressure variation (PPV), are not indicators of actual preload but of relative preload responsiveness. Normal SVV values are less than 10–15% on controlled mechanical ventilation.

Central venous pressure (normal values 2–6 mm Hg) reflects the right atrial pressure. It measures right ventricular end diastolic pressure or right ventricular preload.

Right atrial pressure (RAP) is an indicator of right heart preload; 2–6 mm Hg.

Pulmonary artery pressure (PAP) is a measure of the blood pressure found in the pulmonary artery; systolic: 15–30 mm Hg, diastolic: 5–15 mm Hg.

Systolic pulmonary artery pressure (sPAP) or PAP systolic (normal values 15–30 mm Hg) represents the rapid blood flow from the right ventricle into the pulmonary artery. It occurs with the opening of the pulmonic valve.

Diastolic pulmonary artery pressure (dPAP) or PAP diastolic (normal values 5–15 mm Hg) represents the diminished blood flow from the right ventricle into the pulmonary artery. It occurs with the closure of the pulmonic valve.

Mean pulmonary artery pressure (MPAP) (normal values 7–16 mm Hg) is calculated as: (DPAP × 2) + sPAP.

Pulmonary capillary wedge pressure (PCWP) (normal value 8–12 mm Hg) estimates the left atrial heart pressure and left ventricular end diastolic pressure. It is an indirect indicator of left ventricular filling pressure or preload. When the balloon of the PAC is inflated, a branch of the pulmonary artery is occluded. The pressure that is transmitted by the pulmonary vein is approximately the same as the left atrial pressure, because there are no valves in the lung vasculature that would create a change in pressure between the left ventricle and the pulmonary vein.

Pulmonary vascular resistance (PVR) (normal value is 50–150 dynes/cm^{-5}) is the right heart after load.

Pulmonary vascular resistance index (PVRI) (normal value is approximately 225–285 dynes.sec/cm^5/m^2 is the (MPAP–MPAWP) × 79.9/CI [dynes.sec/cm^5/m^2].

Extravascular lung water index (ELWI) is the water content outside of the lung vasculature; indicates presence of pulmonary edema, which could be of carcinogenic or noncardiogenic origin.

Pulmonary vascular permeability index (PVPI) is the ratio of extravascular lung water to preload and is supposed to be an indicator of pulmonary capillary leakiness.

True mixed venous O_2 saturation or SvO_2 (70–75%), represents how well the tissues are extracting O_2 from the blood. It is drawn from the end of the PAC, being a mixture of blood from the inferior vena cava, the superior vena cava and the coronary circulation having been well-blended in the right ventricle. It is determined by four interacting variables: (i) SaO_2, (ii) CO, (iii) hemoglobin, and (iv) O_2 consumption.

Central venous O_2 saturation or $ScvO_2$ (≥70%) is drawn from the central venous line, generally subclavian or jugular. It measures the relationship between O_2 consumption and O_2 delivery in the body.

Oxygen delivery index (DO_2I) (~800 mL O_2/min-m^2) is the volume of gaseous O_2 pumped from the left ventricle per minute per meter squared BSA.

Oxygen consumption index (VO_2I) (~200 mL O_2/min-m^2) is the volume of gaseous O_2 returned to the right atrium per minute per meter squared BSA.

Global ejection fraction (GEF) (normal values 25–35%).

Global end-diastolic volume index (GEDVI) represents the volumes of the right and left heart at the end of diastole and often reflects left ventricular end-diastolic volume estimated by echocardiography provided that right ventricular dilatation is absent.[21]

Right ventricular stroke work index (RVSWI) (normal value is 10–15 g/m^2/beat) is a measure of the amount of work that the right ventricle does during each contraction. It is a way of evaluating the right ventricle pumping function.

Left ventricular stroke work index (LVSWI) (normal value is 45–75 g/m^2/beat) is a measure of the amount of work the left ventricle does during each contraction. It is a way of evaluating the left ventricle pumping function of the left ventricle.

Arterial O_2 content or CaO_2 (normal value is 17–20 mL/dL) is the actual amount of O_2 found bound to hemoglobin and dissolved in the plasma in each 100 cc of arterial blood.

Arteriovenous O_2 content difference or avDO_2 (normal value is 4.2–5.0 mL/dL) is the difference between the arterial O_2 content and the mixed venous O_2 content (CaO_2 - CvO_2). When an increase in tissue extraction results in the mixed venous O_2 content decreasing, the avDO_2 increases.

Oxygen extraction ratio or O_2ER (normal value is 24–28%) is a reflection of the use of O_2 by the tissues; being the fraction of available O_2 consumed by the tissues.

Alveoli-arterial O_2 difference or AaDO_2 or A-a gradient (normal value is 10–15 mm Hg) a measure of the difference in partial pressure of O_2 between the alveoli and the arteries is indicative of the efficiency of O_2 exchange between the lung alveoli and the pulmonary capillaries.

Q_S/Q_T (% of arteriovenous shunt; normal value is 3–5) measures the amount of shunting being indicative of the extent to which arterial blood is less than maximally oxygenated. It is the blood that is returning to the left heart without being oxygenated.

MINIMALLY INVASIVE CARDIAC OUTPUT MONITORING DEVICES

Minimally invasive CO monitoring devices use one of four main principles to measure CO:[9,22,23]

- *Pulse contour analysis:*
  - *Calibrated:* PiCCO™, LiDCO™
  - *Uncalibrated:* Flowtrac™, PRAM
- *Pulsed Doppler technology:* USCOM®, esophageal Doppler device
- *Applied Fick principle:* NICO
- *Bioimpedance/bioreactance:* ECOM, NICOM.®

Pulse Contour Cardiac Output Monitor (Fig. 1)

The pulse contour cardiac output monitor (PiCCO) method represents an inexpensive, less invasive technology for quantification of CO, intrathoracic blood volume and extravascular lung water. It is less invasive than using PACs since it employs a central line and an arterial line.

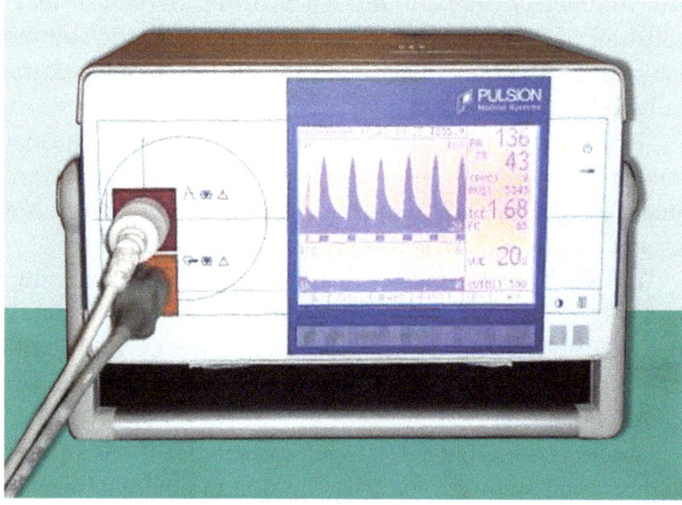

Fig. 1: Pulse contour cardiac output monitor.

A pulse contour analysis assumes that the contour of the arterial waveform is proportional to the patient's SV. By knowing the patient's HR, the CO can be calculated each beat by multiplying the HR by the SV. The variable in this method is the impedance of the patient's aorta and as such the system must be calibrated by using another method of CO measurement.[9]

The PiCCO method is a combination of transpulmonary TD technique and arterial pulse contour analysis. The transpulmonary TD technique requires a central venous line (internal jugular or subclavian site) and an arterial catheter placed in one of the bigger systemic arteries, e.g., the femoral or the axillary artery to determine:

- Thermodilution CO
- Continuous CO using the pulse contour method (CCO)
- Intrathoracic blood volume
- Extravascular lung water.

Now connect temperature connector to one of lumens of central line; the blue temperature probe which is on CO cable connects to this connector and arterial line is connected to flush device and transducer.

The trace of arterial pressure can be obtained from PiCCO monitor to the Spacelabs monitor via exiting white cable from rear of machine. The arterial line is connected to the red temperature connector of CO cable and are screwed together and confirm that venous and arterial access are on separate limb so there is no interference in the results.

To assess SV on a beat-to-beat basis a dedicated thermistor-tipped catheter is placed in the femoral artery is used by pulse contour cardiac monitor. A radial or brachial catheter also can be used.

A central venous line is needed for calibration of cardiac output via transpulmonary TD. The adjustment of individual aortic impedance needs calibration and should be done every 8 hours in hemodynamically stable patients where as in unstable patients it should be done every hour.

The injectate is injected through the central venous line. Transpulmonary TD CO is used to calibrate the CCO derivation by means of pulse contour analysis. The CCO module continuously determines CO by an improved arterial pulse contour analysis without the need of a more invasive PAC. The relationship between blood flow out of the aorta and pressure measured at the end of the aorta (femoral artery or other large artery) is determined by the aortic compliance function. The aortic compliance functions can therefore be characterized by measuring blood pressure and blood flow (CO) simultaneously.

Contraindications

- Restricted arterial access (e.g., following severe burns)
- Unreliable in intracardiac shunts, aortic aneurysms, aortic stenosis, pneumonectomy, extracorporeal circulation. Sources of potential errors that are specific for the transpulmonary TD come from the fact that the

PiCCO estimates the CO of the left heart whereas the PAC TD that of the right side. These should be identical in ideal conditions; however, a discrepancy is encountered in the presence of intracardiac and intrapulmonary shunts
- Incorrect pulse contour analysis may be seen with an intra-aortic balloon catheter or any other ventricular assist device which alters the characteristic arterial waveform.

Lithium Dilution Cardiac Output Monitor (Fig. 2)

The LiDCO hemodynamic monitor is intended for continuous monitoring of CO, via blood pressure, in patients with preexisting peripheral arterial line access. The LiDCO uses lithium dilution to calibrate the system intermittently.[9]

Inj. Lithium chloride in 0.5–2 mL boluses are injected through peripheral or central line to measure lithium concentration by aspirating blood from arterial catheter by using lithium sensitive electrode. Since the electrode has low sensitivity for distinguishing lithium from sodium, a correction factor is applied for sodium plasma levels and a baseline voltage is determined that helps differentiate the concentration of the two cations.

They use the same pulse pressure algorithm to track continuous changes in SV. This algorithm is based on the assumption that the net power change in the system in a heartbeat is the difference between the amount of blood entering the system (SV) and the amount of blood flowing out peripherally.[24]

The main advantage of lithium as an indicator is that it does not naturally occur in plasma and therefore can generate a high signal-to-noise ratio when used with a sensitive electrode, followed by a rapid redistribution time and an insignificant first-pass loss from the circulation.[25]

Indications

- Acute heart failure, history of cardiac disease, complex circulatory situations
- Gram-negative sepsis, drug intoxication, acute renal failure
- Severe hypovolemia and fluid shifts
- Medical emergencies.

Contraindications

- Lack of accuracy in a patient already on lithium treatment
- The use of bolus doses of muscle relaxant drugs in the operative and intensive care setting can interfere with correct readings. They incorporate a positively charged quaternary ammonia ion that can be detected by the sensor and thus lead to an overestimation of the CO. For example, atracurium and rocuronium. But suxamethonium, vecuronium and pancuronium can be used provided that a time interval of 15–30 minutes elapses between their bolus administration and the LiDCOplus™ calibration
- Patients who weigh less than 40 kg (88 lb)
- Patients who are in the first trimester of pregnancy
- Patients with severe peripheral arterial vasoconstriction, aortic valve regurgitation, and with aortic balloon pumps.

Advantages

- The system is safe, accurate and easy to use
- It can be setup in under 5 minutes by a trained nurse or doctor
- It can be used in a conscious patient in perioperative settings
- In many cases, it averts the necessity for an invasive PAC and associated morbidity.

FloTrac™ Monitor (Fig. 3)

This particular system is unique because it does not require central venous access or placement of a PAC to obtain hemodynamic data. The Vigileo/FloTrac™ system utilizes an existing radial or femoral arterial line that is attached to its monitoring unit. The system obtains comprehensive hemodynamic data including CO, CI, SVR, SV, SVI, and SVV.

Calibration is not necessary with this system. The benefits of a noncalibrated system include ease of use,

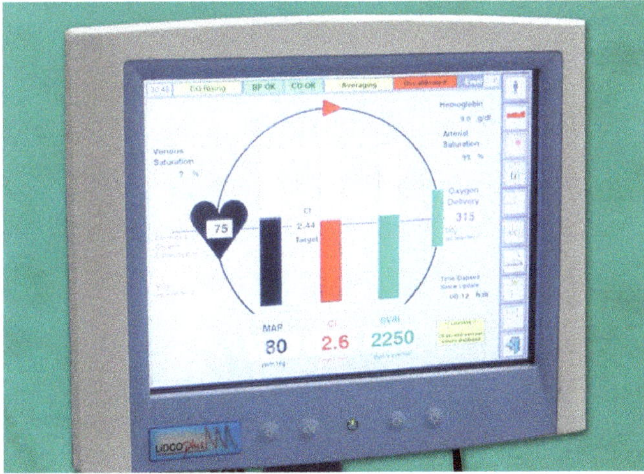

Fig. 2: Lithium dilution cardiac output monitor.

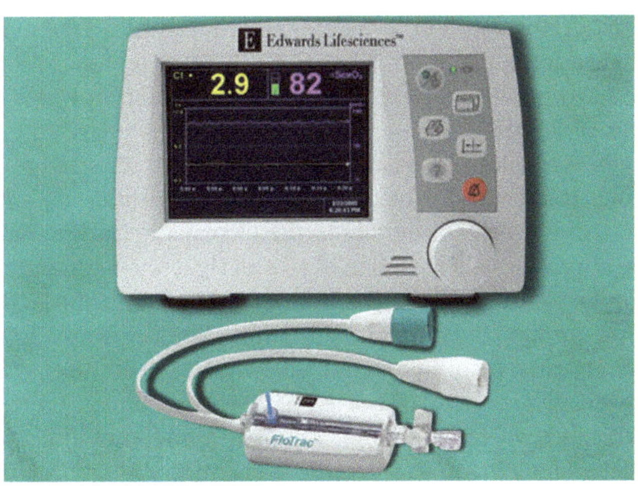

Fig. 3: FloTrac™ monitor.

less invasiveness with decreased risk, a quick setup, and the ability to use the FloTrac™ monitor in many different clinical settings.

The FloTrac™ sensor is a key component for operation of the monitoring system. The sensor replaces the traditional arterial line transducer and provides two pressure cable connections. One pressure cable connection allows for conventional arterial waveform monitoring and the other connects directly to the Vigileo™ monitoring unit. The Vigileo™ monitor is the processing and display unit of the system.[22]

The monitor derives hemodynamic values from mathematical algorithm which analyses the arterial waveform.

The patient data such as age, height, weight, gender is incorporated in this device. The algorithm uses basic hemodynamic principles for the determination of SV from the arterial waveform and includes HR to calculate CO (CO = SV × HR).

The arterial pressure waveform 100 times/s every 20 seconds for 2,000 data points for use in its algorithm by system. The peak of arterial wave form determines heart rate. The three variables are used to calculate SV they are: (i) arterial pulsatility, (ii) resistance, and (iii) compliance.

The monitoring system accounts for changes in vascular tone by internal waveform analysis by employing and including variables such as compliance and vascular resistance.

The pulse pressure is the difference between the systolic and diastolic blood pressure and is comparative to flow. The pulse pressure (arterial pressure) and SV are proportional so, pulse pressure is incorporated in the algorithm to derive hemodynamic data. Stroke volume variation is then measured by the variation of the SV from the mean of the arterial waveform with every beat of the heart.

A simple equation is used for calculation of the SVV value. The maximum SV value is subtracted from the minimum SV value over a specified period of time and then divided by the mean. An SVV greater than 13% may indicate the need for volume replacement and can be investigated with a volume challenge. If the SVV is less than 13%, the SVI must be considered. A normal SVI (40–50 mm Hg) may indicate the need for vasopressor support, a low SVI (<40 mm Hg) may specify the need for an inotrope, and a high SVI (>50 mm Hg) may require a diuretic.

Stroke volume variation is an expected occurrence in which the arterial waveform fluctuates 5–10 mm Hg with spontaneous breathing due to the changes in intrathoracic pressure. A greater variation of 10 mm Hg is known as pulsus paradoxus. Controlled mechanical ventilation produces the same variation but in a reverse manner. The arterial waveform rises during inspiration and falls during expiration. The waveform is reversed due to the positive pressure introduced with mechanical ventilation versus negative pressure with spontaneous breathing. The assessment of SVV is intended to predict fluid responsiveness.

Stroke volume variation is the main focus of the algorithm in guiding preload and/or volume responsiveness. The algorithm guides and assists the anesthesia provider through a series of decisions to obtain fluid optimization verses the need for other interventions, such as vasopressor support, inotropic support or diuretic therapy.

Advantages

Fluid optimization guided by SVV and CO to improve hemodynamics has many benefits such as:

- Decreased length of hospital stay
- An earlier return to bowel function after a major operation
- Decrease in postoperative nausea and vomiting

The balance of fluid optimization is critical in patients because too much or too little fluid may result in devastating consequences perioperatively, such as pulmonary edema, shock or renal failure.

It also provides hemodynamic data without the need for calibration of the system or central venous access.

Indications

Currently, the monitoring system is only recommended for patients that are 100% mechanically ventilated and not spontaneously breathing.

Contraindications

- Arrhythmias can change the arterial pressure waveform and, therefore, alter the SVV and ability to accurately predict fluid responsiveness along with CO
- Elevated levels of positive end-expiratory pressure (PEEP) can erroneously increase SVV and warrant for fluid resuscitation as per the monitor, but may not actually be needed for the patient
- Large changes in vascular tone or vasodilation may also correlate with an increased SVV.

Pressure Recording Analytical Method (Fig. 4)

Pressure recording analytical method (PRAM) is another method to estimate SV continuously without calibration or

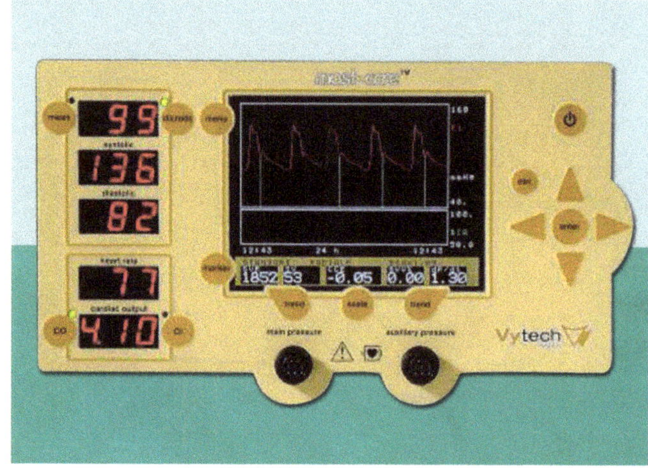

Fig. 4: Pressure recording analytical method.

demographic data. It is based on mathematical assessment of the pressure signal obtained from an arterial line without calibration.[9]

Pressure recording analytical method has been validated so far in humans undergoing cardiac surgery. Similar to other devices that use pulse contour analysis, the accuracy of PRAM derived CO is affected by the quality of the pressure signal and by factors that interfere with the ability to detect a pressure signal (for instance, in patients with aortic valve stenosis or valve insufficiencies).

Stroke volume is proportional to the area under the diastolic part of the arterial pressure wave divided by characteristic impedance. The proportionally factor is usually obtained by calibration with an independent SV measurement (for instance by intermittent TD). With PRAM, SV is calculated for each beat and CO per beat is then derived by multiplying SV with HR of the same beat. Cardiac output is presented as the mean value of 12 beats. In the same screen, it is possible to see parameters related to contractility, flow, preload, and afterload.

Disadvantages

As the internal calibration of PRAM is derived from the morphology of the pressure curve, this makes the method vulnerable to sources of errors related to signal quality and in patients with heart diseases that are suspected to affect the arterial pressure waveform.

Esophageal Doppler (Fig. 5)

Cardiac output can be estimated noninvasively using esophageal or transthoracic Doppler probes. The esophageal Doppler (ED) monitor, which is based on the Doppler effect to measure the velocity of blood flow, was first introduced in the 1970s as a noninvasive means to measure CO. Esophageal Doppler monitoring is undertaken with a single-use probe, which is placed in the esophagus via the mouth or nose. The device generates a low-frequency ultrasound signal, which is reflected by red blood cells traveling down the aorta. By applying the Doppler principle, the reflected signal can be used to determine flow velocity. The aortic diameter is obtained from a built-in nomogram or by direct measurement using M-mode echocardiography.[26] A validated nomogram is used to derive volumetric data such as SV and CO.

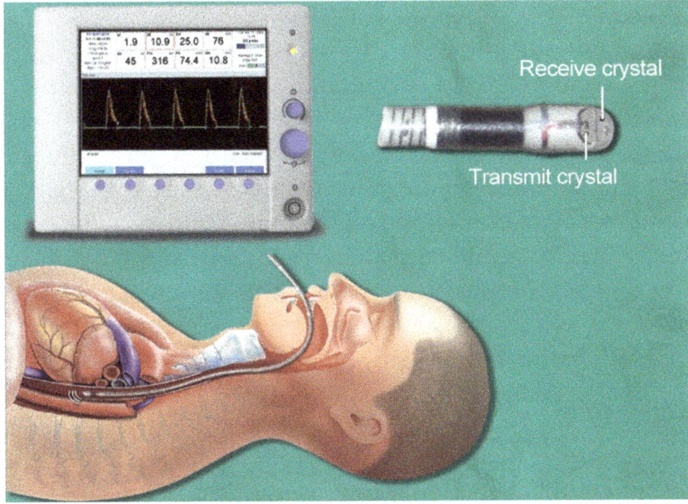

Fig. 5: Esophageal Doppler.

The ED also can measure the corrected flow time (FTc) as a measure of cardiac preload. The FTc is the duration of flow during systole corrected for an HR of 60 bpm and the ability to respond to a fluid challenge is best determined by FTc. Several studies have compared FTc with other indices, such as pulmonary artery occlusion pressure and have found good correlation between the two.[27]

Advantages

- Useful in perioperative hemodynamic optimization studies
- Reduction in complication rates and hospital length of stay.

Disadvantages

- It measures blood flow in the descending aorta and assumes a fixed partition between flow to the cephalic vessels and to the descending aorta. This may not be true in aortic pathology or compression or due to abnormal upper to lower body blood flow distribution
- Doppler probes are smaller than conventional transesophageal echocardiography probes and position may change frequently, thus limiting CCO assessment. Even small misalignments of the ultrasound beam with blood flow will lead to underestimation of flow when using the Doppler equation
- It is an operator-dependent device and 10–12 insertions are required to obtain accurate measurements
- Aortic cross-sectional area is always dynamic in any individual due to changes in pulse pressure, vascular tone, aortic compliance, volume status or catecholamine use. Hence, the use of a nomogram may result in less accurate CO estimation
- The nomogram assumes that the flow is laminar and any turbulent flow in the aorta will reduce measurement accuracy.

Ultrasound Cardiac Output Monitor (Fig. 6)

Alternatively to the esophageal route, the transthoracic approach [ultrasound cardiac output monitor (USCOM)] may be used to assess CO. It targets the pulmonary and aortic valves using Doppler technology accessed via the parasternal and suprasternal windows in order to assess cardiac output completely noninvasively. Validation studies have revealed conflicting results, which could be explained primarily by the inherent problem of variable signal detection.

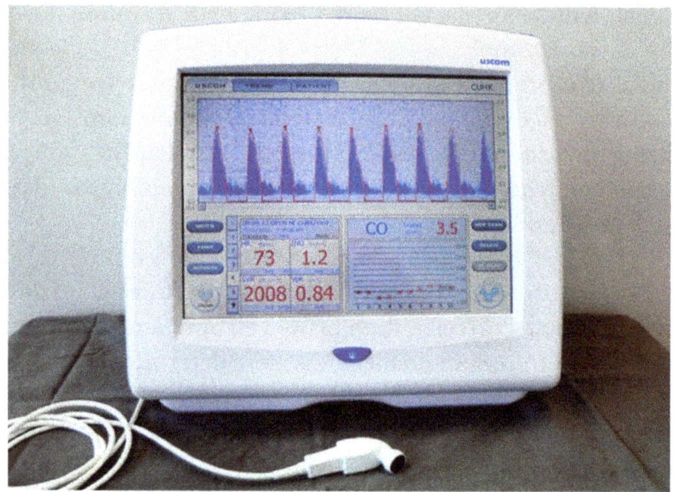

Fig. 6: Ultrasound cardiac output monitor (USCOM).

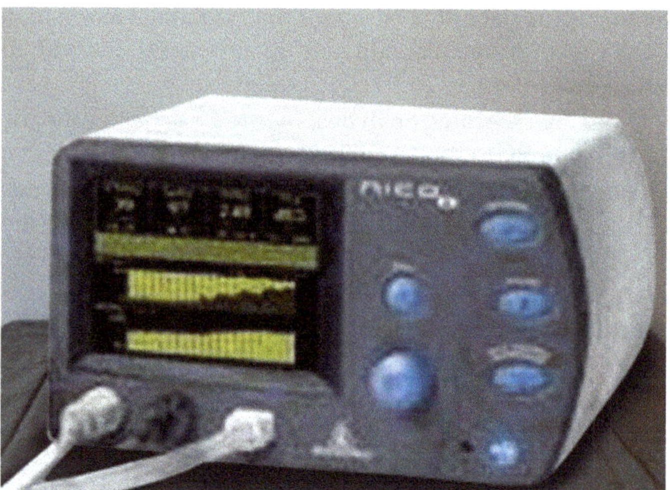

Fig. 7: Noninvasive cardiac output monitor.

The USCOM device is a noninvasive, USCOM designed to measure and record changes in the hemodynamic status of critically ill patients transcutaneously. The USCOM utilizes continuous-wave Doppler ultrasound and can measure both left and right CO.

A transducer is placed on the chest in either the left parasternal position to measure transpulmonary blood flow, or the suprasternal position to measure transaortic blood flow.[23] The flow profile is displayed on the USCOM monitor with the spectral display showing variations of blood flow velocity with time. The USCOM device allows for real time, beat-to-beat quantitative evaluation of 14 CO parameters: CI, cardiac output CO, peak velocity of flow (Vpk), velocity time integral (Vti), HR, ejection time per cent (ET%), SV, SVI, SVV, SVR, SVRI, minute distance (MD), mean pressure gradient (Pmn), and flow time (FT).[28]

Advantages

The device is highly portable, weighing less than 7 kg and is powered by an internal battery.

The primary applications of the USCOM device are in the emergency heart failure, resuscitation, hemorrhage, sepsis, in ICU for postsurgical monitoring, heart failure, myocardial infarction and in pediatrics.

Disadvantages

It takes a much longer time to become sufficiently familiar with the different signal sounds and patterns to recognize when a truly reliable signal has been obtained. Significant experience and psychomotor skill is needed to be able to acquire clinically reliable data.[23]

Noninvasive Cardiac Output Monitor (Figs. 7 and 8)

The noninvasive cardiac output (NICO) monitor system applies Fick principle to carbon dioxide (CO_2) in order to obtain CO noninvasively in intubated, sedated, and mechanically-ventilated patients using a disposable rebreathing loop that is attached to the ventilator circuit.

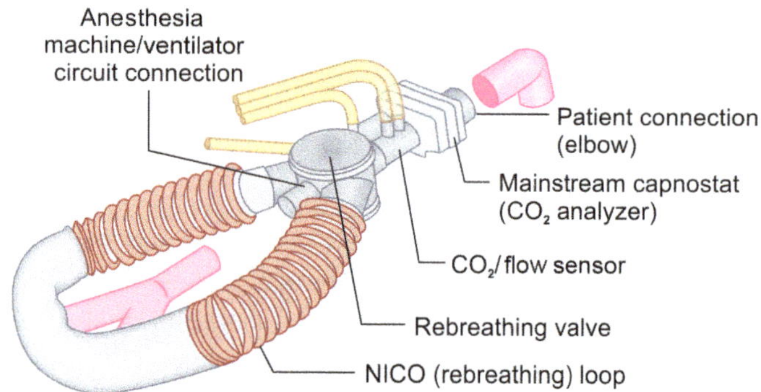

Fig. 8: Noninvasive cardiac output (NICO) connections.

It is unique as it calculates:

- *Alveolar ventilation (MV_{ALV}):* Reflects effective ventilation
- *Carbon dioxide elimination (VCO_2):* Reflects changes in ventilation and perfusion
- *Total dead space to tidal volume ratio (Vd/Vt):* Estimates efficiency of cardiovascular system.

It consists of a mainstream infrared sensor to measure CO_2, a disposable airflow sensor, and a pulse oximeter. CO_2 production (VCO_2) is calculated from minute ventilation and its CO_2 content, whereas the arterial CO_2 content ($CaCO_2$) is estimated from end-tidal CO_2, with adjustments for the slope of the CO_2 dissociation curve and the degree of dead space ventilation. Every 3 minutes, a partial rebreathing state is generated using the attached rebreathing loop, which results in an increased end-tidal CO_2 and reduced CO_2 elimination. Assuming that CO does not change significantly between normal and rebreathing states, the difference between normal and rebreathing ratios are used to calculate CO. Cardiac output is proportional to the change in CO_2 elimination divided by the change in $EtCO_2$ resulting from a brief rebreathing period.[22]

Limitations

- The need for intubation and mechanical ventilation allows this technique to be used in a precisely defined clinical setting in mechanically ventilated patients only

- Not accurate in variable ventilator settings, mechanically assisted spontaneous breathing
- Unreliable in severe chest trauma, significant intrapulmonary shunt, dead-space ventilation, low minute ventilation and high CO
- No studies available in hemodynamically unstable patients
- It only measures the CO and does not provide information on the intravascular volume status or fluid responsiveness.

Electrical Bioimpedance Cardiac Output Monitor (Fig. 9)

The changes in electrical impedance of thoracic cavity occurs during ejection of blood from left ventricle into ascending aorta and is correlated with thoracic electrical bioimpedance. During cardiac ejection, the impedance of tissue remains constant even though blood and tissue impede electric current.

The volume of blood in the chest changes with each SV results change in volume causes changes in impedance, which is detected by electrical patches placed on the neck and thorax. The SV and CO can be calculated with the aid of an algorithm which interprets these changes in thoracic impedance. The pulsatile changes in thoracic blood volume result in changes in electrical impedance. CO is continuously estimated using skin electrodes or electrodes mounted on an endotracheal tube (ECOM) by analyzing the occurring signal variation with different mathematical models.

The impedance is the resistance to the flow of electrical current. The blood and other fluids are excellent conductors of electricity and have low impedance, particularly compared to bone, tissue and air while blood and fluid in the lungs are the most conductive substances in the thorax.

To measure hemodynamic parameters in impedance cardiography the four pair of electrodes and a set of electrocardiography leads are used. Each pair of electrodes can transmit and sense electrode and two pairs are applied to the base of neck on directly opposite and other two pairs are placed at level of the sternal-xiphoid process junction and again directly opposite each other. The upper and lower limits of thorax define upper electrode and distance between is thoracic length.

A high frequency, low amplitude alternating current is introduced through the transmitting thoracic electrodes and the sensing thoracic electrodes measure impedance associated with the pulsatile blood flow in the ascending aorta which occurs during the cardiac cycle. By measuring the impedance change generated by the pulsatile flow and the time intervals between the changes, SV can be calculated.

During systole, there is increase in blood volume, flow velocity and alignment of red blood cells and during diastole there is decrease in blood volume, flow and more random configuration of red blood cell.[29]

Disadvantages

Inaccurate readings in motion artifacts, electrical interference, cardiac arrhythmias, heart and lung pathologies (as chest deformities, pulmonary edema, pleural and pericardial effusions, intracardiac shunts) and foreign bodies (as chest tubes).

Noninvasive Cardiac Output Monitoring (Fig. 10)

The thoracic bioimpedance has been introduced as alternative to bioreactance noninvasive cardiac output monitoring (NICOM). It refers to the electrical resistance, capacitive and inductive properties of blood and biological tissue that induce phase shifts between an applied electrical current and the resulting voltage signal.

The bioreactance technique analyzes the frequency spectra variations of the delivered oscillating current when comparing with bioimpedance. When blood flows out of the heart, phase shifts occur if alternating currents are applied across the patient's chest and it results in a higher

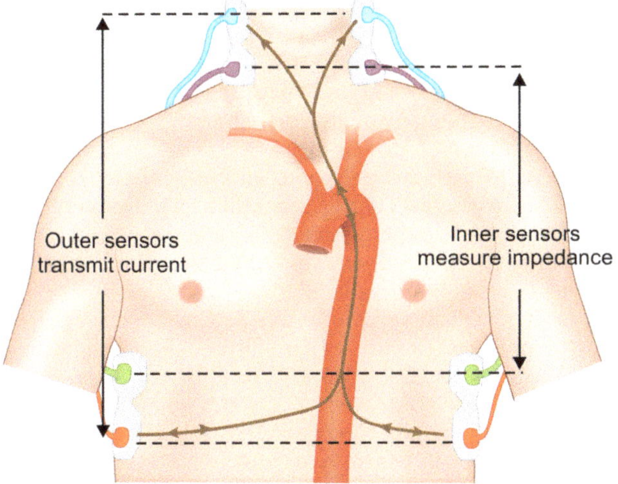

Fig. 9: Electrical bioimpedance cardiac output monitor position of leads.

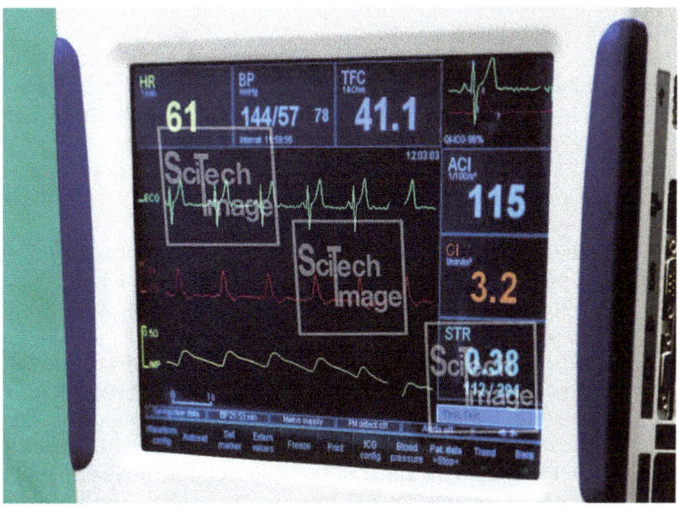

Fig. 10: Noninvasive cardiac output monitoring.

signal-to-noise ratio and thus in an improved performance of the device.

These phase shifts are conceptually like a frequency modulation as used in radio transmission and are measured continuously and relates to almost linearly to blood flow in the aorta. It results in less interfering from the electrical noise, patient movement, respiratory effort, lead placement and body mass index.

In addition to CO, mean bioreactance measurements are indicative of the total thoracic fluid content. Thoracic fluid content is affected by both intravascular and extravascular fluid in the chest cavity and although it does not correlate with pulmonary artery wedge pressure (PAWP), its changes are very reliable indicators of the changes in intravascular or extravascular fluid volume.

Advancing age and perioperative fluid shifts in patients, pulmonary edema, myocardial ischemia and electrical interference may produce errors with CO measurement by bioimpedance.

CONCLUSION

Studies over time have not shown consistent proven survival benefits by the use of any particular hemodynamic monitoring device. The available hemodynamic devices work on different principles and have their inherent issues. The choice of the system to be used would be depended on the institution, the patient care area for which it is intended, the patient-related factors and the preference of the attending physician based on the financial constraints, availability of facilities, clinical presentation and level of available expertise and back up. The different systems may actually supplement each other; a knowledge and training of more than one system would be helpful. Using the trends and numbers generated by the monitors to help guide hemodynamic management strategy is what will improve outcomes.

REFERENCES

1. Rivers E, Nguyen B, Havstad S, et al. Early goal-directed therapy in the treatment of severe sepsis and septic shock. N Engl J Med. 2001;345(19):1368-77.
2. Lopes MR, Oliveira MA, Pereira VO, et al. Goal-directed fluid management based on pulse pressure variation monitoring during high-risk surgery: A pilot randomized controlled trial. Crit Care. 2007;11(5): R100.
3. Gan TJ, Soppitt A, Maroof M, et al. Goal-directed intraoperative fluid administration reduces length of hospital stay after major surgery. Anesthesiology. 2002;97(4):820-6.
4. Noblett SE, Snowden CP, Shenton BK, et al. Randomized clinical trial assessing the effect of Doppler-optimized fluid management on outcome after elective colorectal resection. Br J Surg. 2006;93(9):1069-76.
5. Hamilton MA, Cecconi M, Rhodes A. A systematic review and meta-analysis on the use of preemptive hemodynamic intervention to improve postoperative outcomes in moderate and high-risk surgical patients. Anesth Analg. 2011;112(6):1392-402.
6. Marik PE, Baram M, Vahid B. Does the central venous pressure predict fluid responsiveness? A systematic review of the literature and the tale of seven mares. Chest. 2008;134(1):172-8.
7. Marik PE, Monnet X, Teboul JL. Hemodynamic parameters to guide fluid therapy. Ann Intensive Care. 2011;1(1):1.
8. Connors AF, Speroff T, Dawson NV, et al. The effectiveness of right heart catheterization in the initial care of critically ill patients. SUPPORT Investigators. JAMA. 1996;276(11):889-97.
9. Alhashemi JA, Cecconi M, Hofer CK. Cardiac output monitoring: an integrative perspective. Critical Care. 2011;15(2):214.
10. Prys-Roberts C. The measurement of cardiac output. Br J Anaesth. 1969;41(9):751-60.
11. Stewart GN. The output of heart in dogs. Am J Physiol. 1921; 57:27-50.
12. Stewart GN. Researches on the Circulation Time and on the influences which affect it. J Physiol. 1897;22(3):159-83.
13. Geerts BF, Aarts LP, Jansen JR. Methods in pharmacology: measurement of cardiac output. Br J Clin Pharmacol. 2011;71(3):316-30.
14. Nishikawa T, Dohi S. Errors in the measurement of cardiac output by thermodilution. Can J Anaesth. 1993;40(2):142-53.
15. Swan HJ, Ganz W, Forrester J, et al. Catheterization of the heart in man with use of a flow-directed balloon-tipped catheter. N Eng J Med. 1970;283(9):447-51.
16. Lee AJ, Cohn JH, Ranasinghe JS. Cardiac output assessed by invasive and minimally invasive techniques. Anesthesiol Res Pract; 2011. p. 475151.
17. Reuter DA, Huang C, Edrich T, et al. Cardiac output monitoring using indicator-dilution techniques: basics, limits, and perspectives. Anesth Analg. 2010;110(3):799-811.
18. Marik PE. Noninvasive cardiac output monitors: A state-of the-art review. J Cardiothorac Vasc Anesth. 2013;27(1):121-34.
19. Angelsen BA, Hoem J, Dørum S, et al. High-frequency annular array transesophageal probe for high-resolution imaging and continuous wave Doppler measurements. Transesophageal Echocardiography; 1989. pp. 13-20.
20. Kubicek WG, Karnegis JN, Patterson RP, et al. Development and evaluation of an impedance cardiac output system. Aerospace Med. 1966;37(12):1208-12.
21. Hofer CK, Furrer L, Matter-Ensner S, et al. Volumetric preload measurement by thermodilution: a comparison with transesophageal echocardiography. Br J Anaesth. 2005;94(6): 748-55.
22. Chamos C, Vele L, Hamilton M, et al. Less invasive methods of advanced hemodynamic monitoring: principles, devices, and their role in the perioperative hemodynamic optimization. Perioper Med. 2013;2(1):19.
23. Critchley LA. Minimally invasive cardiac output monitoring in the year 2012. In: Aronow WS (Ed). Artery Bypass. In Tech; 2013.
24. Pearse RM, Ikram K, Barry J. Equipment review: an appraisal of the LiDCO plus method of measuring cardiac output. Crit Care. 2004;8(3):190-5.
25. Siranovic M, Kovac J, Gopcevic A, et al. Constant cardiac output monitoring using the PiCCO and LiDCO methods versus PAK in septic patients: when to do calibration? Acta Clin Croat. 2011;50(2):267-72.
26. National Institute for Health and Care Excellence. (2011) CardioQ-ODM (oesophageal Doppler monitor) to guide intravenous fluid management in patients undergoing surgery, or in critical care. [online] Available from http://guidance.nice.org.uk/MT/80 [Last accessed February, 2014].
27. Lee JH, Kim JT, Yoon SZ, et al. Evaluation of corrected flow time in oesophageal Doppler as a predictor of fluid responsiveness. Br J Anaesth. 2007;99(3):343-8.
28. Thom O, Taylor DM, Wolfe RE, et al. Comparison of a suprasternal cardiac output monitor (USCOM) with the pulmonary artery catheter. Br J Anaesth. 2009;103(6):800-4.
29. Mathews L. Paradigm shift in hemodynamic monitoring. The Internet J Anesthesiol. 2006;11(2).

Entropy

Naina P Dalvi, Nazmeen I Sayed

ABSTRACT

Entropy monitor is a part of monitoring of depth of anesthesia along with somatosensory evoked potentials, bispectral index monitor and Narcotrend-M monitor. The use of electroencephalography-based depth of anesthesia monitors is recommended during any type of general anesthesia in patients considered at higher risk of unintended awareness and patients at higher risk of excessively deep anesthesia.

This chapter deals with the entropy principle and the use of entropy monitor. It also explains the interpretation of the graphs and the readings on the entropy monitor.

INTRODUCTION

Entropy module was introduced in 2003 by the Datex-Ohmeda Company. The product is based on many studies, which show that entropy could be used to characterize the electroencephalography (EEG) and the depth of general anesthesia. The main principle of entropy is that increasing depth of anesthesia causes increase in regularity of the EEG, which is then be inferred by the entropy and used to estimate the depth of anesthesia.[1]

Being aware while under anesthesia is terrifying and infrequent, but not rare. Many research publications indicate an incidence of approximately 1:600 cases in adult practice, with more frequent occurrence during high-risk groups (obstetric, cardiac, and airway surgery), as well as during anesthesia in children.

Patients at higher risk of unintended awareness during general anesthesia:[2]

- Patients with high opiate or high alcohol use
- Patients with airway problems
- Patients with previous experience of accidental awareness during surgery
- Older patients
- Patients with comorbidities.

In these patients, lower levels of anesthetic are often used to prevent adverse effects on the cardiovascular system and these levels can be inadequate.

Patients at higher risk of excessively deep levels of anesthesia:[2]

- Older patients
- Patients with liver disease
- Patients with a high body mass index
- Patients with poor cardiovascular function.

Awareness experiences may frighten patients and can leave a lifetime of residual emotional and psychological problems. Standard clinical practice is cautious and anesthetists may err on the side of safety by administering larger than adequate drug doses in the hope of avoiding awareness. This generous approach to drug dosage may increase the risk of hypotension, delay recovery time, and has the potential to increase other complications.

One of the objectives of modern anesthesia is to ensure adequate depth of anesthesia to prevent awareness without inadvertently overloading the patients with potent drugs.

Vital signs, such as pulse, heart rate, blood pressure, and movement are indirect indicators of consciousness, and along with expired gas analysis of inhalational anesthetic agents, can reasonably prove that the patient is unconscious and not aware of their surroundings. However, the direct measurement of brain activity using a basic EEG can help measure effects of anesthetics more comprehensively. This is because as anesthesia "deepens", there are predictable changes in the EEG, including slowing, synchronicity, and burst suppression, that in the case of bispectral index (BIS) and entropy, are converted to a number expressing the likelihood of awareness.

ENTROPY

Principle

Entropy was defined for the first time by Shannon in 1948 and was further applied to a power spectrum of any signal by Johnson and Shore in the year 1984. Entropy as a physical concept is related to the amount of disorder in a system. The concept of spectral entropy originates from a measure of information called Shannon entropy. When applied to the

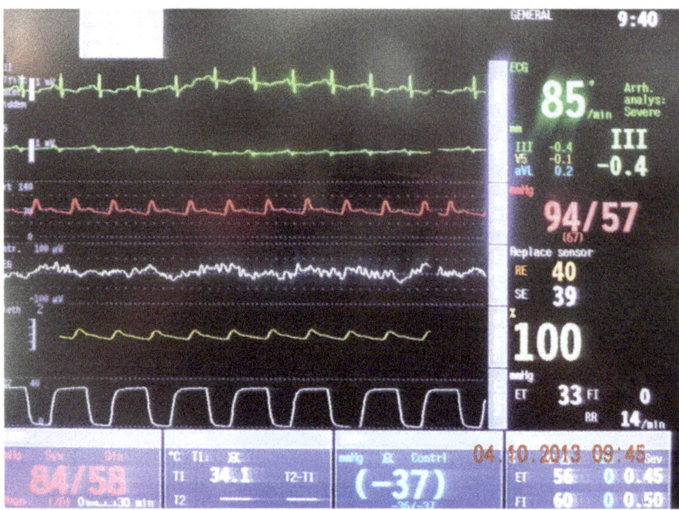

Fig. 1: Entropy monitor.

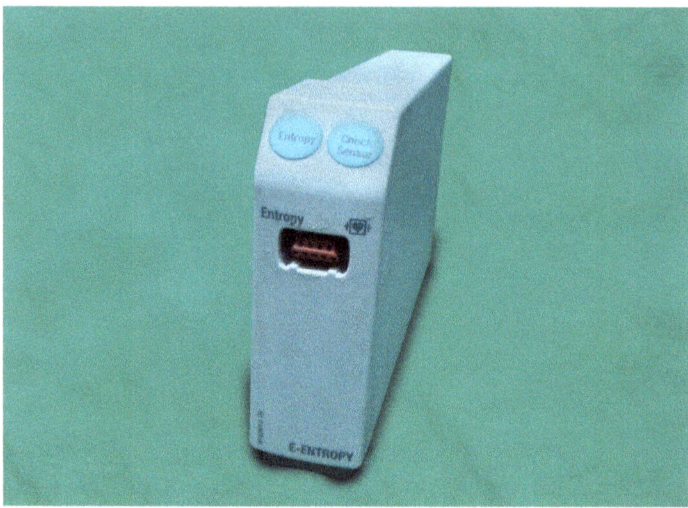

Fig. 2: Entropy module.

power spectrum of EEG, spectral entropy is obtained and it measures the regularity of the frequency distribution.[3]

Entropy monitor is an EEG-based monitor that is used in combination with standard clinical monitoring and clinical skills to indicate the patient's response to anesthetic drugs during surgery **(Fig. 1)**.

Indications

Entropy is indicated for adult and pediatric patients aged 2 years and older within a hospital for monitoring the state of the brain. The measurement can be started, and stopped, at any time during the operation.

Contraindications

There are no absolute contraindications to use of entropy, but the results may be inconsistent in following patients:

- Pediatric patients younger than the age of 2 years[4]
- Those undergoing procedural or conscious sedation
- Seizure activity may also cause interference
- Patients with neurological disorders, traumas, or their sequelae
- When using benzodiazepines, nitrous oxide, or ketamine as sole anesthetic agents
- Psychoactive medication or very high opiate doses may slow down the EEG activity; hence, decreasing its entropy content, even if unconsciousness is not induced by hypnotics.

Entropy is a plug-in module **(Fig. 2)**. Brain and facial muscular activity is recorded using a disposable sensor with three electrodes that are attached to the patient's forehead and a sensor cable that connects the sensor to the entropy module **(Figs. 3 and 4)**.

Next, the digitized signal is put through the artifact detection and removal algorithm **(Fig. 5)**. Then the entropy monitor measures irregularity in spontaneous brain and facial muscular activity, using a proprietary algorithm to process EEG and frontal electromyography (EMG) data.

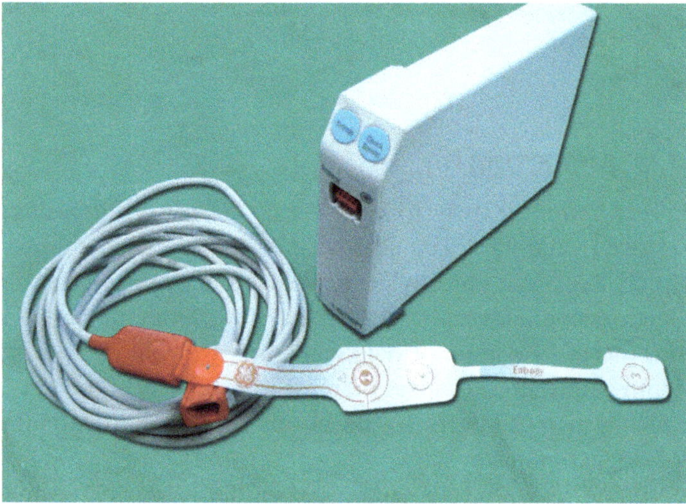

Fig. 3: Entropy module with sensor and cable.

After that, the signal is divided into two frequency bands (0.8–32 and 0.8–47 Hz) of spectral entropy [state entropy (SE) and response entropy (RE)], respectively. The spectral entropy is then calculated from the power spectrum of the particular epoch of the signal within a particular frequency band. The SE scale ranges from 0 (no brain activity) to 91 (fully awake) and should mainly include EEG activity. The RE scale ranges from 0 (no brain activity) to 100 (fully awake) and includes EEG and EMG activity.[3]

Additionally, the monitor performs the burst suppression (BS) analysis and displays the burst suppression ratio (BSR).

Highly irregular signals with variation of wavelength and amplitude over time produce high entropy values and may indicate that the patient is awake.

More ordered signals with less variation in wavelength and amplitude over time produce low or zero entropy values, indicating suppression of brain electrical activity and a low probability of recall.[2]

With majority of anesthetics, with deeper levels of anesthesia, BS occurs first, followed by suppression of EEG

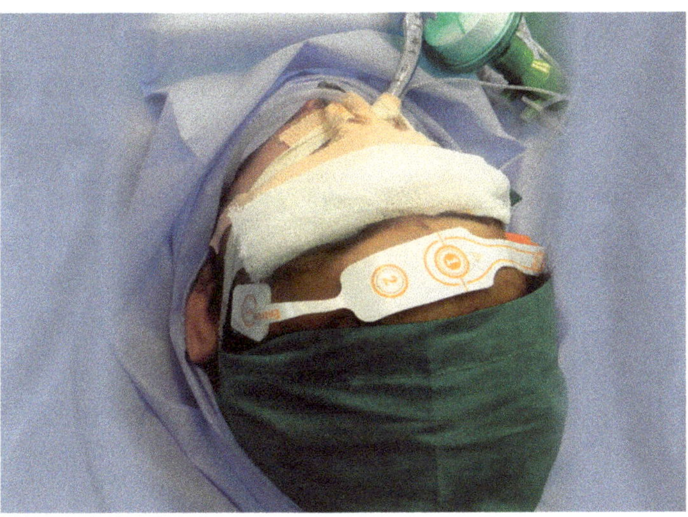

Fig. 4: Site of attachment of entropy sensor.

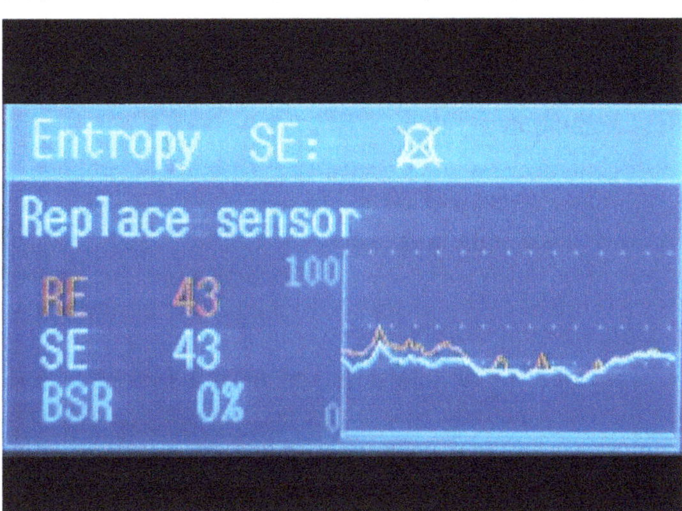

Fig. 6: Adequate anesthesia [response entropy (RE)-state entropy (SE) minimal or no difference]. (BSR: burst suppression ratio)

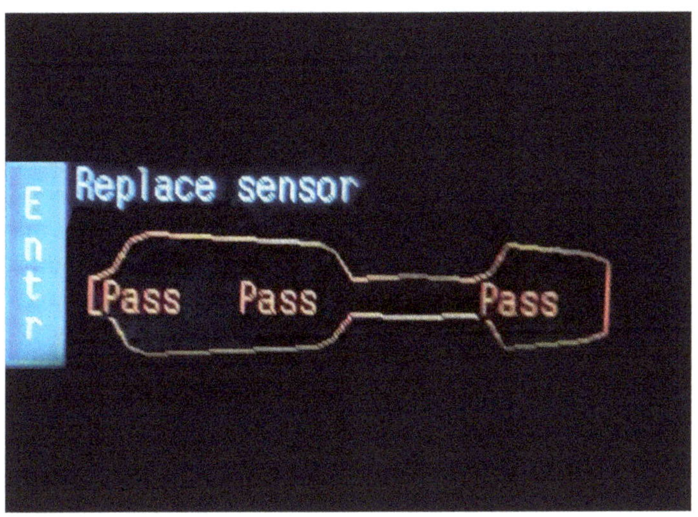

Fig. 5: Checking integrity of sensor.

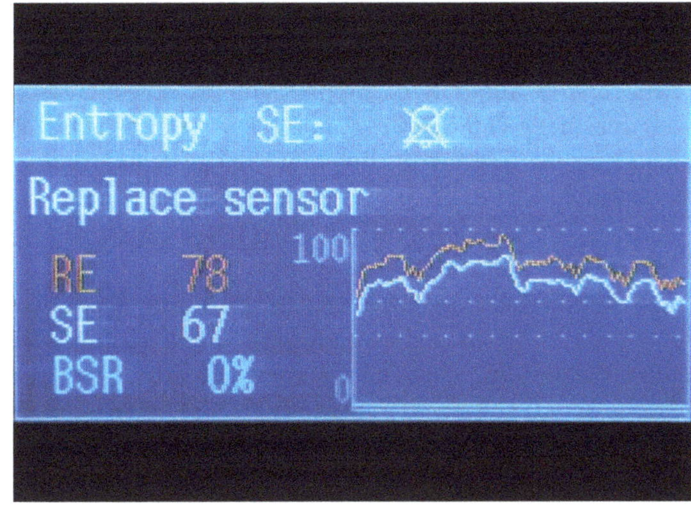

Fig. 7: Inadequate anesthesia [response entropy (RE)-state entropy (SE) >10]. (BSR: burst suppression ratio)

wave forms. The entropy of a completely suppressed signal is zero.

The target range for entropy value is 40–60 **(Fig. 6)**. Response entropy and SE values near 40 indicate a low probability of awareness with recall. At this point, unintended awareness is extremely unlikely; on the other hand, recovery from anesthesia is not unnecessarily prolonged.

While the SE includes information only from EEG, the RE also includes the EMG activity. When the RE and SE values are identical (subtracted value 0–3), the level of anesthesia can be considered "adequate". A slow increase in the difference between the RE and SE values during anesthesia is a sign of frontal muscle EMG activity, which in turn is a sign of "inadequate" anesthesia **(Fig. 7)**. Thus, it is possible to directly evaluate both cortical SE and subcortical RE components providing better anesthetic adequacy.[5]

A difference between SE and RE larger than 10 indicates the presence of significant EMG interference in the EEG signal.[6] It is typical for the RE and SE values to differ during intubation, when it is a case of nociception, and during recovery at the end of anesthesia when the diminishing effect of the drugs on the nervous system can be seen as activation of the frontal muscle.

In conclusion, the monitor does not perform any fusion of the calculated features into a single index like in the BIS.

The usefulness of entropy is limited by sensitivity to artifact, and paradoxical increase during light sedation in the presence of beta activity and during deep anesthesia as a result of BS. To outperform these, entropy monitors include an artifact detection algorithm and need to guarantee a monotonic dose-response relationship, even in the presence of beta activity or burst suppression.[7]

Artifact Detection

Artifact detection algorithm identifies specific artifacts, such as electrocautery, electrocardiogram, pacemaker spikes,

EMG activity or eyeblink events by exceeding a preset threshold value in a certain frequency range.[7]

Beta Activation

Most general anesthetics elicit an increase in EEG frequency band, between 13 and 30 Hz. Therefore, EEG-based depth of anesthesia monitors have to employ mathematical algorithms to compensate for this activation, to prevent this pattern of EEG activation being reported by entropy as arousal.[6]

The entropy module does not have a special feature for high beta activity, assuming that the spectral entropy is monotonically decreasing with increasing anesthetic drug concentrations even with beta activity during light sedation.[7]

Burst Suppression

It represents an EEG pattern frequently seen in healthy brain at deep levels of anesthesia. This pattern is composed of episodes of electrical quiescence (suppression) alternated with high frequency, high amplitude electrical activity (bursts). The duration of suppression periods increases with anesthetic depth. Entropy and BIS have mathematical algorithms that prevent the burst intervals to be interpreted as arousal.[6]

Burst Suppression Ratio

Burst suppression patterns of the EEG are classically quantified as "burst suppression ratio". Burst suppression ratio indicates the ratio of suppressed (isoelectric, flat line) periods in EEG compared to entire epoch of EEG (including both the bursts and the suppressed periods) in 1 minute.[7]

When the measurement range of entropy parameters decrease, the EEG begins to show an increase in the amount of silent periods and is displayed as an increase in BSR percentage. Emergence of BS pattern may indicate very deep anesthesia, hypothermia or ischemia.

When BS sets in, spectral entropy values RE and SE are in principle computed in the same way as they are calculated at lighter levels of hypnosis. The part of the signal that contains suppressed EEG is treated as a perfectly regular signal with zero entropy, whereas the entropy associated with the bursts is computed as usual.

The target value for BSR during general anesthesia, in the absence of requirements for profound levels of anesthesia, is 0%. Higher levels of BS indicate very deep hypnosis or unconsciousness level and are generally a sign of unnecessarily deep anesthesia.

Within the clinical range for entropy, RE and SE values of 40–60, no BS is usually seen. Entropy values are typically below 40 when BS begins to appear during profound levels of anesthesia **(Fig. 8)**.

In entropy monitor, by default RE and SE are seen on the screen. The display of BSR is optional.

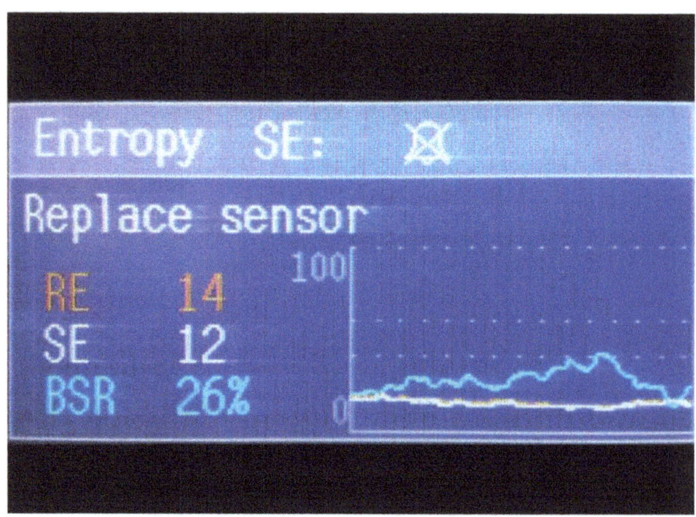

Fig. 8: Too deep anesthesia. (RE: response entropy; SE: state entropy; BSR: burst suppression ratio)

ENTROPY AND ANESTHETIC DRUGS

The functionality of the entropy monitor has been validated for propofol, thiopental, sevoflurane, and desflurane anesthesia. They produce anesthesia by increasing the activity of inhibitory gamma aminobutyric acid type A receptors (GABA-A receptors) in the brain. This is reflected in a general reduction of EEG activity. Exceptions to this rule are ketamine, xenon and nitrous oxide that produce anesthesia by interacting with other brain receptors, mainly, but not exclusively, by inhibiting excitatory N-methyl-D-aspartate brain receptors. These three general anesthetics produce different changes in EEG activity.[6] Therefore, entropy monitoring is not able to reliably assess the patient's depth of anesthesia when ketamine,[8] xenon or nitrous oxide[9,10] are used and may encourage the clinician to deepen the anesthetic, perhaps unnecessarily, when these drugs are used.

The entropy indices are found to be less interfered with the electrocautery unit than BIS during intraoperative period. However, like other monitors measuring consciousness on the basis of EEG, entropy is also unreliable during high dose opioid anesthesia.

It should be taken into account that even when using entropy, a sudden pain stimulus during an operation may unexpectedly change the anesthesia into "inadequate". The difference between the RE and SE values does not necessarily predict a situation like this.

A large multicentric study comparing entropy with classical BIS in terms of reduction of myoelectrical interference and noxious stimuli with EEG signals confirmed that the values of RE and SE were comparable with BIS value, at the onset of unconsciousness during propofol anesthesia. After elimination of myoelectrical activation, all values of RE, SE and BIS decreased significantly, and the three indices were less sensitive to noxious stimuli than cardiovascular responses.[11]

Entropy monitoring-assisted titration of propofol, especially during the last part of the procedures, as indicated by higher entropy values, decreased consumption of propofol, and shorter recovery times in the entropy group.[12] Similarly, compared with standard practice, patients with BIS or spectral entropy monitoring required 29% less sevoflurane.[13]

The entropy monitor was used in patients of a good grade subarachnoid hemorrhage. It was seen that it is a reliable monitor for maintaining depth of anesthesia in these patients.[14]

The entropy measurement is always to be used as an adjunct to other physiological parameters. There appears to be increasing evidence that anesthesia depth monitors like entropy reduces the incidence of unexpected intraoperative awareness and also improve the quality of anesthesia. Entropy ensures shorter recovery time and cost-effective anesthesia in terms of usage of anesthetic agents, but it is expensive, and requires consumables that are to be purchased for every case.[15]

CONCLUSION

Entropy is a very useful tool for monitoring the depth of anesthesia, especially in group of patients who may remain too deep or too light during surgery due to their risk factors. Because of ease of its usage and numeric interpretation, it has gained popularity. But it should be kept in mind that the entropy measurement is always to be used as an adjunct to other physiological parameters.

REFERENCES

1. Morley A. Depth of anaesthesia and neurophysiological monitoring. In: Davey AJ, Diba A (Eds). Ward's Anaesthetic Equipment, 5th edition. Philadelphia: Saunders; 2005.
2. National Institute for Health and Care Excellence (2012). NICE diagnostics guidance 6: Depth of anaesthesia monitors [Bispectral Index (BIS), E-Entropy and Narcotrend-Compact M]. [online] Available from http://www.nice.org.uk/dg6. [Last accessed February, 2014].
3. Kotur PF. Entropy—a new measure of anaesthetic depth. Indian J. Anaesth. 2004;48(3):170-1.
4. Davidson AJ, Huang GH, Rebmann CS, et al. Performance of entropy and bispectral index as measures of anaesthesia effect in children of different ages. Br J Anaesth. 2005;95:674-9.
5. Nunes RR, Almeida MP, Sleigh JW. Spectral entropy: a new method for anesthetic adequacy. Rev Bras Anestesiol. 2004; 54:(3)404-22.
6. Musizza B, Ribaric S. Monitoring the Depth of Anaesthesia. Sensors (Basel). 2010;10:10896-935. [online] Available from www.mdpi.com/journal/sensors. [Last accessed February, 2014].
7. Bruhn J, Myles PS, Sneyd R, et al. Depth of anaesthesia monitoring: what's available, what's validated and what's next? Br J Anaesth. 2006;97:85-94.
8. Hans P, Dewandre PY, Brichant JF, et al. Comparative effects of ketamine on bispectral index and spectral entropy of the electroencephalogram under sevoflurane anaesthesia. Br J Anaesth. 2005;94:336-40.
9. Anderson RE, Jakobsson JG. Entropy of EEG during anaesthetic induction: a comparative study with propofol or nitrous oxide as sole agent. Br J Anaesth. 2004;92:167-70.
10. Sleigh JW, Barnard JP. Entropy is blind to nitrous oxide. Can we see why? Br J Anaesth. 2004;92:159-61.
11. Gao JD, Zhao YJ, Xu CS, et al. Evaluation of entropy for monitoring the depth of anesthesia compared with bispectral index: a multicenter clinical trial. Chin Med J (Engl). 2012;125(8):1389-92.
12. Vakkuri A, Yli-Hankala A, Sandin R, et al. Spectral entropy monitoring is associated with reduced propofol use and faster emergence in propofol-nitrous oxide-alfentanil anesthesia. Anesthesiology. 2005;103:274-9.
13. Verroust N, Masson-Lefoll C, Taylor G, et al. Does monitoring bispectral index or spectral entropy reduce sevoflurane use? Anesth Analg. 2006;103:1469-77.
14. Duncan D, Kelly KP, Andrews PJ. A comparison of bispectral index and entropy monitoring, in patients undergoing embolization of cerebral artery aneurysms after subarachnoid haemorrhage. Br J Anaesth. 2006;96:590-6.
15. Sneyd JR. Depth of anaesthesia monitoring. South Afr J Anaesth Analg. 2012;18(1):27-9.

Somatosensory-evoked Potentials

Rajashree U Gandhe, Chinmaya P Bhave, Neeta V Karmarkar, Amruta A Ajgaonkar

ABSTRACT

Neurophysiological monitoring is an integral part of a multimodal monitoring strategy to help in identification and prevention of neurological damage at a reversible stage.

This chapter focuses on the study of somatosensory-evoked potentials which test the functional integrity of the somatosensory pathway; from the peripheral nerve receptors to the sensory cerebral cortex. The chapter sheds light on the factors influencing the somatosensory-evoked potential recordings and highlights the variety of its applications.

INTRODUCTION

Intraoperative neurophysiological monitoring was first introduced in the mid-1960s.[1] First guidelines for the use and interpretation of somatosensory-evoked potentials (SSEPs) was published in 1987 by the American Electroencephalographic Society [now American Clinical Neurophysiology Society (ACNS)]. These have been modified from time to time.[2-6]

Since its introduction as an intraoperative monitoring test, SSEPs have been extensively used and recommended as an important tool to assess and monitor the neurological integrity especially during neurosurgical procedures. Somatosensory-evoked potentials are a measurement of electrical potentials produced in response to a stimulus. Stimulation site in SSEP is a peripheral nerve and its response is monitored along its course from peripheral receptors to cerebral cortex.

ANATOMICAL CONSIDERATIONS

The somatosensory system consists of five submodalities. They are (i) mechanoception, (ii) proprioception, (iii) visceroception, (iv) nociception, and (v) thermoception. All these help in the continuous perception of sensory information from the skin, musculoskeletal system and viscera.

This system has two major parts: (i) the dorsal column-lemniscal system and (ii) the spinothalamic system as mentioned in **Table 1**[7,8] and the pathways are illustrated in **Figure 1**.[8]

Each of the two systems is divided into four neuronal populations.

First order neurons: Origin in the dorsal root ganglia, the trigeminal ganglion, the midbrain trigeminal nucleus, and the vagal ganglion nodosum.

Second order neurons: Dorsal column nuclei (lemniscal system), dorsal horn of the spinal cord (spinothalamic tract system). These axons cross the midline.

Third order neurons: Ventroposterior nuclei of the thalamus.

Fourth order neurons: Network of somatosensory cortex areas.

TABLE 1: Lemniscal system and spinothalamic tract.

Parameter	*Lemniscal system*	*Spinothalamic tract*
Sensation conducted	• Mechanoception (tactile localization, recognition, vibration, and texture) • Proprioception (joint position, movement, and force)	• Thermoception (warmth and cold sensation) • Nociception (painful stimuli, impending tissue damage) • Visceroception
Nerve morphology	Large, myelinated nerves (I and II or Aa and Ab)	Small diameter, thin myelination (III or Ad) or unmyelinated (intravenous and subcutaneous)
Peripheral terminals	Corpuscular nerve endings in skin, joint or muscle	Free nerve endings in skin, bone, joint, capsule, tendon, muscle, and organs
Conduction velocity	High 30–80 m/s	2–33 m/s (III or Ad) or 0.4–1.8 m/s (intravenous and subcutaneous)
Threshold for electric stimulation	Low threshold. Hence easily activated	High threshold. Not easily activated

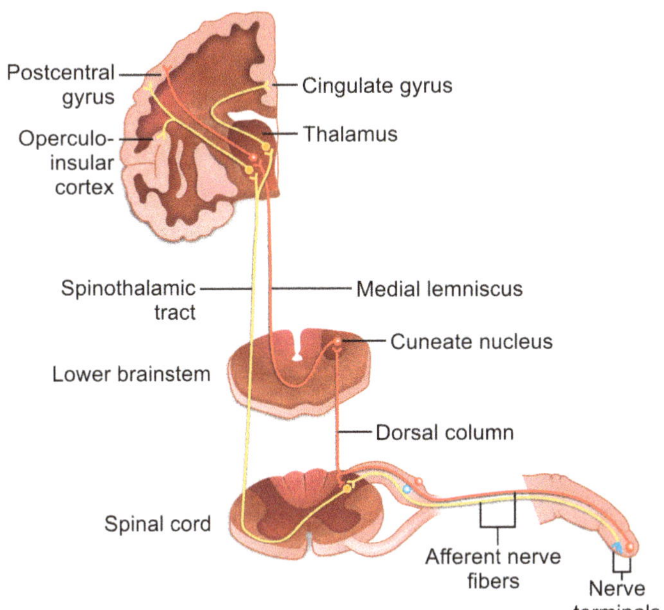

Fig. 1: Schematic diagram of the somatosensory pathway.

Dorsal spinocerebellar tract, postsynaptic dorsal column pathway, and vagus nerve also mediate somatosensory function

RECORDING OF SOMATOSENSORY-EVOKED POTENTIALS

Somatosensory-evoked potentials are responses elicited on stimulating a peripheral nerve. These responses are recorded at standardized points along the pathway of the nerve and are analyzed on the basis of amplitude and latency. For an ideal SSEP recording, it is essential to separate noise. Recommended use of stimulation frequency is between 2 and 5 Hz; though lower (1–3 Hz) can also be used.[1,9]

Somatosensory-evoked potentials data are interpreted after averaging. It averages at least 100 responses to present proper waveform morphology. Hence, a lag period of 30–60 sec, from stimulation to analysis is seen in SSEP recordings.[9]

Recording Sites

Basic Principle

To stimulate distal to the surgical site and to record proximal to the surgical site.

Recording sites include at least one cortical and one subcortical site. For peripheral stimulus, an additional electrode can be placed proximal to the stimulating site but distal to the surgical site.

The location of electrodes is different for the commonly used nerves which are chosen because of identifiable anatomical landmarks and the ease with which the stimulating electrode can be placed near the nerve to be stimulated. Each stimulating electrode has a cathode and anode **(Video 19)**.

For Upper Extremity

Median nerve SSEP: The recording electrodes should be at ipsilateral Erb's point (peripheral); parietal CP3 or CP4-contra lateral and 2 cm posterior to C3 and C4 on 10–20 system of EEG (cortical).

Cathode: 2–4 cm proximal to wrist crease.

Anode: 2–3 cm distal to the cathode.

For Lower Extremity

Tibial nerve SSEP: The recording electrodes should be at ipsilateral popliteal fossa (peripheral); lumbar level (spinal); CPz-midline and 2 cm posterior to Cz on 10–20 system.[1,7]

Cathode: In between the medial malleolus of the ankle and the Achilles tendon just proximal to the malleolus.

Anode: 2–3 cm distal to the cathode.

Stimulating Electrodes

Various types of electrodes can be used to stimulate the peripheral nerves. They include bar electrodes, EEG metal disk electrodes, subdermal needle electrodes, and adhesive surface electrodes.

Waveform Description, Nomenclature, and Interpretation (Fig. 2)

The SSEP waveform that is displayed on the monitor is presented in the form of different montages between the recording electrodes. While describing the SSEP waveform, the terms used frequently are:[9,10]

Onset latency: Time taken from stimulus to onset of the deflection.

Peak latency: Time taken from stimulus to maximum deflection.

Interpeak (peak-peak) latency: Time difference between two similar direction peaks.

Peak-peak amplitude: Sum of amplitudes between an upward and its corresponding downward deflection.

Central conduction time (CCT): Time needed for the signal to travel from the subcortical area to contralateral sensory cortex. It is measured as the difference between N20 and N13.[9]

The waveform is made up of peaks and valleys designated as N or P (N for upward and P for downward deflection respectively). This is followed by a numerical value representing its peak latency (in milliseconds), from the stimulus. Somatosensory-evoked potentials can be classified based upon their peak latencies into short (<30 ms), intermediate (30–75 ms), and long latency (>75 ms) waveforms.[9]

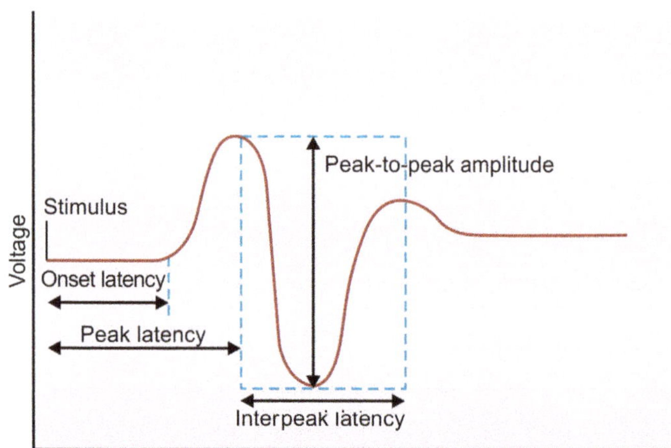

Fig. 2: Schematic representation of somatosensory-evoked potential waveform.

Interpretation of SSEP waveform looks at changes in the amplitudes and latencies with respect to a preoperatively or previously obtained baseline.

Majority studies[1,7] consider a more than 50% decrease in amplitude and more than 10% increase in latency or both to be significant changes for compromised integrity of neurological pathways. While interpreting the changes, reversible causes (anesthesia and physiological factors) should be eliminated.

EFFECT OF ANESTHETICS ON SOMATOSENSORY-EVOKED POTENTIAL

Inhalational Anesthetics

These have a significant effect on cortically recorded SSEPs than subcortical SSEPs. All volatile anesthetics produce a dose-dependent increase in latency and decrease in amplitude along with increased central conduction time.

Studies[1,10] have shown that isoflurane is the most potent while halothane and enflurane are the least potent for causing SSEP changes. Sevoflurane and desflurane have similar effects to isoflurane, but allow the use of higher inhaled concentrations. Subcortical SSEP responses are thought to be resistant to the effects of inhalational agents.

Nitrous Oxide

The use of nitrous oxide (N_2O) should be avoided while recording cortical SSEPs as it produces decrease in amplitude and increase in latency when used alone or with inhalational anesthetic agents. When used in combination with inhaled anesthetic gases, N_2O is shown to affect cortical SSEP at a lower concentration than when inhaled agents are used alone. N_2O may be acceptable when only subcortical or peripheral responses need to be monitored.[1,10]

Intravenous Anesthetics

These affect SSEPs less than inhaled anesthetics. The effect is seen predominantly over the short and intermediate latency components of SSEP. Total intravenous anesthesia (TIVA) is considered ideal for anesthetic administration during SSEP monitoring.

Barbiturates

There is a dose-dependent decrease in amplitude and increased latency of the cortical waveforms than subcortical waves. Cortical SSEP acquisition is possible even at doses that cause isoelectric suppression of the EEG. Redistribution of barbiturates allows SSEP monitoring to be resumed within a short time of their discontinuation.[1,10]

Etomidate

It has effects that are unlike the barbiturates. It causes more than 20% increase in cortical SSEP amplitude with decrease in subcortical SSEP amplitude by 50%. This is thought to be due to increased synchronization at the thalamus due to alterations in excitatory and inhibitory impulses. Also it is associated with higher incidences of myoclonus and patients with myoclonic seizures are shown to have enhanced SSEPs.[10]

Ketamine

It has an effect similar to etomidate on the cortical SSEP amplitude without affecting subcortical waveform latency. However, its effect on intracranial pressure precludes its use in patients with raised intracranial pressures. Addition of N_2O to ketamine decreases the cortical SSEP amplitude.[10]

Propofol

Due to its favorable pharmacological profile, propofol has emerged as the ideal choice for TIVA during SSEP monitoring. It produces decreased amplitude of cortical SSEP with rapid recovery after termination of infusion. The use of propofol in combination with opioids during TIVA has a favorable effect on SSEP than N_2O-opioid or midazolam-opioid anesthesia.[1,10]

Benzodiazepines

Mild-moderate cortical SSEP depression occurs with the use of benzodiazepines. Subcortical and peripheral SSEPs are not affected by both diazepam and midazolam. When combined with opioids or N_2O, Midazolam preserves cortical SSEPs better than inhaled anesthetics.[10]

Opioids

They generally have a very mild effect on SSEP response. The response is even lesser subcortical and peripheral SSEPs. The effect is related to changes in drug concentration with maximal effect seen after administration of a bolus of opioids. As opioids alone are incapable of producing adequate sedation and amnesia, they need to be combined with other anesthetic drugs or agents.[10]

Dexmedetomidine and Clonidine

The α_2 adrenergic agonists have gained popularity due to their benefits during general anesthesia. They are shown to reduce the requirements of general anesthetics. Studies[10] have shown that both dexmedetomidine and clonidine have minimal effect on SSEP responses at doses used for sedation. Clonidine at 10 mcg/kg caused 10% decrease in subcortical amplitude and 2% increase in latency. Due to their minimal effects on SSEPs, both can be used as anesthetic adjuvants.[10]

Neuromuscular Blocking Drugs

These drugs have no direct influence on evoked potential recordings. They, however, improve SSEP acquisition and waveform quality by favorably influencing signal-noise ratio. This is due to their elimination of electromyographic potentials.[10]

Lidocaine

Intravenous administration of preservative free lidocaine will affect cortical SSEP, though not to the extent of hampering intraoperative monitoring.[10]

Regional Anesthesia

Spinal anesthesia blocks the sensory pathway; thereby abolishing SSEP completely. Extremity nerve blocks will also suppress SSEP by blocking peripheral nerves or plexuses. Epidural anesthesia will variably affect lower limb SSEP depending upon the dose and dermatome blocked.[10]

PHYSIOLOGICAL FACTORS AFFECTING SOMATOSENSORY-EVOKED POTENTIAL

Temperature

Patients undergoing surgeries are subject to low ambient temperatures in the operation theater. The net loss of body temperature depends upon the area exposed, duration of surgery, and the operating room temperature. Hypothermia has its effects on drug metabolism, synaptic transmission, and neurotransmitter release. The effect of mild-moderate hypothermia is primarily seen on latency without much reduction in amplitude. The increase in cortical or subcortical latency is linear. Somatosensory-evoked potentials changes are gradual (roughly 0.75–1.5 ms increase in the latency of the N20 waveform for every 1°C decrease in nasopharyngeal temperature).[10]

With mild hyperthermia (39°C), there occurs 5–7% decrease in latency with increased conduction velocity. The latency is prolonged with further increases in the temperature till it becomes irreversible at temperature more than 42°C.

Carbon Dioxide

Induced hypocapnia shortens SSEP latencies by 2–4% without changes in amplitude in anesthetized patients. This may be due to increased neuronal excitability as a result of alterations in the pH, intracellular calcium concentrations, and ionic equilibrium across the nerve membrane.[10]

Hypoxia

Severe or progressive hypoxia leads to decrease in SSEP amplitude and increase in latency. Cortical SSEP waves are considered more sensitive than subcortical or peripheral waves to hypoxia. Changes of SSEP following hypoxia are a result of cerebral ischemia as they correlate with reductions in the level of high energy phosphates.[1]

Blood Pressure

The fall in blood pressure beyond the lower limit of autoregulation results in progressive decrease in amplitude of SSEP without change in the latency. This change is due to cerebral ischemia occurring with fall in blood pressure, which may be reversible or irreversible.[1,10]

APPLICATIONS OF SOMATOSENSORY-EVOKED POTENTIALS

Peripheral Nervous System

Somatosensory-evoked potential helps assess the peripheral nervous system where nerve conduction studies may be inadequate or technically difficult. SSEP responses may be affected by other nerves or nerve roots, which have normal function. It is advisable to use dermatomal SEP (DSEP) which assesses the individual nerve roots and can help accurately localize and warn of any potential damage.

Somatosensory-evoked potential can be used in peripheral nerve repair, position related brachial plexus or ulnar nerve injury; avoidance of neuropraxia during shoulder arthroscopy; sciatic nerve protection during hip surgery.[11]

Spinal Cord and Spine Surgeries

The SSEPs are widely used to assess spinal cord function. It helps identify changes, predict reversibility, and recovery and also is a prognostication tool.[11] Somatosensory-evoked potentials cannot assess spinal cord supplied by the anterior spinal artery and it would require monitoring of motor-evoked potentials (MEP) for complete monitoring of spinal cord function.

Although not disease specific, somatosensory-evoked potentials can identify afferent conduction damage, which occurs as the sequelae to certain disorders. Any pressure over the spinal cord causing its compression, as is seen with cervical spine spondylosis or myelopathy, can be identified by SSEP.

Congenital diseases of the spine like hereditary spastic paraplegia can be identified by abnormal subcortical response to median nerve stimulation in the presence of normal peripheral conduction.[11]

Somatosensory-evoked potentials can also be used to test the effects of metabolic disorders, nutritional deficiencies (Vitamin B_{12}) on spinal cord integrity, and diseases that affect the conduction along the spinal cord like Guillain-Barre syndrome, multiple sclerosis. Somatosensory-evoked potentials shows prolonged latency, decreased amplitude or no response.

Somatosensory-evoked potentials finds many applications as an intraoperative monitoring device during surgeries of the spine.

The most studied spine procedures for applicability of SSEP is pedicle screw fixation and deformity corrections of the spine (scoliosis). Pedicle screw fixation involves bony fusion of the spine with the help of screws inserted into the pedicles.[12] Medial angulation or displacement of the screws will result in direct pressure on the spinal cord and dorsal nerve roots. If not corrected in time, this may result in permanent damage or debility. Somatosensory-evoked potentials helps identify these changes at a reversible stage by showing a decreased amplitude, increased latency or sudden absence of recordings from subcortical electrodes. Return to the baseline value may be correlated with functional improvement.[12]

Excess distraction of the spine during corrective spine surgery may result in waveform changes of the SSEP by the stretching of the spinal cord, dorsal roots and by compromised spinal cord blood supply secondary to vascular compression or hypotensive anesthesia.[12]

In addition to bony surgeries over the spine, SSEP has been used to monitor the function of the spinal cord during the resection of spinal intramedullary tumors,[13] spinal vascular malformations, meningomyelocele correction, and detethering of the spinal cord.[11]

Prognostic value of SSEP is evident in traumatic injury to the spinal cord. Incomplete injuries have been shown to have a better prognosis than complete spine injuries based on the SSEP. Cortical SSEP is absent on stimulation of a nerve below the level of injury. It is abnormal or may be normal in incomplete cord injuries. The level of the injury can be localized by DSEP.[11]

Peripheral Vascular Surgeries

Somatosensory-evoked potentials are useful in carotid endarterectomies,[14] during thoracoabdominal aortic surgeries.[15] Intraoperative SSEP monitoring identifies spinal cord ischemia and could play a critical role in evaluating management strategies like glycemic control, better bypass techniques, intrathecal papaverine, and opiate antagonists.[15]

Brain and Brainstem

As the sensory ascending pathways terminate in the cerebral cortex via the brainstem, diseases and procedures involving them will have an influence on the SSEP values and recording.[11]

Diseases affecting myelination affect the conduction in the central nervous system (CNS) thereby affecting the SSEP waveforms. Ninety percent of multiple sclerosis patients will show abnormal SSEPs. Both upper and lower limb testing is indicated despite lower limb SSEP more likely to have abnormal findings than upper limb SSEP. Most commonly seen feature is increased cortical latency with or without changes in the amplitude. Subcortical SSEP can also be selectively abnormal in multiple sclerosis.[11]

Hereditary Central Nervous System Degeneration

Diseases like hereditary cerebellar ataxia, spastic paraplegias, or Friedreich's ataxia will show delayed CNS conduction or absent mid-latency cortical responses.[11]

Myoclonus

Somatosensory-evoked potential helps classify the type and the origin of myoclonus. As described with etomidate previously, patients with myoclonus show increased amplitude due to enhanced cortical activity. Similar SSEP findings are seen with progressive myoclonic epilepsy, late infantile lipofuscinosis, and photosensitive epilepsy.[11]

Intraoperative (Fig. 3)

Somatosensory-evoked potential helps localize the central sulcus, sensory and motor cortex intraoperatively. It thus helps delineate the limits of safe resection of a mass lesion involving and around these highly important areas. Somatosensory-evoked potentials also helps in functional localization of the thalamus prior to thalamotomy. It is also of use in intracranial vascular surgeries like aneurysm clipping,[16,17] arteriovenous malformation excision resection to prevent or minimize postoperative complications.

Intensive Care Unit

Application of SSEP in the intensive care unit is both diagnostic and prognostic. Altered cortical and subcortical SSEP responses occur in patients in coma. Deeper levels of coma and brainstem death show complete loss of cortical SEP recordings. Prognosis is good in patients with slight abnormal cortical SEP, while is poor in patients with absent cortical SEP recordings.[11]

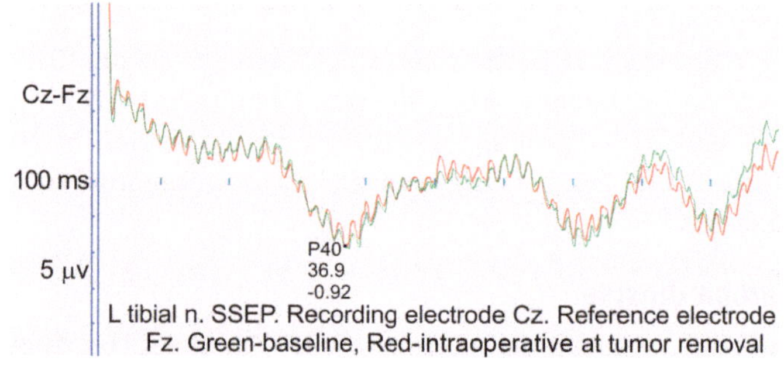

Fig. 3: Intraoperative somatosensory-evoked potential recording.

CONCLUSION

Adequacy of neurologic function is an important goal of anesthesia and critical care. Assessment of neurological function is not possible under anesthesia and in neurologically ill patients. Various modalities for monitoring the neurologic function in these have evolved over past few decades. Neuromonitoring helps in early detection of damage to the neurologic function, and aids in the institution of prompt measures to minimize the neurologic functional damage.

Somatosensory-evoked potential is a neurophysiologic monitor assessing the integrity of the somatosensory pathway. It has found wide applications in the fields of neurology, neurosurgery, and intensive care unit.

REFERENCES

1. Intraoperative monitoring using Somatosensory evoked potentials: a position statement by the American Society of Neurophysiological Monitoring; 2010.
2. American Electroencephalographic Society Guidelines for intraoperative monitoring of somatosensory evoked potentials. J Clin Neurophysiol. 1987;4:397-416.
3. American Electroencephalographic Society Guidelines for intraoperative monitoring of somatosensory evoked potentials. J Clin Neurophysiol. 1994;11:77-87.
4. American Society of Electroneurodiagnostic Technicians (ASET). Position statement on electrodiagnostic technologists in the operating room; 1998.
5. Erwin AC, Erwin CW. Intraoperative evoked potential monitoring-a historical perspective. Am J End Technol. 2000; 40:98-120.
6. International Organisation of Societies for Electrophysiological Technology (OSET). Guidelines for performing EEG and evoked potential monitoring during surgery. Am J End Technol. 1999;39:257-77.
7. Cruccu G, Aminoff MJ, Curio G, et al. Recommendations for the clinical use of somatosensory-evoked potentials: invited review. J Clin Neurophysiol. 2008;119:1705-19.
8. Treede RD. Das somatosensorische system. In: Schmidt RF, Lang F, Heckmann M (Eds). Physiologie des Menschen, 30th edition. Heidelberg: Springer; 2007. pp. 297-323.
9. Waziri AE, Taggard DA, Traynelis VC. Neurophysiology. In: Moore AJ, Newell DW, Lumley J (Eds). Neurosurgery: Principles and Practice. London: Springer-Verlag; 2005. pp. 3-22.
10. Banoub M, Tetzlaff JE, Schubert A. Pharmacologic and physiologic influences affecting sensory evoked potentials-implications for perioperative monitoring. Anesthesiology. 2003;99:716-37.
11. Kraft GH, Aminoff MJ, Baran EM, et al. Somatosensory evoked potentials: clinical uses. SSEP subcommittee chair and members. Muscle Nerve Suppl. 1999;22(8):S111-8.
12. Chung I, Grigorian AA. EMG and evoked potentials in the operating room during spinal surgery. In: Schwartz M (Ed). EMG Methods for Evaluating Muscle and Nerve Function. InTech; 2012. pp. 325-40. [online] Available from www.intechopen.com. [Last accessed May, 2021]
13. Gottfried ON, Gluf W, Qinones-Hinojosa A, et al. Spinal meningiomas: surgical management and outcome. Neurosurg. Focus. 2003;14:1-8.
14. Manninen PH, Tan TK, Sarjeant RM. Somatosensory evoked potential monitoring during carotid endarterectomy in patients with a stroke. Anesth Analg. 2001;93:39-44.
15. Sloan TB, Jameson LC. Electrophysiologic monitoring during surgery to repair the thoraco-abdominal aorta. J Clin Neurophysiol. 2007;24(4):316-27.
16. Lopéz JR, Chang SD, Steinberg GK. The use of electrophysiological monitoring in the intraoperative management of intracranial aneurysms. J Neurol Neurosurg Psychiatry. 1999;66:189-96.
17. Min KT, Kim JH, Shin YS, et al. The monitoring of somatosensory evoked potentials and neurologic complications in aneurysm surgery. Yonsei Med J. 2001;42(2):227-32.

Point-of-care Monitoring Equipment

Indrani Hemantkumar Chincholi

ABSTRACT

The point-of-care testing (POCT), also known as "STAT" laboratory, has revolutionized patient care, especially in critical care, operating room, outpatient departments or emergency room areas. Essential parameters testing and management at or near the site of patient care is a reality and has helped in integrating treatment decisions that improve patient outcomes and reduce patients' criticality, morbidity, and mortality. The results can also be uploaded into the hospital information system. Presently, multiparametric tests can be performed with a single hand held or a desk top monitor with possibility of test selection thereby eliminating unnecessary tests. This chapter deals with some of the common POC tests like hemoglobin, glucose, glycated hemoglobin (HbA1c), arterial blood gas, serum lactate, serum electrolytes, and coagulation tests.

INTRODUCTION

The point-of-care testing (POCT) monitoring equipment have largely been designed to provide tests for patients, who need close monitoring of their essential parameters and fluid balance at or near the site of patient care, such as critical care, operating room (OR), outpatient departments or emergency room.[1] It is also referred to as a "STAT" laboratory, a satellite laboratory, a near-patient instrument, or a bedside testing instrument. Most of the equipment are user friendly and technologically advanced. The most medically informative tests for this application include hemoglobin (Hb), glucose, arterial blood gas (ABG), lactate, serum electrolytes (sodium, potassium, magnesium and ionized calcium), creatinine, thromboelastograph (TEG) to name a few. The POCT scores over "traditional" laboratory testing, as it can expedite results in both conventional and unconventional settings. Even though it may seem to be deceptively simple and reduce the turnaround time (TAT), POCT does not replace traditional core laboratory instrumentation in all patient care situations. It plays a very important role in the treatment and outcome of patient's especially in tests like ABG, serum electrolytes or coagulation wherein delayed results from a conventional laboratory may not reflect the current state of metabolism, electrolyte or coagulation system and may lead to inappropriate treatment. The purpose of POCT is to provide immediate information to physicians about the patient's condition, so that this information can be integrated into appropriate treatment decisions that improve patient outcomes and, reduce patient's criticality, morbidity, and mortality.[2,3] However, QC, i.e., accuracy, performance, and reliability of these instruments is very important and should be addressed. Point-of-care testing may be "connected", i.e., test results are downloaded and recorded readily into the hospital and laboratory information system (HIS/LIS).

Point-of-care testing is estimated to be increasing by at least 10–12% per year overall and upwards to 30% per year in some testing areas. New applications for POCT continue to be explored, which makes this an area to stay abreast in technology, personnel and regulatory standpoints. Even though POCT may seem inexpensive, overutilization and inappropriate test utilization leads to significant increases in cost of care.

POINT-OF-CARE TESTS

Point-of-care test includes but not limited to

- Routine tests
  - Hemoglobin
  - Urea, creatinine, electrolytes
  - Full blood count with platelets, erythrocyte sedimentation rate
  - Glucose
  - Liver function test (complete)
  - Amylase
  - Comprehensive metabolic panel
  - Lipogram
  - HbA1c
  - Microalbuminuria
  - C-reactive protein, procalcitonin
  - International normalized ratio (INR)
  - Prostate-specific antigen and alpha-fetoprotein
- Emergency testing
  - ABG
  - Serum electrolytes (Na, K, Mg, Ca, Cl)
  - TEG

- Serum lactate
  - Oximetry
  - INR
  - D-dimer (Dd)
  - B-natriuretic peptide (BNP)
  - Troponin (Trp)
  - Myoglobin (M)
  - Human immunodeficiency virus-enzyme linked immunosorbent assay (HIV-ELISA)/rapid HIV
  - *Drug testing:* Barbiturates, amphetamines, paracetamol, antidepressants (TAD), opiates, cocaine, methamphetamines, etc.
  - Beta-human chorionic gonadotropin (βhCG)
  - Phencyclidine (PCP).

ADVANTAGES AND DISADVANTAGES OF POINT-OF-CARE TESTING

Advantages[2]

- Reduced therapeutic turnaround time of diagnostic testing
- Unprocessed specimen, e.g., whole blood analysis does not need clotting, centrifugation or aliquoting
- Onsite testing requires fewer steps and exchanges reducing the risk of sample contamination
- Rapid data availability
- It can be performed in a variety of locations
- It can do away with paper due to direct computerization of results
- Reduced preanalytic and postanalytic testing errors
- Self-contained and user-friendly instruments
- Small sample volume for a large test menu
- Shorter patient length of stay
- Convenience for clinicians
- *Close knit working for clinical staff and physician:* As the physician examines the patient and determines the need for testing, POCT can be conducted and medical care can be promptly adjusted
- Ability to test many types of samples (i.e., capillary, saliva, urine)
- *Reduced potential for sample deterioration:* Sample can be immediately tested, instead of being transported for testing.

Disadvantages

- Concerns about inaccuracy, imprecision, and performance (i.e., potential interfering substances)
- Bedside laboratory tests performed by poorly trained nonlaboratorians
- Difficulty in recruiting qualified technicians especially for the evening and night shifts
- Quality management or assurance issues and responsibilities not defined
- Higher cost of POCT compared with traditional laboratory testing even though POCT eliminates transportation and other costs involved in centralized testing. However, the overall cost of care may be lower when POCT is employed, considering the quick availability of results
- Personnel performing POCT may inappropriately use a test kit or device outside of its intended use or the written procedure
- Quality of testing is operator-dependent
- Difficulty in integrating test results with HIS or LIS—lack of connectivity
- Narrower measuring range for some analysts
- Reagent storage is decentralized and widespread, making management of supplies and monitoring of storage conditions problematic
- Documentation of test results, normal range values, units, operator identification, internal control results, etc., may be haphazard and difficult to standardize.

CONSIDERATIONS FOR CHOOSING A POINT-OF-CARE TESTING DEVICE

Technology

It should be appropriate for all patient populations, such as neonates, critical care patients, dialysis patients, and hypotensive patients. There should not be wide differences in results based on specimen type: arterial, venous, and capillary and should be comparable with those of the central laboratory.

Quality Control

Quality control (QC) consists of a combination of electronic and liquid controls and should run from time to time at least once a day. Quality control should be documented.

Reagents

Shelf life and stability at room temperature should be noted. They may need refrigeration.

Training

Comprehensive training should be provided to nonlaboratory operators.

Documentation

The instrument should have the ability to record both patient and quality control results along with operator identification.

Portability

The size of the instrument should be small enough to move from patient to patient. Some POCT tests should be useful in home setting as in glucose or prothrombin time (PT)/INR.

Data Management

The results should be recorded and should be transmitted electronically to the LIS.

Cost-effectiveness

The costs of the instrument, reagents, maintenance contract, etc., should be worth implementing the POCT program.

The impact of POC testing on outcomes in the emergency department (ED), intensive care unit (ICU), OR, and primary care, can be measured in a variety of ways. These include: mortality, morbidity, earlier or more effective intervention, lower cost while maintaining quality, safety, patient or physician satisfaction, and return to normal lifestyle.

POINT-OF-CARE TESTING INSTRUMENTS IN ANESTHESIA AND CRITICAL CARE

Hemoglobin Estimation

This is one of the most commonly performed tests as either part of preoperative workup of the patient, before blood donation, epidemiological studies, and general primary health care or in the critical care. Anemia is very common in pregnant women and malnourished children and can be a significant cause of death. In pregnancy it is associated with increases in stillbirths and low-birth weight babies, and in children it causes stunting and impaired intellectual development. Normal levels vary between 12 and 15 g/dL in women, and 13 and 16 g/dL in men. Hematocrit levels vary between 40 and 54% in men, 37 and 47% in women. Hemoglobin estimation becomes even more valuable when therapeutic decisions need to be made in the perioperative period. These are safe, reliable, accurate, and user-friendly devices. Hemoglobin can be estimated using invasive or noninvasive devices.

Invasive Devices

Point-of-care devices available are either use finger prick or whole blood samples—hand-held, palm sized or bench-top analyzers.

Electronic and portable hemoglobin meters using spectrophotometric technology provide fast Hb results with a high degree of quality and can be operated using battery or mains electricity. This equipment could be imperative in patients with difficult critical venous access, especially neonates and those undergoing chemotherapy due to the low amount of blood (10 μL) required by these devices, as well as in natural disasters or in sports medicine.[4] The use of these POCT devices is the best options in a bleeding patient (e.g., critical hemorrhages in the OR, intensive care patients) for instant Hb estimation. These instruments use capillary blood collected in a special cuvette by the finger stick method. However, arterial or venous blood can also be used and tests performed in them are found to be more accurate as compared to the capillary tests.

The easy to operate system consists of a portable meter that analyses the intensity and color of light reflected from the reagent area of a test strip, ensuring quick and accurate results. The hemoglobin testing system provides results in less than 15 seconds and requires only a single drop of whole blood **(Fig. 1)**.

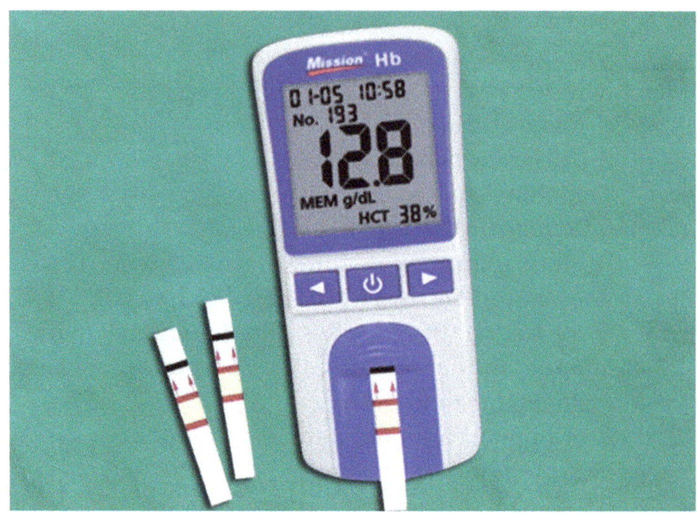

Fig. 1: Hemoglobinometer with test strips.

Components

- 25 test strips
- 25 capillary transfer tubes
- 1 test strip insert
- 1 code chip
- 3 AAA batteries
- 1 carrying case
- 1 user's manual
- 1 quick reference guide.

Hemoglobin and Hematocrit Estimation (Fig. 2)

These can be done with a single test using a portable device using the same technology. This analyzer uses advanced microcuvette system and features a slot at the rear of the sample chamber that allows trapped air to escape. Trapped air in a blood sample will deliver inaccurate results, so by getting it right first time; this system keeps costs and patient discomfort to a minimum. The analyzer's software allows users to link to a personal computer and then transfer data to an information management system.

Instrument Using Color Scale for Hemoglobin Estimation

The hemoglobin color scale (HCS)[5] is a simple, rapid and cheap method for estimating hemoglobin concentration with a finger prick blood sample **(Figs. 3A to C)**. It has been developed for use in resource-poor settings where there is no laboratory. In this method, the color of a drop of blood absorbed onto a filter paper is compared with standard colors on a laminated card, varying from pink to dark red. These colors correspond to hemoglobin levels of 4, 6, 8, 10, 12, and 14 g/dL. Intermediate shades can be identified, allowing

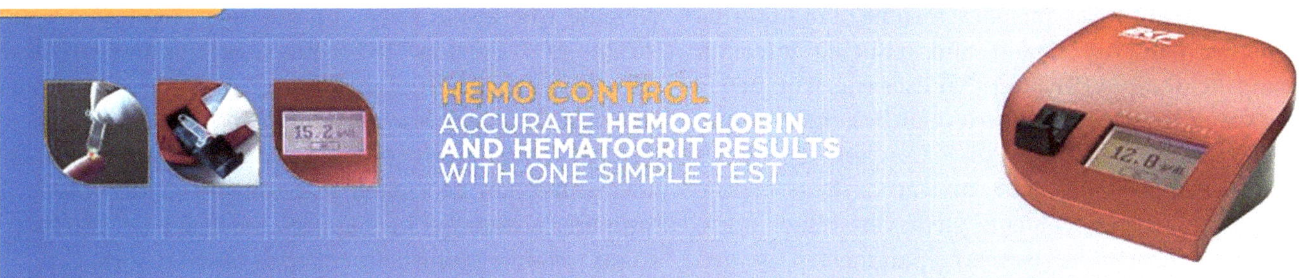

Fig. 2: Hemoglobin and hematocrit estimation.

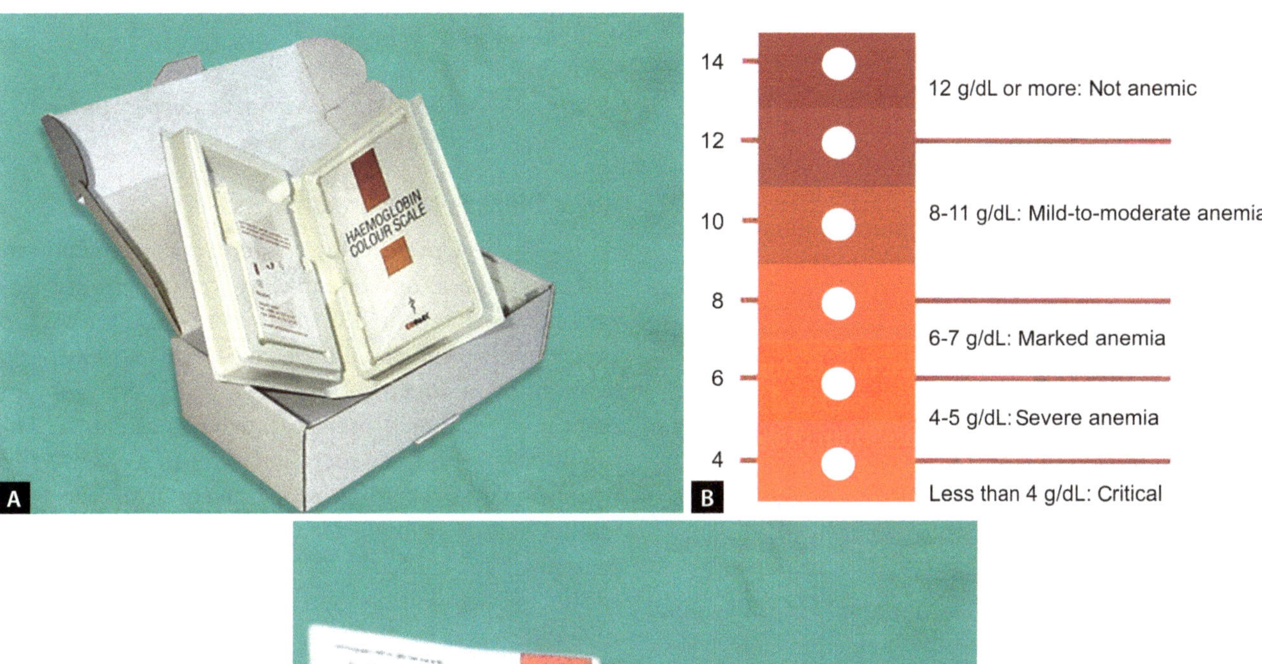

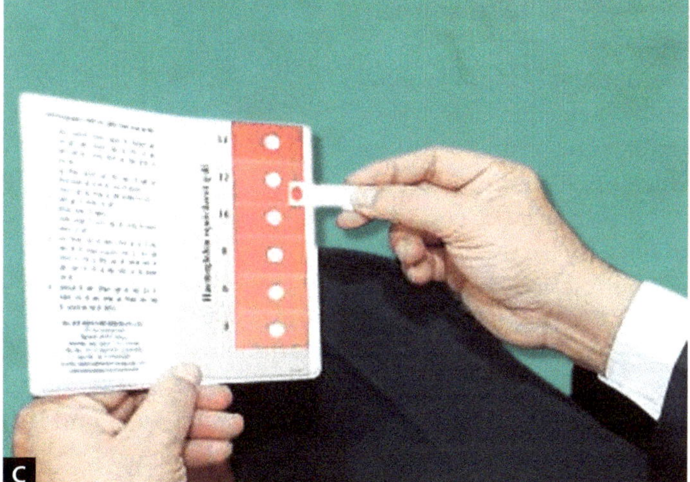

Figs. 3A to C: Hemoglobin color scale.

hemoglobin levels to be judged to 1 g/dL. This is the only method currently available that is affordable for widespread primary care use by the most impoverished countries. For severe anemia, though less accurate by the above method, the scale shows a sensitivity of 95% and a specificity of 99.6%.

The device is simple to use:

1. Place a drop of blood on the test strip provided.
2. Wait about 30 seconds.
3. Match immediately the color of the blood spot against one of the hues on the scale.

The HCS does not require special training, electricity, or battery. It is portable and results are immediate.

Hemoglobin and Hematocrit Estimation Using Blood Gas Analyzer

The blood gas analyzer can be used for a quick and reliable bedside measurement of Hb and hematocrit.[6] The values obtained are reliable and could be of immense use in a modern neonatal ICU. The tests can be done concomitantly with blood gases, alleviating the need for extra blood drawing and therefore decreasing the risk of iatrogenic anemia.

NONINVASIVE MEASUREMENT OF HEMOGLOBIN BY PULSE CO-OXIMETRY

Noninvasive and continuous hemoglobin measurement may be of value in a variety of clinical settings. This method is simple, fast and improves anemia screening or monitoring by eliminating pain, discomfort and reducing infection risk. A hand-held, rapid POC test that uses transcutaneous reflection spectroscopy to measure total hemoglobin and oxygenated Hb is available.[7] Pulse Co-oximetry allows the noninvasive measurement of carboxyhemoglobin, methemoglobin, oxygen content, pleth variability index, along with standard pulse oximetry parameters, oxygen saturation, pulse rate and perfusion index. The pulse Co-oximetry technology uses a multiple wavelength, spectrophotometric sensor that may be an adhesive single use type for continuous monitoring or a reusable finger clip sensor for spot check assessments. This instrument works on the principle of "photoplethysmography (PPG)". A typical Co-oximetry system consists of a light source, a series of lenses, several filters, mirrors that focus the light beams, a sample chamber, a temperature regulated block, a hemolyser, a monochromator and photodiode detectors that emit electrons **(Fig. 4A)**. Basically, it shines light of three different wave lengths onto the finger, and through the tissue of the patient's finger. Once this is done, based on the amount of light transmitted, absorbed and scattered, one can figure out the amount of hemoglobin present in the blood. Hemoglobin has a characteristic absorbance. For estimation of oxygen saturation, the technique is similar to the one used in pulse oximeters. However, a pulse oximeter cannot measure total hemoglobin.

Because the test is noninvasive, it is ideal for prehospital triage decisions, such as hospital selection, etc. This technology can also assist emergency department staff in making diagnosis of anemia which could indicate occult bleeding or other disease processes requiring intervention or therapeutic decisions. This technology is also used in other devices for measuring cardiac output, peripheral vascular disease detection, etc.

In noninvasive there is no benefit of blood collecting, may not be beneficial but fear of needle prick makes sampling difficult[8] whereas in neonate's multiple pricks are required for blood collection. In such cases noninvasive device may decrease risk of exacerbating any underlying anemia. However, for diagnosis of anemia Hb levels are not the only test. A full blood count would be required, and noninvasive device may not be useful. In neonate's regular blood gas sampling is required in ICUs. So, these devices can help to adjust treatment long before getting blood reports.

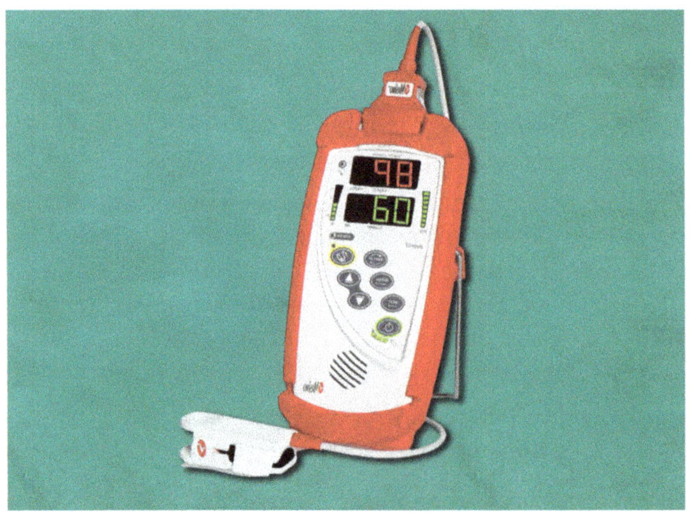

Fig. 4A: Hemoglobin measurement by pulse Co-oximetry.

Three simple steps to use pulse Co-oximetry are **(Figs. 4B to D)**:

1. Place sensor on finger
2. Press test button
3. *Obtain results:* Automatically saved, option to print, e-mail, or manually record.

Blood Glucose Measurement

Blood glucose monitoring evaluates the concentration of glucose in blood and is a critical component of care of the patient. The determination of the concentration of glucose in the blood (venous, arterial, or capillary) is usually performed to monitor or diagnose presence of hyperglycemia (more commonly diabetes mellitus) or hypoglycemia. Diabetes mellitus is a group of metabolic diseases characterized by hyperglycemia resulting from defects in insulin secretion, insulin action, or both. Healthcare expenditure in diabetic patients is probably the maximum as India is the diabetic capital of the world. World Health Organization (WHO) recommends using both the fasting plasma glucose and the oral glucose tolerance test with a 2-hour plasma glucose level of 200 mg/dL (11.1 mmol/L) to establish the diagnosis of type 1 and type 2 diabetes mellitus.

Hospitalized patients with type 1 and type 2 diabetes, are usually treated with a sliding-scale insulin dose with insulin dose determined by recent glucose value. The POC instruments for spot determination of blood glucose are mandatory for this treatment. This is also approved for home use by the US Food and Drug Administration (FDA) for the diagnosis of hypoglycemia but not for treatment of diabetes mellitus.

Many studies have established that the implementation of tight glycemic-control protocols that rely on POC glucose testing improves outcome for critically ill patients.[9,10] In a landmark study Van deer Bergh et al. demonstrated that intensive insulin therapy by maintaining blood glucose at about 110 mg/dL reduced morbidity and mortality in critically ill patients. POC glucose testing obtained by a finger stick capillary blood specimen analyzed on a portable glucose analyzer allows the rapid detection of hypoglycemia in patients on insulin therapy and, thus, can reduce harm. The usual justification for the implementation of POC testing is to decrease the turnaround time and improve patient care. For example, the central laboratory results provided 90 minutes later for a patient whose intravenous (IV) insulin

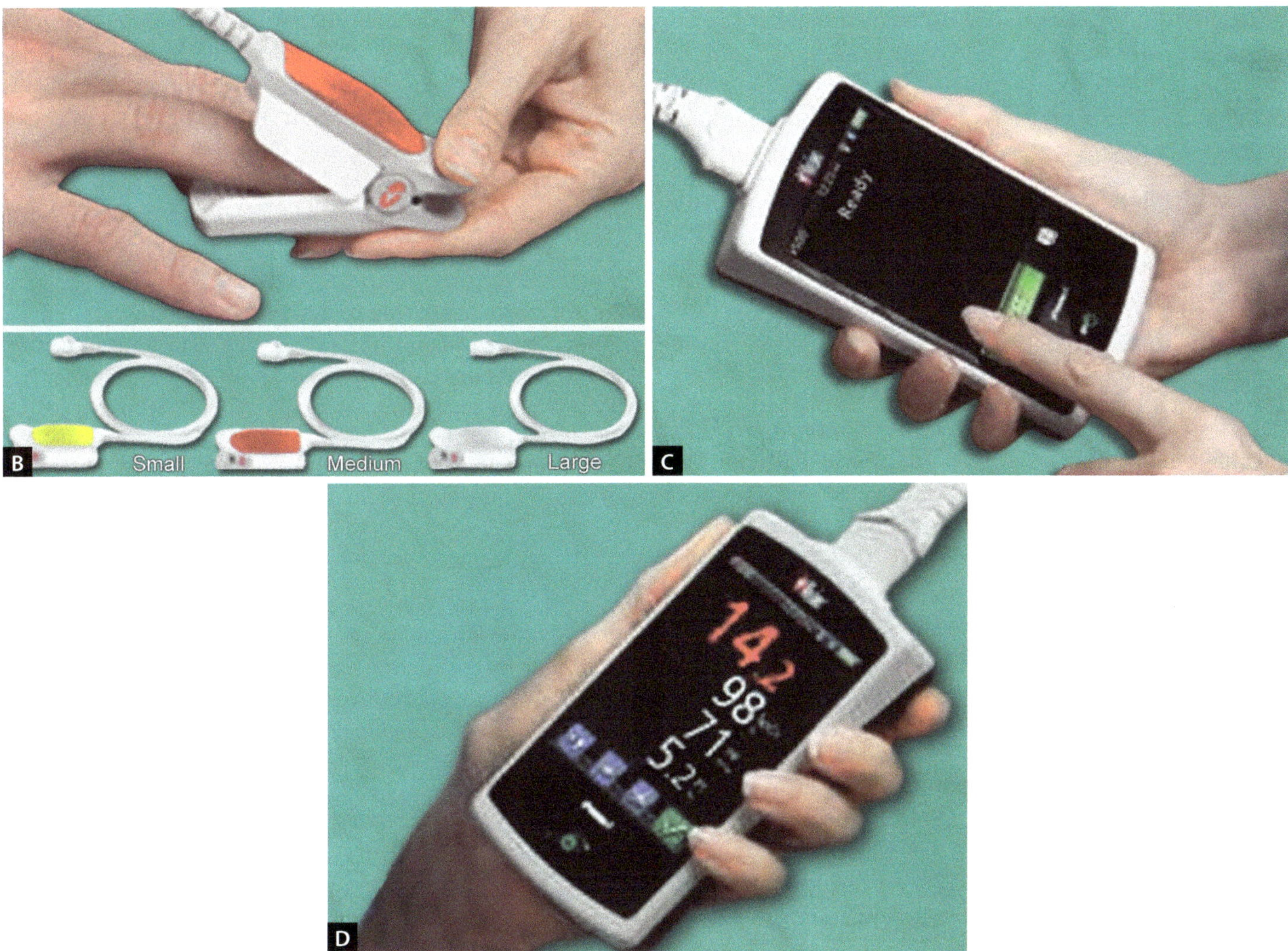

Figs. 4B to D: Three simple steps to use pulse Co-oximetry. (B) Place sensor on finger; (C) Press test button; (D) Obtain results: Automatically saved, option to print, e-mail, or manually record.

drip rate is changed every 60 minutes is of no clinical use in making decisions of change if any of insulin drip rate. Therefore complications related to hypoglycemia (headache, confusion, blurred vision, dizziness and epigastric discomfort to seizures, loss of consciousness, irreversible damage, and even death) or hyperglycemia (irreversible or ischemic brain damage, nosocomial infections, polyneuropathy, and mortality) can be averted.

The three primary biochemical reactions typically used to measure blood glucose values with POC devices are:[11]

1. Glucose oxidase method (color-coded paper)
2. Glucose dehydrogenase method (microcuvette)
3. Hexokinase method.

Specimens from arterial blood have higher glucose levels than venous blood. Plasma glucose concentration is 10–15% higher than blood glucose concentrations. Capillary glucose estimations may show false results in the presence of septic shock, dehydration or ketoacidosis. Patients on medication containing maltose or fructose can get false results in meters utilizing the glucose dehydrogenase method.

Laboratory test—normal/critical (POCT):

- *Glucose (adult/pediatric):* 70–199 mg/dL <60 or >400 mg/dL
- *Glucose (neonate):* 55–115 mg/dL <40 or >150 mg/dL.

The glucose concentration in the blood can be determined in a variety of ways, e.g., by comparing the color of the testing side with a calibrated reference or a color chart or by reflectance photometry.

Gluco-check Using Color-coded Strips[12]

These were used earlier in the hospitals as well as home to determine blood glucose. This involves a pin-prick and placing a drop of blood on the strip and getting a blood glucose reading from "color-coded paper". Reagent strips incorporating enzyme-based compositions contain an indicator which turns a different shade of color, depending on the concentration of glucose in a blood sample that has been applied to the strip. The enzyme glucose oxidase oxidizes glucose to gluconic acid, lactone and hydrogen peroxide. They also contain an oxidizable dye and a substance having peroxidative activity, which is capable of selectively catalyzing oxidation of the oxidizable dye in the presence of hydrogen peroxide. When the blood contacts the strip, it causes, in a reagent impregnated in the strip, a color change that is a measure of the glucose concentration in the blood.

Method: A drop of blood is placed on the test strip for 1 minute. The blood is then wiped off, and then compared to a color chart that gives the range of blood sugar after another minute. The color-coded sheet ranges from blue (negative) to green (trace) to orange (positive).

Glucometer (Fig. 5)

This system is at home or bedside hand-held monitor for glucose estimation. It uses a drop of blood placed on reagent strip or microcuvette to be inserted into a monitor to get glucose value. The test reaction is based on the enzyme glucose dehydrogenase gets glucose converted to gluconolactone. It liberates an electron that reacts with a coenzyme electron acceptor, the oxidized form of the mediator hexacyanoferrate, forming the reduced form of the mediator, hexocyanoferrate. This strip employs the electrochemical principle of biamperometry. The monitor applies a voltage between two identical electrodes, which causes the reduced mediator formed during the incubation period to be reconverted to an oxidized mediator. This generates a small current that is read by the monitor. It is important to make sure the glucose meter is operating correctly by applying QC material to the strip, for home glucometers.

Over the years, the glucose meter has undergone continuous improvements and become vital to the management of critically ill patients, diabetics and recovery after surgery. Newer glucometers are more accurate and gives instant results (<6 seconds) and are almost as good as the laboratory blood analyzers. The later models can also test ketones in the blood. Each cartridge or strip is used once and discarded. Blood glucose meter test strips generally use capillary whole blood as a sample. Laboratory measurements of glucose use plasma as a sample. Some test strips are calibrated to give results that are comparable with laboratory glucose results and these are termed "plasma calibrated". Plasma calibrated test strips give results that are approximately 12% higher than whole blood results **(Fig. 6)**.

Storage and Stability

The monitor, test strips and control solutions should be stored between 14 and 40°C (57–104°F) away from moisture. Test strips should be kept at less than 85% humidity for the most accurate results.

Limitations and Interfering Substances

- Improper handling of the equipment and the test strips (wet, expired or otherwise damaged test strips) can lead to analytical error
- Over manipulation of the patient's fingertip during collection to encourage blood flow; or dilution of the sample by unevaporated alcohol or fluid from IV lines
- Hematocrit levels between 20 and 65% are required for this monitor to provide an accurate result. Blood glucose levels above 200 mg/dL require hematocrits to be 25–55% to provide an accurate result. A blood glucose test instead of bedside glucose test is required if hematocrits do not fall within these ranges
- If yellow mesh is seen on test strip after application of blood on strip within 15 seconds of first sample and if more than further 15 seconds have passed then test result are erroneous so better to repeat test
- Galactose, maltose, or fructose more than 10 mg/dL may give falsely elevated results
- In hypoglycemic patient's the Uric acid concentrations more than 10 mg/dL and uric acid more than 16 mg/dL in euglycemic and hyperglycemic patients (blood sugars >70 mg/dL) may give false high levels

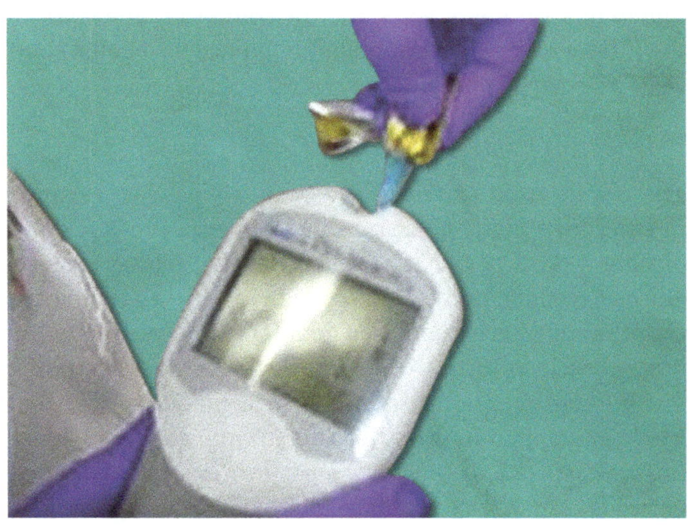

Fig. 5: Glucometer.

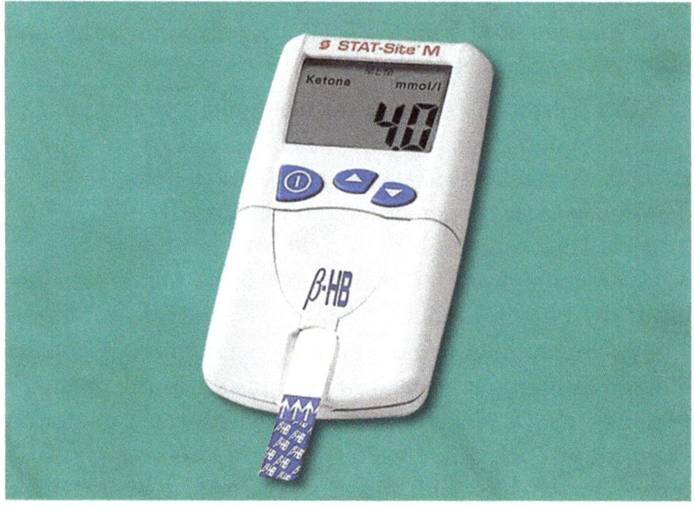

Fig. 6: Glucose and ketone estimation.

- In patients with decreased blood flow, finger stick blood testing may not reflect the patient's true physiological state. For example, severe dehydration caused by diabetic ketoacidosis or the hyperglycemic hyperosmolar nonketotic state, hypotension, shock, or peripheral vascular disease.

Glycated Hemoglobin Analyzer (Fig. 7)

Another POC instrument which incorporates microelectronics, optics and dry reagent chemistry tests HbA1c and hemoglobin.[13] This is finger stick test using less than 10 μL of blood. It contains two dry reagent lateral flow strips with an HbA1c immunoassay test zone on one side and total hemoglobin test zone in the other. Once the blood is added on the strip, the monitor self-activates. An on board microprocessor calculates the percentage of HbA1c from the reflectance's of the test zones. The microprocessor also self-corrects electrical functioning, sample volume, reagent characteristics and optical variations. Tests results are displayed in numeric form within 8 minutes in the liquid-crystal display (LCD) of the monitor.

Future Technology

- *Noninvasive glucose monitoring:* Eliminates skin puncture. There is also a possibility that sweat can be drawn through the skin using a low-level electrical current. Infrared light is being looked to measure glucose through saliva or tears. Noninvasive methods based on Raman spectroscopy and optical coherence tomography (OCT) are under development
- Radiofrequency or modem to the LIS will directly connect POC glucose devices
- Implantable sensor devices (subcutaneous) or central line continuous glucose monitoring (every 1–5 minutes) that last 3–7 days have been approved by the FDA and will allow for even stricter glycemic control with less discomfort for the patient. A transmitter sends information via radio waves to a wireless monitor **(Fig. 8)**.

Arterial Blood Gas and Serum Electrolytes (Figs. 9A and B)

A major concern for ICUs is the maintenance of tissue oxygenation, ventilation, and normal acid base status.[14] Because life-threatening changes in these parameters can occur suddenly, rapid results are often needed for effective monitoring and treatment in the ICU. Not only clinical, but cost advantages are also seen in patients who have had ABG monitoring. Hence, presence of a portable ABG monitor is a necessity in intensive care areas.

The repeated acid base status is needed in neonates on oxygen as high concentration of inhaled oxygen as it can be toxic and damage lungs and eyes. In premature infants, inhalation of lowest possible oxygen concentration is used to maintain arterial oxygen tension (PaO_2) to benefit lung disease. The monitoring the levels of arterial carbon dioxide ($PaCO_2$) and oxygen allows assessment of respiratory competence in intubate patients on artificial ventilation. In addition, the rate or depth of ventilation, ventilator dead space or airway pressure to maintain physiological stability. To help diagnosis of disease the measurement of pH and carbon dioxide pressure of arterial blood concentration and serum electrolytes is necessary. For example, acidosis in diabetes mellitus, the insulin deficiency results in excessive production of ketoacids and lactic acid which lowers extra cellular fluid and blood pH. The, acid base disorders if not treated effectively may side effects such as shock, cardiac arrest, and alkalosis with mental confusion leading to coma.[15]

In neonates or adults on high frequency oscillatory ventilation (HFOV), PaO_2, and $PaCO_2$ changes are needed

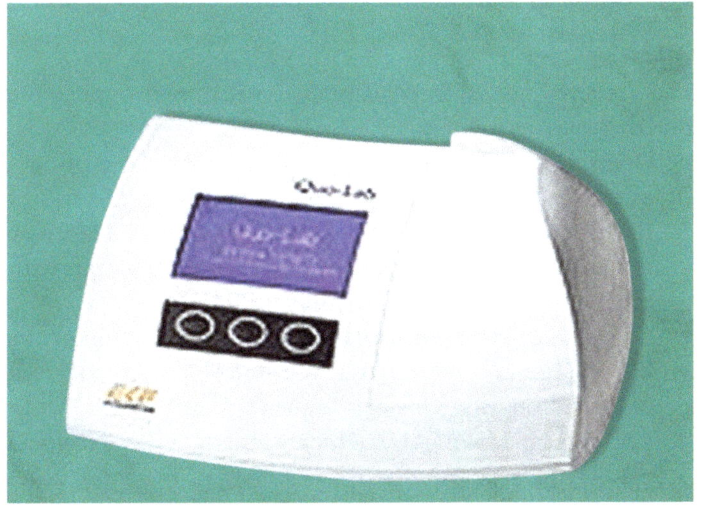

Fig. 7: Glycated hemoglobin estimation.

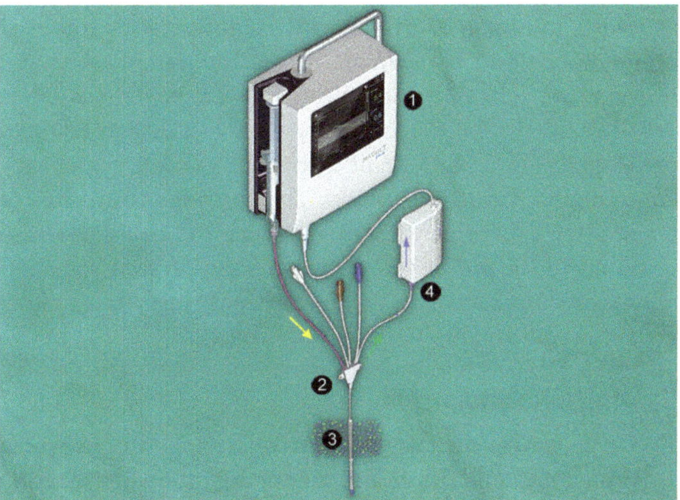

Fig. 8: Central line continuous glucose monitoring. 1. Monitor with syringe compartment; 2. EIRUS central venous catheter; 3. Microdialysis membrane; 4. Sensor (including waste-container) + sensor reader.

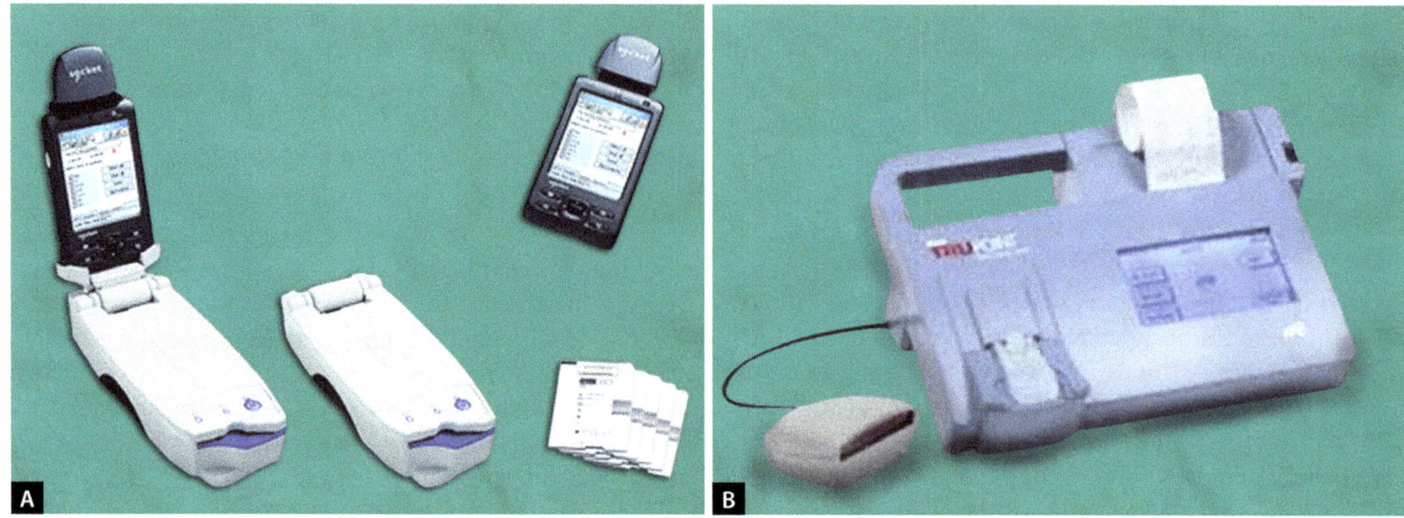

Figs. 9A and B: (A) Arterial blood gas; (B) Serum electrolytes monitors.

to adjust the oscillatory amplitude. For early goal directed therapy (EGDT) in sepsis, pH and central venous oxygen saturation (CvO_2) values are necessary and are obtained by ABG. Most neonatal seizures occur in the presence of acidosis and umbilical cord pH of less than 7.0. Arterial blood gases are also useful in cardiac surgery, and extracorporeal membrane oxygenation (ECMO), etc., each with its own requirements for speed in obtaining results. They have been found useful for prehospital monitoring and trauma resuscitation. Most monitors provide blood gas parameters along with hemoglobin, hematocrit, serum electrolytes (Na, K, Mg, ionized Ca), blood urea nitrogen (BUN), and glucose. Some instruments have the capability to measure oxyhemoglobin, deoxyhemoglobin, carboxyhemoglobin, methemoglobin or sulfhemoglobin.

The POCT blood gas analyzers come with modular design, and state-of-the-art technology featuring large, color touch screen with icons and an integrated video. The sample volume can be as little 0.1 mL of blood. They have clot detection and clearance features. It provides maximum QC with minimal effort. The instrument needs minimal maintenance and measurements are interference free. All of them are portable and battery powered. Many models are available in the market today with vast design features developed for a variety of applications. Most are self-contained and cartridge based. The cartridge comprises of a sampling unit with sensors, reagents and calibrators are required to do the tests. The wash solution and the fluid waste are contained in a wash/waste cartridge. Test results are very rapid and often within 60 seconds.[16]

Specimen Requirements

- Only unfractionated heparin should be used as anticoagulant. Other anticoagulants may significantly alter the results
- It is important that the sample should not be exposed to air during or after its collection. Any bubbles should be expelled from the collection device immediately after sample collection, and the collection device should have an air-tight seal from the time of collection until it is analyzed. Air bubbles in a specimen should be considered a contaminant, as the blood gas values may be affected. Also, air bubbles introduced into an analyzer may cause the sensor to register incorrect results. For these reasons, any sample with froth in it should be considered an unacceptable sample, and, where possible, another sample must be drawn
- Before analyzing the sample, the syringe or the capillary tube should be rolled between your palms and gently inverted several times to mix the sample thoroughly and to distribute the anticoagulant. Blood cells settle during storage, and if the sample is not well mixed before analysis, the results obtained can be falsely decreased or increased
- If the sample is chilled, the mixing time should be increased to ensure that the sample is thoroughly mixed
- Dispose of used sample collection devices as biohazard material.

The technological improvements of modern portable machines are as follows:

- *Compact size:* Modern ABG instruments are compact and user-friendly. Hence, it is easy for hospitals to use them in satellite laboratories and near-patient sites. Few tabletops formats can be converted to portable units with temporary battery power supply
- *Short therapeutic turnaround time:* Treatment delays can be avoided and complications minimized if results are obtained rapidly. This can improve their outcomes and generate cost savings by reducing length of stay in critical care settings
- *Small sample volume:* This is crucial in critically ill patients to minimize and avoid unnecessary transfusions. It is also crucial in young patients, such as

premature infants and neonates who have small total blood volume

- *ABG systems:* They can provide a complete panel of measurements with less than 0.2 mL of blood especially when only one or two analytes (e.g., glucose and lactate) are needed
- *Wide test selection:* They can measure up to 25 parameters simultaneously. Tests include blood gases [partial pressure of oxygen (pO_2), partial pressure of carbon dioxide (pCO_2)], pH, electrolytes (Na^+, K^+, Ca^{++}, Cl^-, Mg^{++}), hematocrit, CO-oximetry (Hb, O_2 saturation, oxyhemoglobin, methemoglobin) and metabolites (glucose, lactate, creatinine, urea nitrogen). Activated clotting time (ACT) Kaolin®, ACT Celite®, PT/INR, cardiac troponin levels (cTnl), creatine kinase-myocardial band (CK-MB) and BNP are other tests
- *Advanced quality management features:* The latest ABG instruments have improved features such as "lock-out" options, automatic QC and electronic QC. The lock-out feature, when activated, allows operators to use the instrument for patient testing only if QC testing has met manufacturer's control ranges and the patient identification and/or operator identification has been entered. Hence, only certified hospital staff can perform and document tests, thereby providing reliable results. Automatic QC features make sure that QC testing is performed routinely. Electronic QC can reduce extra costs associated with purchasing reagents and control materials for QC testing
- *Minimal errors and cost-effectiveness:* Bedside ABG testing potentially could minimize preanalytic and postanalytic errors associated with central laboratory testing, optimizing patient outcome, and saving cost.

Concerns

High/low blood oxygen tension, pH and hematocrit, or high blood levels of medications potentially could cause whole blood methods on hand-held devices to over- or underestimate the glucose measurement which is part of multiparametric testing in these instruments.

Selective testing is not possible in few models. These extra-tests could increase expenditure of supplies (i.e., reagents and disposable sensors, electrodes and cartridges), waste patient blood volume and labor time and subject patients to hazardous use of transfusion services.

Continuous Intra-arterial Blood Gas Monitors (Fig. 10)[17,18]

A new technology that monitors blood gas levels using optical sensors (optodes) is now available from which real-time intra-arterial blood gas (IABG) monitoring is possible.

It is a sterile, disposable, fiberoptic sensor inserted through a 20 gauge (G) arterial catheter. It has a microprocessor-controlled monitor with self-contained calibration unit and detachable display and control panel. The sensor has optical fibers bundled together in a biocompatible package each fiber is of a diameter of human hair.

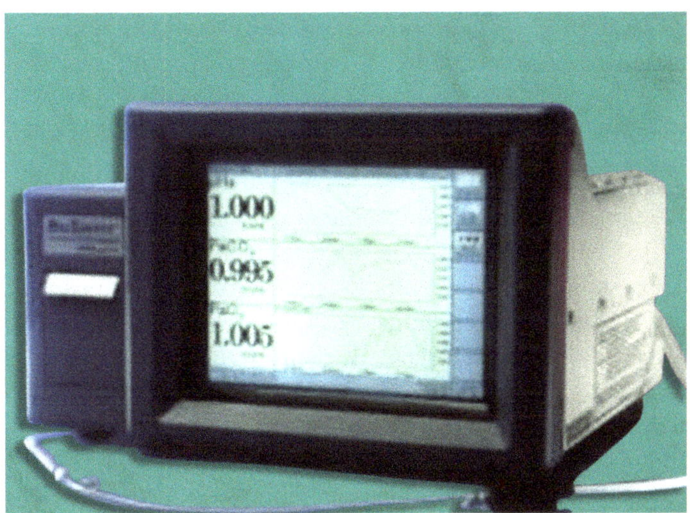

Fig. 10: Continuous intra-arterial blood gas monitor.

The sensing element is at the tip of the optic fibers and displays values every 20 seconds. The display screen provides current numerical values and real-time trends for each parameter, allowing continuous monitoring.

The continuous monitoring provides reliable values of blood gases available online and is crucial for ICU patients.

Serum electrolytes (Na, K, Cl, and ionized Ca) are tested in most ABG analyzers.[19] Some instruments can provide serum magnesium levels in addition. Arterial, venous or capillary blood can be used for testing blood gases or electrolytes.

Clinical Significance

pH: Acidosis (low pH) occurs due to either respiratory failure (high pCO_2) or from metabolic causes (including ketoacidosis, lactic acidosis, severe diarrhea, uremia, hypoaldosteronism, renal tubular disease, drug effects, or poisoning from several specific agents). Alkalosis (high pH) stems from hyperventilation (low pCO_2) or from metabolic causes (including excessive vomiting, potassium depletion, gastric drainage, drug effects, hyperadrenocorticism, or excessive alkali intake). Extreme abnormalities of pH will prompt a potentially life-threatening pathophysiologic state that must be corrected promptly.

pCO_2: The pCO_2 reflects the overall respiratory status. High pCO_2 indicates respiratory suppression or failure, whereas low pCO_2 indicates hyperventilation (which may occur from hypoxia, anxiety, fever, cerebral disease, cirrhosis, or excessive mechanical ventilation). Extreme abnormalities of pCO_2 reflect a potentially life-threatening pathophysiologic state that must be corrected promptly.

pO_2: The pO_2 reflects the ability of the lungs to deliver oxygen to the blood. Hypoxia (low pO_2) may occur despite adequate

respiration due to parenchymal lung diseases (pneumonia, asthma, pulmonary edema, and pulmonary fibrosis) due to pulmonary shunting of blood. Extremely low pO_2 is a potentially life-threatening pathophysiologic state that must be corrected promptly.

Sodium: Abnormal concentrations of Na^+ occur due to deficit or overload of total body water or of sodium itself. These abnormal concentrations arise from diverse clinical conditions, such as congestive heart failure, liver disease (cirrhosis), renal disease, neuropsychiatric disorders (causing abnormal fluid intake), IV fluid therapy, excessive fluid loss (vomiting, diarrhea, heat stroke), drug therapy (diuretics), diabetes mellitus (causing osmotic diuresis), and imbalances of hormones [antidiuretic hormone (ADH), mineralocorticoid, glucocorticoid] that regulate sodium and water excretion. An extremely abnormal plasma sodium concentration may itself directly cause altered mental status, stupor, coma, seizures, brain swelling or dehydration leading to cerebral hemorrhage or ultimately, death. Thus, extreme abnormalities of sodium reflect a potentially life-threatening pathophysiologic state that must be corrected promptly.

Potassium: High concentrations of K^+ commonly stem from renal failure, excessive potassium replacement, drug effects (including some potassium sparing diuretics), hemolytic disease, or crush injury. Low concentrations stem from gastrointestinal loss, dietary insufficiency, or drug effects (most diuretics). Other metabolic imbalances (acid-base, mineralocorticoid, glucocorticoid, insulin effects) can also cause abnormal potassium concentrations. An extremely abnormal plasma potassium concentration causes neuromuscular paralysis, respiratory failure, cardiac arrhythmia, or cardiac arrest. Thus, extreme abnormalities of potassium reflect a potentially life-threatening pathophysiologic state that must be corrected promptly.

Chloride: Cl^- is used most commonly to distinguish high-anion-gap acidosis (ketoacidosis, lactic acidosis, uremia, poisoning from several specific agents) from hyperchloremic acidosis (loss of alkali as in severe diarrhea, hypoaldosteronism, potassium-sparing diuretics, renal tubular acidosis). Changes in plasma chloride concentration tend to parallel those of sodium in the absence of acidosis. Thus, chloride is high in dehydration and low in over hydrated states.

Ionized calcium: Ca^{++} abnormalities typically stem from parathyroid disease, vitamin D imbalance, renal disease, pancreatitis, drug effects, abnormalities of magnesium or phosphorus, malignancy, or sarcoidosis. An extreme hypocalcemia may cause neuromuscular symptoms, tetany, altered mental status, seizures, heart failure, or arrhythmias. Thus, extreme abnormalities of ionized calcium reflect a potentially life-threatening pathophysiologic state that must be corrected promptly.

Future Strategies and Evolving Technologies

- Miniature sensors
- Wireless system that interfaces to an electronic data manager (EDM) and bluetooth printer
- Smart card technology
- 0.1 mL sample volume (very useful in neonates and anemic states)
- Room temperature cartridge storage and consumables
- Storing patient record
- Easy use even by nonlaboratory trained individuals
- Intravenous, intra-arterial, subcutaneous, and transcutaneous techniques, are available or under development for measurement of pO_2, pH, pCO_2, glucose, lactate and electrolytes. Noninvasive techniques are also being developed for analytes in exhaled air, and via the lumen of the gastrointestinal tract.

Blood Lactate

Blood lactate levels help determine whether oxygen uptake (VO_2) is adequate for the needs of aerobic metabolism. Blood lactate monitoring therefore is indirectly used as a marker of tissue hypoxia. Because lactate levels in the whole blood and plasma are equivalent, both measurements are called blood lactate. The normal blood lactate concentration is less than 2 mmol/L but the threshold for an elevated blood lactate is higher at 4 mmol/L. Serum lactate can be elevated in sepsis, shock, liver failure, heavy exercise, etc. Serum lactate more than 4 mmol/L is associated with poor outcome regardless of etiology with few exceptions being salbutamol toxicity and seizures.[20]

A rapid serum lactate results in the ED, OR or ICU can serve patients better. Better outcomes following EGDT in sepsis management has been proven in avoiding multiorgan dysfunction or even death and hence keeping serum lactate below set threshold is part of the management of EGDT. The duration for which serum lactate is elevated (by serial lactate analyses) gives an estimation of oxygen debt. Early recognition of an increase in serum lactate with immediate resuscitation is associated with better outcome. Use of a handheld POC lactate device reduces the time for lactate test results and allow for immediate risk stratification of potentially critically ill patients so that early treatment can be initiated. Patients with acute abdomen, acute myocardial infarction (AMI), asthma, cyanide poisoning, raised intracranial pressure, pulmonary embolism, ECMO, burns, circulatory shock, transfused patients, trauma or following cardiac arrest will need a rapid serum lactate estimation. Similarly, patients undergoing liver or heart transplant, high-risk surgeries, thoracic or abdominal aortic aneurysms, heart surgeries, high-risk neonate/infants, etc., need lactate estimation the poor lactate clearance are found to be a prognostic indicator of poor outcome in trauma.

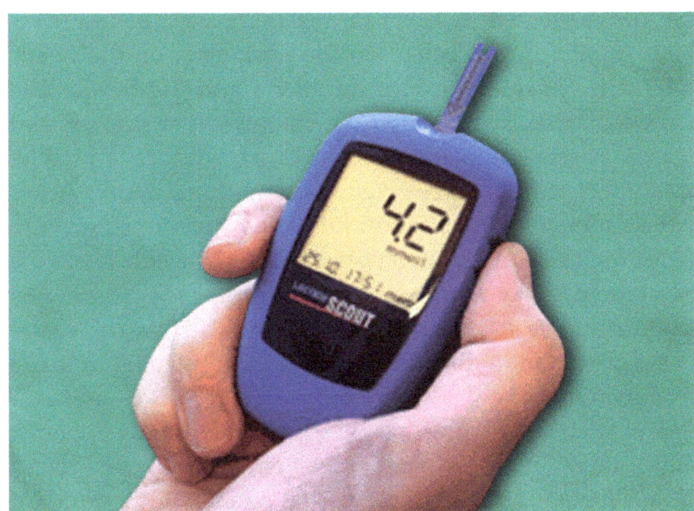

Fig. 11: Serum lactate estimation.

Serum Lactate

Serum lactate can be measured using fingertip POC device with whole venous or arterial blood **(Fig. 11)**. Lactate is currently measured in blood gas analyzers which require much larger sample volume of blood than a standalone blood lactate monitor (100–200 µL vs. 0.6 µL). These portable devices also come with data connectivity with USB and data transfer software.

COAGULATION MONITORING

Perioperative monitoring of blood coagulation is valuable in a large variety of clinical scenarios, e.g., massive hemorrhage, assessment of hyper- or hypocoagulable states, guiding pro- and anticoagulant therapies, and to predict the risk of bleeding during the consecutive anesthetic or surgical procedures. Point-of-care coagulation monitoring devices can overcome many limitations of routine coagulation tests in the perioperative setting.[21] Several technologies for coagulation monitoring are used in outpatient departments, cardiac surgery units, liver surgeries, and intensive care and dialysis units. Principles used for testing for coagulation are listed in **Box 1**. Those tests which utilize viscoelastic properties of blood, e.g., TEG or Sonoclot are useful to determine the cause of bleeding. A surgical cause of bleeding has to be considered when the viscoelastic properties are normal. Plasma, capillary or whole blood is used depending upon the test or the analyzer.

Patients presenting for cardiac surgery may have preexisting platelet defects which can be drug induced or acquired. Platelet count may be reduced in heparinized patients. Cardiopulmonary bypass (CPB) may add to platelet dysfunction. The POC platelet analyzers can assess platelet function rapidly and can measure the effects of antiplatelet therapy. The gold standard to measure platelet function is platelet aggregometry using platelet-rich plasma. However, this technique is labor intensive and time-consuming and hence not applicable for the surgical patient. The POC tests

BOX 1: Principles used for testing for coagulation.

1. Optical detection of clot
2. Mechanical detection of clot
3. Clot impedes flow of metallic particles
4. Iron particles caught in forming clot in magnetic field
5. Fluorescent thrombin substrate
6. Laser photometry to detect changes in blood flow when clot forms

of platelet function are therefore used as they need whole blood, are portable, user friendly, and provide instant results. After CP, the platelet defect is quite profound and is best monitored with viscoelastic whole blood tests, such as thromboelastography.

All platelet function tests are not alike; the etiology of the platelet dysfunction dictates the type of test that can be used to monitor platelet function. Platelet inhibition in patients treated with antithrombotic drugs can be tested using a variety of tests. Platelet function can be assessed in the static phase, dynamic phase, and as a response to an agonist. Static tests of platelet function, such as the measure of β-thromboglobulin release or mean platelet volume, are not valuable measures of platelet function, as the function is captured at a single point in time. Dynamic tests, such as the viscoelastic tests and the response to a platelet agonist, are more valuable tests of platelet function over time. The agonist used in these tests may be thrombin or collagen which tests the platelet response to endothelial injury and thus its ability to mediate hemostasis *in vivo*. Other agonists like adenosine diphosphate (ADP) or arachidonic acid is used in order to test the efficacy of clopidogrel or aspirin, respectively, in inhibiting platelet function.

Point-of-care Platelet Function Tests Using a Platelet Agonist

Platelet Function Analyzer (Fig. 12)

The procedure involves placing of whole blood on test cartridge and vacuum perfuses the blood across a collagen-coated membrane and aperture is created in the membrane in presence of epinephrine or ADP. The force of blood being drawn through vacuum which activates platelets and it promotes adherence and aggregation. The closure time is the time taken for formation of clot inside glass tube and prevent further blood flow. Which depends upon functional platelet GP1b and GPIIb/IIIa, von Willebrand factor, platelet count and hematocrit. The response to epinephrine is suggestive of aspirin-induced dysfunction. In von Willebrand's and uremia, ADP or epinephrine channels accurately detect platelet dysfunction.

Point-of-care Turbidimetric-based Optical Detection System (Figs. 13A and B)

It is used to measure agonist-induced agglutination of whole blood and has mixing chamber which contains platelet agonist Tts, and are activated if they are responsive to agonist.

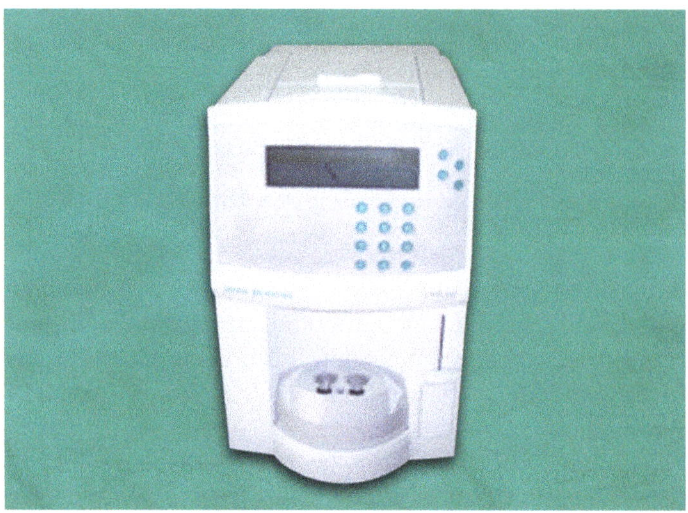

Fig. 12: Platelet function analyzer.

The activated GPIIb/IIIa receptors on the platelets bind to adjacent platelets via the fibrinogen on the beads and cause agglutination of the blood and the beads. The light transmittance through the chamber is measured and increases as agglutination increases. The degree of platelet inhibition can be quantified once antithrombotic drugs effects reduces agglutination. In patients of clopridrogel to determine residual platelet activity this is useful following placement of coronary stent. The aspirin-induced platelet dysfunction is assessed by arachnoid acid cartridge and are more accurate in clopidrogel-induced platelet-induced dysfunction.

An instrument that uses the principle of the "platelet count ratio" to assess platelet reactivity using whole-blood is available. It compares platelet counts in a standard ethylenediamine tetra-acetic acid (EDTA) tube versus

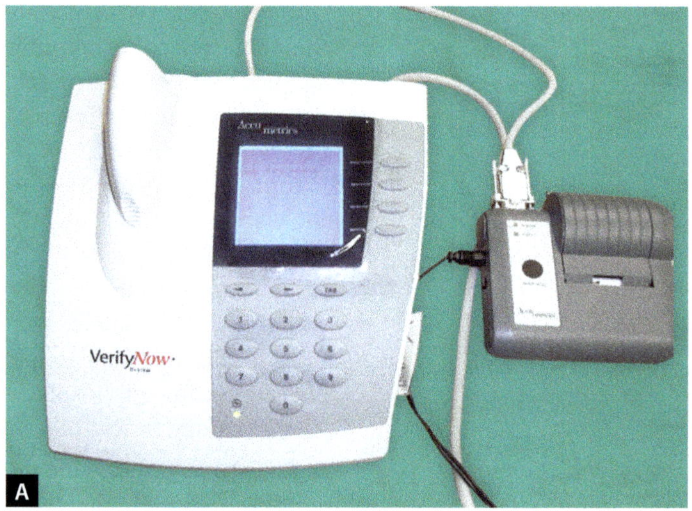

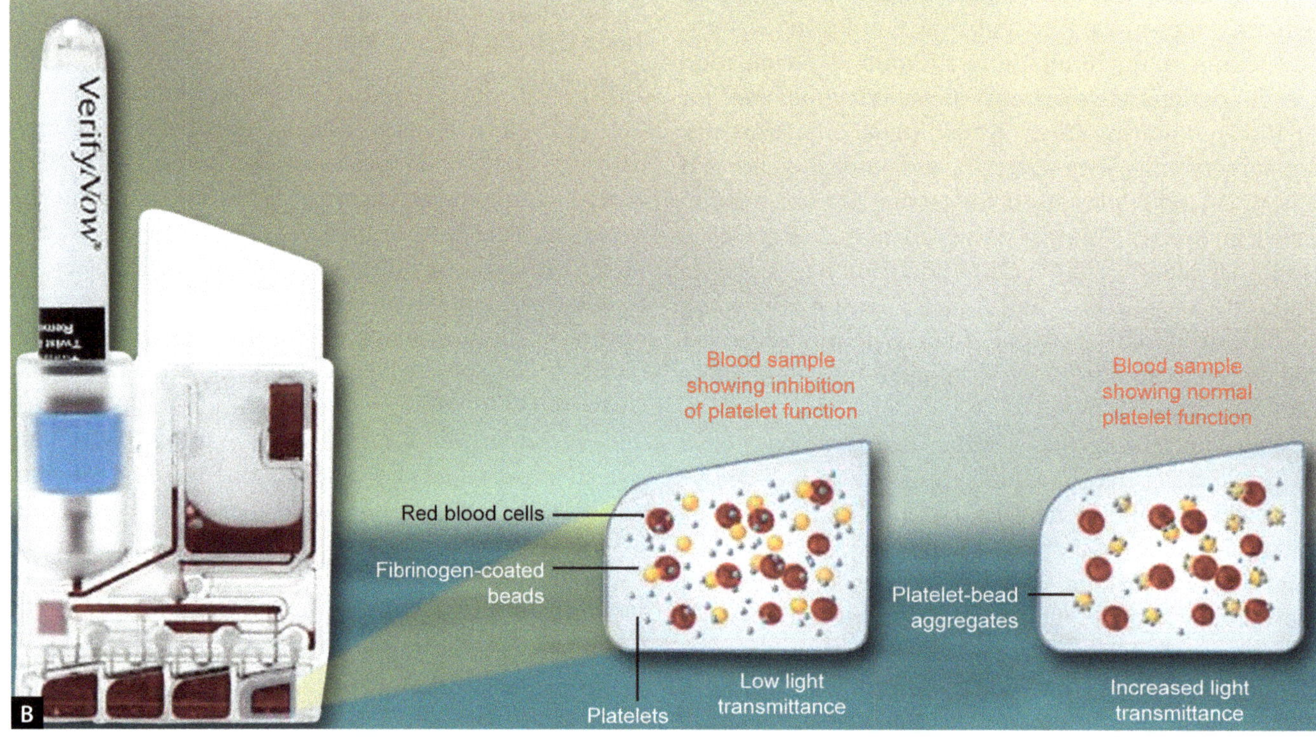

Figs. 13A and B: (A) Platelet function analyzer using optical detection system; (B) The VerifyNow® process.

platelet counts in a citrate tube after aggregation with either ADP or collagen. When blood is added to these agonist tubes, platelets activate, adhere to the tube, and are effectively eliminated from the platelet count. The ratio of the activated platelet count to the nonactivated platelet count is a function of reactivity of the platelets.

The real value in testing the platelet response to a specific agonist is derived from the measure of specific platelet defects that accompany antithrombotic drug therapy. These tests may not be very useful in the presence of gross platelet dysfunction as in CPB and strong agonist like thrombin needs to be used. Hence, viscoelastic tests like TEG are more useful in such conditions of bleeding following CPB.

Impact Cone and Platelet Analyzer (Fig. 14)

The whole blood is exposed to uniform shear stress by the spinning of a cone in a standardized cup. This mimics platelet function testing under physiological blood flow like conditions. Therefore, the pattern of platelet function is more accurate.

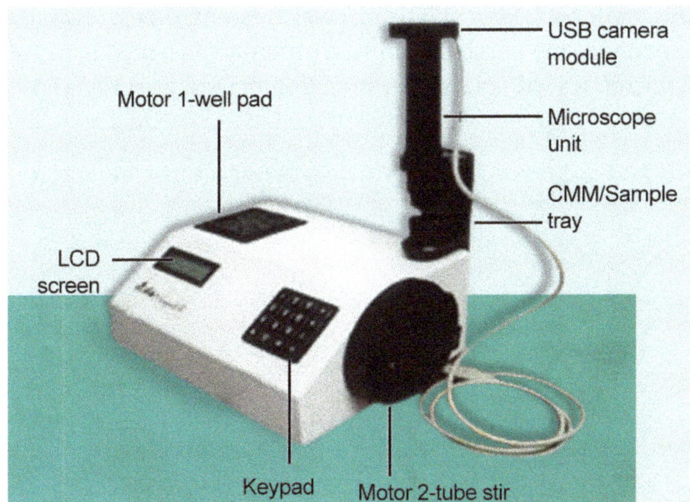

Fig. 14: Impact cone and platelet analyzer. (USB: universal serial bus; LCD: liquid-crystal display; CMM: coordinate measuring machine)

The plasma proteins adhere to the wall surface immediately upon application of blood sample into polystyrene well. They become attractive for platelets which results in adhesion and aggregation on the well surface under flow conditions. After washing of excess blood and staining of adhered platelets, image analyzer quantifies the results. It is expressed as percentage of well surface covered by platelet aggregates and its average size. It is used for hypo- and hyperfunction of platelets and useful to monitoring of congenital hemostatic anomalies.

Viscoelastic Tests of Clot Formation (Sonoclot, Thromboelastograph)

Sonoclot

It tests viscoelastic properties of blood to provide information on coagulation factors, formation of fibrin gel, clot retraction and fibrinolysis. It is done with tubular probe which oscillates up and down within a blood sample.

The viscous force of the blood creates impedance to the ultrasonic vibrating probe as it clots, which is converted to an output signal which is processed by a microcomputer and is reported as the clot signal. The graphic recording of dynamics of clot formation as a Sonoclot signature which yields quantitative results **(Fig. 15A)**, which is the plotted values of clot signal versus time **(Fig. 15B)**.

The quantitative results include a lag period (SonACT) that corresponds to activated clotting time and a wave that occurs because of cross-linkage of fibrin (clot rate). The tracing indicates platelet-fibrin binding, fibrin formation and clot retraction. The clot retraction is a measure of platelet activity and its quantitative parameter is the time to peak.

The Sonoclot can detect hemostasis anomalies such as platelet dysfunction; factor deficiencies of disseminated intravascular coagulation (DIC); anticoagulant effects; hyperfibrinolysis; hypercoagulable states; and to diagnose and treat platelet dysfunction and bleeding disorders after CPB.

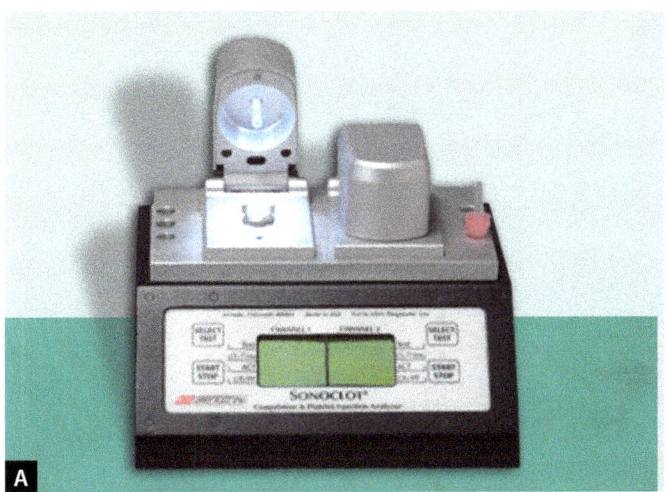

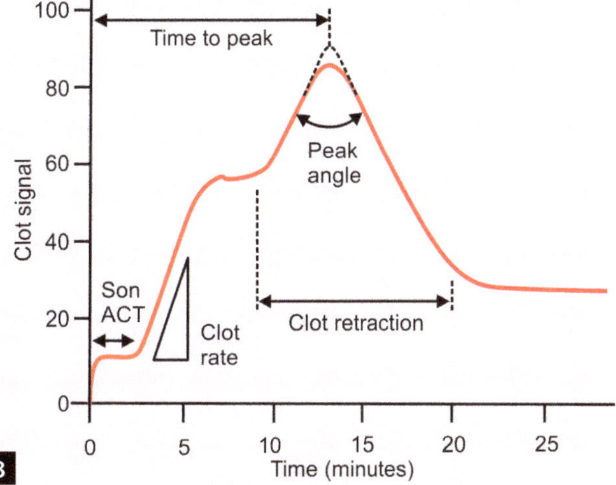

Figs. 15A and B: (A) Sonoclot® analyzer; (B) Graph represents description of the Sonoclot signature and variables.

Thromboelastograph

The TEG was invented in 1948 and uses the viscoelastic properties of blood. This test also provides information from the time of initiation through acceleration, control and eventual lysis. The TEG is extensively used for coagulation monitoring during liver transplantation, cardiovascular surgery, obstetric anesthesia, trauma anesthesia and ICUs. A small amount of blood (0.36 mL) is placed in an oscillating curette and a piston is lowered into the blood sample. The curette oscillates at an arc angle of 4 degree 45 minutes. As clots form in the sample, the fibrin-platelet bonds move the piston relative to the clot strength. A detector records the axis rotation over time and this rotation is drawn into a signature tracing called thromboelastogram.[22] This reveals information about fibrin formation, platelet-fibrin interactions, platelet clot strength, and fibrinolysis. An activator (Celite®, Kaolin®, or tissue factor) is needed because the onset to coagulation varies, and the time to clot formation can conveniently be accelerated so that the test is useful in POC settings. There are five parameters to the TEG tracing that measure different stages of clot development: (i) R, (ii) K, (iii) an angle, (iv) maximum amplitude (MA), and (v) MA60 **(Figs. 16A to C)**. In addition, clot lysis indices are measured at 30–60 minutes after MA (LY30 and LY60). Normal values vary depending on the type of activator used.

The "R value" is a measure of "clotting time (CT)" which is the period of time from the start of the test to the initial fibrin formation, i.e., time from the beginning of the reaction to a 2 mm increase in amplitude. This indicates the initiation of clotting, thrombin formation, and the start of clot polymerization.

The "K value" is the clot kinetics measurement of the speed to reach a specific level of clot strength: the time from beginning of clot formation (the end of R time) until the amplitude reaches 20 mm. This signifies fibrin polymerization and clot stabilization with platelets and factor XIII.

The "a" angle is the angle between the horizontal line in the middle of the TEG tracing and the line tangential to the developing "body" of the TEG tracing at 2 mm amplitude. The "a" angle represents the acceleration (kinetics) of fibrin build up and cross-linking (clot strengthening).

The "MA" reflects the ultimate strength of the clot which depends on the number and function of platelets and their interaction with fibrin. The MA which is a marker for platelet function is the parameter most frequently measured because it correlates with platelet dysfunction in cardiac surgery.

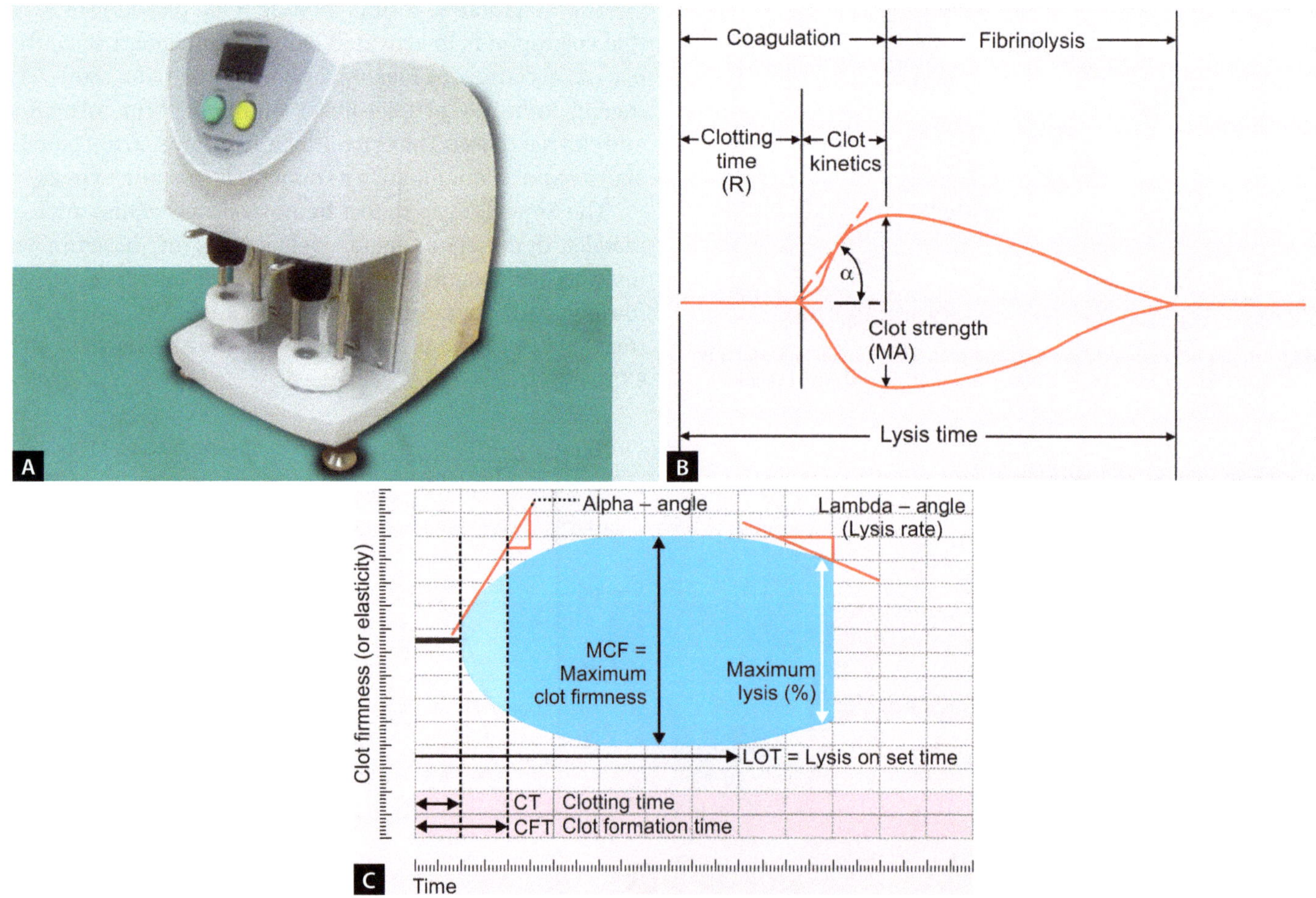

Figs. 16A to C: (A) Thromboelastography analyzer; (B) Waveform output generated by the TEG analyzer; (C) Thromboelastograph.

LY30, or the lysis index at 30 minutes after MA, is increased with fibrinolysis.

Maximum velocity (maxVel)—The maximum of the first derivative of the clot curve.

Time to maximum velocity (t-maxVel)—Time from start of reaction until maxVel is reached.

The "area under curve" is defined as the area under the velocity curve, that is, the area under the curve ending at a time point that corresponds to maximum clot firmness (MA).

A limitation of the TEG is its inability to detect impairment in platelet function induced by antiplatelet agents. Platelet mapping assay is useful to detect antiplatelet agent-induced dysfunction. Use of TEG in cardiac surgery has significantly reduced the use of just whole blood without use of component therapy and eventually helps in less re-exploration rates. The TEG R value determines the quantity of fresh frozen plasma needed to reverse the coagulation defect in the postcardiac surgical patients **(Table 1)**.

TABLE 1: Thromboelastograph-based transfusion algorithm.

Thromboelastograph (TEG) modifications		
TEG variable	***Implication***	***Therapy***
R > 14 mm and < 21 mm	↓Clotting factors	One FFP
R > 21 mm and < 28 mm	↓↓Clotting factors	Two FFP
R > 28 mm	↓↓↓Clotting factors	Four FFP
MA < 48 mm	↓Platelet number/function	One-pooled platelets
MA < 40 mm	↓↓Platelet number/function	Two-pooled platelets
Lys > 7.5%	Increased lysis	Aprotinin

(MA: maximum amplitude; Lys: lysis; FFP: fresh frozen plasma)

Platelet mapping assay: This test is more accurate in patients with antiplatelet medications. It has three cuvettes each containing thrombin, reptilase and arachidonic acid/ADP. The ability of the MA to increase in response to ADP (clopidogrel) or arachidonic acid (aspirin) is a measure of drug-induced inhibition due to their respective pathways. This POC tests correlates with the gold standard test optical aggregometry **(Flowchart 1)**.

ROTEM

Rotational thromboelastometry (ROTEM) evolved from TEG technology and both devices generate output by transducing changes in the viscoelastic strength of a small sample of clotting blood (300 μL) to which a constant rotational force is applied.

A number of cartridges are available and which allow various aspects of hemostasis to be analyzed in real-time. The ROTEM analyzer provides a trace similar to that of the TEG with related parameters including clotting time (CT) and maximum clot firmness (MCF) **(Tables 2 and 3)**.

Both ROTEM and TEG provide a great deal of quantitative data; however, a simple approach to treatment begins with focusing on three questions about clots:

1. How fast?
2. How strong?
3. For how long?

1. *How fast?:* This stage is represented by the left side of the graph labeled clotting time (CT) for ROTEM (or specifically ROTEM's EXTEM test, with re-agents added to isolate the extrinsic pathway of the coagulation cascade), or reaction time (R) for TEG. The time for new clot

Flowchart 1: A simplified treatment-based approach to TEG and ROTEM.

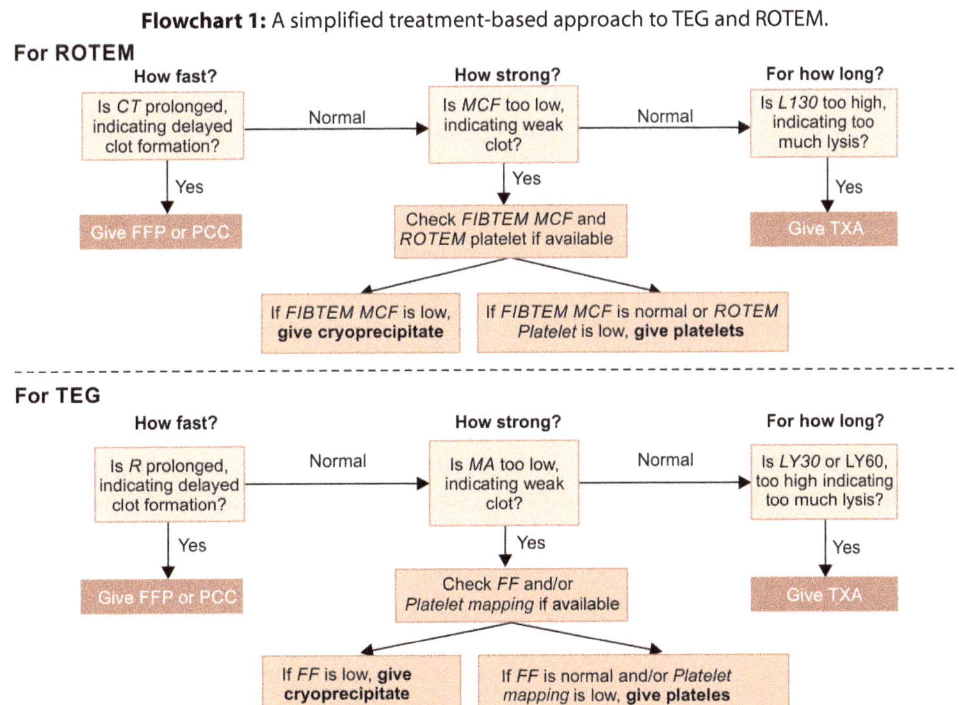

TABLE 2: Rotational thromboelastometry (ROTEM).

Tests	*Interpretation*
INTEM	Contains Phospholipid and ellagic acid as activators and provides information similar to that of the APTT
EXTEM	Contains tissue factor as an activator and provides information similar to that of the PT
HEPTEM	Contains lyophilized heparinase for neutralizing heparin
APTEM	Contains aprotinin for inhibiting fibrinolysis
FIBTEM	Based upon the INTEM but in addition contains Cytochalasin D, a platelet inhibitor which blocks the platelet contribution to clot formation, allowing qualitative analysis of the functional fibrinogen component
ECATEM	Contains Ecarin and so is similar to the Ecarin clotting time. This makes it very sensitive to presence of direct thrombin inhibitors (DTIs)

TABLE 3: Variables measured by the TEG and ROTEM.

Variables	*TEG*	*ROTEM*
Measurement period	–	Reaction Time (RT)
Time from start to when the waveform reaches 2 mm above baseline	R	Clotting Time (CT)
The time from 2 mm above baseline to 20 mm above baseline	K	Clot Formation Time (CFT)
Alpha angle [°]	Slope between R and K	Angle of tangent at 2 mm amplitude
Maximum angle	–	CRF
Maximum strength	Maximal Amplitude (MA)	Maximal Clot Firmness (MCF)
Time to maximum strength	–	MCF-t
Amplitude at a specific time	A30, A60	A5, A10...
Clot elasticity	G	MCE
Maximum lysis	–	CLF
Clot Lysis (CL) at a specific time (minutes)	CL30, CL60	LY30, LY45, LY60
Time to lysis	2 mm from MA	CLT (10% difference from MCF)

formation indicates the cumulative functionality of all the higher-level clotting factors within the coagulation cascade, leading up to the conversion of prothrombin to thrombin. Although there may be a great deal of complexity in this portion of the coagulation cascade, for the purposes of emergent bleeding, we can reduce this entire section to a single numerical value. Prolonged CT or R can be treated with fresh frozen plasma (FFP) or prothrombin complex concentrate (PCC).

2. *How strong?:* This should be thought of as a two-part question, because there are two major components that give a clot its strength—fibrin and platelets. A clot is composed of a platelet plug, reinforced by cross-linked strands of polymerous fibrin chains. A deficiency in either fibrin or platelets will result in a pathologically weak clot. TEG and ROTEM have released technologies capable of measuring platelet functionality directly, specifically TEG's Platelet Mapping Assay or ROTEM Platelet.
   - When assessing clot strength, we are looking at the highest amplitudes within the middle of the graph, namely the maximum clot formation (MCF) in ROTEM, or the maximum amplitude (MA) in TEG. If each of these values is normal, then there is likely no clot strength deficiency. However, if the clot is too weak overall, then we have to assess the two main components separately. Each platform has a devoted test to measure the contribution of fibrin to clot strength—the FIBTEM MCF in ROTEM, or the Functional Fibrinogen (FF) level in TEG. If the FIBTEM MCF or FF test is normal, but the overall clot strength (MCF or MA) is deficient, then we can infer that there is a deficiency in platelet functionality, and these should be repleted accordingly.
   - If the fibrin component has been corrected but the overall clot strength remains deficient, this indicates there must be a concurrent platelet deficiency, which should also be treated. Or alternatively, using the newer technologies, we can measure both fibrin and platelets individually and replete whichever is lacking.
3. *For how long?:* The rightward portion of the graph where the amplitude begins to decrease again, corresponding to the process by which plasminogen converts to the active plasmin and begins breaking down fibrin strands. This gives information on durability of clot or its flimsiness (Fibrinolysis). This process occurs normally in healthy patients, however overactive plasmin causes hyperfibrinolysis, which is a treatable form of coagulopathy. To detect hyperfibrinolysis, we may examine the lysis index at 30 minutes (LI30) in ROTEM, or the lysis at 30 or 60 minutes (LY30, LY60) in TEG. If the bleeding patient's clots are being lysed too quickly, we may treat with tranexamic acid **(Fig. 17)**.

Point-of-care Testing of Heparin Effect

Coagulation management of cardiac surgical patients is complex because of the need to maintain a balance between anticoagulation for CPB and hemostasis after CPB. The antiplatelet drugs can cause impaired platelet function. During CPB, optimal anticoagulation dictates that coagulation is antagonized and platelets are prevented from activation so that clots do not form. The whole process of anticoagulation with heparin, antagonism with protamine, and postoperative hemostasis therapy can be guided by POC tests that assess hemostatic function in a timely and accurate manner.

Heparin and Anticoagulation for Cardiopulmonary Bypass

The most commonly used anticoagulant in clinical use is heparin because it is easy to dose, administer, measure,

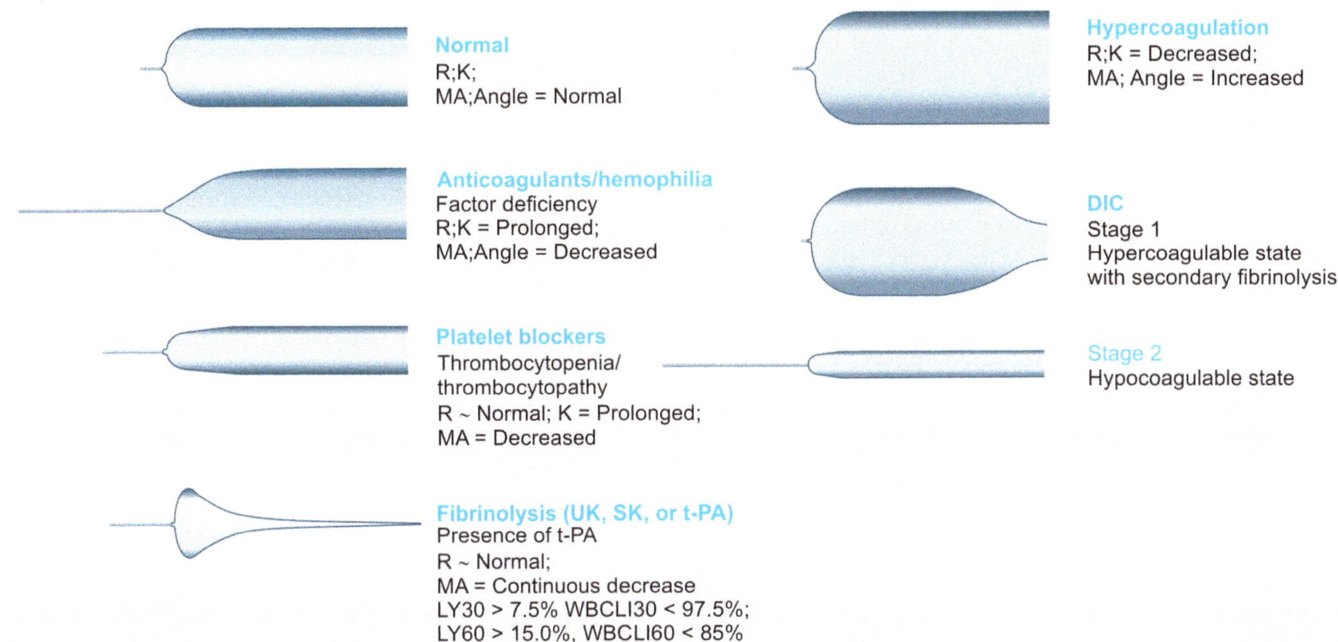

Fig. 17: Thromboelastograph signatures. (MA: maximum amplitude; LY30: lysis in 30 minutes; LY60: lysis in 60 minutes; t-PA: tissue plasminogen activator; DIC: disseminated intravascular coagulation; WBCLI30: white blood cells lysis index in 30 minutes; WBCLI60: white blood cells lysis index in 60 minutes; UK: urokinase; SK: streptokinase)

and reverse. Heparin works by activating antithrombin III (ATIII). Therefore, appropriate levels of levels of ATIII are necessary for heparin to be effective. Activated ATIII inactivates thrombin and other proteases involved in blood clotting, especially factor Xa. Empiric heparin dosing of 300 U/kg has been replaced by the monitored use of heparin, i.e., ACT monitoring.

Activated Coagulation Time Monitoring

Activated coagulation time has been used to monitor heparinization during cardiopulmonary surgery, vascular surgery, in the coronary care unit or for monitoring heparin during renal dialysis. ACT is prolonged in heparinized patients, hypothermia, hypofibrinogenemia, hemodilution, use of aprotinin, lack of coagulation factors or in the presence of qualitative platelet abnormalities.[23] The immediate availability of test results significantly improves clinical care. Also, excessive transfusion, increased morbidity, mortality and excessive hospital costs can be avoided. Standalone ACT testing instruments are available inside the ORs or catheter laboratories. Otherwise, ACT can also be tested as one of the parameters in an instrument, which provides a battery of coagulation tests. To measure ACT, a specimen of whole blood is drawn directly from the patient or from the extracorporeal circuit into a standardized vacuum collection tube containing a particulate coagulation activator such as diatomaceous earth. The test automatically starts with the insertion of the test tube containing blood and coagulation activator. The automated instrument gently mixes the specimen at 37°C and measures the end

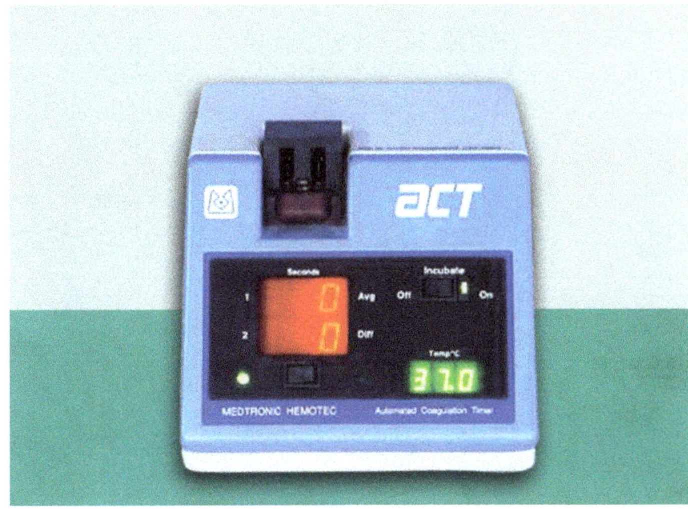

Fig. 18: Activated coagulation time monitor.

point (i.e., blood clot). The activator normally causes the blood to coagulate within about 120 seconds, but heparin prolongs coagulation time in proportion to its concentration in the blood. These devices are reliable and precise for measuring heparin effect as against manual methods **(Fig. 18)**.

Activated Coagulation Time Testing—Modifications

The POC device (Hemachron®) has a precision aligned magnet within a test tube and a magnet detector located within the well. The whole blood is added to activator containing test tube (Celite®, Kaolin®, glass beads, or a combination of these) and put in the well. Once clot begins to form magnet is lifted within the tube and magnet gets displaced form magnet detector. The time clot takes to displace magnet at a given distance is CT.

Another device (Hemotec®) uses a two-chamber cartridge containing kaolin as an activator. In each chamber 0.4 mL blood is placed and a daisy-shaped plunger increases and decreases in the chamber. At the start of clot formation, the rate of descent of the plunger slows down and the decrease in velocity of the plunger is detected by a photo-optical system which signals the end of the test.

The hypothermia and hemodilution during CPB, the poor correlation with anti-Xa measures of heparin activity or concentration are the limiting factor. This is especially true of pediatric patients whose consumption of heparin is increased.

The thrombocytopenia, the presence of platelet inhibitors, platelet membrane receptor antagonists, and the use of the antifibrinolytic aprotinin (Celite® only) are factors altering ACT. The control of heparin anticoagulation and its reversal will reduce blood loss and transfusion requirements in patients undergoing CPB can be reduced.

Cascade Point-of-care System or Heparin Management Test

This uses a completely different technology for measuring the effect of heparin. Disposable cards with celite activator are used to measure heparin activity. This card contains paramagnetic iron oxide particles that move in response to an oscillating magnetic field. When clot formation occurs, movement of the iron oxide particles is decreased. The decreased movement of the particles is detected optically as the sample clots and the result is displayed as PT and as INR. For measuring PT, rabbit brain thromboplastin is used as the activator and for activated partial thromboplastin time (aPTT), aluminum magnesium silicate is used as the activator. Heparin management test (HMT) correlates well with anti-Xa heparin activity in CPB and is more superior to standard ACT.

Point-of-care Monitoring of Prothrombin Time/Activated Partial Thromboplastin Time/International Normalized Ratio (Figs. 19A to C)

Several instruments are available for measuring PT (in seconds) and INRs in specimens collected by capillary

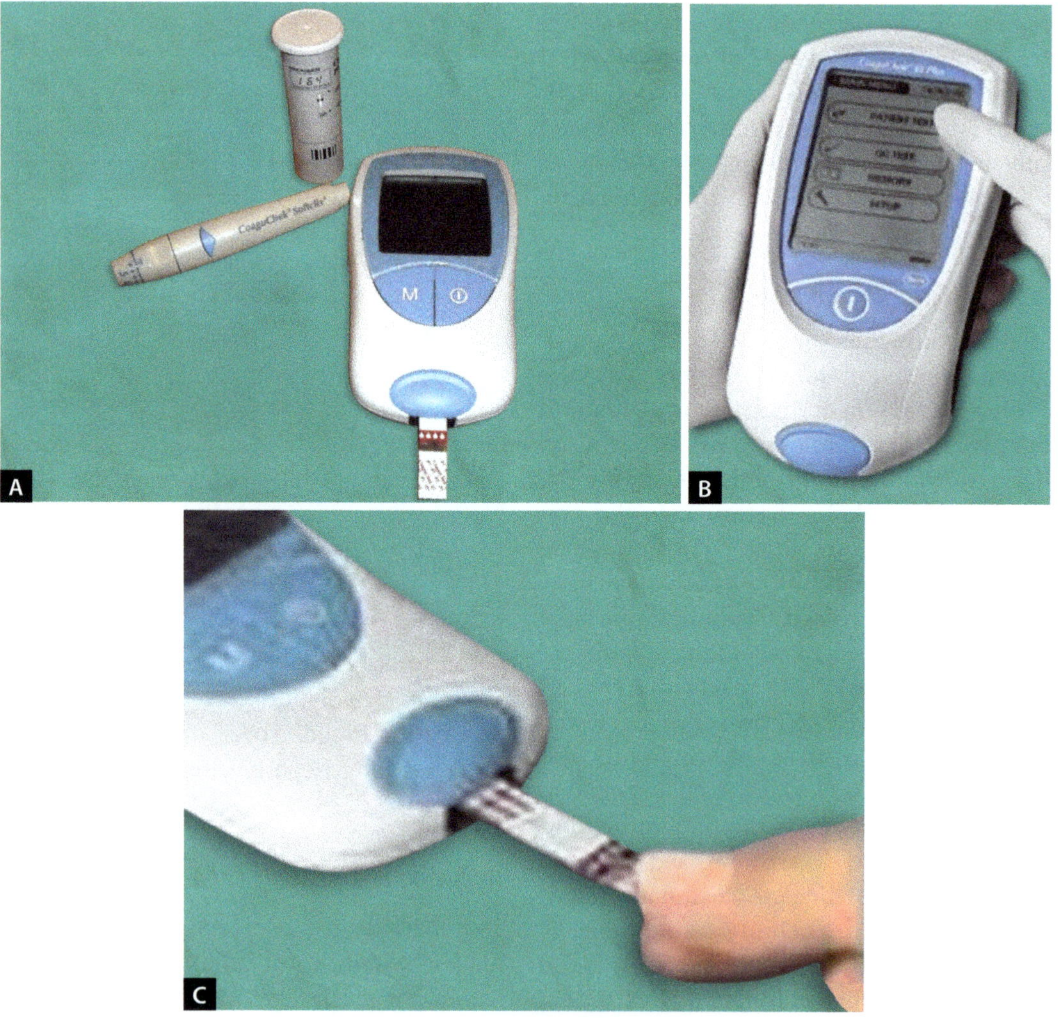

Figs. 19A to C: (A) Prothrombin time monitor; (B) Activated partial thromboplastin time monitor; (C) International normalized ratio monitor.

puncture especially the ones used at home. The control is run simultaneously with each specimen tested or digitalized controls are used by some devices. Performing the tests at home can help adjusting of oral anticoagulant dosages according to physician guidelines resulting in improved anticoagulation.

Current transfusion guidelines for blood-component therapy strongly recommend results of PT and aPTT to guide administration of fresh frozen plasma and cryoprecipitate.[24] Many decisions regarding transfusion of blood products are based on clinical judgment as results from central labs take time. The POCT may help therefore in reducing unnecessary transfusion of blood or its products.

Recently a laser-lancing device has been marketed. This POC monitor uses whole blood sample which is added to a test cartridge that contains a soybean activator and phospholipids. As the sample clots, a laser beam optically monitors the decrease in blood flow, and the resultant CT is displayed in seconds for PT and aPTT, and as a ratio for INR. A very important application of this POC device has been its use in transfusion algorithms to direct transfusion of fresh frozen plasma and platelets.

Whole-blood Point-of-care Analyzer's for Multiparametric Tests

This instrument can measure more than 25 different tests for every sample of blood. Currently available instruments require a small blood volume to perform a test—as little as 2.5 mL for a single measurement on a handheld glucose meter, or as little as 0.4 mL for 1 or 2 measurements, such as glucose and lactate, on a whole-blood analyzer. The analysis time can be as rapid as 15 seconds for a single measurement, or 45 seconds for a multiple parameter test. The latest whole-blood analyzers have the capability of selecting the tests needed thereby eliminating unnecessary tests, which can generate financial losses and waste patient blood.

CONCLUSION

The future will see more and more tests incorporated in POC technology with shorter analysis time, reduced sample volume and bidirectional connectivity of transportable, portable, and hand-held devices. Point-of-care testing undoubtedly will take a more active role in critical care and operation theaters. It will be used more for on-site diagnostic testing and trend monitoring of patient conditions. While POCT may not necessarily replace centralized laboratory testing, it is becoming an important modality for improving patient care and outcomes.

REFERENCES

1. Kost GJ. Goals, Guidelines and Principles for Point-of-Care Testing. Kost GJ (Ed). Principles & Practice of Point-Of-Care Testing, 1st edition. Hagerstwon: Lippincott Williams & Wilkins; 2002. pp. 3-12.
2. Louie RF, Tang Z, Shelby DG, et al. Point-of-care testing: millennium technology for critical care. Lab Med. 2000;31(7): 402-8.
3. England JM, Hyde K, Lewis SM, et al. Guidelines for near-patient testing: haematology. Cline Lab Haem. 1995;17:300-9.
4. Nkrumah B, Nguah SB, Adu-Sarkodie Y, et al. Hemoglobin estimation by the HemoCue® portable hemoglobin photometer in a resource poor setting. BMC Clin Pathol. 2011;11(5):9-15.
5. Paddle JJ. Evaluation of the haemoglobin colour scale and comparison with the hemocue haemoglobin assay. Bull World Health Organ. 2002;80(10):813-6.
6. Chedid C, Rahmani A, Durrani N, et al. Point of care measurement of hemoglobin and hematocrit in newborn infants using a blood gas analyzer. E J Neonatol Res. 2013;3(1):11-6.
7. Lamhaut L, Apriotesei R, Combes X, et al. Comparison of the accuracy of noninvasive hemoglobin monitoring by spectrophotometry (SpHb) and HemoCue® with automated laboratory hemoglobin measurement. Anesthesiology. 2011;115(3):548-54.
8. Lindnor G, Exadaktylos AK. How noninvasive haemoglobin measurement with pulse CO-oximetry can change your practice: an expert review. Emerg Med Int. 2013;2013:701529.
9. Dungan K, Chapman J, Braithwaite S, et al. Glucose measurement: confounding issues in setting targets for inpatient management. Diabetes Care. 2007;30:403-9.
10. Scott M, Bruns D, Boyd J, et al. Tight glucose control in the intensive care unit: are glucose meters up to the task. Clin Chem. 2008;55:18-20.
11. Rebel A, Rice MA, Fahy BG. The accuracy of point-of-care glucose measurements. J Diabetes Sci Technol. 2012;6(2):396-411.
12. Clarke SF, Foster JR. A history of blood glucose meters and their role in self-monitoring of diabetes mellitus. Br J Biomed Sci. 2012;69(2):83-93.
13. Al Ansary L, Farmwr A, Hirst J, et al. Point-of-care testing for HbA1c in the management of diabetes: a systematic review and meta-analysis. Clin Chem. 2011;57(4):568-76.
14. Zaloga GP, Roberts PR, Black K, et al. Hand-held blood gas analyzer is accurate in the critical care setting. Crit Care Med. 1996;24:957-62.
15. Engineer RS, Peacock WF. The use of blood gas analysis in point-of-care patient monitoring. US Resp Disease. 2011;7(2):70-5.
16. Mahutte CK, Sasse SA, Chen PA, et al. Performance of a patient-dedicated, on-demand blood gas monitor in medical ICU patients. Am J Respir Crit Care Med. 1994;150:865-9.
17. Roupie EE. Equipment review: continuous assessment of arterial blood. Crit Care. 1997;1(1):11-4.
18. Barker S, Hyatt J. Continuous measurement of intra-arterial pH, $PaCO_2$ and PaO_2 in the operating room. Anesth Analg. 1991;73: 43-8.
19. Crowley MP. Point-of-Care Testing in the Operating Room. In: Sandberg W, Urman R, Ehrenfeld J (Eds). MGH Textbook of Anesthetic Equipment, 1st edition. Philadelphia: Saunders Elsevier; 2011. pp. 271-82.
20. Glover DB. Understanding blood lactate testing and lactate threshold. [online] Available from www.enduranceworks.net/blog/226. [Last accessed April, 2021].
21. Meybohm P, Zacharowski K. Point-of-care coagulation management in intensive care medicine. Ann Update Intensive Care Emergency Med. 2013:397-412.
22. Thakur M, Ahmed AB. A review of thromboelastography. Int J Periop Ultrasound Applied Technol. 2012;1(1):25-9.
23. Practical-Haemostasis. Activated Clotting Time (ACT). [online] Available from http://www.practical-haemostasis.com. [Last accessed April, 2021].
24. National Committee for Clinical Laboratory Standards. Point-of-care monitoring of anticoagulation therapy; approved guideline. Wayne: Clinical and Laboratory Standards Institute; 2004.

Equipment for Central Neuraxial and Regional Blocks

SECTION 7

Spinal, Epidural, and Combined Spinal-Epidural Anesthesia

Manjari S Muzoomdar, Preeti G More

ABSTRACT

Over the years regional anesthesia with central neuraxial blockade has gained widespread popularity and is commonly used nowadays. Hence, a knowledge of the various techniques to achieve these blocks and needles and catheters used for administering spinal, epidural, or combined spinal-epidural anesthesia is required for a safe and effective central neuraxial blockade. This chapter describes in detail the techniques and the equipment involved in central neuraxial block.

INTRODUCTION

The history of spinal anesthesia (SA) starts way back from the late 1800s. August Bier is credited with administering first spinal anesthetic in 1898. In the course of the last century, materials, diameters and tip geometries of spinal cannulas have been revised and changed. Spinal needles are available in various sizes [from 16 gauge (G) to 30 G], lengths, bevels and tip designs. The sharp cutting with end injection (Quincke's) needle was refined with noncutting blunt (pencil) tipped needles by Whitacre in 1951. These disposable, pencil point with lateral orifice just proximal to the tip of spinal cannulas markedly decreased the incidence of postdural puncture headache (PDPH).

Then came the technique of continuous SA using indwelling spinal catheters. Smaller gauge catheters came in use in 1960s and microcatheters as small as 32 G appeared in the late 1980s. The alleged association of spinal microcatheters with cauda equina syndrome led the Food and Drug Administration (FDA) to prohibit their use in sizes of 27G or smaller.

Epidural anesthesia (EA) was described first in 1921 by Fidel Pagés and again in 1931 by Achille Dogliotti. In 1945, Tuohy introduced the curved tip needle which is still the most commonly used. Disposable epidural sets with catheters are used for continuous epidural techniques in surgery, obstetrics, labor analgesia and postoperative pain control. Sethna and Berde used 5 cm, 19 G, epidural needles for infants and younger children.

Later interests in combining the fast onset of action of intrathecal drugs with the flexibility of continuous EA led to the technique of combined spinal-epidural anesthesia (CSEA). Several manufacturers started marketing combination sets of epidural and spinal needles. Today this technique is being extensively used for all major surgical, orthopedic, plastic, and gynecological procedures and labor analgesia.

CENTRAL NEURAXIAL BLOCKS

The regional blocks involving the spinal (subarachnoid), epidural and caudal spaces are called central neuraxial blocks (CNBs). While they are now an invaluable form of anesthesia and occasionally even an adjunct to general anesthesia (GA), their use is not a new phenomenon.

Excluding the obvious fact that the surgical conditions primarily dictate the type of anesthesia to be given, most operations below the neck can be performed under CNB.

Advantages of Central Neuraxial Blocks[1]

- A decrease in postoperative morbidity and sometimes even in mortality.
- A reduction in the incidence of venous thrombosis and pulmonary embolism
- A decrease in blood transfusion requirement
- A reduction in the incidence of respiratory compromise following thoracic and upper abdominal surgery
- A decreased stress response with positive cardiac benefits such as reduced perioperative and postoperative ischemia.

Despite these proposed advantages of CNB, adverse reactions and complications can occur. These can range from self-limited back soreness to permanent neurological deficits and even death.

SPINAL ANESTHESIA

SPINAL NEEDLES

History

Corning (1885): Leonard Corning is considered the precursor of SA.[2] In 1885, he performed lumbar puncture (LP) in dogs using cocaine. His needle **(Fig. 1)**[3] was made of a flexible material with an introducer and a limiter to keep

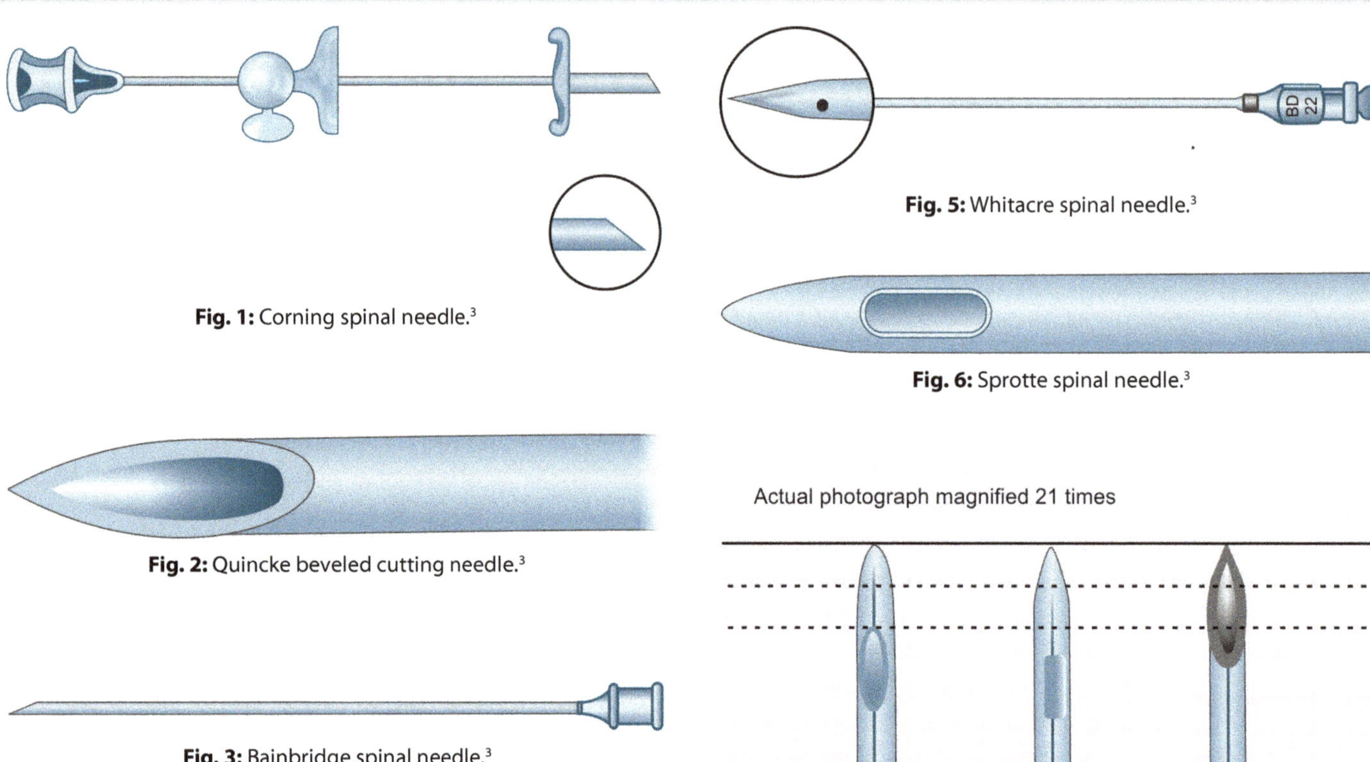

Fig. 1: Corning spinal needle.[3]

Fig. 2: Quincke beveled cutting needle.[3]

Fig. 3: Bainbridge spinal needle.[3]

Fig. 4: Greene atraumatic needle.[3]

Fig. 5: Whitacre spinal needle.[3]

Fig. 6: Sprotte spinal needle.[3]

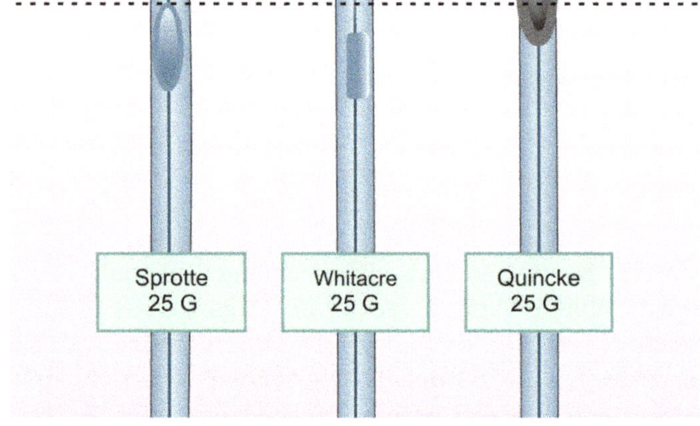

Fig. 7: Sprotte, Whitacre, and Quincke spinal needles.[3]

the equipment fixed whilst approaching to the subarachnoid space. The tip of the needle had a short and sharp bevel.

Quincke (1891): Heinrich Irenaeus Quincke, German physician, demonstrated technique of LP by beveled cutting needle **(Fig. 2)** for drainage of cerebrospinal fluid (CSF) in patients with intracranial hypertension.

Bier (1898): He demonstrated the first spinal anesthetic on himself and suffered from PDPH.[2]

Bainbridge (1900): American physician who described and published a subarachnoid puncture needle **(Fig. 3)** that he used for spinal analgesia in children in 1900.

Greene (1926): He described the use of an "atraumatic needle with thin end" **(Fig. 4)**. This form of needle tip was able to pass between the dural fibers rather than through them. Hence, reported incidence of PDPH was less than 4%.

Whitacre (1951): Whitacre developed conical pointed needles described as "resembling a sharpened pencil" and a distal side orifice next to it. They were popularly called "pencil point needles" **(Fig. 5)**.

In 1950, Whitacre became president of the American Society of Anesthesiologists (ASA).[4]

The Whitacre needle is one of the most currently used for spinal and mostly used in obstetric patients.

After the 1960s emerged the disposable needles, they reduced the chances of contamination caused by residues of detergents and other cleaning solutions used in reusable needles thus reducing serious neurological deficits secondary to SA.

Sprotte (1987): He modified the Whitacre needle into an elongated tip in an attempt to promote a more gradual separation of the dural fibers with a large lateral oval orifice **(Figs. 6 and 7)**.

Design

The standard spinal needle consists of three parts: (1) a hub, (2) cannula ending in a tip, and (3) a stylet **(Fig. 8)**. The stylet is removable and occludes the distal lumen and tip of the cannula.

The tip has a bevel. The tips of the cannulas usually are made of stainless steel and must meet the standards of stiffness, flexibility and resistance to breakage.

Spinal needles come in:
- *Various sizes (from 16 G to 30 G):* The luminal size of the cannula decreases as the size of the needle increases. Hence, bigger the gauge finer the needle and less chances of PDPH
- *Various lengths:* 3½–4 inches (8–10 cm) and 15 cm in obese patients.

They can have sharp or blunt tip with either end injection or side injection and either sharp or blunt bevel edges.

The Quincke-Babcock needle is considered to be the standard spinal needle. It has a small hub, medium bevel length with sharp edges, a sharp tip and end injection. The hub has a Luer-lock connector.

Other needles **(Figs. 9A to D)** available are:
- *Pitkin needle:* Short, sharp bevel and pointed end injection. The stylet also has a short bevel and fits the tip of the cannula
- *Greene needle:* It has a small hub and a Luer-lock connector. There are rounded, noncutting edges to the bevel which is of medium length. The stylet has a rounded tip to fill the opening point of the cannula. The tip has a pencil point with noncutting edges of the bevel which separates rather than cut the dural fibers
- *Whitacre needle:* This is also pencil-pointed needle having a rounded tip, no cutting edges, and the orifice is on one side of the cannula about 2.5 mm proximal to the tip of the cannula with a fitted stylet
  - These Greene and Whitacre needles as they are pencil point, they separate the dural fibers instead of cutting them, thereby reducing the size of the dural puncture, which causes less CSF leak, reduces the incidence of PDPH
- *Quincke needle:* For pediatric use, size—22 G and 25 G (2.25–3.5 cm).

Commonly used disposable Quincke, Whitacre, or Sprotte spinal needles are available in diameters from 22 G to 29 G.[5]

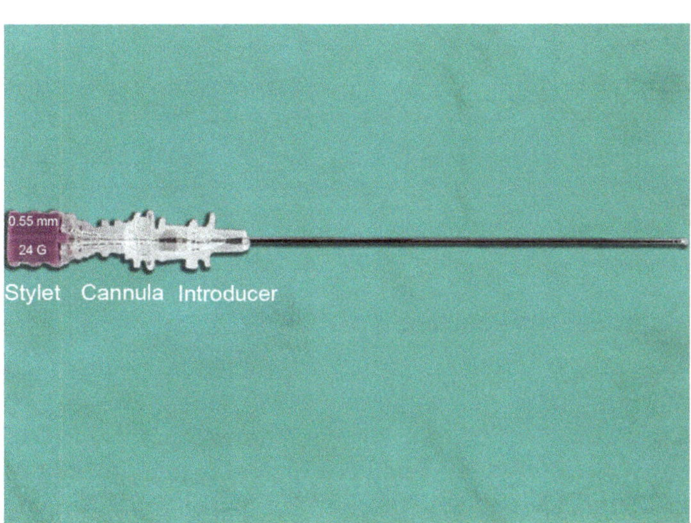

Fig. 8: Sprotte spinal needle with introducer.

SPINAL INTRODUCERS

- They are used for the introduction of fine spinal needles
- They avoid bending and breaking of fine spinal needles
- There are less chances of infection from skin and subcutaneous tissue entering via the tip of fine spinal needles.

Types of Introducers

- Sise introducer—2 inches length (In 1910, Lincoln F Sise invented it)
- Corning introducer
- Lundy introducer.

SPINAL CATHETERS

History

- In 1907, Dean performed continuous SA by leaving spinal needle *in situ*
- In 1940, Lemmon devised an apparatus for continuous SA6
- In 1944, Tuohy introduced no. 4 ureteral catheter through 15 G needle intrathecally

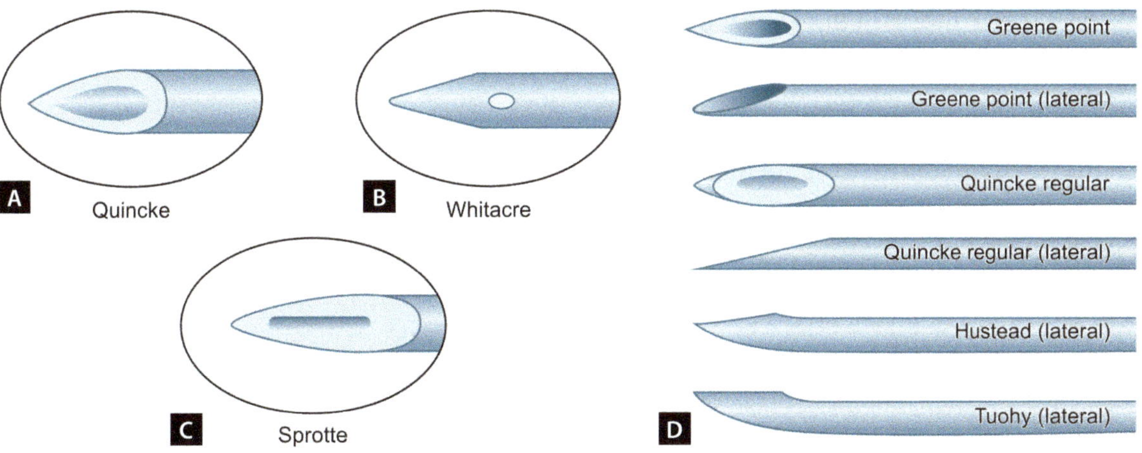

Figs. 9A to D: Various spinal needles.[3,6]

- Continuous SA gained popularity in 1980s with the development of microcatheters (29–32 G)[7]
- In 1987, Hurley reported their use of a 32 G, 36-inch polyamide catheter through a 26 G needle.[6] They are used to give continuous SA
- Portex set made available with size 23 G needle and micro-catheter of 28 G
- Continuous SA set (Intra Long set with Sprotte special cannula) from Pajunk (Germany)
    - Permits controlled guidance of the cannula
    - Rounded edges of the lateral orifice of the cannula prevents catheter cut off
    - Available gauges: Cannula: 21 G, 22 G
      Catheter: 90 cm.

INDICATIONS FOR SPINAL ANESTHESIA

- In lower abdominal, inguinal, urogenital, rectal, gynecological, and lower extremity surgeries
- Obstetrics—cesarean sections.

CONTRAINDICATIONS

Absolute[8,9]

- Patients refusal
- Significant coagulopathy
- Raised intracranial pressure (ICP)
- Infection at the site of puncture
- Valvular heart diseases (severe stenotic or ventricular outflow tract obstruction)
- Severe untreated hypovolemia.

Relative

- Surgical scars
- Spinal deformities (Scoliosis)
- Sepsis
- Neurological deficits or demyelinating diseases
- Uncooperative patient.

Controversial

- Major blood loss
- Previous spinal surgery at the site of injection.

TECHNIQUE OF SPINAL ANESTHESIA[10] (VIDEO 12)

It is difficult to teach a technique by describing it. Only through experience one can obtain a "feel" for the technique. We shall however cover some important and practical points that will be helpful when administering spinal anesthetics.

Preparation

- Explain the procedure in short to the patient. Explain to him the risk and benefit of SA/EA versus GA, sensory and motor block, its reversibility, etc.
- The patient should be attached to the standard monitors including electrocardiogram, noninvasive blood pressure (NIBP), and pulse oximetry. Record an initial set of vital signs
- Secure an intravenous (IV) access with a large bore needle (20 G/18 G) and preload or coload the patient with 1–1.5 L of crystalloid IV solution, depending upon the cardiac, pulmonary and renal status of the patient. Now the patient is ready to receive the spinal anesthetic.

Position for Spinal Injection

There are three positions used for administration of SA:

1. *Lateral decubitus:* Patient is positioned with his back parallel to the long side of the operation theater (OT) table. Thighs are flexed up and neck is flexed forward (foetal position). Patient should be positioned (i.e., head low/head high) to take the advantage of the baricity of the spinal LA in determining the height of the block **(Fig. 10)**.
2. *Sitting:* The patient should be sitting up with his back parallel to the long side of the OT table and his feet supported on a stool (like sitting on a chair). Patient should sit up straight not swaying or slumping to the side, his head flexed, upper arms hugging a pillow over the chest **(Fig. 11)**. Patient should not simply lean forward, he should arch his back to resemble the letter "C". This will maximize the "opening" of the vertebral interspaces **(Fig. 12)**.
3. *Prone:* The prone position is used when the patient will be in this position for the surgical procedure (i.e., rectal, perineal, lumbar procedures). Hypobaric LAs are administered. Patient positions self, lumbar lordosis should be minimized, a paramedian approach is often used.

Projection and Puncture

After proper positioning, the back should be painted and draped. Under sterile measures, feel for the landmarks. A horizontal line drawn between the superior borders of either iliac crests corres-ponds to either L4 vertebral body or L4-L5 interspace **(Figs. 13A and B)**. It may be challenging to palpate these landmarks in the obese or in those with abnormal anatomical curvatures of the spine.

By proper positioning you should have an access to L2-L3, L3-L4, L4-L5, and L5-S1 interspaces.

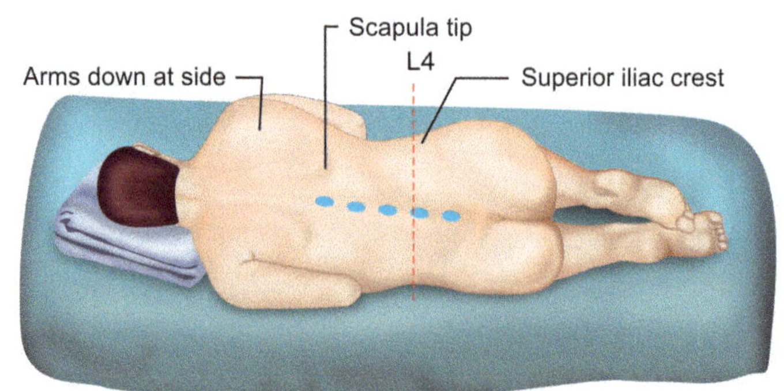

Fig. 10: Lateral decubitus position.

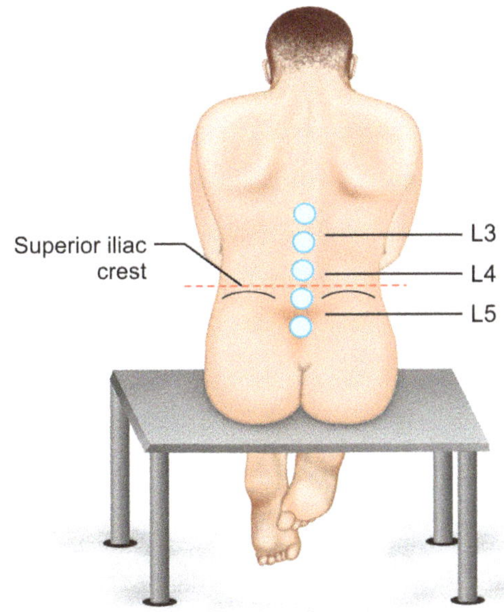

Fig. 11: Sitting position.

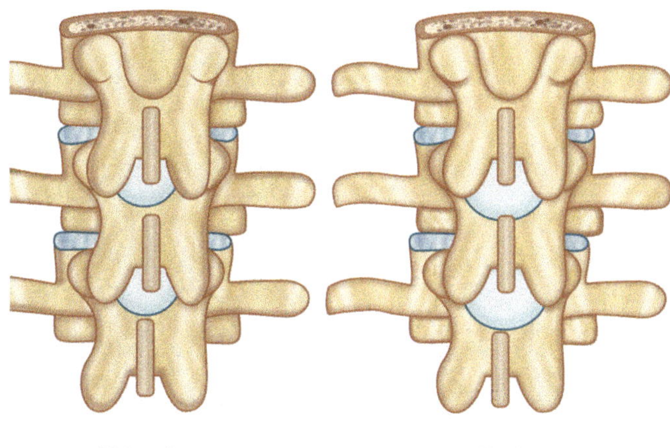

Fig. 12: Extension of the back narrows the intervertebral spaces while flexion of the back opens up or widens the intervertebral spaces.

There are two approaches for accessing the subarachnoid space: (1) the midline and (2) the paramedian approach.

Midline Approach

It offers two advantages:

Anatomic projection is only in two planes, making visualization of the intended trajectory and anatomical structures more apparent. It also provides a relatively avascular plane.

Identify the interspinous ligament in the midline and note the extent of the space cephalad and caudad by feeling the upper and lower spinous processes **(Figs. 14A and B)**.

After local infiltration, introduce the spinal needle in the mid space in 15–20° cephalad direction with bevel parallel to the longitudinal fibers of dura. This helps to reduce cutting of the fibers and enhances tactile sensation as anatomical structures are crossed. Slowly advance the needle. The structures pierced by the spinal needle en route while locating the subarachnoid space from dorsal to ventral are:

- Skin
- Subcutaneous tissue
- Supraspinous ligament
- Interspinous ligament
- Ligamentum flavum
- Epidural space
- Dura.

As the ligamentum flavum and dura are traversed, there will be a distinct "give way" or a "pop" felt for each.

After the second "give way" of dura, the needle is in the subarachnoid space. Now remove the stylet and CSF should appear. One may rotate the spinal needle by 90° in such a way that the bevel becomes cephalad.

- If CSF is not obtained, then assess the needle position and depth. Being off midline is one of the commonest reasons for CSF not coming out. If off midline, remove

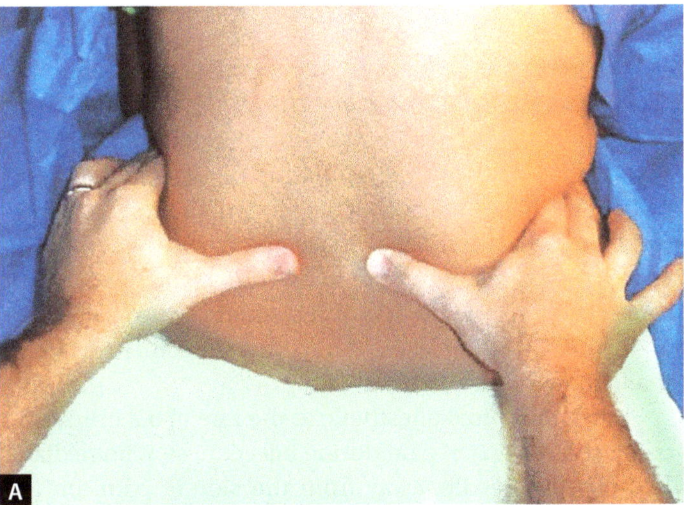

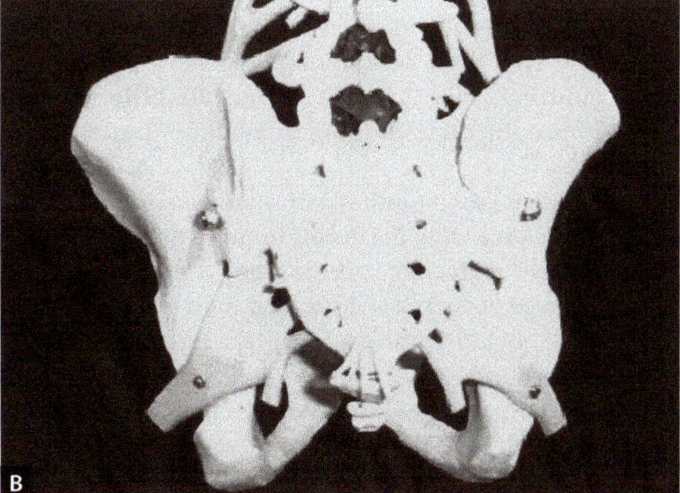

Figs. 13A and B: "Tuffier's" line is a line drawn across the iliac crest that crosses the body of L4 or L4–L5 interspace. This is a helpful landmark for the placement of spinal or epidural anesthetics.

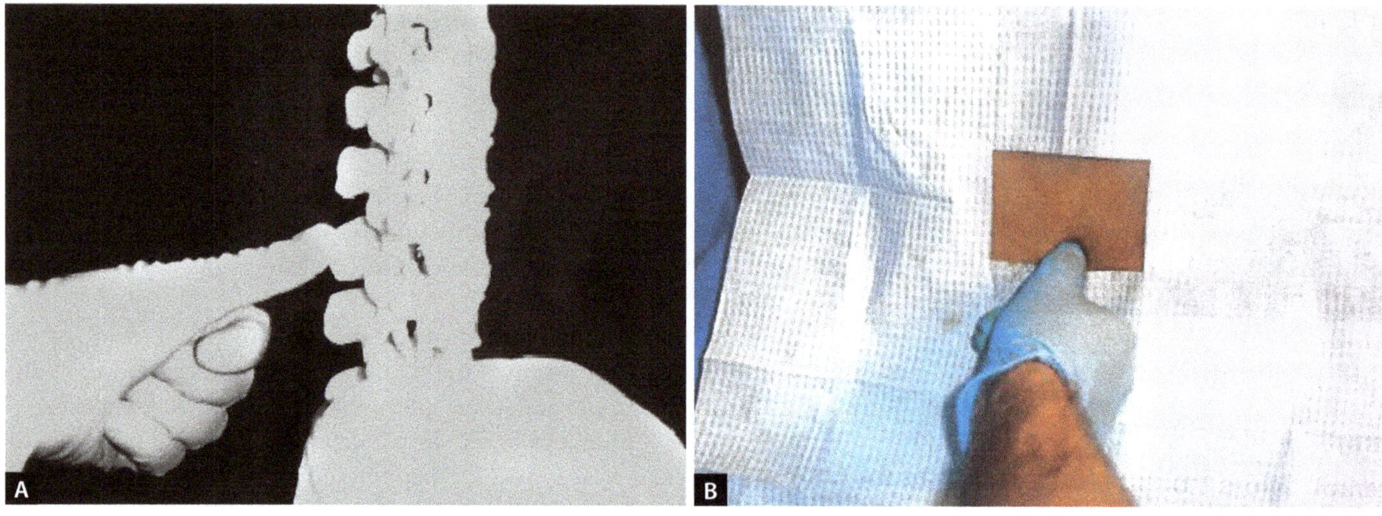

Figs. 14A and B: Palpation of spinous process and intervertebral space.

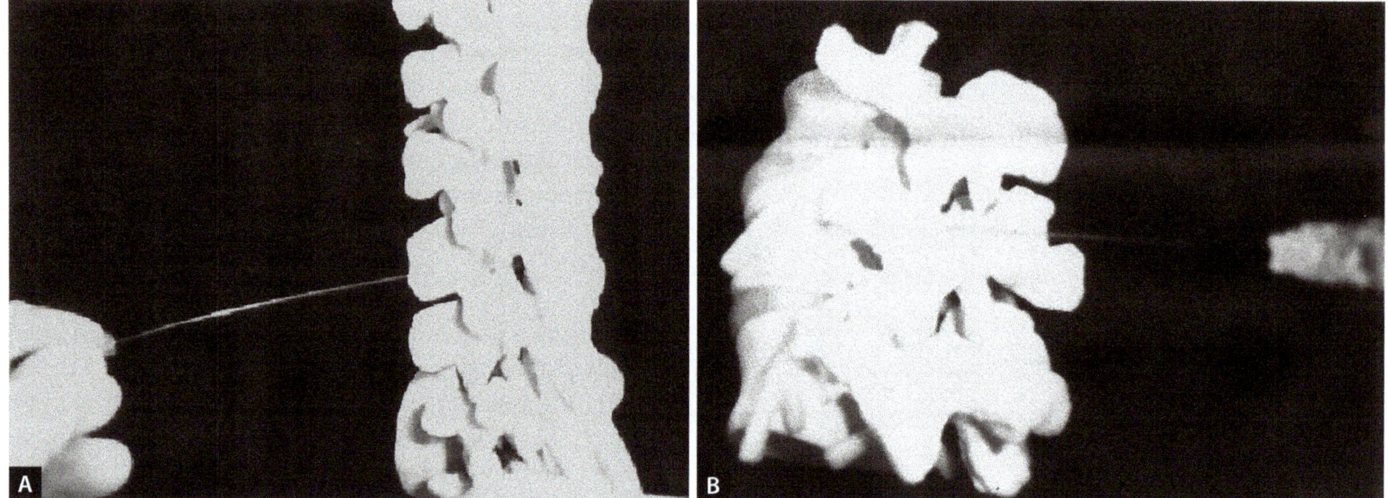

Figs. 15A and B: The spinal needle contacting the spinous processes and the lamina.

the needle and start all over again. The subarachnoid space is about 4–6 cm deep from the skin. So if the needle is not adequately deep, advance the needle further.

- If blood appears from the spinal needle, wait to see if it clears. If it does not clear, reassess the needle position. If the needle is in midline, it could have punctured the epidural vein. Advance the needle little further to traverse the dura, or if not in midline, start all over again
- If the patient gets paresthesia or sharp pain in thigh and legs while advancing the needle, remove the needle and start all over again. If the needle is not in vertical midline and mid-space, then it is not uncommon to encounter a nerve root. Before starting again, make sure that the pain has stopped.
- If bone is encountered, reassess the patient's position and ensure that the needle is in vertical midline and mid-space. If bone is contacted immediately after insertion of needle, the needle may be contacting the spinous process **(Fig. 15A)**. Move the needle slightly caudad. If bone is contacted after further advancement of the needle, the needle may be contacting the lamina of the vertebra **(Fig. 15B)**. Move the needle slightly cephalad. Moving down an interspace may increase the chances of success since the inter vertebral spaces will be larger.

Once the CSF returns, steady the needle and attach the syringe with spinal anesthetic. Gently aspirate CSF into the syringe. You should be able to get good free aspiration of about to ¾ mL of CSF; aspiration of just about a drop of CSF is not enough, as even if the bevel of the spinal needle is partly in the subarachnoid space and partly in the subdural space, you may still be able to aspirate just a little CSF. But then only part of the spinal anesthetic will be deposited in the subarachnoid space and therefore this SA will be inadequate.

Inject the spinal anesthetic at the rate of 0.2 mL/s. If the patient complains of pain during injection, stop immediately. Redirect the needle, away from the side of pain and into the midline. Once the injection is over, place the patient in supine position.

Paramedian Approach

The advantage of the paramedian approach is that by placing the needle laterally the anatomical limitation of the spinous process is avoided. If the puncture is made too far from the midline, then lamina is encountered.

Insert the spinal needle 1 cm laterally from the midline in the line of the mid space 10–15° off the sagittal plane. If the needle is inserted too far cephalad then lamina is encountered. If bone is contacted then redirect the needle little caudad.

As you advance the needle, you will feel the characteristic "give way" or "pop" of dura. With the lateral approach, the needle is inserted further than with the midline approach.

Once CSF is obtained, continue in the same manner as the midline approach.

Monitoring

After successful placement of spinal anesthetic, the patient should be monitored for:

- *Block progression and its complications:* After the LA is injected in the SA space, the LA gets mixed with the CSF and then gets attached to the neural tissue. Once all the LA gets attached to the neural tissue, the spinal anesthesia is fixed and the height of the block is finalized. The time for fixing is different for different local anesthetics. For bupivacaine, it is about 5–7 minutes.
  The Autonomic fibers being thinnest, are blocked first, then the sensory and the motor fibers are last to get blocked. The progression of the autonomic blockade is seen in the form of hypotension and bradycardia. The progression of sensory block can be checked by gently pinching the patient, starting from the lower limbs upwards. The progression of motor blockade can be checked by asking the patient to move lower extremities. Gradually the power in the lower limbs will become zero. The autonomic blockade is about 2 segments/dermatomes higher while the motor blockade is about 2 dermatomes lower than the level of sensory block.
- *Hemodynamics, i.e., blood pressure (BP), pulse rate:* Hypotension is almost inevitable after the spinal injection is done. To prevent or minimize the drop in bp after the spinal injection, preloading/coloading is recommended. IV fluids should be given fast after the injection to correct hypotension. If hypotension is associated with bradycardia which may occur a little later as a result of block progressing upwards and blocking cardiac sympathetic, then IV Atropine or Glycopyrrolate is recommended. One may need to inject vasopressors like phenylephrine (alpha 1 agonist) or ephedrine (alpha 1 and beta agonist) to maintain preload and cardiac output and thus the bp.
  Hypotension is far more pronounced in a patient who is on multiple antihypertensive drugs as compared to a patient who is on no such drugs. The decrease in the preload caused by the calcium channel blockers, the nitrates, and the α1-blockers; the contracted intravascular volume because of the diuretics; the bradycardia with the beta-blockers and the reduction in the afterload caused by the angiotensin-converting enzyme (ACE) inhibitors and angiotensin receptor blockers (ARBs), coupled with the sympathetic blockade caused by the SA can cause a precipitous drop in BP and pulse rate and therefore these patients need a greater amount of IV fluids to maintain BP as compared to nonhypertensives receiving no antihypertensive medicines.
- *Problems with breathing:* If the spinal anesthesia blocks the upper thoracic dermatomes, the intercostal muscles can be paralyzed and the patient may experience difficulty in breathing. The FiO_2 can be increased by using supplemental oxygen via nasal cannula or a face mask. The O_2 saturation should be monitored continuously. A watch on the pattern of respiration (whether the accessory muscles are working or the respiratory rate is increased) can be useful in assessing the severity of the problem.
  Usually the dyspnea settles after a while, once the spinal is fixed. The cervical roots are rarely paralyzed, so the phrenic nerves are spared.
- *Sensorium:* Usually after the spinal anesthesia, the patient is alert and co-operative. If the hypotension and/or bradycardia is very profound then patient may become drowsy for a while, but once the BP and/or pulse rate settles, the patient regains alertness. If any opioid is injected as an additive along with the LA in the SA space then the patient may feel sleepy or drowsy.

Factors Affecting Height of Spinal/Epidural Anesthesia

- *Age:* Height of block achieved is higher in older patients.
- *Height:* Height of block achieved is higher in shorter patients.
- *Volume injected:* Height of block achieved is higher with larger volume injected.
- *Interspace selected:* Height of block achieved is higher with upper or higher interspace.
- *Speed of injection:* Height of block achieved is higher with faster rate of injection. Barbotage while injecting can also achieve higher height of the block.
- *Position of the patient during injection:* Height of block achieved is higher in lateral decubitus position than sitting position.
- *Position of the patient after injection:* Height of block achieved is higher in head low position as the solution in the epidural space and SA space (hyperbaric) will flow under the effect of gravity. The hypobaric solution in the SA space will flow in the reverse direction.
- *Engorgement of epidural veins (gravid uterus, large intra-abdominal tumours compressing IVC), large amount of epidural fat, epidural catheter:* Height of block achieved is higher if any of these is present in epidural space.

DEVELOPMENT OF A DIFFICULTY SCORE FOR SPINAL ANESTHESIA[11]

Multiple attempts at spinal puncture may be hazardous. Accurate preoperative prediction of difficulty adds to the delivery of high quality care. So certain difficulty predictors for SA have been recognized and a grading system with scores has been devised. If every patient is assessed preoperatively and then stratified into categories of the grading system and then given scores, the anesthesiologist will exactly know whether he is dealing with an easy or difficult block. The age of the patient, body mass index (BMI), spinal bony landmarks, spinal bony deformity and radiological characteristics of lumbar vertebrae are the predictors of difficulty. The spinous processes of lumbar vertebrae (spinal bony landmarks) are assigned as easily palpable (clear) or difficult to palpate (unclear); spinal bony deformities include kyphosis, scoliosis and lordosis. Difficult radiological characteristics of the lumbar vertebrae include osteophytes, ligament calcification and narrow intervertebral spaces. Score of 4 is the difficulty score at or above which difficulty is expected. Spinal bony landmarks and radiological characteristics of the lumbar vertebrae are independent predictors of difficulty during SA.

This grading and scoring system for predicting difficulty in spinal block can be easily used for predicting difficulty in epidural block as well **(Table 1)**.

COMPLICATIONS OF SPINAL ANESTHESIA[10,12]

Though rare, complications of SA can be troublesome. They range from transient neurologic symptoms to cauda equina syndrome to backache.

- Nausea/vomiting
- Postdural puncture headache
- Neurological (cauda equina syndrome, anterior spinal artery syndrome)
- Meningitis
- Retention of urine
- Paralysis of 6th cranial nerve
- Subdural block.

Postdural Puncture Headache

Although not life-threatening, PDPH carries substantial morbidity by restricting activities of daily life. It occurs because of leak of CSF from dural puncture with resultant loss of CSF pressure, gravitational traction of brain structures and painful neurovascular response from meninges. Spontaneous resolution of PDPH takes 1–6 weeks.

Postdural puncture headache is common in:

- Young age
- Patients with lesser BMI
- Female gender
- Pregnancy and labor
- Patients with history of recurrent headaches
- Patients with history of previous PDPH.

Postdural puncture headache is:

- Less with fine pencil point spinal needles
- More common in young adults[13] and decreases with increasing age
- Less with use of small diameter spinal needles and with noncutting tips.[2]

Factors contributing to headache after LP are:

- Needle size
- Direction of bevel
- Needle design
- Number of LP attempts.[13]

The noninvasive treatment of PDPH is with bed rest, fluids, analgesics, caffeine and sumatriptan whereas the invasive treatment is epidural blood patch.

Since no effective noninvasive treatment for PDPH exists, we need to concentrate on prophylactic reduction of CSF loss after dural puncture:

- By using small gauge pencil point needles
- By turning cutting bevels longitudinally so that the longitudinal dural fibers are separated and not cut.

Subdural Block[14]

This is a little less recognized complication of SA and EA but not so uncommon. The subdural space is a narrow potential space between the dura and the arachnoid containing a minute amount of serous fluid. It extends into the cranial cavity throughout the distribution of meninges, covering all neural structures. The arachnoid is loosely attached to the dura at certain points where there are a few intercellular joints; so iatrogenic separation of this cellular plane can

TABLE 1: Grading and scoring system for predicting difficulty in spinal block.

Gas	*Scores*			
	0	*1*	*2*	*3*
Age (year)	20–40	41–60	>60	–
Body mass index (kg/m × m)	<22	22–27	>27–34	>34
Spinal bony landmarks	Clear	Unclear	–	–
Spinal bony deformity	No	Yes	–	–
Radiological characteristics of lumbar vertebrae	Easy	Difficult	–	–

A score of ≥4 will be a difficult spinal block

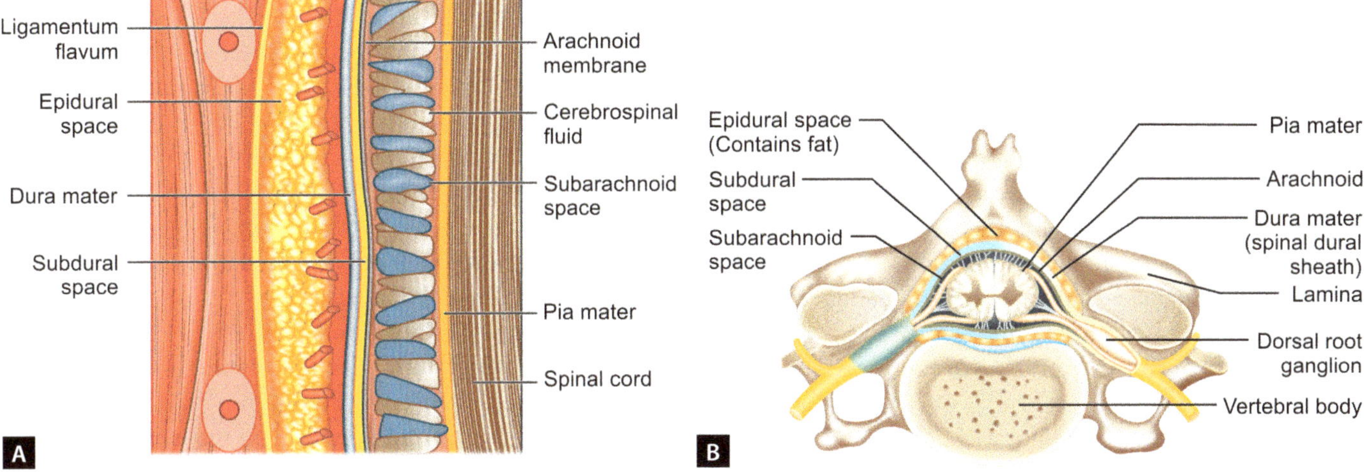

Figs. 16A and B: Subdural space.

occur on application of pressure by mechanical forces such as air or fluid injection or advancing spinal needle.

During subarachnoid anesthesia, the dura mater is intentionally pierced, with the subdural space being traversed before piercing the arachnoid **(Fig. 16A)**. Therefore, the chances of placing the needle in the subdural space with SA may be higher than with the EA. The long-beveled needles used for subarachnoid block may further increase the chance of subdural placement as part of the bevel could be placed in the subarachnoid space and part of it could be in subdural space **(Figs. 16A and B)**. However, some authors believe that subdural localization is more likely with an epidural needle, as the comparatively blunt epidural needle may pierce dura without piercing the arachnoid **(Figs. 16A and B)**.

The predisposing factors for accidental subdural block are:
- Rough handling and rotation of the epidural needle in the epidural space.
- Difficult block
- History of previous spine and back surgery
- History of recent lumber puncture

The clinical presentation may often be attributed to other causes.

The characteristics of the subdural injection are:
- Gradual and delayed onset (10–30 minutes)
- High and extensive sensory block, sometimes even involving the cranial nerves due to extension of subdural space into the cranium.
- The height of sensory block is disproportionate to the volume of LA injected.
- Often the sympathetic and motor fibers are spared.
- Hypotension may occur but is less than that with spinal.
- In worst case scenario, with large volumes of LA injected in subdural space, there can be intracranial tracking of LA leading to respiratory depression, dyspnea with desaturation and loss of consciousness.

The subdural block usually lasts for 2 hours followed by a complete recovery.

Several considerations should be made to minimize unintentional and unrecognized subdural injection.
- Anesthesiologist should be careful when handling Tuohy needle in the epidural space.
- Difficult blocks and previous spine surgery are predisposing factors of accidental subdural injection.
- Once dura is punctured fully or partly with Tuohy needle, it is advisable to choose another interspace if neuraxial block is required.
- During continuous epidural catheter technique, every top up should be given in fractionated manner, as per usual safe practice
- Single orifice catheter is preferable to multiple orifices catheter.

Anesthesiologist should have a high index of suspicion and should be aware of the presentation of subdural block so that it can be diagnosed and managed in time.

USES OF CONTINUOUS SPINAL ANESTHESIA

- Prolonged duration of surgeries under SA.
- All orthopedic, urogenital, perineal, rectal, lower abdominal, and pelvic surgeries.

Advantages

- Profound surgical anesthesia
- In old high-risk patients as small titrated doses of LAs required
- Less systemic toxic effects
- Duration of anesthesia can be prolonged
- Postoperative analgesia with intrathecal opioids.

Complications

- Accidental removal
- Adhesive arachnoiditis
- Infection
- Bleeding
- Neurological (transient neurological syndrome, cauda equina syndrome).[5,6]

EPIDURAL ANESTHESIA

EPIDURAL NEEDLES

History

- *Corning (1901):* First described the epidural space[6]
- *Fidel Pagés (1921):* First used EA in humans[15]
- *Tuohy (1945):* Edward Boyce Tuohy a prominent American anesthesiologist, designed a curved bevel needle tip.[2] This facilitated the introduction of catheters in the epidural space, either cephalic or caudal direction
- Tuohy epidural needle **(Fig. 17)** is most used worldwide to perform punctures and introduction of epidural catheters[15]
- *Curbelo (1949):* Curbelo, Cuban anesthesiologist, was the first to insert a catheter in the epidural space[15]
- *Philip Bromage (1961):* Philip Bromage established conti-nuous epidural technique
- *Sprotte (1989):* He implemented the technique of continuous epidural by conical tip needles. He added a plastic edge to the inner distal face of its needle in order to direct the catheter through the lateral orifice. The needle is conventionally called the Special Sprotte Needle **(Fig. 18)**. Note in the first of it the dashed line corresponding to the distribution of this plastic piece
- Epidural needles are also available as atraumatic conical tip needles similar to that suggested by Sprotte **(Figs. 19 and 20)**
- The epidural needles are designed to allow the passage of epidural catheters through them
- Tuohy needle **(Figs. 21 and 22)** has:
  - A hub which may be without wings or with wings for better control during insertion
  - A shaft with 1 cm markings to measure the depth of the epidural space
  - Tip with a blunt bevel having a curve at 15–30° through which passes the epidural catheter at an angle and not straight hitting dura or spinal canal
  - A plastic stylet.

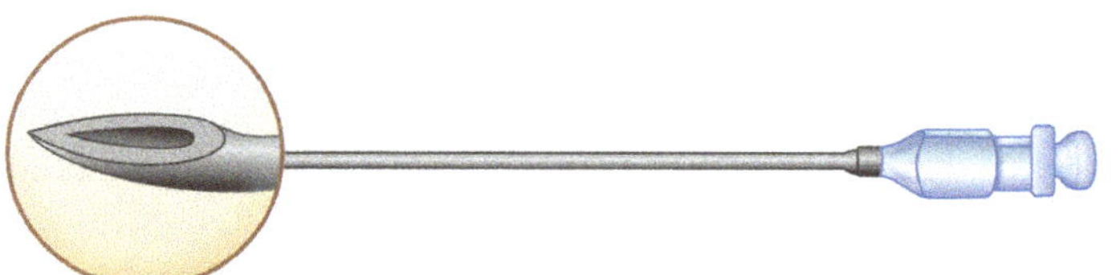

Fig. 17: Tuohy epidural needle.[3]

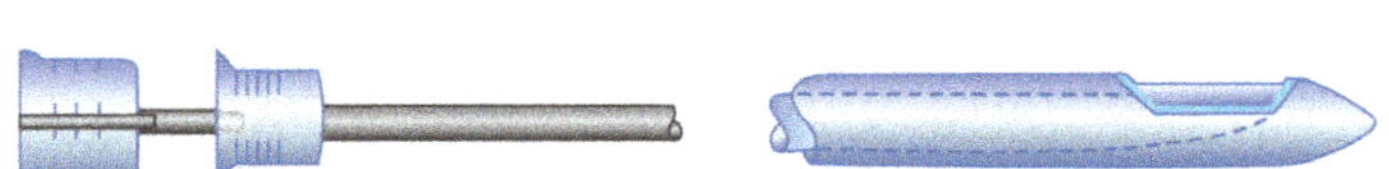

Fig. 18: Special Sprotte needle.[3]

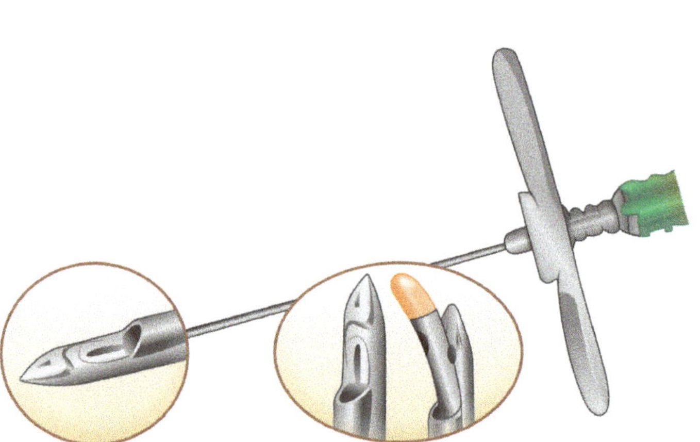

Fig. 19: Sprotte epidural needle (tip with catheter).[3]

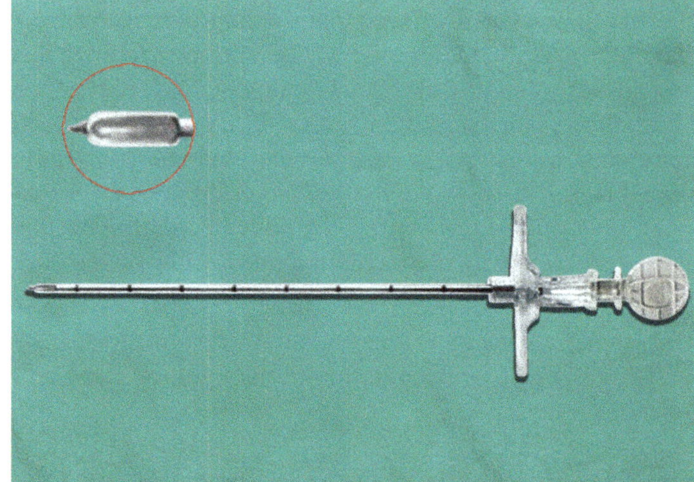

Fig. 20: Sprotte atraumatic epidural needle.[3]

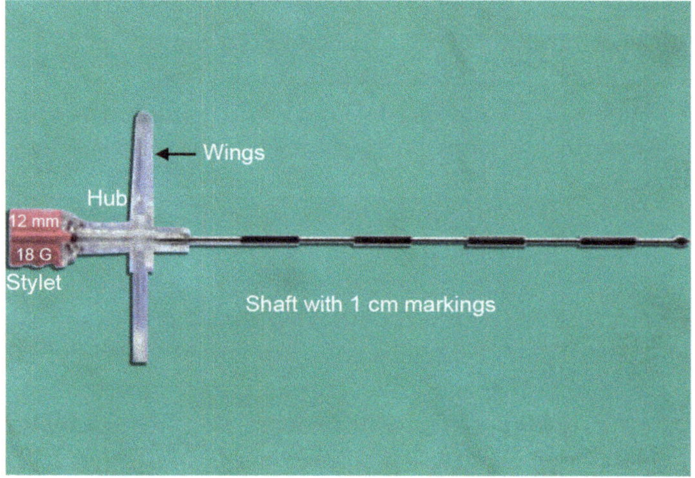

Fig. 21: Tuohy epidural needle: Parts in detail with markings of shaft of needle.

Types of Epidural Needles

- *Tuohy needle:* 10 cm in length, 3½ inch marked with 1 cm gradations. 16 G and 18 G are available. Tip is called Huber's tip. Pediatric 19 G, 5 cm in length with 0.5 cm markings are available. This allows the passage of a 21 G catheter
- *Modified Tuohy needle (Tuohy Hustead needle):* Short length, short rounded tip, and a bevel opening located 2.7 mm from the tip to minimize accidental dural puncture
- *Weiss epidural needle with fixed wings (17 G, 18 G):* It gives stable grip[17]
- *Portex needles:* 16 G (light blue), 18 G (dark blue) sizes
- *Blunt tip epidural needle:*[16] Introduced by Dr Baheti for interventional block. It is 20 G, 15 cm or 6 inches long needle made of stainless steel, which can be repeatedly autoclaved **(Fig. 23)**.

Complications due to Epidural Needles

Accidental dural puncture causing CSF leak leading to PDPH can occur during epidural block. However, epidural needles are also used for interventional procedures like celiac plexus block, lumbar sympathectomy, hypogastric plexus block, etc. Reported complications in the literature are pneumothorax, renal injury, injury to veins, paraplegia, neuralgia, etc. The probable cause for these iatrogenic complications can be sharp tip of the needle resulting in a puncture of internal organ like pleura, peritoneum or vein.[16] The blunt tip needle introduced by Dr Baheti[15] may reduce the complications following such interventional procedures.

EPIDURAL CATHETER (FIG. 24)

- Made up of nylon or polyvinyl chloride
- Radiopaque
- Tip is atraumatic, rounded having lateral holes and closed end Connector with Luer-lock cap **(Fig. 25)**

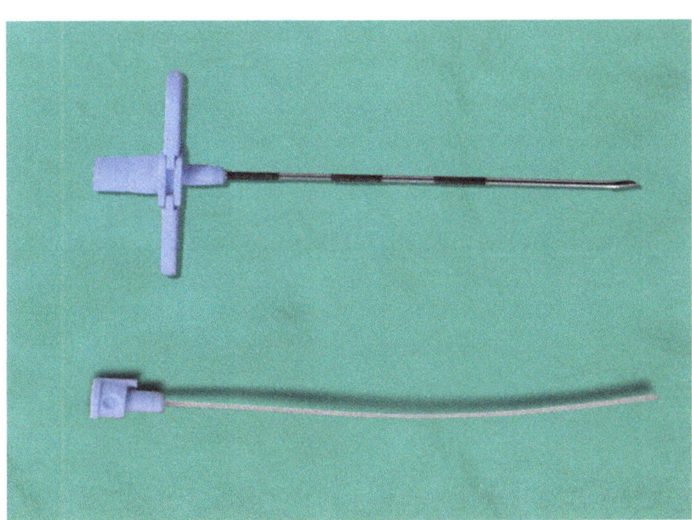

Fig. 22: Tuohy epidural needle with stylet.

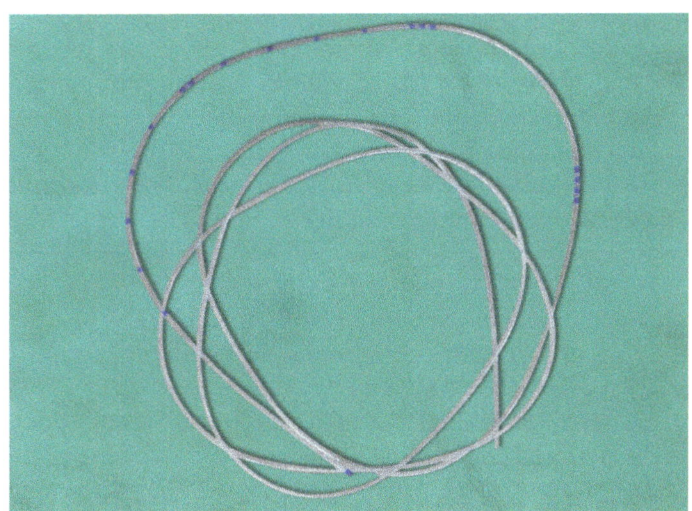

Fig. 24: Epidural catheter.

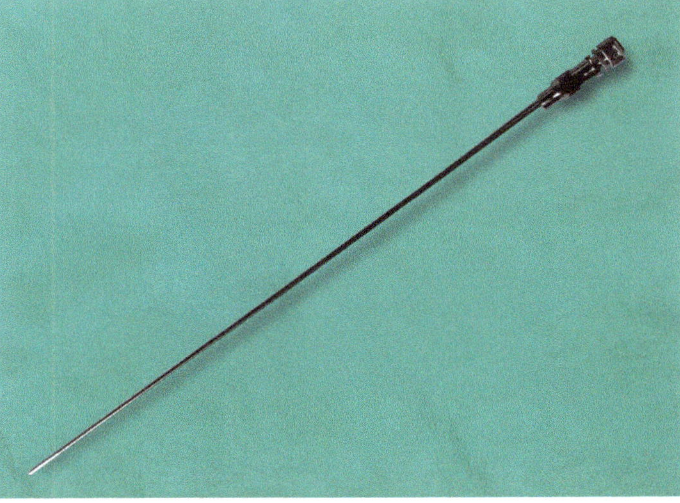

Fig. 23: Blunt tip epidural needle.[17]
Courtesy: Dr DK Baheti.

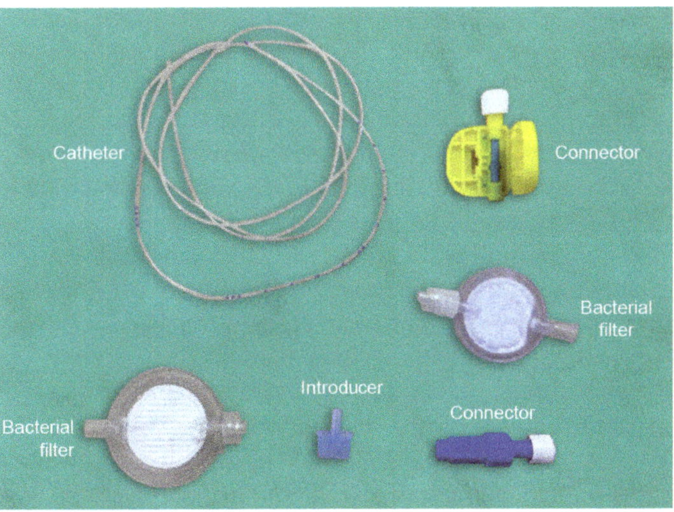

Fig. 25: Epidural catheter, bacterial filters, introducer, connectors.

- *Catheter length:* 90–100 cm with markings at 5 cm, 6 cm, 7 cm, 8 cm, 9 cm, 10 cm, 15 cm, 20 cm from the tip
- Catheter size—16 G, 18 G, 19 G, 20 G available. Bigger the gauge thinner the catheter, it can pass through any size epidural needle. However a 16 G catheter will not pass through a 18G epidural needle
- *Catheter diameter:* 0.9 mm (18 G), 1.1 mm (16 G)
- *Color coded:* Dark blue (18 G), light blue (16 G)
- *Filter:* 0.22 hydrophilic made of micron mesh
- *Loss of resistance (LOR) syringe:* Made of glass or plastic, has a low-resistance plunger to identify the epidural space by the LOR technique. The LOR using saline for catheter placement is the commonly used technique
- Catheter distance from tip to the epidural space is 3–4 cm. The catheter should be advanced only 3–5 cm into the epidural space[17,18]
- Minipacks (Portex) contain epidural needle, epidural catheter, connector, introducer, bacterial filter (0.2 μ), LOR syringe. Ideally for single use, disposable
- A spring wire reinforced flexible catheter[8] allows easy passage, decreases incidence of catheter migration
- Avoid withdrawing the catheter once it has passed the bevel of the Tuohy needle as this can transect the catheter. Therefore, safe to remove both the needle and catheter together[17]
- Continuous epidural set, available from Pajunk (Germany), which consists of:
  - Tuohy cannula for easy insertion
  - Available with metal or plastic stylet
  - Radiopaque catheter for easy guidance
  - Catheter with central opening/lateral opening for even flow of anesthetic
  - *Available gauges:* 17 G, 18 G, 19 G, 20 G, 21 G
  - *Sizes:* 50 cm, 90 cm, 120 cm.

ANATOMY FOR EPIDURAL PLACEMENT[1,19]

- The contents of the epidural space are fat, lymphatics and veins with nerve roots that cross it.
- Veins in the epidural space form a plexus called Batson's venous plexus. These veins connect with the iliac and azygos veins and are significant because of a lack of valves commonly found in veins. It is the lack of these valves in conjunction with a compressed inferior vena cava from a gravid uterus, which results in the venous engorgement of epidural veins found in the parturient.
- The amount of epidural fat and epidural venous engorgement are the two main factors that determine the volume of the LA solution in the epidural space necessary for adequate anesthesia or analgesia.

  The above points (1) and (2) are very important determinants for the amount and volume of LA to be injected in the epidural space of the parturient whose epidural veins are engorged; and in the elderly and the obese patients whose fat content in the epidural space is higher.
- The epidural space is a potential space with crevices or septations which create inconsistent paths that make flow through it less uniform.
- Spinal cord in adults ends at lower border of L1 vertebra while in children it is at the lower border of L3. By the age of 8 years, one can target the same lumbar level for safe epidural placement as in adult, while below the age of 7 years, caudal approach to epidural space is safer.
- The normal curvature of the vertebral column is "lordotic" at cervical and "lumbar" level; while "kyphotic" at "thoracic" and "sacral" level **(Fig. 26)**. The lumbar lordosis is more pronounced in females. Equally importantly, the curvatures of the vertebral column are maintained and "preserved" in the "supine" position.[19]
- When epidural catheter is inserted in an interspace, the tip of the epidural catheter reaches 1 to 1.5 interspace higher (cephalad) than the space of insertion because about 5–6 cm of catheter are kept inside the epidural space. The taller the person, the greater is the height of the vertebral body and therefore the lesser is the height reached by the tip of the epidural catheter in the epidural space cephalad. The shorter the person, the lesser is the height of the vertebral body and therefore the greater is the height reached by the tip of the epidural catheter in the epidural space cephalad. This is because in both the scenarios, about 5–6 cm (i.e., the constant length of the catheter) are kept inside the epidural space.

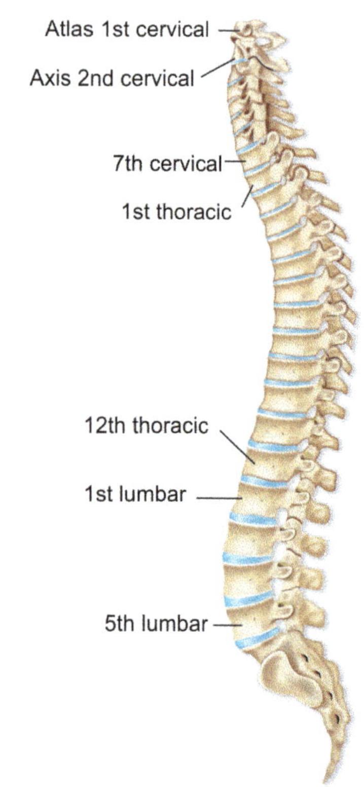

Fig. 26: The vertebral column in standing position. Note the cervical lordosis, the thoracic kyphosis, lumbar lordosis, and sacral kyphosis.

The above points (6) and (7) are of paramount importance, for blocking L2-L3-L4 nerve roots supplying the knee, with epidural anesthetic solution. How and why these points are so very relevant in blocking the knee and the area below the knee, will be explained a little later in this chapter.

TECHNIQUE OF EPIDURAL ANESTHESIA[9] (VIDEO 12)

Preparation and Position

The preparation and position for EA are same as described earlier under the heading "Technique of Spinal Anesthesia".

Projection and Puncture

After proper positioning and sterile preparation, place a wheal with LA at a predetermined site of injection.

Identify the midline and introduce the epidural needle up to ligamentum flavum. In the lumbar area, the depth of the ligamentum flavum from the skin is about 4-6 cm. The average thickness of ligamentum flavum is 5-6 mm.

The structures traversed by the needle are skin, subcutaneous tissue, supraspinous ligament and interspinous ligament. If "LOR" technique is started by attaching the syringe to the epidural needle when the latter is in one of these structures, a false positive may be experienced.

Once the epidural needle is on the ligamentum flavum, remove the stylet and attach the special plastic syringe with a plunger that has a very low resistance (provided in the kit) to the hub of the Tuohy needle.

Once the tip of the needle passes through the ligamentum flavum, it enters the epidural space. The epidural space is very narrow and is sometimes called a potential space, as the ligamentum flavum and the dura are usually closely adjacent. The epidural space therefore has to be identified as the bevel of the Tuohy needle exits the ligamentum flavum, as the dura will be penetrated shortly after, if the needle is advanced any further. (Epidural space in lumbar region is 5-6 mm in width.) To identify this point, a syringe is used to identify the LOR when pressure is applied to the plunger.

Normal saline as well as air can be used in the syringe to identify LOR as the tip of the needle enters the epidural space after crossing ligamentum flavum.

Once the needle enters the ligamentum flavum, there is a distinctive sensation of increased resistance, as this is a dense ligament with a leathery consistency.

Once the needle crosses the ligamentum flavum, and enters the epidural space, there will be smooth injection of saline or air into the epidural space.

Now remove the syringe and gently thread the catheter into the epidural space. It should be advanced till 15-18 cm appear at the hub of the needle. Now remove the needle carefully while noting the marking on the needle. The marking on the needle will show the depth of the needle from the skin to the epidural space. This distance or the depth will determine the length of the epidural catheter to be inserted in the epidural space from the skin. For example, if the needle entered the epidural space at the depth of 6 cm then the 11 cm mark of the catheter should come at the skin so that about 5 cm of catheter is inside the epidural space.

PROBLEMS SOLVING DURING EPIDURAL PLACEMENT

- You may encounter bony resistance everywhere
  - You may use paramedian approach
  - Patient's spine can be kept in greater flexion
- You are unable to thread the catheter
  - Try rotating the needle gently so that the bevel changes its direction. In the authors' opinion, if the epidural space is properly located, i.e., the tip of the Tuohy needle is properly placed in the epidural space, then the catheter does get threaded. If the catheter is not getting threaded, then the epidural space is not properly located. If unsuccessful then relocate the epidural space
- You may get fluid through the needle
  - If you have used saline to locate the epidural space, then wait for a few seconds to see if it stops flowing. If not, it could be a dural puncture. Respite epidural at a different level, give small doses of LA incrementally and observe carefully for SA block
- You may get fluid through the catheter
  - Most likely, catheter has punctured dura and therefore you may continue as SA and remove the catheter immediately after the surgery
- Patient gets pain on insertion of catheter
  - A brief sensation of "electric shock" is common, but it disappears. If it persists then remove the catheter and relocate the epidural space
- You may get blood in the epidural catheter
  - This indicates that the catheter is in the epidural vein. Withdraw catheter slowly by 1-2 cm, ensure that at least 2-3 cm are still inside the epidural space. Flush the catheter with saline. If there is no blood on aspiration, catheter may be used carefully making sure the following:
    - Aspirate catheter for all subsequent doses
    - All doses are given in small increments
    - Monitor the patient for early signs of LA toxicity.

Test dose before injecting the full dose of LA through the catheter is a must. Test dose consists of 3 mL of 2% lignocaine (preservative-free) with 1:200,000 epinephrine. Lignocaine (60 mg) injected intrathecally will give rise to SA and epinephrine (15 μg) injected intravascularly will give rise to an increase in heart rate (HR) by 20% or more. BP may be elevated or remain normal. If test dose is negative then incremental doses of 5 mL of LA every 5-7 minutes should be injected via the catheter to avoid catastrophes.

Differences between spinal and epidural anesthesia have been given in **Table 2**.

COMPLICATIONS OF EPIDURAL NEEDLES

- *Epidural hematoma:* To reduce epidural hematoma, use smallest needle possible, do not thread an epidural further than 5 cm, minimize recurrent passes, abort the technique if difficulty should be suspected[12]
- Postdural puncture headache—due to accidental dural puncture[11,12,16]
- Backache
- Epidural abscess.

COMPLICATIONS OF EPIDURAL CATHETERS

- Kinking, shearing, breaking, knotting (internally or externally)[20]
- Blockage by blood clot, debris
- Accidental dural puncture and CSF leak
- Accidental epidural vein insertion
- Difficulty in insertion due to nerve root obstruction
- Infection.

Continuous epidural analgesia is given in chronic pain, acute postoperative pain, cancer pain with the help of infusion devices and patient-controlled analgesia (PCA) pumps.[16] Epidural catheters are used for labor analgesia.

FAILED EPIDURAL

- Incorrect primary placement of the catheter[21]
- Secondary migration after correct placement of catheter
- Suboptimal doses of LAs and opioids
- Disconnection
- If a single orifice catheter is used, it can lie laterally or anteriorly in the epidural space, putting the LA more on one side and produce a unilateral block. Hence, multi orifice catheters are considered better than single orifice catheters[21]
- Occasionally manufacturing errors may occur, such as faulty markings on the epidural catheter which can lead to wrong depth of placement.[22]

TABLE 2: Differences between spinal and epidural anesthesia.

	Spinal	*Epidural*
1.	Simple to perform	Difficult to perform
2.	Has rapid onset of action	Has slower onset of action
3.	Requires small doses of LA	Requires larger doses of LA
4.	Gives reliable analgesia and muscle relaxation	At times, does not provide reliable analgesia and muscle relaxation
5.	Has shorter duration of action	Because of epidural catheter, prolongation of duration of block is possible
6.	Inability to extend the height of the block once fixed	Extension of the height of the block is possible
7.	Can cause precipitous drop in BP	Drop in BP is gradual
8.	Inability to provide postoperative analgesia	Ability to provide postoperative analgesia

(LA: local anesthetic; BP: blood pressure)

COMBINED SPINAL–EPIDURAL ANESTHESIA

COMBINED SPINAL–EPIDURAL NEEDLES

History

- *Soresi (1937):* He described it for the first time as "episubdural". He first injected a dose of LA epidurally, then advanced the same needle intradurally and then injected the spinal dose of LA
- *Curelaru (1979):* He performed first combined SA and EA. He used dual puncture technique, first inserted a epidural catheter through a Tuohy needle and then a dural puncture, one to two lumbar segments distally using a 26 G spinal needle. He called it the double-segment or double-space technique
- *Bainbridge (1981):* He described successful use of double-space technique for elective cesarean section
- *Coates and Mumtaz (1982):* He used the "needle-through-needle" technique **(Fig. 27)**
- First an epidural puncture is performed and the needle is leased in the space. Then another needle longer than the first is inserted in the subarachnoid space. Again it was not described, the use of special needles except for the use of a longer spinal needle than usual
- *Hanaoka (1986):* He developed a special combined spinal-epidural (CSE) needle. It was a standard Tuohy-Huber needle with another orifice aligned with its longest longitudinal axis close to its distal end. This orifice, called "back hole", passed the spinal needle inserted through the interior of the epidural needle **(Fig. 28)**
- This was needle-through-needle technique.

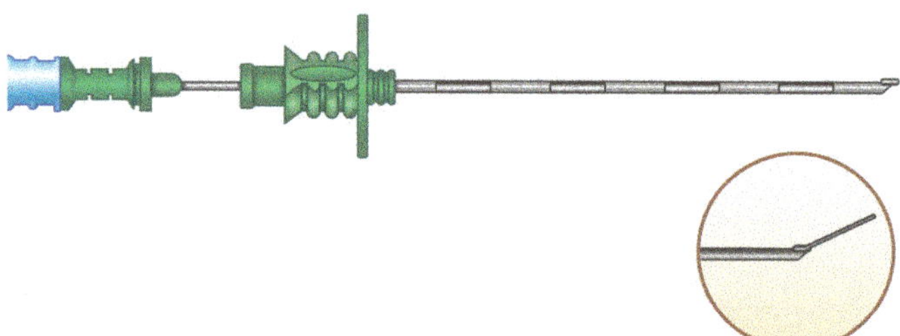

Fig. 27: Needle-through-needle (combined spinal-epidural).[3]

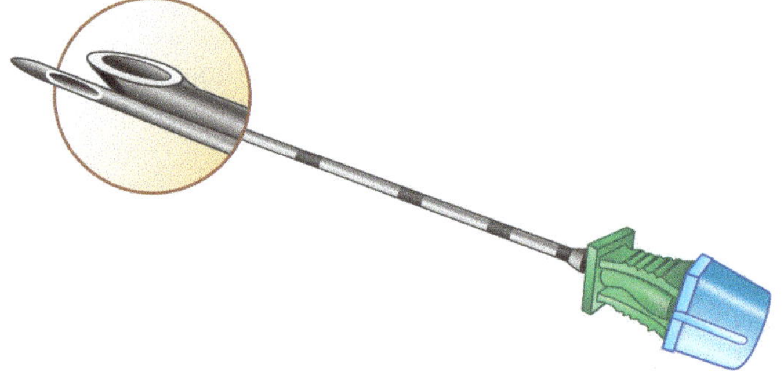

Fig. 28: Hanaoka combined spinal-epidural needle.[3]

Types of Combined Spinal-Epidural Needles

- Tuohy needle with an additional aperture, back eye or hole in the distal curve which allows the passage of 26 G spinal needle (needle-through-needle technique). A 26 G spinal needle, 12 cm length passes through a 16 G Tuohy needle.
- *Double lumen Tuohy needle with a straight tube:* A short 20 G guide tunnel is welded onto the lateral side of Tuohy needle through which a 25 G spinal needle can be inserted. The epidural catheter is inserted as usual through the needle before the subarachnoid block.
- *Portex "Secure" CSE needle* ***(Figs. 29A and B)****:* Epidural needle has markings on its hub starting from 0, in the increment of 0.5 mm, till 15 mm. Even numbers are written against the markings.

Spinal needle has corresponding notches on and under its hub. When the spinal needle is introduced through the Tuohy needle, the hub of the spinal needle lies over the hub of the Tuohy needle. Once the dura is punctured, the spinal needle which has a locking mechanism, can be locked over the Tuohy needle so that the displacement of the spinal needle is prevented while injecting, thus avoiding failed or patchy subarachnoid block **(Video 12)**.

Combined spinal-epidural set, available from B Braun company, which consists of:

- 18 G epidural needle with 27 G (needle-through-needle which is Whitacre spinal needle)
- 20 G epidural catheter
- Spinal needle extends 1.2 cm outside the epidural needle.

Epi Spin Lock

- CSE set **(Figs. 30 to 32)** from Pajunk (Germany)
- *Available guages of epidural needles:* 16 G, 17 G, 18 G, 19 G, 20 G, 21 G. Size: 90 mm
- *Spinal cannulae sizes:* 22 G, 24 G, 25 G, 27 G, 29 G Newly designed fixation system.

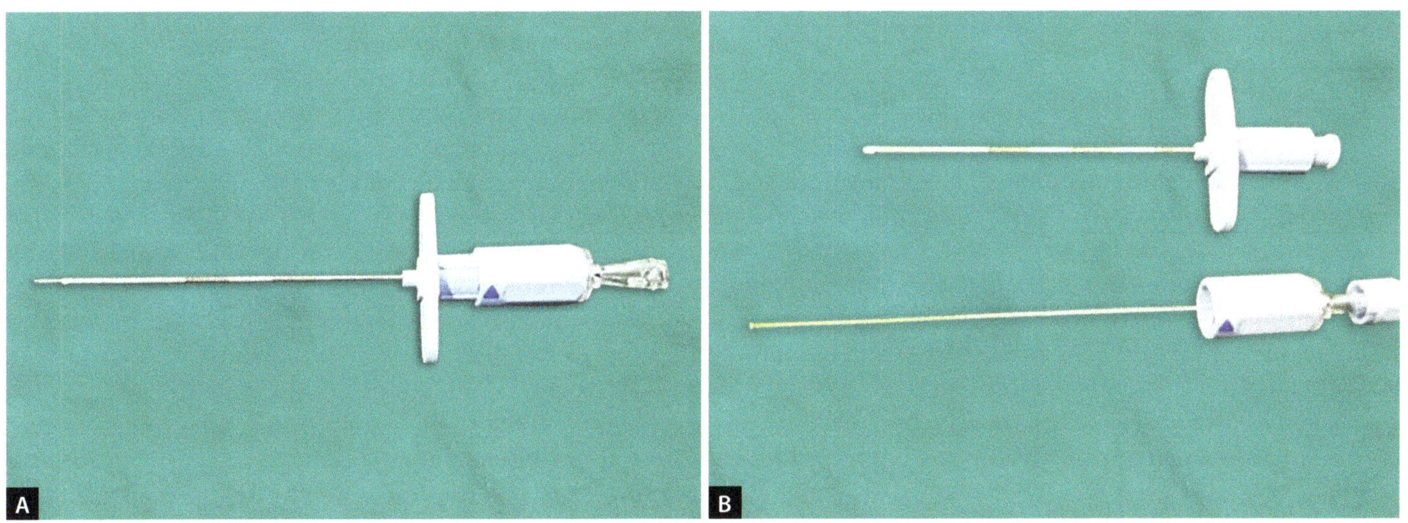

Figs. 29A and B: (A) Combined Portex spinal epidural needle, spinal needle jutting out through the epidural needle; (B) Portex combined spinal epidural needles.

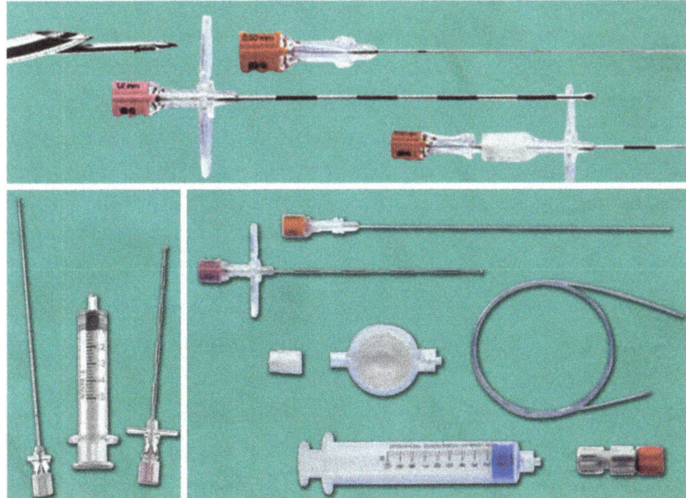

Fig. 30: Combined spinal epidural needle (Pajunk company).

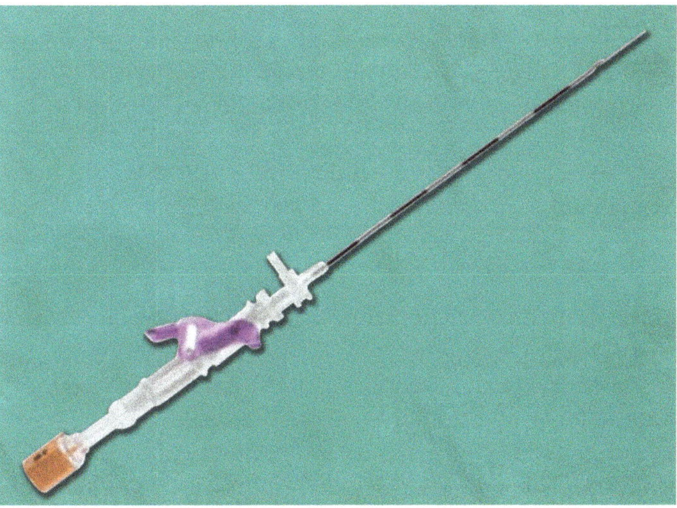

Fig. 31: Combined spinal-epidural needle (EpiSpin lock Pajunk company).

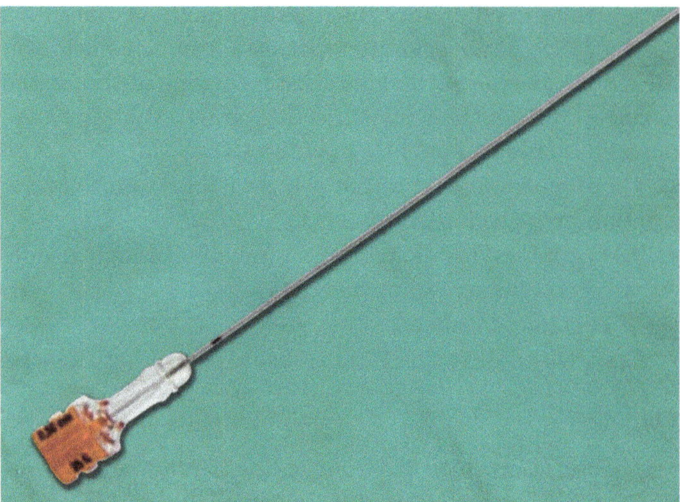

Fig. 32: EpiSpin lock Sprotte spinal needle for CSE (Pajunk company).

- Visual indication of the puncture depth and hence precise puncture
- Sprottes spinal needle can be locked in the desired position.

ADVANTAGES OF COMBINED SPINAL–EPIDURAL ANESTHESIA

- Rapid onset, reliable and profound block due to spinal
- Prolongation of duration of block using epidural catheter
- Sequential block can be given
  Lesser volume of LA is injected in the SA space and then height of the block is increased to the desired level by injecting the LA in the epidural space via the epidural catheter. This technique assures blockage of ONLY the desired number of segments, thus the undesired effects of a high block like hypotension and bradycardia are avoided.
- Postoperative analgesia for pain relief.

DISADVANTAGES OF COMBINED SPINAL–EPIDURAL ANESTHESIA

- Difficulty in passing the epidural catheter after spinal LA is given in needle-through-needle single space technique
- Displacement of epidural catheter in subarachnoid space[2,20]
- Time consuming if technical difficulties like in obese patients.

INDICATIONS

- Orthopedics—especially hip and knee replacements, lower limbs surgeries
- Gynecological, urogenital, rectal, perianal, pelvic, upper and lower abdominal surgeries
- Microvascular surgeries of lower limbs
- In labor analgesia (walking epidural) with intrathecal opioids and later continued with epidural doses of bupivacaine if cesarean section required.

SALIENT FEATURES OF COMBINED SPINAL–EPIDURAL ANESTHESIA (VIDEO 12)

Although the introduction of continuous EA has revolutionized the intraoperative and postoperative management, especially in long surgical cases, the CSEA technique has given a new dimension to regional anesthesia.

In 1981, Brownridge used CSEA technique using two interspaces. In 1982, Coates advocated CSEA technique in single intervertebral space and in 1986, Narinder Rawal started giving sequential CSEA blocks.

Thus CSEA began its journey way back in 1981 and over the last three decades it has progressed immensely to become one of the most versatile regional anesthesia techniques.

Combined spinal-epidural anesthesia preserves advantages of both SA and EA and if used sensibly also minimizes or eliminates their drawbacks.

Combined spinal-epidural anesthesia can be given by three methods:

1. Single-segment "needle-through-needle" method
2. Single-segment/double-barrel method
3. Double-segment method.

The present day anesthesia practice recommends the use of single-segment "needle-through-needle" technique over double-segment technique because:

- It causes less discomfort and trauma to the patient
- With it, there is 50% decrease in morbidity associated with intervertebral space penetration (backache, epidural vein puncture hematoma, infection) in contrast to two level penetration.

Let us enumerate the practical points showing distinct advantages of the single-segment "needle-through-needle" method over other methods.

- Since in the double-segment method, the higher interspace is used for insertion of epidural catheter and the lower interspace for spinal, it is either a high epidural or a low spinal. The hemodynamic alterations will be certainly greater with a high epidural. With the single level needle-through-needle method, an ideal and lower interspace for both spinal and epidural can be chosen to minimize the hemodynamic alterations. This point is very relevant in obstetrics where labor analgesia is given to the parturients. In case of those parturients who land up with caesarean section, the epidural route would be used for anaesthesia and the higher interspace used for epidural insertion would give rise to a higher height of block giving rise to a lot of undesirable hemodynamics alterations in the form of hypotension and bradycardia, which can be detrimental to the foetus.
- The lumbar curvature of the spine being lordotic and the thoracic curve being kyphotic, placement of epidural catheter is very important for blocking the L2–L3–L4 nerve roots as they emerge out at the highest point (peak) of lumbar lordosis to supply the knees.

In the epidural space, the tip of the catheter introduced at the L2–L3 interspace will reach around L1 cephalad. So, in supine position, under the effect of gravity, the epidural solution emerging from the tip of the catheter at L1 will flow towards the thoracic kyphosis, instead of flowing upwards and backwards towards the lumbar lordosis. So, as a result, the lower thoracic roots, and not the L2–L3–L4 nerve roots get blocked **(Figs. 33A to E)**. This effect is more pronounced in the females, who are shorter and have a steeper lumbar lordosis as compared to the males (**Fig. 34**, also refer to points 6 and 7 of "Anatomy of Epidural Placement"). So, for knee replacement surgery, the quality of intraoperative anesthesia and postoperative analgesia with the epidural route with this particular placement of the catheter will be poor, particularly when the action of the combined SA wears off. (It commonly is seen in bilateral knee replacement surgeries, where the first knee can be completed under SA but for the second knee, SA wears off and the EA is ineffective. It is also seen in revision knee replacement surgery where the operative time exceeds spinal time).

Please note **(Figs. 33A to E)**, in the epidural space, the flow of the LA solution emerging from the tip of the catheter at different levels. In the supine position, under the effect of gravity, the flow of the solution from the tip of the catheter at T12, L1, L2 is towards the thoracic kyphosis.

So, for the surgeries of the knee, it is very important to use the L4–L5 interspace for the introduction of epidural catheter so that after keeping length of 5–6 cm of the catheter in the epidural space, the tip will reach around L3.

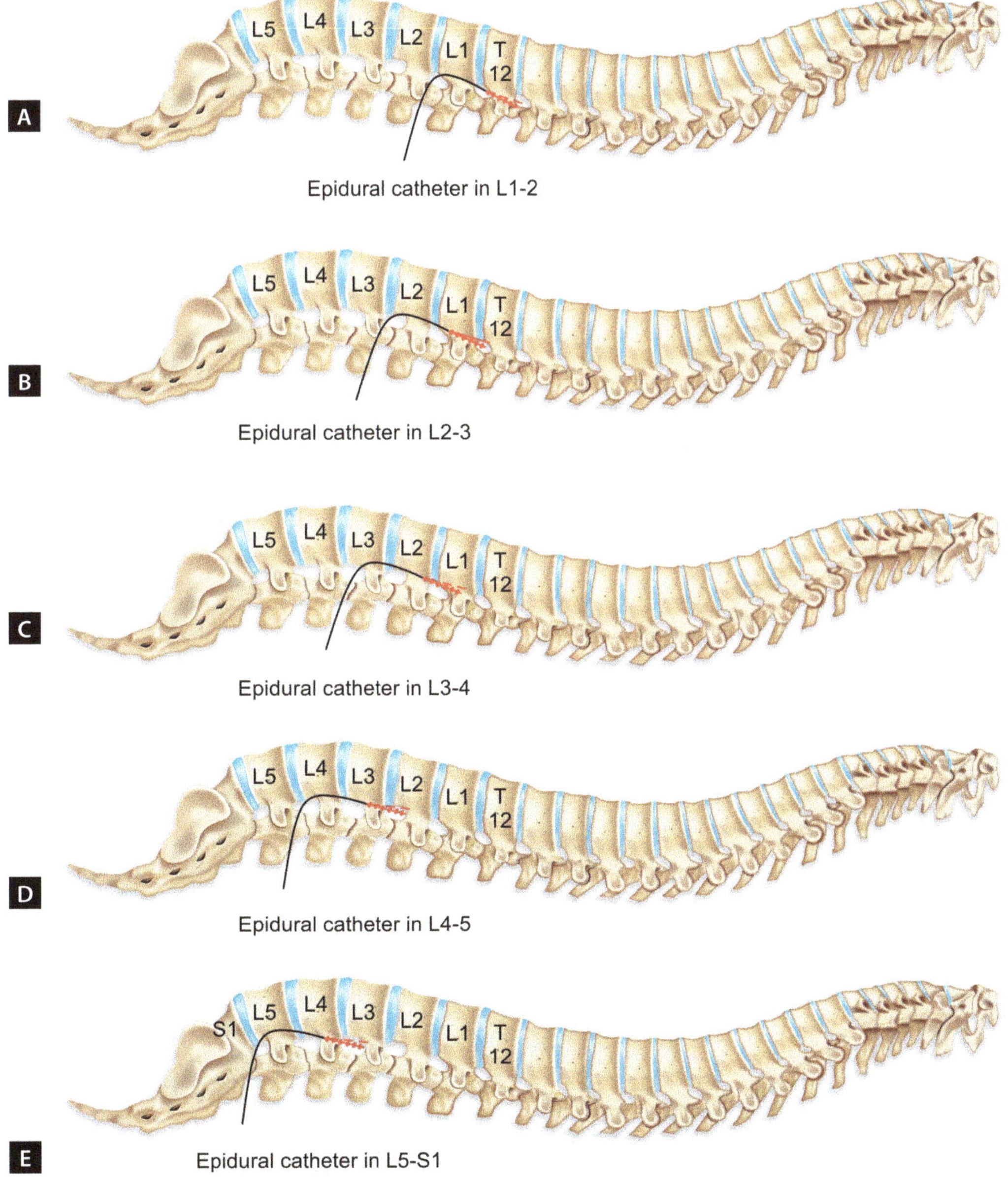

Figs. 33A to E: Insertion of the catheter in the epidural space at different intervertebral spaces like A. L1–L2; B. L2–L3; C. L3–L4; D. L4–L5; E. L5–S1. Please note, in the epidural space, the flow of the LA solution emerging from the tip of the catheter at different levels. In the supine position, under the effect of gravity, the flow of the solution from the tip of the catheter at T12, L1, L2 is towards the thoracic kyphosis.

Now the solution emerging from the tip of the catheter at L3 will properly soak the L2–L3–L4 nerve roots and thus block them effectively **(Figs. 33A to E)**.

With double-segment technique, if epidural catheter is inserted in L4–L5 interspace, then spinal will have to be given in L5–S1 interspace which may not be very easy technically. If epidural catheter is introduced in any space higher than L4–L5, then epidural will not act well for knees and surgery below knee as explained earlier.

With single level needle-through-needle technique, the ideal L4–L5 interspace can be used for both the epidural and spinal so that the tip of the epidural catheter remains in vicinity of L3.

For the surgeries of the tibia and ankle, the tip of the epidural catheter should reach around L4 so that the epidural solution trickles towards sacral kyphosis under the effect of gravity in supine position and the desired sacral roots can be blocked. But most of the times, surgeries of tibia and ankle get over within the spinal time and therefore this problem of "epidural not acting well once spinal wears off" is not seen in these cases.

- Conditions like osteoarthritis of knee and hip (these patients always have secondary changes in spine because of faulty weight-bearing axis); spinal deformities like scoliosis, kyphosis, exaggerated lumbar lordosis, Lis thesis and canal stenosis; obesity and old age make our entry into spinal and epidural spaces difficult. With double-segment technique, one has to successfully locate the spaces twice which could be a difficult task in these patients.

  With single level needle-through-needle technique, once the epidural space is located, i.e., Tuohy needle is in the epidural space, the spinal needle just has to be advanced through the Tuohy needle for locating the subarachnoid space. The spinal needle will encounter only one and single resistance and that is of dura. The whole tract is open as the epidural needle works as an introducer. Once dura is punctured, CSF will flow out **(Video 12)**.
- There is a specific purpose of the markings present on the hubs of the Tuohy needle and spinal needle of the Portex CSE set **(Figs. 35A and B)**. When the spinal needle is advanced through the Tuohy needle placed in the epidural space, for locating the subarachnoid space, only one resistance of dura is encountered and dura is punctured. At that moment of "give way" of dura, one must note down the number on the hub of the Tuohy needle. The number tells you the depth of dura and width of the epidural space. In case you are not happy

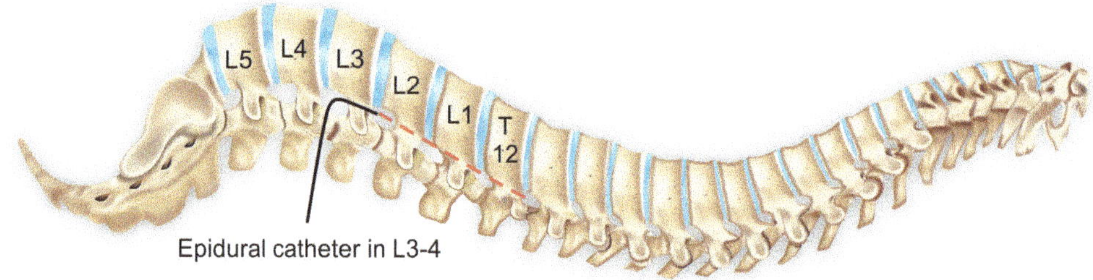

Fig. 34: Steep lumbar lordosis in a female.
Note the ease with which the local anesthetic solution in the epidural space will flow towards the thoracic kyphosis, in supine position, under the effect of gravity, especially when the tip of the catheter is reaching T12, L1 and L2.

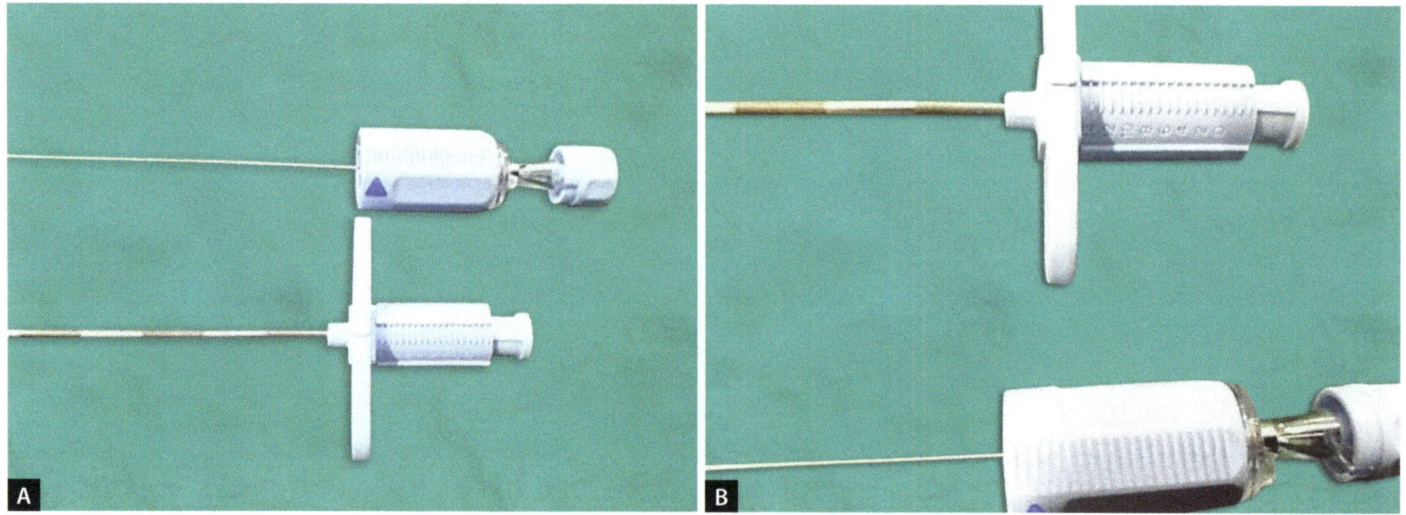

Figs. 35A and B: Note the even numbers written on the hub of the epidural needle and the notches on the hub of the spinal needle.

with the free flow of CSF on aspiration and you want to relocate the subarachnoid space, you will exactly know, till what depth you need to advance the spinal needle through the Tuohy needle to puncture dura. Also, equally importantly, you will be able to advance or withdraw the spinal needle through the Tuohy needle ½ a mm by ½ a mm, to establish a free flow of CSF. Location of subarachnoid space is so very accurate and precise with single-segment needle-through-needle technique that the spinal given by this method rarely fails or is patchy as compared to the spinal given by a plain spinal needle **(Video 12)**.

Causes of Failure to Locate Subarachnoid Space with Single-segment Needle-through-needle Technique (Figs. 36A to D)[12]

- Spinal needle falls short
- Spinal needle tents the dura instead of puncturing it
- Tuohy needle enters the lateral epidural space. Therefore, spinal needle also enters the lateral epidural space and therefore cannot come in contact with the dura to puncture it.

Problems with Epidural Catheter[10]

Problems are encountered in the insertion and placement of epidural catheter, most commonly in orthopedic patients, especially in those with bilateral osteoarthritis of hip and knee, as they have secondary changes in the spine.

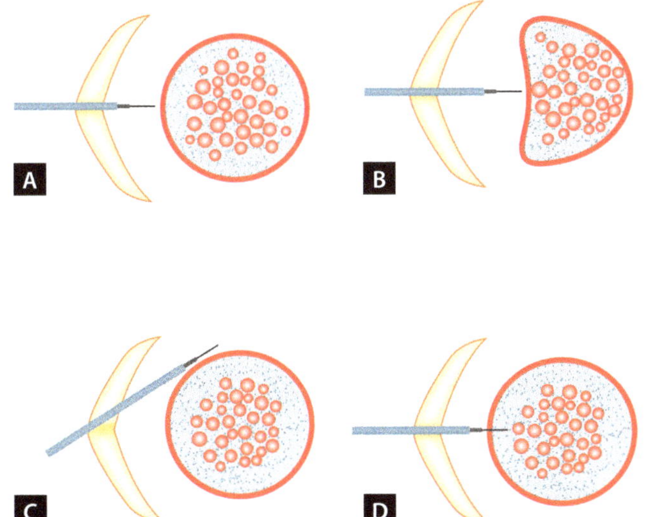

Figs. 36A to D: Various possibilities for combined spinal-epidural block: (A) The spinal needle falls short or the epidural space is too wide, i.e., greater than 1.5 cm or 15 mm. You can advance the Tuohy needle a little more in the epidural space and then introduce the spinal needle for location of subarachnoid space; (B) The spinal needle tents the dura without puncture; (C) The epidural needle has got deviated from the midline and has entered the lateral epidural space. As a result, the spinal needle which is passing through the Tuohy needle has also entered the lateral epidural space and therefore cannot puncture dura and enter the subarachnoid space. This is the most common situation, especially with spinal deformity; (D) This shows the correct technique with successful dural puncture.

- If the epidural space is located laterally, i.e., the Tuohy needle is in the position as shown in **Figure 36C**, then epidural catheter also enters the lateral epidural space
- The catheter takes path of the least resistance, so even if the epidural space is located in the midline, the catheter can still enter the lateral epidural space.

In both these situations, the catheter remains in the proximity of either sided roots, right or left. This will lead to more intense block on the side where the catheter is lying, because those roots are in closer contact with the epidural solution. To make this unilateral block effective for the surgery of the opposite side, the following may be done:

- One can turn the operation table on the side of the inadequate block and then inject LA solution so that under the effect of gravity LA may act on opposite roots (dependent side).
- One can inject a larger volume of LA, so the opposite roots receive adequate dose
- For lower limb surgery, in this situation, for postoperative analgesia, the patient can be nursed in lateral decubitus position on the side of surgery so that epidural infusion is effective enough to relieve pain.

To summarize, the SA and EA, especially the CSEA, are the versatile neuraxial anesthetic techniques with an expanding area of indication. They can be used in the perioperative setting as the sole anesthetic, or in combination with GA. The key to maximizing the advantages while minimizing the disadvantages of these techniques is to become familiar with the anatomical, physiological, pharmacological and technical aspects of block placement.

FACTORS AFFECTING HEIGHT OF EPIDURAL ANESTHESIA

Factors that affect the height of EA are fewer and less predictable than SA. They are as follows:

- Volume of local anesthetics
- Age
- Height of the patient
- Gravity.

Volume of Local Anesthetics

Placement of an epidural catheter at an appropriate level is essential. An epidural should be placed at an appropriate level that corresponds to the dermatome level of the intended surgical procedure since epidural produces a segmental block. The rule of thumb for dosing an epidural is 1-2 mL of LA per dermatome segment. For example, if an epidural catheter is placed at L4-L5, and for surgical purpose a T4 sensory block is required, then dose the patient with 12-24 mL of LA. There are 4 lumbar dermatomes (L1-L4) and 8 thoracic dermatomes (T12-T4), so a total of 12 dermatomes. Therefore, 12 × 1-2 mL/dermatome = 12-24 mL of LA solution is required. Since the dose may be variable from patient to patient, it is important to dose the epidural in increments while continually assessing block progression.

Age

As the patients age, less LA is required to achieve the same level of block as their younger counterparts. This is due to change in size and compliance of the epidural space.

Height of the Patient

Height of the patient plays a role in determining epidural block height. The shorter the patient, the lesser is the LA solution required to achieve the same level of anesthesia as a tall patient. For example, a person of 5 feet 3 inches tall needs 1 mL/dermatome of LA to achieve a block height of T10, then a person of 6 feet 2 inches tall would need 2 mL/dermatome of LA to reach the same block height.

Gravity

Positioning the patient after injection of LA into the epidural space affects its spread and height of block because LA will flow under the effect of gravity. For example, if the patient is turned in right lateral decubitus position after the injection of LA in epidural space, the drug will flow towards the right side under the effect of gravity and the block could be denser and higher on right side.

DRUGS AND DOSAGES FOR EPIDURAL ANESTHESIA

Lidocaine

Lidocaine is the prototypical amide LA. For EA, concentrations of 1.5–2% are commonly used. Epinephrine will prolong the duration of lidocaine by 50%. The addition of preservative-free fentanyl (50–100 µg) will accelerate the onset of analgesia and create a more potent/complete block.

Strengths of lignocaine with their time of onset and duration of block when injected epidurally are given in **Table 3**.

Bupivacaine

Bupivacaine is a long-acting amide LA. For EA, the most common concentrations are 0.5–0.75%. Concentrations for analgesia range from 0.125 to 0.25%. Epinephrine (1:200,000) will prolong the duration of action of bupivacaine, but is not as reliable as with lidocaine and mepivacaine. Bupivacaine in concentrations of 0.75% should not be used for obstetric anesthesia. The FDA's recommendation in 1983 occurred after several cardiac arrests were reported related to inadvertent IV injection. Bupivacaine (in addition to etidocaine) is more likely to impair the myocardium and conduction than other LAs during inadvertent IV injection. Patients are difficult to successfully resuscitate due to bupivacaine's high protein binding and lipid solubility, which allow it to accumulate in the cardiac conduction system, resulting in refractory reentrant arrhythmias.

Strengths of bupivacaine with their time of onset and duration of block when injected epidurally are given in **Table 4**.

NEURAXIAL ANESTHESIA AND THROMBOPROPHYLAXIS

Patients receiving antithrombotic or antiplatelet therapies are at a higher risk for developing spinal-epidural hematoma with neuraxial anesthesia.

Risk factors for epidural bleeding are:

- Coagulation disorders
- Antithrombotic or fibrinolytic therapy
- Use of any agent interfering with different components of coagulation
- Difficult vertebral or spinal cord anatomy
- Difficult or traumatic catheter insertion
- Lack of guidelines.

Quick Reference Guide

Neuraxial anesthesia in the patient receiving thromboprophylaxis (based on second Consensus Conference on Neuraxial Anesthesia and Anticoagulation, 2002).

Antiplatelet medications: No contraindication with nonsteroidal anti-inflammatory drugs (NSAIDs); discontinue ticlopidine 14 days, clopidogrel 7 days, glycoprotein (GP) IIb/IIIa inhibitors (eptifibatide, tirofiban and abciximab) 8–48 hours prior to surgery.

Unfractionated heparin, SC: No contraindication, consider delaying heparin until after block if technical difficulty anticipated.

TABLE 3: Dosages of lidocaine for epidural anesthesia.

Agent	*Concentration*	*Onset*	*Sensory block*	*Motor block*	*Plain solution*	*1:200,000 epinephrine*
Lidocaine	1.5%	Intermediate, 15 minutes	Dense	Mild-to-moderate	80–120 minutes	120–180 minutes
Lidocaine	2%	Intermediate, 15 minutes	Dense	Dense	–	–

TABLE 4: Dosages of bupivacaine for epidural anesthesia.

Agent	*Concentration*	*Onset*	*Sensory block*	*Motor block*	*Plain solution*	*1:200,000 epinephrine*
Bupivacaine	<0.25%	Slow	Dense	Minimal-to-moderate	–	–
Bupivacaine	0.5–0.75%	Slow	Dense	Mild-to-dense	165–225 minutes	180–240 minutes

Unfractionated heparin, IV: Heparinize 1 hour after neuraxial technique, remove catheter 2–4 hours after last heparin dose; no mandatory delay if traumatic.

Low-molecular-weight heparin (LMWH), twice daily dosing: LMWH 24+ hours after surgery, remove neuraxial catheter 2 hours before first LMWH dose.

LMWH, single daily dosing: First dose: 6+ hours after surgery, second dose: 24+ hours after the first dose. Neuraxial catheter may be safely maintained; catheter removed 10–12 hours after LMWH and 2–4 hours prior to next dose; postpone LMWH 24 hours in cases of traumatic placement.

Warfarin: Warfarin therapy must be stopped ideally 4–5 days before the scheduled procedure. Prior to neuraxial technique, document normal international normalized ratio (INR); remove catheter when INR is less than 1.5 (initiation of therapy).

Thrombolytics: No data on safety interval for performance of neuraxial technique or catheter removal; follow fibrinogen level.

Herbal therapy: No evidence for mandatory discontinuation prior to neuraxial technique, be aware of potential drug interaction.

In certain medical conditions like valve replacement surgery or recent coronary artery stenting, patient cannot be off the oral anticoagulant (warfarin) or the antiplatelet medication (clopidogrel) even for a day. In such a situation, the warfarin or clopidogrel is stopped as per the guideline and patient is put on LMWH which is continued till the previous day of surgery and is stopped 24 hours prior to neuraxial block.

Simultaneous use of more than one agent influencing different components of the clotting system is not recommended as it may increase the risk of epidural hematoma formation.

It is recommended to use epidural solutions that minimize sensory and motor block to facilitate detection of signs and symptoms of cord compression in the postoperative period. Close postoperative monitoring of neurologic function is a must.

CAUDAL EPIDURAL (VIDEO 12)

It is a technique of giving epidural block via the sacral route. It is the most common type of pediatric regional block used today. Caudal block is a useful adjunct to GA in most procedures performed below the umbilicus in children and is safe method for postoperative analgesia in children for these surgeries. Caudal epidural block is not commonly given in adults because:

- Lumbar and thoracic epidural spaces are easier to access in the adults than is the caudal space
- Sacral hiatus and other landmarks are more difficult to identify and the caudal space is more difficult to enter with increasing age as the sacral bones begin to fuse and the sacrococcygeal ligament gets calcified
- Epidural fat is loose in texture in children and it becomes fibrous close meshed texture in adults. Therefore, caudal LA spread in children is predictable, while in adults it is not predictable
- In the parturient in labor, there is an increased risk of injecting LA into the fetus with a caudal block due to the level of foetus and the level of needle insertion site being in close proximity.

Indications

- Pediatric surgeries like hypospadias repair, circumcision, orchidopexy, inguinal hernias, anal procedures, orthopedic procedures for lower extremities
- In adults, for all anorectal procedures like hemorrhoidectomy, transurethral operations and operations on the lower limbs.

Anatomy and Landmarks[23]

The anatomy of the lumbosacral epidural space in infants and small children is slightly different from that in adults. The sacrum is a large triangular bone formed by the fusion of the five sacral vertebrae. It articulates above with the 5th lumbar vertebrae and below with the coccyx. The sacral hiatus is formed due to the nonfusion of the laminae of the 5th and sometimes the 4th sacral vertebrae in the midline **(Figs. 37A and B)**. The sacral cornua are the large bony processes which are the tubercles of the inferior articular processes of the 5th sacral vertebra.

The coccyx lies immediately caudal to the sacral hiatus. The hiatus is covered by the sacrococcygeal membrane. These landmarks are easily identifiable and palpable in infants and prepubertal children due to the absence of sacral pad of fat.

The sacral canal runs through the length of the sacral bone and follows its curvature.

The boundaries of the sacral canal are as follows:

- Superiorly, it is continuous with the lumbar vertebral canal Inferiorly lies the sacral hiatus, closed by the posterior Sacrococcygeal membrane
- Anteriorly bound by the bodies of the sacral vertebrae
- Posteriorly bound by the fusion of the laminae
- Laterally situated are the four sacral foramina which divide in the form of a Y into the anterior and posterior sacral foramina.

Sometimes fibrous strands occur in the canal which divides the epidural space into compartments. This is responsible for failure to produce adequate, uniform analgesia with LAs.

The contents of the sacral canal are dural and arachnoid sacs, sacral nerves, blood vessels, lymphatics and alveolar tissue. The dural and the arachnoid sacs usually terminate

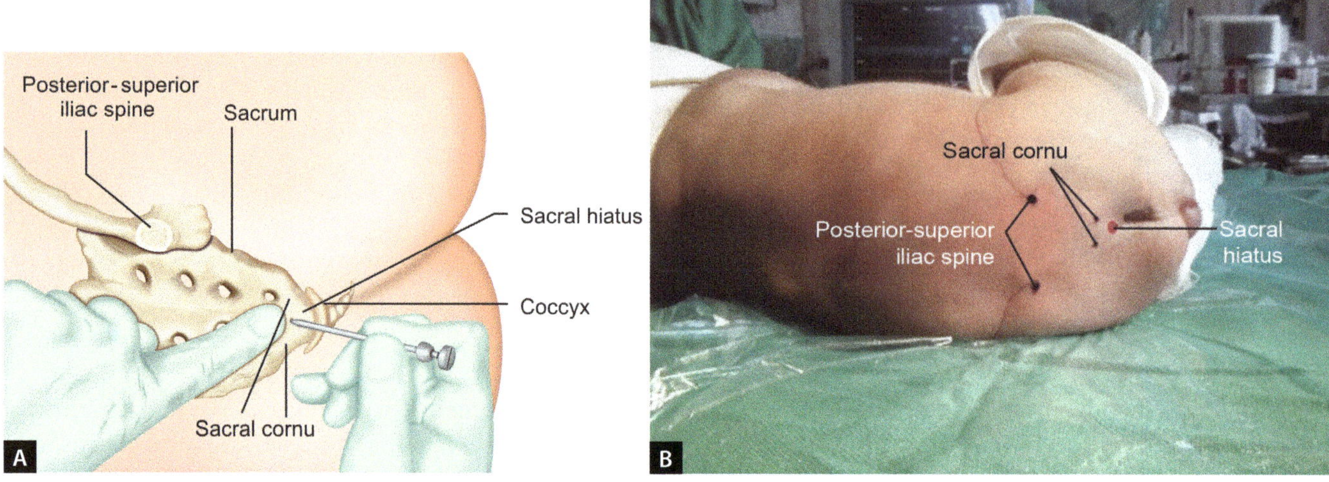

Figs. 37A and B: Sacral anatomy and landmarks.

at the level of the 2nd sacral vertebrae in adults, they may extend to the 3rd or 4th sacral vertebrae in infants, hence the distance between the sacral hiatus and the end of the dura is relatively short in them.

The average capacity of the sacral canal is 34 mL in males and 32 mL in females.

The average length is 10–15 cm.

Technique (Figs. 38A to C)

- An IV cannula is inserted
- The lateral position with flexion of hip joints is commonly used for giving a caudal epidural block as the identification of landmarks is easier. Care should be taken to avoid over flexing the hips, as this can make the landmarks more difficult to palpate
- The sacral hiatus and the posterior superior iliac spines form an equilateral triangle pointing inferiorly. First palpate for the tip of the coccyx and then moving up, about 3–3.5 cm above, the sacral hiatus can be felt as a depression in the skin using a firm pressure by the left index finger. It is always above the intergluteal fold
- With patient in lateral position, all aseptic precautions are taken and a wheal is raised over the hiatus between the sacral cornua, using a 25 no. needle with LA. Then using a 1–1.5 inch needle (22 G/23 G hypodermic needle, scalp needle or cannula) with a syringe containing the appropriate volume of the LA kept attached to the needle, the caudal space is approached. The needle is kept exactly in the midline, is first inserted through the sacrococcygeal membrane making an angle of 45° to the skin. A distinct "pop" or "click" is felt as the sacrococcygeal membrane is punctured. Once through the membrane the needle is depressed a further so that the needle shaft is almost parallel to the skin. The bevel should face anteriorly and advanced 2–3 mm to enter the caudal space **(Figs. 38A to C)**. Avoid further advancement to prevent piercing the anterior sacral wall and puncturing the dura. After confirming the absence of any blood or CSF on aspiration, a test dose of the LA solution can be injected into the caudal space. If there is blood on aspiration then reposition the needle. If CSF appears then abandon the procedure. Following a negative test dose and in the absence of pain on injection, the definitive dose should be injected slowly in small repeated increments. Single shot needles or cannulas are withdrawn following injection. For continuous block, the catheter is passed and strapped in position or can be tunneled subcutaneously under the skin **(Fig. 38D)**.

Drugs and Dosages Used[8,23,24]

Most commonly used drugs include lidocaine 1% and bupivacaine 0.25%.

Bupivacaine has a longer duration of action than lidocaine and is used more often.

Drugs used for caudal injection should come from single use ampoules and should be preservative-free.

There are three important variables that determine the quality, duration and the extent of the caudal block:

1. Volume of the drug
2. Total dose of the drug
3. Concentration of the drug.

Various studies have been done and show that age, weight and height were all important in determining the dosage of LAs. Bromage and Schulte-Steinberg studied the factors,[24] affecting the volume of LA for caudal block. Both their formulas approximately simplify to:

Dose = Age × 0.1 mL/dermatome × number of dermatomes to be blocked

Using this formula, they found that using 1% lidocaine or 0.25% bupivacaine solutions, a volume of approximately 0.1 mL/segment/year of age was effective in prepubertal children. Thus to produce analgesia up to the umbilicus in a 5-year-old child, the dose required would be 0.1 × 13 (segments) × 5 (years) = 6.5 mL.

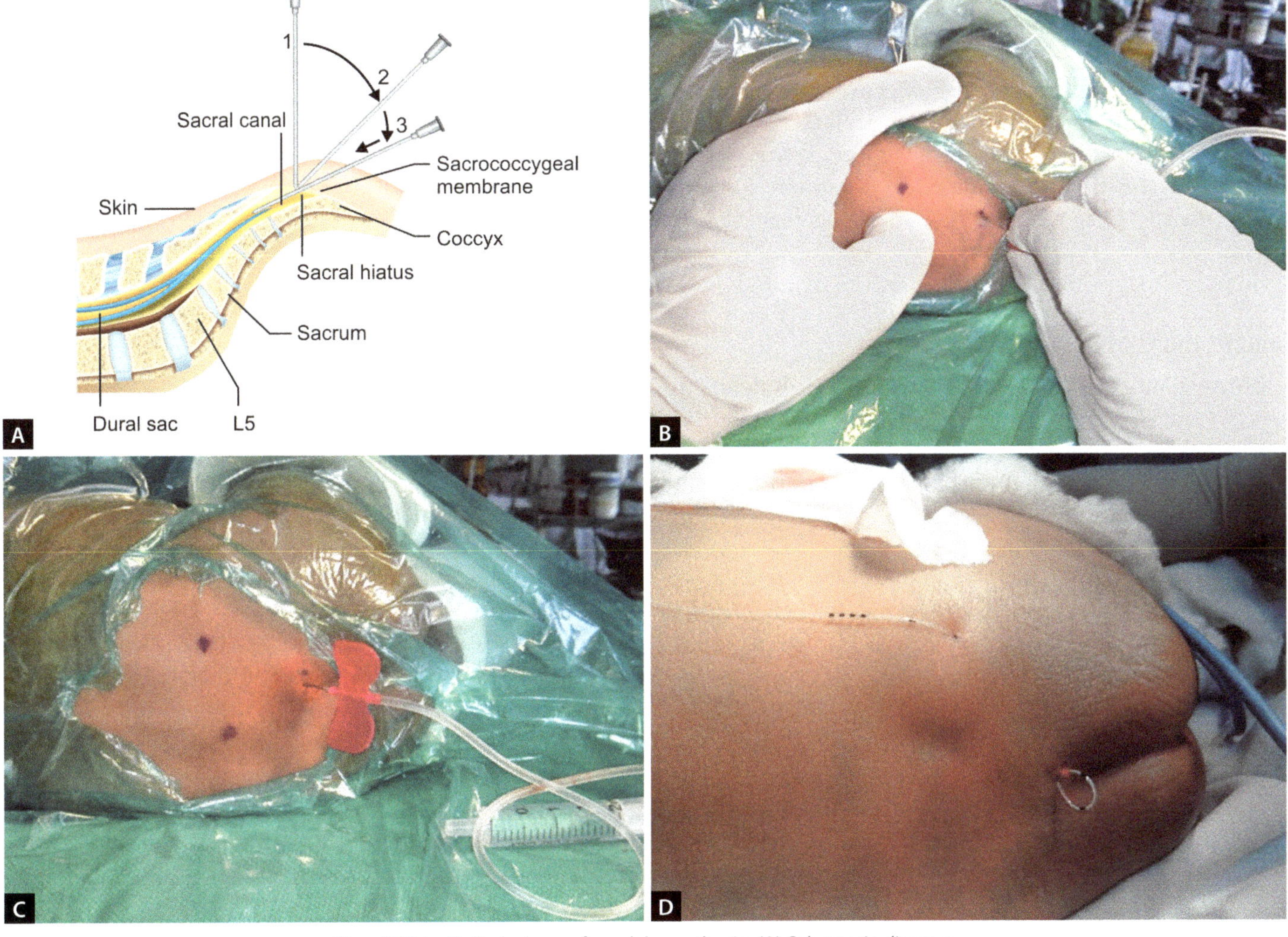

Figs. 38A to D: Technique of caudal anesthesia: (A) Schematic diagram; (B and C) Single shot with scalp needle; (D) Continuous with catheter.

Similarly Takasaki[24] and colleagues studied the dose requirements for caudal anesthesia in a large series of infants and children. They concluded that for patients ranging in age from newborn to 7 years, the segmental dose requirements correlated better with body weight than with age.

Dose = Weight × 0.056 mL/segment anesthetized

Thus using this formula, the volume required in the same 5-year-old child to produce a 13-segment block, assuming the body weight to be 20 kg would be

Dose = 13 (segments) × 0.056 × 20 (kg) = 14.56 mL which is more than double the volume calculated according to Schulte-Steinberg.

Thus, a volume of 0.5 mL/kg would give adequate sacral block; 1 mL/kg is used for lower thoracic block and 1.25 mL/kg to reach up to the mid thoracic region.

For caudal analgesia, lower concentrations (0.125%, 0.25%) of bupivacaine would suffice. Higher concentrations (0.5%, 0.75%, 1%) would give a motor block. The total dosage should be checked to avoid toxic doses.

As per Armitage formula the dosages are:

- 0.5 mL/kg for a lumbosacral block
- 1 mL/kg for a thoracolumbar block
- 1.25 mL/kg for a midthoracic block
- 0.25% bupivacaine up to a maximum of 20 mL.

Maximum dose:

- Bupivacaine—3 mg/kg
- Lidocaine—5 mg/kg
- Lidocaine with epinephrine (1:200,000)—7 mg/kg.

Most commonly used drugs include lidocaine 1% and bupivacaine 0.25%.

Bupivacaine has a longer duration of action than lidocaine and is used more often.

Other drugs like ropivacaine (0.25%)[25] and levobupivacaine (0.25%, 0.5%, 1%) can be used. Adjuvant drugs like opiates, clonidine and ketamine can be added to the LAs to prolong the duration of the analgesia without side effects such as motor block[26] and also for effective postoperative pain relief.

Opioids like morphine (30–75 μg/kg) and fentanyl (1–1.5 μg/kg) are used. Combinations of bupivacaine or ropivacaine (0.1–0.125%) along with fentanyl 1–3 μg/kg can be given as continuous infusion via catheters at the rate of 0.1–0.3 μg/mL/h.

Clonidine (1–2 μg/kg) gives effective analgesia and prolongs the duration of action of bupivacaine.

In adults, undergoing anorectal procedures, a dose of 15–20 mL of 1.5–2.0% lidocaine with or without epinephrine is usually effective. Fentanyl 15–20 μg may also be added.

In poor-risk patients, lower doses will be required.

Complications of Caudal Block

- Intravascular and intraosseous injection leads to systemic toxicity, grand mal seizures and/or cardiac arrest. Neonates present with respiratory distress. This can be prevented by repeated aspirations, slow injection and constant assessment of the patient for clinical signs.
  There can be difficulty in ruling out inadvertent intravascular injection of test dose in children because:
  - Veins may collapse on aspiration, giving false-negative response
  - As baseline HR would be high after atropine premedication, HR response with epinephrine may be negative. However, arrhythmias can occur with higher dose of epinephrine.
- Local anesthetics toxicity.
  There can be difficulty in eliciting signs and symptoms of LA toxicity in children because:
  - Pain or agitation on injection may be confused as central nervous system (CNS) toxicity
  - If caudal is given as supplement to general anesthesia, GA would suppress signs and symptoms of toxicity
- Hematoma formation
- *Intrathecal injection:* Extreme care must be taken to avoid this as "total spinal block" will occur if the dose for a caudal block is injected into the subarachnoid space. Unconsciousness, apnea and hypotension will rapidly result. Management includes IV fluids, use of vasopressors, taking charge of airway and ventilation
- Urinary retention
- Motor blockade
- Rectal perforation. If this occurs then contamination of needle and spread of infection is extremely dangerous
- "Sepsis" which can be avoided if strict asepsis is maintained.

Advantages of Caudal Block

- Good postoperative pain relief
- Useful along with GA in pediatric patients, reduces the requirements of analgesics, inhalational agents and muscle relaxants.

Disadvantages of Caudal Block

- Difficulty of positioning the child while performing the block
- Technical difficulties if anatomy is distorted
- Time consuming
- Pain on injection. Children may need to be sedated or under light GA
- Lack of success and control of the height of the block
- Inadequate block and muscular relaxation
- Infection, if proper asepsis and cleaning of the site of injection not done.

EPIDUROSCOPY

Epiduroscopy[27] can be performed for visualization of epidural fibrosis, granulation tissue, neovascularization, etc. Epiduroscope is introduced into caudal epidural space through steerable catheter or introducer. Flexible fiberoptic endoscope is used for epiduroscopy.

Flexible fiberoptic endoscope **(Fig. 39)** used for epiduroscopy is 0.9 mm in external diameter and 125 cm long. Magnification is 40x and has a resolution of 10,000 pixels. It has a standard 32 mm eyepiece that couples to the video coupler. The distal tip incorporates the micro lens assembly.

Video-guided catheter (VGC) or steering device **(Fig. 40)** is radiopaque and guides the flexible fiberoptic endoscope in the epidural space. The VGC is 2.7 mm in external diameter. It has two 1.3 mm working channels with a two-way steering mechanism and a radiopaque tip. The two working channels can be used; one for the fiberscope, the other for saline flush/instrumentation. There are two side ports that terminate with standard female Luer locks. One side port is used for saline infusion and to monitor the epidural space pressure and the other port is left open to air to act as a vent

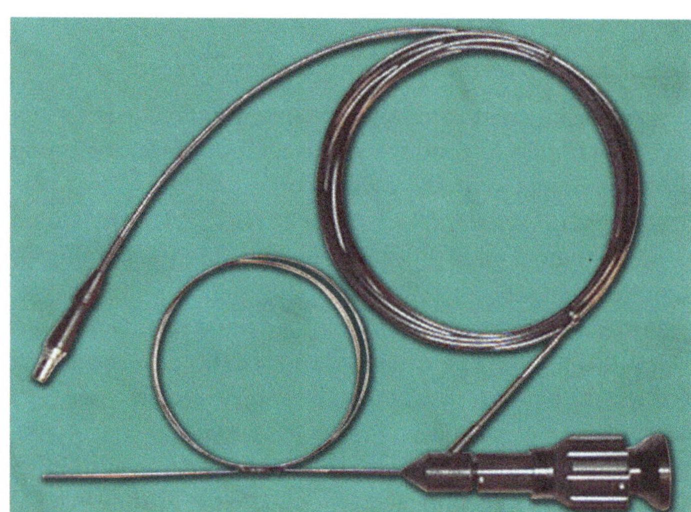

Fig. 39: Epiduroscope.

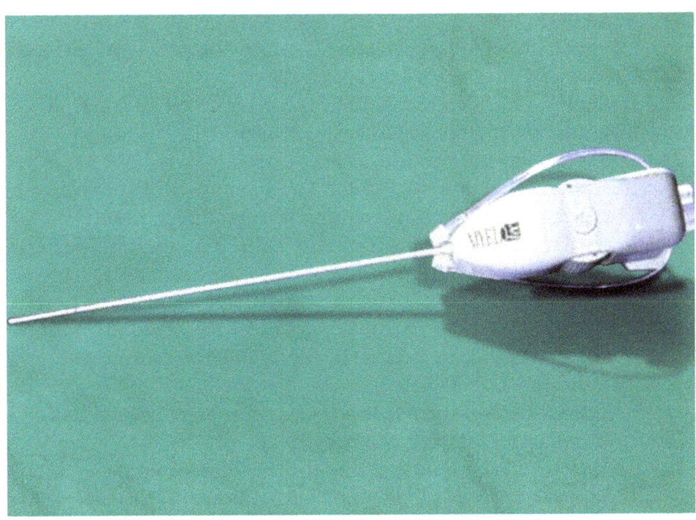

Fig. 40: Video-guided catheter.

for excess saline thus preventing excessive rise in epidural pressure.

Accessory port: This port contains a Tuohy-Borst adapter, duck-bill valve and side port channel. These ports are used to pass accessories through the working lumen of the catheter, i.e., fiberoptic scope, instruments. Handle assembly houses the steering mechanism and is used to hold and direct the VGC. Steering dial controls the steering mechanism that manipulates the tip of the VGC and thus the fiberscope can be directed in two different directions. This is exactly like using a fiberoptic bronchoscope. Video-guided catheter shaft is a flexible shaft with steerable tip. Video-guided catheter distal tip is radiopaque tip and can be viewed under fluoroscopy.

Technique of Epiduroscopy

Under aseptic precaution and under fluoroscopic control epiduroscope is introduced into caudal epidural space through steerable catheter or introducer. The catheter is then maneuvered closer to epidural scarring. An epidurogram is done to see filling defect indicating area of scarring or fibrosis. Thereafter, hyaluronidase is injected with reasonable force to hydrolyze excess ground substance in epidural scar tissue thus allowing diffusion of LA and corticosteroid to target area.

SADDLE BLOCK

It is the anesthesia of those parts of the patient's body that would touch a saddle if the patient was to ride a horse, i.e., the buttocks, perineum and the inner side of both thighs.

Indications

The indications for saddle block are:
- Rectal surgeries like hemorrhoidectomy, fistulectomy Perineal surgeries
- Obstetrics—suture of episiotomy.

Technique

After giving a spinal injection in the same way as described earlier in the chapter, the patient is made to sit for 5 minutes so that the hyperbaric spinal LA settles to the lowest point of dural sac with gravity. The volume of the spinal anesthetic injected is very little, i.e., 1.5–2 mL of 0.5% sensorcaine (0.8–1 mL of 5% lignocaine in earlier days). After 5 minutes of the injection, the spinal LA gets fixed to the lower sacral nerve roots. Then the patient is turned into supine position and then into desired position (lithotomy/prone).

The advantage of this saddle block is that there is a great amount of hemodynamic stability as very few spinal nerve roots are blocked.

CONCLUSION

Spinal, epidural, CSE, caudal, and saddle block are used routinely by anesthesiologists all over the world. These techniques have evolved from single shot to continuous techniques. Along with LAs adjuvants are used, especially to prolong the effect of the block and to use them for postoperative pain relief. The techniques are also used in patients receiving antiplatelet and antithrombotic agents. These techniques are not devoid of complications. It is, therefore, extremely important to know the dosages, appropriate timings and contraindications for these techniques.

REFERENCES

1. Bauer M, George JE, Seif J, et al. Recent advances in epidural analgesia. Anesthesiol Res Pract. 2012;2012:309219.
2. Barash PG, Cullen BF, Stoelting RK. Clinical Anesthesia, 5th edition. Philadelphia: Lippincott Williams and Wilkins; 2006.
3. Spinal and epidural needles. [online] Available from www.cothon.net/Anestesia-Obstetrica/Neuroaxial needles [Last accessed March 2014].
4. Bause GS, Edmonson JM. Special article: Anesthesia and analgesia. 2012;115:1414.
5. Brown DL. Regional Anesthesia and Analgesia, 1st edition. Philadelphia: WB Saunders; 1996.
6. Davies NJ, Cashman JN. Lee's Synopsis of Anaesthesia, 13th edition. Oxford: Butterworth Heinemann; 2006.
7. Hurley RJ, Lambert DH. Continuous spinal anesthesia with a microcatheter technique: preliminary experience. Anesth Analg. 1990;70:97-102.
8. Morgan GE, Mikhail MS, Murray MJ. Clinical Anesthesiology, 4th edition. New York: Lange Medical Books/McGraw-Hill; 2008.
9. Mulroy MF, McDonald S, Bernards CM, et al. A Practical Approach to Regional Anesthesia, 4th edition. Baltimore: Lippincott Williams and Wilkins; 2009.
10. Brown DL. Spinal, epidural and caudal anesthesia. In: Miller RD (Ed). Miller's Anesthesia, 6th edition. Philadelphia: Elsevier Churchill Livingstone; 2005.
11. Atallah MM, Demian AD, Shorrab AA. Development of a difficulty score for spinal anaesthesia. Br J Anaesth. 2004;92: 354-60.
12. Liu SS, McDonald SB. Current issues in spinal anesthesia. Anesthesiology. 2001;94:888-906.

13. Halpern S, Preston R. Postdural puncture headache and spinal needle design. Anesthesiology. 1994;81:1376-83.
14. Agarwal D, Mother M, Tyagi A, et al. Subdural block and the anaesthetist. Anaesth Intensive Care. 2010;38:20-6.
15. Bacon DR. The historical narrative: tales of professionalism? Anesthesiol Clan. 2008;26:67-74.
16. Baheti DK. Use of new modified needle with blunt tip for neurolytic sympathetic block in abdominal malignancies—Abstracts, 11th World Congress on Pain: IASP Press; 2005. pp. 489-90.
17. Al-Shaikh B, Stacey S. Essentials of Anaesthetic Equipment, 3rd edition. Philadelphia, USA: Churchill Livingstone, Elsevier; 2007.
18. Spinal, epidural and caudal anaesthesia In: Miller R. Miller's Anesthesia, 7th edition. Philadelphia: Elsevier Churchill Livingstone; 2010.
19. Standring S. Gray's Anatomy: The Anatomical Basis of Clinical Practice, 41st edition; 2015.
20. Hermanides J, Hollmann MW, Stevens MF, et al. Failed epidural: causes and management. Br J Anaesth. 2012;109(2):144-54.
21. Segal S, Eappen S, Datta S. Superiority of multi-orifice over single-orifice epidural catheters for labor analgesia and cesarean delivery. J Clin Anesth. 1997;9:109-12.
22. Goebel A, Ovenden K, Glynn C. Incorrect distance markings on an epidural catheter. Br J Anaesth. 2003;91:610.
23. Spinal analgesia: intradural and extradural. In: Atkinson RS, Rushman GB, Davies NJ (Eds). Lee's Synopsis of Anaesthesia, 11th edition. Oxford: Butterworth-Heinemann Ltd.; 1993.
24. Rice LJ, Broadman LM, Hannallah RS. Regional anaesthesia in pediatric patients. Advances in Anaesthesia. 1989;6:303-7.
25. De Negri P, Ivani G, Tirri T, et al. New drugs, new techniques, new indications in pediatric regional anesthesia. Minerva Anesthesiol. 2002;68:420-7.
26. Lönnqvist PA, Morton NS. Postoperative analgesia in infants and children. Br J Anaesth. 2005;95(1):59-68.
27. Baheti DK, Deshpande A, Patil V. Epiduroscopy—an interventional pain management for post laminectomy pain—a first case report from India—Bombay Hospital Journal. 2002;44(2):296-7.

Peripheral Nerve Stimulators/ Locators, Needles, and Catheters

Aparna A Nerurkar, Devangi A Parikh

ABSTRACT

The peripheral nerve block involves location of a nerve or a nerve bundle and injection of local anesthetic around the nerve to block its conduction. The methods currently in use are paraesthesia elicitation, nerve stimulation, only ultrasound or nerve stimulation with ultrasound. Nerve stimulators have sought to add an objective end-point to nerve location. The total charge applied to stimulate the nerve is guided by the intensity (I) of the current and the duration (t) of the square pulse of the current. The stimulus needs to be strong enough and it needs to be applied for sufficient time to produce an action potential to depolarize the nerve. Motor nerves have a shorter chronaxie than sensory nerves. This implies that it is possible to stimulate a motor nerve but not the sensory nerve by using a current of smaller chronaxie (shorter time), which is applicable in the practical use of the peripheral nerve stimulator. An appropriate motor response, corresponding to the motor innervation of the nerve to be blocked, has shown to improve the success of a block. Nerve stimulators are designed to be constant current generators with monophasic square wave of current with a sharp rising time of short pulse width, e.g., 50–100 µsec with 1–2 Hz stimulation. The ability of the nerve stimulator to deliver accurate current output and the integrity of the stimulator needle return electrode circuit is of utmost importance for both the block success and safety of the procedure. Newer advancements like sequential electric nerve stimulation (SENSe) and percutaneous electrode guidance (PEG) may tackle some of the shortcomings of conventional nerve stimulators.

The insulated needles which are coated with a layer of nonconducting material over the entire length of the needle just barring the tip prevent nerve injury. Continuous peripheral nerve blockade serves to provide prolonged anesthesia in long duration surgeries. Needle and catheter assemblies are available as cannula over needle design, catheter through needle design and the recent catheter over the needle design. Catheters can be nonstimulating or stimulating. Nerve injury due to direct needle trauma, intraneural injection, underlying nerve pathology and/or surgical factors is one of the dreaded complications. Local anesthetic systemic toxicity is another feared complication. Peripheral nerve catheters are prone to complications ranging from difficult placement, removal, entrapment and infection.

There are no guidelines exists for the practice of peripheral nerve blocks and future efforts should be directed and targeted for more objective nerve localization techniques, injection pressure monitoring devices and better diagnostic modalities to detect complications. The results of these efforts will be crucial for the safe and successful practice of peripheral nerve blockade.

INTRODUCTION

The growing interest in regional anesthesia has led to considerable innovations in the field of peripheral nerve blockade. Peripheral nerve block involves location of a nerve or a nerve bundle and injection of local anesthetic around the nerve to block its conduction. Various techniques are used to achieve this aim. The methods currently in use are paraesthesia elicitation, nerve stimulation, only ultrasound or nerve stimulation with ultrasound.

Success of any nerve block depends upon precise localization of the nerve, which also reduces the amount of local anesthetic agent required. Elicitation of paraesthesia with or without the use of nerve locator,[1] and recently the aid of ultrasound[2] are in use for exact localization of nerve.

Historically, nerve blocks were performed using anatomical landmarks as a guide to insertion of the needle and then elicitation of paraesthesia. This technique is being practiced in many centers even today. While locating the nerve using this technique, the patient experiences a "pin and needles" or an "electric shock" like sensation when the needle touches the nerve. The disadvantage of using this technique is the risk of damage to nerve when the needle touches it. Also the success rate is less as it relies on the patient's subjective sensation, and there is no definitive objective response that can guarantee the accurate location of the nerve. Uncooperative patients pose greater difficulties. The sensation of paraesthesia and blind manipulation of nerve block needle is uncomfortable and unacceptable to some patients. Thus injury to nerve, multiple pricks, large amount of local anesthetic, and high incidence of incomplete block are the main disadvantages of elicitation of paraesthesia technique.[3]

The objective of nerve stimulators is to have end-point to nerve location which is done by applying a small amount of direct current to the needle, that is transmitted to the nerve to produce a motor response.

The thorough knowledge of anatomical landmarks is necessary for use of nerve stimulators and decreases risk of paresthesia technique.

In addition, use of ultrasonography has provided tremendous help for nerve blocks techniques. It has improved visualization of the nerve plexuses which decreases the chances of injury and increased success rates. The basics of ultrasound and ultrasound-guided blocks will be covered in the next chapter "Ultrasound-guided Blocks".

HISTORY

Kulenkampf[4] in 1911 described brachial plexus block and Perthes[5] located it by electrical stimulation although it was crude and cumbersome. Pearson in 1955 demonstrated electrical stimulation of nerves with an insulated needle.[6] In 1962, Greenblatt and Denson[7] devised a portable transistorized nerve stimulator with variable current output. This has increased use of nerve stimulators in regional anesthesia. Wright in 1969, reported use of the block-aid monitor[8] for nerve blocks. To start with noninsulated needles were used but soon it was replaced by insulated one.

ELECTROPHYSIOLOGY[9,10]

In order to use nerve stimulation effectively, it is important to know the electrophysiological principles guiding them. The following information is based on theoretical as well as practical concepts of nerve stimulation which are routinely accepted. However, there are a few discrepancies and conflicting concepts in nerve stimulation.[11]

Neurons, like any other cell in the body, are in a resting state with a negative electric potential inside the cell relative to the outside. This is called the resting membrane potential and is about 70 mV. When a neuron is stimulated, a transient change in the ion permeability of the membrane (an increase in sodium conductance) occurs. If the stimulus is strong enough it depolarizes the membrane sufficiently to set off an action potential **(Fig. 1)** which then propagates along the nerve to stimulate the muscle and cause a contraction. Also depending on the characteristic of the electric impulse, the motor or sensory or both nerve fibers could be stimulated.

Total Charge

The total charge (Q) applied to stimulate the nerve is guided by the intensity (I) of the current and the duration (t) of the square pulse of the current.

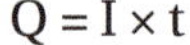

$$Q = I \times t$$

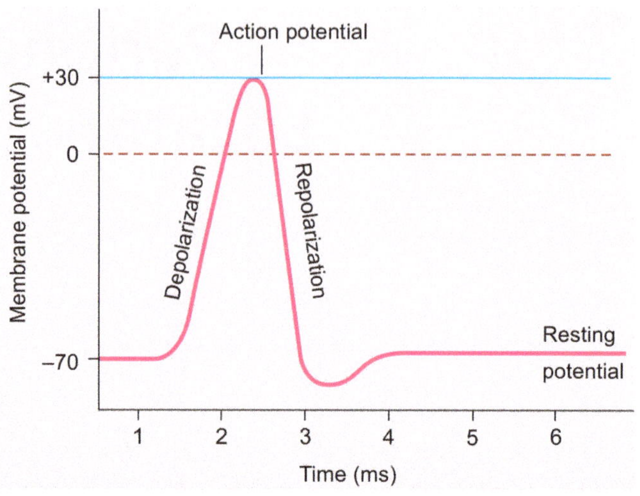

Fig. 1: Action potential.

If the stimulus is not strong enough, even if it is applied for a long time it will not produce an action potential. Conversely if a strong stimulus is applied for only a very short time it will not produce an action potential. Thus, it can be said that the stimulus needs to be strong enough and it needs to be applied for sufficient time to produce an action potential to depolarize the nerve.

Current

The minimum current intensity required to initiate an action potential in the nerve is called the rheobase (Ir). It is expressed by the relationship

$$I = Ir\,(1 + C/t)$$

Chronaxie

It is the length of time the current must be applied to the nerve to initiate an impulse when the current intensity is twice the rheobase. This terminology is used to describe the excitabilities of different nerve fibers. The chronaxie (C) varies in different nerves depending on their sensitivities and their refractory period. The larger the nerve fiber, the shorter the chronaxie. Faster conducting nerves like Aα motor nerve fibers have a smaller chronaxie due to a shorter refractory period than the slower conducting sensory nerves like Aδ or the unmyelinated C sensory nerve fibers. Motor nerves have a shorter chronaxie than sensory nerves **(Table 1)**. This implies that it is possible to stimulate a motor nerve but not the sensory nerve by using a current of smaller chronaxie (shorter time), which is applicable in the practical use of the peripheral nerve stimulator (PNS).

However, the patient may still experience some sensory stimulation such as tingling. Recent data has suggested that, factors like withdrawing and repositioning the stimulating needle, exaggerated motor response and use of high intensity current rather than pulse width are responsible for patient discomfort during nerve block.[13-15]

TABLE 1: Chronaxie of different nerves.[12,13]

	Nerves	Chronaxie time (ms)
Unmyelinated	C	0.40
Myelinated	Aδ	0.17
Myelinated	Aα	0.05–0.10

The threshold current is the lowest current which produces a motor response. A value between 0.2 and 0.5 mA has been suggested to ensure a successful block.[16] It suggests the proximity of the needle to the nerve; however, it cannot be taken as a reliable indicator. Ultrasound-guided blocks have demonstrated that it is possible to be in close proximity to the nerve yet be unable to elicit motor responses, the incidence of which may be as high as 13.5%.[17]

Distance

For effective nerve stimulation, the relationship between current intensity and distance from nerve is governed by Coulomb's law.

$$I = k\,(i/r^2)$$

(I) is the current intensity, (k) is a constant, (i) is the minimum current from the needle tip, and (r) is the distance of stimulus source from the nerve. It is evident that the current intensity is inversely proportional to the square of its distance from the nerve. Hence, while depolarizing a nerve, the farther the nerve from the stimulating electrode, higher the current stimulus required.[12]

Polarity

Polarity of nerve stimulation plays an important role in the success of nerve blocks. Most peripheral nerve block stimulators have the cathode (negative electrode) as the stimulating electrode connected to the needle and the anode (positive electrode) to the patient's skin. With this arrangement significantly less current is required to elicit a motor response as the negative current immediately reduces the voltage outside the membrane, decreases the voltage gradient across it and causes depolarization.[13,18] If the needle is connected to the positive electrode then the nerve will get hyperpolarized. Therefore, a larger current will be needed to depolarize the nerve and obtain a response.

Frequency

The ideal electric parameters for comfortable stimulation are 1–2 Hz. A higher frequency gives more frequent feedback to the operator, but often causes greater discomfort to the patient. If too low a frequency is used then there is a risk of nerve damage between current impulses. There is also a risk of missing the nerve between two stimuli.

PERIPHERAL NERVE STIMULATORS

Elicitation of paraesthesia is an all or none phenomenon, i.e., either the needle contacts the nerve or does not. Electrical nerve stimulation gives a window for graded information useful for locating the nerve, depending on the motor response. There is room to manipulate the needle rather than groping in the dark as by the paraesthesia technique. A nerve stimulator is indispensable in performing a successful peripheral nerve block.

The use of nerve stimulation to locate peripheral nerves was first suggested by von Perthes as early as 1912; however its use has been extensive only in the last two decades. The use of nerve stimulator with a variable current output was first introduced by Greenblatt and Denson.[7] With renewed interest in regional anesthesia, many nerve stimulators have evolved with better functions and accuracy in locating nerves. However, these specialized nerve stimulators contain complex and sophisticated electronics with various functions and features which may confuse the practitioner. An ideal PNS for regional anesthesia should be designed to serve that purpose only, i.e., stimulate and locate the nerve, be simple to operate, reliable, and user-friendly.

Ideal Electrical Characteristics of a Peripheral Nerve Stimulator

Constant Current Generator

Nerve stimulators are designed to be constant current generators, i.e., the current between the anode and cathode of the nerve stimulator is kept constant irrespective of the impedance or resistance of the tissue surrounding the nerve. The impedance of tissues, needles, connecting wires and grounding electrodes may vary (e.g., 1–20 kOhm). The constant current design of the stimulator incorporates automatic compensation in voltage output for changes in tissue or connection impedance during nerve stimulation, assuring accurate delivery of the specified current. The current output can range from 0.01 to 5 mA. It is controlled by digital means or an analog dial on the PNS or a foot paddle connected to it. Remote controlled knobs to manipulate the settings are also available.

Current Wave Form

Monophasic square wave of current with a sharp rising time should be used. Current flows in one direction only. A prolonged subthreshold stimulus or a slow rising current reduces nerve excitability by inactivating sodium conductance (accommodation of nerve fibers).[19]

Pulse Width

A short pulse width, e.g., 50–100 µsec corresponds to chronaxies of alpha fibers, triggering muscle twitches rather than causing pain on stimulation. Low intensity current with a short pulse width is the ideal combination for stimulating a nerve with a motor response which is not uncomfortable to the patient. A longer pulse width (300 µsec to 1 msec) with a low intensity current, may stimulate sensory nerves and therefore elicit a paraesthesia during stimulation.[12,15]

Stimulating Frequency

Traditionally, PNS have had 1 Hz stimulation, meaning 1 pulse per second. However, 2 Hz stimulation capability is clinically advantageous, since it allows faster manipulation of the needle.

Digital Display of Actual Flowing Current

The ability to read the current being delivered is of utmost importance, since the current intensity at which the nerve is stimulated gives the operator an approximation of the needle-nerve distance; 0.5 mA or less indicating intimate needle-nerve relationship. The stimulator design should allow for change in the current intensity in increments of 0.01 mA.

Safety Features

Circuit disconnection alert, impedance alerts, low battery and malfunction alerts should be available. Leads should be clearly marked to avoid confusion as to which is cathode and which is anode. In modern machines stimulators can only connect to the cathode of nerve stimulator. The site on the patient's skin where the anode is attached is immaterial if a constant current nerve output stimulator is used.[13] Stimulators that can deliver only low-output stimulation and are not capable of monitoring neuromuscular blockade are preferable. This is because stimulators designed for neuromuscular monitoring operate at currents much higher than necessary and are not recommended for peripheral nerve localization. Presence of this feature can make things much more confusing.

Remote Control Operated

Hand or foot controlled to eliminate the need of an assistant.

A typical PNS has the following parts depicted in **Figure 2**.

Tracer II (LifeTech Inc.) has the foot pedal **(Fig. 3)** current control capability.

Stimuplex® DIG (B Braun) has a handheld remote facility **(Fig. 4)**.

Multi Stim sensor (Pajunk®) **(Fig. 5)** has additional feature of percutaneous localization and identification of nerves with the aid of a stimulation handle, the percutaneous electronic guidance (PEG)-electrode.

Multi Stim switch **(Fig. 6)** indicates patient resistance thereby permits the instant detection of intraneural, intravascular and intrathecal cannula placement, which can be corrected immediately. A switch-over function enables the practitioner to either select the catheter or the cannula for the stimulation.

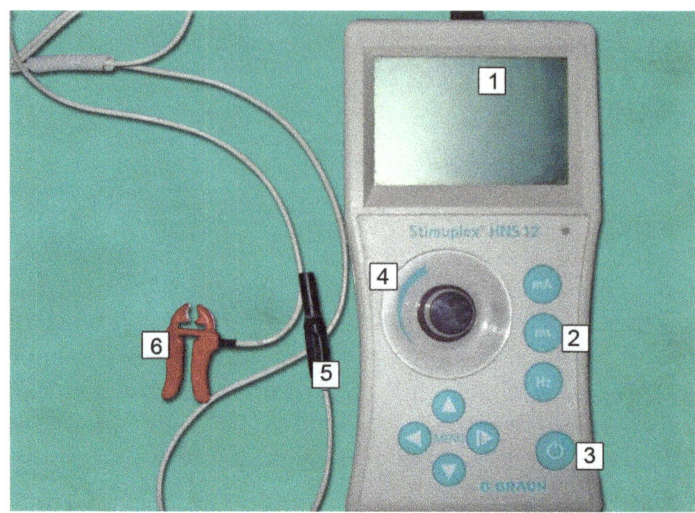

Fig. 2: Peripheral nerve stimulator. 1. Screen displaying the set and delivered current and other features like frequency and duration of stimulus; 2. Buttons to alter current, duration of stimulus and frequency; 3. On/off button; 4. Dial to increase and decrease the settings; 5. Black color cathode connected to the needle; 6. Red-colored anode terminal which is connected to the electrocardiogram (ECG) electrode on the skin of the patient remote from needle insertion.
Courtesy: B Braun.

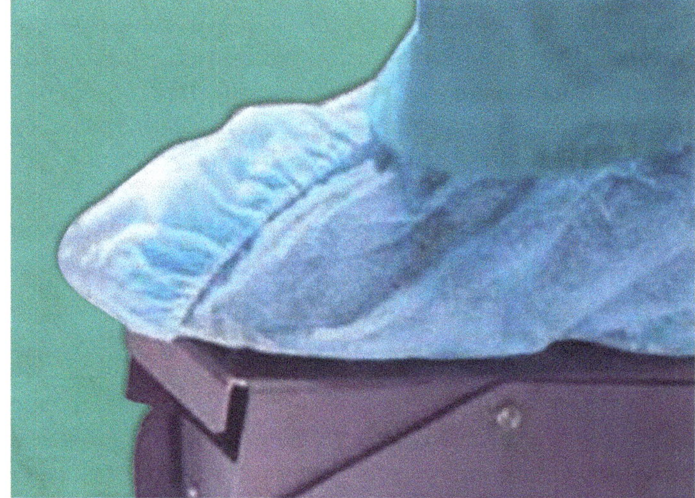

Fig. 3: Foot pedal remote control.

NS 272 (Fisher and Paykel) has a nerve locator with a stimulator to monitor neuromuscular blockade.

Nerve Stimulator Components[20]

The **Figure 7** shows the standard block circuit of the modern peripheral nerve stimulator.

Clock Reference

The clock reference is the synchronizing mechanism of the nerve stimulator. It is a crystal oscillator that produces an accurate, high frequency clock signal. This clock signal is then fed to the microcontroller as input and is used to control its functions. The type of microcontroller decides the specific frequency of the oscillator.

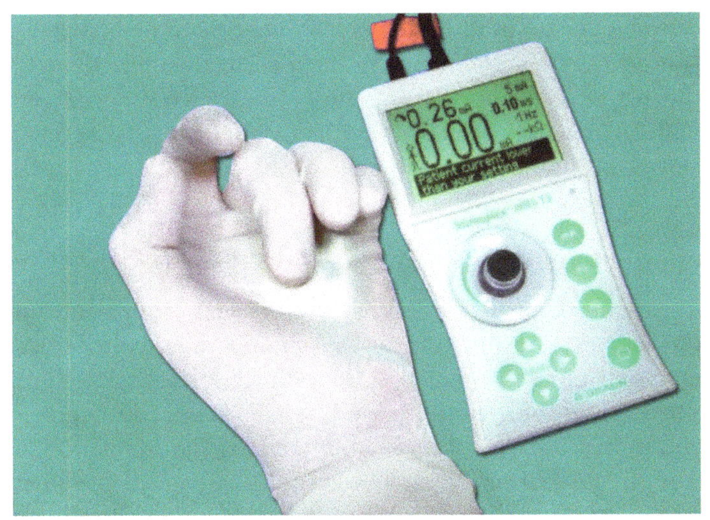

Fig. 4: Handheld remote control.
Courtesy: B Braun.

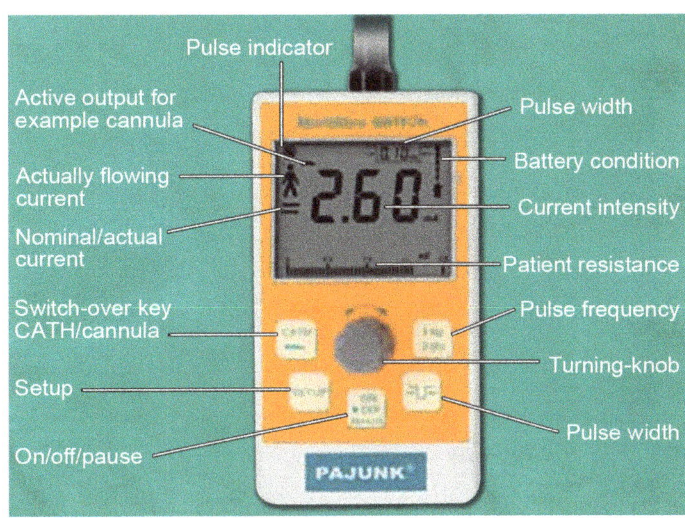

Fig. 6: Multi Stim switch.
Courtesy: With permission of Pajunk®.

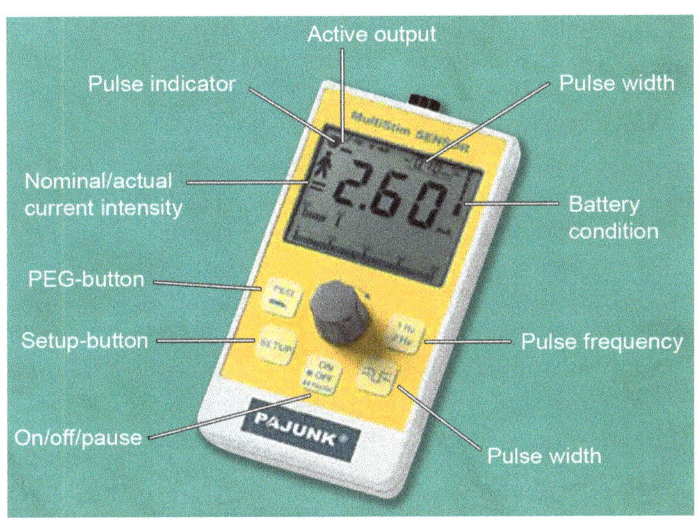

Fig. 5: Multi Stim sensor.
Courtesy: With permission of Pajunk®.

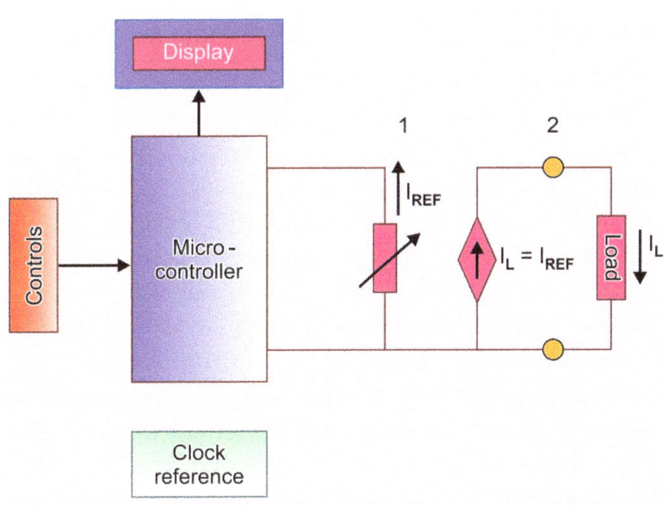

Fig. 7: Peripheral nerve stimulator (PNS) circuitry. 1. Current reference generation; 2. Constant current generation.
Courtesy: B Braun.

Microcontroller

It functions as the most important part of the nerve stimulator. It is very essential to select a low power microcontroller as most of the stimulators run on battery power. The microcontroller receives input from the controls, and as per the inputs it changes the current, frequency and the pulse width. It relays the same to the display, so that the user is aware of the new settings.

Constant current generator: Ideally, constant current source should deliver the same current irrespective of the impedance (resistance) load connected to it. In nonavailability constant current source, a current generator is used. It provides a reasonably stable current over a wide range of impedance loads. This is achieved by generating a progressively higher voltage output as the impedance between the electrodes is increased.

Controls: On a nerve stimulators three sets of controls are available: (1) frequency, (2) pulse width and (3) current. These controls can be analog or digital, and it increases or decreases the value of the controlled parameter.

Current reference generator: It is a voltage source and low tolerance potentiometer controlled by the microcontroller using a series a command pulses which tells it to increase or decrease the value.

Display: It is usually a standard liquid crystal display (LCD) **(Fig. 8)** which uses less current and is more versatile than the light emitting diode (LED) displays. It shows the value of current, frequency and pulse width. Additionally some

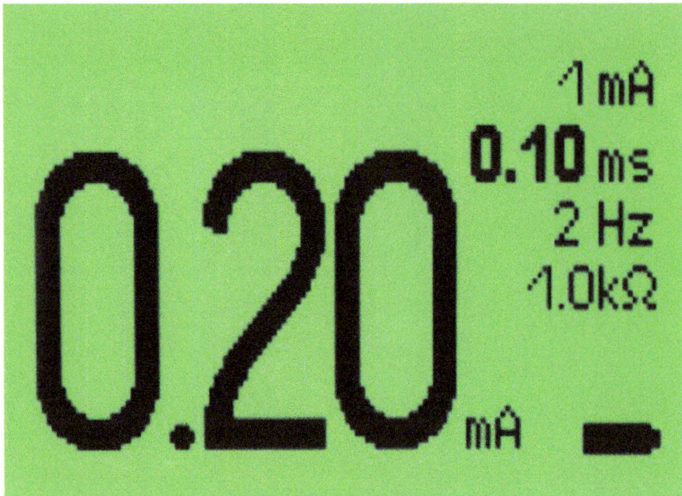

Fig. 8: Display.

models may also have displays depicting low battery level, needle disconnect and abnormal impedance.

Steps in Using a Peripheral Nerve Stimulator (Video 14)

The equipment needs to be checked prior to starting. The desired initial current (1–2 mA), pulse duration (0.1 ms) and frequency (2 Hz) need to be set. The needle is connected to the cathode of the machine and the anode is connected to the patient via an electrocardiograph (ECG) electrode which is placed on the patient. The local anesthetic syringe is connected to the flexible tubing of the needle and the tubing is flushed with local anesthetic solution or saline which acts like a stylet and prevents tissue entering the needle.

The point of needle insertion is determined by anatomical landmarks. It is important to make sure the circuit is complete as soon as the needle is inserted. The machine may have a flashing light or audible beep or some other mechanism to indicate that the circuit is complete. The needle approach and direction should be anatomically correct to maximize the chances of correct localization and minimizing complications. The needle is then advanced in the direction towards the nerve until distinct muscle contractions occur in the innervated area. The current is then reduced gradually till motor response is seen at roughly 0.5 mA. The displayed current on the nerve stimulator is noted. For peripheral nerve location, 2–5 mA currents increase sensitivity but specificity is achieved by successful stimulation at a lower current. A current between 0.2 and 0.5 mA is accepted as ideal threshold current. Stimulation at currents above 0.5 mA may result in block failure as the needle may be farther away from the nerve.[21] The stimulation of nerve at currents below 0.2 mA suggest that the needle tip is in the nerve and there is a danger of intraneural injection.[13]

The negative aspiration confirms that needle is not intravascular. Now inject local anesthetic in increments of 5 mL without moving the needle tip. After injection of 0.5–1 mL the motor twitch should disappear which is either due to mechanical displacement of the nerve from the needle (Raj test) or due to change in the electrical conductivity of the nerve. The signs such as failure of the twitch to disappear, pain on injection, solution requiring high injection pressures suggests intraneural placement of the needle tip, in such case withdraw needle tip by (0.5–1 mm).

Clinical Pearls while Using a Nerve Stimulator

The ability of the nerve stimulator to deliver accurate current output and the integrity of the stimulator needle return electrode circuit is of utmost importance for both the block success and safety of the procedure. In clinical practice, it is common for a clinician to fail in locating the nerve due to some technical problem; however this technical problem goes unrecognized and multiple manipulations of the needle are done to locate the nerve leading to repeated unsuccessful attempts and thereby increasing chances of complications. To avoid this it may be recommended that

- Clinicians should be familiar with how the nerve stimulator indicates proper current delivery and failure to deliver set current (disconnect alarm). They should verify the absence of disconnect alarm as soon as needle is inserted in the skin
- High quality skin electrodes should be used. The skin electrode should be visibly and palpably inspected to ensure that the conducting gel is present and not desiccated
- Usually there is an indicator (flashing light or audible beep) which indicates that the circuit is complete. While administering block one should periodically check the LCD indicator to ensure this and also that set current is delivered.

RECENT DEVELOPMENTS IN NERVE STIMULATION

With the available nerve stimulators, there is very precise localization of the nerve as close to the needle as possible. However, while searching for the nerve, motor response may be abolished by even the tiniest fine movements of the needle the leaving the practitioner clueless. Newer advancements like sequential electric nerve stimulation (SENSe) and percutaneous electrode guidance (PEG) may tackle some of the shortcomings of conventional nerve stimulators.

Sequential Electric Nerve Stimulation

Most of the nerve stimulators function on a fixed pulse duration (0.1 ms or 0.2 ms). New nerve stimulators have been innovated where the pulse duration can be adjusted; however one can use only one fixed pulse duration at any given time. This ensures more patient safety and improved clinical efficiency. Urmey and Grossi[22] used a nerve stimulator programmed to deliver SENSe. The stimulator generated alternating sequential electric pulses of differing pulse duration at a frequency of 3 Hz.

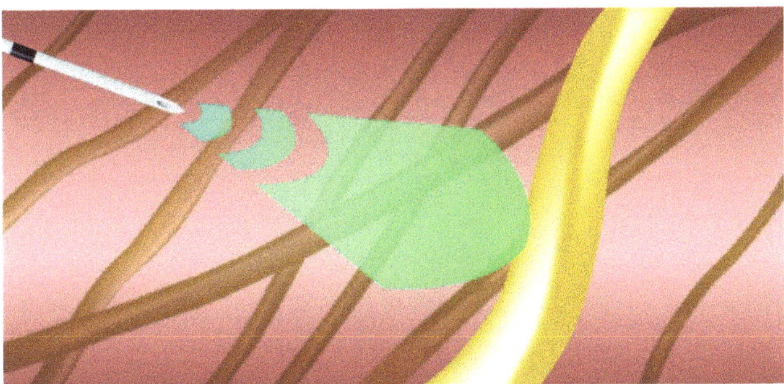

Fig. 9: Sequential electric nerve stimulation (SENSe) step 1—one muscle twitch is visible and this indicates that the needle is in the direction of the nerve.
Courtesy: B Braun.

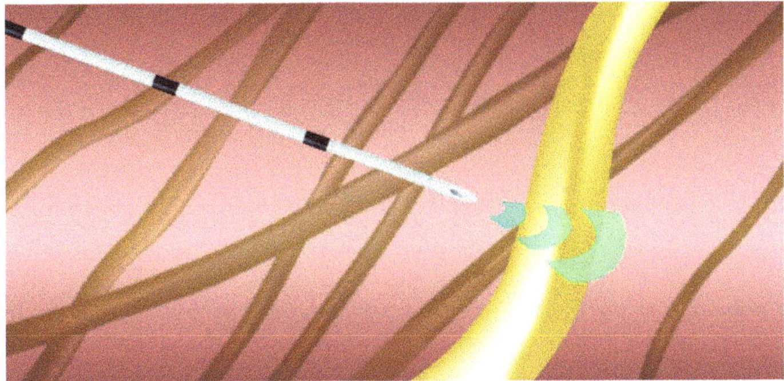

Fig. 11: Sequential electric nerve stimulation (SENSe) step 3.
Courtesy: B Braun.

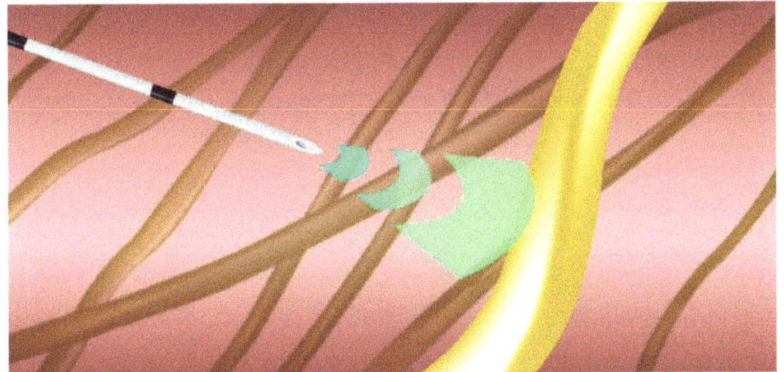

Fig. 10: Sequential electric nerve stimulation (SENSe) step 2.
Courtesy: B Braun.

The commercially available B Braun Stimuplex® HNS 12 with SENSe[23] uses a sequence of two fixed impulse duration of 0.1 ms along with a third longer impulse duration. This results in getting the first twitch already at a distance from the nerve and requires less adjustment to amperage control, while maintaining a visual feedback. It also incorporates a built in programmed attenuation of the third impulse in response to decreasing amperage, to eliminate strong contractions as the needle is close to the nerve.

From the alternating sequence of three impulses, the third longer impulse stimulates the nerve already at a distance **(Fig. 9)**.

The stimulation needle is further advanced toward the nerve while SENSe maintains the motor response. Current strength adjustments lead to definite reductions in third impulse **(Fig. 10)**.

At the threshold set of approximately 0.3 mA all three muscle twitches are visible as all the three impulses elicit a motor response **(Fig. 11)**.

If the muscle twitch has been lost the third longer impulse helps to easily find it again. Thus SENSe allows easier and more reliable nerve localizations for better blocks.

REGIONAL BLOCK NEEDLES

Pearson introduced the use of insulated needles for peripheral nerve blocks.[6] Montgomery and colleagues demonstrated that ordinary uninsulated needles could also be used to localize nerves, with higher current.[24]

Insulated needles are coated with a layer of nonconducting material (e.g., polytetrafluoroethylene or silicon) over the entire length of the needle just barring the tip. There are needles which have a pin-point electrode tip, in which both the shaft and the bevel are coated and only the tip conducts current, thereby enabling more precision in localization. These types of needles may be associated with a higher success rate.[16]

Uninsulated needles are bare metallic needles that transmit the current throughout the entire length of the shaft. They have a much larger conducting area in contrast to insulated needles. This results in lesser current density at the tip of the needle. This mechanism demands a higher threshold current, usually more than 1 mA to stimulate a nerve.[25] With these needles it may be more difficult to accurately localize the nerve. These needles are connected to the nerve stimulator by an alligator clip **(Figs. 12A and B)**. They are slowly losing favor as insulated needles are being used.

The **Figure 13** shows that current leaks all through the shaft of the needle in case of uninsulated needles. Also in the case of insulated needles as the current only comes out of the tip, means that it gives more focus on the position of the nerve in relation to the tip. As the needle moves away from the nerve there is a rapid increase in the stimulating current with an insulated needle as opposed to a more gradual change in the noninsulated needles. With a noninsulated needle, the motor response may only be elicited after the needle tip is beyond the nerve due to current leaking from the shaft.[25]

Needle Designs

A wide variety of needles are available for peripheral nerve blocks **(Fig. 14)**.

The type of needle chosen by the practitioner depends on the block performed, the size of the patient and individual preference.[26-28]

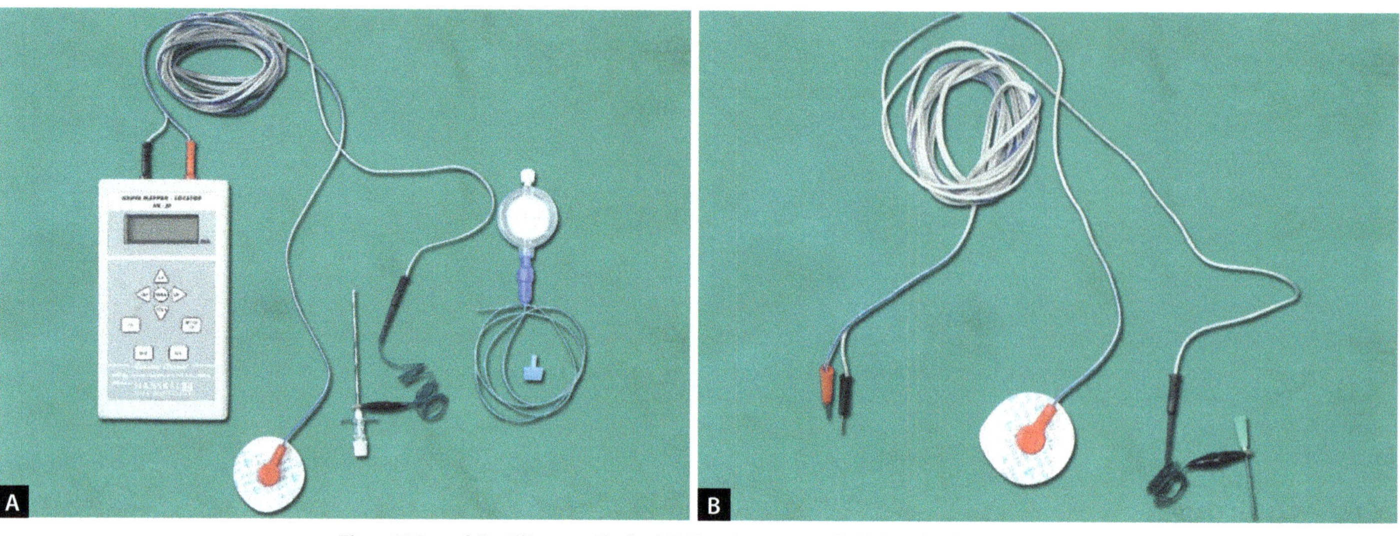

Figs. 12A and B: Alligator clip for (A) Continuous; and (B) Single shot blocks.

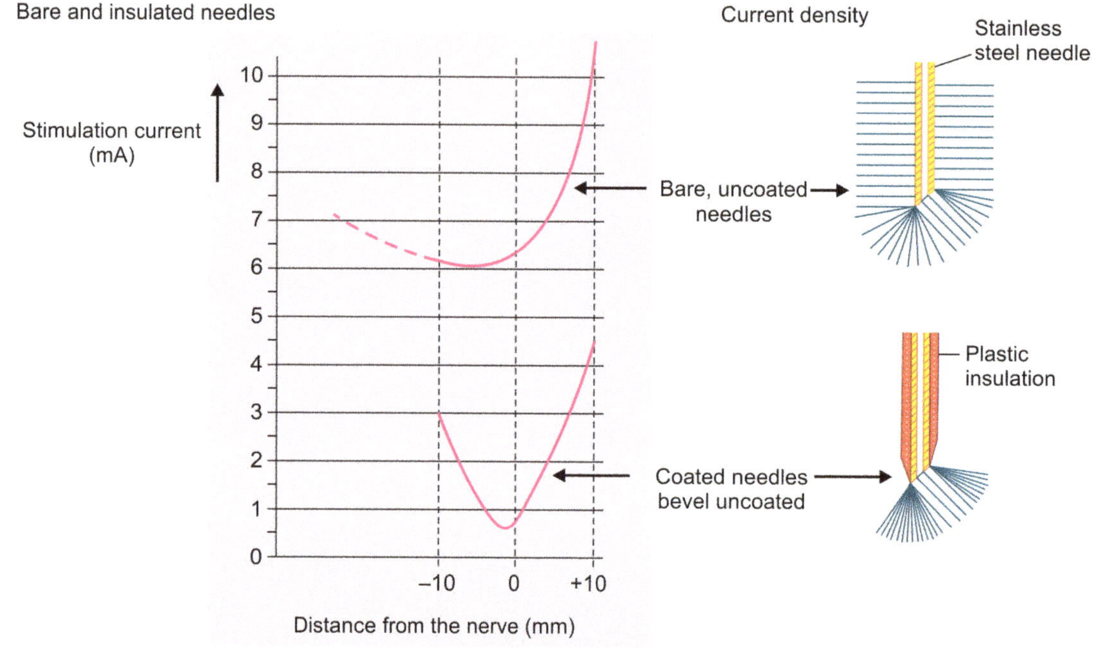

Fig. 13: Insulated versus noninsulated needles.
Courtesy: B Braun.

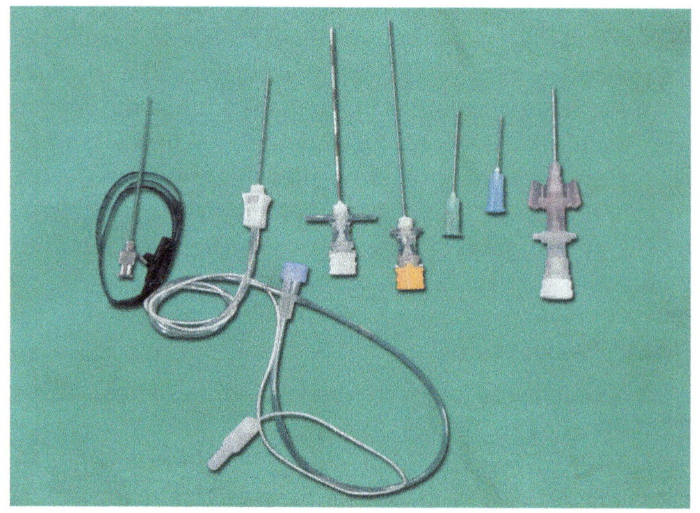

Fig. 14: Variety of needles for peripheral nerve block.

Parts of the Insulated Needles

- The needle is insulated along the shaft except for the tip
- There is a comfortable finger grip attached at the proximal end of the needle
- There is a wire attached to the needle which connects it to the stimulator. This wire is soldered to the needle shaft and has an appropriate connector for the nerve stimulator
- There is a long clear extension tubing integral to the needle shaft which facilitates injection of local anesthetics and also for early detection of blood
- The needle typically has a bevel ranging from 15 to 45° with different manufacturers and makes
- Markings on the needles in centimeters are helpful in determining the depth of the needle from the skin.

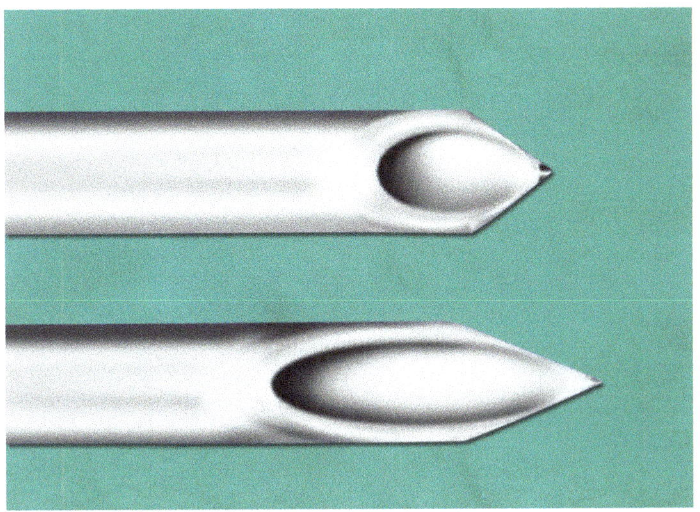

Fig. 15: The 15° and 30° bevels.

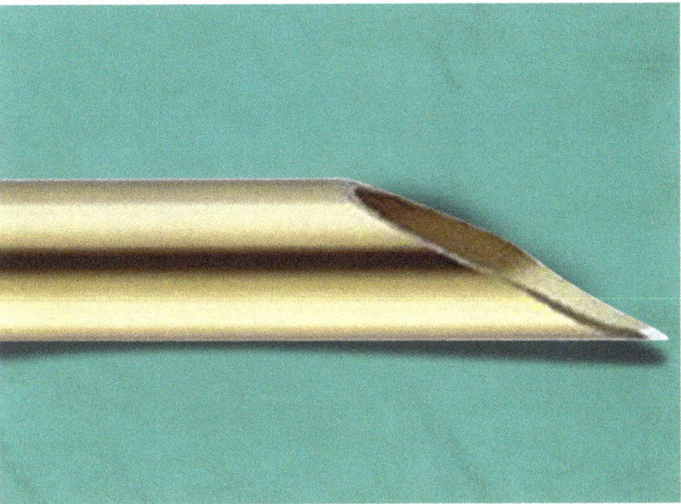

Fig. 16: Facet tip bevel.
Courtesy: With permission of Pajunk®.

Needle Tip

The most commonly used needle tip design is the pencil-point or short, blunt-bevel needle design which are claimed to cause less injuries during nerve blocks. Currently there is lack of evidence to recommend a needle design which may not be implicated in nerve injury. In fact whether the needle design is directly responsible for nerve injury or not is also a subject of debate. In spite of this research, workers presents arguments for choice between long bevel (cutting, sharp) and short bevel (blunt, pencil-point) needles. Proponents of pencil-point or short bevel designs believe that blunt needles are less likely to injure and cut nerves.[29,30] In contrast proponents of long bevel needles think that its design allows for smooth passage through tissue planes and results in better control than the "popping" motion associated with blunt needles.[31,32] Most anesthesiologists believe that the short, blunt bevel is less likely to penetrate or cut nerves.

The design of needle tip also guides anesthesiologists to structures which are penetrated while locating a nerve. Blunt, short bevel needles offer more resistance and thus give a better feel as the needle passes through tissue layers than do sharper long beveled needles. In an in vitro study, anesthesiologists preferred needles that offered moderate resistance and enhanced feel with the tissue penetration.[33]

For single shot deep nerve or major plexus blocks, short and blunt beveled insulated needles can be used. Sharper and smaller gauge needles (24 G or 25 G) are often used for transarterial axillary block, superficial nerve blocks and field blocks like hernia blocks, penile block. If a block does not require stimulation (e.g., paravertebral block) a 22 G Tuohy or a Quincke's spinal needle can be used.

Commonly available insulated needles include Stimuplex® A and D (B Braun) which have a short blunt bevel at an angle of 15° or 30° **(Fig. 15)**.

Nano Line (Pajunk®) is available as a facet tip **(Fig. 16)** as well as Sprotte tip bevel **(Fig. 17)**.

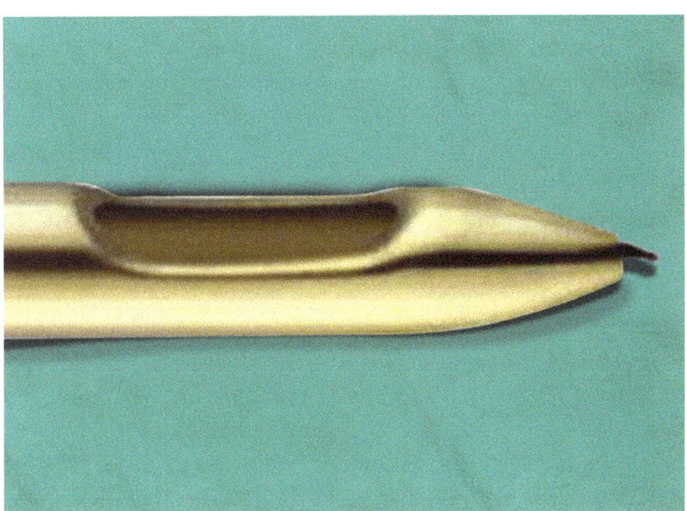

Fig. 17: Sprotte tip bevel.
Courtesy: With permission of Pajunk®.

Needle Length

An appropriate length of the needle is of paramount importance in conduct of a successful block. Too short a needle will not reach its targeted depth. Too long needles pose their own problems as they are difficult to manipulate and there is always a subconscious tendency on the part of the anesthesiologist to insert it deeply if the nerve cannot be located. Generally, longer needles are used to access deep-set nerves (e.g., sciatic nerve) or in obese patients. These needles cannot be sterilized and they are one time use only. The **Figure 18** shows various stimulating needle sizes that are available.

Needle Gauge

Choice of the gauge of the needle depends whether the block is single shot or continuous, patient profile and availability. It is preferable to use a smaller gauge needle to reduce the risk of tissue trauma and discomfort. However, smaller gauge

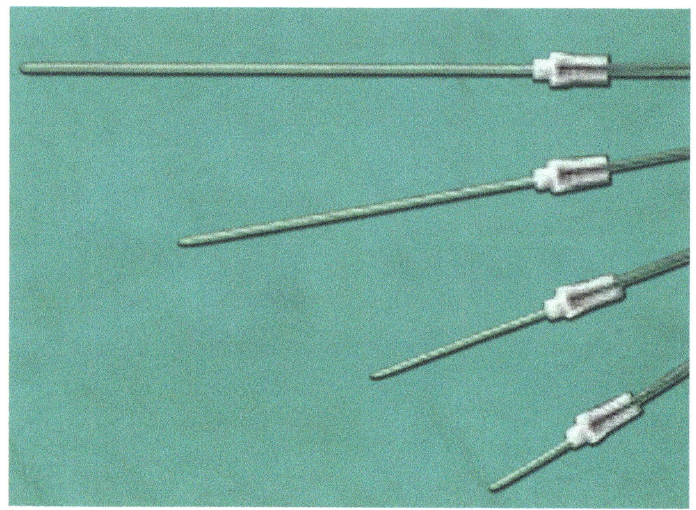

Fig. 18: Various sizes of stimulating needle.
Courtesy: B Braun.

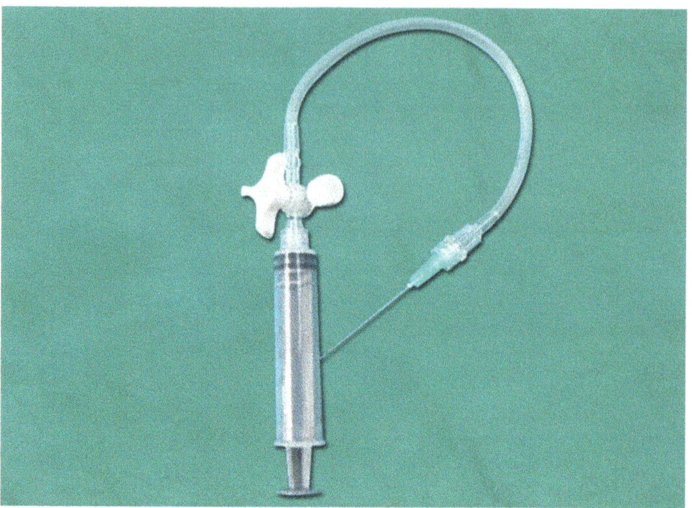

Fig. 19: Prefixed extension tubing with bivalve.

needles bend more easily. It is also more difficult to inject local anesthetics, assess injection pressure and resistance, and detect intravascular placement. 24 G or 25 G needles for superficial blocks and 22 G needles for major conduction and deeper blocks may be preferred. When longer needles are used for deeper blocks, e.g., sciatic nerve or infraclavicular, 21 G needles may be preferred to avoid the problem of bending the needle.

Accessories

Extension tubing attached to the locating needle are desirable as they aid the anesthesiologist in aspiration for detection of intravascular placement. They are helpful in changing syringes without moving the needle. One of the common reasons for block failure despite adequate motor response is displacement of needle while injecting the drug and this is avoided by the extension tubing. Most commercially available needles have preattached extension tubing. In cases where hypodermic needles were previously used, a 10 cm extension tubing prefixed with a bivalve was attached as shown in **Figure 19**.

Transcutaneous Stimulus and Percutaneous Electrode Guidance

It is often difficult to elicit motor response of the desired nerve despite sound anatomical knowledge and marking of exact landmarks. Anatomical landmarks vary from patient to patient and do not always correlate with the underlying nerves. Also anatomical landmarks are sometime difficult to mark accurately. This leads to frequent manipulations causing discomfort and probably injuries. To avoid this, techniques such as transcutaneous and percutaneous nerve stimulation have been introduced to prelocalize the nerves.

Transcutaneous Electrical Stimulation

A current of higher intensity (5–20 mA) can be used transcutaneously to stimulate and prelocalize nerves before needle insertion. Ganta and colleagues[34] used a modified electrocardiographic electrode 0.5 cm in diameter with adherent coupling gel in interscalene block for prelocalization. This electrode was attached to a nerve stimulator. Transcutaneous stimulation can also be used for sensory paresthesia's as described by Shannon and colleagues[15] for lateral femoral cutaneous nerve. In contrast to the short pulse duration desired in stimulating needles, transcutaneous stimulation benefits from a longer pulse duration. Longer pulse duration allows for motor response at lower amperage.

Percutaneous Electrode Guidance of the Block Needle

Percutaneous electrode guidance uses the principle of transcutaneous nerve stimulation to prelocate the plexus or nerves prior to needle insertion and manipulation. Urmey and Grossi[35] reported the first clinical case of peripheral nerve blocks using PEG technique. In contrast to transcutaneous technique, the cutaneous electrode used is sterile, electrically shielded, and cylindrical with a minute, smooth (1 mm) metallic tip. This electrode can be used to indent the skin and the underlying subcutaneous tissue towards the nerve. This maneuver decreases the tissue electrical impedance by condensing underlying subcutaneous tissues and shifting adipose tissue laterally. Indentation also minimizes the sphere of current diffusion, maximizing the electric conductance. It also reduces the distance between the skin and the targeted nerve, improving accuracy. A current between 1.2 and 8.2 mA is applied to locate peripheral nerves in adult patients. At the point of maximal motor response with minimal cutaneous probe amperage the cutaneous stimulator is turned off and a standard nerve stimulator needle is passed through the probe to the nerve. The nerve stimulator then transmits minimal current (usually starting from 0.5 mA) to the stimulating needle to objectively locate the nerve. Minimal transcutaneous stimulation current in mA correlated directly with the measured needle depth beyond the probe tip.[35] Thus, PEG has a net effect of causing motor response with minimal discomfort to the patient.

Scientific Fundamentals Underlying Percutaneous Electrode Guidance

The transcutaneous electric nerve stimulation is
- Directly proportional to current amplitude
- Directly proportional to pulse duration
- Inversely proportional to electrode to nerve distance
- Inversely proportional to electric impedance (resistance of surrounding tissues).

Procedure[36]

The electrode sites are prepared with a degreasing agent (e.g., alcohol) to decrease the skin resistance and enhance the transcutaneous conduction of electricity. The stimulation is usually begun with a current of 5 mA when a stimulus of longer duration is used (e.g., 1 ms) or up to 20 mA when a stimulus of shorter duration is used (0.1 ms). Once a distal response specific to the nerve under localization is elicited, the current is lowered to the minimal intensity at which this response is still seen or felt. The point on the skin at which the stimulation is elicited with the minimal possible current is labeled as the approximate position of the nerve (plexus). During the localization the electrode is continuously and firmly pressed against the skin to shorten the skin nerve distance and decrease the resistance of the skin electrode interface. A standard commercial nerve stimulating needle is then physically guided by the electrode towards the nerve. Since much of the location is done by the probe, which indents the skin towards the nerve, the stimulating needle tip typically travels only a short distance to the nerve **(Fig. 20)**.

In some patients, stimulation with a current of significantly greater intensity than 5 mA may be necessary to evoke a motor response. In these patients, a higher output nerve stimulator (e.g., the one for neuromuscular monitoring) can be used. The current is set at 15–20 mA and applied via an alligator tip; the current is decreased as the motor response is established.

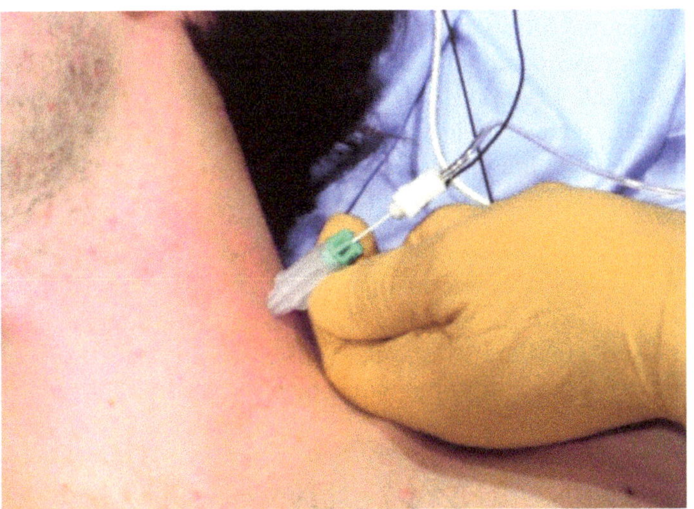

Fig. 20: Use of percutaneous electrode guidance.
Courtesy: B Braun.

Limitations

Surface nerve prelocation provides only a rough estimate of the location of the nerve or a plexus, and needle repositioning as reangling is often necessary to locate the nerve.

CONTINUOUS PERIPHERAL NERVE BLOCKADE

Introduction

Continuous peripheral nerve blockade serves to provide prolonged anesthesia in long duration surgeries. It also gives the additional benefit of extended postoperative pain relief. This technique involves inserting a catheter along the neural bundle. With the advent of peripheral nerve stimulators, ultrasonography, it is easier to place the catheters accurately and reliably at their desired site of action.

Continuous peripheral nerve blockade (CPNB) avoids the risks and side effects of prolonged general anesthesia and central neuraxial blockade. Analgesia is also superior to parenteral opioid and avoids their unwanted side effects like nausea, vomiting, sedation and respiratory depression.[37] The quality of analgesia is comparable to epidural analgesia but devoid of side effects like hypotension, urinary retention and pruritus.[38] CPNB aids in early mobilization thereby decreasing the incidence of deep vein thrombosis and lessens the incidence of postoperative cognitive dysfunction. In some centers, CPNB is given in major trauma patients immediately after initial stabilization to decrease the stress response to tissue trauma.[39] The only limitation is the limited or almost nonavailability of appropriate CPNB equipment in the last century.

History

The earliest report of CPNB was given by Ansbro[40] in 1946 with a blunt needle connected to an injection tubing and a syringe. In 1951, Sarnoff and Sarnoff[41] published the use of catheter for phrenic nerve block. Regional anesthesia practitioners have assembled intravenous access and spinal epidural equipment **(Fig. 21)** to create their own CPNB apparatus.

They have even created their own insulated needles using a larger gauge cannula over a smaller gauge needle,[38,42] or the Seldinger technique,[43] etc. However, these systems had their own limitations—the cannula rarely fitted appropriately over the needle, multiple steps from identifying the nerve to threading the catheter were required which increased the risk of misplacement of catheter. Moreover, there were concerns of neurological complications using long bevel needles, and therefore recommendations to use short bevel needles.[31]

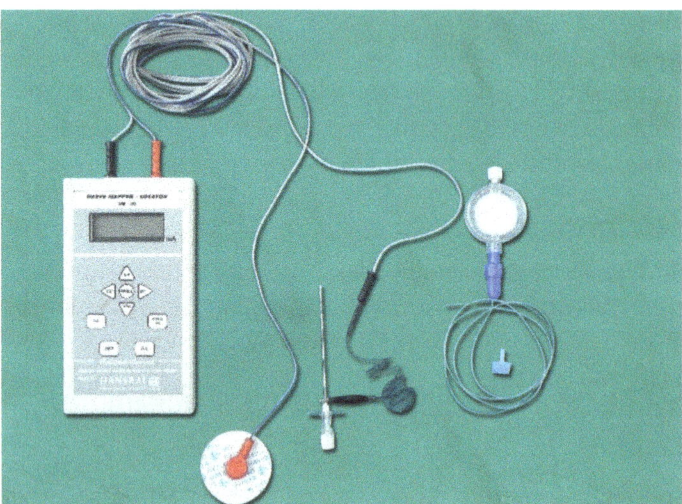

Fig. 21: Epidural equipment for continuous peripheral nerve blockade.

These limitations led to the development of conventionally acceptable CPNB equipment.

Equipment

Peripheral Nerve Stimulator

It is preferable to use a PNS for continuous blocks. The details of its characteristics and functioning have been discussed earlier. In cases where self-assembled insulated needles or regular Tuohy epidural needles are used, a nerve stimulator with alligator clips-cathode connection may be required.

Needles

In most cases, insulated needles are used for better precision. For continuous blocks the needle must be large enough to allow the passage of catheter. Currently most anesthesiologists prefer to use an 18–19 G needle which allows passage of a 20 G catheter.

Cannula over needle design: These assemblies include a cannula over a short beveled needle. The first commercially available equipment for CPNB included this design and it was the original Contiplex® A (B Braun). It had an 18 G needle which was short beveled (32°) and a 20 G catheter (40 cm) long. This was later modified to Contiplex® D model which additionally included an integrated wire for nerve stimulation and connection tubing for simultaneous injection and aspiration. The Contiplex® A and D were very popular and used in 1990s.[44-49]

Contiplex D® needle (bevel 15° or 30°) is available in various sizes and lengths (22/20 G and 54/110 mm). Contiplex S® has an 18 G needle, 20° bevel and catheter insertion directly through the needle with simultaneous aspiration through side port. Miniset (Pajunk®) has 21/24 G needles with either a Sprotte® or facet tip. This design was considered useful in pediatric cases.

The main limitation of this design was that there were multiple manipulations required to insert the catheter, thereby increasing risk of infection and malpositioning of catheter.

Catheter through needle design: This system was devised to address the concerns over the previous system. Contiplex® Tuohy system (B Braun) serves to provide for a single operator use.[50] There is an 18 G insulated Tuohy needle coated with polytetrafluoroethylene along its entire length except at a pin-point area at the distal tip. This needle was designed with a Huber tip to facilitate placement of catheter in a direction parallel to the nerve **(Fig. 22)**.

There is also a 50 cm extension tubing like the previous devices and facilitates immobile needle technique. The luer-lock head has a hemostasis valve and a central diaphragm that allows the passage of catheter through a port separate from where injection and aspiration occur. This eliminates the need for equipment disconnection and reduces chances of needle movement and catheter misplacement. The length of the catheter is 100 cm, made of polyamide nylon, it has centimeter gradations up to 20 and there are three distal orifices with a closed tip. A 40 cm stimulating wire is permanently attached to the needle and connects to the PNS. This product is widely used and published.[51-53] The Plexolong system (Pajunk®) **(Fig. 23)** also contains an 18 G needle, is radiopaque with a styletted epidural catheter, stimulating wire and detachable injection tubing.[54,55] There is a large catheter threading device which keeps the catheter in a sterile coil. The catheter stylet was devised to impart additional rigidity and easy insertion. They offer different needle tip designs like Tuohy, Sprotte®, Facet tip (30° and 45°). 21 G pediatric set is also available. Prolong system (LifeTech) also has a short bevel Tuohy tip with no catheter stylet.

Catheter over the needle design: Contiplex® C is a patented innovation of B Braun, which combines the advantage of single technique block plus continuing anesthesia through catheter. It has a highly echogenic catheter prethreaded over an insulated long cannula. The cannula with catheter is inserted through the skin under neurostimulator and/or ultrasonographic guidance till desired end-point is obtained. The bolus dose is given through cannula which is then removed to leave the catheter in place which can be used for continuous block.

Catheters: Catheters can be nonstimulating or stimulating. There are basically four types of catheters for continuous peripheral nerve blocks.[56]

1. *20 G epidural catheter:* They are nonirritating, flexible, and generate minimal friction on passage through needles. Graduated markings and radiopacity help in confirming placement and insertion depth. Multi-orifice catheters have a closed distal tip and three distal openings 0.5, 1.0, and 1.5 cm from the tip. Single orifice catheters have a single opening at the distal end of the catheter.

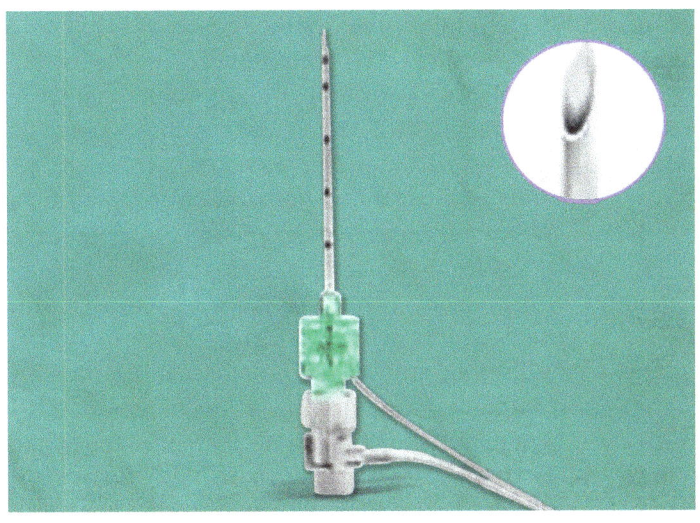

Fig. 22: Contiplex® Tuohy needle.

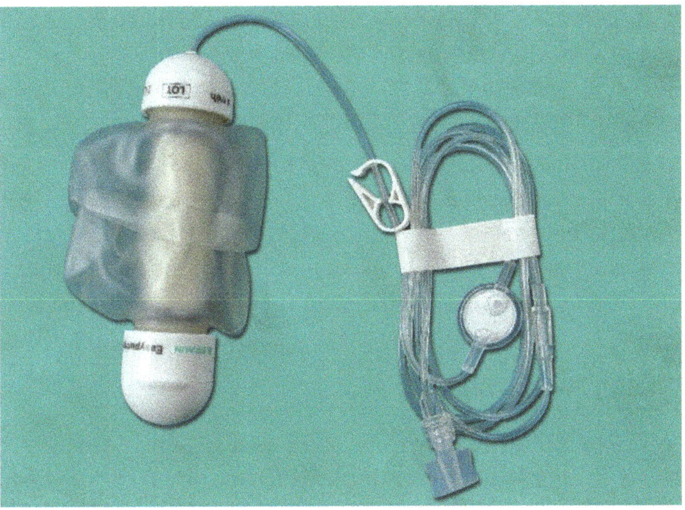

Fig. 24: Elastomeric pumps.

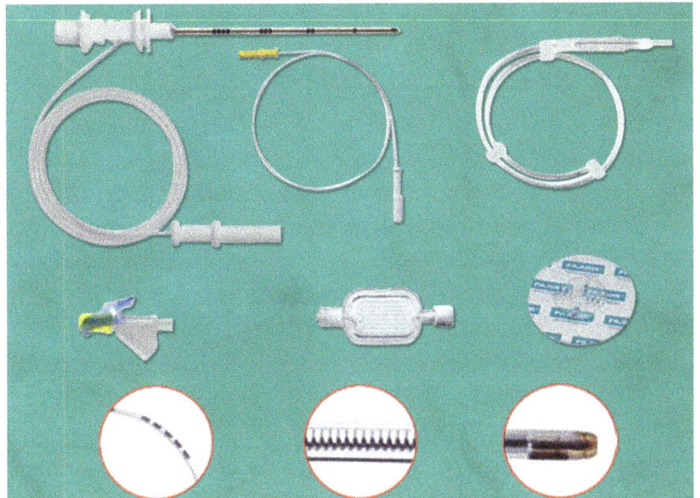

Fig. 23: Plexolong system.
Courtesy: With permission of Pajunk®.

2. *20 or 21 G styletted epidural catheter:* These catheters may help in easier advancement. However, use of these catheters may result in greater tissue trauma. A case report mentions shearing of catheter when stylet was removed.[57]
3. *20 G catheter to be threaded over a wire using Seldinger technique:* This technique is not very commonly used.
4. *Stimulating catheter:* These catheters conduct current to their distal end and thereby confirm appropriate perineural placement. StimuCath™ (Arrow international)[58] has a 17 G or 18 G insulated Tuohy needle in various sizes. There is 5 mm long uninsulated segment at the distal needle tip. The needle is insulated with a thin wall of polyester. Initially there was an alligator clip which connected the nerve stimulator to the proximal end of the needle or the catheter. Recently there is an addition of the integrated stimulating wire attached to the needle. There is also an integrated detachable tubing. Kick, et al.[59] described another stimulating catheter (Stimulong catheter set, Pajunk®). It consists of a 20 G, single hole, 400 mm polyamide catheter with a 405 mm indwelling removable conducting stylet. The metal wire stylet is insulated with Teflon coating along its length except at the distal 0.3 mm. The proximal end has a plug to allow connection to a nerve stimulator. Subsequent modification has involved incorporation of an integrated wire within the catheter (Stimulong Plus, Pajunk®).[60]

Infusion pumps: The continuous catheters are connected to infusion pumps intraoperatively to prolong the duration of anesthesia and postoperatively for analgesia. Elastomeric pumps **(Fig. 24)** provide a constant infusion rate only (2/5/7/10/12 mL/h) depending on the manufacturer.

They could be univariate (single fixed infusion rate) or multivariate (multiple infusion rates) which can give flexibility to alter the rate of infusion. Patient-controlled analgesia (PCA) pump an electronic pump which controls the basal rate and also provides additional boluses with variable lockout times can be used.

Evaluation of stimulating versus nonstimulating catheters: There are limited studies comparing the two though intuitively stimulating catheters should have a higher success rate. Initial study[61] in human volunteers demonstrated increased success rates with stimulating versus nonstimulating catheters. Similarly, Pham Dang et al.[60] reported 0% failed block rates when stimulating catheters were used. However, they unable to obtain any stimulation through the catheter in nearly 5% of all the patients, which would bring the overall failure rate closer to that of nonstimulating catheters. The practical advantages of the stimulating catheter, as reported by previous investigators, were not obvious in a study conducted by Jack et al.[62] In terms of outcome measures such as pain scores and morphine consumption, they found no significant differences between stimulating and nonstimulating catheters. Another study[63] found no significant difference in primary block success rates with both catheters, however secondary block failure rates were higher with nonstimulating C catheters.

Continuous Catheter Placement Techniques

The continuous peripheral nerve block is an advanced regional anesthesia technique and adequate experience with the single shot technique is mandatory to ensure its safety and efficacy. Steele and colleagues[50] described the catheter placement techniques for the nonstimulating catheter and Sanofi[64] for the stimulating catheter.

Nonstimulating Catheter Technique

In this technique, the nerve is located using an insulated needle and needle tip is advanced closer to the nerve. After desired motor response at the desired current amperage, the local anesthetic is injected through the extension tubing that is attached to the needle. This is called as "primary block". Now after removal of the needle the catheter is passed through the cannula. Injection of drug through the catheter is called as "secondary block".

It is a reliable technique and simple to perform. The only limitation is the catheter is placed without confirming the tip position which makes it difficult to predict success rate of secondary block. This disadvantage has been overcome using a stimulating catheter.

Stimulating Catheter Technique or Sarnoff Technique

The nerve stimulator is attached to an insulated 17–20 G stimulating needle which is advanced till a brisk motor response is obtained at 0.4–0.5 mA. Now hold needle in steady position (do not inject local anesthetic agent) and disconnect nerve stimulator from the needle and attached to the proximal end of the stimulating catheter. Then the catheter is advanced through the needle to elicit a similar motor response as obtained before. The catheter is advanced beyond the needle tip, while aiming to maintain the similar motor response. If the desired motor response disappears, then the catheter is withdrawn back in the needle, the needle is manipulated clockwise, counterclockwise, inward or outward, seeking the optimal motor response. The nerve stimulator remains connected to the catheter while manipulating the needle, because the catheter in the needle essentially converts stimulation to itself to stimulation through the needle. Once the desired stimulation is obtained the catheter is advanced 3–5 cm along the chosen nerve. This technique leads to more accurate placement of catheter. Also both the bolus dose and the continuous injection of the local anesthetic are injected through the catheter, thereby providing a lower risk of secondary block failure.

Fixation

Securing the catheter is as important as the procedure of locating the nerve and inserting it. It is ideal to secure the catheter perfectly and eliminate the chance of accidental dislodgement. There are two techniques: one where the catheter is tunneled and second is without tunneling. If the catheter is not tunneled it is held steady and the needle is removed carefully just like epidural needle. The catheter is secured using a benzoin skin preparation followed by a sterile transparent adhesive tape or dressing. If the catheter is expected to be kept in place for more than 3 days then it should be tunneled. Tunneling decreases the chance of dislodgement and infection. It can be done using the Tuohy needle itself or an intravenous cannula. All patients with CPNB catheters should have a documented daily inspection of catheter site and vital parameters. One must confirm the desired infusion rate, lock out time, bolus drug and the volume of local anesthetic remaining and rule out local anesthetic toxicity. If catheter is in sciatic nerve, then the heel should be elevated off the bed at all times, so that pressure ulcers do not form.

Requirements to Conduct a Safe Block

With the growing popularity of PNBs, the one big obstacle in conducting regional anesthesia is the delay in operation room time. The availability of a designated area to perform the regional anesthesia namely "the block room" will expedite the flow of the operating room, reduces the delay and enhances residents' teaching.[65] Armstrong et al.[66] reported that brachial plexus block when performed in the block room can significantly reduce the total anesthesia time when compared to brachial plexus performed in the operating room.

Regional anesthesia is usually performed in a designated area with proper equipment. This area could be a separate operation theater or a separate area with standard monitoring equipment, oxygen, suction, airway, emergency hemodynamic equipment, adequate staff and availability of appropriate transport facility to the operation theater after the procedure is done.[67,27] Advanced cardiac life support facility, medications, inotropes, intralipid to treat local anesthesia toxicity should be available. All the patients undergoing regional anesthesia should be monitored like general anesthesia. Proper informed consent and detailed documentation of nerve block procedure, level of consciousness, vital signs (pulse oximeter, heart rate, ECG, respiratory rate) are essential. The area should have adequate lights. Regional blocks are performed in sterile conditions. Medical personnel should wear a mask, cap and sterile gloves. A sterile gown is also desirable.

Regional Anesthesia Equipment Storage Cart

A typical block table for PNB is shown in **Figure 25**.

General Considerations[68]

- The most qualified person should assign a coordinator who can facilitate and maintain the quality of safe practice

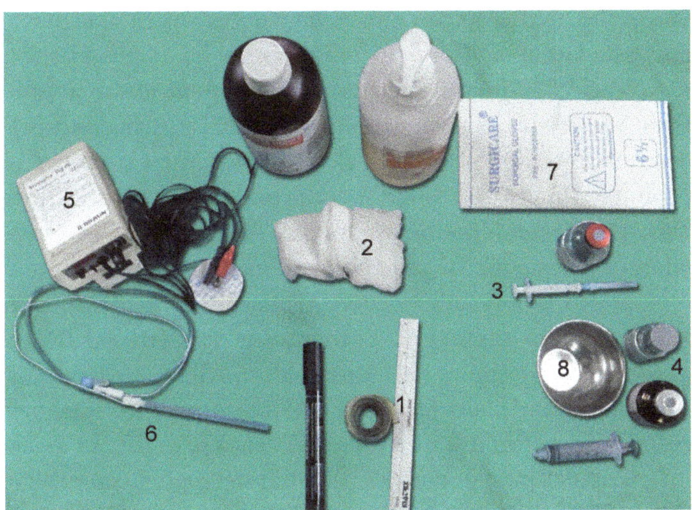

Fig. 25: Block tray. 1. Ruler and marking pen for measuring and marking landmarks; 2. Gauze pieces for cleaning with Beta scrub followed by spirit swabs; 3. 25 G hypodermic needle attached to syringe to anesthetize the skin for needle puncture; 4. Local anesthetic; 5. Peripheral nerve stimulator with skin electrodes; 6. Stimulating needles; 7. Sterile gloves; 8. Bowl to hold calculated volume of LA to be aspirated and injected with a 5-mL syringe.

by direct supervision with keeping up the records of each block in a log book

- The digital library made available where the images and videos which can be reviewed at later in case of abnormal finding such as incorrect placement of the needle or unequal distribution of the local anesthetics. Russon, et al. reported a case of intraneural injection of the musculocutaneous nerve while reviewing the static images at the end of the day[69]
- Follow-up detection of delayed complications, pain control by acute pain service team.

COMPLICATIONS

As mentioned before, patients undergoing surgery under peripheral nerve block should be monitored as carefully as a patient under general anesthesia. After completion of block they should be monitored closely for at least 30 minutes to see any signs of local anesthetic toxicity. There could be immediate complications due to intravascular administration or sometimes complications may occur typically 20 minutes following injection. This is because the serum local anesthetic levels typically peak around that time after absorption. Patients receiving PNB should be reminded to avoid using the blocked extremity for at least 24 hours and that protective reflexes and proprioception could be diminished or absent for at least 24 hours.

Nerve Injury

Peripheral nerves can be damaged by direct injury to the nerve by the needle or catheter. However, there is a lack of reliable and consistent data about the incidence of nerve injuries after peripheral nerve block. Retrospective studies estimate an incidence of 0.5–1%, however one prospective study estimates an incidence of up to 10–15%.[70] The incidence varies as per the definition of nerve injuries. An incidence of 1.5/10,000 has been reported for permanent nerve damage.[71] Most of the injuries are usually transient, subclinical and present as minor neuropathies. The incidence of transient paranesthesia may be as high as 8–10% in the days following the block.[72,73]

Anatomical Considerations

Direct needle trauma is associated with significant nerve injury if the needle penetrates the perineurium and enters the fascicle. Individual nerve fibers are enveloped by endoneurium, which are then organized into fascicles surrounded by perineurium. These fascicles are embedded within the stromal tissue and surrounded by epineurium. So, it is evident that it is possible to penetrate the nerve (epineurium) but still be extrafascicular. This is a very important concept as intraneural extrafascicular injection do not necessarily yield postoperative injury.[74]

Resistance to Injection

Assessing resistance to injection while performing PNB is a common practice. Studies suggest that perineural injections are associated with low injection pressures (<15–20 psi). In contrast, high injection pressures (>20 psi) are associated with intrafascicular injections and as such carry a risk of neurological injury.[75] Intraneural but extrafascicular injection occurs quite commonly in practice.[74] This usually results in block of fast onset and long duration rather than neurological injury. However while we are administering block we only rely on subjective sensation of resistance to injection. This is very crude and unreliable. The future needle syringe designs may incorporate an inline pressure monitors to avoid injection force to avoid intraneural injection. It is our practice to inject local anesthetic using a 5-mL syringe rather than a bigger syringe to judge the subjective resistance to injection.

Monitoring Depth of Needle Insertion

Monitoring the depth of needle insertion is important to avoid too deep an injection for, e.g., spinal cord in interscalene block[76] or pneumothorax with supraclavicular block.[76,77] The recently suggested standardized block documentation procedure requires clinicians to document the depth at which the needle was inserted. It is desirable to use a needle with markings on the shaft, and the clinician should also have an appropriate knowledge of the right length of the needle required for the specific block.

Pain on Injection

Pain on injection has always been thought as a warning sign for intraneural injection. It has usually been suggested that blocks should be avoided in anesthetized patients or patients who are heavily premedicated. However, there are case reports which suggest that pain on injection is not a reliable as a sole warning of nerve injury as it may present only a minority of cases.[78-80] Also a certain discomfort on injection which is commonly known as pressure paraesthesia coined by Winnie[81] is normal and hints at a successful block. In clinical practice it is difficult to differentiate when pain-paraesthesia is a normal phenomenon and when it is an ominous sign of intraneural injection.[82]

Intensity of Stimulating Current

The optimal current intensity in localizing the nerve is controversial. Most authors suggest that nerve stimulation with current intensity of 0.2–0.5 mA indicates intimate needle nerve placement. They also opine that stimulation with current intensity of less than or equal to 0.2 mA may be associated with intraneural placement. Also it may happen that motor response to nerve stimulation may be absent even when the needle is inserted intraneurally. Nerve injuries do occur despite extensive use of nerve stimulators which indicates that stimulators are only rough guides.[70] This mainly happens because the current from the needle tip flows in all directions apart from towards the nerve, mainly along the path of least resistance. A small change at the needle tip tissue interface may make the current flow away from the nerve along the path of least resistance. This may result in cessation of motor response even if the needle is close to the nerve or intraneurally. This explains the current interest in ultrasound-guided nerve block.

Needle Choices

Standard needles have a tip angle of around 14° and are known as "sharp" needles. It is frequently recommended to perform regional block with short bevel needles with an angle of 30–45°. This recommendation is mainly based on the suggestion by Selander and colleagues[83] that the risk of perforation of a nerve fascicle is significantly lower when a short bevel needle was used as opposed a long bevel. This concept was challenged by Rice et al.[32] According to these authors it is more difficult to penetrate a nerve fascicle with a short bevel needle than with a sharp needle, but should this occur, the lesions are more severe. Although this topic of needle design remains controversial, practitioners and manufacturers are both comfortable with short beveled needles.

Use of Epinephrine

Epinephrine containing local anesthetic solutions may theoretically produce nerve ischemia by vasoconstriction of the epineural and perineural blood vessels. Prolonged exposure, high doses, high concentrations, positioning are known to cause transient or permanent neurological injury. Once the neurological injury has occurred, it has been suggested that addition of epinephrine or a pre-existing neurologic condition predisposes the patient to the neurotoxic effects of local anesthetics (double crush concept). Also an intraneural intrafascicular injection can cause a prolonged increase in endoneural pressure, which in turn can lead to endoneural ischemia. The addition of vasoconstrictor agents theoretically enhances ischemia in view of reduced blood flow.[83] There is no substantial evidence validating the same and epinephrine is used safely for a long time. The 2010 American Society of Regional Anesthesia and Pain Medicine (ASRA) practice guidelines recommends the use of epinephrine in nerve blocks as an intravascular marker considering that the benefits outweigh the risks in majority of the patients.[84] In our practice, a solution containing epinephrine in a concentration of 1:400, 000 is used.

There are other common causes of nerve injury which include surgical compression, stretch or ischemia, tourniquets and improper positioning. Pre-existing nerve pathology can contribute to nerve damage. Postoperatively the nerves can be damaged by a tight cast or splint, wound hematoma or surgical edema.

Pre-existing Nerve Pathology

Patients with underlying nerve pathology are more susceptible to complications like prolonged duration of block and increased neurotoxicity to local anesthetic agents. This may be related to increased sensitivity of already damaged nerves, e.g., in diabetic neuropathy, neurotoxic chemotherapy.[80] A pre-existing neurological injury should always be documented.

Tourniquet Neuropathy

Tourniquet-induced neuropathy can range from mild neuropraxia to permanent neurological injury.[85] Higher tourniquet inflation pressures (>400 mm Hg) was associated with an increased risk of transient nerve injury.[86] Current recommendations for appropriate use of tourniquet include a maximum of 150 mm Hg greater than the systolic blood pressure and deflation of the tourniquet every 90–120 minutes.[85]

Compressive Hematoma

Compressive hematomas leading to neuropathy may be secondary to needle manipulations when performing blocks, specifically if the patient is on anticoagulants.[87] However, these neuropathies usually resolve completely.[88,89]

Local Anesthetic Systemic Toxicity

Vigilance while performing the block procedure and prompt intervention at the earliest sign of local anesthetic toxicity form a very important role in successful management.

Treatment is mainly supportive by administering supplemental oxygen, maintenance of airway and ventilation, control of convulsions using sedation, and anticonvulsants as well as pharmacological treatment of cardiovascular effects. Lipid emulsion has been first used for treatment of bupivacaine and mepivacaine toxicity in 2006.[90] Its use has been subsequently reported in case reports where ropivacaine and levobupivacaine was used.[91,92] Lipid emulsion has become a standard, early in the management of local anesthetic systemic toxicity (LAST). The ASRA recently published an advisory on LAST that reviews the history, prevention, diagnosis and treatment of this condition.[84,93]

Complication with Peripheral Nerve Catheters

Peripheral nerve catheters (PNCs) are prone to complications ranging from difficult placement, removal, entrapment, and infection.

Complications while Placement

Nerve localization, threading of catheter may be difficult, or the local anesthetic may not spread adequately after catheter insertion. If threading of the catheter is difficult, there may be inadvertent vascular puncture and further complications. Nerve stimulation and ultrasound offer high success rates for PNC placement. Site of insertion and operator skill also determine successful catheter placement. When catheter insertion is difficult, a bolus of normal saline 20 mL can be injected through the needle to ease insertion.[94] However, saline use can abolish the motor response should a nerve stimulator-based technique or a stimulating catheter is used. Dextrose solutions may preserve nerve stimulation.[95]

Inadvertent Catheter Removal

Catheters can get removed accidentally if they are not fixed properly. Tunneling and suturing have been recommended to prevent this complication. Many centers use skin adhesives 2-octyl cyanoacrylate (Dermabond®) instead of sutures to fix catheter.[96] This binds to the epidermis and sloughs off naturally. It may cause minor abrasions if removed early. There have been case reports where tunneling has caused catheter cutting when the tunneling needle was moved in the skin.[97] There have been reports where the catheter was cut at the time of removal while sutures were being cut.[98] All these possibilities should be borne in mind by the clinician while managing PNCs.

Entrapment of Catheter

This issue can occur if the catheter has got knotted, looped or kinked. Though this complication is rare it has been recommended that superficial catheters be advanced 3 cm past the needle tip and deeper catheters should be advanced 5–10 cm beyond the needle tip.[99]

Infection

The incidence of localized inflammation (0–13.7%), local infection (0–3.2%), abscess formation (0–0.9%) are low.[100] The incidence of bacterial colonization of PNC is high ranging from 7.5 to 57%. Femoral and axillary catheters have the highest rate of colonization, popliteals have a low rate.[94] Factors affecting the bacterial colonization include ICU admission, trauma, diabetes mellitus, catheter more than 48 hours, males, and absence of antibiotics; independently increase the risk of infection.[100]

Clinicians can decrease the infection rate by following strict asepsis and application of chlorhexidine skin disinfectant. Tunneling, use of bacterial filters and transparent dressings contribute to preventing infection. Single dose of antibiotic at the time of placement and subsequent administration postprocedure up to 24 hours is advisable to prevent infection. There should be also strict aseptic handling while loading and changing infusion pumps and while handling catheters in the ward.

Accidental Vascular Puncture

This complication may occur during difficulty in threading catheters or if the patient is on anticoagulants. Ultrasound guided placements may reduce these complications. If there is a hematoma at insertion site then it would be worthwhile to remove the catheter as the hematoma may serve as a nidus for bacterial seeding.

RECOMMENDATIONS FOR SAFE CONDUCT OF PERIPHERAL NERVE BLOCK[101]

- Aseptic technique
- Use of short bevel insulated needles
- Needle of appropriate length for each block technique
- Surface localization using nerve mapper or PEG in patients with difficult anatomy to decrease the number of needle manipulations
- Needle should always be advanced and withdrawn slowly. With a frequency of 1 Hz or 2 Hz there is no current delivery in between pulses, so inadvertent nerve puncture may not be detected
- Smaller doses of local anesthetic (5 mL) should be administered with repeated aspiration to prevent intravascular administration
- Operational nerve stimulator is an absolute requirement
- Avoid forceful and fast injections to prevent intravascular and intraneural injections
- Do not inject when patient complains of pain
- Do not exceed the toxic dose of local anesthetic and the choice of local anesthetic should be guided by the surgery required and the safety profile of local anesthetic
- It is preferable to avoid blocks in anesthetized patients, and if the need be an experienced person preferably under ultrasound guidance should be done

- Avoid repeating a block after a failed block as neuro stimulation may not be possible, hence chances of complications widen
- The ASRA third consensus conference in regional anesthesia and anticoagulation recommends that patients undergoing deep plexus or peripheral nerve block be treated with the same guidelines as those pertaining to neuraxial techniques[102]
- With regards to nerve injury ASRA states,[103] "no nerve localization or monitoring technique has been shown to be clearly superior in terms of reducing the frequency of clinical injury. These techniques include paraesthesia seeking, peripheral nerve stimulation, and defined minimal or maximal milliamperage for acceptance of motor response, ultrasound guidance or monitoring of injection pressures." The same report concluded, "peripheral nerve injury associated with regional anesthesia is likely caused by combination of insults to the nerve's internal milieu. However, the exact sequence and relative importance of these insults remain unknown." Whether one modality, such as ultrasound by itself, will have enough impact on the "combination of insults" in order to reduce the incidence of nerve injuries appears questionable. In addition, given the previously mentioned low overall incidence, which will require larger size investigations, this evidence might be extremely difficult to obtain and might never become available.

CONCLUSION

The importance of meticulous care, patient selection, experience, follow-up, careful documentation cannot be overemphasized for PNB. The American Society of Anesthesiologists practice guidelines have made practice of general anesthesia safer. However, such guidelines do not exist for the practice of PNBs. Future efforts should be directed and targeted for more objective nerve localization techniques, injection pressure monitoring devices and better diagnostic modalities to detect complications. The results of these efforts will be crucial for the safe and successful practice of peripheral nerve blockade.

REFERENCES

1. Sia S, Bartoli M, Lepri A, et al. Multiple injection axillary plexus block. A comparison of two methods of nerve localization nerve stimulation versus paraesthesia. Anaesth Analg. 2000;91: 647-51.
2. Marhofer P, Greher M, Kapral S. Ultrasound guidance in regional anaesthesia. Br J Anaesth. 2005;94:7-17.
3. Kaufman BR, Nystrom E, Nath S, et al. Debilitating chronic pain syndromes after presumed intraneural injections. Pain. 2000; 85:283-6.
4. Kulenkampf D. Anaesthesia of the brachial plexus (German). Zentralbl Chir. 1911;38:1337-50.
5. Perthes von FA. Über leitunganasthesisb unter zuhilfenahme elek-trischer reizung. Munch Med Wochenschr. 1912;47:2545-8.
6. Pearson RB. Nerve block in rehabilitation. A technique of needle localization. Arch Phys Med Rehabil. 1955;36:631-3.
7. Greenblatt GM, Denson JS. Needle nerve stimulator-locator: nerve blocks with a new instrument for locating nerves. Anaesth Analg. 1962;41:599-602.
8. Wright BD. A new use for the block-aid monitor. Anesthesiology. 1969;30(2):236-7.
9. Ganong WF. Excitable tissues: Nerve. In: Ganong WF (Ed). Review of Medical Physiology, 22nd edition. New Delhi: Tata McGraw-Hill; 2008. pp. 51-64.
10. Guyton AC, Hall JE. Membrane potentials and action potentials. In: Guyton AC, Hall JE (Eds). Textbook of Medical Physiology 12th edition. Philadelphia: WB Saunders; 2011. pp. 57-70.
11. Hadzic A. Peripheral nerve stimulators: cracking the code one at a time. Reg Anesth Pain Med. 2004;29:185-8.
12. Pither CE, Raj PP, Ford DJ. The use of peripheral nerve stimulators for regional anaesthesia. A review of experimental characteristics, technique, and clinical applications. Reg Anesth. 1985;10:49-58.
13. Hadzic A, Vloka JD, Claudio RE, et al. Electrical nerve localization. Effects of cutaneous electrode placement and duration of stimulus on motor response. Anesthesiology. 2004;100:1526-30.
14. Koscielnaik-Nielson ZJ, Rassmussen H, Jepson K. Effect of impulse duration on patient's perception of electrical stimulation and block effectiveness during axillary block in unsedated ambulatory patients. Reg Anesth Pain Med. 2001;26:428-33.
15. Shannon J, Lang SA, Yip RW, et al. Lateral femoral cutaneous nerve block visited. A nerve stimulator technique. Reg Anesth Pain Med. 1995;20:100-4.
16. Hadzic A, Vloka J. Peripheral nerve stimulators and nerve stimulation. In: Hadzic A, Vloka J (Eds). Peripheral nerve blocks: principles and practice, 1st edition. New York: McGraw-Hill; 2004. pp. 43-50.
17. Sites BD, Spence BC, Gallagher J, et al. Regional anaesthesia meets ultrasound: a speciality in transition. Acta Anaesthesiol Scand. 2008;52:455-66.
18. Tulchinsky A, Weller RS, Rosemblum M, et al. Nerve stimulator polarity and brachial plexus block. Anesth Analg. 1993; 77:100-3.
19. Kimura J. Facts, fallacies and fancies of nerve stimulation techniques. In: Kimura J (Ed). Electro diagnosis in diseases of nerve and muscle: Principles and Practice, 2nd edition. Philadelphia: FA Davis; 1989. pp. 139-66.
20. Hadzic A, Urmey W. Fundamentals of nerve stimulation. In: Hadzic A, Urmey W, Gerhard R (Eds). Dual Guidance: A Multimodal Approach to Nerve Location, 1st edition. Germany: B. Braun Mlungu AG; 2008. pp. 25-36.
21. Magora F, Rozin R, Ben-Menachem Y, et al. Obturator nerve block: an evaluation of technique. Br J Anesth. 1969;41:695-8.
22. Urmey W, Grossi P. Use of sequential electrical nerve stimuli (SENSe) for location of the sciatic nerve and lumbar plexus. Reg Anesth Pain Med. 2006;31:463-9.
23. B Braun. Sharing expertise. Stimuplex® HNS 12: nerve stimulator for peripheral nerve blocks. [online] Available from http://www.bbraun.com/cps/rde/xchg/bbraun-com/hs.xsl/products.html?id=00020742770000000022&prid=PRID00001835. [Last accessed March, 2014].
24. Montgomery SJ, Raj PP, Nettles D, et al. The use of the nerve stimulator with standard unsheathed needles in nerve blockade. Anesth Analg. 1973;52:827-31.
25. Ford DJ, Pither CE, Raj PP. Comparison of insulated and uninsulated needles for locating peripheral nerves with a peripheral nerve stimulator. Anesth Analg. 1984;63:925-8.
26. Hadzic A, Vloka J. Equipment and patient monitoring in regional anaesthesia. In: Hadzic A, Vloka J (Eds). Peripheral nerve blocks: principles and practice 1st edition. New York: McGraw-Hill; 2004. pp. 29-41.

27. Raj PP, Johnston M. Organization and function of the nerve block facility. In: Raj PP (Ed). Textbook of Regional Anaesthesia. Philadelphia: Churchill Livingstone; 2002. pp. 162-75.
28. Plancarte RS, Mayer FJM. Monitoring in regional anesthesia. In: Raj PP (Ed). Textbook of Regional Anesthesia. Philadelphia: Churchill Livingstone; 2002. pp. 176-99.
29. Sprotte G, Schedel R, Pajunk H. An "atraumatic" universal needle for single shot regional anaesthesia: clinical results and a 6-year trial in over 30,000 regional anaesthesia [German]. Reg Anaesth. 1987;10:104-8.
30. Galindo A, Galindo A. Special needle for nerve blocks. Reg Anesth. 1980;5(2):12-3.
31. Selander D, Dhuner KG, Lundborg G. Peripheral nerve injury due to injection needles used for regional anaesthesia: an experimental study of the acute effects of needle point trauma. Acta Anaesthesiol Scand. 1977;21:182-8.
32. Rice AS, McMahon SB. Peripheral nerve injury caused by injection needles in regional anaesthesia: influence of bevel configuration, studied in a rat model. Br J Anaesth. 1992;69: 433-8.
33. Sardesai AM, Denny NM, Herrick MJ, et al. A study of the characteristics of single-injection insulated block needles in a biological model. Reg Anaesth Pain Med. 2004;29:476-9.
34. Ganta R, Cajee R, Henthorn R. Use of a transcutaneous nerve stimulator to assist interscalene block. Anesth Analg. 1993; 76:914-5.
35. Urmey W, Grossi P. Percutaneous electrode guidance (PEG). A noninvasive technique for prelocation of peripheral nerves to facilitate nerve block. Reg Anaesth Pain Med. 2002;27:261-7.
36. Robards C, Hadzic A. Injection and Current Delivery Monitoring. In: Hadzic A (Ed). Textbook of Regional Anaesthesia and Acute Pain Management. China: McGraw Hill; 2007. pp. 625-30.
37. Smith BE, Fischer HB, Scott PV. Continuous sciatic nerve block. Anaesthesia. 1984;39:155-7.
38. Serpell MG, Millar FA, Thompson MF. Comparison of lumbar plexus block versus conventional opioid analgesia after total knee replacement. Anaesthesia. 1991;46:275-7.
39. Balavenkatasubramanian J. Continuous peripheral nerve block: Future of regional anaesthesia? Indian J Anaesth. 2008; 52(5):506-16.
40. Ansbro FP. A method of continuous brachial plexus block. Am J Surg. 1946;71:716-22.
41. Sarnoff SJ, Sarnoff LC. Prolonged peripheral nerve block by means of indwelling plastic catheter. Treatment of hiccup. Anesthesiology. 1951;12(3):270-5.
42. Prosser DP. Adaptation of an intravenous cannula for pediatric regional anaesthesia. Anaesthesia. 1996;51(5):510.
43. Rosenblatt RM. Modified Seldinger technique for continuous interscalene brachial plexus block. Reg Anesth. 1981; 6:82.
44. De Andres J, Bellver J, Barrera L, et al. A comparative study of analgesia after knee surgery with intra-articular bupivacaine, intra-articular morphine, and lumbar plexus block. Anesth Analg. 1993;77(4):727-30.
45. Pere P. The effect of continuous interscalene brachial plexus block with 0.125% bupivacaine plus fentanyl on diaphragmatic motility and ventilatory function. Reg Anesth. 1993;18(2):93-7.
46. Guzeldemir ME, Ustunsoz B. Ultrasonographic guidance in placing a catheter for continuous axillary brachial plexus block. Anesth Analg. 1995;81(4):882-3.
47. Pham Dang C, Meunier JF, Poirier P, et al. A new axillary approach for continuous brachial plexus block. A clinical and anatomic study. Anesth Analg. 1995;81(4):686-93.
48. Lucas MA, Harrop-Griffiths AW. Interscalene patient controlled analgesia. Anaesthesia. 1997;52(3):263-4.
49. Mezzatesta JP, Scott DA, Schweitzer SA, et al. Continuous axillary brachial plexus block for postoperative pain relief. Intermittent bolus versus continuous infusion. Reg Anesth. 1997;22(4):357-62.
50. Steele SM, Klein SM, D'Ercole FJ, et al. A new continuous catheter delivery system. Anesth Analg. 1998;87(1):228.
51. Klein SM, Grant SA, Greengrass RA, et al. Interscalene brachial plexus block with a continuous catheter insertion system and a disposable infusion pump. Anesth Analg. 2000;91(6):1473-8.
52. Klein SM, Greengrass RA, Grant SA, et al. Ambulatory surgery for multi-ligament knee reconstruction with continuous dual catheter peripheral nerve blockade. Can J Anesth. 2001;48(4):375-8.
53. Denny NM, Barber N, Sildown DJ. Evaluation of an insulated Tuohy needle system for the placement of interscalene brachial plexus catheters. Anaesthesia. 2003;58(6):554-7.
54. Casati A, Borghi B, Fanelli G, et al. Interscalene brachial plexus anesthesia and analgesia for open shoulder surgery: A randomized, double blinded comparison between levobupivacaine and ropivacaine. Anesth Analg. 2003;96(1):253-9.
55. Dadure C, Raux O, Gaudard P, et al. Continuous psoas compartment blocks after major orthopedic surgery in children: a prospective computed tomographic scan and clinical studies. Anesth Analg. 2004;98:623-8.
56. Chelly JE. Equipment. In: Chelly JE, Casati A, Fanelli G (Eds). Continuous Peripheral Nerve Techniques: An Illustrated Guide. London: Mosby; 2001. pp. 37-42.
57. Lee BH, Goucke CR. Shearing of a peripheral nerve catheter. Anesth Analg. 2002;95(3):760-1.
58. Wehling MJ, Koorn R, Leddel C, et al. Electrical nerve stimulation using a stimulating catheter: what is the lower limit? Reg Anesth Pain Med. 2004;29(3):230-3.
59. Kick O, Blanche E, Pham Dang C, et al. A new stimulating stylet for immediate control of catheter tip position in continuous peripheral nerve blocks. Anesth Analg. 1999;89(2):533-4.
60. Pham Dang C, Kick O, Collet T, et al. Continuous peripheral nerve blocks with stimulating catheters. Reg Anesth Pain Med. 2003;28(2):83-8.
61. Salinas FV, Neal JM, Sueda LA, et al. Prospective comparison of continuous femoral nerve block with nonstimulating catheter placement versus stimulating catheter-guided perineural placement in volunteers. Reg Anesth Pain Med. 2004;29:212-20.
62. Jack NTM, Liem EB, Vonhögen LH. The use of stimulating catheters for total knee replacement surgery-preliminary results. Br J Anaesth. 2005;95(2):250-4.
63. Dhir S, Ganapathy S. Comparative evaluation of ultrasound guided continuous infra clavicular brachial plexus block with stimulating catheter and traditional technique: a prospective randomized trial. Acta Anaesthesiol Scand. 2008;52(8):1158-66.
64. Boezaart AP, deBeer JF. Accurate placement of a catheter for selective continuous interscalene brachial plexus nerve block. World Congress of Anaesthesiologists, Sydney, Australia; 1996.
65. Martin G, Lineberger CK, MacLeod DB, et al. A new teaching model for resident training in regional anaesthesia. Anesth Analg. 2002;95:1423-7.
66. Armstrong KP, Cherry RA. Brachial plexus anesthesia compared to general anesthesia when a block room is available. Can J Anesth. 2004;51:41-4.
67. Neal JM, McMahon DJ. Equipment. In: Brown DL (Ed). Regional Anaesthesia and Analgesia. Philadelphia: WB Saunders; 2005. pp. 159-72.
68. Mohammed AH, Dawlatly AE. How to set up a regional anaesthesia service? Saudi J Anesth. 2011;5(2):217-8.
69. Russon K, Blanco R. Accidental intraneural injection into the musculocutaneous nerve visualized with ultrasound. Anesth Analg. 2007;105:1504-5.
70. Liguori GA. Complications of regional anaesthesia: nerve injury and peripheral neural blockade. J Neurosurg Anaesthesiol. 2004;16:84-6.
71. Auroy Y, Benhamou D, Bargues L, et al. Major complications of regional anaesthesia in France: the SOS Regional Anaesthesia Hotline Service. Anesthesiology. 2002;97:1274-80.

72. Liu SS, Zayas VM, Gordon MA, et al. A prospective, randomized, controlled trial comparing ultrasound versus nerve stimulator guidance for interscalene block for ambulatory should surgery for postoperative neurological symptoms. Anesth Analg. 2009;109:265-71.
73. Fredrickson MJ, Kilfoyle DH. Neurological complication analysis of 1,000 ultrasound guided peripheral nerve blocks for elective orthopedic surgery: a prospective study. Anaesthesia. 2009;64:836-44.
74. Sala-Blanch X, Pomes J, Matute P, et al. Intraneural injection during anterior approach for sciatic nerve block. Anesthesiology. 2004;101:1027-30.
75. Vloka J, Hadzic A, Mulcare R, et al. Combined popliteal and posterior cutaneous nerve of the thigh blocks for saphenous vein stripping in outpatients: an alternative to spinal anaesthesia. J Clin Anaesth. 1997;9:618-22.
76. Benumof J. Permanent loss of cervical spinal cord function associated with interscalene block performed under general anesthesia. Anesthesiology. 2000;93:1541-4.
77. Gerancher J, Viscusi E, Liguori G, et al. Development of a standardized peripheral nerve block procedure form. Reg Anesth Pain Med. 2005;30:67-71.
78. Bhananker S, Domino K. What actions can be used to prevent peripheral nerve injury? In: Evidence Based Practice of Anesthesiology, 2nd edition. Philadelphia: Elsevier; 2004. pp. 210-8.
79. Bashein G, Robertson H, Kenndey W. Persistent phrenic nerve paresis following interscalene brachial plexus block. Anesthesiology. 1985;63:102-4.
80. Gillespie J, Menk E, Middaugh R. Reflex sympathetic dystrophy. A complication of interscalene block. Anesth Analg. 1987; 66:1316-7.
81. Winnie A. Interscalene brachial plexus block. Anesth Analg. 1970; 49:455-66.
82. Barutell C, Vidal F, Raich M, et al. A neurological complication following interscalene brachial plexus block. Anaesthesia. 1980; 35:365-7.
83. Selander D, Sjostrand J. Longitudinal spread of intraneurally injected local anaesthetics. An experimental study of the intial neural distribution following intraneural injections. Acta Anesth Scand. 1978;22:622-34.
84. Neal JM, Bernards CM, Buterworth JF, et al. ASRA practice advisory on local anaesthetic systemic toxicity. Reg Anesth Pain Med. 2010;35:152-61.
85. Urban MK. Anaesthesia for Orthopaedic Surgery. In: Miller R, Eriksson LI, Fleisher LA, Weiner-Kronish JP, Young WL (Eds). Miller's Anaesthesia, 7th edition. Philadelphia: Churchill Livingstone; 2010. pp. 2241-60.
86. Fanelli G, Casati A, Garancini P, et al. Nerve stimulator and multiple injection technique for upper and lower limb blockade: failure rate, patient acceptance, and neurological complications. Anesth Analg. 1999;88:847-52.
87. Adam F, Jaziri S, Chauvin M. Psoas abscess complicating femoral block catheter. Anesthesiology. 2003;99:230-1.
88. Klein S, D'Erole F, Greengrass R, et al. Enoxaprin associated with psoas hematoma and lumbar plexopathy after lumbar plexus block. Anesthesiology. 1997;87:1576-9.
89. Weller R, Gerancher J, Crews J, et al. Extensive retroperitoneal hematoma without neurological deficit in two patients who underwent lumbar plexus block and were later anticoagulated. Anesthesiology. 2003;98:581-5.
90. Rosenblatt MA, Abel M, Fischer GW, et al. Successful use of a 20% lipid emulsion to resuscitate a patient after a presumed bupivacaine-related cardiac arrest. Anesthesiology. 2006;105: 217-8.
91. Litz RJ, Popp M, Stehr SN, et al. Successful resuscitation of a patient with ropivacaine-induced asystole after axillary plexus block using lipid infusion. Anaesthesia. 2006;61:800-1.
92. Foxhall G, McCahon R, Lamb J, et al. Levobupivacaine-induced seizures and cardiovascular collapse treated with intralipid. Anaesthesia. 2007;62:516-8.
93. Weinberg GL. Treatment of local anaesthetic systemic toxicity (LAST). Reg Anesth Pain Med. 2010;35:188-93.
94. Cuvillon P, Ripart J, Lalourcey L, et al. The continuous femoral nerve block catheter for postoperative analgesia: bacterial colonization, infectious rate and adverse effects. Anesth Analg. 2001;93:1045-9.
95. Pham Dang C, Lelong A, Guilley J, et al. Effect on neuro stimulation of injectates used for perineural space expansion before placement of a stimulating catheter: normal saline versus dextrose 5% in water. Reg Anaesth Pain Med. 2009;34:398-403.
96. Klein SM, Nielsen KC, Buckenmaier CC, et al. 2-Octyl cyanoacrylate glue for the fixation of continuous peripheral nerve catheters. Anesthesiology. 2003;98:590-1.
97. Rose GL, McLarney JT. Retained continuous lumbar plexus block catheter. J Clin Anesth. 2009;21:464-5.
98. Despond O, Kohut GN. Broken interscalene brachial plexus catheter: surgical removal or not? Anesth Analg. 2010;110: 643-4.
99. Rudd K, Hall PJ. Knotted femoral nerve catheter. Anaesth Intensive Care. 2004;32:282-3.
100. Capdevila X, Bringuier S, Borgeat A. Infectious risk of continuous peripheral nerve blocks. Anesthesiology. 2009;110:182-8.
101. Deschner S, Borgeat A, Hadzic A. Methods and means of decreasing the risk of neurological complications associated with nerve blocks. In: Hadzic A (Ed). Textbook of Regional Anaesthesia and Acute Pain Management. China: McGraw Hill; 2007. pp. 985-6.
102. Horlocker TT, Wedel DJ, Rowlingson JC, et al. Executive summary: regional anaesthesia in the patient receiving antithrombotic or thrombolytic therapy. Reg Anesth Pain Med. 2010;35:102-5.
103. Neal JM, Bernard CM, Hadzic A, et al. ASRA practice advisory on neurological complications in regional anaesthesia and pain medicine. Reg Anesth Pain Med. 2008;33:404-15.

Ultrasound-guided Blocks

Manoj R Shahane

ABSTRACT

Ultrasound-guided regional anesthesia has developed over last 20 years into an advanced branch of anesthesiology. Physics behind the ultrasonography (USG) technology and its applied use to visualize the peripheral nerve is discussed in this chapter. Ultrasound-guided peripheral nerve block procedures are discussed in details. Optimization of the use of USG technique to enhance and improve the efficacy of the peripheral nerve blocks is elucidated.

INTRODUCTION

Regional anesthesia is vaguely defined as "loss of sensation in a region or a part of the body produced by application of an anesthetic agent to all or some of the nerves supplying that region."

HISTORY AND EVOLUTION OF REGIONAL ANESTHESIA

Regional anesthesia is a very old and well-studied branch of anesthesiology. James Young Simpson reviewed benefits of local anesthesia in 1848 many years before it was formally used. It was even before his time, people have attempted peripheral nerve blockade with ancient techniques like apocryphal, and nerve compression.[1] Sir Benjamin Richardson had experimented with the effects of cold to produce numbing effect. He used ether spray as a local anesthetic prior to cocaine.[2] Viennese ophthalmologist Karl Koller was the first physician to use cocaine for ophthalmic surgery. He published his successful use of local anesthesia in eye surgery in 1884.[3] As cocaine's side effects and addictive potential became known, researchers started looking for newer local anesthetics. Niemann formulated benzoic acid, which was a derivative of cocaine. German researchers derived multiple local anesthetics from 1900–1930.[4] Lidocaine, an amide local anesthetic was invented in 1940s with less allergic potential compared to ester local anesthetics. William Halsted and his associate John Hall were the pioneers of conduction block. They injected local anesthetic in the region of ulnar nerve in forearm and musculocutaneous nerve of the leg.[5] In 1891, Francois-Frank coined the term "blockade" for infiltration of nerve trunk in any part. He also confirmed that the effect is seen in both sensory and motor fibers.[6]

With the development of different regional anesthesia techniques like intravenous regional, spinal, epidural anesthesia over past 100 years, current techniques like brachial plexus blocks and lower extremity blocks with multiple approaches were devised during first decade of the 20th century. Ultrasound technology and its use for peripheral nerve blockade were described in early 1970s. In 1990s, as we saw further advances in ultrasonography (USG), technology, the interest and use of USG-guided nerve blocks was more widespread. In this chapter we will focus on the most common USG-guided nerve blocks namely, brachial plexus nerve block with various approaches and lower extremity nerve blocks like femoral and popliteal nerve blocks.

BASIC PRINCIPLES AND PHYSICS OF ULTRASOUND

Physics of Ultrasound

Ultrasound waves are mechanical sound waves that traverse through the body tissues. These waves can be generated when an electric field is applied to multiple piezoelectric crystals in a transducer. Electrical stimulation of these crystals causes mechanical distortion thus making them vibrate. These vibrations thus produce the sound waves and the addition of all these waves generated on the surface of the transducer creates the USG beam.

The USG waves emitted from the transducer are transmitted into the body, reflected off the tissue interface and returned to the transducer. Once the transducer receives the sound waves back it converts them to an electrical signal, which is processed and displayed as an image on the screen. This conversion is also called as piezoelectric effect. This image can be displayed in a number of modes.

- Amplitude mode A
- Brightness mode B
- Motion mode M.

Among these B mode is the commonly used in USG-guided regional anesthesia.

Tissue Factors

Ultrasound signal once passes through the tissues can get attenuated as the depth of penetration increases. The signal can also get reflected due to scattering of the waves. Adjustment in different modalities like gain, frequency of the sound waves, focus of the beam, angle of the beam does minimize the adverse impact of the image. Detailed discussion of these adjustments is out of the scope of this chapter and should be reviewed separately.

Tissue Echogenicity

Bright image returned form the USG probe is labeled hyperechoic. Bone, diaphragm, gallstones, pericardium are examples of hyperechoic tissues.

Weaker, diffuse reflections are labeled as hypoechoic. Solid organs are hypoechoic.

No reflection is labeled as anechoic. Fluid and blood filled structures are anechoic **(Table 1)**.

Transducer Selection

A higher frequency (10–12 MHz) transducer is better suited to visualize superficial structures. These transducers have limited depth of penetration usually less than 4–5 cm.

A lower frequency (<7 MHz) transducer is better for deeper structures. A transducer with a curvature has better field coverage than the straight one.

ULTRASOUND-GUIDED NERVE BLOCK TECHNIQUE

Equipment Selection and Optimizing Image

- Ultrasound machine menu and user manual should be reviewed in detail
- Transducer frequencies, proper adjustment of depth, focus and gain should be properly set
- Precaution should be taken not to increase the gain excessively
- It is also important to have focus at or slightly below the level of the target structure **(Video 15)**.

Preparing a Transducers

- Place sterile gel on top of the transducer and cover it with the sterile sheath covering. Wrap a rubber band around the transducer surface. Avoid any wrinkles or trapped air that could impede full contact. Apply ample sterile gel onto the skin surface to optimize the visualization

TABLE 1: Tissues and image types.

Tissues	*Image type*
Nerves	Hyperechoic or hypoechoic
Muscles	Hypoechoic with hyperechoic lines or markings
Bones	Hyperechoic lines with hypoechoic shadow
Blood vessels	Anechoic

- Adhesive dressing (Tegaderm™, 3M) can be used instead of sterile sheath for a single shot nerve blocks as it is more economical.

Preparing Patient

- Proper documentation, consent, and site to side verification are done prior to the nerve block
- Minimal sedation is administered to the patient, taking care that a constant communication is maintained with the patient
- Sterilize the skin surface thoroughly with an antiseptic solution.

Nerve Block Technique

- Place the sterile drape over the procedure field
- Place the covered USG probe over the sterile field
- Use the sterile USG gel on the skin to enhance the image
- Infiltrate local anesthesia with a 25 G needle under USG guidance
- Once the nerve bundle or sheath is visualized with the USG probe, 20 G stimulating nerve needle is used
- The nerve stimulator is kept at around 0.8–1.0 mA at 1 Hz at the beginning. As the needle is advanced under USG guidance, the twitch for the correct dermatome is checked
- Once the desired twitch is elicited, the current should be reduced down to 0.4 mA at which the twitch should be very weak or disappear entirely thereby confirming the needle position near the sheath and not in the nerve bundle. This will avoid inadvertent intraneural injection
- The local anesthetic solution is then administered under USG guidance with drawing back every 5 mL to check for an intravascular injection
- Leave few mL of the local anesthetic solution in the syringe which can be used to assist in the catheter threading
- Catheter is then advanced through the top of the needle. The depth of the catheter at skin varies from patient to patient. If one is having trouble threading a catheter, small volume of the local anesthetic solution is flushed as you are advancing the catheter
- Catheter position is checked with a combination of local anesthetic and few mL of air. This once injected will create a snow effect on USG, which can give us a rough idea of about the location of the catheter
- Catheter is then secured to the skin using occlusive dressing
- Patient can be sent home with a continuous pneumatic or electrical pump filled with local anesthetic solution usually with a more dilute concentration at a prefixed rate. The common solution used in US is 0.2% ropivacaine (optical isomer of bupivacaine) at 6–8 mL per hour for about 3 days

- The patients and their family members are educated about the care of an insensate extremity and local anesthesia toxicity
- Routine telephone follow-up is done after the patient discharge. Patient is asked to remove the catheter at home
- Two distinct approaches can be used to insert the nerve block needle. The stimulating needle can be inserted: (1) in-plane or (2) out-of-plane in relation to the USG probe

In-plane Approach

In this approach, the nerve block needle is inserted few inches away from the transducer, both the needle and the transducer in the same plane as shown in **Figure 1**:

- In-plane technique is better for needle visualization as the entire needle including the needle tip can be visualized
- As the tip of the needle is seen on the monitor, it is easy to deposit the local anesthetic solution as close to the sheath as possible thereby reducing the requirement of larger volume injections
- Lower volume also helps minimizing the spread of local anesthetic in the surrounding tissues thereby reducing chances of unwanted side effects
- In-plane approach for threading a catheter may pose slightly increased level of difficulty due to the angle it needs to thread and advance the catheter

Out-of-Plane Approach

In this approach, the nerve block needle is inserted perpendicular to the USG probe as seen by the **Figure 2**:

- In this approach, the needle is advanced perpendicular to the USG probe making the needle visualization difficult
- The best way to ascertain the position of the needle is by injecting a small volume of local anesthetic solution and checking the spread on the monitor
- This technique is easier in trained hands where needle visualization is not a problem

Catheter threading is much easier in this approach compared to in-plane approach.

ULTRASOUND IMAGE GALLERY

See **Figures 3 to 6**.

OPTIMIZATION OF THE NERVE BLOCK

Following factors are very helpful in augmenting the success of the block:

- Needle approach
- Needle handling and body ergonomics
- Comfortable handling preferred
- Would recommend using both hands (learn to be ambidextrous!).

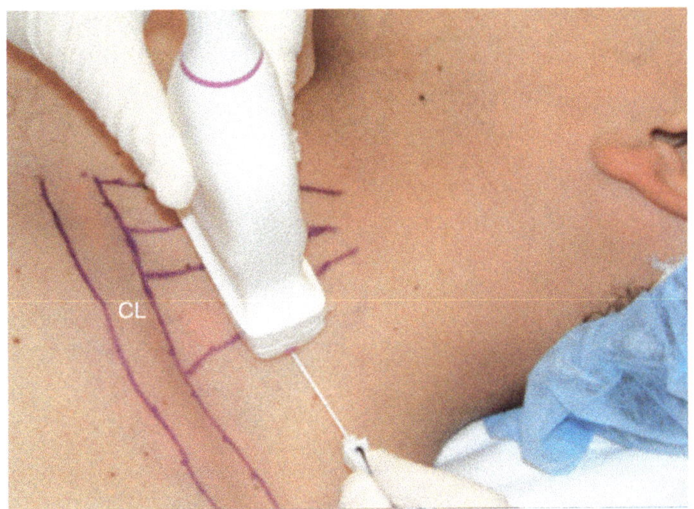

Fig. 1: In-plane interscalene approach. (CL: clavicle)
Courtesy: Dr Chan, Ultrasound Imaging for Regional Anesthesia.

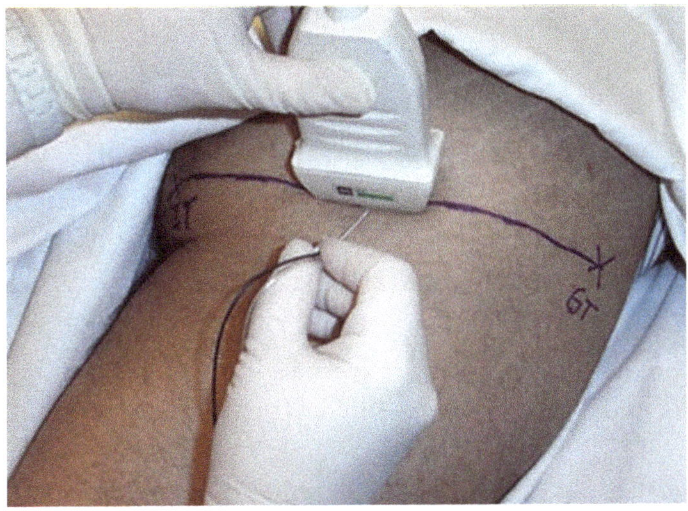

Fig. 2: In out-of-plane approach, the nerve block needle is inserted perpendicular to the ultrasound probe.
Courtesy: New York Society of Regional Anesthesia.

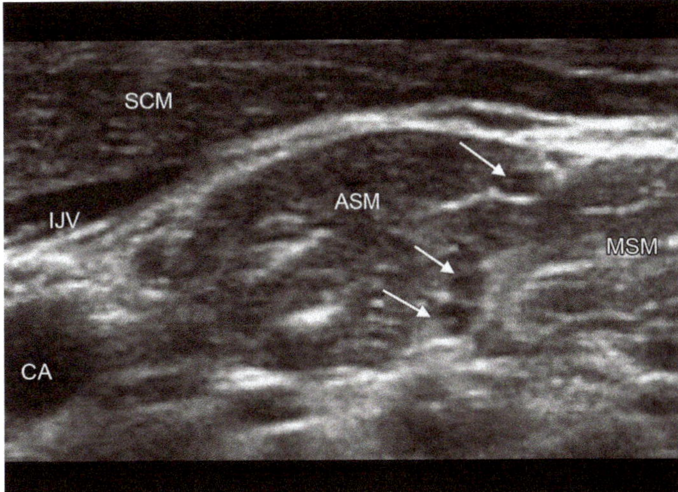

Fig. 3: Interscalene ultrasound image. (ASM: anterior scalene muscle; MSM: middle scalene muscle; SCM: sternocleidomastoid muscle; CA: carotid artery; IJV: internal jugular vein)
Courtesy: Dr Vincent Chan, Ultrasound Imaging for Regional Anesthesia.

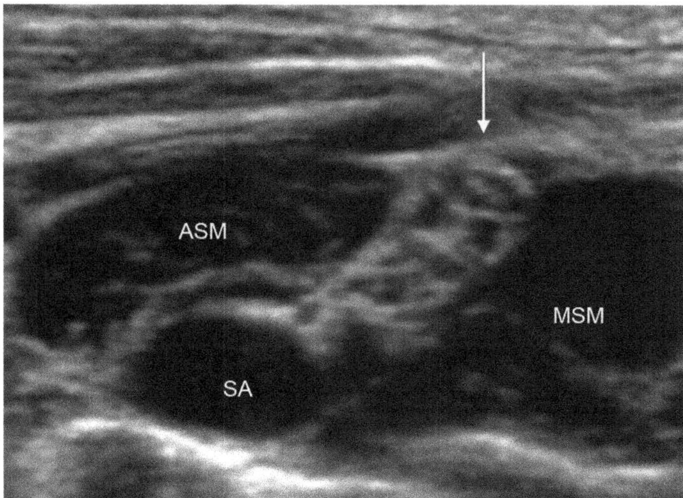

Fig. 4: Supraclavicular region ultrasound image. (ASM: anterior scalene muscle; MSM: middle scalene muscle; SA: subclavian artery)
Courtesy: Dr Vincent Chan, Ultrasound Imaging for Regional Anesthesia.

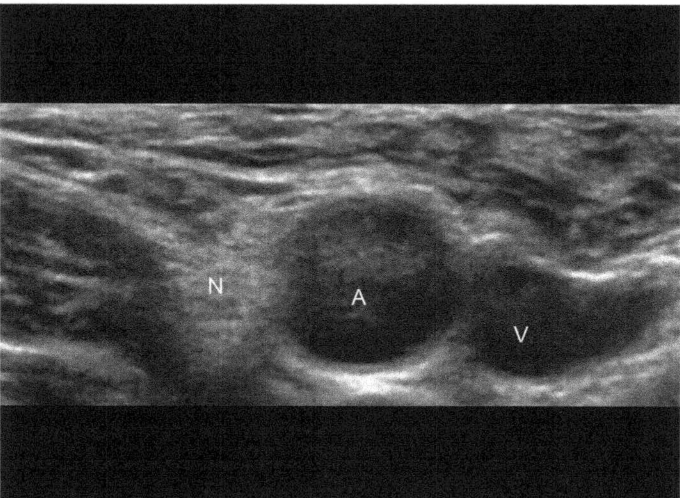

Fig. 5: Femoral nerve region ultrasound image. (A: femoral artery; V: femoral vein; N: femoral nerve)
Courtesy: Dr Vincent Chan, Ultrasound Imaging for Regional Anesthesia.

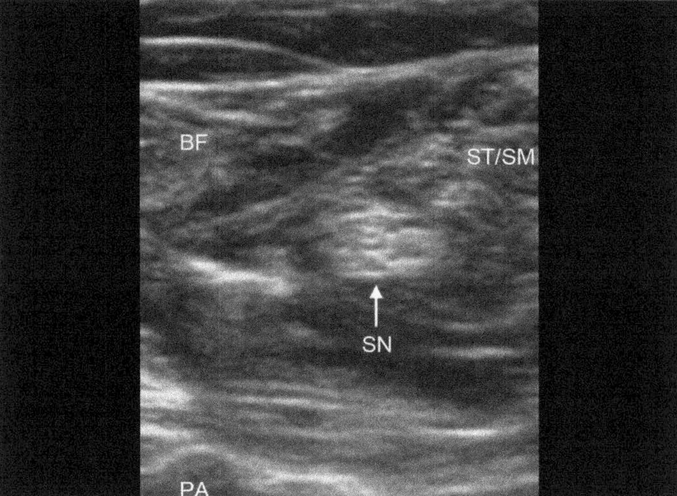

Fig. 6: Popliteal nerve region ultrasound. (SN: sciatic nerve; ST/SM: semitendinosus/semimembranosus muscle; PA: popliteal artery; BF: biceps femoris muscle)
Courtesy: Dr Vincent Chan, Ultrasound Imaging for Regional Anesthesia.

- Stay upright and save your back
- Hold transducer close to the contact surface
- Proper hand and arm positioning with good support
- Needle localization
- Three dimensional visualization necessary
- Needle tip wiggle to locate "out-of-plane" needle location
- Hydrolocation technique
- Possible multiple injections depending on the spread
- Avoid direct nerve contact
- Look for "donut sign" after local anesthesia injection.

DECISION-MAKING PROCESS

- Few factors a physician should consider before performing the ultrasound-guided nerve block:
  - Is this patient a candidate for the block?
  - History of diabetes mellitus/neuropathy/brachial plexopathy
  - Does the patient want a catheter? "Don't push it"
  - Does the patient understand all the possible side effects and complications?
  - Obese and big structured patients have higher incidences of shortness of breath on lying flat hence may not be very good candidates for nerve block
  - Subjective difference in bolus and continuous infusion effects. Patients will experience difference in the quality of continuous bolus paresthesia and pain relief compared to the dilute continuous infusion at home. They should be educated about this beforehand.
- How do I get better at doing the nerve blocks?
  - What will make me better?
  - Regional courses?
  - Books?
  - Videos?
  - Handholding (literally!)?
  - Practice, practice, practice.

CONCLUSION

Ultrasound-guided peripheral nerve blocks is a newer technique that has helped transform the nerve block technique. USG-guided nerve blocks have shown to improve block success rates[7,8] onset times and duration,[9] lowers local anesthesia dose requirements.[10,11] Detailed discussion about various approaches, different nerve blocks are out of the scope of this chapter. Continuous practice with the USG is a key in the success of the nerve block technique. Future advances in USG technology and newer local anesthetic drugs will surely improve and refine the technique in near future.

REFERENCES

1. Vandam LD. Early American anesthetists: the origins of professionalism in anesthesia. Anesthesiology. 1973;38(3): 264-74.

2. Greene NM. A consideration of factors in the discovery of anesthesia and their effects on its development. Anesthesiology. 1971;35(5):515-22.
3. Koller C. On the use of cocaine for producing anaesthesia on the eye. Lancet. 1884;2:990-2.
4. Covino B. One hundred years plus two of regional anaesthesia. Reg Anesth. 1986;11:105.
5. Hall RJ. Hydrochlorate of cocaine. NY Med J. 1884;40:643-4.
6. Francois Franke CA. Action paralysant locale de la cocaine sur les nerfs et les centres nerveux: applications a la technique experimentale. Arch Physiol Norm Pathol. 1892;24:562.
7. Chan VW, Perlas A, McCartney CJ, et al. Ultrasound guidance improves success rate of axillary brachial plexus block. Can J Anaesth. 2007;54(3):176-82.
8. Williams SR, Chouinard P, Arcand G, et al. Ultrasound guidance speeds execution and improves the quality of supraclavicular block. Anesth Analg. 2003;97(5):1518-23.
9. Marhofer P, Sitzwohl C, Greher M, et al. Ultrasound guidance for infraclavicular brachial plexus anaesthesia in children. Anaesthesia. 2004;59(7):642-6.
10. Casati A, Baciarello M, Di Cianni S, et al. Effects of Ultrasound guidance on the minimum effective anaesthetic volume required to block the femoral nerve. Br J Anaesth. 2007;98(6): 823-7.
11. Sandhu NS, Bahniwal C, Capan LM. Feasibility of an infraclavicular block with a reduced volume of lidocaine with sonographic guidance. J Ultrasound Med. 2006;25(1): 51-6.

Infusion and Syringe Pumps

Smita D Sharma

ABSTRACT

The drug delivery in anesthesia practice can range from simple injection with a syringe to highly sophisticated equipment. The computers and feedback mechanism aid in using the optimum dose of a drug in the operation theater for anesthesia and in the intensive care unit.

The syringe pump is one of the infusion pumps and is the most common gadget used in practice. Infusion pumps are categorized into manual and automated pumps. All the advances are around automated pumps. The target-controlled infusion (TCI) pump which is an open loop system has been popular for years. The most recent development is the closed loop system. These will probably serve as the pharmacological component of robotic anesthesia. While science will keep progressing it is important for the practicing anesthetist to understand pharmacokinetics and pharmacodynamics of drugs and be fully informed about doses and regimes. In addition, care should be taken to be familiar with safety concerns and maintenance of equipment used in clinical practice.

INTRODUCTION

The infusion and syringe pumps are a part of routine anesthesia care in public and corporate hospitals. However, these devices have a history of only about 30 years. The technology is moving rapidly to find the ideal anesthesia and drug delivery solutions with the help of the computer.

HISTORY

In 1628, William Harvey discovered systemic circulation. He described that venous blood was transported to the arterial circulation and thus to the organs via the heart. This led to the first intravenous (IV) injection which was administered by Sir Christopher Wren in 1656. He injected opium intravenously into dogs and humans and rendered them unconscious. However, the concept of injectable anesthetics was introduced by Pierre Cyprien Ore in 1874. He administered chloral hydrate intravenously for a surgical procedure. There has been a steady progress in technology and in 1981 Helmut Schwilden developed the first computerized infusion device. He demonstrated the ability to attain desired plasma levels of an intravenous anesthetic drug by using a computer-controlled infusion pump, based on the pharmacokinetics of a drug.[1] This led to a new era of IV drug delivery devices. The Cardiff Palliator was the first commercially available patient-controlled analgesia (PCA) pump in 1976.

UNDERSTANDING PHARMACOKINETICS

The aim of any anesthetic is to provide smooth induction and to be able to maintain the adequate depth of unconsciousness and analgesia for the required duration of the surgical procedure. While the induction of anesthesia in most cases barring a few is with the use of IV drugs, the maintenance of anesthesia is with the help of both inhalational and IV agents. There is an increasing trend towards using total intravenous anesthesia today and hence the need to use these drugs in their optimum doses.

For the maintenance phase of anesthesia intermittent boluses result in excessive drug effect at the time of bolus and inadequate drug effect just before the next bolus. These fluctuations in drug concentration can be overcome using continuous infusion. This technique allows for the use of just the right amount of drug to achieve the therapeutic blood or plasma drug concentration. However, to maintain a given target, concentration drug must be delivered at the same rate that is exiting the body.

The dose requirement for any drug can be calculated from a pharmacokinetic model which exists for every IV drug. Pharmacokinetic models are mathematical descriptions of how the body disposes off the drug. The general pharmacokinetic model of drug disposition in anesthesia considers each bit of drug independently and analyses its contribution by means of a polyexponential decay over time. The mathematical formula for this is depicted below.[2]

$$C(t) = I(t) * \sum_{i=I}^{n} A_i e^{-\lambda_i t}$$

where, $C(t)$ = plasma concentration at time t

$I(t)$ = Drug input (bolus or infusion)

Σ = Summation

n = Integer, i.e., no. of exponentials (compartments)

A_I = Coefficient

λ_i = Exponent

With the help of this complex formula which works with the amount of drug given, plasma concentration, half-life and pharmacokinetic disposition function researchers have calculated the standard bolus and infusion rates. The details of these pharmacokinetic calculations would be available in standard textbooks and are beyond the scope of this article. These calculations have made it possible for us to deliver drugs very accurately with the help of the infusion delivery system.

INFUSION PUMPS

An external infusion pump is a medical device used to deliver fluids into a patient's body in a controlled manner. There are different types of infusion pumps, which are used for a variety of purposes and in a variety of environments. Infusion pumps can deliver fluids in large or small amounts, and may be used to deliver nutrients or medications such as anesthetic agents, insulin or other hormones, antibiotics, chemotherapy drugs, and pain relievers. Infusion pumps may be stationery, i.e., bedside or ambulatory.

Types of Infusion Devices

Infusion devices can be classified into:

- Manual delivery systems
- Automated delivery systems.

Manual Delivery Systems

These consist of all the devices which deliver drugs or IV fluids at a rate that is determined by the physician. They can be further classified into:

- *Controllers:*
  - A simple IV set with its controlling C air clamp is the most basic infusion delivery system
  - Dial a flow **(Fig. 1)**.

  While infusing a solution through a controller there is a variation in the amount delivered depending on gravity. In other words, as the height of the device and its distance from the IV line changes the rate of infusion changes. The rate of infusion in the dial a flow significantly alters due to the raising or lowering of the height of the IV stand. This makes this device and its dial setting not so accurate. However, it is economical, less bulky and do not require electrical supply or battery for its use.

- *Positive displacement pumps:* These are devices that deliver IV fluids or drugs accurately at a fixed predetermined rate that is not influenced by the effect of gravity. Their mechanism of action is by positive displacement of fluid with the help of a motor. Positive displacement pumps have either a peristaltic or a piston mechanism. The various types of positive displacement pumps are:
  - *Drip rate pumps:* These pumps use drip sensor attached to IV set to count drops to achieve control of infusion rate. The speed of pumping mechanism is under feedback control from a drip sensor/counter. The limitation of its accuracy is because 1 mL of fluid may be equivalent to 10, 15, or 20 drops
  - *Volumetric pumps* **(Fig. 2)**: These pumps overcome limitations associated with variation in drop size. They use either a piston type action or peristaltic pumping action on an accurately made section of tube which forms part of a special administration set
  - These special administration sets increase the cost of each infusion. They also need special IV tubing of

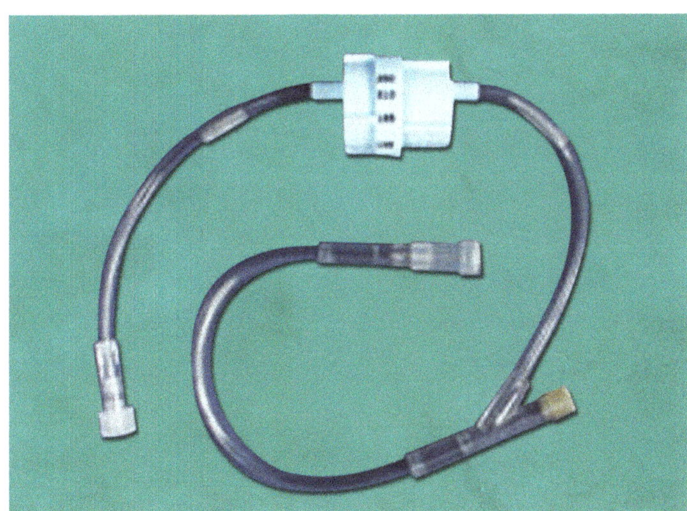

Fig. 1: Dial a flow.

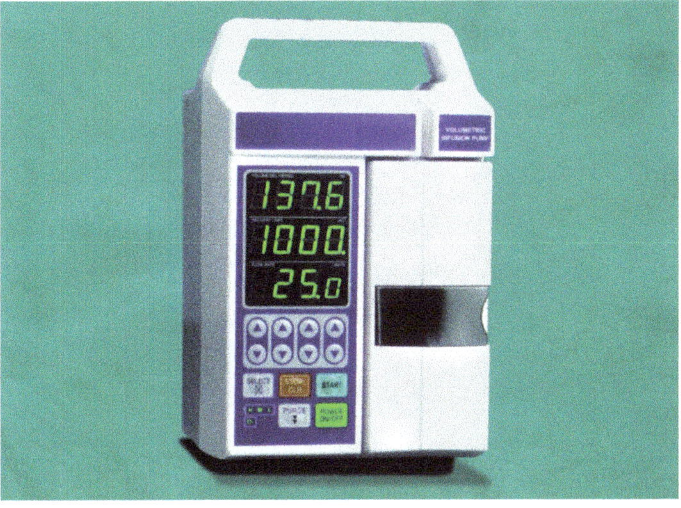

Fig. 2: Volumetric pump.

standard size which is 2–4 times more expensive than normal tubing. However, the pumps are calibrated in mL/h and are capable of precise regulation of the set flow rates. Volumetric infusion pumps can calculate the volume of fluid with the microprocessor-based calculations, considering the size of the drop produced and the standardized diameter of the tubing. Both drip rate pumps and volumetric pumps are useful for accurate IV fluid administration in pediatric and adult population.

- *Syringe pumps* **(Figs. 3 and 4)***:* The most commonly used pumps for the administration of IV drugs are positive displacement syringe pumps that utilize a gear reduction mechanism and lead screw. These pumps are extremely accurate and have the convenience of not requiring specialized tubing. Drugs are delivered from the syringe through a simple IV pressure line. The main parts of the syringe pump are the control panel, display panel, and a driving unit. At the most basic level the operator sets up the infusion rate at mL/h.

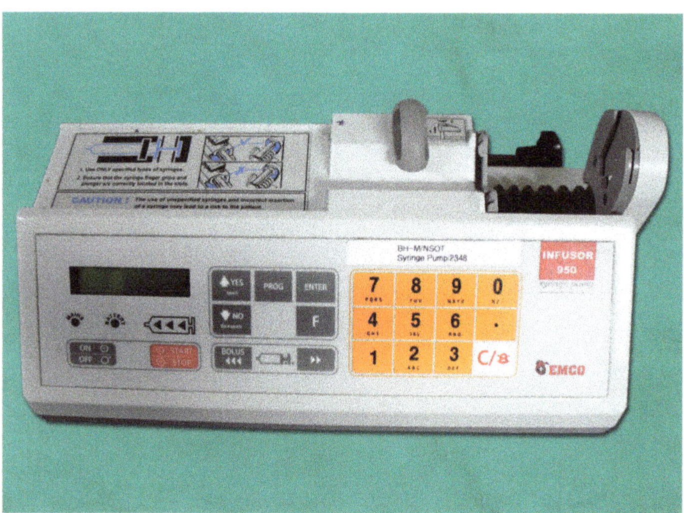

Fig. 3: Basic syringe pump.

As these pumps developed, several new additional features were inbuilt into them:

- Bolus dose
- Syringe size recognition
- Occlusion alarms
- Near empty and empty syringe alarm
- Multisyringe pumps
- Two-staged drug delivery—loading dose followed by maintenance regime[3]
- Dose calculator—the physician feeds in the weight of the patient, drug concentration and infusion rate in dose/unit of weight/unit time. The syringe pump calculates the infusion in volume/unit time
- Drug libraries—these display the drug name, class of drug, suggested doses and safe limits
- Infusion or withdrawal syringe pumps for blood samples
- Disposable ambulatory syringe pumps—these are elastomeric pumps. They are used for short-term use for acute postoperative pain or chronic pain and can deliver drugs through epidural and IV route **(Fig. 5)**
- Very recently a computer-assisted personalized sedation system for endoscopy suites has been given US Food and Drug Administration premarket approval. This device will be used to give low dose propofol. Currently it is under trial and is to be used under the supervision of anesthetist until its safety is approved. This device is to be used for (American Society of Anesthesiologists) Grade 1 and 2 patients only. It automatically detects and responds to signs of over-sedation (oxygen desaturation and low respiratory rate/apnea) by stopping or reducing delivery of propofol, increasing oxygen delivery, and automatically instructing patients to take a deep breath.

Automated Delivery Systems

This is also known as target-controlled anesthesia or target-controlled drug delivery. These are mechanical or electronic devices that deliver and adjust doses on their own based

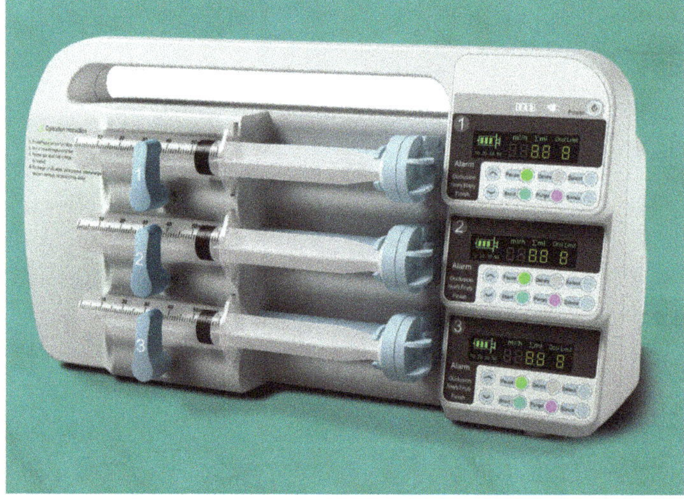
Fig. 4: Multisyringe pump.

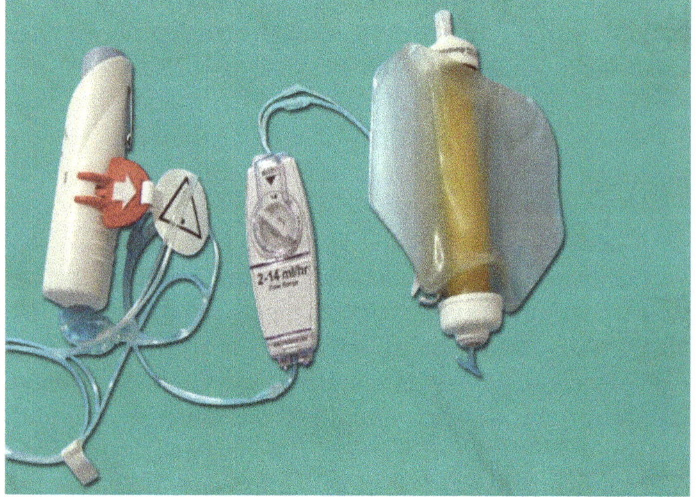

Fig. 5: Ambulatory postoperative analgesia pump (epidural).

on the preset criteria decided by the clinician. The desired target such as plasma drug concentration or a clinical response such as bispectral index is fed into the system and the drug dosages are preprogrammed.

Automated delivery systems can be:
- Open loop system
- Closed loop system.

Open loop drug delivery systems: Open loop systems are used when the feedback signal cannot be readily measured and clinical judgment is required to assess the drug effect. Hence, drug is delivered at a rate decided by the mathematical model which calculates the predicted plasma concentration for a dose. This model works very well for injection of insulin or other hormones and chemotherapy.

The open loop system use for induction and maintenance of anesthesia is the target-controlled infusion (TCI).[4] The first drug to be used with TCI is propofol.

A TCI is an infusion controlled in such a manner as to attempt to achieve a user defined drug concentration in a body compartment of interest or tissue of interest. This concept was first suggested by Kruger Thiemer in 1968. Other researchers worked on it for over a decade. Today TCI has become a routine in the western world.

While manual infusion systems are simple and work well it is not always possible to titrate the drug in a controlled manner to respond to changing anesthetic and surgical requirements. It is, therefore, not possible to manipulate the concentration of a drug in a predictable way during surgery and volatile supplementation may be required to produce satisfactory anesthesia. This led to the development of computer control of administration of drugs.[5]

The computer is programmed with the mathematical solution to the patient's pharmacokinetic model for a drug. The model operates in real time to generate the infusion rates calculated to achieve and maintain the theoretical target blood concentrations selected by the anesthetist. A TCI system can rapidly achieve and maintain a desired concentration at the effect site making it as convenient as the use of a vaporizer. With TCI, induction and maintenance are a continuous process with a single agent and hence the ease of control of anesthesia is improved as compared to conventional infusion techniques. TCI equipment are user-friendly and it does not take the operator too long to get used to it and start preferring it over manual infusions. TCI work very well for propofol and fentanyl and its other synthetic analogs.

Closed loop drug delivery systems: These are devices that measure the drug effect and adjust the drug dosage to produce the accurately desired response. This considers the patient's physiological and pharmacological response to a given dose and hence the infusion rate is tailor made to the individual need. Closed loop systems reduce the necessity of minute to minute intervention in infusion rates by the anesthetist. For a closed loop system to work completely it should receive feedback regarding consciousness, analgesia, the degree of muscle relaxant, and hemodynamic parameters. These are called control variables. Bispectral index measures the depth of anesthesia, train of four measures the muscle relaxant adequacy and hemodynamics are easily measured. What remains is a quantitative measurement of pain. One of the recent successful methods is the Analgoscore™ and this can be incorporated.[6]

The computer is fed with a preset ideal value. It then measures the actual patient value and calculates the variation which is called "error signal". The computer algorithm calculates the amount by which the set infusion should be modified to achieve the preset value. These systems deliver the exact number of anesthetic drugs and aid the timely extubation of the patient.

Researchers are in the process of manufacturing and using ideal closed drug delivery systems and are coming close to it.[7]

Other applications of closed loop delivery systems:
- Closed loop drug delivery systems are also very useful for optimal maintenance of blood pressure at a desired level using a vasopressor or an antihypertensive as need be[8]
- Closed loop fluid administration systems can be used to optimize fluid volume replacement
- Another example of closed loop drug delivery in medicine is feedback driven insulin pumps.

Patient-controlled analgesia (PCA) pumps: PCA can be considered a type of closed loop infusion system where the patient provides the input signal to control the administration of the analgesic drug **(Fig. 6)**.[9] The patient who is considered an integral part of the closed system provides the actual versus desired values of pain relief. The patient demands the analgesic with the press of a button. With a PCA, the patient is protected from overdose by the caregiver, programming the PCA to deliver a dose at set intervals.

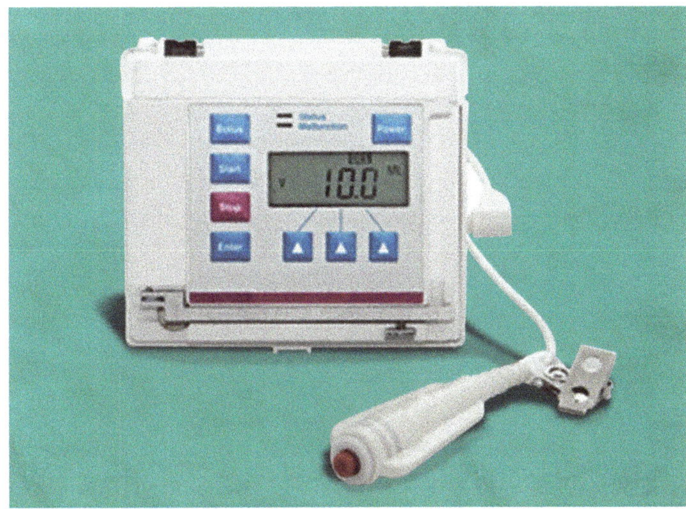

Fig. 6: Patient-controlled analgesia pump.

If the patient presses the button sooner than the prescribed intake, pressing the button does not operate the PCA. (The PCA can be set to emit a beep telling the patient a dose was "not delivered"). Dosage is also controlled when the patient is too sedated to press the button; preventing the patient from receiving needless doses and is safe from overdosing.

Patient-controlled analgesia pumps can be used for acute postoperative pain or for chronic pain. They can inject the drugs intravenously or epidurally and are available for the ambulatory patient also.

Common drugs dispensed by the PCA pump are:

- Morphine
- Pethidine
- Fentanyl
- Alfentanil
- Sufentanil
- Remifentanil
- Ketamine in combination with morphine
- Tramadol.

Some advancements in infusion pumps are MRI compatible pumps, remote-controlled pumps and infusion/withdrawal pumps. Withdrawal pumps have a feature that permits automatic withdrawal of fluid and blood sample and unattended filling of syringes. Ambulatory syringe pumps are nowadays used for parkinsonism and parenteral nutrition helping patients to live their routine lives while receiving medication or therapy.

Common Drugs Administered by Infusion Devices

To summarize, the various types of drugs that are dispensed with the help of the drug delivery systems are:

- Anesthetics
- Analgesics
- Inotropes
- Antihypertensive
- Insulin
- Chemotherapy
- Epidural analgesia
- Patient-controlled analgesia drugs
- Hormones
- Treatment at home or rehabilitation centers provides a whole new market for syringe pumps.

Anesthetic Drugs Infused by Syringe Pumps

As we have seen anesthetic drugs and narcotics are routinely administered by the practicing anesthetist using these infusion delivery systems both in the operation theater and the intensive care unit (ICU). The standard doses both for the onset of action and maintenance regimes should be known and applied for optimal patient care. The following are the doses of drugs to be used by the manual delivery systems **(Table 1)**:

- Lower doses are used for:
  - Elderly patients
  - Sick and hemodynamically compromised patient
  - For sedation regimes
- Higher doses may be used for mechanical ventilation of patients
- For the pediatric population, the drug dose response depends on multiple factors such as age, total body water content, volume of distribution, protein binding and redistribution. In addition, they are more sensitive to drugs acting on the heart, respiratory systems, brain and neuromuscular junctions. Hence, some drugs require relatively higher doses and some lower and this fact has to be understood and studied for each drug.

SAFETY CONCERNS AND OTHER PROBLEMS ASSOCIATED WITH INFUSION DELIVERY SYSTEMS

Syringe and infusion pumps deal with IV drugs and hence mishaps can occur within minutes. Mishaps involving the

TABLE 1: Dosage regimes for commonly used drugs.

Name of drug	*Onset of action*	*Peak action*	*Bolus dose*	*Continuous infusion dose*
Propofol for anesthesia	30–45 seconds	1.6–2.2 minutes	1–2.5 mg/kg	50–150 µg/kg/min
Propofol for sedation	30–45 seconds	1.6–2.2 minutes	0.25–1 mg/kg	25–100 µg/kg/min
Fentanyl	1–2 minutes	3.6 minutes	1–2 µg/kg	0.5–2 µg/kg/h
Sufentanil	0.45–60 seconds	5.6 minutes	0.5–5 µg/kg	0.01–0.05 µg/kg/min
Alfentanil	45 seconds	1.4 minutes	50–150 µg/kg	0.5–3 µg/kg/min
Remifentanil	30–60 seconds	1.6 minutes	0.5–1 µg/kg	0.1–0.4 µg/kg/min
Midazolam	30–60 seconds	2.8 minutes	25–50 µg/kg	0.25–1.00 µg/kg/min
Lorazepam	1–2 minutes	15–20 minutes	20–40 µg/kg	0.25–1.00 µg/kg/min
Ketamine	30 seconds	1–2 minutes	1–4.5 mg/kg	0.1–0.3 mg/kg/min
Dexmedetomidine	5–8 minutes	10–20 minutes	1 µg/kg over 10 minutes	0.2–0.7 µg/kg/h
Atracurium	90 seconds	2–2.5 minutes	0.4–0.6 mg/kg	0.3–0.6 mg/kg/h
Cisatracurium	1–1.5 minutes	1.5–2 minutes	0.15–0.2 mg/kg	0.06–0.1 mg/kg/h
Rocuronium	1.35 minutes (for 0.6 mg/kg/min)	30 seconds to 2 minutes (dose dependent)	0.6–1.2 mg/kg	0.3–0.6 mg/kg/h

use of infusion systems have led to deaths and near-fatal drug overdoses in healthcare organizations worldwide. Common mishaps are:

- Dosing errors
- Inaccurate delivery rate
- Backflow into syringe pump
- Mixing of drugs in delivery tube
- Accidental purging of dangerous cardiac drugs
- Instruction errors
- Alarm failure
- Failure of operating staff to understand information provided by alarms
- Battery failure
- Sparks and fires
- Infection
- Mobile phones theoretically interfere with the function of syringe pumps. It is recommended to keep mobile phones at a distance of at least one foot away from the diameter of the pump.[10]

It is the duty of practicing anesthesiologists and physicians to report inaccurate or inefficient syringe pumps and moral obligation of manufactures to withdraw defective products.

Alarms

Even the most basic syringe pump today has alarms and their proper function is of vital importance. Conversely the failure of alarms can be disastrous. Alarm systems should give the information for:

- Occlusion
- No delivery of drug
- Near empty syringe
- Wrongly fitting syringe
- Air in the tubing's.

An important point to be made here is that while alarms should be loud in ICU setup, they should be low volume or muted in the operation theater as they create unnecessary panic among the surgical team.

Cleaning of the Syringe Pumps

As per hospital-acquired infections guidelines syringe pumps come in the category of semicritical items and hence require to be kept disinfected.

While much literature is not available on cleaning of syringe pumps, a review of operating manuals recommends that syringe pumps be cleaned with a disposable cloth dampened with warm water and a general-purpose detergent. Then it can be dried with another dry disposable cloth. Alcohol-based solutions should not be used on a syringe pump. For continuous infusions in the ICU syringes should be changed every 24 hours to prevent growth of organisms.

CONCLUSION

The infusion pumps are the safe and effective means of administering IV fluids and drugs accurately. Advances in pharmacokinetics and biomedical engineering have made it possible to have a tight control of anesthetic depth and hemodynamics in operative and critically ill patients. Acute and chronic pain can be treated today with optimal doses and reduced side effects. However, machine and medication errors are a distinct possibility. There is a responsibility on the manufacturer to adhere to exacting standards of accuracy and inbuilt safety. Similarly, the anesthesiologist and physician also must not in any way compromise on their vigilance in the monitored care of patient. In addition, it is the duty of the practitioner to report malfunctioning of infusion devices and the manufacturer to withdraw such a product. Infusion pumps when used with care add value to quality healthcare for the patient.

REFERENCES

1. Schwilden H. A general method for calculation the dosage scheme in linear pharmacokinetics. Eur J Clin Pharmacol. 1981;20(5):379-86.
2. Glass PSA, Shafer SL, Reves JG. Intravenous Drug Delivery Systems: Miller RD (Ed). Miller's Anaesthesia, 7th edition. Philadelphia: Churchill-Livingstone. 2010. pp. 829-30.
3. Wagner JG. A safe method for rapidly achieving plasma concentration plateaus. Clin Pharmacol Ther. 1974;16(4):691-700.
4. Ting CH, Arnott RH, Linkens DA, et al. Migrating from target-controlled infusion to closed-loop control in general anaesthesia. Comput Methods Programs Biomed. 2004;75(2):127-39.
5. White M, Kenny GN. Intravenous Propofol anesthesia using a computerized infusion system. Anesthesia. 1990;45(3):204-9.
6. Hemmerling TM, Charabati S, Salhab E, et al. The Analgoscore: a novel score to monitor intraoperative nociception and its use for closed-loop application of remifentanil. J Comput. 2009;4: 311-8.
7. Hemmerling TM, Arbeid E, Wehbe M, et al. Evaluation of a novel closed-loop total intravenous anesthesia drug delivery system: a randomized controlled trial. Br J Anaesth. 2013;110(6): 1031-9.
8. Emura KU, Ugimachi MS, Uemura K, et al. Automated cardio-vascular drug infusion system to control hemodynamics. Adv Biomed Engg. 2013;2:32-7.
9. Scherpereel P. Patient-controlled analgesia. Ann Fr Anaesth Reanim. 1991;10(3):269-83.
10. Hans N, Kapadia FN. Effects of mobile phone use on specific intensive care unit devices. Indian J Crit Care Med. 2008;12(4):170-3.

Miscellaneous

SECTION 8

How to Interpret X-rays, CT Scan, and MRI in Clinical Anesthesia Practice

Abhijit A Raut, Prashant S Naphade

ABSTRACT

The radiological investigations are commonly done in preoperative workup of patients and in intensive care units. Anesthetist's should be aware of basic interpretation of common radiological investigation, including chest X-ray, computed tomography, and magnetic resonance imaging. In this chapter, we have provided the systematic approach in the interpretation of chest X-ray and common related pathologies of brain and thorax on cross-sectional imaging.

INTRODUCTION

The various radiological investigations are performed in day-to-day anesthesia practice and basic knowledge of radio anatomy and technical details apart from advantages, limitations, and contraindications of these tests are essential for correct interpretation. In this chapter, we are discussing about chest radiography and cross-sectional imaging [computed tomography (CT) and magnetic resonance imaging (MRI)]. which will be helpful for pain physician and better patient care.

CHEST X-RAY

The chest X-ray (CXR) is the most common radiological investigation. The careful observation, sound understanding of chest anatomy, and the principles of physiology and pathology and systematic approach to review CXR are essential to gain the optimum diagnostic information. The purpose of this section is to highlight normal CXR findings and demonstrate common pathologies seen on the CXR. Detailed evaluation of technical factors of CXR is beyond the scope of this book. However, important technical parameters are described in this section apart from few important radiological signs.

One must know that air appears lucent (dark) on CXR while soft tissue appears gray and that of fat appears dark gray. The calcification and metallic densities are brighter on the X-ray.

Posterior-anterior or Anterior-posterior Radiograph

The posterior-anterior (PA) radiograph is the most routinely performed projection in standing position, while anterior-posterior (AP) radiograph is performed for the evaluation of sick patients who are unable to stand. The AP radiograph leads to magnification of anterior structures, i.e., clavicles, sternum, and cardia with resultant widening of superior mediastinum and an apparent cardiomegaly is seen due to increased distance from the film as compared to PA radiograph.

Adequate Inspiration

Ideally, the film is taken at the peak of inspiration. In inspiratory film, anterior ends of first six ribs are visible above the left dome of diaphragm. Poor inspiratory efforts lead to apparent cardiomegaly and prominence of bronchovascular margins in lower zones simulating atelectasis **(Figs. 1A and B)**.

Rotation

In a normal CXR, medial ends of both clavicles are equidistant from the spinous process. If the patient is rotated toward right side, medial end of right clavicle will be distant from spinous process as compared to medial end of left clavicle and the right lung will appear more lucent compared to left. This may lead to unusual prominence of right brachiocephalic artery and superior vena cava, which may simulate a mediastinal mass.

The systemic approach is important for correct interpretation of CXR and suggested following approach while evaluation of CXR.

Airway: The airway appears lucent. Trachea is often seen in the right paramedian region because of left-sided aortic arch. The upper limits of coronal and sagittal diameters of trachea are approximately 25–27 mm in men and 21–23 mm in women. The right paratracheal stripe should be less than 5 mm in thickness; widening of tracheal stripe indicates paratracheal lymph nodes, neoplasm and pleural effusion **(Fig. 2)**.

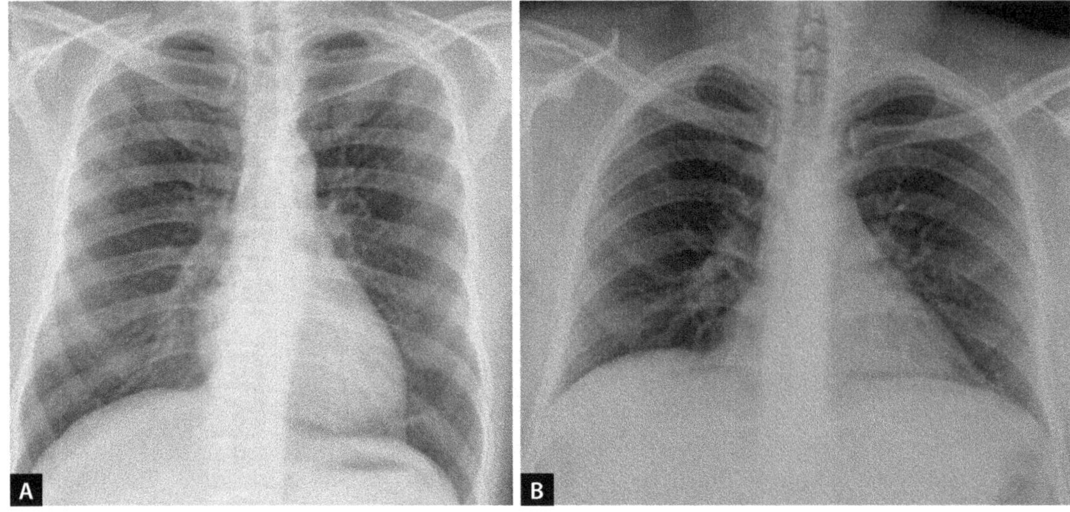

Figs. 1A and B: Normal inspiratory and expiratory chest X-ray. Note anterior ends of first six ribs are visible above the left dome of diaphragm in the inspiratory film. In the expiratory film, spurious cardiomegaly is seen.

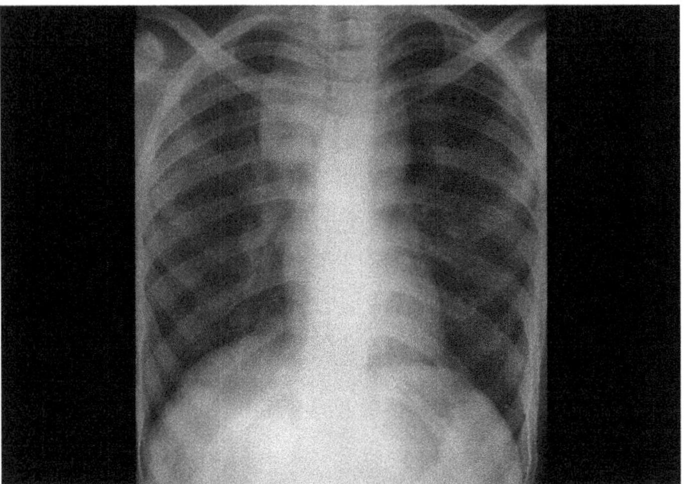

Fig. 2: Posterior-anterior radiograph of chest reveals thickening of right paratracheal stripe secondary to enlarged lymph nodes.

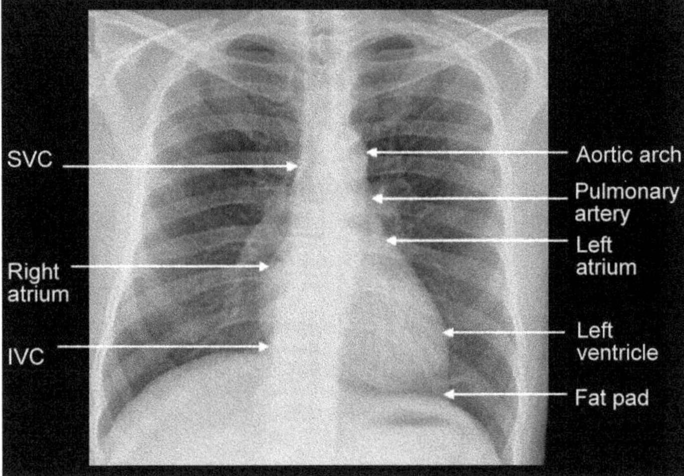

Fig. 3: Posterior-anterior radiograph of chest demonstrating mediastinal contours. (SVC: superior vena cava; IVC: inferior vena cava)

The carina is located at fourth thoracic vertebral level during expiration and at sixth thoracic vertebral level during inspiration. The widening of carina occurs if the carinal angle exceeds 60–75°, mostly due to left atrial enlargement or adenopathy.

Lung parenchyma: Conventionally, the lung parenchyma on the CXR is divided into three zones: (i) upper, (ii) mid, and (iii) lower zones, which do not correspond to the anatomical lobes. The upper zone is above the superior edge of the second rib and a horizontal line joining its anterior end to the midline. The mid zone is between the second and fourth ribs. The remaining lung fields below the fourth rib constitute the lower zone. The lung fields should be equally translucent on both sides at the same level.

Mediastinum: Central dense shadow seen on CXR compromises mediastinum, heart, spine, and sternum. The left outline is formed from superiorly to inferiorly by the left brachiocephalic vein, the aortic knuckle, the left main pulmonary artery, the left atrial appendage and left ventricle. The right border is formed by the right brachiocephalic vein, the superior vena cava and right pulmonary artery, and the right atrium and inferior vena cava **(Fig. 3)**.

Hilum evaluation: The hila (lung roots) consist of major bronchi, pulmonary veins, and arteries. The left hilum is at higher level than right because the left pulmonary artery which is located above the right main bronchus. Right hilum should never be higher than left hilum. Both hila are of similar size, density, and shape and prominence of hilum can result from rotation. In upper lobe collapse, hilum is elevated while lower lobe collapse results in depression of hilum.

Heart: The maximum transverse diameter of the heart should be half or less compared with the maximum transverse thoracic diameter. A cardiothoracic ratio of more than 50% represents cardiomegaly in adults **(Fig. 4)**.

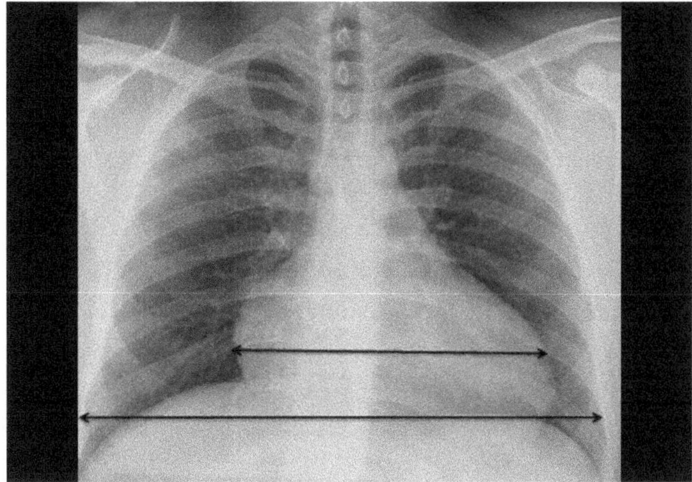

Fig. 4: Posterior anterior radiograph of chest reveals cardiomegaly. Cardiothoracic ratio is ratio of maximum transverse diameter of heart and maximum transverse thoracic diameter between the inner borders of ribs above the level of diaphragm.

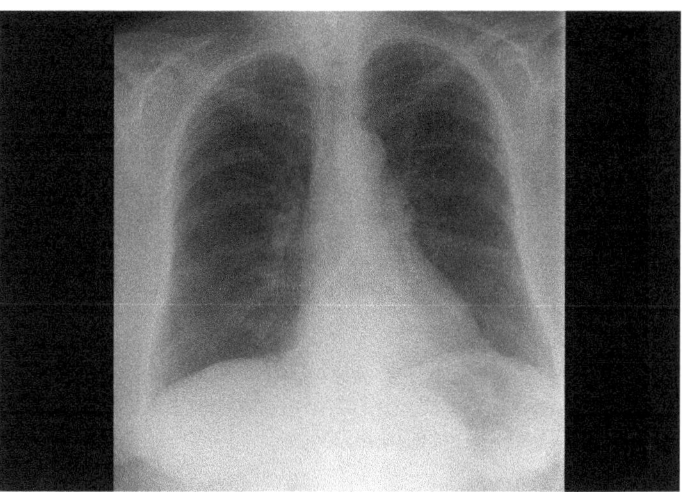

Fig. 6: Chest X-ray showing hiatal hernia, retrocardiac double density is seen secondary to hiatal hernia.

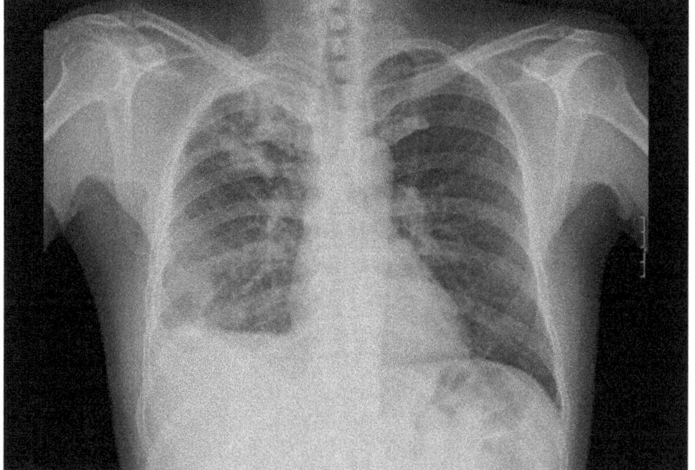

Fig. 5: Chest X-ray showing right-sided pleural effusion. Right costophrenic angle blunting is seen with flattening of the diaphragm secondary to right-sided pleural effusion. Also note the infiltrations in the right upper lobe with pleural thickening in Koch's infection.

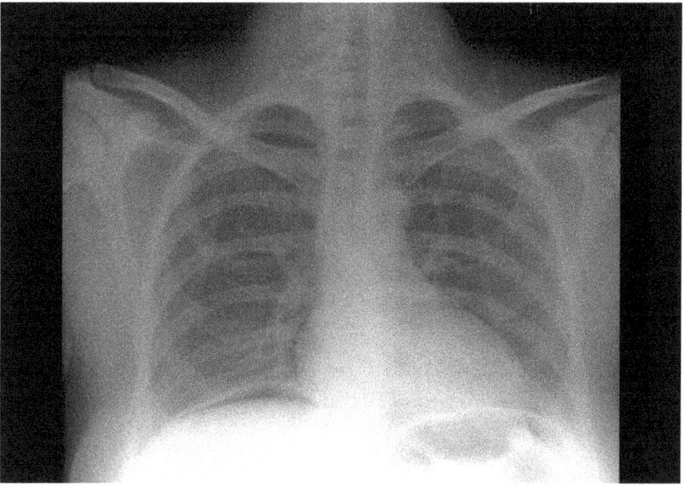

Fig. 7: Lucency beneath the right dome of diaphragm suggests free intraperitoneal air secondary to perforation of hollow viscus.

Pleura and fissures: Pleura is visible only when it is thickened or filled with fluid or air. The costophrenic and cardiophrenic angles should be sharp and clear. Costophrenic angle gets obliterated when there is at least 150–200 cc pleural effusion is present **(Fig. 5)**.

Diaphragm: Right diaphragm is higher than left one by 3 cm, as heart pushes the left diaphragm down and liver pushes the diaphragm up.

Bony thorax: Ribs, scapula, clavicles, and thoracic vertebrae are to be looked for texture, erosions, destruction, associated soft tissue mass, and possible fracture, which are seen in common pathologies like infection, metastasis, and fractures.

The ribs are always counted from their posterior ends. The transverse processes of the thoracic vertebrae are directed upward while those of cervical vertebrae are directed downward in PA view. A cervical rib can be easily detected by identifying down sloping transverse process of C7 vertebra.

Soft tissue evaluation: Breast should be evaluated for asymmetry. Absence of breast shadow may be suggestive of mastectomy.

Chest X-ray evaluation cannot be completed if following areas are not looked for:

- *Retrocardiac area:* Lower lobe collapse and hiatal hernia **(Fig. 6)**
- Below the diaphragm—to see for pneumoperitoneum **(Fig. 7)**
- *Lung apex:* Tubercular infiltrates, pancoast tumor.

Role of Lateral Radiograph of Chest

The lateral CXR can confirm or exclude the equivocal findings detected on frontal radiographs and can provide location in anteroposterior plane of mediastinal and lung masses.

Retrosternal and Retrocardiac Space

Normally, retrosternal and retrocardiac lucency are equal in size and lucency. The retrosternal lucency is lost in anterior mediastinal masses while it is increased in chronic obstructive pulmonary disease. The retrocardiac lucency is lost in lower lobe diseases and pleural effusion.

The thoracic vertebrae should appear increasingly *blacker* as we move toward caudal aspect. If it does not follow this rule, lower lobe consolidation, mass or effusion are the possible causes **(Figs. 8A and B)**.

Diaphragm

Both domes of diaphragm should be clearly demarcated except for anterior part of left diaphragm. The obliteration of the margin of diaphragm suggests lower lobe disease or pleural effusion.

Hilar Assessment

The irregular lumpy bumpy appearance and increased density suggest hilar mass.

Radiographic Appearance of Common Pathologies

Silhouette Sign

The silhouette sign is a misnomer, rather this sign should be called the "loss of silhouette" sign. If an intrathoracic radio-paque lesion is in anatomic continuity with the margins of heart of aorta will obscure that border. For example, if right heart border is obliterated by a mass lesion, then the mass lies in right middle lobe, anterior mediastinum or anterior part of pleural cavity **(Figs. 9A and B)**.

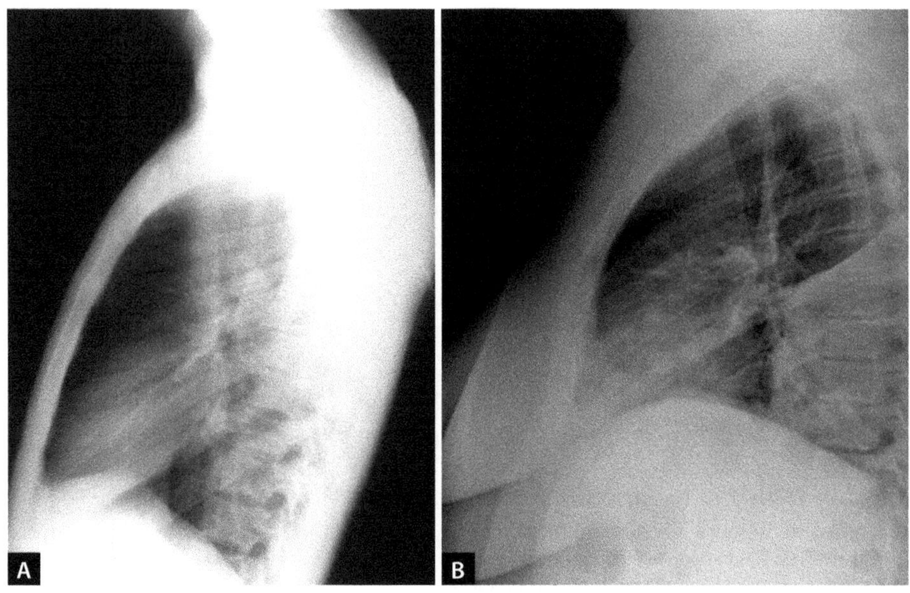

Figs. 8A and B: (A) Normal lateral chest X-ray; to note the lower thoracic vertebrae are more lucent as compared to upper thoracic vertebrae; (B) Reveals the lower thoracic spine to be more opaque due to collapse of left lower lobe.

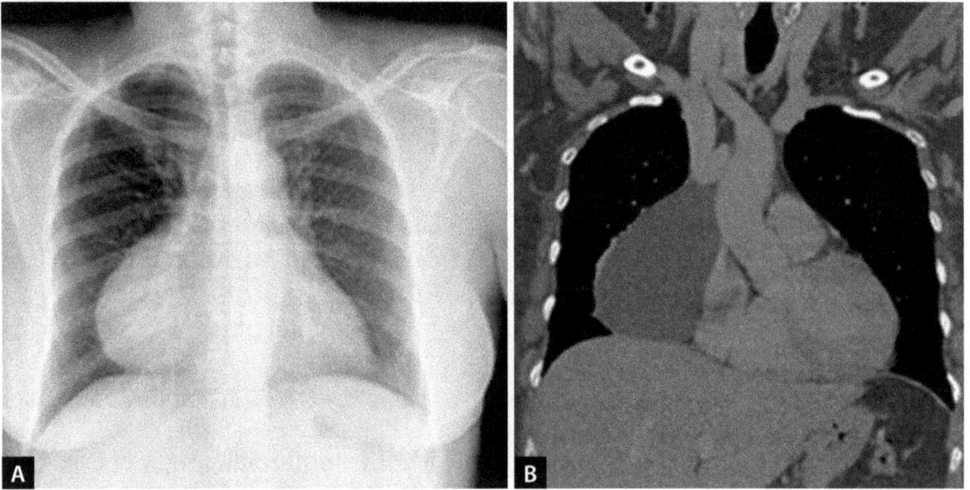

Figs. 9A and B: Chest X-ray and coronal multiplanar reformation image of chest CT showing right heart border obliteration secondary to pleuropericardial cyst located in the anterior mediastinum (Silhouette sign).

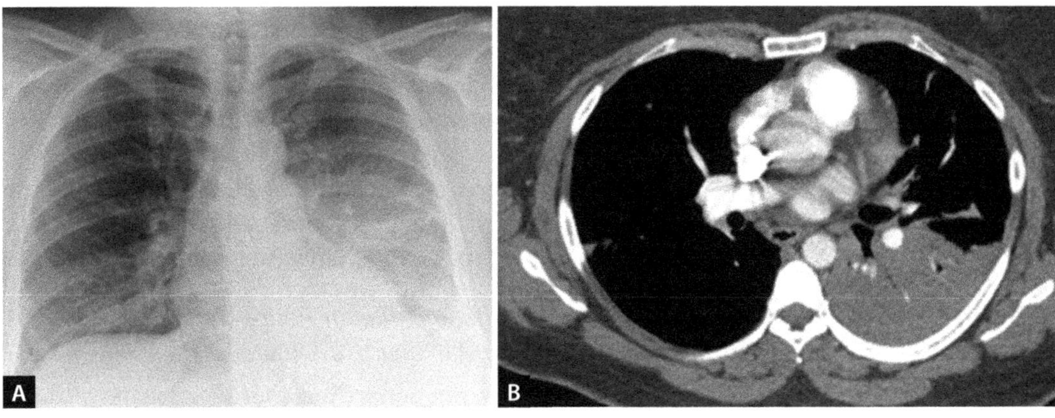

Figs. 10A and B: Chest X-ray and axial CT scan showing opacification of left lower lobe due to left lower lobe consolidation.

Consolidation

The replacement of alveolar air by fluid, blood or soft tissue present as consolidation. The patent airways in between the alveoli are seen as air bronchogram. Here, correlation with clinical history is required for appropriate diagnosis. Whenever air bronchogram is seen, differentials include pneumonia, pulmonary edema, aspiration pneumonia, pulmonary hemorrhage, bronchoalveolar cell carcinoma, and lymphoma **(Figs. 10A and B)**.

Collapse

The hallmark of collapse is loss of volume of affected segment or lobe and presents as opacity with or without air bronchogram. There are three types of collapse, which includes obstructive collapse (bronchogenic carcinoma, mucous plug, and foreign bodies), passive collapse (pleural effusion and pneumothorax) and fibrosis (tuberculosis and pulmonary fibrosis).

The direct signs of collapse include displacement of the fissures with the convexity toward the collapsed lobe, crowding of bronchovascular markings and increased opacity of the collapsed lobe. Increased opacity may not be appreciable in many cases because of compensatory hyperexpansion of the adjacent lobe, which overlaps the collapsed lobe.

The indirect signs of collapse include shift of the mediastinum and hilum superiorly or inferiorly, tracheal shift, elevation of the dome of the diaphragm, crowding of the ribs and compensatory hyperexpansion of the adjacent lobe or opposite lung. If air bronchogram is seen in a collapsed lung, it means that the etiology is nonobstructive. However, the absence of air bronchogram does not necessarily indicate obstruction on a chest radiograph.

Right upper lobe collapse: The trachea and mediastinum will shift toward right side, right hilum and horizontal fissure show superior displacement, and compensatory hyperinflation is seen in the right middle and lower lobes **(Fig. 11)**.

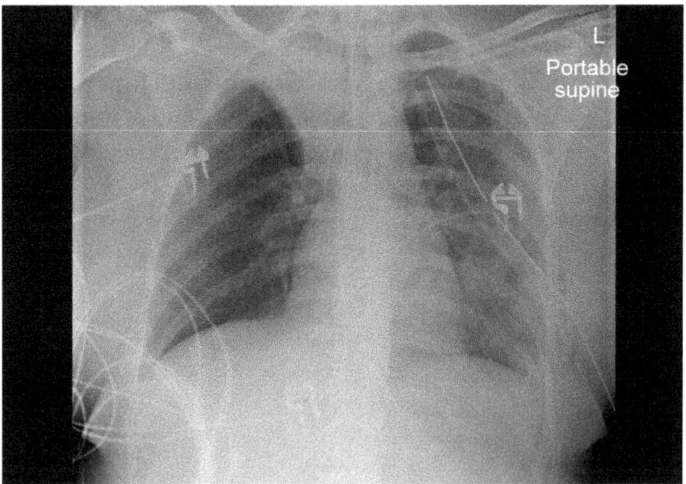

Fig. 11: Chest X-ray reveals right upper lobe collapse. Also note shift of trachea and mediastinum to right and rest of the right lung is more lucent due to hyperinflation.

Right middle lobe collapse: It is a special case as no significant sign of volume loss, displacement of hilum will be seen. It may or may be perceived as white shadow. However, it causes blurring of the adjacent right heart border (Silhouette sign).

Left lower lobe collapse: A triangular white shadow is seen superimposed on the heart. Inferior displacement of left hilum is seen associated with obscuration of borders of left descending pulmonary artery and adjacent part of diaphragm. Left upper lobe will appear blacker due to compensatory hyperinflation **(Fig. 12)**.

Alveolar versus Interstitial Disease

The alveolar pathologies present with fluffy, ill-defined, coalescing opacities. The presence of air bronchogram and segmental/lobar distribution strongly suggests alveolar disease. The interstitial pathologies present as reticular-nodular shadowing, peripheral septal thickening, or loss of lung volume in case of extensive changes.

Pulmonary edema: Cardiogenic pulmonary edema presents with cardiomegaly, bilateral basal septal thickening, confluent alveolar shadows and pleural effusion. However, noncardiogenic pulmonary edema [acute respiratory distress syndrome (ARDS)] shows no apicobasal gradient with absence of cardiomegaly and pleural effusion. The shadows of ARDS are likely to remain on follow-up radiographs despite clinical improvement while there is rapid radiographic clearance in cases of cardiogenic edema **(Figs. 13A and B)**.

Pleural effusion: It is white meniscus causing blunting of costophrenic angle with lateral margin being higher than medial margin. A loculated pleural effusion can be seen anywhere along the pleural cavity and complete white out of lung and shift of mediastinum toward opposite is seen in massive effusion.

In supine position (AP radiograph), pleural effusion leads to whiter ipsilateral lung as compared to contralateral lung **(Fig. 14)**.

Pneumothorax: It is black stripe devoid of vascular markings parallel to the lateral chest wall in erect position **(Fig. 15A)**. In supine position, deep dark anterior cardiophrenic and lateral costophrenic sulci can be seen with radiolucent upper abdomen. Air in the pleural space collects adjacent to lung base in supine position and causes black sharp margins of adjacent diaphragm and cardiac border. Whenever there is doubt about pneumothorax, imaging in expiration can increase the conspicuity of pneumothorax. The tension pneumothorax is a surgical emergency and classic radiographic signs include pneumothorax associated with flattened, depressed ipsilateral diaphragm and shift of mediastinum toward opposite side **(Fig. 15B)**.

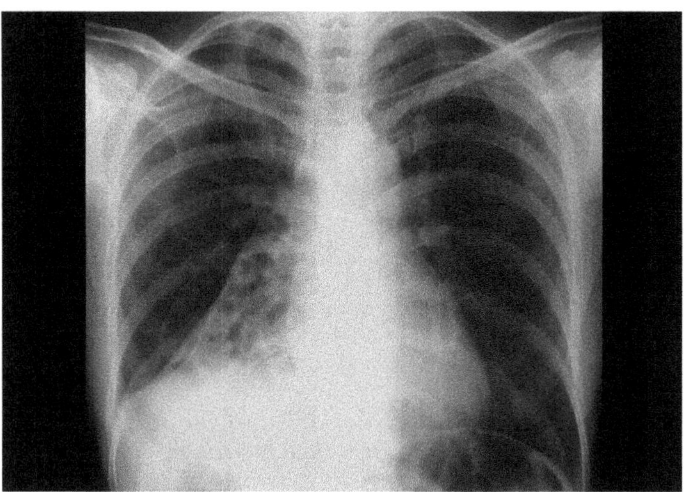

Fig. 12: Posterior-anterior radiograph of chest reveals right lower lobe consolidation with partial collapse and bronchiectatic changes.

Differentiation of Peripheral Pulmonary, Pleural, and Extrapleural Masses

The pulmonary mass forms an acute angle with the adjacent pleura while the pleural and extrapleural masses form obtuse angle. In cases of extrapleural lesions (infection, metastasis, fracture), adjacent rib destruction is usually seen.

LINES AND TUBES (TABLE 1)

The portable AP radiograph of chest are usually taken after insertion of catheters and drainage tubes for assessment of appropriate position and to rule out procedure related complications. The lines and tubes should also be checked on every CXR done for other indications **(Figs. 16 and 17)**.

COMPUTED TOMOGRAPHY SCAN

The CT scan is acquisition of thin cross-sectional images of the body and reformatting in multiple planes. The images are obtained by rotating X-ray source and detector along the gantry providing the attenuation. Here, based upon the attenuation map, digital grayscale image composed of pixels is generated as per the average attenuation coefficient of the corresponding voxels in the cross section.

The Hounsfield unit (HU) is the CT number, which represents average CT attenuation coefficient of tissues within the voxel. HUs of water and air are constant while the HUs of other tissues are dependent upon kilovoltage (kVp) and energy of X-ray beam. Most current CT systems display

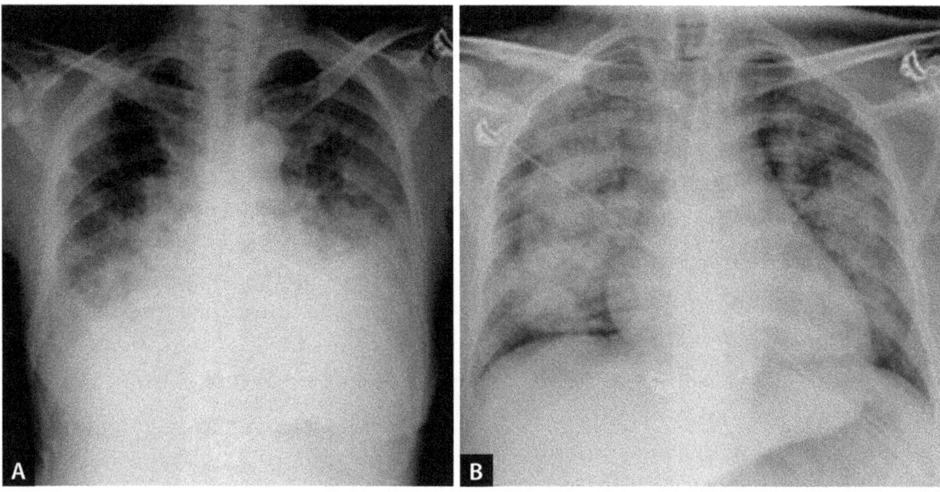

Figs. 13A and B: (A) Chest X-ray (CXR) showing cardiogenic pulmonary edema; to note cardiomegaly, basal pleural effusion and ground glass opacities; (B) CXR showing noncardiogenic pulmonary edema in acute respiratory distress syndrome case with bilateral fluffy opacities. To note absence of pleural effusion and cardiomegaly.

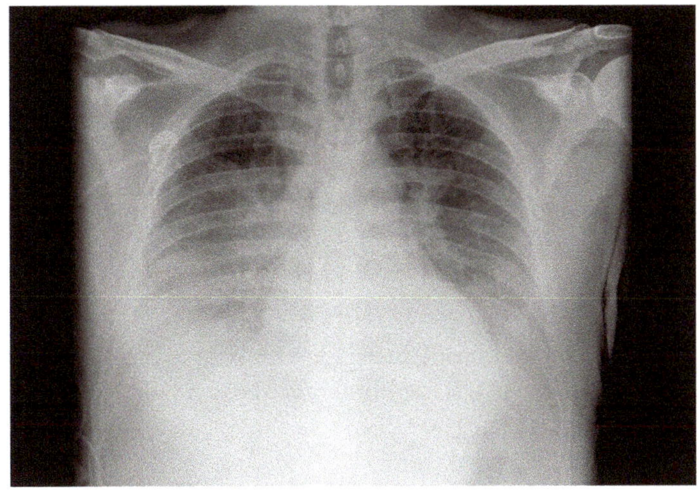

Fig. 14: Pleural effusion in supine position; generalized increased opacity of lower and mid zones is seen.

commonly 4,096 levels of gray corresponding to HU—1,024–3,071. However, inability of human eyes to distinguish between different levels of gray is up to 50. Therefore, windowing is used to display selective HU range more effectively. Generally, windowing is chosen automatically depending on protocol. However, it can be changed as per requirement **(Table 2)**.

As compared to plain radiographs, superimposition of structures is avoided in CT scan imaging and provides better contrast resolution. With the help of multidetector CT scanner, images can be acquired in single breath hold.

Common Methods of Display

Multiplanar Reformats

It displays images in coronal, sagittal, and oblique planes as per the requirement **(Figs. 18A and B)**.

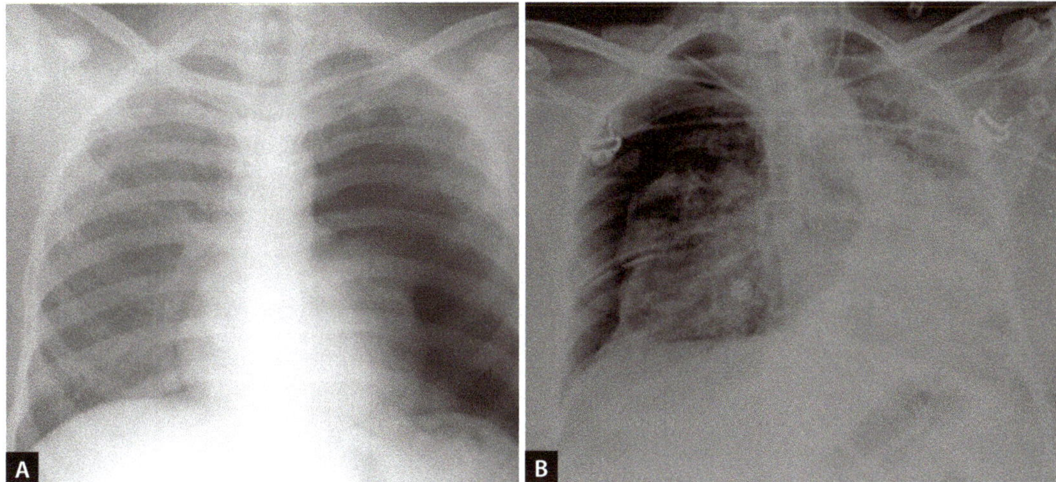

Figs. 15A and B: (A) Increase lucency with absence of vascular markings on left side secondary large left sided pneumothorax; (B) Chest X-ray showing right-sided pneumothorax with flattening of right dome diaphragm and shift of mediastinum to left-side suggestive of tension pneumothorax.

TABLE 1: Lines and tubes on chest X-ray with their appropriate locations.

Tubes	***Appropriate position***
Nasogastric tube	Tip of tube (white) should be at least 10 cm distal to gastroesophageal junction. This ensues side holes lie in the stomach
Nasoenteric tube	Tip of tube should be distal to pyloric sphincter, typically beyond fourth part of duodenum
Endotracheal tube	5–7 cm above the carina in neutral position (up to 2 cm caudal and cranial displacement of tip occurs in neck flexion and extension, respectively). Other landmarks include midway position between vocal cords and carina or at the level of medial ends of clavicles. Caudal displacement of endotracheal tube in right bronchus may lead to ipsilateral hyperinflation and contralateral collapse
Tracheostomy tube	Several centimeters above the carina midway between stoma site and carina. Its walls should be parallel to the tracheal walls without distending the tracheal walls
ICD tubes	Tip and side holes should be inside the pleural cavity. In case of pleural effusion, tube is directed posteroinferiorly while in cases of pneumothorax, it is directed anterosuperiorly
CVP line	Tip of CVP line should lie distal to distal venous valve and in brachiocephalic vein or SVC and proximal to venoatrial junction. The junction of brachiocephalic vein and SVC is at the level of right first intercostal space. SVC and atrial junction is at the level of lower border of bronchus intermedius
Swan-Ganz catheter	Tip should be within 2 cm of mediastinal outline between main and inter lobar pulmonary arteries
Pacemaker	Single chamber pacemaker can be in right atrial appendage directed anteriorly or right ventricular apex abutting the myocardium. Dual chamber pacemakers have leads in right atrium and right ventricular apex. In case of biventricular pacing, third electrode is seen in coronary sinus for left ventricular pacing

(ICD: intercostal drainage; CVP: central venous pressure; SVC: superior vena cava)

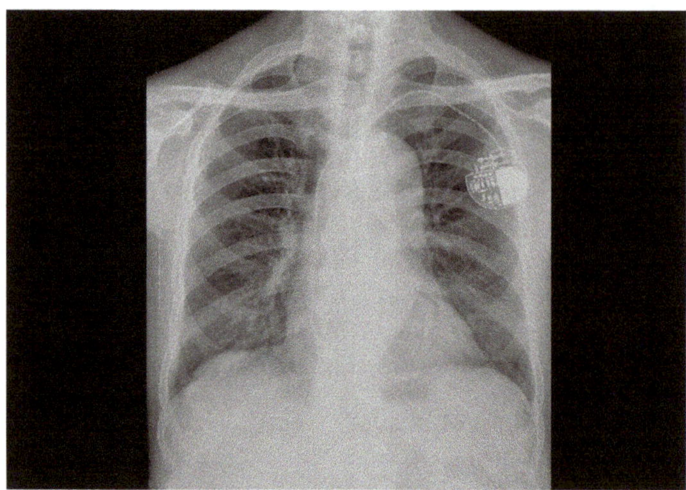

Fig. 16: Chest X-ray showing pacemaker device; to note the tip of the catheter in the right ventricle.

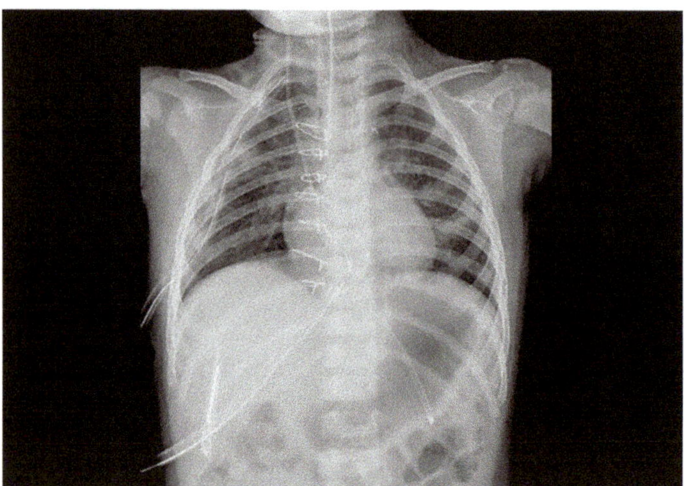

Fig. 17: Chest X-ray reveals intercostal drainage catheter in the right hemithorax and tip of Ryle's tube in the stomach bubble. Endotracheal tube is reaching up to carina extending toward right main bronchus and requires repositioning.

TABLE 2: Attenuation values (HU) of various tissues in human body and their appearance on gray scale CT image.

Tissues	HU	
Air	–1,000	Black
Fat	–60 to –120	↓
Lungs	–400 to –800	↓
Water	0	↓
Intraluminal blood	20–30	↓
Brain	25–45	↓
Muscle	45–65	↓
Blood clot/acute hematoma	50–80	White
Bone	500–1,500	

(HU: Hounsfield unit)

Maximum Intensity Projection

It displays maximum HU along each projection ray in a volume of given thickness. Commonly used for CT angiography **(Figs. 19A and B)**.

Minimum Intensity Projection

It displays minimum HU along each projection ray in a volume of given thickness. Commonly used for demonstration of tracheobronchial tree.

Three-dimensional Surface Rendering

Used for displaying the surface of scanner structures.

Virtual Endoscopy

It is a surface rendering technique for displaying the intraluminal surface of tracheobronchial tree and colon.

Three-dimensional Volume Rendering

It is a three-dimensional representation of given volume with different colors. It is commonly used in angiography to display its relationship with adjacent structures and in cases of fractures **(Figs. 20A and B)**.

Common Pathologies on Head Computed Tomography

The CT scan is the modality of choice for detection of acute hemorrhage. Acute hematomas appear whiter (hyperdense) on CT scan and appear isodense to hypodense (progressively blacker) with increasing chronicity.

Extradural Hematoma

Acute extradural hematoma (EDH) appears as biconvex extra axial (outside the brain parenchyma) hyperdense collection most commonly in temporoparietal regions due to rupture of middle meningeal artery. It is associated with adjacent fractures in most cases. It does not cross the sutures **(Fig. 21)**.

Subdural Hematoma

Acute subdural hematoma (SDH) appears as crescent-shaped hyperdense collection most commonly in frontoparietal regions due to rupture of bridging cortical veins. In contrast to EDH, SDH can cross the sutures **(Figs. 22A and B)**.

Subarachnoid Hemorrhage

Most common causes include trauma and aneurysmal rupture. The linear hyperdensity of blood attenuation extending along the sulci and basal cisterns and sylvian fissure represent subarachnoid hemorrhage and further evaluation with CT angiography can excellently demonstrate the ruptured aneurysm **(Fig. 23)**.

Intraparenchymal Hematomas

Acute intraparenchymal hematomas can be caused by trauma, hypertensive, venous infarct, hemorrhagic transformation of ischemic arterial infarct and amyloid angiopathy. In case of trauma, hemorrhagic contusions are seen typically

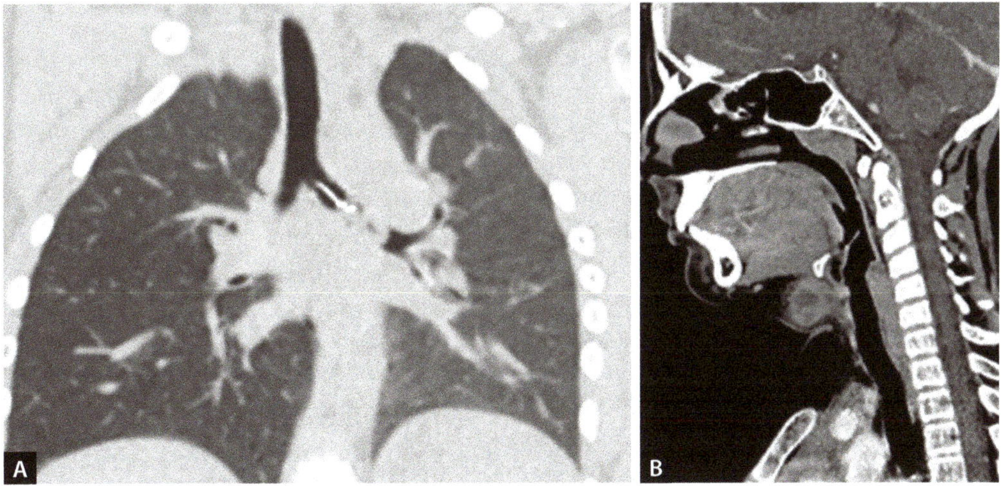

Figs. 18A and B: (A) Coronal multiplanar reconstruction reveals hyperdense foreign body at the level of origin of left main bronchus; (B) Sagittal reconstruction of neck reveals the relationship of infected thyroglossal cyst with airway.

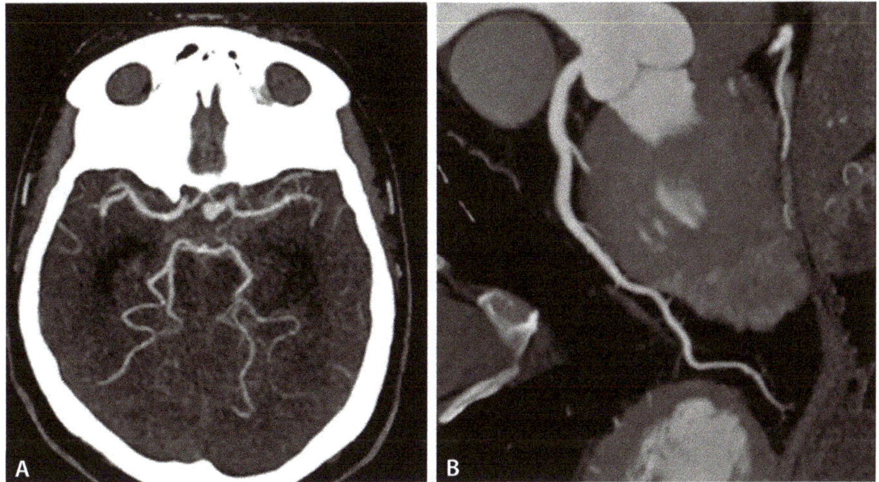

Figs. 19A and B: (A) Maximum intensity projection (MIP) images demonstrating saccular aneurysm arising from supraclinoid internal carotid artery on the left side; (B) MIP image from CT coronary angiogram reveals normal right coronary artery.

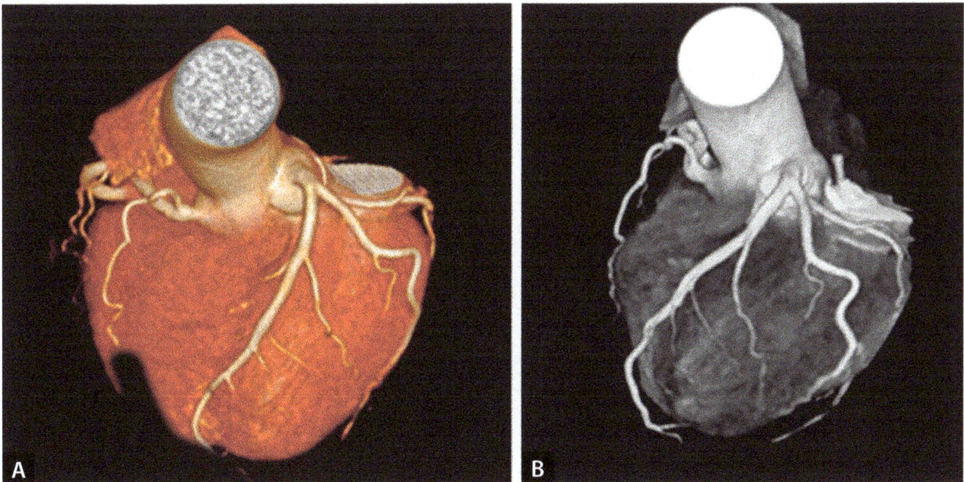

Figs. 20A and B: Volume rendered image showing left main coronary and its branches.

in basal frontal and anterior temporal lobes. Hypertensive hematoma typically occurs in putamen, thalami, pons and cerebellar hemispheres **(Fig. 24)**. The venous hemorrhagic infarct causes hemorrhage in the territory of occluded venous sinus. The hemorrhagic transformation in ischemic infarct is seen in the specific arterial territory and occurs in cases of large infarcts and in patients with anticoagulation therapy.

Infarct

Acute ischemic infarct appears as wedge-shaped hypodense lesion involving cortical and subcortical white matter and occurs in the territory supplied by blocked vessel. As the infarct evolves cerebral edema develops which appears as loss of gray-white interface and effacement of adjacent sulci **(Fig. 25)**. The primary role of CT is to exclude intracranial hemorrhage or hemorrhagic transformation of infarct. The CT perfusion and angiography can be done at the same time which can be helpful in treatment planning. The intravenous thrombolytic therapy can be performed within 4.5 hours while the intra-arterial thrombolysis can be performed up to 6 hours. The chronic infarct appears as low-density area of gliosis with prominence of adjacent sulcal spaces and ventricles due to atrophy.

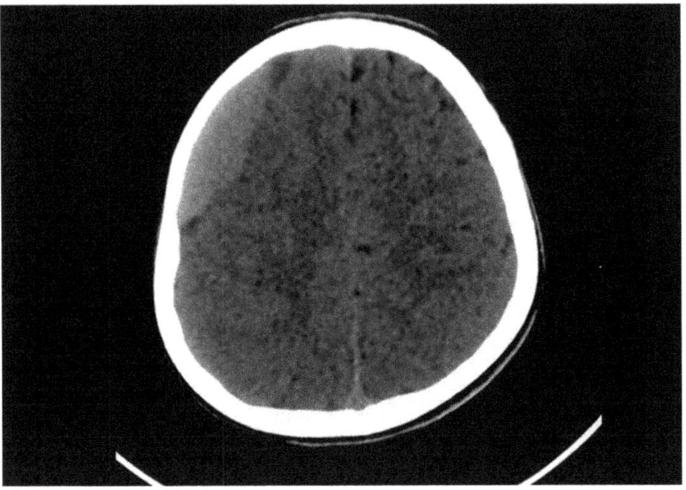

Fig. 21: Axial and coronal reconstructed computed tomography images reveal right frontal biconvex hyperdense collection of blood density causing mass effect on the cortical sulci suggestive of acute extradural hematoma.

Evaluation of Trachea

Axial CT scan with multiplanar reconstructed images provide accurate noninvasive evaluation of the trachea compared to bronchoscopy. Further in case of high-grade tracheal obstruction, visualization of distal airways is possible with CT scan as conventional bronchoscopy is not feasible. Tracheobronchomalacia, tracheal stenosis, and extrinsic tracheal compression can be detected on multiplanar CT **(Figs. 26A to C)**.

Interstitial Lung Disease

A high-resolution CT scan is the modality of choice in diagnosis of interstitial diseases. The interstitial lung diseases appear as interlobular and intralobular interstitial thickening predominantly in subpleural basal regions associated with traction bronchiectasis. The nonspecific interstitial pneumonia reveal, associated patchy ground glass opacities and honeycombing is seen in usual interstitial pneumonia (idiopathic pulmonary fibrosis) **(Figs. 27A and B)**.

Pneumothorax

In supine position, air in the pleural cavity collects anteromedially adjacent to the heart and can be missed on portable AP radiographs. In case of suspicious cases, CT can solve the problem. Even a case of small pneumothorax can enlarge and become symptomatic if patient is on positive pressure ventilation.

The pleural effusion is low density, fluid in the pleural cavity and high density, fluid (40–75 HU) in pleural cavity is seen in case of hemothorax.

The pulmonary contusions are patchy alveolar opacities in nonsegmental distribution immediately after the injury. Appearance of these opacities after 24 hours suggests

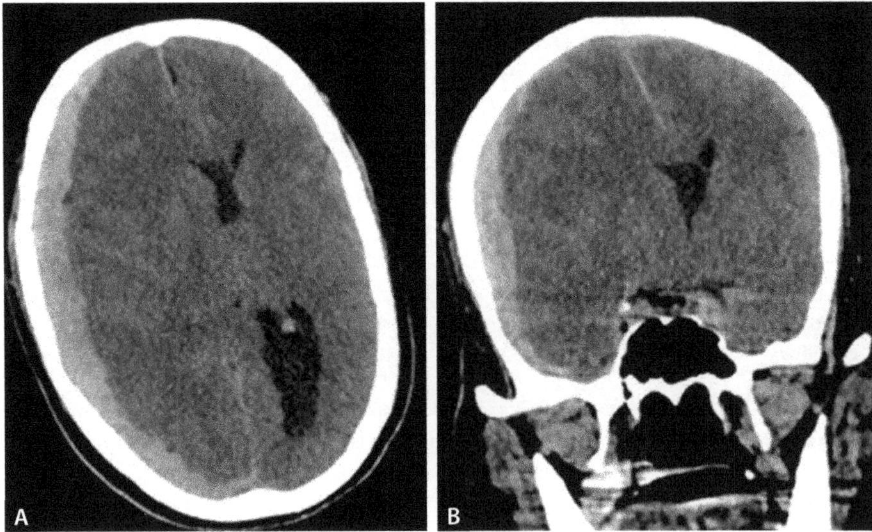

Figs. 22A and B: Axial and coronal reconstructed CT images reveal right frontoparietal extraxial crescent-shaped blood density causing mass effect on the cortical sulci with compression of ipsilateral lateral ventricle and subfalcine herniation suggestive of acute subdural hematoma with mass effect.

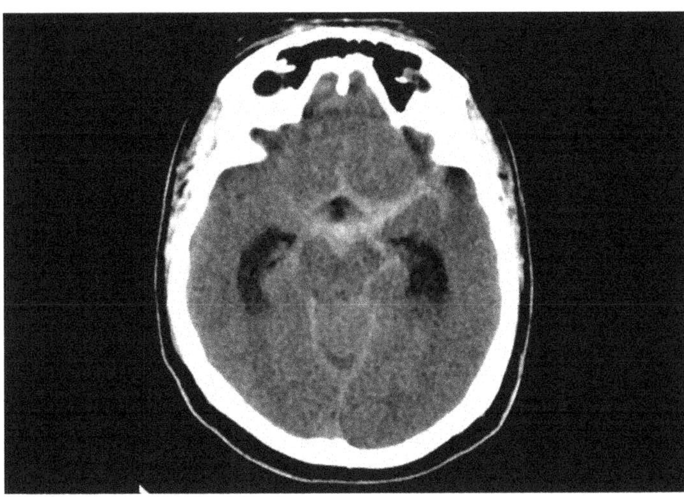

Fig. 23: Computed tomography axial image reveals hyperdensity in the basal cisterns suggestive of subarachnoid hemorrhage.

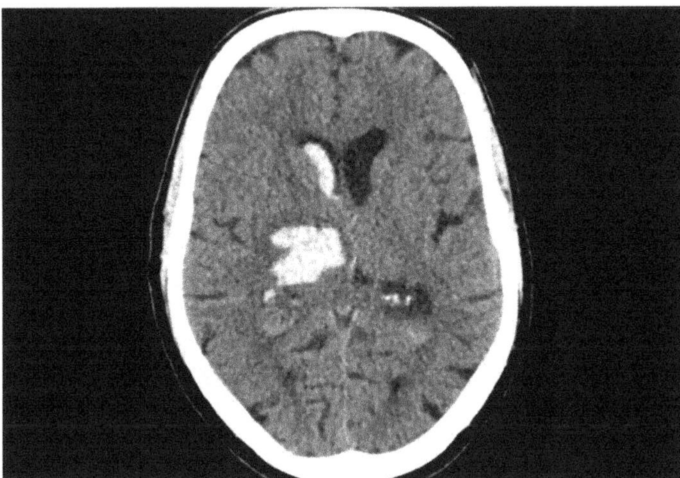

Fig. 24: Computed tomography axial image reveals hyperdense hemorrhage in the right thalamus with intraventricular extension suggestive of acute hypertensive hematoma.

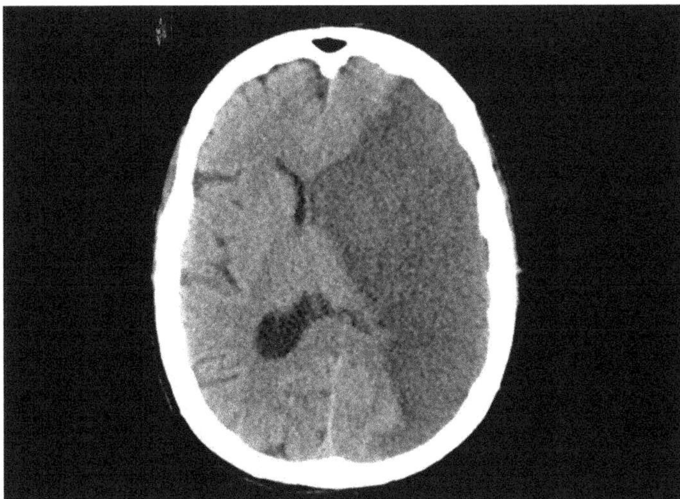

Fig. 25: Computed tomography (CT) axial CT image at the level of frontal horns reveals a large wedge-shaped hypodense area in the left frontal temporal and gangliocapsular region causing mass effect suggestive of acute infarct. No hemorrhage is seen within the infarct.

other pathologies like aspiration pneumonia, ARDS, and fat embolism.

The tracheobronchial injuries are suspected on CT scan in cases of pneumomediastinum and persistent pneumothorax despite intercostal drainage placement. The tracheal injuries cause subcutaneous emphsysema in the neck and bulging/herniation of ET tube balloon through the defect in intubated patients.

Flail Chest

The flail segment with paradoxical motion occurs in three or more contiguous rib fractures associated fractures occurring at two or more places. It usually represents significant thoracic trauma and may require mechanical ventilation.

MAGNETIC RESONANCE IMAGING

The reconstruction of MRI image is done by placing the patient in the magnet and transmitting a radiofrequency wave toward and receiving the emitted radiofrequency waves from the patient. It actually measures the hydrogen content of body and assigning it an appropriate shade of gray. Currently, superconducting electromagnets of 1.5 or 3 T are used. Increasing the magnetic field strength in term of tesla leads to increased MR signal and quality of images.

The advantages of MRI include: Superior soft tissue contrast; multiplanar imaging without repositioning the patient; noncontrast angiogram and venogram are possible and no radiation is required. Further, with advanced MR sequences, such as diffusion can diagnose acute infarct within minutes.

The disadvantages of MRI include—expensive as compared to CT, possibility of claustrophobia, loud noise by the MRI scanner and degradation of image quality by movement (not suitable for uncooperative patients).

Contraindications include—pacemaker, cochlear implant, ferromagnetic aneurysm clips, and metallic foreign body near the eye. The ferromagnetic structures are not allowed in the scanner room. The magnetic field is always present in MRI scanner room, irrespective of patient being scanned or not. The metallic objects should not be brought in the scanner room unless they are clearly marked as MR compatible.

Common MRI sequences include T1, T2, diffusion and gradient sequences.

How to Identify T1-weighted and T2-weighted Sequences

On T2-weighted (T2W) images, fluid appear bright while gray matter appears relatively brighter compared to white matter. On T1-weighted (T1W) images, fluid and cerebrospinal fluid appears dark while gray matter is gray and white matter is bright **(Figs. 28A and B)**.

Most of the pathologies are seen hyperintense, i.e., bright on T2 and hypointense, i.e., dark on T1W images and show postcontrast variable enhancement **(Figs. 29A and B)**. Air and cortical bones appear black on both T1W and T2W images.

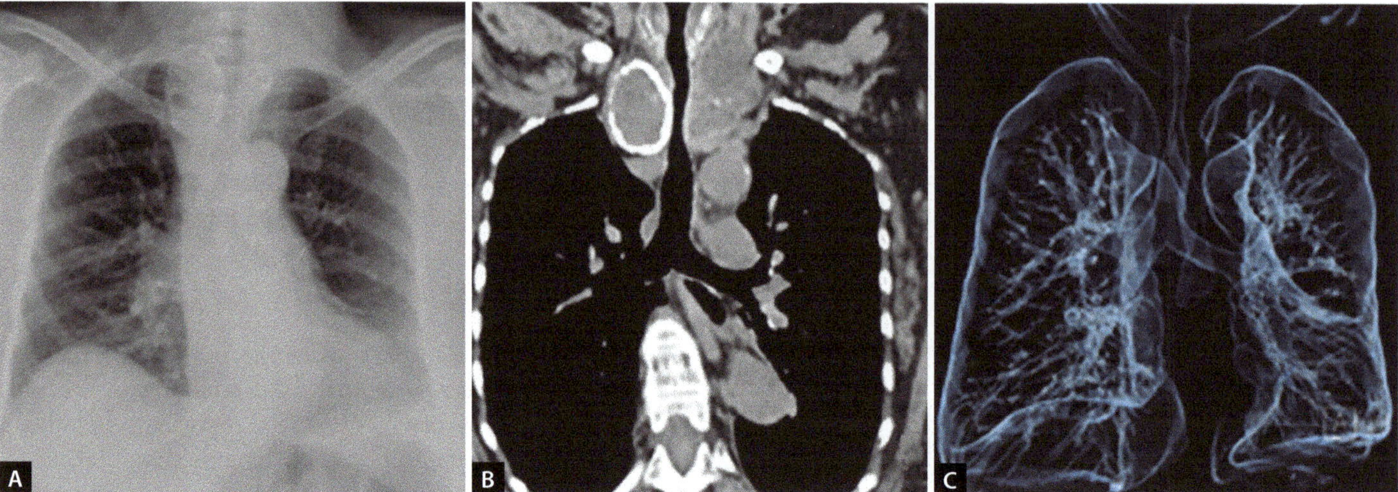

Figs. 26A to C: Chest X-ray reveals bilateral paratracheal soft tissue density masses with peripheral calcification. (A) On computed tomography images, peripheral calcified mass lesion is seen in contiguity with the thyroid gland. Note compression and mass effect on the trachea (B) virtual bronchoscopy reconstructed image (C) excellently demonstrates the tracheal narrowing.

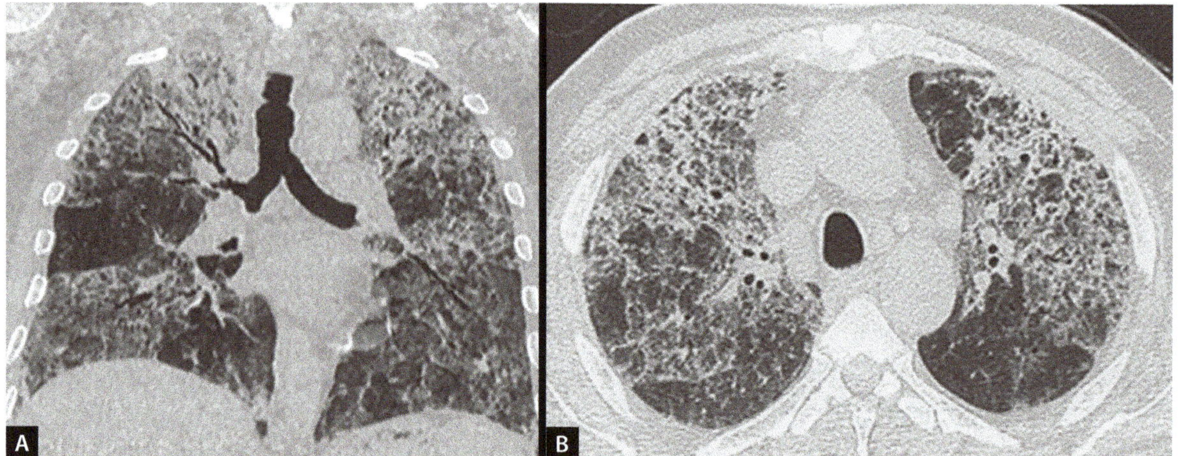

Figs. 27A and B: Coronal reconstructed and axial computed tomography images of thorax reveal extensive fibrotic changes associated with traction bronchiectasis in a case of idiopathic pulmonary fibrosis.

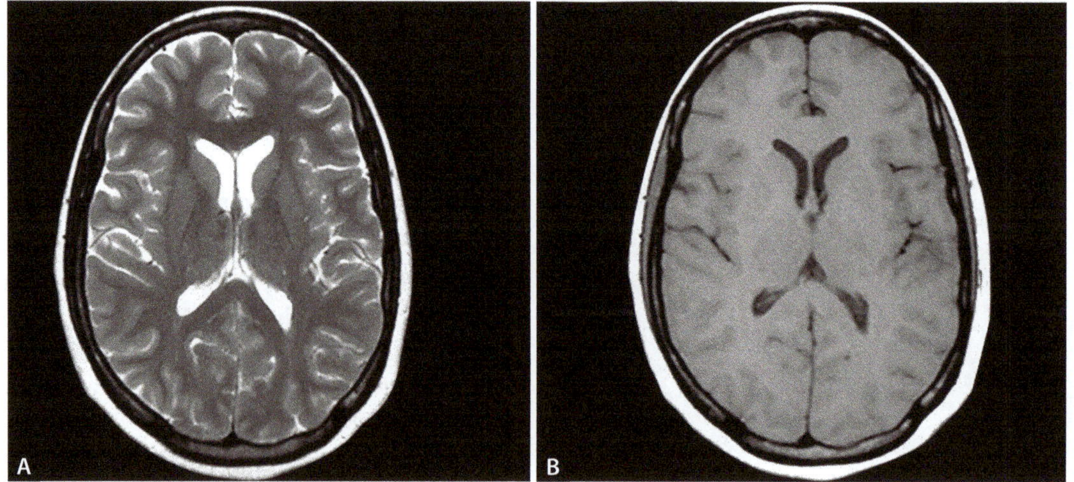

Figs. 28A and B: T2-weighted axial image of brain. (A) It reveals normally hyperintense cerebrospinal fluid (CSF) and slightly dark appearance of white matter; (B) T1-weighted axial image of brain reveals hypointense CSF and hyperintense white matter (normal appearance of brain on T2 and T1 images).

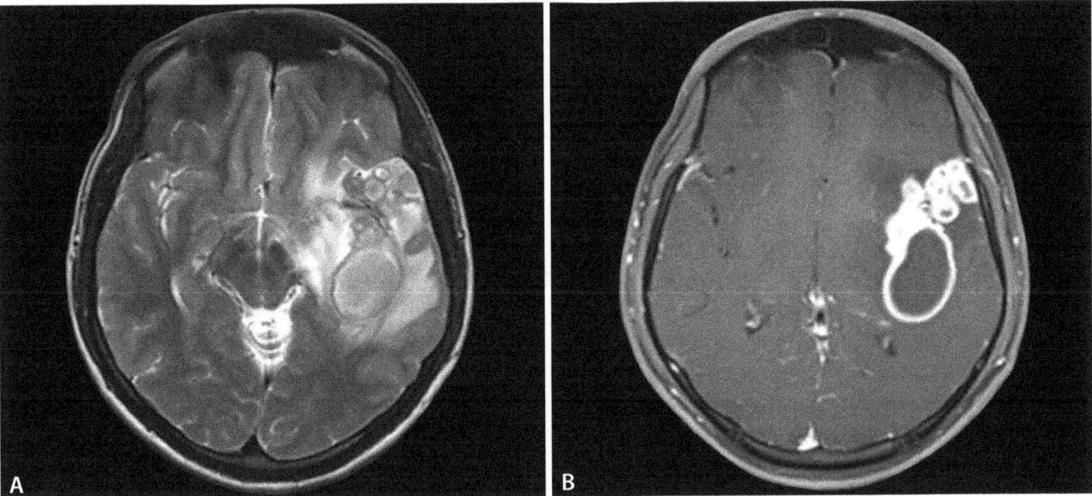

Figs. 29A and B: T2-weighted axial image of the brain. (A) It reveals multiple rounded T2 hypointense lesions in left temporal lobe with adjacent moderate hyperintense white matter edema; (B) These lesions reveal peripheral enhancement on postcontrast scan suggestive of tuberculomas.

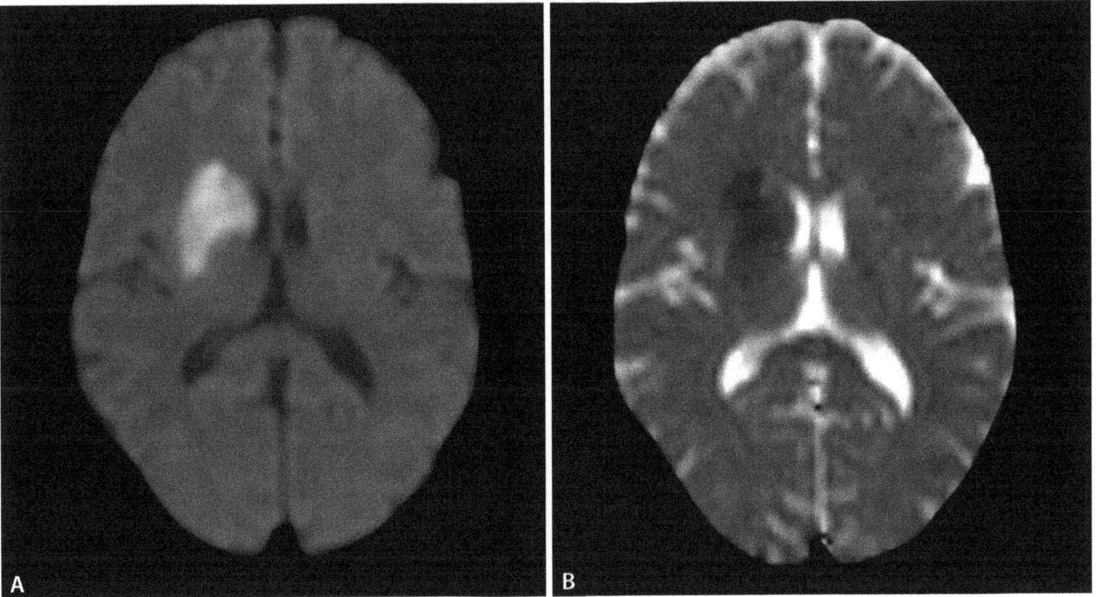

Figs. 30A and B: Axial diffusion (A) and apparent diffusion coefficient (ADC) (B) images of brain reveal restricted diffusion (bright) in right basal ganglia with corresponding darkening on ADC image suggestive of acute infarct in right middle cerebral artery territory.

Diffusion-weighted images (DWI) detect acute infarct as soon as it is developed. Acute infarct shows restriction of diffusion, which is bright on DWI and appears dark on apparent diffusion coefficient (ADC) map **(Figs. 30A and B)**. Other common causes of restricted diffusion include pyogenic abscess, epidermoid cyst, herpes encephalitis, late subacute hematoma, and lymphoma.

Gradient images are evaluated for hypointense (black) areas, which represent hemorrhage or calcification. In acute infarct, hemorrhagic transformation can be assessed on these images. In multiple diffuse axonal injury microhemorrhages in gray-white matter interface, corpus callosum and brainstem are detected on gradient images.

Acute ischemic infarct is seen as a bright area (restricted diffusion) following vascular territory with corresponding black area on ADC images. On conventional T2W images, acute infarct appears as T2 hyperintense cortical edema with loss of gray-white differentiation following vascular territory and may not be apparent for up to 2–6 hours. Chronic infarcts reveal T2 hyperintense gliosis without any restricted diffusion. Postcontrast perfusion MRI along with DWI can differentiate irreversibly damaged infarcted brain parenchyma and salvageable brain parenchyma (penumbra) with thrombolytic therapy. Further MR angiogram can localize the site of thrombosis and provides road map of arterial anatomy in case of intra-arterial thrombolysis is required.

Intracranial hematomas have varied appearance on MR depending upon the age of hematoma **(Figs. 31 and 32; Table 3)**.

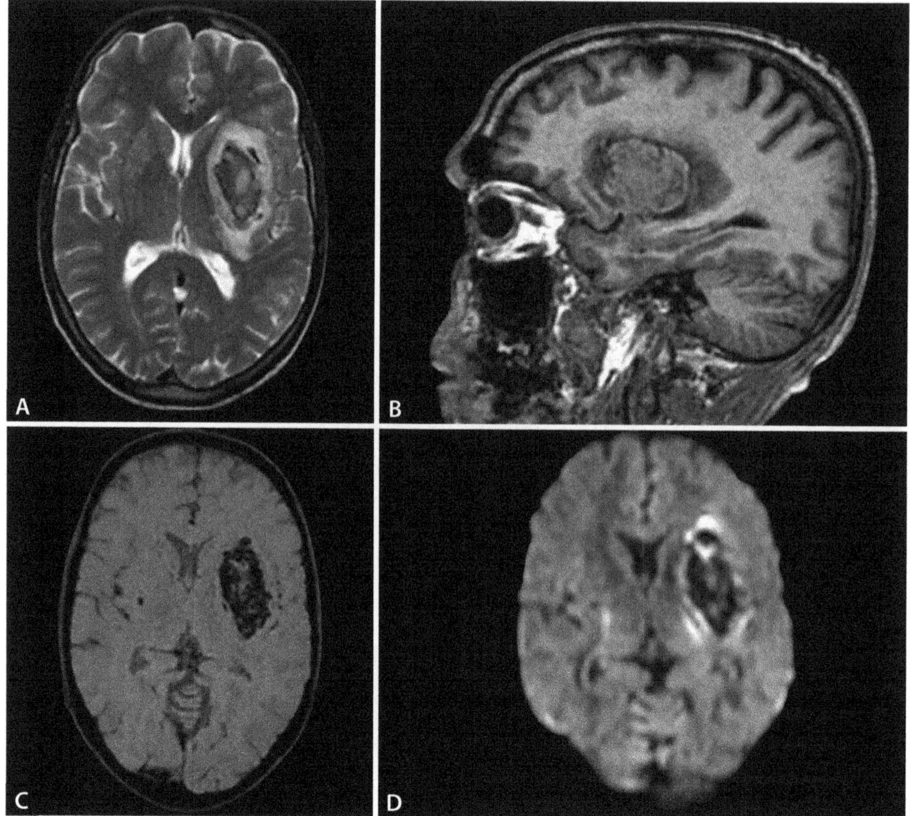

Figs. 31A to D: A well-defined oval T2 hypointense (A) and T1 isointense (B) lesion is seen in left basal ganglia with mild adjacent edema. It shows extensive hypointense areas within on gradient images (C) suggestive of acute hypertensive hematoma; (D) No significant restriction of diffusion is seen.

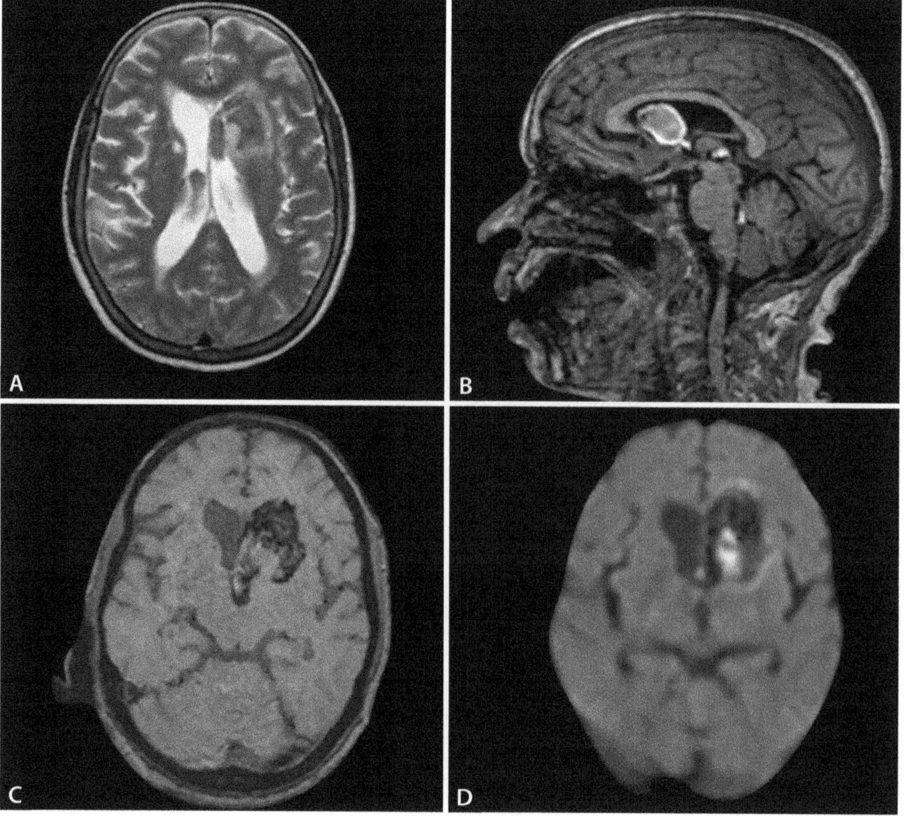

Figs. 32A to D: A well-defined oval T2 hypointense (A) and T1 hyperintense (B) lesion is seen in left corona radiata and basal ganglia with mild adjacent edema. It shows extensive hypointense areas within on gradient images (C) suggestive of early subacute hematoma. Mild restriction of diffusion is seen (D).

TABLE 3: Magnetic resonance imaging appearance of intracranial hematomas of different ages on common MR sequences.

Stage of hematoma	*T1*	*T2*	*DW*
Hyperacute (<24 h)	Isointense	Hyperintense	–
Acute (1–3 days)	Isointense	Hypointense	–
Early subacute (>3–7 days)	Hyperintense	Hypointense	–
Late subacute (1–4 weeks)	Hyperintense	Hyperintense	Appear bright
Chronic (>4 weeks)	Hypointense	Hypointense	–

CONCLUSION

There are various radiological investigations that are often performed for diagnostic purpose. The accurate interpretation influences patient management especially in emergency hours. With increasing availability of sophisticated imaging modalities, it is the responsibility of referring physician to ask for the appropriate investigation to get correct diagnosis. A cross-sectional imaging although gives detailed information, but problems related to the availability and cost of the investigation can arise.

Even today plain CXR is the first line of investigation and is cost-effective and apart from basic anatomy and pathology knowledge it is essential to have basic technical information before reading any radiological investigation.

BIBLIOGRAPHY

1. Allisy-Roberts PJ, Williams J. Farr's Physics for Medical Imaging, 2nd edition. USA: Saunders Ltd; 2007.
2. Benjamin F. Chest Roentgenology, 3rd edition. USA: WB Saunders Co; 2007.
3. de Lacey G, Morley S, Berman L. The Chest X-Ray: A Survival Guide, 1st edition. USA: Saunders Ltd; 2012.
4. Hunter TB, Taljanovic MS, Tsau PH, et al. Medical devices of the chest. Radiographics. 2004;24(6):1725-46.
5. Jain SN. A pictorial essay: Radiology of lines and tubes in the intensive care unit. Indian J Radiol Imaging. 2011;21(3): 182-90.

Equipment for Anesthesia in Remote Locations

Aparna A Nerurkar, Devangi A Parikh

ABSTRACT

The remote location anesthesia presents many challenges to anesthesiologists. The limited space, unfamiliar environment, safety hazards in these areas, and often limited equipment test the skills of the anesthesiologists. These remote areas are often specifically designed for imaging or for a particular specialty with minimum consideration to patient or anesthetic needs.

The radiology suites, e.g., cardiac catheterization laboratory, interventional radiology, digital subtraction angiography, computed tomography scanning (CT scan), magnetic resonance imaging (MRI); gastroenterological procedure rooms; psychiatric wards for electroconvulsive therapy are some examples of remote location anesthesia. Standard equipment with modified placement can be used in almost all these areas.

The MRI suite merits special consideration due to the unique challenge of a strong magnetic field affecting standard ferromagnetic equipment. Special "MRI safe" or "MRI conditional" equipment needs to be used.

The non-MRI compatible anesthesia machines and other equipment can be modified for use in a magnetic field by replacing their ferromagnetic components or by keeping them away from the core of the magnet or by securing them firmly to the floor or wall or using wall mounted machines. Magnetic resonance imaging-compatible anesthesia machines and equipment made largely of stainless steel, brass, aluminum, and plastic are available.

The nonferrous oxygen and nitrous cylinders having an aluminum body with brass fittings are preferred. Sufficiently long Bain circuits, T-piece systems or circle absorbers can be used. Most of the routine airway devices can be used with special precautions. Batteries of routine laryngoscopes are of concern and require alternative arrangement. Inadvertent cable loops or various monitor probes may cause burns. Careful positioning, use of insulating material like foam, careful avoidance of coiling of pulse oximeter and electrocardiography cables, etc., are to be followed. Other monitors like capnograph, blood pressure monitors, etc., can be used with longer tubings. It should be remembered that the defibrillator cannot be brought into the MRI area.

INTRODUCTION

Anesthesia for patients undergoing procedures at remote locations is challenging. The greatest challenge lies in providing anesthesia of operating room standards to a patient in a nonoperating room environment. The American Society of Anesthesiologists (ASA) has issued guidelines as early as October 2003, for remote location anesthesia. These were amended in 2008 and apply to all anesthesia care involving anesthesiology personnel, for procedures intended to be performed in locations outside an operating room.[1] Guidelines have also been issued by other organizations like Association of Anaesthetists of Great Britain and Ireland, American College of Radiology, Medicines and Healthcare Products Regulatory Agency.[2-4]

The data from the ASA closed claims database suggests that anesthesia at remote locations poses a significant risk to the patient.[5-7] Indian reports regarding complications at these locations are also emerging.[8,9] Many of these locations expose the patient and provider to multiple hazards. The limited space, unfamiliar environment, and safety hazards in these areas, especially CT scan and MRI suites can dictate, which techniques or equipment can or cannot be used. Also, these remote areas are often specifically designed for imaging or for a particular specialty. There is minimum consideration to patient needs or needs of the practitioners required to provide patient care.

DEFINITION OF REMOTE LOCATIONS

The remote locations, by definition, include areas where anesthesiologists may be required to administer anesthesia or sedation outside the operating theaters. These areas may be:

- Radiology suites, e.g., cardiac catheterization laboratory, interventional radiology, digital subtraction angiography, computed tomography scanning (CT scan), magnetic resonance imaging (MRI)

- Endoscopy suites—gastroenterological procedures
- Psychiatric wards for electroconvulsive therapy
- Burns procedure room
- Dental chair
- Renal unit for lithotripsy
- Gynecology procedures room for oocyte retrieval
- Radiation therapy unit.

The standard equipment can be used in almost all these areas. Only the placement needs to be different keeping in mind the ergonomics of those particular areas. The footprint of the scanners, fluoroscopy units, etc., is generally big and floor-space for anesthetic machines, monitors and other equipment is limited.

SPECIAL CONSIDERATIONS WITH MAGNETIC RESONANCE IMAGING

The MRI suite merits special consideration due to the unique challenges it presents. The strong magnetic field exerted by the scanner affects the standard ferromagnetic equipment. Special equipment has therefore been developed for use in the MRI suite. The problems associated with this remote area have been well documented[10-12] right from the first known publication in 1984.[13]

Ferromagnetism

Ferromagnetism is the basic mechanism by which certain materials (such as iron) form permanent magnets, or are attracted to magnets. Thus "ferromagnetic" refers to an element that can become magnetized when exposed to an external magnetic field. It is important to understand that not all ferromagnetic objects contain iron, and not all iron-containing (or ferrous) objects are ferromagnetic. "Ferro" refers to iron which is the most common example of ferromagnetism but other ferromagnetic elements include nickel, cobalt, some of the rare earth metals (e.g., gadolinium) and minerals like lodestone. Conversely, stainless steel is mostly iron, but the chromium, nickel and carbon in the alloy alter its magnetic properties. The most common form of stainless steel is called "austenitic" and is nonferromagnetic.

Problems with Equipment in the Magnetic Resonance Imaging Suite

There are three types of energy in the MRI suite that can affect monitors and equipment and thus anesthetic delivery.

Static Magnetic Field

First is a powerful static magnetic field which is always on. Depending on the scanner it has a strength of 1.5/3 tesla (15,000/30,000 times greater than the magnetic field of the earth's surface respectively). One tesla is equal to 10,000 gauss. Small objects such as paper clips and hairpins have a terminal velocity of 40 mph when pulled into a 1.5 T magnet. They can thus become dangerous projectiles sufficient to injure or kill anyone in their path, pose a serious risk to the patient and anyone else in the scan room. The force with which projectiles are pulled toward a magnetic field is proportional to the mass of the object and distance from the magnet. Even surgical tools such as hemostats, scissors and clamps, although made of a surgical stainless steel, are strongly attracted to the main magnetic field. The magnetic field can cause larger objects to trap or crush a patient or staff member. Foreign bodies in the eye may become dislodged,[14] leading to vitreous hemorrhage. Implanted pacemakers, defibrillators, and other devices may be inactivated, reprogrammed, dislodged, or converted to an asynchronous mode by the magnetic field.

Radiofrequency Pulses

The second form of energy is in the form of radiofrequency (RF) pulses that cause magnetic resonance by super-energizing cells that then emit RF signals. This can lead to potentially nonuniform power dissipation within the patient and a corresponding increase in temperature. The main concerns occur with field strengths greater than 2 T. The specific absorption rate is used to measure this heating. The US Food and Drug Administration (FDA) limit is 0.4 W/kg averaged over the whole body. The specific absorption rate may be reduced by changing the pulse sequence, decreasing the number of slices, lengthening the repeat time, decreasing the RF scale, and switching to a smaller transmitter coil. In practice, significant patient heating is only encountered in infants.

The real danger lies in the focused heating of conductive materials. Radiofrequency heating creates a risk of severe and rapid burns from any conductive material left on the patient's skin. This includes monitor probes, RF coils, loops of cable, etc. Therefore, contact with the metal in clothing, RF coils, electrocardiography (ECG) leads, and other equipment must be avoided.

Time-varied Magnetic Field Gradients

The third form of energy consists of time-varied magnetic field gradients that encode the emitted RF to produce 2-dimensional and 3-dimensional images. These are small and dynamic magnetic fields which are manipulated rapidly during image acquisition. They can induce a current sufficient to stimulate the peripheral nerve and muscle cells, sometimes causing discomfort. Medical MRI scanners apply limits on gradient field manipulation to avoid the more extreme consequences of induced currents such as limb movement or ventricular fibrillation. This form of energy has no direct impact on anesthetic equipment but the switching gradient fields produce acoustic noise. This is typically above the safe level of 85 dB. This can lead to hearing loss, especially during long scans, and mandates the need for ear protecting devices for patients regardless of whether they are anesthetized or not. Staff members also need to protect the ears to prevent noise-induced hearing loss.

The strength of the magnetic field diminishes as the distance from the magnet bore increases. The strength of the field is described by gauss lines that define the strength of the field at different distances from the magnet. The gauss line indicates a perimeter around the MR scanner within which the static magnetic field generated by the machine is more than 5 gauss. Beyond this line, the static field is below 5 gauss and is considered safe for healthcare providers who are regularly exposed to such fields. Equipment that needs to be placed in the vicinity of the scanner should be sorted as per its compatibility with the gauss lines.

What is Ideal Magnetic Resonance Imaging Equipment?

The primary requirement of the equipment used in the MRI suite is that the magnetic field must not affect the equipment and that the equipment must not interfere with the imaging process. Also the equipment must pose no danger to the patient either by spontaneous movement within the magnetic field or overheating. MRI compatible equipment has therefore been especially developed for this purpose. The equipment is made compatible by minimizing the iron content, where replacing iron possible with aluminum, plastic or steel, so that devices can be safely brought into the scanner room. Other safe metals include nickel, alloys, tantalum, and titanium. If compatible equipment is not available, all efforts must be made to bolt the equipment tightly to the floors and walls so as to prevent spontaneous movement. Use of wireless probes, equipment, etc., and careful placement of wires ensuring that coils are avoided can tackle the problem of overheating. The safe proximity to the magnet can vary from device to device and devices should be located as per their compatibility. Some devices can be placed directly next to the scanner.

CLASSIFICATION OF EQUIPMENT AS PER COMPATIBILITY

Any equipment near MRI suite is broadly divided into three categories:[15]

1. MRI safe
2. MRI conditional
3. MRI unsafe.

Magnetic Resonance Imaging Safe

"Magnetic resonance imaging safe" denotes equipment which presents no safety hazard to patients or personnel when it is taken into the MRI scanning room, provided that instructions concerning its use are correctly followed. This does not, however, guarantee that it will function normally and not interfere with the correct operation of the MRI imaging equipment, with degradation of image quality.

The equipment that is designated as "MRI compatible" is MRI safe, functions normally in the MR environment, and does not interfere with the correct operation of the MRI imaging equipment providing instructions concerning its proper use are correctly followed. The device or implant is completely nonmagnetic, nonelectrically conductive, and non-RF reactive, eliminating all of the primary potential threats during an MRI procedure.

Magnetic Resonance Imaging Conditional

The "MR conditional" equipment poses no hazard in a specified MR environment during specific conditions of use. The device or implant may contain magnetic, electrically conductive, or RF-reactive components that are safe for operations in proximity to the MRI, provided the conditions for safe operation are defined and observed. The conditions of use may include limits on static field strength, spatial gradient, and rate of change of magnetic field, RF fields, and specific absorption rate, or configuration of the equipment itself. Since the MRI scanners vary with regard to the magnetic fringe field, and also their operating range for other critical parameters, the use and placement of MR conditional equipment must be considered separately for each scanner in association with advice from the local MRI technician and in consultation with the biomedical engineer.

Magnetic Resonance Imaging Unsafe

The "MR unsafe" equipment is the equipment which is known to pose a hazard in all MR environments. Such equipment generally contains ferromagnetic material and poses a clear and direct threat to persons and equipment within the magnet room.

It is important to know that this terminology (i.e., MR safe, MR conditional, and MR unsafe) has not been applied retrospectively. Thus, implants and devices that have received FDA approved labeling prior to December 2005 using the terms "MR safe" or "MR compatible" are not included in this terminology.[16] MRI-related labeling may thus be different for "older" versus "newer" implants, or those that have undergone retesting. Also evolving MRI machines may be of greater strength than the conditions under which device was tested.

Thus, prior testing, reading the literature supplied by the manufacturer, and/or MRI-related labeling by a recognized body, such as the FDA is essential prior to using any equipment in the MRI suite. A list of equipment, implants, pacemakers and other devices, with type of compatibility for MRI is also available for free use on the website[17] www.mrisafety.com. Some of the devices whose status is unknown can be verified on this site. It is also advisable to consult the manufacturer or biomedical personnel with expertise in MRI regarding such devices. A strong magnet may be kept in the MRI suite to confirm magnetic status of equipment. A new breed of ferromagnetic detectors developed specifically for screening patients and objects entering the MRI suite have been made available recently. These specialized metal detectors give an alert on magnetic materials that may become missile-threats in proximity to the MRI magnet. In fact, screening forms[18] are also available to minimize the possibility that MRI unsafe equipment or objects are taken into the vicinity of the scanner. The MRI compatible equipment should be clearly labeled to distinguish it from the standard equipment which should not be taken into the restricted area.

Equipment Required in Magnetic Resonance Imaging

The equipment and monitors required in the MRI suite are ideally equivalent to an operating theater setup and include MRI safe/compatible:

- Anesthesia machine
- Monitors
- Basic anesthesia equipment
- Resuscitation equipment
- Other equipment.

Anesthesia Machine

As per ASA guidelines, "in any location in which inhalational anesthesia is to be administered, there should be an anesthesia machine equivalent in function to that employed in operating rooms and maintained to current operating room standards."[1]

The anesthesia machines can be modified for use in a magnetic field by replacing their ferromagnetic components.[19] Non-MRI compatible anesthesia machines can also be used by keeping them 20–30 feet away from the core of the magnet or by securing them firmly to the floor or wall or using wall-mounted machines. Currently, manufacturers offer MRI-compatible machines made largely of stainless steel, brass, aluminum and plastic. The AESTIVA®/5 MRI machine **(Fig. 1)** offers an additional feature in the form of a physically integrated magnetic field strength monitor (Gauss Alarm). Green light is shown when monitor is sampling and magnetic fringe field is less than 275 gauss, amber light when magnetic fringe field is 275–300 gauss and red light with audio alarm when magnetic fringe field is more than 300 gauss.

Philips MRI 508 and Dragger FABIUS® MRI are some of the other machines available. The position of the machine in the suite should be determined by a biomedical engineer.

The early generation vaporizers were not accurate in the MRI suite, due to malfunctioning of the bimetallic strip temperature compensation. Modern generation vaporizers (e.g., Tec 5, Tec 7) can be used as they function accurately within the magnetic field. Floating vaporizers may become projectile hazards.[20]

The anesthetic circuit needs to be very long (6 m) to allow for rotation of the table into the MRI coil. A coaxial Mapleson D (extended Bain) system with 10 m long tubes,

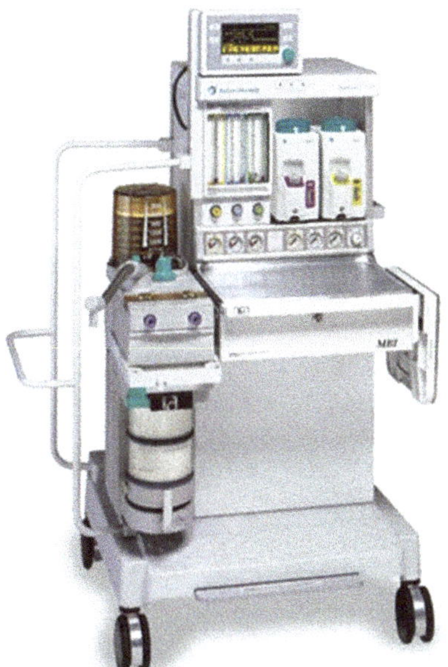

Fig. 1: AESTIVA®/5 MRI with Gauss alarm. *Source:* GE Healthcare.

circle absorbers with long plastic tubing's have successfully been used in MRI suites. A modified T-piece system with 10 m long fresh gas flow tube can be used for both spontaneous and controlled breathing. Care should be taken to exclude positive end expiratory pressure (PEEP) valves that contain metal springs. Magnetic resonance imaging compatible PEEP valves are available. The Ambu® disposable PEEP valve has been tested in MR conditions up to 3 tesla.

It should be remembered that all the connections to the machine and monitor must be kept neatly together to prevent accidental disconnection.

Gas Cylinders

Molybdenum steel-based gas cylinders are unsafe and multiple incidents of oxygen and nitrous oxide cylinders being pulled to the magnet have been reported **(Figs. 2 to 4)**.[21-23]

The oxygen cylinder acting as a flying projectile has resulted in a fatality in 2001.[24] Nonferrous oxygen and nitrous cylinders having an aluminum body with brass fittings are preferred. They may be marked 3 AL or 3 ALM. Each cylinder should be checked with a strong hand magnet before being bought into the theater. Ideally, they should be fitted to the machine when the machine is outside the theater for additional safety.

Flow meters made of brass fittings are available for use in the MRI suite.

Ventilators

The nonferromagnetic ventilators that work on compressed oxygen are available for use in the MRI suite. Fluidic ventilators work well in the MRI environment. Most MRI compatible machines come with ventilators capable of delivering both conventional and newer modes of ventilation.

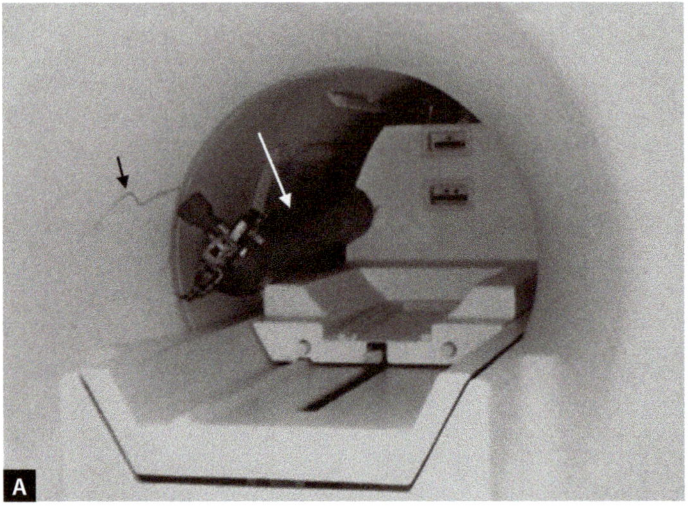

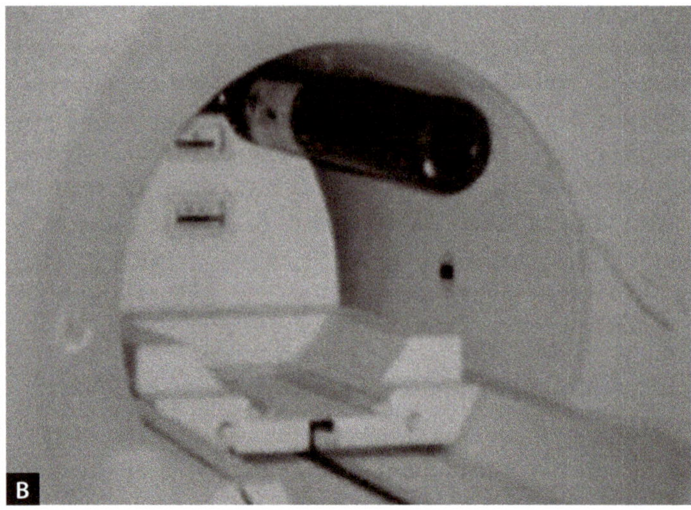

Figs. 2A and B: Oxygen cylinder in magnetic resonance imaging bore.
Courtesy: www.simplyphysics.com.

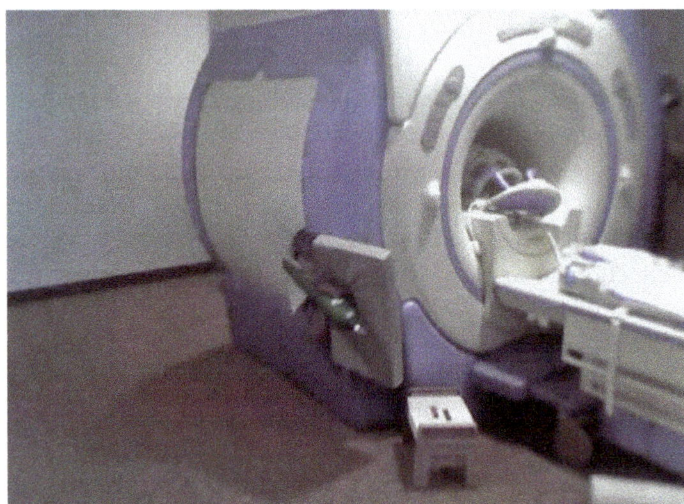

Fig. 3: Oxygen cylinder outside magnetic resonance imaging.
Courtesy: www.simplyphysics.com.

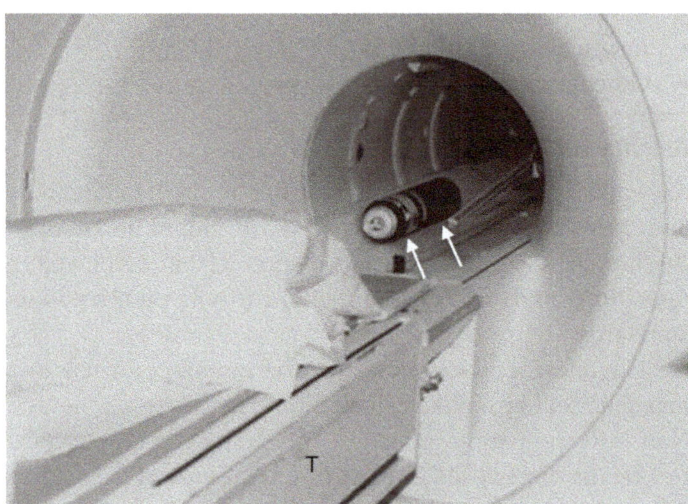

Fig. 4: Nitrous oxide cylinder in magnetic resonance imaging
Courtesy: www.simplyphysics.com.

Monitors

All the monitoring equipment must be appropriately shielded and rated to work within the defined magnetic fields. Sources for monitoring systems available in the magnet room should consist of isolated duplex power circuits with filtered alternating current to filter noise artifacts from interfering with the images. Monitors plugged into these outlets should be located as far from the core of the magnet as possible, beyond the gauss line. Also, they should be free of ferromagnetic material and RF shielded. If unshielded electrical equipment is used it will need to be unplugged from power during scanning as the MRI images will otherwise be degraded.

Also one needs to be aware of the risk of inadvertent cable loops causing burns[25] or probe induced burns due to various monitors.[26] To prevent patients from experiencing excessive heating and possible burns in association with MR procedures, the guidelines[27] by Institute for Magnetic Resonance Safety, Education, and Research recommending careful positioning, use of insulating material like foam, careful avoidance of coiling, etc., are to be followed. Wireless pulse oximeter probes and ECG cables can be used.

Pulse Oximetry

The standard pulse oximeters are preferably not used in the MRI suite due to electromagnetic interference leading to burns to extremities.[28,29] These are caused by the induction of current within a loop of wire in the presence of magnetic flux with resultant heating of the wires. If conventional oximeters are to be used, the sensor should be placed on the extremity as distant to the magnet bore as possible, the sensor wires should be free of coils and parallel to the magnet bore, and the digits should be protected with clear plastic wrap.

The MRI compatible pulse oximeters using heavy fiber optic cables may be preferred. The fiberoptic cables cannot be looped and do not get overheated. However, they are quite fragile and expensive.

Electrocardiography

Electrocardiography is difficult within a static magnetic field. Maximum voltage charges are induced in any column of conducting fluid thus blood flow through the aorta itself can create voltage potentials. The superimposed potentials are greatest in ST segments and T waves of leads I, II, V1, V2, and increase with field strength. Spike artifacts that mimic R waves are often produced because of the changing magnetic fields of the imaging gradients. ST segments cannot be analyzed as when the patient is being scanned, there is often the appearance of ST segment elevation on the ECG.

The changes in the ECG waveform are present even in filtered systems designed for MRI use and make it impossible to reliably monitor for ischemia or to interpret arrhythmias.

The ECG electrodes may cause burns **(Fig. 5)**.[30,31] The leads should be braided together and must not be placed directly on the patients' skin in case they heat up. The ECG electrodes are placed only about 20 cm apart and can only give approximations of leads I, II, and III. Electrocardiography cables are coaxialized to avoid any coils, as a current is induced in the coil due to the changing magnetic field which can lead to burning of the skin. A small towel folded and placed on the patient's chest to avoid contact with the skin can be used as an extra precaution.

The nonmagnetic ECG electrodes are available which incorporate four electrodes in a single, easy to use disposable patch with a large electrode contact area to provide optimal ECG performance. They are available in adult and neonatal sizes. Nonmagnetic electrodes with the added advantage of four individual pads having large, wet gel contact area allowing for optimal cardiovascular placement, with electrodes and lead wires developed specifically for cardiovascular MRI are also available.

Capnography

The mainstream capnometry sensors cause image interference. Side stream monitors can be used with long gas sampling tubing's and monitor placed beyond the gauss line. Long sampling tubing may result in mixing of end-tidal gas with dead space gas. As a result, end-tidal measurements may not be accurate, although they are adequate for apnea monitoring and for trends. Long tubing may also give rise to a long lag time (up to 20 seconds). Infrared monitors analyzing end-tidal carbon dioxide will give rapid detection of loss of ventilation and circuit disconnection.

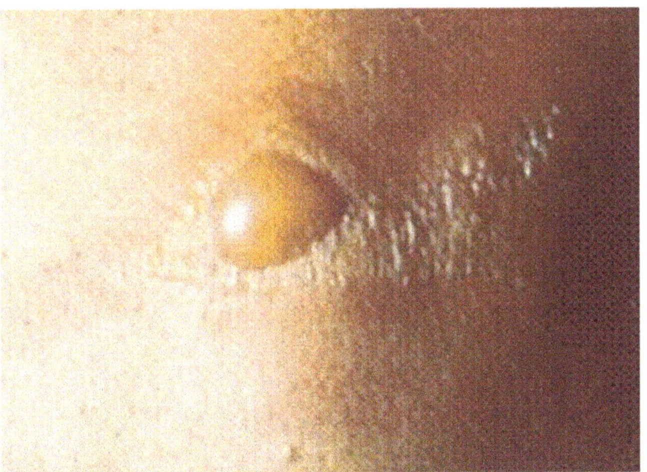

Fig. 5: Burns due to electrocardiograph lead.
Courtesy: www.simplyphysics.com.

Blood Pressure

The conventional manual sphygmomanometers can be adapted for use during MRI by replacing all ferromagnetic components with brass, aluminum, or plastic pieces. The automated oscillometric blood pressure monitoring can be used, as it is based on pneumatic principles which avoid electromagnetic interference.[32] The extra-long tubing's and plastic connectors can be used to add the required length.

A standard arterial line can be placed and conventional disposable transducers placed outside the gauss line for invasive blood pressure monitoring. Disposable transducers are not likely to get damped from the extra-long tubing's as they have a predictably high natural frequency.

Temperature

As the standard temperature probes made of metal are conductive they can heat up and harm the patient.[33] Fiberoptic temperature probes with optical sensor technology based on the fluorescence decay time of a special thermosensitive phosphorescent (phosphor) sensor, located at the end of a fiberoptic cable can be used. The fiberoptic probes are relatively small. Fiberoptic probes (as small as 0.5 mm diameter) are available. The probe is not suitable for insertion to a body cavity so it is placed in the axilla.

Nerve Stimulator

The peripheral nerve stimulators with the box placed outside the gauss line can be used.

Multiparameter Monitors

The MRI compatible multiparameter monitors are available. This technology combines modalities, such as pulse oximetry, ECG, noninvasive blood pressure monitoring, temperature monitoring, capnometry and anesthetic agent analysis as well as invasive pressure monitoring. Wireless ECG and SpO_2 feature shorter cables designed to increase efficiency. Shorter cables also reduce the risk of cable heating and are less prone to damage.

Magnetic Resonance Imaging Compatible Basic Anesthesia Equipment

Laryngoscopes

The plastic handles, blades have been used. Whereas, the usual stainless-steel blade, bulb, and handle are compatible but the batteries are ferromagnetic. The lithium batteries have been used. A remote fiberoptic light source can be used. The specially designed, lightweight, low-magnetic signature fiberoptic laryngoscopes with brighter, whiter xenon light are available with carbon zinc battery packs which are MRI conditional.

Endotracheal Tubes/Laryngeal Mask Airways/I-gels

The plain endotracheal tubes (ETTs) or laryngeal mask airways (LMAs) are made of compatible material but the valves often contain a ferrous spring. This lightweight spring can distort the MRI image.[34] The valve of the ETT should be therefore taped to the ETT to keep it as far away from the imaging area as possible. Alternatively, the pilot balloon tubing can be knotted and the spring cut off.

The LMA may not be suitable if MR spectroscopy is performed because the resonance of some silicone-containing materials compromises interpretation of the scans. MRI compatible LMAs are available. I-gels have also been safely used in the MRI suite.[35]

The tracheal and tracheostomy tubes with metal reinforced shafts can be used safely if the area of interest of the scan is not in the close vicinity of the tube shaft. The nonclinical testing of these devices has demonstrated that they are MR conditional. A patient with this implant/device can be scanned safely immediately after placement under the following conditions:

- Static magnetic field of 3 tesla or less
- Maximum spatial gradient magnetic field of 720 gauss/cm or less (other values for the spatial gradient magnetic field may apply if properly calculated)
- Maximum MR system reported whole-body-averaged specific absorption rate (SAR) of 3 W/kg for 15 minutes of scanning (per pulse sequence).

With reference to temperature rise, in nonclinical testing, the implant/device produced a temperature rise of less than or equal to 3.0°C at a maximum MR system-reported whole-body-averaged SAR of 3 W/kg for 15 minutes (per pulse sequence) of MR scanning in a 3 tesla MR system using a transmit/receive body coil.

The reinforced LMAs or intubating LMAs are unsuitable for use in MRI as they cause excessive artifact.

Suction Equipment

The MRI compatible suction machines are available. Wall-mounted secure suction can also be used. Many of the modern anesthesia machines adapted for MRI have integrated patient suction units.

Resuscitation Equipment

Cardiac Arrest

The defibrillator cannot be brought into the MRI area. The patient needs to be moved out of the MRI area into either the anesthetic room or a designated area, should a defibrillator be needed. The resuscitation bags without metallic valve components are to be used.

Other Equipment

Patient Warming

The convection-based forced warm air blowers cannot be used due to the electrical interference they would create during scanning and the risk of magnetic attraction.

The heated water blankets, light weight and flexible thermal gel mats which are made of 100% medical grade soft silicone gel material are available. They are placed directly onto the surgical table and they are designed to mold to the contours of the patient's body thus maximizing surface contact, ensuring safe and effective warming. Warming is achieved by utilizing 12 V technology and the system is turned off during the imaging sequences. Also during this time, the material maintains its core temperature for up to 30 minutes. The fluid warmers should not be used unless absolutely needed as they cause interference with the imaging.

Syringe Pumps

The intravenous pump systems with unique nonmagnetic ultrasonic motor providing safe dependable fluid delivery are available. The Space Station™ **(Fig. 6)** from B Braun which is a casing station made of shielded aluminum housing accommodating up to four normal infusion pumps at a time with capacity to detect and trigger acoustic and optical alarms about strength of magnetic field are also available.

The other equipment's routinely used include trolleys, IV poles, chairs, etc., which must all be carefully checked for compatibility as accidents have been known to happen **(Figs. 7 and 8)**.

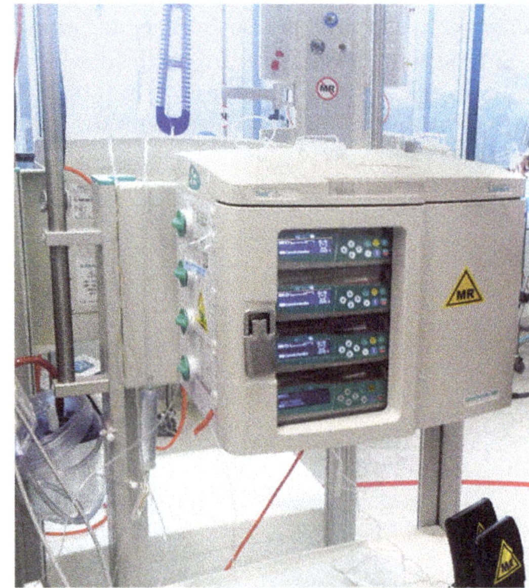

Fig. 6: Space Station™.
Courtesy: B Braun

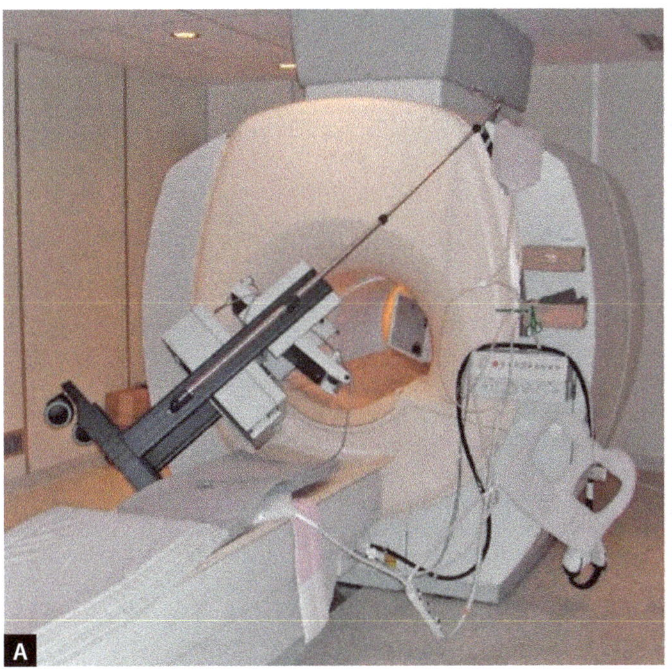

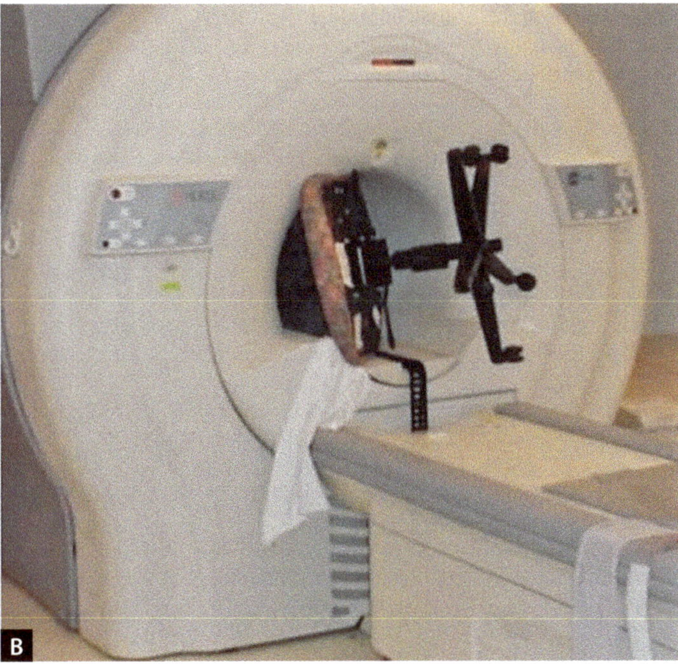

Figs. 7A and B: Intravenous pole and chair in magnetic resonance imaging.
Courtesy: www.simplyphysics.com.

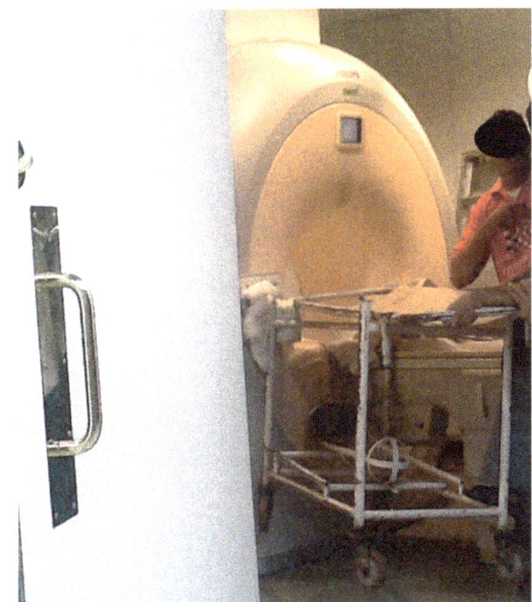

Fig. 8: Trolley stuck to magnetic resonance imaging.

The equipment should be labeled as per their MRI suitability as per the labeling mentioned earlier. Some equipment may be only available in non-MRI compatible form, e.g., diathermy or cautery machines. In this case great care must be taken to avoid them from coming close to the magnet. As with anesthesia machines, all such devices must be tethered to the wall or pendant to ensure that they cannot get to close to the magnet. The wheeled devices should have brakes as well (e.g., instrument trolleys) but this may not be always possible. Other equipment, which is used mainly for patient and provider comfort include ear protecting devices to tackle acoustic noise, MRI eyewear with prism glasses for tackling claustrophobia, MRI carts for storage of equipment, etc.

OTHER CONCERNS

Helium Escape

When a superconductor is used to maintain the main static magnetic field, the cryostat typically contains around 1,000 L of liquid helium within a few degree Celsius of absolute zero. In the event of a spontaneous or emergency field shutdown, known as a quench, the liquid helium expands to gas and must be vented very rapidly. The MRI suite is designed to vent this outside the building via a quench pipe but, if this fails or becomes blocked, some or all of the gas may enter the suite necessitating rapid evacuation.

CONCLUSION

The remote location anesthesia presents many challenges. Placement of equipment and devices is a problem in most of the locations. Magnetic resonance imaging presents unique challenges due to the magnetic field. Specialized equipment, equipment with suitable modifications, and meticulous care can smoothen the conduct of anesthesia in this location.

REFERENCES

1. American Society of Anesthesiologists. Statement on non-operating room anesthetizing locations. Standards and Practice Parameters Committee. ASA House of Delegates; 2003. (Amended on October 22, 2008)
2. Association of Anaesthetists of Great Britain and Ireland. Safety in magnetic resonance units: an update. Anaesthesia. 2010;65(7):766-70.
3. American College of Radiology. ACR Guidance Document for Safe MR Practices: 2007. AJR. 2007;188:1447-74.

4. Medicines and Healthcare Products Regulatory Agency. Devices bulletin: safety guidelines for magnetic resonance imaging equipment in clinical use. London: MHRA; 2007.
5. Metzner J, Posner KL, Lam MS, et al. Closed claims analysis. Best Pract Res Clin Anaesthesiol. 2011;25(2):263-76.
6. Metzner J, Posner KL, Domino KB. The risk and safety of anesthesia at remote locations: the US closed claims analysis. Curr Opin Anaesthesiol. 2009;22(4):502-8.
7. Robbertze R, Posner KL, Domino KB. Closed claims review of anesthesia for procedures outside the operating room. Curr Opin Anaesthesiol. 2006;19(4):436-42.
8. Mufti S, Sheikh MA, Hakim A, et al. A "Near-Miss Lethal Accident Case" in MR Suit of a Tertiary Care Hospital. Case Rep Radiol. 2011;2011:793570.
9. Agarwal A, Singhal V, Dhiraaj S, et al. Head injury from an MRI compatible pulse oximeter. Anaesthesia. 2005;60:1042-52.
10. Reddy U, White MJ, Wilson SR. Anaesthesia for magnetic resonance imaging. Contin Educ Anaesth Crit Care Pain. 2012; 12(3):140-4.
11. Jayaraman L, Sethi N, Sood J. Anaesthesia outside the operating theatre. Update in Anaesthesia. 2009;25(1):37-41. [online] Available from: www.anaesthesiologists.org. [Last accessed May, 2021].
12. Manninen HP. Anaesthesia outside the operating room. Can J Anaesth. 1991;38(4): R126-9.
13. Geiger RS, Cascorbi HF. Anesthesia in an NMR Scanner. Anesth Analg. 1984;63:622-3.
14. Kiliç A, Avcu S, Tekïn S, et al. MRI-induced migration of retained metallic foreign body in the eye. Ophthalmic Surg Lasers Imaging. 2010;9:1-3.
15. Clauson D. ASTM standards in action, promoting the safe use of MRI technology. [online] Available from http://www.astm.org/standardization-news/features/promoting-safe-use-of-mri-technology-ma12.html. [Last accessed March, 2014].
16. Shellock FG, Woods TO, Crues JV. MR labeling information for implants and devices: explanation of terminology. Radiology. 2009;253(1):26-30.
17. Shellock FG. MRI Safety Premier information resource for magnetic resonance safety. [online] Available from www.mrisafety.com. [Last accessed March, 2014].
18. Institute for Magnetic Resonance Safety, Education, and Research (IMRSER). (2001). Magnetic resonance screening form for individuals. [online] Available from http://www.imrser.org. [Last accessed March, 2014].
19. Rao CC, McNiece WL, Emhardt J, et al. Modification of an anesthesia machine for use during magnetic resonance imaging. Anesthesiology. 1988;68(4):640-1.
20. Zimmer C, Janssen MN, Treschan TA, et al. Near-miss accident during magnetic resonance imaging by a "Flying Sevoflurane Vaporizer" due to ferromagnetism undetectable by handheld magnet. Anesthesiology. 2004;100(5):1329-30.
21. Chaljub G, Kramer LA, Johnson RF, et al. Projectile cylinder accidents resulting from the presence of ferromagnetic nitrous oxide or oxygen tanks in the MR suite. Am J Roentgenol. 2001; 177(1):27–30.
22. Colletti PM. Size "H" oxygen cylinder: accidental MR projectile at 1.5 Tesla. J. Magn Reson Imaging. 2004;19(1):141-3.
23. Simply physics. (2008). Danger! Flying Objects! [online] Available from http://simplyphysics.com/flying_objects.html. [Last accessed March, 2014].
24. Chen DW. Boy, 6, dies of skull injury during MRI. The New York Times. (NY region); 2001.
25. Knopp MV, Essig M, Debus J, et al. Unusual burns of the lower extremities caused by a closed conducting loop in a patient at MR imaging. Radiology. 1996;200(2):572-5.
26. Kanal E, Shellock FG. Burns associated with clinical MR examinations. Radiology. 1990;175(2):585.
27. Institute for Magnetic Resonance Safety, Education, and Research (IMRSER). (2001). Guidelines to prevent excessive heating and burns associated with magnetic resonance procedures. [online] Available from http://www.imrser.org/PaperPDFRecord.asp?WebRecID=102&PgName=Guidelines&WebRecID=&sb_SummaryTitle. [Last accessed March, 2014].
28. Bashein G, Syrory G. Burns associated with pulse oximetry during magnetic resonance imaging. Anesthesiology. 1991;75(2): 382-3.
29. Brown TR, Goldstein B, Little J. Severe burns resulting from magnetic resonance imaging with cardiopulmonary monitoring. Risks and relevant safety precautions. Am J Phys Med Rehabil. 1993;72(3):166-7.
30. Keens SJ, Laurence AS. Burns caused by ECG monitoring during MRI imaging. Anaesthesia. 1996; 51:1188-9.
31. Kugel H, Bremer C, Püschel M, et al. Hazardous situation in the MR bore: induction in ECG leads causes fire. Eur Radiol. 2003;13(4):690-4.
32. Patteson SK, Chesney JT. Anesthetic management for magnetic resonance imaging: problems and solutions. Anesth Analg. 1992; 74(1):121-4.
33. Hall SC, Stevenson GW, Suresh S. Burn associated with temperature monitoring during magnetic resonance imaging. Anesthesiology. 1992;76(1):152.
34. Grady RE, Perkins WJ. An unexpected cause of magnetic resonance image distortion: the endotracheal tube pilot balloon. Anesthesiology. 1997;86(4):993-4.
35. Taxak S, Bhardwaj M, Gopinath A. The I-gelTM-A promising airway device for magnetic resonance imaging suite. J Anaesthesiol Clin Pharmacol. 2012;28(2):263-4.

Role of Anesthetist in Preventing Nosocomial Infections

Vaibhavi Baxi, Dwarkadas K Baheti

ABSTRACT

Nosocomial infections (NIs) are among the common medical complications involving hospitalized patients. There are multiple factors that affect the incidence of NI, some of which are preexisting and nonmodifiable, whereas some other modifiable factors that can be optimized in the perioperative period.

This chapter discusses the role of anesthesiologist in preventing NIs and outlines the preventive strategies such as use of aseptic measures, prophylactic antibiotics, preventing contamination of intravenous medicines, cautious use of intravenous fluid, prevention of hypothermia, adequate glycemic control, and measures to prevent ventilator-associated pneumonia (VAP) and urinary tract infection (UTI).

INTRODUCTION

Nosocomial infections (NIs) also known as hospital-acquired infection are one of the common perioperative complications in hospitalized patients. NIs such as respiratory or urinary tract infection (UTI), bacteremia, enteritis, and intravenous cannula-related infections can affect tissue oxygen delivery or enzyme function. This will impair production of oxygen free radicals. All these factors help bacteria to survive so that infection sets in.

The factors such as age, American Society of Anesthesiologists (ASA) status, and preoperative preparation of site of operation, hematoma formation, anastomotic leak and poor surgical technique, choice of antiseptic, difficult or extensive surgery, immune suppression, comorbidities, and colonization by *Staphylococcus aureus* can increase incidence of surgical site infections (SSIs).

Impact of NIs adds to functional disability and emotional stress of the patient and in some cases, leads to disabling conditions that reduce the quality of life. NIs are one of the leading causes of death.[1] The economic costs are considerable.[2,3]

The increased length of stay for infected patients is the greatest contributor to cost.[4] Coella et al.,[5] showed that the overall increase in the duration of hospitalization for patients with surgical wound infections was 8.2 days, ranging from 3 days for gynecology to 9.9 for general surgery, and 19.8 for orthopedic surgery. Prolonged stay not only increases direct costs to patients or payers but also indirect costs due to lost work. The increased use of drugs, the need for isolation, and the use of additional laboratory and other diagnostic studies also contribute to costs.

Nosocomial infections add to the imbalance between resource allocation for primary and secondary health care by diverting scarce funds to the management of potentially preventable conditions.

DEFINITION

The National Nosocomial Infections Surveillance (NNIS) System defines an NI as a localized or systemic condition that results secondary to an infectious agent or its toxin, provided that it was not present or incubating at the time of admission to the hospital. NIs are defined and classified based on clinical findings, laboratory results, and other diagnostic studies. The bacterial NIs usually become evident after 48 hours of admission which is the typical incubation period.[6]

The following two conditions are also considered to be NIs:

1. Infection that is acquired in the hospital but does not become evident until after hospital discharge.
2. Infection in a neonate that results from passage through the birth canal.

The following conditions are not considered to be NIs:

- Infection associated with a complication or extension of infection already present on admission, unless a change in pathogen or symptoms strongly suggests the acquisition of a new infection.
- In an infant, an infection that is acquired transplacentally (e.g., toxoplasmosis, rubella, cytomegalovirus, or syphilis) and becomes evident at or before 48 hours after birth.[7]

During the beginning of infection control procedures, recommendations were made for high-risk situations.

However, it was recognized that such situations were often unknown or unpredictable. It was hence recommended that these procedures be adopted as routine measures. Subsequently these became known as "universal" precautions to be applied in all situations. More recently, the terminology has changed to "standard" precautions.

EPIDEMIOLOGY AND REVIEW OF LITERATURE

The incidence of NI, a major health issue, is on a rise affecting every one of ten admitted patients. The incidence is rising with increasing use of implantable medical devices, invasive medical, and surgical procedures.

According to a literature review of national or multicenter studies published from 1995 to 2008, the overall prevalence of NI in developed countries varies between 5.1 and 11.6%. The European Centre for Disease Prevention and Control reported an average prevalence of 7.1%. The estimated healthcare-associated infections incidence rate in the United States was 4.5% in 2002. Studies conducted in healthcare settings in developing countries report hospital-wide NI rates markedly higher than those in developed countries. Hospital-wide prevalence rates vary from 5 to 19%, but most studies report values higher than 10%.[8] Intensive care unit (ICU) patients are at a greater risk of NI with use of mechanical ventilation, invasive procedures, and immune compromised status. The European Prevalence of Infection in Intensive Care Study, involving over 4,500 patients, demonstrated that the NI prevalence rate in ICU was 20.6%.[9]

PATHOGENS COMMONLY ASSOCIATED WITH NOSOCOMIAL INFECTIONS

Nosocomial infections may be caused by viral, bacterial, or fungal pathogens. Gram-positive cocci—*S. aureus*—is the most predominantly-associated pathogen in NI. *Pseudomonas aeruginosa, Enterobacter cocci, Escherichia coli, Klebsiella pneumoniae,* and *Candida albicans* are the others implicated as causative pathogens for NIs.

TYPES OF NOSOCOMIAL INFECTIONS

Common NIs are bloodstream infection, pneumonia, e.g., ventilator-assisted pneumonia, SSI, gastrointestinal infection, skin infection, and most frequent being the UTI. The route of transmission may be direct or indirect contact, airborne or droplet transmission, or common vehicle transmission, e.g., medications, medical devices, and equipment.

PREVENTION OF NOSOCOMIAL INFECTIONS

Prevention of nosocomial infections requires following integrated, monitored program with following key features:

- Washing of hand and use of glove
- Aseptic practice and isolation strategies
- Sterilization and disinfection practice
- Control of environmental risk for infection
- Protection of patients from antimicrobials
- Adequate nutrition
- Minimize risk of infection from endogenous procedures
- Use of antimicrobial use and surveillance of infection
- Identifying and controlling outbreaks of infection
- Prevention of infection of staff members
- Enhancing staff care practices
- Continuing of staff education

It is responsibility of healthcare professional for infection control of doctors, nurses, therapist, pharmacist, engineers, and others.

The protocols to prevent NI should be strictly followed by all medical personnel, nursing staff, and paramedical staff at every stage of treatment, i.e., from admission to the discharge.

FACTORS THAT INFLUENCE THE RISK OF NOSOCOMIAL INFECTION

Patient Characteristics

- Poor nutritional status
- Uncontrolled diabetes
- Altered immunity, e.g., human immunodeficiency virus/acquired immunodeficiency syndrome (HIV/AIDS), chemotherapy
- Comorbidity
- Obesity
- Smoking
- Lengths of hospital stay (exposure to resistant organisms)
- Old age
- Patient in critical care unit

Perioperative Factors

- Operation theater ventilation: Positive pressure, air changes, and air filtration
- Prophylactic antibiotics
- Instrument processing
- Use face mask and aseptic measures by operation theater personnel
- Operation theater traffic
- Operation theater personnel hand hygiene
- Hypothermia
- Fluid management
- Blood and products transfusion

Surgical Factors

- Site and type of surgery—less tissue handling and less contaminated wound lessen the risk of infection
- Duration of surgery—infection rate almost doubles with every passing hour of surgery
- Use of medical devices/implants
- Preoperative shaving increases the risk by 5–10 times by providing growth of multiple microorganisms, so trimming hair would be better

- Skin preparation—alcohol-based antiseptic solution over a wide area around the incision site minimizes the risk of infection
- Surgical drains—preferably closed suction drain through a separate stab wound
- Postoperative incision wound care

Anesthesia-associated Factors

- Types of anesthesia (general anesthesia vs. regional anesthesia)
- Invasive procedures, e.g., central venous catheter (CVC)
- Anesthesia circuits
- Use of multidose vials
- Disinfection of airway devices such as laryngoscope blades
- Use of inhalational gases
- Rapid patient turnover
- Fluid management
- Glycemic control
- Adequate postoperative pain relief

SUGGESTED PROTOCOL FOR PREVENTION AND REDUCTION OF INCIDENCE OF NOSOCOMIAL INFECTIONS

To increase awareness about NIs, it is important to implement and improve measures to minimize the risk of transmission of infection to hospitalized patients. One needs to focus on the following strategies to prevent the NIs.

Hand Hygiene

Hand washing is one of the most important techniques in the prevention of cross infection. The transient microorganisms acquired by contact with patients, other healthcare workers, or contaminated surfaces are more often responsible for NI can effectively remove by routine hand wash with soap and clean water as they live in upper layers of skin. The resident microorganisms living in the deeper layers of the skin and hair follicles are less likely to cause infection.

Alcohol-based antiseptic hand scrubs contain 60–90% alcohol, antiseptic, e.g., povidone-iodine 5–10% and chlorhexidine 2–4%, has residual action and an emollient (to protect the skin). They are fast acting, effective, and remove transient flora and some resident microorganisms. The effective washing of hand before direct patient contact will result in significant reduction in the carriage of potential pathogens and decrease the incidence of preventable NI.

Anesthetists must ensure that hand hygiene becomes an indispensable part of their clinical culture.[10] Gloves are not a substitute for hand hygiene.

Asepsis and Skin Preparation

Preoperative skin preparation with an appropriate antiseptic decreases skin microbial colony counts. The principles of asepsis should be followed when placing intravascular devices, e.g., CVCs, spinal, or epidural anesthesia catheters, and while administering intravenous drugs.

A long-acting antiseptic solution with quick onset, minimal toxic effects, and effective against a wide range of microorganisms without getting deactivated with organic material (blood and body fluids) would be ideal. Commonly used solutions include povidone-iodine, chlorhexidine gluconate with or without isopropyl alcohol, an iodophor preparation in isopropyl alcohol, and isopropyl alcohol alone. The aqueous 70–92% alcohol solutions have germicidal activity against bacteria, fungi, and viruses, but spores can be resistant. Alcohol is readily available, inexpensive, and remains the most effective and rapid-acting skin antiseptic, however, one potential disadvantage of the use of alcohol in the operating room is its flammability.

Povidone-iodine (5–10%) is a germicidal compound that relies on its continual release of iodine which penetrates the cell wall and alters protein synthesis. Addition of isopropyl alcohol further increases the release of iodine. Disadvantages of povidone-iodine is its delayed onset, limited duration of action, local skin reactions (such as erythema and urticaria), and neutralization of its effect by organic fluids. Chlorhexidine gluconate (0.5–4%) is a potent broad-spectrum germicide that efficiently alters cell wall permeability, immediately precipitating components of the cell membrane and cytoplasm. The addition of isopropyl alcohol further accelerates these bactericidal effects. It is effective against nearly all nosocomial yeasts and bacteria (gram-positive and gram-negative); effect lasts for several hours, remains effective in presence of organic fluids and induces fewer (and less severe) skin reactions than other compounds.

Both povidone-iodine and chlorhexidine solutions are Food and Drug Administration (FDA) approved for skin preparation before surgery but not so far for regional anesthesia in view of lack of clinical testing. The Material Safety Data Sheet registered with the FDA does not describe adverse neurologic or central nervous system events after recommended povidone-iodine and chlorhexidine use. The chlorhexidine 0.5% in 80% ethanol significantly reduces the likelihood of catheter and site colonization and maximizes the rapidity and potency of bactericidal activity when compared to other solutions. Therefore, alcohol-based chlorhexidine solutions should be considered the antiseptic of choice before regional anesthetic techniques (grade A recommendation).[11]

Antibiotic Prophylaxis

The prophylactic use of antibiotic minimizes the risk of infection by inhibiting the growth of contaminating bacteria and their adherence to prosthetic implants. As per Centers for Disease Control and Prevention (CDC) guidelines for prevention of NIs (1999), prophylaxis antibiotics should be timed so that a bactericidal concentration of the drug is established in serum and tissues by the time the skin is incised (CDC recommendation category IA).

Hence, prophylactic antibiotic should be administered intravenously 30 minutes before skin incision, at least 10 minutes before inflation of tourniquet to achieve appropriate tissue concentration. In patients undergoing cesarean section, the initial dose should be administered immediately after the umbilical cord is clamped. The choice of antibiotic should cover the common pathogens (e.g., *S. aureus*, streptococci) and should be directed against the most likely infecting organism for a specific surgery or procedure. In case of prolonged surgeries (>3 hours) and those associated with major blood loss; repeat dose of antibiotics should be considered. The microbiologist should be consulted regarding which antibiotics to use to be both effective and to minimize the development of resistant strains.[11]

Asepsis during Invasive Procedures

The risks and benefits associated with subclavian, jugular, and femoral catheterization must be considered with respect to each patient's medical and surgical conditions before insertion of a CVC. The subclavian site is associated with fewer CVC-related blood stream infections when compared with the internal jugular and femoral sites.

The strict adherence to aseptic technique and barrier precautions are essential for the prevention of infection. The ASA[10] recommends cleansing the skin site with an appropriate antiseptic, such as 70% alcohol, 10% povidone-iodine, 4% chlorhexidine, or 2% tincture of iodine, before catheter insertion.

The handling of catheter and subsequent catheter dressings require a surgical hand wash. The multilumen catheters are associated with a higher risk of infection than single-lumen catheters.

The ultrasound guidance during insertion may reduce CVC-related infections due to fewer needle insertions and increased speed of insertion, with reduced incidence of hematoma formation. The ASA also recommends use of disposable transducers and a sterile gauze or transparent dressing to cover the catheter site to lower rate of skin colonization. Antibiotic-coated CVCs have been recommended in adults if the CVC is expected to remain *in situ* longer than 5 days.

The CDC guidelines (1999) recommend—thorough hand washing to prevent cross contamination before any regional anesthetic technique, alcohol-based antiseptic solution to provide maximal antimicrobial activity with extended duration, and use of maximal barrier precautions especially surgical masks to reduce the likelihood of site contamination from microorganisms grown in the upper airway of clinicians.

An epidural micropore bacterial filter prevents foreign material from gaining access to epidural space in addition to filtering the bacteria from the perfusing solution. The use of bacterial micropore filters is generally not recommended during short-term epidural catheterization (<24 hours) or perineural catheter infusions (grade B). The epidurals catheter should generally be removed within 72 hours or tunneled as the incidence of infection increases sharply after this time. The inserting of nerve block catheters in ultrasound guidance and distant from the surgical site may reduce the possibility of infection.[12]

Thermoregulation

The hypothermia is known to impair immune response. Perioperative hypothermia causes vasoconstriction and further impairs subcutaneous tissue oxygen tension by triggering thermoregulatory vasoconstriction in anesthetized patients, resulting in poor neutrophil function and reduced collagen deposition in healing wounds. Hypothermia itself may delay healing and predispose patients to wound infections. The maintaining of normothermia intraoperatively is likely to decrease the incidence of infectious complications in patients undergoing colorectal resection and shorten their duration of hospitalization.

Andrea et al.,[13] found surgical wound infections in 18 of 96 patients assigned to hypothermia (19%) but in only 6 of 104 patients assigned to normothermia (6%, $p = 0.009$). This study confirms that hypothermia also directly impairs immune function normothermia (involving warming with forced air and fluid to a mean temperature of 37 ± 0.3°C). The mean (±SD) final intraoperative core temperature was 34.7 ± 0.6°C in the hypothermia group and 36.6 ± 0.5°C in the normothermia group ($p < 0.001$). The sutures were removed a day later in the patients assigned to hypothermia than in those assigned to normothermia ($p = 0.002$), and the duration of hospitalization was prolonged by 2.6 days (approximately 20%) in the hypothermia group ($p = 0.01$).

Deacock[14] reported that heat retention by using passive systems such as plastic wraps and reflective wraps during anesthesia does help in prevention of hypothermia. An increase in heat gain above heat loss was noted in all patients during prolonged surgery with wraps along with other routine methods of heat loss prevention.

Therefore, it is advisable to monitor patient's core temperature and keep them warm especially for surgeries of long duration. The use of thin plastic wrap, thermal blanket, and warm intravenous solutions does help in preventing hypothermia **(Fig. 1)**.

Types of Anesthesia

In comparison to general anesthesia, the neuraxial anesthesia is associated with less incidence of NIs as there is immune modulation because of improved tissue oxygenation by vasodilatation. Improved postoperative analgesia helps patients to cough and clear secretions more efficiently.

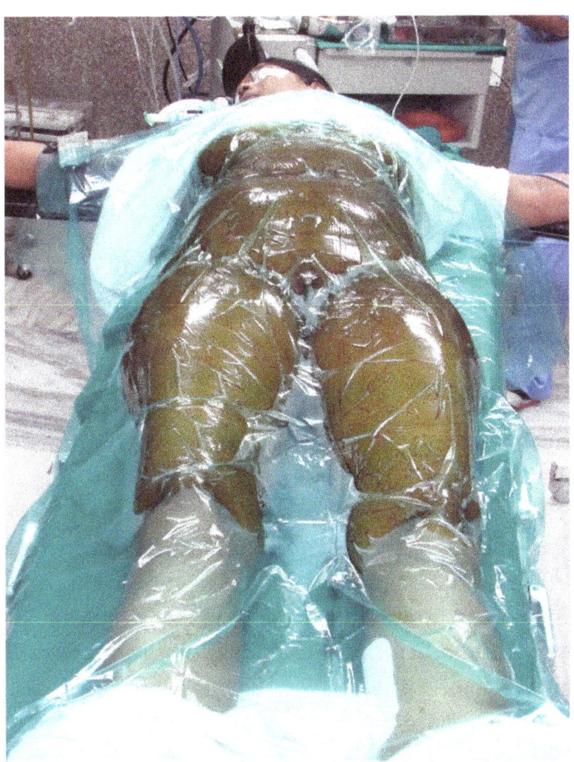

Fig. 1: Patient covered with thin plastic.

The endotracheal intubation by disrupting the ciliated tracheal epithelium results in defect in mucociliary transport and a local inflammatory response and the intubation may also transfer microorganisms from the pharynx to the tracheobronchial tree. In addition, the high concentration (dry) oxygen and inhalational gases also impair the mucociliary function. The Enigma trial revealed that avoidance of inhaled nitrous oxide intraoperatively reduced the incidence of postoperative infection among other postoperative complications.[15] The opioids such as morphine, fentanyl, and remifentanil used during general anesthesia are associated with suppression of the immune system.

Glycemic Control

There are many deleterious effects of acute hyperglycemia such as decreased vasodilatation, impairment in reactive endothelial nitric oxide generation, increased expression of leukocyte and impaired neutrophil chemotaxis, and phagocytosis. The after effects are increased inflammation vulnerability, and dysfunction of multiple organs. Lipshutz and Gropper[16] have reported direct relationship between tight glycemic control between 4, 5, and 6 mmol/dL and reduction in blood-borne infection and hospital mortality in cardiac surgery patients.

It is further suggested about the dilemma about lax blood sugar control may be at expense of increase in number of episodes of hypoglycemia which is a cause of clinical concern in these patients. To be on safer side, it is advised to maintain blood glucose below 10 mmol/dL and avoid variation in blood glucose.

Fluid Management

Till date, to compensate the preoperative fasting, intraoperative fluid losses, optimization of hemodynamic variables, and maintaining of urine output in surgical patients, a liberal fluid approach was used. This leads to the patient being significantly fluid positive perioperatively resulting in detrimental effects including wound site infection and postoperative pneumonia. Although the subcutaneous tissue requires little total oxygen, the prevention of infection is critically dependent on adequate perfusion[17] and right oxygen delivery is to the maintenance of an adequate perfusion state such as euvolemia.[18]

The hypothesis that aggressive fluid administration would better maintain subcutaneous perfusion and wound oxygen tension was tested in a randomized, double-blind trial. Arkilic[17] in 56 patients undergoing elective colon surgery did randomized trial of traditional of fluid management (8–10 mL kg/h 1 intraoperatively and 1 h postoperatively) or aggressive fluid management (10 mL/kg bolus followed by 16–18 mL kg/1 h intraoperatively and 1 h postoperatively). And in addition, fluid was given to both groups in a 3:1 ratio to replace blood loss and for urine output <1 mL kg 1/h or blood pressure <70% of baseline.

In a randomized trial, the aggressively hydrated group had statistically higher intra- and postoperative tissue O_2 tension and no data of incidence of SSIs.[19] In another study, there was no statistical difference in the incidence of SSI or wound healing scores with aggressive versus traditional fluid management.[20] Lang et al.,[21] used hydroxyethyl starch intra- and postoperatively decrease the amount of crystalloid to maintain hemodynamics and urine output while increasing tissue oxygen tension. In same study, colloid group showed 54% increase in tissue oxygen tension and in crystalloid group it was 29%.[22]

The evidence suggests that aggressive fluid management with hydroxyethyl starch does improve tissue oxygenation and no incidence of increase incidence of SSI.

However, aggressive fluid management decreases pulmonary function and bowel edema leading prolonged return of gastrointestinal function seen in some surgical patients.

It is necessary to maintain euvolemia while aggressive fluid resuscitation.

It is common practice with perioperative physicians to administer intravenous fluids to replace fasting deficits, third space losses, and blood loss to maintain cardiac output, blood pressure, and urine output. One needs to maintain mild-to-moderate total body hypovolemia is well tolerated in healthy adults as interstitial fluid moves into the intravascular space to help to preserve cardiac output. This will preserve urine output and hemodynamic stability while leaving the subcutaneous tissue relatively hypovolemic.

There is some evidence for improved outcomes because of goal-directed therapy which requires invasive monitoring such as central venous pressure, pulmonary artery occlusion pressure, or stroke volume via esophageal Doppler probes. However, all these measures need not reduce postoperative infection.

Opioid-induced Immunosuppression

The opioids such as morphine, fentanyl, remifentanil, and meperidine, and to a lesser extent methadone have the tendency to suppress the immune system. However, certain drugs, such as oxycodone, buprenorphine, and hydromorphone, have no significant effects on the immune system, but tramadol, due to its complex mechanism of actions, does have immune-enhancing properties.

Opioid-induced immune suppression makes patients more vulnerable to infection, especially after surgery, trauma, or both, even lead to decreased tolerance to malignant disease with increased likelihood of secondary deposits and there is an increased chance of HIV infection in drug abusers.[23]

In immune compromised patients with chemotherapy, the use of opioid may put them at further risk of increase in immunosuppressive activity.

It is advised to avoid using known immune suppressive opioid analgesic in critically ill and immunosuppressive patients.

Prevention of Contamination of Medicine

To overcome rapid patient turnover, often, only portions of single-dose ampoules/multidose vials of multiple drugs are given to each patient during anesthesia (e.g., propofol, midazolam, rocuronium, etc.). The drug left behind in open ampoules may get contaminated with airborne microorganisms/nonsterile glass fragments. The use of sterile needles and syringes to aspirate the contents of an ampoule or vial is recommended by ASA.

When appropriate sterile precautions have been used consistently, an uncontaminated multidose vial may be used until the expiration date. Aseptic technique should be used each time the multidose vial is punctured which includes cleansing the rubber stopper with alcohol before puncture. The preservative-free ampoules/vials/prefilled syringes do not contain any bacteriostatic agent and are intended for a single patient as a single dose. These medications should be drawn up just before administration and any remaining contents should be discarded.

Medications from one syringe must not be administered to another patient even if the needle on the syringe is changed as removing the needle from a syringe creates a siphoning effect that aspirates the needle contents into the syringe. Medications drawn up in syringes should be discarded within 24 hours.[24]

Propofol being a lipid emulsion supports bacterial growth which rapidly increases after 6 hours of inoculation. Unused propofol in syringes, vials, or administration tubing should be discarded at end of procedure or within 6 hours after opening an ampoule. Intravenous line administering propofol should be flushed every 6 hours and at end of procedure to remove residual propofol.

The stopcocks should be kept free of blood and covered by a sterile cap or syringe when not in use. The intravenous injection ports should be cleaned with an appropriate disinfectant prior to entry.[24]

At the end of each patient's anesthetic, all used syringes and needles should be discarded immediately in an appropriate puncture-resistant container.

Anesthetic Equipment

The revised anesthetic policy recommends rigorous implementation of standard (universal) precautions. Any instrument or device that comes into contact with patient's blood and body fluids (vascular needles and catheters, regional block needles, and catheters) should be preferably disposable and if reusable should be cleaned and sterilized. The parts of equipment that encounter mucous membranes (face masks and laryngoscope blades) or become contaminated with respiratory secretions (breathing circuits and connectors) should undergo high level disinfection.

Microorganisms get carried by the anesthetic gases from the equipment to the patient and vice versa. Greater contamination of the anesthetic circuit is usually at the parts closest to the patient. Soda lime may filter the bacteria but fails to kill many other organisms including *Mycobacterium tuberculosis* and bacillus species which survive prolonged exposure.[25] Use of disposable circuits and bacteria/viral filters will reduce the potential risk of transmission of bacterial and viral infections.

If corrugated tubings are being used due to financial constraints, then the tubings should be washed with soap and water and dried after every patient use. Also, they should be disinfected in 2% glutaraldehyde and then washed with water and dried before use at least once in a day.[26] Heat-moisture exchange devices and bacterial filters optimize heat and moisture output, and thus reduce condensation in the tubing and minimize the risk of bacterial growth. They also have bacterial and viral retention properties.

Ultrasound

The ultrasound has been in use in anesthesia for vascular access, regional analgesia, and transesophageal echocardiography. During the use of ultrasound, infection control measures are needed for both the technique and for the equipment.

Ultrasonography by anesthetists could pose a unique risk of hospital-acquired infection to patients. These machines are often transported from room to room in the operating suite.

The ultrasound equipment can be categorized into noncritical (contact only with intact skin), semicritical (contact with mucous membranes or nonintact skin), and critical (contact with internal organs or body cavities). Medical equipment with critical and semicritical exposure (transesophageal and transrectal probes) require sterilization or high-level disinfection (thorough cleaning followed by immersion in chlorine dioxide or orthophthalaldehyde and then rinsing). Noncritical exposure requires only low-level disinfection (removal of ultrasound gel and then cleaning of the transducer).

General hygiene during scanning is of paramount importance and should include hand hygiene prior to applying gloves and commencing scanning. When using the ultrasound probe in a semicritical or critical environment, a sterile protective probe cover should be used.[27] This in theory obviates the need for high-level disinfection. However, inadvertent sheath breeches can occur, potentially resulting in probe contamination.

High-level disinfection is warranted for procedures such as real time imaging to guide needles into vessels and around nerves as it could result in semicritical exposure of the probe. When performing a needle procedure a sterile probe cover should be used.

Cross infection of the device keyboard is prevented by using a dedicated hand to interact with the keyboard or by using a disposable keyboard cover or by using an assistant.

Gel contamination can be minimized by using single-use sterile gel sachets for all except noncritical uses, although single-use gel containers/packets are recommended even in noncritical applications.

On completion of the procedure, the operator should remove the probe cover (without contaminating the probe) and then his or her gloves. Gel and debris are removed from the probe with a dry towel and then the probe is cleaned with detergent-impregnated wipes or washed with soap and water.[28] Application of a disinfectant spray/wipe to the probe can be considered (70% isopropyl alcohol).

This cleaning process is an effective way of removing bacteria and preventing NI. The ultrasound machine should be stored in a dry clean room. If the probe has been contaminated with blood or body fluids a high-level disinfection should be performed.

Prolonged Mechanical Ventilation

Nosocomial pneumonias associated with mechanical ventilation are termed VAP. Approximately 8–28% of patients receiving prolonged (>48 hours) mechanical ventilation develop VAP.[29] It is associated with major morbidity, prolonged intensive care, increased healthcare costs, and high attributable mortality.

The potential strategies to prevent VAP include noninvasive ventilation as intubation bypasses natural host defenses such as cough reflexes, mucociliary clearance, and provide access to oronasopharyngeal bacteria to lower respiratory tract. If intubation is a must, then orotracheal intubation should be preferred, instead of nasotracheal intubation, as the latter has been associated with both VAP, sinusitis with common bacteria. The focus should be on interventions such as regularly assessing endotracheal cuff pressure, performing endotracheal suctioning, draining ventilator tube condensate, avoiding gastric overdistention, semirecumbent position to reduce the extent of aspiration, appropriate use of heat and moisture exchangers, regular hand cleaning with soap or alcohol disinfectant, and on minimizing the duration of mechanical ventilation by minimizing sedation and use of weaning protocols. Maintaining cuff pressure of endotracheal tubes at ≥20 mm Hg reduces the passage of contaminated secretions pooled above the endotracheal cuff into the trachea. The endotracheal tubes with a dorsal lumen to allow drainage or continuous subglottic suctioning of pooled secretions above the cuff are available. Strategies to reduce the risk of VAP also include eradicating the oropharyngeal and/or intestinal microbial colonization such as chlorhexidine oral care, selective gut decontamination, a rotational schedule for empirical antibiotic administration and the use of sucralfate, H_2 antagonists, or proton-pump inhibitors to reduce the acidity of gastric secretions which in turn reduces bacterial overgrowth.[30]

Prevention of Nosocomial Urinary Tract Infections

The UTI accounts for almost 40% of all NIs,[31] most of which are associated with urinary catheters. Several practices have been evaluated to prevent hospital-acquired UTI, first of which includes catheterizing only if necessary and removal of catheter when not required. If the use of catheter is deemed necessary, care should be taken to minimize unnecessary manipulation, prevent trauma, and maintain the system close and patent. Urinary catheter should be inserted by a trained and competent person with aseptic precautions using sterile equipment, appropriate antiseptic solution, and generous sterile lubricant. Maintain a sterile and closed urinary drainage system. The antimicrobial urinary catheters are available to be used in patients at high risk for infection. External catheters, e.g., condom catheters/suprapubic catheters, can be used when appropriate. The portable bladder ultrasound scanners have been used to measure urinary retention to detect the need for urinary catheterization. Because the risk of infection increases as the duration of catheterization increases, perhaps the best infection prevention strategy would be to use computer-/nurse-based reminders to alert the physician regarding catheter status of their patients. In a Taiwanese ICU, a nurse-based reminder, in which nurses were instructed to remind physicians to remove unnecessary urinary catheters, demonstrated a reduction in the duration of catheterization (7 vs. 4.6 days) and UTI rates (11.5 vs. 8.3 cases per 1,000 catheter days; p = 0.009).[32] Routine prophylactic antibiotics for urinary catheterization is not recommended, as it increases the risk of emergence of resistant bacteria unless otherwise clinically indicated.

IMPLICATIONS OF NOSOCOMIAL INFECTION

Nosocomial infection is a leading cause of morbidity and mortality especially in critical care setting. It has direct impact on cost of medical care for the healthcare system, increases the length of hospital, causes loss of productive hours for the patient due to chronic illness, and also increases resistance of microorganisms to antimicrobials. NIs such as bloodstream infection (sepsis) and VAP have a more severe impact than others in terms of mortality and extra costs.

CONCLUSION

It is the responsibility of anesthetist and all medical personnel to adopt methods of minimizing NIs to make it cost effective. During surgery, the patients are more vulnerable so anesthetists and other operating room personnel can play a vital role in preventing of NIs. The anesthetist and all concerned personnel should take utmost care and precaution during the perioperative period to limit the risk of infection.

REFERENCES

1. Ponce-de-Leon S. The needs of developing countries and the resources required. J Hosp Infect. 1991;18(Suppl):37681.
2. Plowman R. The socioeconomic burden of hospital-acquired infection. London: Public Health Laboratory Service and the London School of Hygiene and Tropical Medicine; 1999.
3. Wenzel RP. The economics of nosocomial infections. J Hosp Infect. 1995;31:7987.
4. Pittet D, Taraara D, Wenzel RP. Nosocomial bloodstream infections in critically ill patients. Excess length of stay, extra costs, and attributable mortality. JAMA. 1994;271:1598601.
5. Coella R, Glenister H, Fereres J, et al. The cost of infection in surgical patients: A case study. J Hosp Infect. 1993;25:23950.
6. Garner JS, Jarvis WR, Emori TG, et al. CDC definitions for nosocomial infections. In: Olmsted RN (Ed). APIC Infection Control and Applied Epidemiology: Principles and Practice. St. Louis: Mosby; 1996. pp. A1A20.
7. Garner JS, Jarvis WR, Emori TG, et al. CDC definitions for nosocomial infections. Am J Infect Control. 1988;16:2840.
8. WHO. Burden of healthcare associated infection worldwide factsheet. Systematic review. Geneva: WHO; 19952008.
9. Louis V, Bihari MB, Suter P, et al. The prevalence of nosocomial infections in intensive care units in Europe. European Prevalence of infection in Intensive care (EPIC) study. JAMA. 1995;274:63944.
10. Infection Control in Anaesthesia. Anaesthesia. 2008;63(9): 1027-36.
11. Hebl JR. The importance and implications of aseptic techniques during regional anesthesia. Reg Anesth Pain Med. 2006; 31(4):31123.
12. Gifford C, Christelis N, Cheng A. Preventing postoperative infection: Anaesthetist's role. Continuing Educa Anaesth Crit Care Pain Adv. 2011;11(1):1516.
13. Kurz A, Sessler DI, Lenhardt R. Perioperative normothermia to reduce the incidence of surgical-wound infection and shorten hospitalization. Study of Wound Infection and Temperature Group. N Engl J Med. 1996;334(19):120915.
14. Deacock S. Heat retention using passive systems during anaesthesia: Comparison of two plastic wraps, one with reflective properties. Br J Anaesth. 1997;79:7669.
15. Myles PS, Leslie K, Chan MT, et al. Avoidance of nitrous oxide for patients undergoing major surgery: A randomized controlled trial. Anaesthesiology. 2007;107:22131.
16. Lipshutz AK, Gropper MA. Perioperative glycemic control: An evidence-based review. Anesthesiology. 2009;110:40821.
17. Hopf HW, Hunt TK, West JM, et al. Wound tissue oxygen tension predicts the risk of wound infection in surgical patients. Arch Surg. 1997;132:9971004.
18. Jonsson K, Jensen JA, Goodson WH III, et al. Assessment of perfusion in postoperative patients using tissue oxygen measurements. Br J Surg. 1987;74:2637.
19. Arkilic CF, Taguchi A, Sharma N, et al. Supplemental perioperative fluid administration increases tissue oxygen pressure. Surgery. 2003;133:495.
20. Kabon B, Akca O, Taguchi A, et al. Supplemental intravenous crystalloid administration does not reduce the risk of surgical wound infection. Anesth Analg. 2005;101:154653.
21. Lang K, Boldt J, Suttner S, et al. Colloids versus crystalloids and tissue oxygen tension in patients undergoing major abdominal surgery. Anesth Analg. 2001;93:4059.
22. Nisanevich V, Felsenstein I, Almogy G, et al. Effect of intraoperative fluid management on outcome after intraabdominal surgery. Anesthesiology. 2005;103:2532.
23. Budd K, Shipton E. Acute pain, the immune system and opio immunosuppression. Acute Pain. 2004;6:12335.
24. Samuel CH, Morris B, Lyndon JB, et al. Recommendations for infection control for the practice of anaesthesiology, 2nd edition, United States: American Society of Anaesthesiologists; 1999.
25. Duse AG. Nosocomial pulmonary infections related to anaesthesia. SAJCC. 1999;15(2):223.
26. Richard VS, Mathai E, Cherian T. Role of anaesthetic equipment in transmitting nosocomial infection. J Assoc Physicians India. 2001;49:4548.
27. Shokoohi H, Armstrong P, Tansek R. Emergency department ultrasound probe infection control: Challenges and solutions. Open Access Emerg Med. 2015;7:19.
28. Waseem AM, Syed HI, Mohd. Salim AK, et al. Cleaning methods for ultrasound probes. J Coll Physicians Surg Pak. 2008;18(5): 2869.
29. Cook DJ, Kollef MH. Risk factors for ICU-acquired pneumonia. JAMA. 1998;279(20):16056.
30. Steven MK, Jonathon DT. Ventilator-associated pneumonia: Diagnosis, treatment, and prevention. Clin Microbiol Rev. 2006; 19(4):63757.
31. Klevens RM, Edwards JR, Richards CL, et al. Estimating health care associated infections and deaths in U.S. hospitals, 2002. Public Health Rep. 2007;122:1607.
32. Huang WC, Wann SR, Lin SL, et al. Catheter-associated urinary tract infections in intensive care units can be reduced by prompting physicians to remove unnecessary catheters. Infect Control Hosp Epidemiol. 2004;25:9748.

Simulators in Anesthesia

Nandini M Dave

ABSTRACT

Simulation in medicine is gaining widespread acceptance as a teaching tool and as an adjunct for competency testing and continuing training. Simulation allows personnel to practice and learn principles in a controlled environment that will better prepare them for the safe administration of health care to patients. This chapter focuses on the equipment available for simulation in anesthesiology teaching and training.

INTRODUCTION

Simulation refers to the recreation of something real by imitation. A simulator is a device or product that is used in simulation.

Medical simulators were introduced in the early 1960s, in the form of manikins designed to aid in teaching mouth-to-mouth resuscitation, and the first computer-controlled simulators were seen in the mid-1960s.[1]

The aviation industry provided the impetus for the development of simulators in anesthesia. Anesthesia practice involves multiple tasks which require a high degree of vigilance, and procedural, monitoring, and decision-making skills in a complex environment; all of which are affected by simultaneous interactions between members of the team. In anesthesia, serious complications need to be diagnosed quickly and corrected; also one requires to practice skills in crisis management without causing harm to real patients.[2]

ADVANTAGES OF SIMULATORS[3-5]

They simulate a high degree of reality:

- No risk for a real patient
- Tasks/scenarios can be created to demand
- Skills can be practiced repeatedly
- Allows for practice on clinically rare scenarios
- Videotaping allows for review
- Simulation can be stopped or restarted for teaching
- Transfer of training from classroom to real situation is enhanced.

SIMULATOR FIDELITY

Fidelity is the extent to which the appearance and behavior of the simulator or simulation matches the appearance and behavior of the simulated system.[6] The level of fidelity required depends on the type of task and stage of training, and influences skills transfer. Simulators are typically described as low, intermediate, or high fidelity based on this attribute. Fidelity could be physical fidelity (the device replicates physical aspects of the human body), environmental fidelity (the simulation room looks like an operating room), equipment fidelity (the clinical equipment works like or is the real thing), or psychological fidelity (the simulation evokes behaviors similar to the real situation).

CLASSIFICATION OF SIMULATORS

Simulators have been categorized as follows:[7-9]

- Part task trainers
- Computer-based systems
- Virtual reality and haptic systems
- Simulated patients
- Simulated environments
- Integrated simulators
    - Instructor-driven
    - Model-driven.

Part Task Trainers

These are designed to replicate only part of the environment and resemble anatomical areas of the body, e.g., models used to train basic skills, such as intubation, or venipuncture. They are relatively inexpensive.

Computer-based Systems

Computer systems can be used to model aspects of human physiology or pharmacology, simulated tasks or environments and allow interaction with these through a computer interface.

The focus is on learning and on using the information to make treatment decisions and it also provides feedback to the student allowing independent learning.

Virtual Reality and Haptic Systems

It is the ultimate computer-based technology and it presents virtual objects or environments to all human senses which are identical to their natural counterpart.

Haptic (touch) feedback produces a feeling of resistance while using instruments within the simulated environment, which creates the illusion of coming into physical contact with the model, e.g., flexible fiberoptic intubation trainer.

Simulated Patients

Simulated patients are lay people who are trained to portray specific conditions, often in a standardized manner. They are the highest "fidelity" simulators and its use is excellent for teaching communication and interpersonal skills.

Simulated Environment

It is recreating the working environment so multidisciplinary teams can work together, e.g., operating room which gives learners an opportunity to examine their roles within a team.

Integrated Simulators

These are a combination of part or whole body manikins linked to computers. The computer programs drive the manikin to produce physical signs and feed physiologic signals and data to patient monitoring systems. Model-driven (high fidelity) simulators are lifelike manikins with computer programs driven by scientifically derived complex mathematical models of respiratory and cardiovascular physiology and extensive pharmacological modeling.

The Medical Education Technologies, Inc. Human Patient Simulator, Emergency Care Simulator, PediaSim are examples of commercially available high-fidelity simulators.

Model-driven simulators make the dynamic interaction and feedback less operator-dependent and hence more complex scenarios can be undertaken. Due to their complexity, model-driven simulators are very costly, both in terms of purchase and running costs.

"Instructor-driven (intermediate fidelity)" simulators combine part or full body manikins with less complex computer programs, e.g., Laerdal SimMan®. The computer software produces physiological signals that are displayed on a computer screen rather than standard clinical monitor and an instructor is required to adjust signs to reflect patient responses.

Cumin and Merry classified simulators based on three features: (i) How the user interacts with the simulator, (ii) its simulated physiology, and (iii) its use **(Table 1)**.[9]

TABLE 1: Attributes of simulators according to the classification proposed by Cumin and Merry.

Interaction	*Physiology*	*Used for teaching*
Hardware-based	No physiology	Knowledge
Screen-based	Script-controlled	Cognitive skills
Virtual reality-based	Model-controlled	Psychomotor skills

INTERACTION

Screen-based Simulators

A screen-based simulator runs on a computer with no additional hardware. Users interact with it through conventional devices (such as its keyboard or mouse), e.g., Gas Man®, used to simulate the uptake and distribution of anesthetic gases in the body. Screen-based simulators are good devices to acquire technical skills. The advantage of screen-based simulators over hardware-based simulators is their low cost. Screen-based simulators can more readily be used by a trainee alone, without the need for a tutor or actors, which also reduces cost. The disadvantage of screen-based simulators is that they cannot be used to practice psychomotor skills or teamwork.[10]

Hardware-based Simulators

It is also called mannequin-based simulator (commonly used synonyms are full-scale simulator, hands-on simulator, realistic simulator, high-fidelity simulator). The trainees interact in much the same way they would interact with a real patient. The control logic is manipulated through an instructor/operator's station that allows the instructor to create specific patients, select and implement abnormal events and faults, and monitor the progress of the simulation session. It is common to obtain detailed records of the simulation and the actions taken from video and audio recording of the personnel working in the replicated clinical environment. Mannequin-based simulators would probably provide better training for behavioral aspects of crisis management, such as communication, leadership, and interpersonal conflicts **(Table 2)**. Hardware-based simulators usually require more space, as well as other equipment (such as anesthetic machines and defibrillators). The ongoing costs, such as repairs and maintenance, are therefore higher for hardware-based simulators.

Virtual Reality Simulators

Virtual reality refers to a set of techniques in which one interacts with a synthetic (virtual) environment that exists solely in the computer. Using virtual reality, parts or all of the patient and environment are presented to the user by three-dimensional representations with or without "touch" to create a more "immersive" experience. A screen-only simulator could be viewed as a very limited virtual reality simulator.

TABLE 2: Functionality of current mannequin-based (high fidelity) simulator systems.[6,11,12]

Clinical area	*Features and functions*
Airway	• Appropriate pharyngeal, glottic, and bronchial anatomy • Placement of face mask, ETT, LMA, LT, combi tube • Laryngospasm, tongue and airway swelling, cervical immobility, jaw closure, breakable teeth • Cricothyrotomy, transtracheal jet ventilation
Head	• Eyelid movement, pupil dilation, and reaction to light or medications • Patient voice and sounds, such as coughing and vomiting (through built-in loudspeaker) • Palpable carotid pulses • Cyanosis by blue light • Tearing
Chest	• Physiologic and pathophysiologic heart and breath sounds • Spontaneous breathing with chest wall movement • Bronchospasm • Adjustable pulmonary compliance and airway resistance • Pneumothorax • Needle thoracotomy and chest tube placement • Defibrillation, transthoracic pacing • Chest compressions
Extremities	• Palpable pulses • Cuff blood pressure measurement • Modules for fractures and wound modules • Intravenous line placement • Thumb twitch in response to peripheral nerve stimulation • Arm movement • Representations of tonic-clonic spells
Monitoring (waveforms or numeric)	ECG (including abnormalities in morphology and rhythm), SpO_2, invasive blood pressure, CVP, PAP, PCWP, cardiac output, temperature, CO_2, anesthetic gases (may have actual uptake and distribution of agents)
Automation	Quality of chest compressions, ventilation rate and volume, defibrillation and pacing (including energy measurement), respiratory gas analyzer, drug recognition

(ETT: endotracheal tube; LMA: laryngeal mask airway; LT: laryngeal tube; ECG: electrocardiogram; CVP: central venous pressure; PAP: positive airway pressure; PCWP: pulmonary capillary wedge pressure)

PHYSIOLOGY

Some simulators have no physiological attributes. Others have computer programmable physiological interactions, e.g., an increase in blood pressure following a fluid bolus. Script-controlled physiology depends on a set of commands (a script) specifying physiological responses. Model-controlled physiology depends on the use of mathematical models to determine the physiological responses to various interventions.

USE FOR TEACHING

A simulator may be used to teach skills (psychomotor or cognitive) or to impart knowledge.[13,14]

The range of commercially available technologies used in medical simulation range from simple part-task training models to highly sophisticated computer-driven models. No single system is the best choice for all uses, so the decision about the type of simulator required must be based on the objectives and needs of the application.

CONCLUSION

Simulation is an educational technique that allows interactive activity by recreating all or part of a clinical experience without exposing patients to the associated risks. Many applications have been found for simulators in anesthesia including teaching and training, evaluation, and research. The range of medical simulator devices continues to grow with technological advances. These range from simple part-task training models to highly sophisticated computer-driven models. Appropriate simulators must be chosen to address identified key skills or techniques.

REFERENCES

1. Chopra V. Anesthesia simulators. In: Aitkenhead AR (Ed). Quality Assurance and Risk Management in Anaesthesia. Bailliere's Clinical Anaesthesiology International Practice and Research. London: Baillière Tindal; 1996. pp. 297-315.
2. Kurreck MM, Fish KJ. Anesthesia crisis resource management training: an intimidating concept, a rewarding experience. Can J Anaesth. 1996;43(5 Pt 1):430-4.
3. Wong AK. Full scale computer simulators in anesthesia training and evaluation. Can J Anaesth. 2004;51(5):455-64.
4. Hunt EA, Shilkofski NA, Stavroudis TA, et al. Simulation: translation to improved team performance. Anesthesiol Clin. 2007;25(2):301-19.
5. Forrest FC, Taylor MA, Postlethwaite K, et al. Use of a highfidelity simulator to develop testing of the technical performance of novice anaesthetists. Br J Anaesth. 2002;88(3):338-44.
6. Rall M, Gaba DM, Dieckmann P, et al. Patient simulation. In: Miller RD (Eds). Miller's Anesthesia, 7th edition. Philadelphia: Churchill Livingstone Elsevier; 2010.
7. Good ML, Gravenstein JS. Anesthesia simulators and training devices. Int Anesthesiol Clin. 1989;27(3):161-8.
8. Maran NJ, Glavin RJ. Low- to high-fidelity simulation—a continuum of medical education? Med Educ. 2003;37(Suppl 1): 22-8.
9. Cumin D, Merry AF. Review article: Simulators for use in anaesthesia. Anaesthesia. 2007;62(2):151-62.
10. Nyssen AS, Larbuisson R, Janssens M, et al. A comparison of the training value of two types of anesthesia simulators: Computer screen-based and mannequin-based simulators. Anesth Analg. 2002;94(6):1560-5.
11. Milton S. Hershey Medical Center. PSU simulation. [online] Available from http://www.hmc.psu.edu/simulation/sim_list/sim_list.html. [Last accessed November, 2017].
12. CAE Healthcare. METI. [online] Available from http://www.meti.com. [Last accessed November, 2017].
13. Seropian MA. General concepts in full scale simulation: Getting started. Anesth Analg. 2003;97(6):1695-705.
14. Leblanc VR. Review article: Simulation in anesthesia: state of the science and looking forward. Can J Anesth. 2012;59(2):193-202.

Maintenance, Safety, and Hazards

SECTION 9

Cleaning and Sterilization of Anesthetic Equipment

Nandini M Dave

ABSTRACT

Anesthesia equipment is a potential vector for transmission of disease. Single use equipment must be used whenever appropriate. The reusable equipment must undergo decontamination, disinfection, and sterilization as indicated. The choice of method depends on the infection risk associated with their use and manufacturer's recommendations must be followed for all types of equipment.

INTRODUCTION

In order to ensure that the practice of anesthesia is as safe as possible for patients, anesthetists and other healthcare workers, it is imperative that infection risks to all parties be minimized. The effective use of disinfection and sterilization procedures is important in preventing healthcare-associated infections. The numerous published articles documenting infection after improper reprocessing of reusable medical equipment have emphasized the requirement for all healthcare services to use appropriate disinfection and sterilization techniques.[1-4] Where appropriate, single use disposable equipment will remove the difficulties of reuse and decontamination procedures. The use of such equipment is to be encouraged. There are problems, however, of cost, storage and disposal of single patient use devices and for certain pieces of equipment there is no feasible disposable alternative.[5]

SOME TERMINOLOGIES[6]

- *Antimicrobial:* A chemical capable of destroying or inhibiting the growth of microorganisms
- *Antiseptic:* A chemical germicide that has antimicrobial activity and that can be safely applied to living tissue
- *Asepsis:* A process that prevents contact with microorganisms
- *Bioburden:* The population of viable infectious agents contaminating an object
- *Cleaning:* Removal of foreign material from an item
- *Decontamination:* The removal of microorganisms and unwanted matter from contaminated materials or living tissue
- *Disinfection:* Process capable of destroying most microorganisms but, as ordinarily used, not bacterial spores
- *Sterilization:* Process capable of removing or destroying all viable forms of microbial life, including bacterial spores
- *Universal precautions:* Use of protective barriers and workplace practices to reduce the risk of exposure to any body fluid that may contain contagious microorganisms.

TABLE 1: Spaulding's classification of medical equipment and required level of reprocessing.

Classification	*Definition*	*Level of processing/ reprocessing*
Critical equipment	Equipment/device that enters sterile tissues, including the vascular system	Cleaning followed by sterilization
Semicritical equipment	Equipment/device that comes in contact with nonintact skin or mucous membranes but do not penetrate them	Cleaning followed by high-level disinfection (as a minimum) Sterilization is preferred
Noncritical equipment	Equipment/device that touches only intact skin and not mucous membranes, or does not directly touch the patient	Cleaning followed by low-level disinfection

The Spaulding's classification divides medical equipment into three categories based on degree of risk of infection involved with their use (**Table 1**).[7]

Critical Items

The items that penetrate the skin or mucous membranes or are in contact with normally sterile areas of the body. These items assigned to the critical items category present a high risk of infection if the item is contaminated with any microorganism, including bacterial spores. Thus, it is critical that objects which enter sterile tissue or the vascular system be sterile.

For example, vascular and regional block needles and catheters.

Semicritical Items

The semicritical items contact mucous membranes and nonintact skin but do not break the blood barrier. Ideally, semicritical items should be sterile. However, high-level disinfection is an acceptable standard of care when sterilization is not practical.

For example, endoscopes, laryngoscope blades, face masks, oxygen masks, oral and nasal airways, resuscitation bags, breathing tubes and connectors, esophageal stethoscopes, reusable rectal, nasopharyngeal and esophageal temperature probes.

Noncritical Items

The noncritical items meet intact skin. Since intact skin is an effective barrier to most microorganisms, these items need only cleaning followed by intermediate- or low-level disinfection.

For example, precordial stethoscopes, blood pressure cuffs and tubing, pulse oximeter sensors and cables, electrocardiogram cables and electrodes, reusable skin temperature probes, temperature monitor cables, carbon dioxide absorber assemblies, the exteriors of the anesthesia machine, ventilator, humidifiers, scavenging system, intravenous fluid pumps, monitors, and equipment carts.

CLEANING[6,8]

This refers to the general removal of debris (dirt, blood, saliva, and other body secretions) from equipment. It reduces amount of organic matter that contributes to proliferation of bacteria and viruses. All medical instruments and devices must be cleaned as a first step to decontamination. One cannot achieve disinfection or sterilization without precleaning. As organic material dilutes disinfectants, bioburden must be reduced for processes to be effective.

Steps in cleaning include:

- *Removal of visible soil:* An initial water rinse or soaking with a specialized product (e.g., a protein-dissolving solution) prevents blood coagulation on the device and removes gross debris. One may need to disconnect or separate instrument parts. After soaking long enough to loosen organic matter, it should be thoroughly scrubbed inside and out
- *Rinsing:* After cleaning, rinsing should be performed to remove soil and residual detergent and to keep it from resettling on the equipment
- *Drying:* The cleaned item should be thoroughly dried. This is important because a humid environment may encourage the growth of certain organisms. If a liquid chemical agent is to be used, water on the equipment will dilute the agent and make it less effective. If water droplets remain on equipment that is to be gas sterilized, ethylene oxide will dissolve in the water and form ethylene glycol, which is toxic.

The cleaning may be accomplished manually or mechanically using a washing machine. Equipment that have crevices, lumens, and other hard-to-reach areas can be treated in an ultrasonic cleaning system after gross soil has been removed. In an ultrasonic cleaner, high-frequency sound waves passing through a solvent produce submicroscopic bubbles, which collapse on themselves, generating tiny shock waves that knock debris off surfaces.

The cleaning should be performed in a designated location that is separated from other parts of the facility to minimize inadvertent personnel exposure. The ventilation and air-conditioning systems should be designed to minimize spreading contaminants to adjacent spaces. The personnel should wear protective attire and manufacturer's instructions should be followed to determine the appropriate cleaning methods and agents to be used without damaging the equipment.

DISINFECTION

This is defined as the process that eliminates many or all pathogenic microorganisms with the exception of bacterial spores from inanimate objects. This is generally accomplished by the use of liquid chemicals or wet pasteurization.

The efficacy of disinfection depends on:[6]

- Previous cleaning of the object
- Type and level of microbial contamination
- Concentration of and exposure time to the germicide
- Physical configuration of the object (e.g., crevices, hinges, lumens)
- Temperature and pH of the disinfection process
- Biocidal agents being appropriate for the items being disinfected.

The manufacturer's recommendations should be followed to achieve disinfection and to avoid medical device damage.

Use correct dilution—more is not better! Use correct contact time and temperature.

The Centers for Disease Control and Prevention (CDC) classifies disinfection into three levels:[9]

1. *High-level disinfection:* A procedure that kills all organisms with the exception of bacterial spores and certain species, such as the Creutzfeldt-Jakob prion. Most high-level disinfectants can produce sterilization with sufficient contact time
2. *Intermediate-level disinfection:* A procedure that kills vegetative bacteria, including *Mycobacterium tuberculosis*, most fungi, and viruses but not bacterial spores.
3. *Low-level disinfection:* A procedure that kills most vegetative bacteria (but not *M. tuberculosis*), some fungi, and viruses but no spores.

Disinfection and Sterilization Methods[6,8,10]

Pasteurization

Pasteurization or hot water disinfection refers to the process in which equipment is immersed in water at an elevated temperature (but below 100°C) for a specified time. The contact time is inversely related to temperature, CDC guidelines refer to pasteurization as a high-level disinfection process.

Breathing tubes, reservoir bags, face masks, airways, laryngoscope blades, stylets, Y-pieces, elbows, adaptors, and ventilator bellows can be disinfected by pasteurization.

The advantage of pasteurization is that the lower temperature is less damaging to equipment than the higher temperatures employed during autoclaving. There are no toxic fumes or residues. It is simple, inexpensive, and reliable. The main disadvantage is that the treated equipment is wet and must still be dried and packaged, during which time it may again become contaminated. The heat may damage some materials.

STERILIZATION

It is the complete elimination or destruction of all forms of microbial life. It is accomplished by either physical or chemical processes.

- Steam sterilization
- Dry heat sterilization
- Chemical sterilization
- Ethylene oxide sterilization
- Radiation sterilization
- Plasma gas (vaporized hydrogen peroxide) sterilization.

Steam Sterilization or Autoclaving

Steam sterilization or autoclaving utilizes saturated steam under pressure. It is the most widely used and economical sterilization technique. Increasing the temperature reduces the time needed to achieve sterilization. The equipment to be sterilized is cleaned, and then is packaged in a material easily penetrated by steam. After sterilization, the packaging material prevents recontamination during subsequent handling and storage.

By convention, sterilization cycles have been standardized at a few temperature-time relationships. The lowest temperature for a sterilizer is 121°C (250°F). The cycles may also be programmed at 132°C (270°F), 134°C (275°F), or 145°C (285°F), depending on the sterilizer. In general, wrapped items should be sterilized for 30 minutes and unwrapped items for 20 minutes at 121°C. Flash sterilization allows items to be steam sterilized for immediate use. The items to be processed are usually unwrapped. The time and temperature will depend on the sterilizer and the configuration of the load. The processed items are transferred immediately from the autoclave to the point of use, usually the surgical field.

Steam Sterilization Monitoring

Mechanical indicators: These include gauges and displays. The mechanical monitors indicate time, temperature, and pressure. They only indicate if the autoclave machine is working properly. They are not indicators of sterility.

Chemical indicators: These change color with timed exposure to steam, e.g., autoclave tapes. They are used to show that equipment has gone through sterilization process and are not indicators of sterility. The chemical indicators can detect failures or errors in packaging, pack density, loading, insufficient humidification, and inadequate exposure time at the selected temperature, or sterilizer malfunction. The advantages are that they are inexpensive, and they can be read as soon as the packs have been opened.

Biological indicators: The biological indicators are standardized preparations of spores that are placed in the most difficult-to-sterilize locations in the load. They are indicators of sterility and demonstrate whether bacterial spores on test strips or in vials/containers have all been killed. The drawback is the time needed for incubation.

Advantages of Autoclaving

- Destruction of all bacteria, viruses, and spores
- Quick, reliable and economical
- Ease of use
- Absence of toxic products or residues.

Disadvantages[11]

- Some equipment may be damaged due to steam
- Blunting of cutting edges, metal surface corrosion, and shortened life of electronic components.

Dry Heat Sterilization

Dry heat is used for items that might be damaged by moist heat. This technique is time consuming; however, it is effective and does not corrode metal and sharp instruments.

Chemical Disinfection and Sterilization

Chemical disinfection or sterilization involves immersing an item in a solution that contains a disinfectant. This method is especially useful for heat-sensitive equipment. It can be accomplished by automated equipment, which provides a cycle of cleaning, disinfection, rinsing, and sometimes drying.

The time required for different chemical agents to function effectively varies depending on concentration of the disinfectant, temperature, pH and the bioburden. A longer contact time may achieve sterilization. The examples include glutaraldehyde, ortho-phthalaldehyde (OPA or Cidex® OPA), quaternary ammonium compounds, phenolic compounds derived from carbolic acid, ethyl or isopropyl alcohol, iodine compounds, peroxyacetic acid, chlorine compounds, hydrogen peroxide, formaldehyde.

The chemical disinfectants may be inactivated in the presence of organic matter; thorough cleaning of the item must occur for the agent to be effective. The choice of disinfectant and process depends on whether low, intermediate or high level, disinfection is indicated. The disinfectant must be compatible with the particular equipment. It must be used in the appropriate concentration, and have sufficient contact with all surfaces of the item for an appropriate length of time.

Advantages

- Quick, economical, simple
- Useful for equipment that does not require sterilization but does require high-level disinfection.

Disadvantages

- It is not suitable for all equipment
- Risk of contamination exists because prepackaging is not possible
- Sterility is not guaranteed
- Issues with personnel exposure.

Gas or Ethylene Oxide Sterilization

Ethylene oxide kills bacteria, spores, fungi, and viruses. It penetrates into crevices and through permeable bags. Before packaging, items must be disassembled to allow free movement of gas. It is not degraded by organic soil but will not penetrate blood and other dried protein material. The equipment should, therefore, be cleaned thoroughly and rinsed. Items for gas sterilization must be free of water droplets and should be air dried and wrapped. A relative humidity between 35 and 70% and a temperature between 18 and 22°C throughout the processing and storage facility are recommended. The items are then loaded loosely onto wire baskets or metal carts and loaded into the sterilizer. The necessary sterilization time will depend on the concentration of ethylene oxide, temperature and the humidity. The time generally ranges between 1.5 and 6 hours in automatic sterilizers. Up to 12 hours may be required. Physical, chemical, and biological indicators are used to monitor the effectiveness of the sterilization process. The final step in the process is aeration to reduce ethylene oxide to a level safe for both personnel and patient use. Aeration may be done passively in air (ambient aeration) or actively in a mechanical aerator.

Complications

The residual gas from sterilized items can cause skin reactions and laryngotracheal inflammation, hemolysis on exposure to blood, sensitization and anaphylaxis.[12] For personnel involved in the sterilization process, acute exposure to significant levels of ethylene oxide can provoke an irritant response with upper respiratory complaints, eye irritation, headache, and coughing. With higher concentrations, nausea, vomiting, diarrhea, increased fatigability, memory loss, drowsiness, dizziness, lack of coordination, chest discomfort, shortness of breath, and convulsions may occur. Respiratory paralysis and peripheral nerve damage have been reported after massive exposure. Chronic exposure can affect the eyes (corneal burns, cataracts, epithelial keratitis), the central and peripheral nervous system, and skin (irritant and allergic reactions). Respiratory infections, anemia, and impaired cognitive function may occur. Ethylene oxide is a recognized mutagen and carcinogen and may adversely affect the reproductive system.

Advantages

- Reliable, effective
- It can be used for items which would be damaged by heat or moisture
- Items can be prepackaged, so danger of recontamination is eliminated.

Disadvantages

- Expensive
- Long cycle time
- Personnel exposure, risk of fires, explosions.

Radiation Sterilization

This process uses gamma radiation and with sufficiently large exposure, all microorganisms, including bacterial spores and viruses are killed.

Advantages

- Thermosensitive equipment can be sterilized
- Items can be prepackaged prior to sterilization.

Disadvantages

- Expensive
- Not practical for everyday use items.

Plasma Gas Sterilization

Plasma is matter excited to a higher energy state than its gaseous form, referred to as the fourth state of matter, consisting of reactive ions, electrons, and neutral atomic and molecular particles. These reactive particles interact with the molecules that are essential for the metabolism and reproduction of living cells, thus causing sterilization and hydrogen peroxide is commonly used.[3] Items are cleaned, dried and prepacked and introduced into the sterilizer. The sterilization process is a microprocessor-controlled cycle. The cycle time varies with the sterilizer model.

Advantages

- Reliable, effective method
- Heat sensitive items can be sterilized

- Processing time is short
- No toxic residue, so no risk to personnel.

Disadvantages

- Small size of sterilization chamber
- Certain items, e.g., cellulose materials, paper, linens, powders, liquids, and implants cannot be processed.

CONSIDERATION OF INDIVIDUAL ITEMS (TABLE 2)

The choice of decontamination method will depend on a number of factors, including the nature of the contamination, the time required for processing, the heat, pressure, moisture, and chemical tolerance of the item, the availability of processing equipment, and the risks associated with the decontamination method. The manufacturer's instructions should be studied and followed carefully.

Most anesthetic machines and breathing systems are contaminated to a minor degree with microorganisms. Equipment that is in direct contact with the patient (laryngoscopes and masks) becomes more heavily contaminated. All anesthetic equipment that comes into contact with a patient's body fluids (including saliva) must be changed, cleaned and disinfected before use on another patient. This includes equipment that has come into indirect contact with the anesthetist's hands, which may be contaminated with blood, saliva or other body fluid. Additionally, unused items introduced into the anesthetic work-field should be regarded as dirty and reprocessed.

CONCLUSION

Anesthetic equipment is a potential vector for transmission of disease and precautions against transmission of infection between patient and anesthetist or between patients should be a routine part of anesthetic practice. Single use equipment should be utilized where appropriate. The choice of equipment and/or the level of disinfection or sterility required of reusable items is assessed against the risk posed to patients of transmission of infection during any procedure in which the equipment is used. Anesthetists must comply with local theater infection control policies which must be in accordance with internationally accepted guidelines for infection control.

TABLE 2: Infection control guidelines for anesthesia equipment.[1,13-16]

Equipment	*Action*	*Comment*
Face masks	Single patient use or sterilized	Pasteurization, EO, autoclaving, chemical sterilization can be used
Airways	Single patient use or sterilized	Pasteurization, chemical sterilization, EO, plasma sterilization can be used. Rubber airways may be autoclaved
Tracheal tubes	Single patient use	–
Laryngeal masks	Single patient use or sterilized	Autoclaving; 40 uses maximum
Catheter mounts/angle pieces	Single patient use	Metal components can be autoclaved
Breathing systems and Y-piece	Disposable; or high-level disinfection	Change weekly provided new bacterial/viral filter used with every patient; change earlier if visibly contaminated or after infectious patient Reusable tubes can be pasteurized or subjected to chemical disinfection
Bougies	High-level disinfection or single use	–
Laryngoscope blades	Sterilized or single patient use	Blades may be sterilized with EO, steam, plasma, or treated with liquid chemicals. Laryngoscope handles to be disinfected
Flexible endoscopes	Sterilized or high-level disinfection	Chemical or EO sterilization
Stylets	Disposable or sterilized	Autoclaving, EO, plasma or chemical sterilization
Oxygen mask	Single patient use	–
BP cuffs	Cleaned	Cleaned when visibly contaminated or at end of the day. Periodic chemical disinfection or EO
Stethoscopes	Cleaned	Alcohol swab
Resuscitation equipment	Sterilized or single patient use	–
Anesthesia workstation and related equipment	Cleaned and disinfected	At the beginning and end of the day; in between cases if visibly contaminated. Top surface to be provided with a clean cover for every case
Gas cylinders	Cleaned and disinfected	–
Anesthesia ventilator	Cleaned, sterilized	External surface treated similar to anesthesia machine. Bellows and internal parts can be subjected to EO or autoclaving
Absorber	Disassembly, cleaning, disinfection	Autoclaving, EO or chemical disinfection depending on manufacturer's recommendation
Reservoir bags	Disposable or high-level disinfection	Chemical disinfection or EO sterilization
Scavenging equipment	Cleaned and disinfected	Periodic chemical disinfection of hoses

(EO: ethylene oxide; BP: blood pressure)

REFERENCES

1. Baillie JK, Sultan P, Graveling E, et al. Contamination of anaesthetic machines with pathogenic organisms. Anaesthesia. 2007;62:1257-61.
2. Ballin MS, McClusky A, Maxwell S, et al. Contamination of laryngoscopes. Anaesthesia. 1999;54:115-6.
3. Miller DM, Youkhana I, Karunaratne WU, et al. Presence of protein deposits on 'cleaned' re-usable anaesthetic equipment. Anaesthesia. 2001;56:1069-72.
4. Hall JR. Blood contamination of anesthesia equipment and monitoring equipment. Anesth Analg. 1994;78:1136-9.
5. Lees DE. To reuse or not to reuse, that is the question. ASA Newslett. 1992;56:13-5.
6. Dorsch JA, Dorsch SE. Cleaning and sterilization. In: Dorsch JA, Dorsch SE (Eds). Understanding Anesthesia Equipment, 5th edition. Philadelphia: Lippincott Williams & Wilkins; 2008. pp. 956-1002.
7. Centers for Disease Control and Prevention. (2008). Guideline for disinfection and sterilization in healthcare facilities. [online] Available from http://www.cdc.gov/hicpac/Disinfection_Sterilization/2_approach.html. [Last accessed November, 2017].
8. King TA, Cooke RP. Cleaning, disinfection and sterilization. In: Davey JA, Diba A (Eds). Ward's Anaesthetic Equipment, 6th edition. London: Elsevier; 2012. pp. 429-37.
9. Rutala WA. Disinfection and sterilization of patient-care items. Infect Control Hosp Epidemiol. 1996;17:377-84.
10. Favero MS. Principles of sterilization and disinfection. Anesth Clin North Am. 1989;7:941.
11. Bucx MJL, Veldman DJ, Beenhakker MM, et al. The effect of steam sterilization at 134°C on light intensity provided by fibrelight Macintosh laryngoscopes. Anaesthesia. 1999;54:875-8.
12. Moneret-Vautrin DA, Laxenaire MC, Bavoux F. Allergic shock to late and ethylene oxide during surgery for spina bifida. Anesthesiology. 1990;73:556-8.
13. Kyi MS, Holton J, Ridgway GL. Assessment of the efficacy of a low temperature hydrogen peroxide gas plasma sterilization system. J Hosp Infect. 1995;31:275-84.
14. American Society of Anesthesiologists Committee on Occupational Health of Operating Room Personnel. Recommendations for infection control for the practice of anesthesiology; 1998.
15. Association of Anaesthetists of Great Britain and Ireland. Infection control in anaesthesia. Anaesthesia. 2008;63:1027-36.
16. Berry AJ. Infection control in anesthesia. Anesth Clin North Am. 1989;7:967-81.

Anesthesia: Safety and Prevention of Hazards and Accidents

Pradnya C Kulkarni

ABSTRACT

The anesthesiologist's prime concern is safety of patient and personnel working in operation room areas. The concerns regarding safety of patients are equipment malfunctions, errors of medications, errors in performance of anesthesiologist's, or any other member of the team. Environmental safety issues like electricity hazards, fire and explosions, transmission of diseases, accidents, and radiation affect both.

The higher incidence of chemical dependence, addictions, and performance errors due to chronic fatigue, stress, and chronic exposure to anesthetic gases are causes of concern for healthcare professionals. The hospital administration should focus on improving safety and try to strike a golden mean between cost and safety.

INTRODUCTION

Anesthesiologists have always performed a key role in achieving high standards of safety for patients in perioperative period. About 6–7 decades ago, death under anesthesia was considered inevitable in certain situations. In 1949, this view was challenged by Robert Macintosh, "deaths due to anesthesia can frequently (many times) be attributed to failure of anesthetist (or his equipment)".[1]

Since then, increasingly anesthesiologists have substantially contributed toward patient safety, major share of it is due to advancements in engineering, technology, and pharmaceutical progresses. Addressing the problem of human error[2] and emphasis on continued medical education plays a vital role. To minimize the gap between best practice and actual care offered to patients, lies the continuous process of identifying problems and analyzing failures.

It is very important for anesthesiologist to realize that knowledge about safety is as relevant to anesthesia practice as understanding of basic medical subjects like anatomy, physiology, and pharmacology, etc.[2] The anesthesia safety has widened its spectrum to patients, anesthesiologist, surgeons, assistants, nursing staff, other medical professionals, technical staff, and other nonmedical staff [healthcare professionals (HCPs)]. The area for which anesthesiologist is concerned regarding safety is extended to not only operative rooms, but also recovery rooms, intensive care, emergency medicine department (casualty), pain clinics, magnetic resonance imaging (MRI) suit, computed tomography (CT) scan, radiation therapy department, cardiac catheterization laboratories, endoscopy department, etc.

It is the right of the patient to expect safety and protection from harm in perioperative period. The goal should be as an anesthesiologist, to identify potential hazards, source of accidents so as to reduce the occurrence of adverse incidents in perioperative period.

Safety issues can be considered as:
- Pertaining to patients
- Pertaining to HCP
- Common in both (patients and HCP).

Patients Safety

- Equipment malfunction
- Errors
- Medication errors
- Performance errors
- Team work failure.

Healthcare Professional Safety

- Theater pollution—control of trace gas levels
- Radiation hazard
- Chemical dependence
- Stress and chronic fatigue.

Patient and Healthcare Professionals Both

- Electricity hazards
- Fire and explosion hazards
- Laser hazards
- Magnetic resonance imaging suit hazards
- Transmission of diseases
- Accidents and injuries.

DEFINITIONS

Accident

It is an unfortunate incident that happens unexpectedly and unintentionally typically resulting in damage or injury.

Hazard

It is a potential source of danger or risk.

Adverse Incident

It is an event that causes or has the potential to cause unexpected or unwanted effects involving the safety of patients, users, or other persons.

Critical Incident

It is a reporting technique. It is applied in medicine to identify the causes of errors. First reported its use in anesthesia is by Cooper et al.[3] in 1978. They examined errors and equipment failure in anesthesia practice. In last 3 decades, critical incident reporting has been widely adopted in anesthesia to identify causes of adverse outcomes. Many departments and institutes collect the data and analyze, which can be used to modify guidelines, protocols, and for judging performances. This can also be used for training purposes. In the original report critical incident was defined as an occurrence that could have led (if not corrected or discovered in time) or did lead to an undesirable outcome ranging from increased length of hospital stay to death, it must also involve error by a member of anesthetic team or failure of anesthetic equipment to function, occur while patient is under anesthetic care, be described in clear detail by an observer or member of anesthetic team and be clearly preventable. Some authors include nonpreventable causes or nonanesthetic causes or some may include only the incidents which have adverse outcome to make the definition confusing. Therefore, unambiguous and self-explanatory term "real or potential adverse effect" has been proposed.[4]

Analyzing critical incidents has a very important role in identifying risks, potential source of damages, and help forming base for improving safety.[5] Noticing the cause that is occurring very frequently can point to the defect in functioning or designing of an equipment.[6]

Reporting and analysis of critical incident has two major disadvantages:

1. Conscientious and sincere reporter may be labeled as poor performer; this in due course of time can lead to underreporting
2. Apathy and underreporter may be fallaciously labeled as good performer which result in continuation of faulty or risky practices and failure of improvement in safety.

SAFETY ISSUES: PATIENT

Equipment Malfunction

Many studies have shown that human errors are more common than equipment failures but equipment failure still forms a major share of critical incidents. These are failure of breathing circuits, oxygen (O_2) delivery problems, misconnections, disconnections, development of high or low pressures in breathing circuits, major or minor leaks in circuits, delivery of hypoxic mixtures, carbon dioxide (CO_2) retention (hypercapnia), incorrect delivery of inhaled anesthetic agents, inhalation of foreign substances, malfunction of monitoring devices, suction apparatus, monitoring alarms malfunction, physical damage to patient due to machine, and falling of heavy equipment's on patient are all reported. The constant breakthroughs in engineering and technology enable manufacturers to incorporate many safety features in modern anesthesia machines and monitors. The electromagnetic interference due to devices such as cell phones, papers, and internet can cause interference in working of monitors and alarm systems, etc.

Medication Error

The medication error has proved to be a constant problem despite considerable efforts has consistently resisted improvement.[7-9] The standardize technical advances in delivery systems, color-coding of labels, checking of medication using barcodes, and conforming to key principles of safe drug administration is the only factor that has proven to be beneficial in reduction of medication errors.[10] The formal checking and rechecking of medication to be administered is the most recommended and highly safe practice.

Error

By definition, it means unintentional action causing harm or unintentional use of a wrong plan to achieve aim or failure to carry out a planned action as intended. The chances of error are greatly increased by violation of norms.[11,12]

Violation

A deliberate but not necessarily reprehensive deviation from those practices appreciated by the individual as being required by regulations or necessary or advisable to achieve an appropriate objective while maintaining safety and the ongoing operation of the device or system.[7,8] The violation leads to errors or violations magnify damage due to errors, e.g., violating speed limit by a vehicle increases its chance of driver to make error that may lead to accident. The high speed may be the cause of accident and magnified damage.

Teamwork Failure—Error

The failure of team in communication and/or suboptimal performance of any team member may cause wastage of time, waste of resources, tension, procedural errors and adverse incidences, or critical error can lead to unfavorable outcome or even death.[13,14] The failure to communicate has led to grave consequences, e.g., operation on wrong patient, wrong side, and wrong operation, etc. The administration of medication to patient with known allergy is the most common communication failure error. Anesthesiologist performs an important task of coordinating the team comprising of diverse professional groups.

HEALTHCARE PROFESSIONALS

Control of Trace Gas Levels

Healthcare professionals working in operating room (OR) and anesthesia areas are constantly exposed to low concentrations or trace levels of anesthetic gases/vapors. Some of the feared health problems are:

- Spontaneous abortions in HCPs
- Spontaneous abortions in spouses of HCPs
- Birth defects in babies born to HCPs
- Infertility
- Cancer—various
- Impaired performance
- Liver disease
- Kidney diseases
- Hematological abnormalities (leukemia)
- Alteration in immune responses (change in immunological profile)
- Neurological problems (polyneuropathy causing tingling numbness, muscle weakness)
- Cardiac diseases (hypertension, arrhythmias)
- Suicidal tendencies
- Substance abuse causing morbidity and mortality
- *Miscellaneous:* Bone and joint diseases, ulcers, ulcerative colitis, gallbladder diseases, migraine headache, fatigue, asthma, laryngitis, ophthalmic hypersensitivity, conjunctivitis, exacerbation of myasthenia gravis, and skin ulcers, etc.

The evidence that is currently available that exposure to trace gases can be harmful to personnel working in OR areas is inconclusive.[15] There are many epidemiological prospective and retrospective studies, studies on human volunteers, and large number of animal studies have failed to prove cause-effect relationship.[16] It is important to know all the pertinent information on the supposed and proposed risks of prolonged exposure and many ways of reducing the exposure risks.[17] The department of occupational health can educate the HCPs and provide guidelines, which may prove useful in minimizing occupational exposure risks,[18] due to constant concern and persistent controversy of this issue. The American Society of Anesthesiologists (ASAs) Committee on occupational health of OR personnel convened a task force on trace anesthetic gases. After analyzing all the available data at the time, ASA task force concluded that there was no proof of an association between occupational exposure to waste anesthetic gases and adverse health effects.[19] Many anesthesiologists have modified their techniques or anesthesia practice to minimize the exposure to trace gas levels. There is continuous debate on this issue that has got a considerable impact on the decision making of anesthesiologists about their anesthesia practices.[20]

The focus lies on four main areas to minimize concentration of waste anesthetic gases to minimum, with reasonable cost and efforts:

1. Leaks in equipment's breathing systems
2. Operating room ventilation systems
3. Various techniques of gas administration and anesthesia
4. Scavenging systems.

Leaks in Breathing Systems and Equipment

The minor leaks are unavoidable, but major leaks should be identified and corrected. Regular servicing of anesthesia machine equipment will minimize leaks and systematic checking of anesthesia machine (high pressure, intermediate pressure, and low-pressure system) at the beginning of the day, and quick general checkup in between cases is advised.

Room Ventilation System

The room ventilation systems which recirculate the same air are not effective in removing waste anesthetic gases and do not reduce OR pollution, the noncirculating systems are efficient in reducing OR pollution.

A turnover of 20 exchanges per hour is recommended to prevent bacteria from setting on OR surfaces. At the time of planning and construction of operation theater the placement of anesthesia machine should be near room ventilation system and provision for scavenging system for evacuation of waste anesthetic gases.

Work Practices

The work practices adopted by anesthesiologists can help in reducing OR pollution with anesthetic waste gases. These are:

- Checking of anesthesia machines thoroughly prior to induction of each case
- Efficient and correct use of scavenging system
- Holding tightly a properly fitting face mask, will reduce risk of leaks and lessen the escape of anesthetic gases to ambient air
- Meticulous filling and emptying of vaporizers to avoid spillage
- Use of low-flow anesthesia techniques
- Use of cuffed endotracheal tubes versus supraglottic airway, which have higher portion of leaks
- Use of techniques, such as total intravenous anesthesia/ regional anesthesia, complete avoidance of nitric oxide (N_2O), etc.
- Do not use N_2O and inhalational agents to check machine. N_2O and anesthetic agents are started only when breathing circuit is connected to cuffed endotracheal tube.

Scavenging Systems

The scavenging by definition, mean the collection and removal of waste or expired anesthetic gases from OR. As the supplied anesthetic gases are far more than that are necessary for patient to remain anesthetized and to reduce waste anesthetic gases polluting OR, the scavenging is a very efficient mean.

Scavenging systems are of two types:
1. *Active:* In this, suction is applied to actively suck gases, however, it has danger of low or high pressure being transmitted to patient circuit.
2. *Passive:* In this, waste anesthetic gases flow passively from valves on expired tubing through room ventilation, through exhaust grill in OR.

Passive scavenging has possibility of only positive pressure buildup due to some obstruction to flow of exhaust gases.

There are two distinctly different scavenger interfaces: (i) open and (ii) closed. Open interfaces are safe for patient and hence are incorporated in many newer anesthesia machines.

The components of scavenging systems are:
- Gas collection assembly [tubes connected to adjustable pressure-limiting (APL) valve and vent relief valve]
- Transfer tubing 19 mm or 30 mm (mostly in yellow color codes)
- Scavenging interface
- Tubing for gas disposal (carries gas from interface to disposable assembly)
- Gas disposable assembly (active or passive, active is common).

The open interface has no valves and is open to atmosphere (there is provision for allowing both positive and negative pressure relief). These should be used only with active systems. The open interfaces are safe for patient as no pressure is applied to the airway of patient in case of failure of scavenger but they are inferior in controlling trace gas levels and increases risk of occupational exposure to trace gases and this risk increases further by their incorrect use. Closed interface has valves and require appropriate vacuum adjustments to keep reservoir bag adequately filled (neither flat nor over distended) as needed.

Hazards of scavenging system are:
- *Pressure alteration of breathing systems:*
  - *Excess positive (high) pressure buildup:* Barotraumas occurs due to resistance to transfer or occlusion of gas disposable tubing. Occlusion can be caused by equipment's pressing on it like anesthesia machine, trolleys, etc., from outside. Occlusion can occur from inside by water, foreign materials or insects, etc., blocking it
  - Negative pressure applied to breathing circuits is a possibility when active disposal system is used with fully open APL valve
- *Misassemble or misconnection:* It can happen, although scavenging system has connectors of 19 mm or 30 mm as against to 15 mm or 22 mm connections (universal connections) of breathing circuits, misconnection can happen by using adaptors or sticking tapes. These mistakes which mostly occur due to ignorance lead to serious complications
- The accidental administration of high concentration of inhaled anesthetic agent may get unnoticed as strong smell (odor) may get masked due to efficient scavenging system. Monitoring of inspired and expired concentration of volatile anesthetic agents will offer protection against these mishaps
- Occasionally, low minute volume or disconnection alarms may become inactive as atmospheric air can get sucked into the breathing circuits when scavenging is in use.

Monitoring of Exposure to Trace Gases

It is necessary as anesthesiologists are usually most vulnerable personnel for exposure to waste anesthesia gases is maximum in terms of time and intensity.[21]

Places of Monitoring

These are OR, air-condition exhausts, grills, and area just outside OR door are frequent sites for sampling air. The instantaneous, time weighted, or continuous are three methods of sampling of ambient atmosphere of operation theater, for estimation of intensity of exposure to trace gases of theater personnel. The education of HCP, meticulous maintenance of anesthesia machine, proper use of scavenging system, and focus on correct anesthesia practices are principle ways to reduce exposure.

RADIATION

The radiations to which HCPs are exposed are of two types:
1. Ionizing radiation (X-rays, radioactive isotopes, etc.)
2. Nonionizing radiation (lasers).

Ionizing Radiation[22]

It is vital to know the harmful effects of exposure to ionizing radiation and their stringent preventive measures. Areas in which anesthesiologists work routinely, has risk of radiation exposure, such as urological, orthopedic operations. Cardiac catheterization laboratory, interventional procedures in radiology department, radiation therapy department, department of nuclear medicine, and interventional pain treatment procedures need anesthesiologist's services. The exposure of HCPs to radiation comes from scattered X-rays from patients and equipment's. The continuous fluoroscopy has more radiation than single exposure X-ray and radiation exposure from scattered rays depends on distance from the source and is inversely proportional to square of the distance.

As Low as Reasonably Achievable

As no amount of radiation is safe, minimizing radiation exposure is the goal of as low as reasonably achievable (ALARA) concept.[23] The safe limit of maximum yearly occupational radiation exposure is 5 rem (Roentgen equivalent man; rem is a unit of measurement of radiation exposure). Limits are different in pregnancy. Rem is essentially a measure of the biologic damage from radiation, adjusted to apply to all tissues. It is difficult to quantitatively determine ALARA concept.

As low as reasonably achievable concept is considered under three basic divisions:

1. Planning and installation of protective measures at the time of construction of radiation areas
2. Training, teaching, and promoting awareness in the personnel regarding necessity and importance of minimizing radiation exposure. The written guidelines and policies should be available to all
3. Protective measures like lead apron, shields, thyroid shield, protective goggles, and lead gloves should be easily available. Their use should be strictly imposed and encouraged.

Protection of Personnel from Radiation Exposure

- Radiation monitoring
- Understanding harmful effects of radiation exposure
- Protective measures taken to shield from harmful effects of radiation.

Radiation monitoring: Devices available are—

- *Pocket dosimeter:* It is most sensitive instrument, easily damageable, which can be inaccurate in inexperienced hands and this dosimeter does not give permanent record of levels of exposure
- *Film badge:* These are most convenient and can be worn on neck or apron, etc.
- *Thermoluminescent dosimeters* ***(Fig. 1)****:* They are cheap, are seated in teflon to avoid damage, small, and hence could be easily incorporated in jewelry, etc. They can be read directly and are accurate. They have wide range of exposure and resemble human tissue. These are the most commonly used monitoring devices currently.

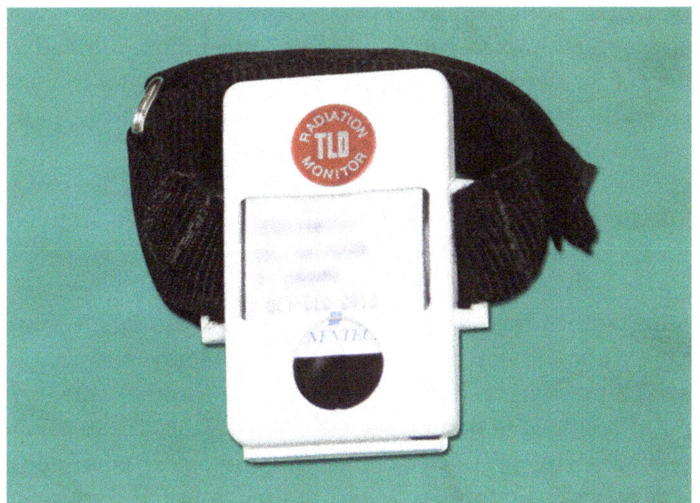

Fig. 1: Thermoluminescent dosimeter badge—with user name.

It is important to note that badges should never be exchanged among personnel and clearly marked for identification. They are returned to laboratory at regular intervals (mostly 3 monthly) for processing under standard conditions.

Harmful effects of radiation exposure: As no radiation is safe, it is always harmful to tissues. The amount and nature of any damage depends on radiation quality, the dose quantity that is absorbed, area of tissue exposed, duration (acute/chronic), or time period of exposure.

The radiation damage or injury is of three types:

1. *Local effects:* Small occupational exposures do not have local skin changes, but exposure of many years can cause chronic skin changes like skin erythema, dry skin, cracking or ulceration, and very rarely cancer induction. A highly radiosensitive structure is optic lens and can cause lens opacities (focal or general, premature cataract formation)
2. *General effects:* Chromosomal abnormalities, blood dyscrasias like changes in lymphocytes, leukocytes, and platelets, etc., increase chances of causing leukemia, shortening of life span are few of many proposed general effects of radiation
3. *Pregnancy:* Radiation exposure during pregnancy is hazardous to conceptus (embryo + fetus). In animal studies with large radiation dose gestational exposure can cause malformation of baby (microcephaly, anencephaly, heart defects, etc.) but human equivalents are not conclusive.

For patients, day 10 rule is followed. From 1st day of menstruation to 10 days is considered to be safe period for elective (planned) radiological studies as the chance of pregnancy is minimal. The recommended exposure limits for pregnant personnel are 0.5 rem (5 mSv) for entire gestation and not more than 0.05 rem (0.5 mSv) in any 1 month.[24] Complete avoidance of radiation, if possible, is desired during pregnancy.

The genetic hazard is most serious problem of radiation exposure, genes particularly in the chromosomes of sex cells are extremely vulnerable. The radiation damage to the genetic material is expressed as chromosomal aberration and gene mutation.

Protective measures: Three general principles are—

1. *Exposure time:* As minimum as possible
2. *Distance:* As much as possible
3. *Lead barrier:* As many as available.

Emphasis on importance of protective measures and frequent revisions of safety precautions ensures maximum cooperation of personnel.

For personnel working in radiation areas:
- Minimize the period, like by avoiding repeat studies[25]
- Anesthesiologist may stand in control room or behind protective drape/glass barrier or behind operator as away as possible from fluoroscopy
- Adopt anesthesia techniques which will allow anesthesiologist to maintain distance from patient (avoid manual ventilation techniques, bag mask anesthesia, etc.)
- Use protection, e.g., lead protective apron, special lead shield for gonads, protective goggles, lead protective thyroid collar, gloves, etc.
- Do not hold patient for radiological examination or procedures. Restrainers, straps, and safety belts can be used for that purpose
- When working in radiology department, always wear a film badge or thermoluminescent dosimeter. If female HCP is planning pregnancy, avoid radiation completely.

For departments:
- On all doors, having access to radiographic and fluoroscopic rooms, an official yellow warning sign reading "caution, radiation area" should be prominently displayed **(Figs. 2 and 3)**.
- All equipment concerned with radiation and personal protective devices should be regularly checked and serviced. They should be always kept in optimum working condition
- Name and emergency contact details of person concerned with radiation safety should be prominently displayed in radiation areas
- Regular teaching, training of personnel, and carrying out continuous educational activities in department with emphasis on minimizing radiation exposure and improving radiation safety are of great benefit.

The danger of ionizing radiation in the well-controlled radiological procedure is nil, if all the personnel make full use of the all protective devices, equipment's, and constantly bear in mind ALARA principle.

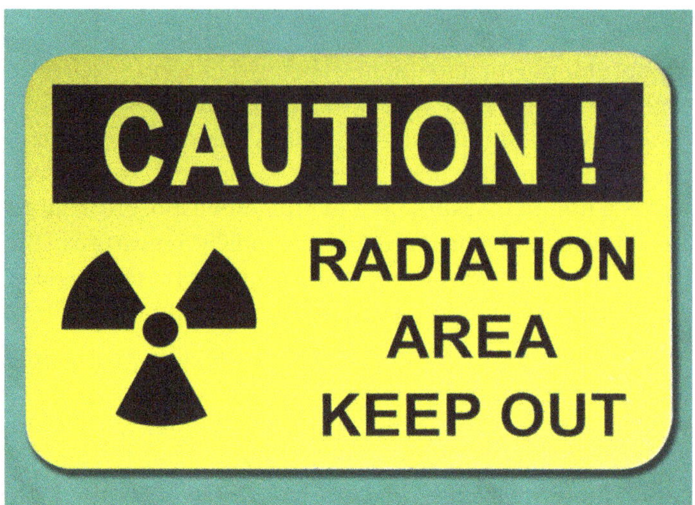

Fig. 2: Official yellow radiation warning sign.

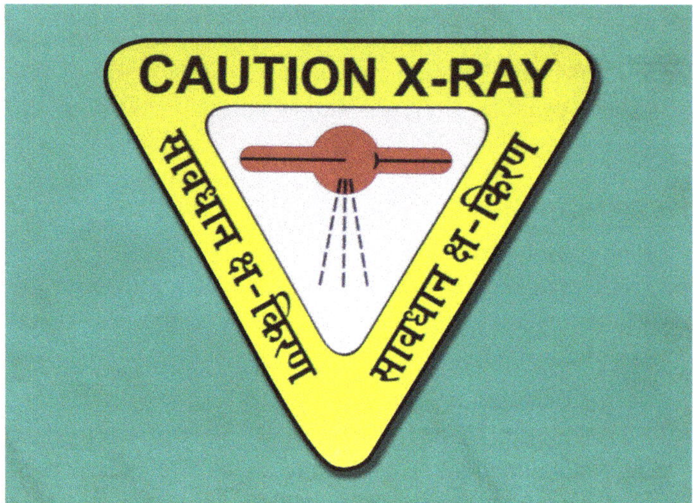

Fig. 3: Radiation warning sign in regional language.

CHEMICAL DEPENDENCE

The prevalence of drug abuse among anesthesiologists is estimated to be roughly 1–2%,[26-28] and commonly cited causes are high levels of stress, easy availability or access to drugs, and knowledge of pharmacology of drugs.[29] Identification of problem is generally delayed due to medical knowledge used to hide it. The death may be the first symptom and early identification, appropriate intervention, and proper treatment are important. Along with treatment and strict adherence to follow-up many can continue to practice their profession.[30]

STRESS AND FATIGUE

Being workaholic is a virtue in medical practice and doctors take pride in working long hours. The factors such as long working hours, working constantly in odd shifts, working without proper breaks, inadequate sleep, and inadequate recreation leads to stress and fatigue. The incidence is high among anesthesiologist and the shortage of personnel is perpetual problem. The period between 2 AM and 7 AM and late afternoon are identified as maximum vulnerable period for sleep[31] and are vulnerable for maximum human errors. It is strongly recommended to enforce work hour regulations.

Some factors that have constantly proven to cause stress are difficult anesthesia cases, frequent night calls, strained professional relationships, and noncooperation from peers, etc. In addition, the domestic problems like divorce, bereavement add to the stress. The effective and adequate communication, interactive sessions, adequate time and proper access for recreational facilities, and adjustments in work hours will help in reducing stress and fatigue.[32] The effective management of stress, at times psychological counseling will improve performance and minimize human errors in some.

LIGHT AMPLIFICATION BY STIMULATED EMISSION OF RADIATION

The use of light amplification by stimulated emission of radiation (LASER) is well established in ophthalmic surgery, plastic surgery, urology, head and neck surgery, airway surgery, neurosurgery, gastrointestinal surgery, and major vascular surgery. The laser causes nonionizing electromagnetic radiation. LASER produces ultraviolet light, visible light, or infrared light. The commonly used lasers in medical practice are CO_2, neodymium-doped yttrium aluminum garnet (Nd:YAG), potassium titanyl phosphate, and argon.

Light amplification by stimulated emission of radiation equipment's are classified in four groups **(Table 1)**.

The commonly used in surgical practice are classes III and IV.

Hazards of Laser

Patient

- Misdirected laser beam can cause perforation of viscous or blood vessels causing bleeding
- Venous air embolism—known with Nd:YAG lasers
- Inadvertent injury to patient's eye
- Burns due to heat generated locally.

Healthcare Professionals

- *Eye injury:* Eye injuries, such as eye damage in form of corneal burns, retinal burns, destruction of macula, optic nerve cataract, etc., seen in HCP due to direct exposure or reflected radiation. The suitable protective eyewear (goggles) must be worn **(Fig. 4)**. The type of protection provided by the filter is marked on the frame of the goggles and must be checked for specificity of the type of laser being used. Laser protective eyewear should be worn by all personnel present in OR as scattered laser beams are equally damaging to eyes. Intensity of scattered laser beams does not significantly reduce for long distances. The visibility of monitors and anesthesia machine should be checked preoperatively as some goggles diminish or blur vision. Do not use broken or shattered goggles
- *Plume:* The vapor and cellular debris caused by laser is called plume.[32] It is harmful when inhaled. Human immunodeficiency virus (HIV)/human papillomavirus (HPV) is found in plume. Although no case of transmission of infection is reported and damage to lungs of operator is very rare, the smoke (plume) should be actively removed by suction or scavenged out of operation theater[33]
- *Fire:* Airway and OR fire is the most dreaded complication of lasers.[34,35] The incidence of airway fire or anesthetic mixture catching fire is approximately 0.5%; however, fire can result from either direct laser illumination and ignition or reflected laser rays. Sometimes tissue particles bloom from surgical site or cottonoids or gauze pieces used can catch fire. If accidently laser beam strikes unprotected endotracheal tube carrying high O_2 concentration anesthesia gas mixture, tube can ignite and fire can start intraluminal. It is called "blowtorch fire".

TABLE 1: Classification of light amplification by stimulated emission of radiation equipment's.

Class I	Totally enclosed with extremely low output
Class II	Low risk—minimal risk to eye
Class III	• Power 1–5 mw—moderate risk to eye • Power 5–500 mw—potentially hazardous to eyes and skin
Class IV	• Continuous mode and power output >500 mw • Great risk to eye, skin, and fire hazard

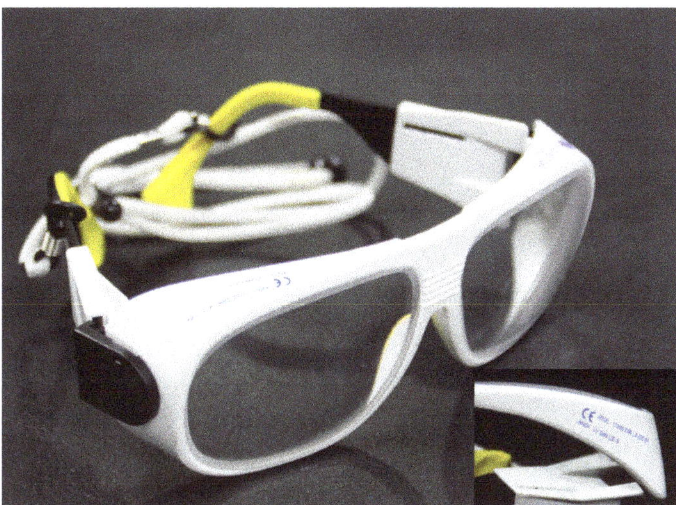

Fig. 4: Laser protective eyewear (goggles), the type of protection provided by the filter is marked on the frame (see inset).

Following measures are taken to minimize complication of airway fire:

- Inspired concentration of O_2 should be as low as possible preferably less than 30%, avoid N_2O and inhalational agents in high concentration
- Endotracheal tube cuff may be filled with cold saline, tinged blue with methylene blue to keep temperatures at the operation site low, dissipate heat, and detect cuff rupture
- Electrosurgical forceps should be kept away from patient as much as possible. Remove from surgical site when not in use
- Laser safe endotracheal tubes should be used
- Instruments should be matt finish and avoid instruments with bright shining surfaces
- Laser plumes from surgical area should be removed by strong active suction.

Laser safe endotracheal tubes are available like Bivona® (Foam cuff®), Xomed laser shield tube, and flexometallic stainless steel double cuff endotracheal tube (Mallinckrodt), red rubber tubes are wrapped with aluminum or copper tapes. The silicon endotracheal tubes, Sheridan® laser tracheal tube,

Oswal-Hunton tube, Merocel® laser guard, and laser tubes silicon tubes are safe. The polyvinyl chloride endotracheal tubes are not safe for laser surgery. All available tubes are reasonably safe to use in airway laser surgery, but none have been specially recommended.

Airway fire: In case of airway fire, all personnel in OR must act in quick and orderly manner. Each person must know what to do and this practice drill should have been practiced earlier and revised at regular intervals.

- Operator/surgeon should promptly detect and remove source of fire and inform OR personnel
- Anesthesiologist should instantly stop ventilation and disconnect circuit and stop O_2 supply to breathing circuit
- The flaming tube should be removed and immersed in bucket of water to extinguish fire. As precaution bucket of water must always be kept ready in OR when laser airway surgery is performed
- After confirming fire inside has completely extinguished, anesthesia should be continued with intravenous agents, and patient ventilated by bag and mask
- Damage should be assessed by direct laryngoscopy, rigid or flexible laryngoscopy, or bronchoscopy and further treatment carried on.

International safety norms for use of lasers in OR are formulated.

Precautions that are followed universally:

- Personnel working in OR should be educated about safe use and side effects of lasers
- A sign board stating use of lasers in OR should be displayed prominently on OR door **(Fig. 5)**
- Provide adequate protection for eyes to all personnel and patient
- Operator/surgeon must be trained in safe use of lasers
- Regular checks to keep laser machines, fibers, and personnel protective devices in optimum working conditions
- Safety officer who is incharge of lasers should be available in case of any troubleshooting.

Anesthesiologist should choose utmost safe anesthesia techniques, follow safety norms, and keep continuous vigilance on laser use.

MAGNETIC RESONANCE IMAGING

Magnetic resonance imaging is used to obtain superior images without ionizing radiation. Majority of patients cooperate for the study but in few like children, critically ill intensive care unit (ICU) patients, patients with involuntary movements, claustrophobic patients, etc., sedation or general anesthesia may be required. As MRI study is not painful and immobile patient is the only requirement and sedation technique generally suffices. But rarely patients may need general anesthesia.

Magnetic Resonance Imaging Hazards

Patient

Ferromagnetic substances are the ones which contain iron, iron oxide, iron coating alloys, nickel, and cobalt. Depending on site, size of object, and position in respect to magnetic field rotational (torque) and/or translational (attraction) forces act on them.[36]

- *Ferromagnetic substances outside patient's body:* Freely moving objects get pulled toward the magnet with alarming speed (missile or projectile effect). This can injure patient, personnel, or may damage equipment's **(Fig. 6)**. Common ones are watches, scissors from nurse's pockets, keys, hairpins, mobile phones, loose coins, jewelry, stethoscopes, etc.
  - All persons entering MRI scan room must be thoroughly checked for internal and external ferromagnetic substances
  - Warning signs should be clearly displayed in prominent areas

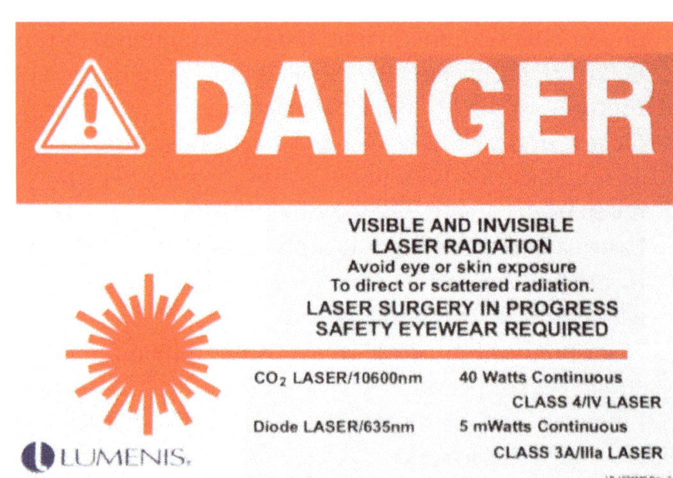

Fig. 5: Laser warning sign.

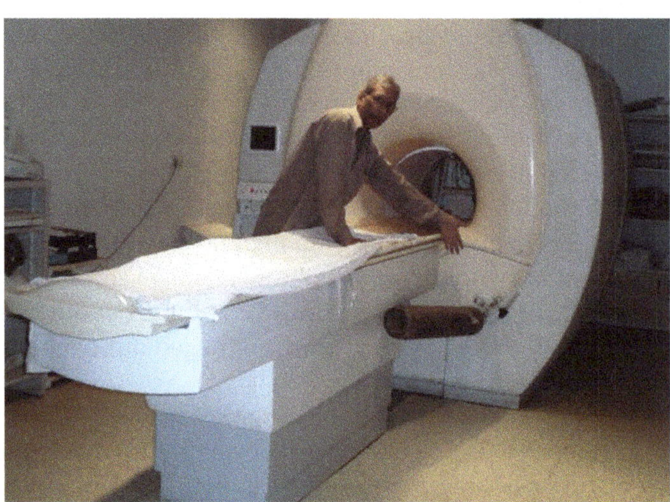

Fig. 6: Accidental collision of full oxygen cylinder to magnetic resonance imaging machine.

- An extensive list of all possible items and clear guidelines about their safety inside MRI suit should be available in department to avoid confusion and mistakes regarding ferromagnetic nature of objects.
- *Ferromagnetic substances inside patient's body:* These are implanted or inserted ferromagnetic objects, such as aneurysm clips, cardiac pacemakers, and foreign bodies embedded in vital organs like eye, indwelling catheters, etc. The newer implants and pacemakers are safe, as they are made up of nonferromagnetic substances. Some cochlear implants and cardioverters may be safe. The equipment malfunction due to MR interference can pose problem to patients and compromise their safety
- Electrocardiography (ECG) leads, cables, sensors, wires, surface, coils, skin staples, etc., can get heated during MR study and cause burns
- Hypothermia can occur especially in small children undergoing long studies.

Patient's safety in MRI can get compromised because of inaccessibility of patient.[37] It may cause problems in airway management, monitoring of patient, intravenous access, etc. Loud noise may interfere with detection of audible alarms.

Note: Powerful magnetic field keeping the oxygen cylinder suspended horizontally in air.

Healthcare Professionals

Since the availability of MRI, the anesthesiologist's work in MRI is infrequent and data regarding hazards due to prolonged exposure are insufficient. Although there is no known evidence and it is advisable for females to avoid MR area, for the 1st trimester. The continuous and prolonged exposure to loud noise of MRI machine can cause hypertension and can damage hearing.

The demonstrated noise level in MRI suit on an average is about 92 decibels. The use of earplugs or headphones by all present will minimize the effect of noise pollution. As MR suits are not equipped with scavenging, trace gas levels may be high. Very rarely, liquid helium which surrounds the superconducting solenoid escapes in MRI suit, at that time atmosphere may contain low O_2 levels leading to hypoxia. This problem can be detected early if O_2 sensors are installed in MRI suits. The detailed understanding of limitations, risks involved, and problems encountered are mandatory for safe anesthesia practice in MR suite.

ELECTRICITY

Electrical Hazards in Operating Room

It is vital for all personnel to understand principles of electrical supply to OR and its inherent hazards. As almost all equipment's used in ORs have electric supply such as anesthesia machine, ventilators, monitors, drug delivery systems (syringe pumps), body warming devices, overhead theater lights, electrosurgical cautery, and suction apparatus, etc.

There are four major ways in which mains electrical supply can be hazardous to patient and/or HCP:

1. Electrocution—shock
2. Electric burns
3. Electrochemical effects
4. Fire and explosions.

Electrocution or Shock (Macroshock)

The effect of shock on humans depends on tissue resistance (R), current (I), potential difference (V), current frequency, current pathway and time (duration), and also on current density.

The thermal energy delivered to the body tissues depends on the power (P) dissipated.

$$V \times I = I2R$$

Where V: potential difference, I: current, and R: tissue resistance.

The electrical resistance of mucous membrane is the least and is highest in skin of sole or very hard callus of hands and soles. The water or moisture or sweat on skin reduces the resistance of skin markedly, i.e., by approximately 10 times than dry skin. The pathological effect of electric shock is directly proportional to the current. At 50 Hz frequency, current of 1 mA causes tingling sensation; pain is caused at roughly 5 mA; 15 mA can cause severe joint and muscle contractions. The "let go threshold" for 50 Hz frequency is about 30 mA, currents above 30 mA cause respiratory muscle contractions, which leads to asphyxia and death. The higher currents about 70–100 mA cause multifocal premature ventricular contraction, cardiac failure, local burns, and ventricular fibrillations. Any current above 1,000 mA causes extensive burns and charring.

The sudden death due to ventricular fibrillation is more likely if current passes through heart horizontally and damage to cardiac muscles is more likely if current passes through heart vertically **(Fig. 7)**.[38]

Microshock

A very small amount of electric current passing through the body also can interfere with normal functioning of muscles and nerves and minimum of 50 mA current is needed to cause ventricular fibrillation. The modern surgical, medical, and critical care procedures, such as pulmonary artery catheterization, central venous catheter placements using "P" wave guidance, dialysis catheter insertion, etc., involves placement of electrodes within or very near heart. Due to this proximity of placement of leads from the heart, extremely small current can cause ventricular arrhythmias, fibrillation. This is called microshock, even stray potential or inductive small currents can cause microshocks.

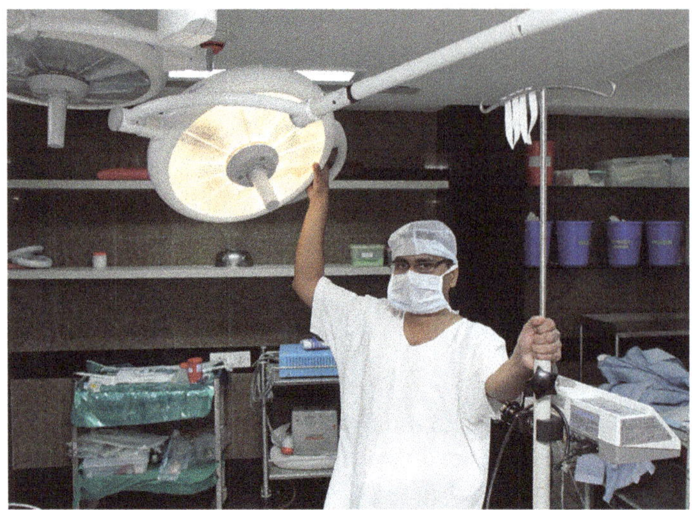

Fig. 7: Possibility of macroshock faulty technique. Ventricular fibrillation: Current passing through heart horizontally.

Capacitative coupling can occur when the electrosurgical current induces stray currents on the other nearby conductions. This phenomenon happens only in alternating current (AC). Although this is generally insignificant, in certain unusual circumstance it can cause severe burns. For example, use of non-MRI compatible pulse oximeter in MRI can cause finger burns.[39] In laparoscopic surgeries if active electrode of electrosurgical cautery is in contact with a noninsulated metal instrument, e.g. laparoscope and if this laparoscope is passed through a metal cannula (electrically energized), current can flow to patient's abdominal wall. If laparoscope is passed through a nonconductive cannula, current can pass to any piece of bowel or abdominal organs which may cause burns. The capacitative coupling can be minimized but cannot be eliminated.

Electric Burns

As current passes through body or skin, heat is generated, depending on the amount of heat generated and area, burns may result.

Enormous heat generated by electric currents can cause two harmful effects:

1. Electric burns
2. Fire and explosion in OR.

Electrical burns are most common with electrosurgical units (ESUs) (diathermy/cautery).

- Unipolar/monopolar electrosurgery (UPES) (unipolar cautery/diathermy/monopolar cautery)
- *Bipolar electrosurgery (bipolar cautery/diathermy):* The difference in unipolar and bipolar electrosurgery is path taken by the electric current. In electrosurgery, electric current is applied by the operator via electrode to body tissues that burn and cut or burn and coagulate the tissues.

In UPES, this current passes through entire body of patient and is collected outside surgical field by a wide, large area to which a well-lubricated and properly gelled grounding pad is applied. This pad is also called dispersing electrode or cautery plate.

In bipolar electrosurgery (BPES) or bipolar cautery, this current from one electrode passes to the tissues for a very small distance and returns back through another electrode only few millimeters away. Bipolar electrosurgery has two pencil point electrodes which resemble forceps. These can be used in patients with cardiac pacemakers, automatic implantable cardioverter defibrillators (AICDs) with reasonable safety, with due caution.

In unipolar/monopolar electrosurgery if grounding pad (dispersing electrode) is small, not gelled well, applied over small area, or contact is minimum due to bony prominence the current has to pass through small area. This increases resistance and heat is generated, which causes burns. If grounding pad is not applied properly or is defective or not applied at all, current will pass through alternate pathway like ECG leads, monitoring cables, etc., and cause local burns in that area. Unipolar/monopolar electrosurgery is unsafe for use in neurosurgery and patients with pacemaker, therefore, should be avoided.

Protection of patient from shock: This can be done by installing small isolating transformer whose output is isolated carefully from the earth in the circuit of equipment running on electricity that is connected to patient. This can enhance patient safety. In this case, patient circuit is completely earth free or fully floating and equipment enclosure can be earthed.

The other method is to install a current operated earth leakage circuit breaker. It operates at low earth leakage currents; its action is very fast and is cheap. Their use has greatly diminished the risk of serious electric shock to patients. The use of equipment working on battery is safe and batteries may be charged by electricity between patients.

The equipment used in medical practice is classified to make sure electrical safely norms are appropriately applied.

- *Class I:* Common household equipment with single insulation
- *Class II:* Equipment with double insulation
- *Class III:* Work at power source less than 24V AC. Less chances of micro- and macroshock.

All three types of equipment are subdivided into type B, type BF, and type CF with increasing safety measures.

The most common source of electric burns is electrosurgery or diathermy or cautery.

The electric burns due to electrosurgery can occur due to:

- Accidental pressing of paddle or footswitch
- Inadequate contact of grounding pad/plate to surface of body

- Any organ or part of it can infarct if vascular supply of the organ is compromised by monopolar electrosurgery, e.g., testes elevated from body on the spermatic cord by monopolar electrosurgery during surgery generates unintentional areas of high current density and compromise blood supply to testes
- *Absent grounding plate:* In case of absent grounding plate electric current is completed via OR table, ECG leads, monitoring cables, temperature probes, and Doppler probes causing severe burns.

Precautions During use of Electrosurgical Unit

- Avoid using ESU in areas where high concentration of O_2 is present, e.g., during tracheostomy
- Should be in standby mode when not in use
- Preferable to use bipolar ESU as it requires less voltage compared to unipolar ESU
- Electrosurgical unit should be activated by operator, only when its tip is in direct vision
- Minimum power setting that is required must be used, if higher than standard power settings are required. Electrosurgical unit should be sent for checking for faults
- Minimize clutter at foot spaces to reduce chances of accidentally pressing footpad of ESU
- Electrosurgical unit should be used very cautiously with metallic cannulas in laparoscopic surgeries
- Electrosurgical unit probe should be safely kept away when not in use and its tip cleaned regularly.

Precautions for use of Prejellied Dispersing Electrode (Cautery Pad/Cautery Plate)

- It should be checked prior to application of jelly
- It should be applied to clear, dry, and nonhairy area with good contact to large skin surface as near surgical area as possible
- Damaged, outdated, old, or already opened ones should be discarded
- It should be of appropriate size (it is available in infant, neonate, and pediatric sizes). Do not cut to reduce its size
- Should never be reused
- Electrocardiography electrodes must be applied as far as away as possible to avoid alternate currents passing.

Preventive maintenance of all electrically operated medical equipment, careful attention to electrical contacts of patient, and understanding significance of electric alarms and taking appropriate action are key methods to minimize electricity hazards in OR areas.

Standard Precautions to be taken in Operating Room

To minimize accumulation of static electricity:

- A metal chain whose at least three links are in contact with the ground is dangled from the anesthesia machine to the floor
- Footwear worn by the OR personnel should have conducting material and should be of specified resistance in compliance with standard norms
- All medical equipment which are mobile including anesthesia machine must be in contact with ground.
- All anesthesia equipment like masks and breathing circuits should have conducting material. This is extremely important, especially when flammable anesthetic agents are used
- Regular maintenance of all electrical equipment and other items is vital.

Knowledge of electrical safety is must for anesthetist, as timely identification of problem will prevent it from escalating and goes a long way in avoiding major catastrophes like severe burns, fire, and explosions.

Fire and Explosions

In the days when chloroform, ethyl chloride, and ether were used as anesthetic agents, fires in OR was a greater danger than it is now with modern anesthetic techniques being used.

Still, fires do occur in OR areas with devastating results in rare occasions. Patients are always at greater risks of harm due to their inability to get away quickly.

Operation theater fires fall in three categories:

1. Fire involving patient directly or something inside patient catches fire
2. Fire initiated and sustained by electricity—mainly electrical equipment catching fire
3. Fires in OR rooms—surgical drapes or any other substrate catches fire.

Presence of three factors is necessary for fires to occur:

1. Combustible material (fuel)
2. Oxidants that support combustion (oxidizer)
3. Source (ignition source).

These three things form a "fire triangle" or "fire triad". Presence of all three in correct proportion under right conditions cause fire.

Chemical combination of combustible material with O_2 causes burning, this when takes place in a confined space leads to dangerous rise in pressure. The rapid liberation of heat and sudden escalation of pressure result in explosions, which are more damaging. In order to minimize the risk or danger of fire, a detail study of all three components of fire triangle is required. The best strategy to deal with fire is to prevent them from happening and meticulous efforts are needed to make sure that all three components of fire triangle do not come together.

Ignition source: All electrically operated instruments are source of ignition and should be used correctly. All instructions in operating manuals should be followed and techniques of using the instrument must fit the recommendations of the manufacturer.

- Electrosurgical unit (cautery/diathermy) is most common source of ignition[40]
- Equipment with high potential to become ignition source is laser machine.

Important precautions needed to be taken while using lasers are:

- Lasers must be used only by professionals who are trained and certified in laser operations
- Laser machine must be kept on "standby" mode when not in use
- Protocols for using lasers should be developed and followed correctly
- Operator must avoid accidental firing of laser beam when laser beam is not directed on operation site
- Laser must not be used blindly
- Regular checkup and proper maintenance of laser machine is mandatory
- Use of lasers should be monitored by safety officers who are trained in safety issues regarding use of lasers
  - *Fiberoptic light source:* The end of fiber optic cable can generate heat enough to start fire and should never be put on patient or drapes. Judicious use and meticulous precautions are required to prevent burns and fires[41]
  - Heaters and humidifiers, defibrillators, suction apparatus, all electrical hubs, and monitors can become source of ignition. When faulty, these equipment can cause sparks
  - Accumulation of static electricity on the floor of OR, any equipment can cause spark and become source of ignition.

Fuels:

- *Endotracheal tubes:* Laser safe endotracheal tube use is highly recommended when airway laser is used. The filling of cuff with ice cold saline will lower temperature rise in surgical area. The use of wet towels, sponges, ice cold saline, soaked cottonoids, and pledges will prevent ignition of these materials. The water soluble lubricating jelly can be used to coat facial hair, eyebrows, beard, and moustaches to avoid burns
- *Preparation solution:* Water-based preparation solutions are preferred as decontaminants to alcohol containing solutions. If alcohol containing solutions are used, use minimum and avoid pooling.[42]
  In situations where fire risks are high such as airway laser surgery, fire resistant drapes can be used to reduce risk of drapes catching fire
- Combustible substances like excessive drapes, ether bottles, wrappers, and covers should be removed from operation theater at regular intervals to reduce the load of combustible substances or fuel in OR.

Oxidizer: Use of oxidizer can be minimized or totally avoided to reduce chances of fire like:

- Nitrogen, helium, or air can be added to O_2 in fresh gas flows to reduce concentration of O_2 in inspired gases to minimum which will maintain adequate oxygenation of the patient
- In cases where risk of fire is high, e.g., airway laser surgery, N_2O should also be avoided as it supports combustion
- Avoid leak of high concentration of O_2, e.g., leak around the cuff of endotracheal tube
- Pneumatic cuffs and tourniquets should not be inflated with O_2 or N_2O
- Avoid high O_2 concentrations to be accumulated around patient, e.g., excessive O_2 use in nasal cannula, face mask, bag and mask ventilators. This can cause pockets of high O_2 concentration areas under the drapes
- *Inhalational agents:* Cyclopropane, ether, and ethyl chloride are explosive in anesthetic concentrations, but are no longer used. N_2O, halothane, trichloroethylene (Trilene), isoflurane, sevoflurane, and desflurane are not flammable at atmospheric pressure. N_2O supports combustion. Halothane at a very high concentration (which is not used clinically) is flammable in O_2.

Zone of risk: When patient is under anesthesia, certain areas near patient or anesthesia machine or breathing circuits are likely to contain highly explosive gaseous mixtures. These areas are considered as "zone of risk". When the flammable anesthetic agents were used whole OR area it was considered as zone of risk. However, with newer non-flammable anesthetic agents are in use, zone of risk is considered to be 25 cm around gas pathways of anesthetic machines and breathing systems.

Near the zone of risk:

- All anesthetic tubing should have antistatic impregnations (e.g., carbon impregnations) or should be antistatic
- All anesthetic machines, trolleys, monitors, and movable items must have antistatic base, bottom, or wheels
- Operating room flooring should be antistatic
- Electrical switches in OR should be spark proof and enclosed and electric sockets which captures the plug (which does not allow it to be pulled out when in ON position). All plugs should be removed in "OFF" position **(Figs. 8 and 9)**.
- All electrical outlets should be 40 cm above ground in OR.
- Anesthetic equipment should be classified as, anesthetic proof (AP) and anesthetic-proof category G (APG) depending on distance they can be used from flammable gas that can escape from breathing systems:
  - *Anesthetic proof:* Instruments with AP mark can be used within distance of 5–25 cm, and it is temperature should not exceed 200°C.

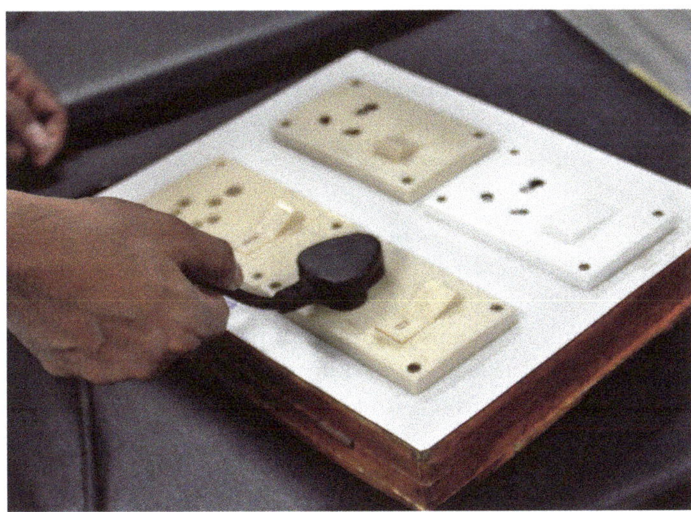

Fig. 8: Wrong method, yanking wire with switch "on".

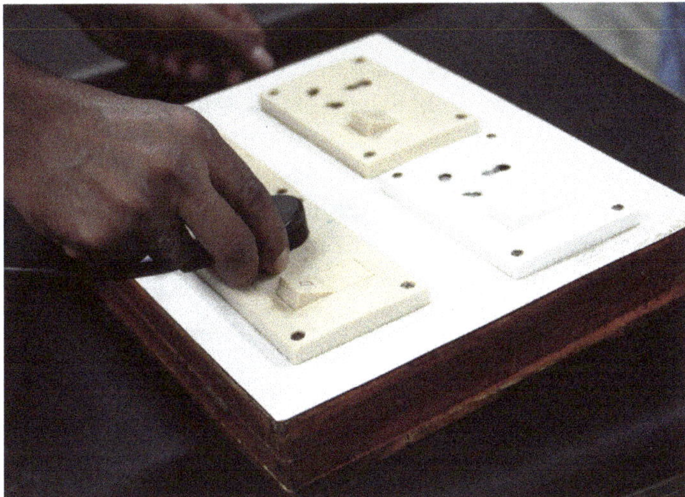

Fig. 9: Correct method of removal of plug when switch is "off".

- *Anesthetic-proof category G:* Instruments with APG mark can be used within 5 cm and temperature not more than 90°C, when ignition energy should not exceed 1 μ J for both.

Reported incidents of fire in OR is higher in certain situations and these are considered very high potential for fire hazard. They are:

- Airway
- Body cavity
- Surgical drapes
- Pressure regulators
- Electrosurgical units.

Airway fire is most common when lasers are used and during tracheostomy with use of cautery. All three angles of fire triangle are present:

1. *Ignition source:* ESU/laser
2. *Fuel:* Endotracheal tube, gauze, etc.
3. High concentration of O_2.

Body cavity: Intraperitoneal fires can occur due to gas escaping from obstructed bowels and during laparoscopic surgeries.[43] Any spark caused during defibrillation can cause fire when high concentration of oxygen is used by face mask for a critically ill patient.

Fires in pressure regulator: The risk of fires in pressure regulator can be reduced by giving detail attention to operating them.

The precautions during operating of pressure regulator are:

- Avoid contamination of pressure regulator with grease, oil, alcohol, etc.
- Cracking of cylinder—opening slowly and briefly in the beginning
- Opening of cylinder should be very slow to allow heat to dissipate which is generated by sudden decompression of gas
- Cylinder should be handled strictly as per recommendations of the manufacturer.[44]

OPERATING ROOM FIRES: ACTION RACE

- *R:* Rescue the patient—small fires can be extinguished with saline or smothered
- *A:* Activate fire alarm and intimate fire department (brigade)
- *C:* Confine fire—shut O_2 supply. If needed, shut electric supply and doors
- *E:* Extinguish fire and evacuate OR personnel at the earliest.

Fire Extinguishers

Fire extinguishers are used as per fuel and location and extent of fire:[45]

- *Class A fires:* Ordinary combustibles, cloth, paper, and plastics
- *Class B fires:* Flammable liquids or gases
- *Class C fires:* Electrically energized fires.

Types of Fire Extinguishers (Fig. 10)

- *Carbon dioxide:* Carbon dioxide extinguisher can be used for all types of fires. They are heavy and bulky. These extinguishers emit a fog of CO_2 gas with liquid and solid particles that rapidly vaporize to cool and control fire
- *Water:* These are more effective in class A fires. They are difficult to use
- Halon fire extinguishers are very effective, but are not easily available and are costly. Halon is a halogenated agent which was used in fire extinguishers in OR for many years. It is not used anymore due to environment concerns.

Steps to Operate Fire Extinguisher: PASS

- *P:* Pull the pin—this will allow discharge of extinguisher
- *A:* Aim at the base of the fire—it should hit the fuel and not flames. Extinguisher on flames will pass across and go waste

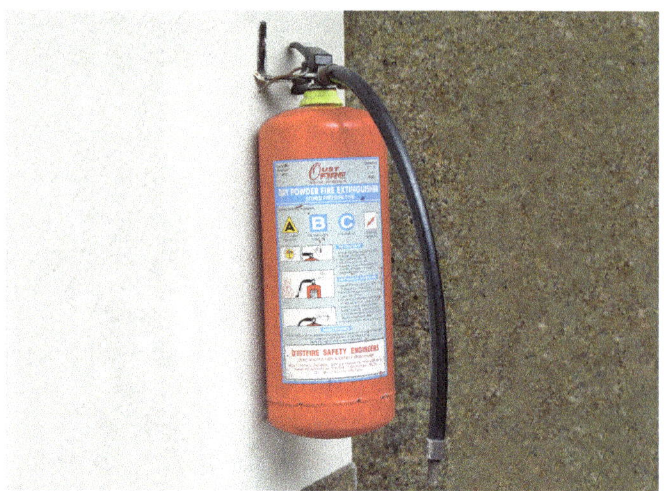

Fig. 10: Fire extinguisher.

- *S:* Squeeze top handle or lever—this depresses the button which releases pressurized extinguishing gas from the extinguisher
- *S:* Sweep from side to side maintaining distance till fire is completely under control. Keep strict vigilance on the area in case fire gets reignited.

Note: Which type of fire and user instructions on the cylinder?

Fire Control Plan

- "A" plan should be in place in OR and personnel working must be trained and should have regular practice of fire drills
- Operating room personnel must know location of fire alarms, fire extinguishers, and gas shutoff valves
- Evacuation procedure should be known to all OR personnel and strictly adhered to in emergency situation
- Immediate call for help—local and fire brigade.

The fire brigade should be notified immediately at slightest doubt of ability to handle the situation before fire reaches enormous scale causing loss of lives and extensive damages.

In case of fires with electrical equipment, electrical supply should be immediately shutoff.

- First thing is to shutoff O_2, N_2O, and all anesthetic gases, maintain anesthesia with air ventilation and intravenous agents. If necessary, O_2 cylinders, patient, and OR personnel should be evacuated and doors to OR should be closed to contain fire and smoke. The electricity and O_2 main supply should be shutoff where appropriate
- The hands on training and experience of using fire extinguisher should be mandatory for all personnel working in OR areas.

Cause of fire should be investigated and incidence reported.

TRANSMISSION OF DISEASES

There is always higher risk of acquiring infections for the personnel in OR due to close proximity with patients. Three routes of transmission of infection are: (i) airborne, (ii) bloodborne, and (iii) direct contact.

The bloodborne route is most common, significant, and complex due to invisible nature and ignorance about its mode of transmission.

Patient

The causes of transmission are transfusion of infected blood and use of contaminated needles, instruments due to reusing, faulty guidelines, and improper sterilization techniques. Transmission from infective HCP to patients is reported but is extremely uncommon.

Healthcare Professional

Most common mode of transmission from patient to HCP is through needlestick injury.[46]

Needlestick Injury

The needlestick injury is a percutaneous puncture wound by needle tip or any other sharp object or instrument. There are millions of incidents of needlestick injuries reported annually in the world and multiples of this number still goes unreported. There is risk of transmission of bacteria, protozoa, other viruses, and prions, but transmission of hepatitis B, hepatitis C, and HIV/acquired immunodeficiency syndrome (AIDS) is of maximum concern. The risk of transmission after exposure is greatest with hepatitis B, with 37–62% seroconversion and 22–31% clinical hepatitis B infection. The hepatitis C has a moderate risk of 1.8% but some newer studies are reporting it, as low as 0.5%, HIV has lower risk of 0.3%. The estimated risk of transmission of infection after single needlestick injury per 1,000 is roughly 300 (30%) for hepatitis B, 30 (3%) for hepatitis C , and 3 (0.3%) for HIV.

Prevention of Needlestick Injury

- *Engineering controls:* Use of needles and syringes with safety devices, vacutainers, etc. **(Fig. 11)**.
- *Administrative controls:* Training of personnel in how to remove needle caps, avoidance of passing sharp instruments from hand to hand, holding needles, and fixing scalpel blades with forceps. The preventive measures include use of blunt tip needle sutures for suturing fascia or for regional procedures, in addition blunt tip needles used or various blocks greatly reduces its complications,[47] avoiding multitasking when using sharps, calming patient down to avoid sudden jerks during procedures, avoiding bending, breaking and resheathing needles with both hands, learning single-handed needle resheathing technique, emptying sharps container when three-fourths full, and use of complete personal protective gear while handling and disposing sharps, etc.

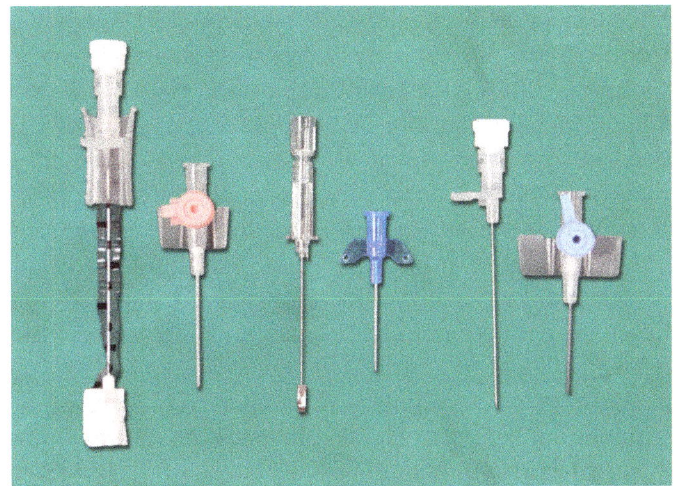

Fig. 11: Intravenous cannula without and with safety devices.

Management of Needlestick Injury

- Affected area should be thoroughly rinsed, washed with soap and water. If eyes are involved then irrigate with sterile saline and use of antibiotic eye drops is advised
- Efficacy of milking of blood from puncture site to minimize quantity of infected blood entering body is controversial and not recommended
- Report incidence to emergency department
- Infective status of the source should be checked if not already known
- Laboratory tests should be performed on the recipient for baseline studies of HIV, hepatitis panel [hepatitis A virus immunoglobulin M (IgM), hepatitis B surface antigen (HBsAg), hepatitis B core IgM, and hepatitis C virus (HCV)] and in immunized individuals, hepatitis B surface antibodies.
  - Where indicated, initiation of postexposure prophylaxis (PEP) as soon as possible, preferably within 1 hour of exposure.
  - Strict adherence to follow ups at base, 6 weeks, 12 weeks, 6 months, and in special cases at 1 year.[48]

Hepatitis B: There is dramatic decrease in incidence of hepatitis B and subsequent morbidity and mortality after the introduction of an effective vaccine.[49] The rate of seroconversion after parenteral inoculation by contaminated percutaneous injuries depends on infectivity of the host and magnitude of the contact with the blood and which on an average is 40%.[50] It is imperative for HCP who are seronegative to be actively immunized with hepatitis B vaccine for effective preexposure prophylaxis against infection. The vaccine is effective in 90% of recipients. The unvaccinated personnel should be passively vaccinated by hepatitis B immunoglobulins (HBIGs), if hepatitis B virus (HBV) exposure is suspected with HBsAg positive source and series of three injections of HBV vaccine should be started simultaneously. Both together have efficacy of approximately 85–90%.

The effectively vaccinated personnel can be either:

- *Responders (seroconvert):* Hepatitis B surface antigen serum level greater than 10 mIU/mL, or
- *Nonresponders (nonzero converted):* Hepatitis B surface antigen serum level less than 10 mIU/mL. The nonresponders are treated like unvaccinated person. If respondent status is not known or undetermined, such personnel are treated by both HBIG and HBV vaccines.

Hepatitis C: Principally transmitted by blood, predominantly transmitted to patients by infected blood transfusion. Chronic hepatitis develops in about 85% who get accidentally infected with HCV, roughly 20% deteriorate to cirrhosis of liver, and about 3% develop hepatocellular carcinoma. The effective PEP is not available, but some evidence shows benefits in treatment with interferon. The early detection and early intervention in chronic cases is recommended to halt further deterioration.

Human immunodeficiency virus/acquired immunodeficiency syndrome: The most likely route of occupation-related HIV infection for anesthesiologist and other HCP is injury from infected needle. Risk is higher with injuries caused by wide bore hollow needles with visible infected blood with deep intramuscular inoculation. The minimum dose or amount of contaminated blood required to cause infection in humans is unknown but the likelihood of development of antibodies to HIV is increased with increase in volume of inoculums and the concentration of viral particles or viral load.[51] Strictly adhering to protocol of universal precautions is absolutely mandatory. As very few occupational exposures result in HIV transmission, the PEP guidelines are laid down by weighing relative risk of exposure and toxicity of the PEP drug treatment. The risk of transmission of HIV infection increases with percutaneous exposure, high viral load, or viral titers, i.e., patient in late stage of disease, hollow wide bore needle, and visible blood on the contaminated sharps.

The PEP must begin as soon as possible, preferably within 24 hours, since no time period is known after which PEP is shown not to be beneficial, it can be initiated even after 1 week after exposure but efficacy may reduce with increasing time between exposure and PEP. Routinely, a basic two antiretroviral drug regimen for 4 weeks is advised but in high-risk cases three drug regimen is recommended, which has higher toxicity.

Airborne Diseases

Airborne contamination is mainly derived from the personnel in the OR and their activities. The bacterial count in OR is influenced by number of personnel present, ventilation, and airflow. Proper design and ventilation of OR is the most important means of controlling airborne contamination and thus preventing airborne infections in OR. The vertical laminar flow is the most effective way to control microbe levels in the entire OR. And compared to conventional

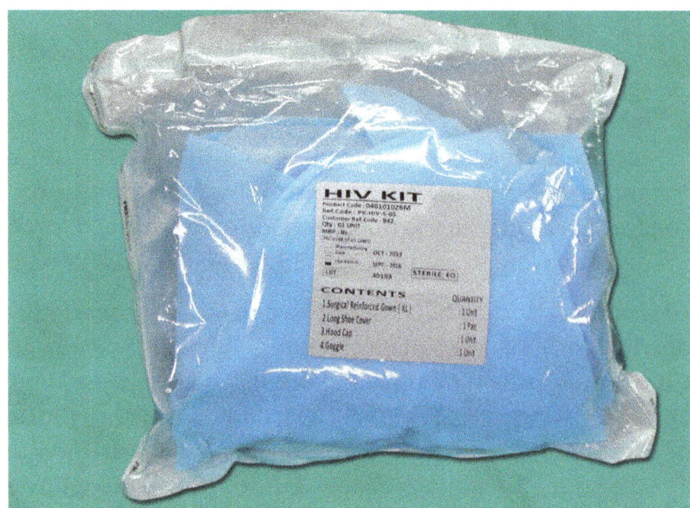

Fig. 12: Sterile pack of personal protective equipment kit.

turbulent ventilation, vertical laminar flow can decrease the number of postoperative infections substantially. In laminar airflow, the entire air mass circulates in one direction and displaces the existing air over the operation area. The first crucial step in vertical laminar flow is when incoming air is blown straight down through high-efficiency particulate absorption (HEPA) air filters which filters air of dust, fungus, microorganisms, etc. The efficiency of HEPA filters is 99.99% of all particles above 0.3 μm in size **(Fig. 12)**. A downward airflow prevents air masses from mixing in the work area. About 10–20% of air is vented out of room and replaced by fresh air. Rest of the air in the room is circulated, filtered with the replacement air, and blown back into the room. This way increased amount of fresh air is not needed, which keeps energy costs down. Laminar flow system can be tailor made for specific OR requirements, but basically it contains vertical airflow unit with HEPA filter and two suction units with prefilters which are placed at the bottom of OR on two opposite walls. By reducing transmission of airborne infections and diseases, vertical laminar flow is more cost effective as it reduces postoperative morbidity and mortality and also safeguards HCP.

Tuberculosis

In early 1990s, the report of transmission of multiple drug-resistant tuberculosis (TB) from patient to patient and to HCP, TB infection was a cause of grave concern. The comprehensive guidelines are issued to prevent spread of multidrug-resistant TB (MDR-TB). The extensively drug-resistant TB (XDR-TB) has emerged in last 5 years, and is on the rise with around 13% prevalence in metropolitan cities in India whose general hotspots are large slums and low socioeconomic housings. The incidence of MDR-TB and XDR-TB is more common in immunocompromised patients like patients with HIV infection, uncontrolled diabetics, and those on immunosuppressing drugs. Primarily, focus is on identification and treatment of patients with TB, development of engineering controls, such as room filters, ventilation, isolation facilities, proper utilization of protection devices, and comprehensive educational programs for HCP. TB infection spreads by small droplets of size 1-5 μm, these droplets become airborne when patients with pulmonary TB coughs, sneezes, speaks, laughs, etc. The infectivity increases greatly with higher concentration of infected droplets and longer duration of exposure. This droplet may remain suspended and viable in air for long periods; they are suspended at an average height of 3–6 feet.[52]

The maximum exposure occurs at the time of the extubation and intubation. The infective exposure is most while performing bronchoscopy.

Factors under consideration in prevention of airborne infections:

- *Control of environment:* It includes exhaust ventilation and general ventilation. High-efficiency particulate absorption, ultraviolet germicidal irradiation (irradiation of the air in the upper portion of the room or within ducts or within recirculating units).
- *Respiratory protection:* Use of N95 masks. These masks have ability to filter particles greater than 1 μm size with more than 95% efficacy up to inspiratory flow rate of 50 L/min. For the mask to be effective, it should have a proper tight fit on the face and should have a clean filter.

Severe Acute Respiratory Distress Syndrome

This disease was first identified in China in 2002. It is caused by coronavirus with single-stranded ribonucleic acid. It initially causes flu-like symptoms like fever, chills, myalgia, headache, and dry irritant cough. The mortality is approximately 9.8% and rises to 25–30% in elderly above 70 years and pregnant patients. The spread of the disease is through respiratory secretions, body secretions, and direct contact. The precautions in the form of environment and respiratory controls like in case of TB are needed to prevent spread. Other diseases where transmission is a risk is swine flu, plague, and scrub typhus which have shown recent resurgence.[53] Significant but rare transmissions like in cases of bovine spongiform encephalopathy (BSE) or Creutzfeldt-Jakob disease (or mad cow disease) appropriate precautions should be taken.

Preventing Measures: For Contact and Bloodborne Transmissions

- Protective equipment's like gloves, gowns, and eye shields should be available at no cost at all to HCPs who have potential to encounter infected blood or secretions or blood products **(Figs. 13 to 15)**
- There should be standard handwashing facilities, which are easily accessible to all HCP

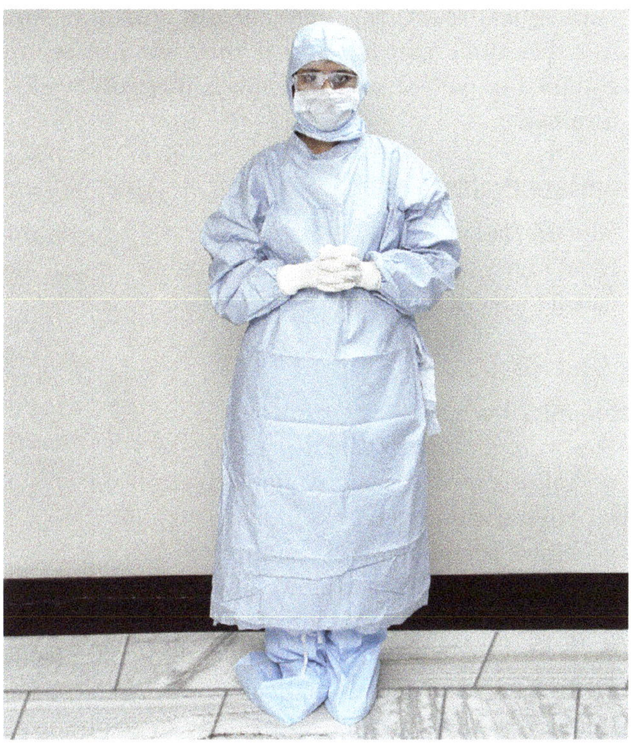

Fig. 13: Personal protective equipment kit.

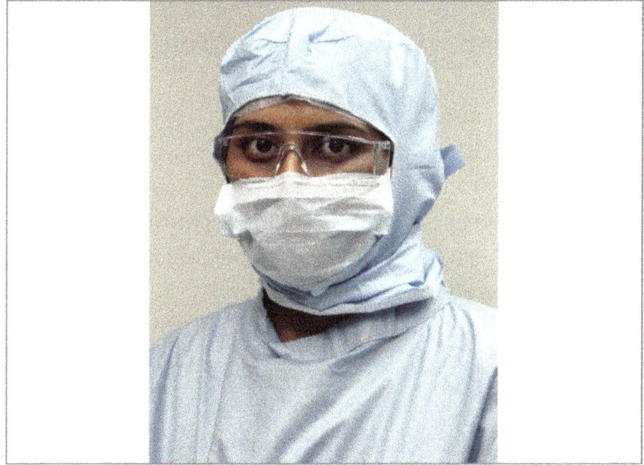

Fig. 14: Personal protective equipment: Protective goggles covering sides also.

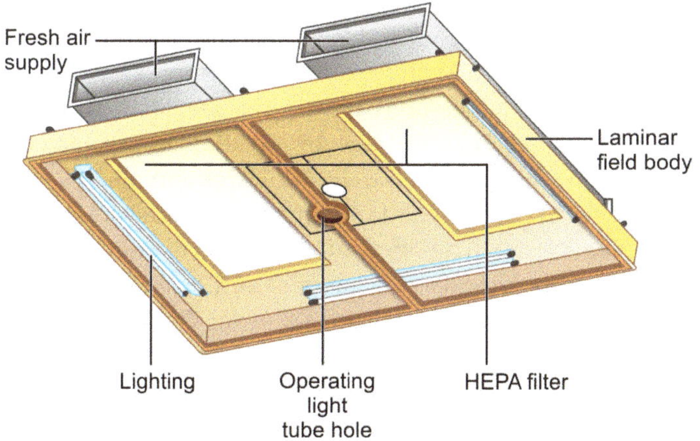

Fig. 15: High-efficiency particulate absorption (HEPA) filter.

- Appropriate containers to store and dispose of contaminated material should be provided enough in number, at minimal efforts
- Education and training about proper handling and disposal of contaminated material should be mandatory to all HCPs
- In case of any accidental exposure to contaminated material (like needlestick injuries) PEP must be implemented without delay. Guidelines regarding further follow-up and management must be issued
- In case of diseases for which vaccines are available, HCP should be freely vaccinated
- In situations where safe and effective alternatives are available (sharps, needles, and knifes), use of unsafe instruments can be eliminated (use of special intravenous cannula, blunt tip, needles, etc.).
- Lapse in concentration and fatigue are known to increase risk of exposure to contaminants by percutaneous injuries.

UNIVERSAL PRECAUTIONS

A series of guidelines for HCP who have contact with patient's blood, blood products, and body fluids are available. Since no symptoms or signs conclusively reflect the presence of bloodborne pathogens, all patient's blood, body fluids should be considered potentially infective. The same precaution should be taken for all patients. Therefore, these guidelines are called universal precautions.

Universal precautions guidelines are composed of two levels:

1. Standard precautions
2. Transmission-based precautions (used as per known or suspected infection with pathogen).

Standard Precautions

These precautions are used for all patients:

- Needles should be disposed off in a puncture proof container. They should not be broken, recapped, or bent
- *Barrier precautions:* Even if there is no visible blood or nonintact skin/mucosa of operator or patient, barrier precautions such as use of gloves, gown, and protective eyewear are used when there is potential contact with patient, blood, blood products, body fluids, secretions, excretions, etc. (except sweat) is anticipated
- All specimens should be handled as if they are infected
- Meticulous handwashing is advised with proper handwashing techniques after removal of gloves even if there is no visible blood or secretions on hand
- During resuscitations, equipment for airway management should be easily available that will obviate need for mouth to mouth or mouth to nose respiration.

Transmission-based Precautions

These precautions are as follows: When patients are known to be infected with highly pathogenic agents or epidemically significant diseases. These are followed in addition to standard precautions:

- *Airborne precautions:* Where fine airborne particles or droplets (size <5 μm) transmit diseases (e.g., measles, rubella, and TB). Several air filtration and air handling techniques are needed
- *Droplet precautions:* When disease which are transmitted by droplets of size greater than 5 μm (e.g., *Haemophilus influenzae* type B, meningitis, and *Mycoplasma pneumoniae*) precautions to limit the spread of droplets are taken
- *Contact precautions:* Certain diseases (e.g., herpes simplex virus, conjunctivitis) are spread by contact, skin to skin, hands, or contact indirectly through fomites, contact precautions are applied.

Transmission of diseases from patient to HCP and patient to patient is a real danger. The four major effective strategies for protection of HCP from transmission of diseases are:

1. Meticulous following of standard precautions and specific precautions in case of highly infective diseases
2. Effective immunization wherever applicable, e.g., hepatitis B, influenza vaccination, etc.
3. Easy and cost-free provision of personal protective equipment (PPE)
4. Postexposure prophylaxis and follow-up management.

ACCIDENTS CAUSING PHYSICAL DAMAGE IN OPERATING ROOM AREAS

Patient[54]

- *Improper positioning of the patient:* It is the most common cause of injury to body parts, nerves, etc., especially in prolonged surgeries. Close attention to positioning will reduce this risk
- *Fall:* Falling of the patient from operation table or recovery room trolley happens mostly in children and elderly patients. Lack of attention of any team member while shifting the patient or patient turning on side or leaning over trolley during vomiting or patient made to sit on side of trolley or stand besides trolley to help void urine (especially in male patients) are some of frequent causes of patient's fall. Use of side railings, straps, following proper lifting and shifting procedures, and close watch on patients can reduce chances of fall
- *Objects or items falling on patient:* Intravenous stands, improperly placed monitors or other equipment carelessly placed over anesthesia machines, and loose parts of OR lights are some reported objects causing harm by falling
- During transport, through narrow corridors injury to extremities can happen if they are not securely confined or patient suddenly splays them especially on turnings.

Healthcare Professional[55]

- Slip/trip/fall
- Head injury by banging head on OR lights
- Fall of heavy equipment.

Slip/Trip/Fall

Commonly, this hazard can result from:

- *Wet or contaminated floors:*
    - Saline slippage or intravenous bottles leaks
    - Floor cleaning products
    - Blood, secretions, and vomitus
    - Condensation due to faulty air conditioner
- Obstruction or accumulation of debris
- Hoses, cords, electrical wires, breathing circuits, and defibrillators wires lying on the floor
- Inadequate illumination, especially in neurosurgery, laparoscopic surgeries.

Prevention

- Avoid running, walking with items which obstruct your view
- Use of slip-resistant footwear
- Minimizing clutter on floor
- Proper illumination of OR areas
- Use of warning sign boards such as "caution—wet floor"
- If dust or floor mats are used, they should be fixed to avoid curling edges
- Use of guard rails or hand rails where appropriate.

CONCLUSION

In 1999, Institute of Medicine published a report "to err is human".[14] This put a spotlight on deaths that were caused by preventable medical errors. The medication error was the most frequent cause of death followed by surgical errors. Since most high-risk period for patient is perioperative period, errors in OR areas have disproportionately led to more harm to patient than any other errors elsewhere in hospital. All hospitals must have a special focus on issues regarding safety in OR areas by creating safety culture. While designing patient safety initiatives, human factors, technological changes, and training of personnel are crucial incorporations.[56,57] The safety must be a never ending quest. The perioperative safety of patients and HCPs working in OR areas can be improved by use of modern technology, improvements in training (simulation techniques of training have proved to be a very effective tool),[58] changing attitudes of HCP, setting high standards of clinical practice, regular checks and audits, and the most important of all is "constant diligent vigilance".[59] In times, when efforts are being made to reduce cost of medical treatment, safety should never be compromised.

REFERENCES

1. Macintosh RR. Deaths under anaesthetics. Br J Anaesth. 1949;21(3):107-36.
2. Weller JM, Merry AF. I. Best practice and patient safety in anaesthesia. Br J Anaesth. 2013;110(5):671-3.
3. Cooper JB, Newbower RS, Long CD, et al. Preventive anesthesia mishaps: A study of human factors. Anesthesiology. 1978;49(6):399-406.
4. Derrington MC. Critical incidences in anaesthesia. In: Walker JS (Ed). Quality and Safety in Anaesthesia. London: BMJ Publishing Group; 1994. pp. 105-28.
5. Aitkenhead AR. Head injuries associated with anaesthesia. A global perspective. Br J Anaesth. 2005;95(1):95-109.
6. Suzuki T, Yoshimitsu K, Muragaki Y, et al. Intelligent operating theater: technical details for information broadcasting and incident detection system. J Med Biol Eng. 2013;33(1):69-78.
7. Kothari D, Gupta S, Sharma C, et al. Medication error in anaesthesia and critical care: A cause for concern. Indian J Anaesth. 2010;54(3):187-92.
8. Mahajan RP. Medication errors: can we prevent them? Br J Anaesth. 2011;107(1):3-5.
9. Wheeler SJ, Wheeler DW. Medication errors in anaesthesia and critical care. Anaesthesia. 2005;60(3):257-73.
10. Jenson LS, Merry AF, Webster CS, et al. Evidence-based strategies for preventing drug administration errors during anaesthesia. Anaesthesia. 2004;59(5):493-504.
11. Reason J. Human Error, 1st edition. Cambridge: Cambridge University Press; 1990.
12. Merry A, McCall SA. Errors, Medicine and the Law. Cambridge: Cambridge University Press; 1991.
13. Lingard L, Espin S, Whyte S, et al. Communication failures in the operating room: an observational classification of recurrent types and effects. Qual Saf Health Care. 2004;13(5):330-4.
14. Schimpff SC. Improving operating room and perioperative safety: background and specific recommendations. Surg Innov. 2007;14(2):127-35.
15. American Society of Anesthesiologists (ASAs). (1999). Waste Anesthetic Gases: Information for Management in Anesthetizing Areas and the Postanesthesia Care Unit (PACU). [online] Available from www.cdc.gov/niosh/docket/archive/pdfs/niosh-064/0064-010199-mcgregor_ref2.pdf. [Accessed October, 2017].
16. Sass-Kortsak AM, Purdham JT, Bozek PR, et al. Exposure of hospital operating room personnel to potentially harmful environmental agents. Am Ind Hyg Assoc J. 1992;53(3):203-9.
17. Arnold WP. Application of OSHA standards to waste anesthetic gases. ASA News Lett. 1992;56(8):23.
18. Leckey JH. Anaesthetic pollution in the operating room: A notice to operating room personnel. Anesthesiology. 1980;52(2):157-9.
19. Waste anesthetic gases: Information for the management in anaesthetizing areas and postoperative care units (PACUs). American Society of Anesthesiologists: Task force on trace anesthetic gases; 2004.
20. Sheraton TE, Gildersleve CD, Hall JE. The use of nitrous oxide in paediatric anaesthetic practice in the United Kingdom: A questionnaire survey. Anaesthesia. 2007;62(1):62-6.
21. Gray WM. Occupational exposure to nitrous oxide in four hospitals. Anaesthesia. 1989;44(6):511-4.
22. McGowan C, Heaton B, Stephenson RN. Occupational x-ray exposure of anaesthetists. Br J Anaesth. 1996;76(6):868-9.
23. Selman J. The Fundamentals of X-Ray and Radium Physics, 8th edition. Springfield: Charles C Thomas Publisher Ltd; 1994.
24. Bushong SC. Radiologic Science for Technologists: Physics, Biology and Protection, 4th edition. St Louis: Mosby; 1988.
25. Kivinitty K, Lahiti R, Lahde S, et al. Radiation doses from X-ray units used outside radiology department. Health Phys. 1980;38(3):419-21.
26. Ward CF, Ward GC, Saidman LJ. Drug abuse in anesthesia training programs. A survey: 1970 through 1980. JAMA. 1983;250(7):922-5.
27. Gravenstein JS, Kory WP, Marks RG. Drug abuse by anesthesia personnel. Anesth Analg. 1983;62(5):467-72.
28. Baird WL, Morgan M. Substance misuse amongst anaesthetists. Anaesthesia. 2000;55(10):943-5.
29. Gallegos KV, Brown CH, Veit FW, et al. Addiction in anesthesiologists: drug access and patterns of substance abuse. QRB Qual Rev Bull. 1988;14(4):116-22.
30. Menk EJ, Baumgarten RK, Kingsley CP, et al. Success of reentry into anesthesiology training programs by residents with a history of substance abuse. JAMA. 1990;263(22):3060-2.
31. Gordon NP, Cleary PD, Parker CE, et al. The prevalence and health impact of shiftwork. Am J Public Health. 1986;76(10):1225-8.
32. Thomas NK. Resident burnout. JAMA. 2004;292(23):2880-9.
33. Dasgupta D, Bakshi V, Jain A. Anaesthesia for Laser Surgery of Oral Cavity, Pharynx, Larynx and Trachea, 2nd edition. Baddi: Cachet Pharmaceuticals Pvt Ltd; 2011. pp. 66-90.
34. Patel KF, Hicks JN. Prevention of fire hazards associated with use of carbon dioxide lasers. Anesth Analg. 1981;60(12):885-8.
35. Snow JC, Norton ML, Saluja TS, et al. Fire hazards during CO_2 laser microsurgery on the larynx and trachea. Anesth Analg. 1976;55(1):146-7.
36. Menon DK, Peden CJ, Hall AS, et al. Magnetic resonance for the anaesthetist. Part I: Physical principles, applications, safety aspects. Anaesthesia. 1992;47(3):240-55.
37. Peden CJ, Menon DK, Hall AS, et al. Magnetic resonance for the anaesthesist. Part II: Anaesthesia and monitoring in MR units. Anaesthesia. 1992;47(6):508-17.
38. Tucker RD, Ferguson S. Do surgical gloves protect staff during electrosurgical procedures? Surgery. 1991;110(5):892-5.
39. Dempsey MF, Condon B. Thermal injuries associated with MRI. Clin Radiol. 2001;56(6):457-65.
40. A clinician's guide to surgical fires. How they occur, how to prevent them, how to put them out. Health Devices. 2003;32(1):5-24.
41. Taylor IR. Hazards of laparoscopic surgery. Br J Anaesth. 1999; 82(4):651.
42. Haggerty R. (2002). Report into the Operating Theatre Fire Accident 17 Aug 2002. Waitakere Hospital Waitemata District Health Board: Final Report 29 September 2002. [online] Available from: www.medsafe.govt.nz/downloads/alertWaitemata.pdf. [Accessed October, 2017].
43. Macdonald AG. A brief historical review of non-anaesthetic causes of fires and explosions in the operating room. Br J Anaesth. 1994;73(6):847-56.
44. Srivastava U. Anaesthesia gas supply: Gas cylinders. Indian J Anaesth. 2013;57(5):500-6.
45. National Fire Protection Association. NFPA Guide to Portable Fire Extinguishers. Quincy: National Fire Protection Association; 2003.
46. Tait AR, Tuttle DB. Prevention of occupational transmission of human immunodeficiency virus and hepatitis B among anesthesiologists: A survey of anesthesiology practice. Anesth Analg. 1994;79(4):623-8.
47. Baheti DK. Use of new modified needle with blunt tip for neurolytic sympathetic block in abdominal malignancies. 11th World congress on pain: IASP Press; 2005. pp. 489-90.

48. Panlilio AL, Cardo DM, Grohskopf LA. Updated U.S. Public Health Service guidelines for the management of occupational exposures to HIV and recommendations for postexposure prophylaxis. MMWR Recomm Rep. 2005;54(RR-9):1-17.
49. Lamphear BP. Trends and patterns in the transmission of bloodborne pathogens to health care workers. Epidemiol Rev. 1994;16(2):437-50.
50. Gerberding JL. Management of occupational exposures to blood-borne viruses. N Eng J Med. 1995;332(7):444-51.
51. Kessler HA, Bick JA, Pottage JC, et al. AIDS: Part I. Dis Mon. 1992; 38(9):633-90.
52. Tait AR. Occupational transmission of tuberculosis implications for anesthesiologists. Anesth Anal. 1997;85(2):444-51.
53. Bhaskar SB. Esoteric infections and anaesthesiologist: Need for self protection. Indian J Anaesth. 2013;57(2):115-6.
54. Contractor S, Hardman JG. Injury during anaesthesia. Contin Edu Anaesth Crit Care Pain. 2006;6(2):67-70.
55. Stanford University, Department of Environmental Health and Safety. (2008). Slip, Trip, and Fall Prevention Guide. [online]. Available from: www.ehs.stanford.edu/topic/general-workplace-safety/slip-trip-and-fall-prevention. [Accessed October, 2017].
56. Smith AF, Arfanis K. 'Sixth sense' for patient safety. Br J Anaesth. 2013;110(2):167-9.
57. Shelton CL, Smith AF. III. In pursuit of excellence in anaesthesia. Br J Anaesth. 2013;110(1):4-6.
58. Moppett I, Sevdalis N. II. From pilots to Olympians: Enhancing performance in anaesthesia through mental practice. Br J Anaesth. 2013;110(2):169-72.
59. Abelsohn J. Unusual accidents and incidents of anaesthesia. SA Med J. 1960;34:216-9.

Corona/COVID-19: Anesthetic Scenario in Corona Pandemic

SECTION 10

COVID-19: Pathophysiology and Management

Harprit Kaur Madan, Pallavi Kharat

ABSTRACT

The current COVID-19 pandemic created unprecedented situations that served to challenge and motivate medical professionals especially the anesthesiologists. The daunting numbers, the attempts to prevent transmission and the mortality involved demand a special section devoted to this pandemic. This section attempts to review the pathophysiology, the management, the equipment involved and the ventilatory strategies adopted during this pandemic.

INTRODUCTION

By the end of 2019, a novel highly infectious coronavirus was identified as the cause of a cluster of pneumonia cases in Wuhan; a city in the Hubei Province of China.[1,2] As it rapidly spread, resulting in an epidemic throughout China, it escalated into a global pandemic. In February 2020, the World Health Organization designated the disease as COVID-19.

As a global crisis, COVID-19 is challenging healthcare systems worldwide. The sheer numbers were daunting. The total number of cases in India touched approximately ten million till January, 2021. Caused by a novel beta-coronavirus, COVID-19 is also known as Severe Acute Respiratory Syndrome Coronavirus 2 (SARS-CoV-2). Depicting a wide spectrum of clinical severity, COVID-19 infection ranges from being asymptomatic to fatal. Although clinical and laboratory characteristics of COVID-19 patients have been well characterized, the pathophysiological mechanisms underlying the disease's severity and progression remain unclear. Thus, there is a significant lacuna in the understanding of the complete pathophysiology of COVID-19-related lung injury.

VIRAL STRUCTURE

Coronavirus are enveloped positive-stranded RNA viruses of -30 kb. They are divided into four genera; α, β, γ and δ depending on their genomic structure. α and β are commonly found infecting mammals.

The viral body is made up of four structural glycoproteins: the spike (S), membrane (M), envelope (E), and nucleocapsid (N) proteins.[3,4] The S protein protrudes from the cell, and is responsible for viral binding and penetration into the host cell. The spike protein S consists of two subunits S1 and S2. S1 is related to binding with the host cell, whereas S2 is related to fusion of viral and host cell membranes.[3,5,6] The M, E, and N proteins are critical for viral particle assembly and release **(Fig. 1)**.

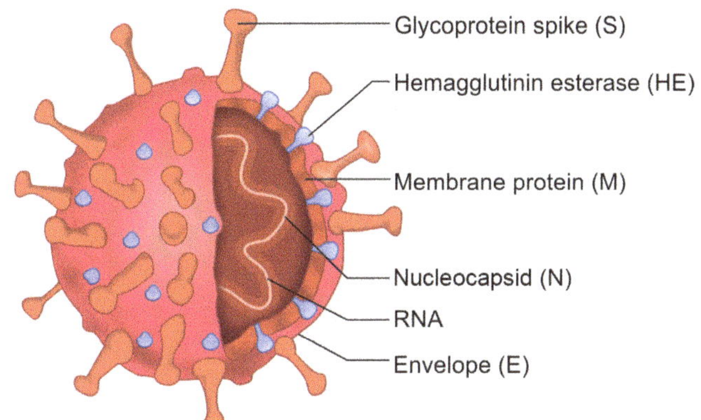

Fig. 1: Structure of Corona virus.

VIRAL TRANSMISSION

COVID-19 virus mainly spreads from person to person through contact, via the respiratory droplet transmission.

The infection occurs when aerosols or droplets from infected person come in contact with mucosal surface of eyes, mouth and nose of the host.[7-11] Exposure for prolonged period with an infected person at a distance of less than 6 feet or for more than 15 minutes increases the chances of its transmission.

Airborne transmissions occur in clinicians and healthcare workers during aerosol-generating procedures, e.g., endotracheal intubation and extubation, nebulization, suctioning, noninvasive ventilation, high frequency nasal cannula oxygenation and bronchoscopy.[12,13] The transmission also takes place via fomites through used clothes, utensils and equipment of an infected person.

Viral Shedding and Period of Infectiousness

The potential to transmit SARS-CoV-2 begins prior to the development of symptoms and is highest early, in the course of illness; the risk of transmission decreases thereafter. The duration of the symptom onset postexposure to an infected person is 5–6 days, and the maximum can scale up to 14 days. During this period, the virus is present in the nasal mucosa and even if the patient is asymptomatic, it can be highly contagious.

Transmissions after 7–10 days of illness is rather unlikely.[7]

CLINICAL PRESENTATION[1,10,14]

Presentations of COVID-19 have ranged from being asymptomatic to mild symptoms, to severe critical illness and even mortality. Typical symptoms include fever, dry cough and shortness of breath. The critical disease includes acute respiratory distress syndrome (ARDS), sepsis, septic shock, cardiac disease, thromboembolic events, such as pulmonary embolism and multiorgan failure.

There are other gastrointestinal symptoms such as nausea, vomiting, abdominal pain and diarrhea. Neurologically-related symptoms observed are anosmia (loss of smell) and dysgeusia (loss of taste), ischemic or hemorrhagic stroke, dizziness, headache, musculoskeletal disturbance, altered mental state, Guillain-Barré syndrome or acute necrotizing encephalopathy.

Cardiovascular events with COVID-19 include myocardial injury, especially in patients with severe infections, myocarditis and myopericarditis with reduced systolic function, cardiac arrhythmias and heart failure.

Ocular manifestations such as conjunctival hyperemia, chemosis, and increased secretions, have also been reported.

Children frequently have mild disease as compared to adults, with few or no symptoms.

PATHOPHYSIOLOGY

The life cycle of the virus consists of attachment, penetration, biosynthesis, maturation and release. Viruses attach themselves to host cell receptors and enter the cell.

COVID-19 infection can be divided into three phases, that correspond to different clinical stages of the disease **(Fig. 2)**.

Binding of SARS-CoV-2 spike (S) glycoprotein to the ACE-2 receptor

↓

Viral entry via membrane fusion or endocytosis

↓

Uncoating: Release of viral genomes in the cell

↓

RNA replication: Viral RNA enters the nucleus to create new RNA strand

↓

New viral RNA integrates and enters into endoplasmic reticulum (Nucleocapsids)

↓

Nucleocapsids released as Golgi bodies into cytoplasm

↓

New viral particles are released out of cell by exocytosis

↓

New viral particles infect the surrounding cells and are released as respiratory droplets

Fig. 2: Life cycle of SARS-CoV-2.

Stage 1: Asymptomatic State

Viral invasion: The virus enters the nasal cavity via respiratory aerosols or droplets which bind to the epithelial cells of the nasal mucosa. The S protein of the COVID virus binds to the angiotensin-converting enzyme 2 (ACE-2) receptors found in epithelial cells of nasal cavity and undergo a protease cleavage by transmembrane serine protein. ACE-2 receptors are functional receptors for SARS-CoV and are found in abundance in the pulmonary epithelial cells. ACE-2 are also found in other organs like small intestines, kidneys, heart, thyroid, testis, and adipose tissue; thus these organs can be affected during COVID viremia.[11,15,16]

This phase usually lasts for 5–6 days with limited immune response. The reverse transcription-polymerase chain reaction (RT-PCR) value for the viral RNA predicts the viral load and its subsequent infectivity and clinical course. Even if the viral load is minimal, the host can be infectious and the virus can be detected by nasal swab at this stage. It is found that patients on ACE inhibitors and ACE receptor blocking drugs have large number of ACE receptors available for viral attack, thus making them more susceptible to the COVID-19 infection.

Stage 2A: Upper Airway and Conducting Airway Response[16,17]

The virus propagates and migrates down the respiratory tract along the conducting airways, where it triggers an immune and inflammatory response, manifesting as clinical signs and symptoms of COVID-19. The immune response is generated via release of interferons (IFN β and INF λ) and chemokine ligand 10 (CXCL-10). Most patients develop this stage and are later treated by their own immune response. The patient presents with fever, cough, malaise and throat pain.

2B: Lower Respiratory Tract[10,16-19]

After the fusion with the host membrane, the virus enters the alveolar epithelial cells and the viral contents are released inside. The viral RNA enters the nucleus and undergoes replication with the help of enzyme RNA polymerase and the formation of negative stranded RNA occurs from a single stranded positive RNA.

The N protein of the virus attaches to the genomic RNA and the M protein helps it to integrate with the endoplasmic reticulum of the host cell. Thus, these newly produced nucleocapsids are transported to the lumen of endoplasmic reticulum and are evacuated as Golgi bodies to the exterior of the cell by exocytosis. These new viral particles then infect the surrounding epithelial cells and can also be transmitted via respiratory droplets. Disease progression is not only due to the viral load but also due to the consequences of dysregulated immune-mediated injury.

At this time, the disease COVID-19 is clinically manifested. The level of CXCL-10 may be predictive of the subsequent clinical course.

Stage 3: Hypoxia, Ground-glass Infiltrates, and Progression to ARDS[10,16-19]

About 20% of the infected patients progress to stage 3 disease and develop pulmonary infiltrates. The virus reaches the gas exchange units of the lung and infects the alveolar type II cell. The alveolar epithelial cells undergo apoptosis with the generation of further viral particles that infect other adjacent alveolar cells causing further lung damage.

The continuous ongoing lung damage, cellular destruction, and release of cytokines and inflammatory markers such as interleukins, tumor necrosis factor, monocyte chemoattractant protein-1 (MCP-1) and macrophage inflammatory protein-1α (MIP-1α) lead to 'cytokine storm'. This storm acts as a chemoattractant for neutrophils, CD4 helper T cells and CD8 cytotoxic T cells, which then begin to get sequestered in the lung tissue. Further cell invasion eventually leads to severe acute respiratory distress syndrome.[11] There may be profound lymphopenia as the virus infects and kills T lymphocyte cells. The virus inhibits lymphopoiesis and increases lymphocytoapoptosis. There will be a rise in markers of inflammation C-reactive protein (CRP), ferritin and interleukin-6 (IL-6) levels.

The pathological result of COVID-19 is diffuse alveolar damage with fibrin rich hyaline membranes and a few multinucleated giant cells. The aberrant wound healing may lead to more severe scarring and fibrosis than other forms of ARDS.

EXTRAPULMONARY INVOLVEMENT

Initiation with pulmonary involvement and progression to multiple organ system is the classical feature seen in severe cases of COVID-19. This extrapulmonary involvement could be due to unrestrained inflammation.

Involvement of Hematology and Coagulation System[20-22]

Critically ill patients without other risk factors for thrombosis can experience various thrombotic events, including microvascular thrombosis, venous and pulmonary thromboembolism, and acute arterial thrombosis.

The cytokine storm due to immune dysregulation is presented as a hypercoagulopathy state along with prolonged prothrombin time, PT/aPTT levels, elevated D-dimer and fibrinogen levels and thrombocytopenia. Patients develop disseminated intravascular coagulation during severe COVID-19 infection.

Complement activation leads to pulmonary tissue damage and microvascular injury.

Immune cell infiltration, secondary to the release of cytokines further leads to endothelialitis (inflammation of endothelial cell) and increased vascular permeability causing procoagulant effects, leading further to overt the disseminated intravascular coagulation (DIC).

Coagulopathy is also stimulated by neutrophils that are attracted by the activated endothelial cells, further releasing more cytokines, triggering further thrombosis.

Pulmonary thrombosis is commonly seen in patients with highly raised inflammatory markers; clinically, they present with refractory hypoxemia, V/Q mismatch, increased pulmonary shunting and a high chest tomography severity score (CTSS).

Cardiovascular Complications

Cardiovascular injury is seen in severe cases of COVID-19 infection. Elevated levels of cardiac markers like cardiac troponins and brain natriuretic peptide (BNP) are found in these patients. Elevated cardiac markers are correlated to raised inflammatory markers. Cytokine storm has been found to affect cardiac cells causing endothelial cell reprogramming.

Clinically, the patients present with arrhythmias, bradycardia, myocarditis, cardiac failure and cardiomyopathy; this could be due to respiratory failure or stress-induced cardiomyopathy. There are limited studies supporting direct infection of cardiac tissue by virus.[23,24]

Renal Complications

Impairment of renal function is observed in cases of severe COVID-19 infection. ACE-2 receptors widely present in kidney, makes the renal tissue more susceptible to the infection. A microscopic examination of the renal tissue of postmortem specimen has shown virally invaded tubular epithelium and podocytes. This leads to mitochondrial dysfunction, acute tubular necrosis and protein leakage. Along with direct infection, cytokine release, thrombosis and ischemia lead to further kidney injury.

Clinically, patients present with oliguria, anuria, acute kidney injury, raised blood urea nitrogen and raised creatinine, need renal replacement therapy as well as extracorporeal membrane oxygenation (ECMO).[25,26]

Hepatic Complications

There is no evidence that the direct infection of hepatocytes is the cause of liver involvement in COVID-19 patients. Some studies have demonstrated the presence of ACE-2 receptors on cholangiocytes, signifying direct bile duct damage. Liver injury can be drug-induced or can be due to hypoxia.

Systemic inflammatory responses causing T cell-induced hepatic necrosis could be one of the causes of hepatic damage.[27,28]

Clinically, patients have elevated levels of aspartate aminotransferase (AST), alanine aminotransferase (ALT), amyloid, elevated bilirubin and elevated gamma glutamyl transferase (GGT).

Gastrointestinal Complications

Gastrointestinal (GI) manifestations of COVID-19 infection are commonly seen and are associated with the direct infection of the enterocytes by the viral particles. There are evidences proving the isolation of SARS-CoV-2 RNA from GI epithelial cells. This causes the dysfunction of cells in ileum and colon.[28,29]

Clinically, patients present symptoms of fever, nausea, vomiting, loose motions and abdominal pain.

Pancreatic Complications

Acute diabetes is observed in many patients with COVID-19 and this could be due to damage done to endocrine pancreas. ACE-2 receptors have also been found in exocrine and endocrine parts of the pancreas.[30,31]

Viral-induced pancreatic dysfunction, immune dysregulation, vasculopathy and coagulopathy have all been linked to pancreatic damage.

Patients show raised amylase or lipase levels and high blood sugar levels with metabolic ketoacidosis in severely infected COVID-19 patients. It has been reported that diabetic patients with diabetic retinopathy were prone to more serious COVID infections.[31,32]

Central Nervous System Complications

Neurological damage could be due to the viral invasion in the endothelial cells of blood capillaries via the ACE-2 receptors.

The loss of taste and smell is due to direct damage of supporting cells of olfactory epithelium, olfactory bulb and altered ACE-2 signal transmission.

Central nervous system (CNS) manifestations could be due to respiratory or metabolic acidosis or multiorgan damage.

The clinical manifestations of neurological involvement include headache, giddiness, confusion, ataxia, stroke, Guillain-Barré syndrome and anosmia/hyposmia as well as loss of taste (ageusia).[33,34]

COVID-19 INFECTION IN CHILDREN

In contrast, COVID-19 can present with much milder symptoms in the pediatric population as compared to adults. The lower incidence could be due to lower expression of ACE-2 receptors on well-differentiated ciliated epithelial cells and a different response to SARS-CoV infection in pediatric population as compared to adults. The increased inflammatory response in the form of cytokine storm is not seen in children.[1]

The clinical presentation affects children in a milder form such as common cold, cough, fever, and very few develop severe symptoms such as breathlessness and the requirement of oxygen support.

COVID-19 IN PREGNANCY

Some studies have suggested that the physiological immune adaptations that occur in pregnancy prevent the hyperinflammatory phase of COVID-19. There is evidence of miscarriage, placental involvement and pre-eclampsia. Further research is needed to clarify the involvement in pregnant patients. Clinically, many pregnant patients present with pregnancy-induced hypertension, thrombocytopenia, coagulopathy, disseminated intravascular coagulopathy and acute kidney injury. Maternal COVID-19 is believed to be associated with low risk for vertical transmission.[35,36]

Cutaneous Complications

Multisystem inflammatory response presents with various cutaneous eruptions like Kawasaki disease and is seen in adults with COVID-19 infection.[37]

Psychiatric Complications

The isolation from relatives to halt the transmission with prolonged stay in intensive care leads to development of anxiety, fear of death, agitation, aggression, mania, depression and hallucinations in most of the patients of COVID-19 illness.

These patients should be treated with empathy, psychiatric counseling and antidepressants to calm them down.

Geriatric Complications

Elderly individuals are particularly at risk because of their diminished immune response and reduced ability to repair the damaged epithelium. The elderly also have a reduced mucociliary clearance, and this may allow the virus to spread to the gas exchange units of the lung more readily.[16]

ANESTHESIA IMPLICATIONS

Anesthesia for a COVID positive patient presents the anesthetist with a triad of responsibilities. The first is to manage the patient, keeping in mind the morbidity involved. Second, to prevent transmission of infection to all the healthcare providers. Finally, it is essential to prevent the contamination of the anesthesia machine and other anesthesia equipment.

Training: Training of the healthcare workers for proper donning and doffing of the personal protection kit and the N95 mask is mandatory.

Personal protection equipment (PPE) for healthcare workers doing aerosol-generating procedures: Appropriate PPE and respirator mask N95 or filtering face piece (FFP3) for health care workers doing the aerosol-generating procedures should be provided.

Protection of anesthesia equipment[13]*:* Only the necessary equipment should be kept in the operating room (OR) during aerosol-generating procedures in patients with COVID-19, to prevent unnecessary contamination and need for disinfection. Backup or emergency equipment should be kept immediately outside the OR and brought in as required by an assistant who is wearing appropriate PPE.

Surface contamination: Care must be taken to prevent contamination of the external parts of the anesthesia machine and other anesthesia equipment. Anesthesia machine, monitors and sonography machines can be covered with plastic sheets to reduce bioburden. The removal and disposal of such protective drapes should be done with utmost care since the possibility of contamination of personnel, equipment, or the operation theater still exists.

Contamination of the internal components of the anesthesia machine: The anesthesia machine, breathing circuit and its connection to the gas analyzer should be protected from becoming a source of infection for subsequent patients via the anesthesia machine. Viral filters with the highest viral filtration efficiency (VFE) are recommended. Two filters are recommended in the circuit, one at the expiratory end and one at patient end.

Decontamination: Routine cleaning of the anesthesia machine and reusable equipment should be performed. Disposables, including the anesthesia breathing circuit, reservoir bag, mask, forced air warming blanket, and any other disposable equipment should be disposed as contaminated waste.

The gas sampling tubing should be changed after use in a COVID-19 positive patient. There is no evidence that the soda lime carbon dioxide (CO_2) absorber needs to be changed after a COVID-19 positive case since it is protected by the filters in the breathing circuit and is highly alkaline and likely viricidal.

Preoperative COVID Screening

All patients who are scheduled for surgery should be tested for COVID-19 within 2 weeks prior to surgery.

INVESTIGATIONS

Blood Investigations

- *Complete blood count (CBC):* Shows decreased white blood cells (WBCs), lymphopenia, thrombocytopenia. Neutrophil: lymphocytes ratio (NLR)> 3.3 is associated with severe COVID infection.
- *Sugars:* High sugar levels are seen in diabetic as well as in nondiabetic COVID patients.
- *Liver function test (LFT):* Elevated alanine and aspartate transferase (ALT/AST).
- *Renal function test (RFT):* Raised creatinine and blood urea nitrogen (BUN).
- Elevated prothrombin time (PT), D-dimer and International normalized ratio (INR).
- Inflammatory markers-elevated CRP, IL-6, LDH, and ferritin levels are seen in moderate to severe COVID patients.

Radiology

- X-ray chest shows bilateral patchy opacities.
- HRCT chest shows bilateral ground-glass consolidation, cavitation, calcification and fibrosis. It is a gold standard for diagnosis with high sensitivity. CO-RAD Score and CT severity score are highly useful to assess the severity of disease and its prognosis **(Table 1)**.

Newer Diagnostic Tests

- *Reverse transcriptase loop-mediated isothermal amplification:* It is similar to RT-PCR and uses constant temperatures. It is a rapid test and result is available in 30 minutes.
- *Lung ultrasound:* It is used at some centers. It has a lower efficiency than CT scan. B lines are seen in COVID-19 positive patients.

Molecular Testing

- COVID RT-PCR taken by nasopharyngeal swab (poor sensitivity).

TABLE 1: CO-RAD Scoring for COVID-19 disease.

CO-RADS Score	*HRCT findings*	*Suspicion of lung involvement in COVID-19 infection*
CO-RADS 1	Normal CT or findings of non-infectious origin	Very low level of suspicion
CO-RADS 2	CT findings of lungs typical of infectious origin	Low level of suspicion
CO-RADS 3	• Findings suggestive of pulmonary involvement that can be due to other viral pneumonias • Homogeneous ground-glass opacities, secondary pulmonary lobules and/or interlobular septal thickening	
CO-RADS 4	Ground-glass opacities without contact with visceral pleura	High level of suspicion
CO-RADS 5	• Ground-glass opacities, with or without consolidation, close to visceral pleura, includes fissures and multifocal bilateral distribution • Typical crazy paving pattern and reverse halo signs	Very high level of suspicion
CO-RADS 6	All above features	COVID RT-PCR positive

- Rapid antigen test (SARS-CoV antigen testing) taken by nasopharyngeal swab-short processing time but less sensitive.
- COVID antibody testing—high titers are suggestive of immunity.

MANAGEMENT OF COVID-19

Treatment of COVID-19 is mostly symptomatic or supportive depending on the symptoms presented by the patients. Disease is divided into mild, moderate or severe grade according to the symptoms of the patients.[7,14,38-40]

Asymptomatic Phase

These are patients with COVID-19 RTPCR positive but clinically asymptomatic. They are advised self-isolation at home or at quarantine centers. They are started on zinc and vitamin C and D supplementation for boosting immunity. They are told to monitor oxygen saturation levels and to report to COVID care centers in case they develop any symptoms.

Mild Disease

These patients have symptoms of fever, running nose and cough. They have SpO_2 levels between 94 and 97% on room air.

Patients are admitted in dedicated COVID care center and started on oxygen therapy with nasal cannula or face mask.

They are started on treatment with tab hydroxychloroquine (HCQ) 400 mg two times a day on day 1 followed by 200 mg two times a day for 4 days (after ECG assessment for QT interval). They are also started on vitamin C and D, zinc supplements and tab ivermectin, tab acetaminophen and good hydration.

Patients with hypertension, chronic obstructive airway disease, kidney failure, and ischemic heart disease require special care.

Moderate Disease

This is the category of patients that maintain saturation between 90 and 94% on room air. These patients need to be isolated to prevent viral transmission. These patients are admitted and are intensely monitored for oxygen saturation levels, ECG, chest X-ray and ABG.

They are started on high concentration oxygen masks (nonrebreathing masks) at flows of 15 L/min. If they are still not maintaining saturation or have a respiratory rate >30/min, persistent dyspnea or deterioration in clinical condition, they are started on HFNO therapy (high frequency nasal oxygenation) or noninvasive ventilation (NIV masks).

The oxygen flow rate in HFNO is 30–40 L/min and needs to be altered as per patient's requirement. HFNO is not advised if the patient is drowsy, hypercapnic or there is no improvement at flow rate of 50 L/min and FiO_2 of >70%. Also, it is associated with aerosol generation so it should be used in negative pressure environment.

Patients who do not improve with 70 L/min flow of HFNO are put on noninvasive ventilation (BIPAP). NIV is given via a face mask with bilevel pressures for improvement in oxygenation. Moderate disease patients are started on tab HCQ 400 mg two times a day on first day followed by 200 mg two times a day for next 4 days. Injection methylprednisolone 0.5–1 mg/kg is started intravenous for 3 days along with anticoagulation with low molecular weight heparin (LMWH) given subcutaneously. Antibiotics are given to treat any secondary bacterial infections. High dose injectable vitamin C 200 mg/kg in 4 divided doses has proved to be beneficial in moderate to severely affected cases.

Severe Disease

These are the patients with oxygen saturation below 90% and have ARDS. They are started on noninvasive ventilation with BiPAP. Invasive ventilation with endotracheal intubation is instituted if there is no improvement in oxygenation or there is development of hypercapnia, hemodynamic instability or multiorgan failure. Endotracheal intubation is done by a skilled person wearing PPE, N95 mask, gloves and face shield. Mechanical ventilation is started with low tidal volume and high respiratory rate in view of ARDS. Prone ventilation is recommended in cases of refractory hypoxemia but requires adequate manpower. High PEEP and sigh maneuvers are used for lung recruitment. In cases of refractory hypoxemia with shock, the extracorporeal membrane oxygenation (ECMO) is recommended. ECMO provides improvement in oxygen levels in severe cases but is available at very few centers, besides being expensive. Lung transplant is the treatment for patients that recover from COVID ARDS with fibrotic lung and poor lung function **(Table 2)**.

Septic Shock Management

Patients with severe ARDS eventually develop septic shock and multiorgan failure. Patients present with hypotension, tachycardia, oliguria/anuria, raised WBC counts, raised lactate levels and hyperthermia. Patients usually require mechanical ventilation with vasopressor support of noradrenaline. Broad-spectrum antibiotics are started to combat secondary infections. Renal replacement therapy (RRT) is recommended for patients with irreversible renal failure.

OTHER MODALITIES OF TREATMENT

Corticosteroids: Steroids are considered for patients with ARDS or hypoxemia not responding to oxygen therapy. Injection methylprednisolone is given in 0.5–1 mg/kg/day dose and up to 1–2 mg/kg/day for severe cases. Dexamethasone is also found to be effective.

TABLE 2: Indicators of severe SARS-CoV-2 disease.

Sr. No.	Indicators of severe COVID infection
1.	Dyspnea at rest or with minimal activity (talking, sitting), SpO_2 on room air <92%, tachypneic, escalating oxygen requirement
2.	Impairment of consciousness
3.	Hemodynamically unstable (systolic blood pressure <100 mm Hg)
4.	Raised WBC, lymphopenia, high NLR ratio, thrombocytopenia and low hemoglobin
5.	Extensive chest X-ray infiltrate with rapid worsening from baseline
6.	Elevated prothrombin time, raised D-dimer, fibrinogen and fibrin degradation products (FDP)
7.	Elevated AST, ALT, raised bilirubin, hypoalbuminemia
8.	Hypokalemia and hypocalcemia
9.	High sugar levels
10.	• Elevated troponin I and creatine kinase-myocardial band (CK-MB) • Elevated brain natriuretic peptide (BNP), and troponin T
11.	Raised C-reactive protein (CRP), interleukin-6 levels (IL-6) , ferritin levels
12.	Raised erythrocyte sedimentation rate (ESR) and lactate dehydrogenase (LDH)
13.	Elevated procalcitonin and lactate levels
14.	Elevated creatine kinase and myoglobin levels

Inhaled steroids: Ciclesonide, an inhaled steroid, has antiviral and anti-inflammatory effect against SARS-CoV-2 and hence is being used to treat moderate to severe cases of COVID pneumonia, in doses of 200 μg twice a day.

Antiviral Drugs[38-40]

- *Remdesivir:* Remdesivir acts by blocking the action of viral RNA-dependent RNA polymerase which leads to reduced production of viral RNA. It is given in loading dose of 200 mg intravenous over 1–2 hours on day 1 followed by 100 mg intravenous daily for 5–10 days. It is not advised to give injection remdesivir in children, pregnant females and patients with hepatic and renal disease.
- *Lopinavir/Ritonavir (LPV/RTV):* Lopinavir acts by inhibiting the viral protease action. It was found to be effective in the Middle-East respiratory syndrome and so it was initially used as a treatment option for COVID-19. However, no significant advantage of LPV/RTV was seen along with the usual therapy of COVID.
- *Oseltamivir (Tamiflu):* Oseltamivir which had been used earlier for influenza outbreaks, has now been used in treating COVID-19 cases in a dose of 75 mg two times a day for 5 days. But there is no evidence of its efficacy against corona virus.
- *Favipiravir (Fabiflu):* Favipiravir gets converted into ribofuranosyl triphosphate by inhibition RNA-dependent RNA polymerase. It is recommended in a dose of 1800 mg two times a day on day 1 followed by 800 mg two times a day for next 14 days. It is effective in decreasing the viral load.

Immunomodulatory Drugs

Tocilizumab

Tocilizumab, monoclonal antibody against IL-6 was highly favored as a treatment in severe cases with a risk of cytokine storm. It is already accepted as a treatment for autoimmune diseases like rheumatoid arthritis. Its target of action is IL-6 receptors and, therefore, it has been used in moderate to severe cases of COVID-19 with rising inflammatory markers, patients in cytokine storm and refractory hypoxemia. It is given in a dosage of 8 mg/kg (maximum 800 mg) in 100 mL normal saline slowly over 1–2 hours. There is no advantage in giving second dose of Tocilizumab. On the contrary it leads to severe immunosuppression and can flare up secondary bacterial and fungal infections. Studies have shown decreased mortality in patients with severe COVID-19 infection after Tocilizumab.[41]

Newer immunomodulators—following are the newer immunomodulators in trial.

- Bruton's tyrosine kinase inhibitors—acalabrutinib, ibrutinib, zanubrutinib
- Janus kinase inhibitors—baricitinib, ruxolitinib, tofacitinib

Hydroxychloroquine and Chloroquine

Hydroxychloroquine is a derivative of chloroquine with better safety profile and has been found to reduce the viral load. Its antiviral action is synergized with azithromycin but can lead to prolongation of QT interval with resultant arrhythmias. It is also found to have immunomodulatory response and can supress the cytokine storm. The dose of HCQ is 400 mg two times a day on day 1 followed by 200 mg two times a day for next 4 days.

Chloroquine is an antimalarial drug with immunomodulatory and antiviral action. It blocks the viral invasion by increasing the endosomal pH needed for viral fusion and for receptor glycosylation. It is given in doses of 500 mg two times a day. It is found to reduce the viral pneumonia and thus cause symptomatic improvement.[38-40]

Antifibrotic Agents

Pirfenidone: 5-methyl-1phenyl-2-[1H]-pyridone is an antifibrotic agent used to treat moderate to severe pulmonary fibrosis caused due to COVID infection. It inhibits apoptosis, down regulates ACE receptors and decreases inflammation and reduces oxidative stress. It protects the pneumocytes from SAR-CoV-2 infection and cytokine storm. It requires LFT monitoring.[42]

Antibiotics

Antibiotics are generally not recommended in viral infections but macrolides like Azithromycin have an anti-inflammatory effect on the airways and have been used in COVID-19 infection.

Injection amoxicillin with clavulanic acid is used to treat secondary infections in patients with moderate to severe disease or in high-risk patients.

Therapeutic Plasma Exchange

Therapeutic plasma exchange (TPE) is a blood purification technique. TPE removes toxins of larger molecular weight and deleterious inflammatory cytokines responsible for cytokine storm syndrome and ARDS in COVID-19 severely ill patients. It can be used as an adjuvant therapy in critically ill patients.[43]

Plasma Therapy

Convalescent plasma is obtained from a treated COVID patient. This contains antibodies and can be used for treating patients with either severe infection or with increasing oxygen requirement. Only a person with high antibody titers can be a potential plasma donor. ABO compatibility and cross matching with donor plasma needs to be done. Dose for plasma therapy is 4–13 mL/kg that is approximately 200 mL slowly over 2 hours. It should be given for 2 consecutive days.[7]

Anticoagulants Drugs

COVID-19 patients are at high risk for thromboembolism. Prophylactic anticoagulant like LMWH is given in a dose of 40 mg subcutaneously once a day. Unfractionated heparin can be used in renal failure patients. Factor Xa inhibitors like fondaparinux and apixaban are being used for COVID-19 patients with elevated D-dimer levels.[44]

CORONA VACCINE

Covaxin by Bharat Biotech and Covishield by Astra Zeneca are the two vaccines that have cleared clinical trials in India and their regular use has started.[45]

CONCLUSION

A chronological sequence of the current COVID-19 pandemic observed from the perspective of an anesthetist is akin to watching a battle epic from the front row. Several factors combined to catapult the anesthetist to a position of frontline warrior in this struggle. Anesthetists were the logical choice for the management of COVID intensive care units given their expertise in ventilator therapy. They were at high risk as they performed procedures with aerosolization specially airway management and suction. Anesthesiology as a speciality fails to capture the public eye in our country but this pandemic offered us an opportunity to demonstrate our expertise not only as critical care physicians but also as leaders and managers.

REFERENCES

1. Yuki K, Fujiogi M, Koutsogiannaki S. COVID-19 pathophysiology. A review. Clinical Immunology. 2020;215:108427.
2. Ksiazek TG, Erdman D, Goldsmith CS, et al. A novel coronavirus associated with severe acute respiratory syndrome. New England Journal of Medicine 2003;348(20):1953-66.
3. Cascella M, Rajnik M, Cuomo A, et al. Features, evaluation and treatment coronavirus disease (COVID-19). In Stat pearls. Treasure Island (FL): Stat Pearls publishing; 2020.
4. Bosch BJ, Van der Zee R, De Haan CA, et al. The coronavirus spike protein is a class I virus fusion protein: structural and functional characterization of the fusion core complex. J Virol. 2003;77(16):8801-11.
5. Rabi FA, Al Zoubi MS, Kasasbeh GA, et al. SARS-CoV-2 and Coronavirus disease 2019: what we know so far. Pathogens. 2020;9(3):231.
6. Bosch BJ, van der Zee R, de Haan CA, et al. The coronavirus spike protein is a class I virus fusion protein: structural and functional characterization of the fusion core complex. J Virol. 2003;77:880111.
7. Parasher A. COVID-19: Current understanding of its pathophysiology, clinical presentation, and treatment. Postgrad Med J; 2020. pp. 2020-138577.
8. Liu J, Liao X, Qian S, et al. Community transmission of severe acute respiratory syndrome coronavirus 2, Shenzhen, China. Emergency Infectious Disease. 2020;6(6):1320-3.
9. Chan J, Yuan S, Kok K, et al. A familial cluster of pneumonia associated with the 2019 novel coronavirus indicating person-to-person transmission: a study of a family cluster. The Lancet. 2020;395(10223):514-23.
10. Huang C, Wang Y, Li X, et al. Clinical features of patients infected with 2019 novel coronavirus in Wuhan, China. The Lancet. 2020; 395(10223):497-506.
11. Bohn MK, Hall A, Sepiashvili L, et al. Pathophysiology of COVID-19: Mechanisms underlying disease severity and progression. Physiology (Bethesda). 2020;35(5):288-301.
12. Burke RM, Midgley CM, Dratch A, et al. Active monitoring of persons exposed to patients with confirmed COVID-19: United States, January–February 2020. MMWR Morb Mortal Wkly Rep March 6;69(9):245-246.
13. Ong SW, Tan YK, Chia PY, et al. Air, surface environmental, and personal protective equipment contamination by severe acute respiratory syndrome coronavirus 2 (SARS-CoV-2) from a symptomatic patient. JAMA. 2020;323(16):1610-2.
14. Thevarajan I. Buising KL, Cowie BC. Clinical presentation and management of COVID-19. Med J Aus. 2020;213(3): 134-9.
15. Hoffmann M, Kleine-Weber H, Schroeder S, et al. SARS-CoV-2 cell entry depends on ACE2 and TMPRSS2 and is blocked by a clinically proven protease inhibitor. Cell. 2020;181:271-80.e8.
16. Mason RJ. Pathogenesis of COVID-19 from a cell biology perspective. Eur Respir J. 2020;55(4):2000607.
17. Xu Z, Shi L, Wang Y, et al. Pathological findings of COVID-19 associated with acute respiratory distress syndrome. Lancet Respir Med. 2020;8:420-2.
18. Tay MZ, Poh CM, Rénia L, et al. The trinity of COVID-19: immunity, inflammation and intervention. Nat Rev Immunol. 2020;20:363-74.
19. Tian S, Hu W, Niu L, et al. Pulmonary pathology of early-phase 2019 novel Coronavirus (COVID-19) pneumonia in two patients with lung cancer. J Thorac Oncol. 2020;15:700-4.
20. Magro C, Mulvey JJ, Berlin D, et al. Complement associated microvascular injury and thrombosis in the pathogenesis of severe COVID-19 infection: A report of five cases. Transl Res. 2020;220:1-13.
21. Iba T, Levy JH. Inflammation and thrombosis: roles of neutrophils, platelets and endothelial cells and their interactions in thrombus formation during sepsis. J Thromb Haemost. 2018;16:231-41.
22. Connors JM, Levy JH. COVID-19 and its implications for thrombosis and anticoagulation. Blood. 2020;135:2033-40.

23. Guo T, Fan Y, Chen M, et al. Cardiovascular Implications of Fatal Outcomes of Patients with Coronavirus Disease 2019 (COVID-19). JAMA Cardiol. 2020;5(7):811-8.
24. Inciardi RM, Lupi L, Zaccone G, et al. Cardiac involvement in a patient with Coronavirus disease 2019 (COVID-19). JAMA Cardiol. 2020;5:819.
25. Chu KH, Tsang WK, Tang CS, et al. Acute renal impairment in coronavirus-associated severe acute respiratory syndrome. Kidney Int. 2005;67:698-705.
26. Su H, Yang M, Wan C, et al. Renal histopathological analysis of 26 postmortem findings of patients with COVID-19 in China. Kidney Int. 2020;98:219-27.
27. Chai X, Hu L, Zhang Y, et al. Specific ACE2 expression in cholangiocytes may cause liver damage after 2019-nCoV infection. BioRxiv; 2020;931766.
28. Cha MH, Regueiro M, Sandhu DS. Gastrointestinal and hepatic manifestations of COVID-19: A comprehensive review. World J Gastroenterol. 2020;26:2323-32.
29. Xiao F, Tang M, Zheng X, et al. Evidence for gastrointestinal infection of SARS-CoV- 2. Gastroenterology. 2020;158:1831-33.e3.
30. Wang F, Wang H, Fan J, et al. Pancreatic injury patterns in patients with Coronavirus Disease 19 pneumonia. Gastroenterology. 2020;159(1):367-70.
31. Cole SA, Laviada-Molina HA, Serres-Perales JM, et al. The COVID-19 pandemic during the time of the diabetes pandemic: Likely fraternal twins? Pathogens. 2020;9:389.
32. Drucker DJ. Coronavirus infections and Type 2 diabetes-shared pathways with therapeutic implications. Endocr Rev. 2020;41:457-70.
33. Vaira LA, Salzano G, Fois AG, et al. Potential pathogenesis of ageusia and anosmia in COVID-19 patients. Int Forum Allergy Rhinol. 2020;10(9):1103-4.
34. Jasti M, Nalleballe K, Dandu V, et al. A review of pathophysiology and neuropsychiatric manifestations of COVID-19. J Neurol; 2020. pp. 1-6.
35. Golden TN, Simmons RA. Maternal and neonatal response to COVID-19. Am J Physiol Endocrinol Metab. 2020;319(2): E315-9.
36. Baergen RN, Heller DS, Goldstein JA. Placental pathology in COVID-19. Am J Clin Pathol; 2020. p. 101.
37. Sachdeva M, Gianotti R, Shah M, et al. Cutaneous manifestations of COVID-19: report of three cases and a review of literature. J Dermatol Sci. 2020;98:75-81.
38. World Health Organization. Clinical management of COVID-19: interim guidance, 27 May 2020. Geneva: WHO, 2020. [online] Available from https://apps.who.int/iris/ handle/10665/332196. [Last accessed May, 2021].
39. Wang M, Cao R, Zhang L, et al. Remdesivir and chloroquine effectively inhibit the recently emerged novel coronavirus (2019-nCoV) in vitro. Cell Res. 2020;30:269-71.
40. Gao J, Tian Z, Yang X. Breakthrough: chloroquine phosphate has shown apparent efficacy in treatment of COVID-19 associated pneumonia in clinical studies. Biosci Trends. 2020; 14:72-3.
41. Zhang C, Wu Z, Li JW, et al. The cytokine release syndrome (CRS) of severe COVID-19 and Interleukin-6 receptor (IL-6R) antagonist Tocilizumab may be the key to reduce the mortality. Int J Antimicrob Agents; 2020. p. 105954.
42. Seifirad S. Pirfenidone: A novel hypothetical treatment for COVID-19. Med Hypotheses. 2020;144:110005.
43. Sarfraz A, Singh-Makkar S, Sarfraz Z, et al. (2020) Therapeutic Plasma Exchange and COVID-19: A Rapid Review. J Clin Immunol Immunother. 2020;6:041.
44. COVID-19 Treatment Guidelines Panel. Coronavirus Disease 2019 (COVID-19) Treatment Guidelines. National Institutes of Health. [online] Available from https://www.covid19treatment guidelines.nih.gov/ [Last accessed April, 2021].
45. ICMR. (2020). COVID-19 Vaccine. [online] Available from https://vaccine.icmr.org.in/covid-19-vaccine [Last accessed April, 2021].

Masks and Other Equipment in COVID-19

Naina P Dalvi, Sunil Gvalani, Maithili Thakur

ABSTRACT

The coronavirus disease 2019 (COVID-19) pandemic altered the approach to the management of acute respiratory distress syndrome (ARDS). Prevention of aerosol spread became the prime concern. Equipment preferences changed as updates about the pathophysiology and effective treatment of the disease arrived. High-flow nasal cannula (HFNC) and noninvasive ventilation (NIV) emerged as the preferred options while invasive ventilation was reserved for refractory cases. Use of personal protective equipment (PPE) while managing COVID patients became the norm.

This chapter discusses the equipment used extensively in COVID patients, but not described elsewhere in this book. The implications of other common equipment utilized for COVID management are also elucidated with the hope that every anesthetist will be oriented with this equipment.

INTRODUCTION

The coronavirus disease 2019 (COVID-19) pandemic presented the anesthesiologist with unfamiliar and challenging scenarios. Ventilators were in short supply and elective procedures were cancelled to reserve ventilators for COVID patients. Anesthesia machines were used as intensive care unit (ICU) ventilators in certain parts of the globe. Aerosol generating procedures (AGPs) became a threat and noninvasive ventilation (NIV) offered an attractive alternative so long as exhalation was filtered to prevent aerosolization. Anesthesiologists, although acknowledged as experts in oxygen therapy, were called upon to optimally utilize the entire spectrum ranging from the Hudson's mask, nonrebreather mask (NRBM), high-flow nasal cannula (HFNC), bilevel positive airway pressure (BiPAP) and finally intubation and invasive ventilation. This chapter attempts to present a rational use of the diverse equipment used in the management of COVID patients.

CLASSIFICATION OF EQUIPMENT

Equipment needed for COVID-19 management can be broadly classified as follows:

- *Equipment for oxygen therapy:*
  - *Oxygen source:*
    - Oxygen cylinder
    - Oxygen concentrator
  - *Oxygen delivery:*
    - Nasal cannula
    - Masks—Hudson mask, Venturi mask, and NRBM
    - HFNC
    - Noninvasive ventilation—continuous positive airway pressure (CPAP) and BiPAP machine with NIV mask
    - Ventilators
    - Extracorporeal membrane oxygenator (ECMO)
- *Equipment related to intubation*:
  - Laryngoscope with disposable blade
  - Video laryngoscope
  - Heat and moisture exchanger (HME) filter
  - Closed suction catheter system
- *Personal protective equipment (PPE)*

Several equipment enlisted here have been discussed elsewhere in this book. Their significance related to COVID-19 management will be highlighted here.

Equipment for Oxygen Therapy

Oxygen Source

Oxygen cylinder (Refer Chapter 4): Oxygen therapy plays an extremely important role in the management of COVID. Depending on the number of beds allotted to COVID patients, the liquid oxygen and oxygen cylinder supply should be arranged, as both low-flow and high-flow oxygen devices are used.

Oxygen concentrator ***(Figs. 1A and B)****:* During the COVID pandemic, hospitals were overcrowded due to the increasing number of COVID-19 patients. The availability of medical oxygen support was crucial and challenging. Oxygen concentrators also known as pressure swing adsorption (PSA) plants help to produce oxygen at the point of use, thus avoiding problems regarding accessibility and transportation.[1,2]

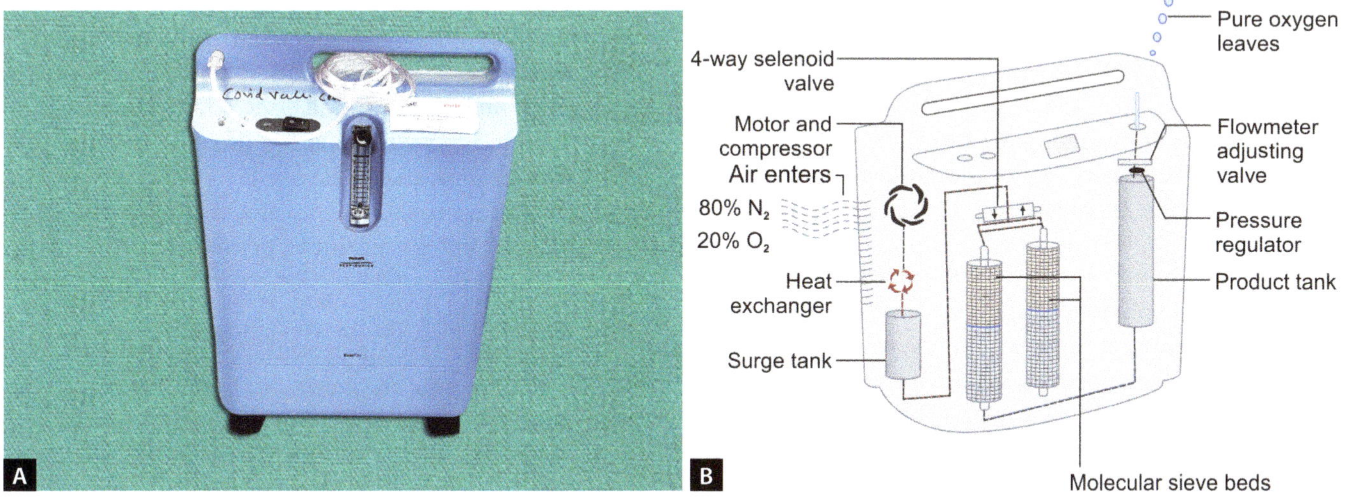

Figs.1A and B: (A) Oxygen concentrator; and (B) Working principle of oxygen concentrator.

These devices may be small, planned to provide oxygen to a single patient (i.e., portable), supply oxygen to an anesthetic machine or these can be large enough to supply oxygen for a medical gas pipeline system.[3]

Oxygen concentrators yield concentrated oxygen from air (consisting of 78% nitrogen, 21% oxygen, 1% argon, and a variable amount of water vapor). By removing nitrogen and water vapor, these supply 95% oxygen and 5% argon.[4]

This chapter discusses the portable oxygen concentrator.

- *Working principle*[3]

  An oxygen concentrator functions on the principle of differential adsorption under pressure of other gases in the atmosphere onto the surface of an adsorbent material, termed zeolite, and a family of aluminosilicates. Oxygen is not adsorbed by the zeolite and hence passes freely through it into a product (accumulator) tank, ready for later use.

  A portable oxygen concentrator has a compressor and a sieve bed filter. The atmospheric air is drawn and pressurized through a compressor. Thereafter, the compressed air is redirected through the sieve bed filters made of zeolite, which selectively retain the nitrogen and water vapor from the air leaving a high concentration of oxygen for delivery to the patient.

  Oxygen concentrators contain two or more zeolite columns, used in succession. Once the cycle of adsorption is complete, the second zeolite column is used for adsorption. Simultaneously, the first column is depressurized by applying a slight vacuum in the opposite direction, causing removal of the adsorbed nitrogen. This sequential switch between the columns is made by a time switch with cycles of around 20 seconds, thereby allowing sequential adsorption-desorption process known as pressure swing adsorption ensuring continuous supply of oxygen. The product (accumulator) tank acts as a reservoir of oxygen. Portable concentrators use a flow metering device to control the flow of product gas. The flow and pressure can be controlled for measured and continuous release of oxygen.

  The maximum achievable concentration of oxygen is around 95%. Argon is concentrated to 5% once all the nitrogen has been removed. Personal oxygen concentrators may supply up to 5–10 L/min oxygen. The typical noise level while operating is around 40 db.
- *Uses:*[1]
  - Most mild COVID-19 cases which do not require ventilatory support can be treated by oxygen therapy facilitated by oxygen concentrator. Such patients can receive oxygen from the safety and comfort of their homes using these devices.
  - It can be combined with a draw-over vaporizer, air compressor, breathing system, and ventilator to form an anesthesia delivery system.
  - Larger concentrators may be used as a backup to the primary hospital oxygen supply or as a main oxygen supply in remote hospitals with unreliable oxygen delivery.
- *Advantages:*[1]
  - It is a portable and cost-effective device for supplying oxygen at home as compared to oxygen cylinders and piped oxygen supply systems.
  - It is self-contained, relatively easy to install and maintain.
  - Contaminants such as sulfur dioxide, ethylene oxide, and exhaust hydrocarbons are filtered by the molecular sieve and released back into the atmosphere.
- *Disadvantages:*[1]
  - The system will stop producing oxygen in case of power failure. These can be powered by backup generators.
  - The oxygen concentrators deliver a maximum of 5–10 L/min which may be inadequate to treat critically ill COVID-19 patients.

- Regular servicing of the compressor is required. It is necessary to clean the air intake filters at the regular intervals.

- *Safety:*[1]
  - Explosion with high concentrations of oxygen can occur; hence home users should keep it away from open flames, heat sources, or electrically-operated devices.
  - The air should not be contaminated by fumes or other atmospheric pollutants.
  - Interruption of oxygen flow can occur due to mechanical or electrical malfunctions.

As per clinical management of COVID-19: Interim guidance by World Health Organization (WHO),[5] adults and children with severe respiratory distress, obstructed breathing, convulsions, and shock should receive emergency airway management and oxygen therapy targeting oxygen saturation (SpO_2) ≥ 94%.

Once stabilized, their SpO_2 should be maintained >90% in nonpregnant adults and children, and ≥92–95% in pregnant women using appropriate delivery devices such as nasal cannula (for rates up to 5 L/min); Venturi mask (for flow rates 6–10 L/min); and face mask with reservoir bag (for flow rates 10–15 L/min).

Oxygen Delivery (Refer Chapter 21)

Nasal cannula: Nasal cannulae are variable flow devices with plastic tubes shaped as two prongs which help to deliver oxygen into the nasal cavities, when connected to an oxygen source. They deliver fraction of inspired oxygen (FiO_2) of 0.24–0.4 at oxygen flows of 1-6 L/min, however, higher flows may cause nasal irritability and crust formation. Use of nasal prongs or nasal cannula is preferred in young children, as these are better tolerated.

Aerosol generation:[6,7] In stable patients using nasal cannula flows of 1 L/min, aerosol can spread up to 0.3 m, while in patients with respiratory distress using higher flows of 5 L/min, it can spread up to 0.42 m. Aerosol spread can further increase to 0.8 m with coughing and sneezing.

Recommendation:[7] In mild-to-moderate symptomatic patients, nasal cannula can be used at flows of 4–6 L/min, with the patient's face covered with N95 or equivalent face mask to prevent spread of infection.

Masks:

- *Hudson mask/simple mask:*[7] Simple Hudson face mask delivers FiO_2 of 0.35–0.5 at flows of 5–8 L/min and is used for the short duration of oxygen therapy in post-anesthesia care units.

  Aerosol generation: In stable patients on Hudson face mask requiring 4 L/min of oxygen flows, aerosol can spread up to 0.2 m. However, in patients with respiratory distress requiring flows ≥10 L/min, the aerosol spread can occur >0.4 m.

  Recommendations:
  - Hudson mask can be used only in cooperative patients with mild-to-moderate respiratory distress.
  - Open nebulizers should be avoided; rather a metered-dose inhaler with spacer device or manual in-line nebulization should be used.
  - Due to increased risk of aerosol spread with Hudson mask, hypoxic patients on nasal prongs may be directly escalated to *nonrebreathing masks*, skipping Hudson masks.

- *Venturi mask:*[6] If nasal cannula or Hudson mask cannot provide adequate oxygenation, a Venturi mask should be used. Supplemental oxygen by Venturi mask allows more precise FiO_2 (between 24 and 60% oxygen) to be delivered using an air/oxygen entrainment device (Venturi). Each FiO_2 level is achieved with a color-coded Venturi, which specifies the requisite oxygen flow rate. Oxygen flow rates vary from 3 to 15 L/min.

  Aerosol generation: Venturi masks generate aerosol up to 0.4 m at FiO_2 of 0.24 and up to 0.33 m at FiO_2 of 0.4.

  Recommendations: Exhalation filters can be used to reduce the spread of aerosol.

- *Nonrebreather mask:*[6] NRBM is a low-flow device consisting of a face mask connected to a reservoir bag filled with a high concentration of oxygen. NRBM should be used, if oxygen therapy with a 60% *Venturi* mask is insufficient. NRBMs deliver FiO_2 above 0.8 at flow rates approaching 15 L/min. These have an additional one-way valve that prevents room air entrainment and rebreathing of exhaled gases. The reservoir bag must always remain inflated to prevent hypercapnia by maintaining flow rates of at least 8–10 L/min.

  Nonrebreather masks offer a safe way to provide supplemental oxygen to COVID-19 patients as they help to limit the spread of aerosol.

  Aerosol generation: NRBMs cause aerosol spread of only up to 0.1 m.

  Recommendations:[7]
  - Exhalation filters can be used to limit the spread of aerosol.
  - Combined nasal cannula at 6 L/min and NRBM at 12–15 L/min may be considered in patients remaining hypoxic after NRBM alone.

High-flow nasal cannula **(Fig. 2)**:[8] Oxygen is typically delivered via low-flow systems (e.g., nasal cannulae or masks) or high-flow systems (e.g., Venturi masks and nonrebreathers). If SpO_2 is not maintained with these masks, then HFNC is used in COVID patients. HFNC reliably delivers warm and humidified oxygen at high flows through nasal cannulae.

- *Components of HFNC system:*
  - *An air/oxygen blender:* The pressurized oxygen and surrounding air is regulated by a flow meter and blender.

- *Humidifier:* A sterile distilled water reservoir is attached to humidifier for humidification of gases.
- *A warmed inspiratory circuit:* Insulated and/or heated circuit maintains temperature and relative humidity and prevents condensation **(Fig. 3)**.
- *Nasal prongs:* Custom-made soft, nonoccluding nasal cannula with prongs is used for oxygen delivery. There are different sizes of cannulae available, depending on the outer diameter. They are small, medium, and large allowing 50 L/min, 70 L/min, and 80 L/min flow. Infant and pediatric size cannulae allow lower flows (20–25 L/min). There is a separate adaptor available for tracheostomy patients. The nasal cannula should snuggly fit into the patient's nares and prevent entrainment of room air around the cannula. A maximum flow rate for each cannula size corresponding to the size and age of the patient is decided by the manufacturer.

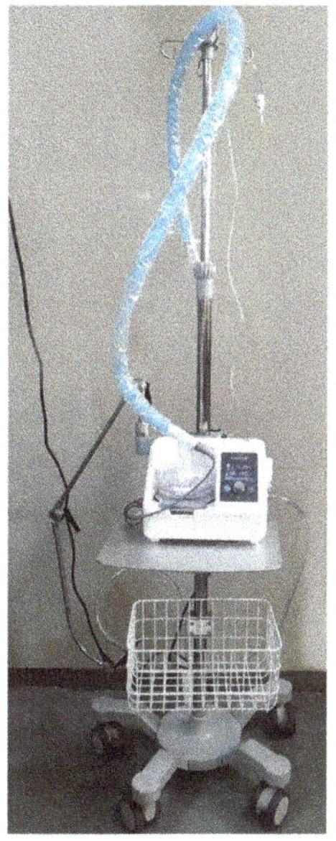

Fig. 2: High-flow nasal cannula (HFNC) machine.

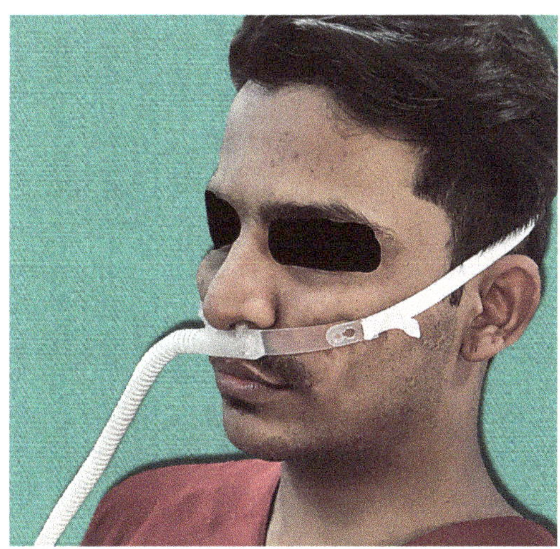

Fig. 3: High-flow nasal cannula (HFNC) .

In HFNC, the FiO_2 may be adjusted from 0.21 to 1.0, flow rates may be as high as 60 L/min in adults, gases can be heated up to 37°C and humidification approaches 100%.

- *Mechanism of action:*
  - *Warming and humidification:* Warming inspired oxygen and heating it to core temperature is more effective than low-flow rates. HFNC is better at heating and humidifying inspired oxygen at high-flow rates (typically >40 L/min) than conventional high-flow systems such as Venturi masks or nonrebreathers (flow rate typically 10–15 L/min) or low-flow systems (flow rates typically <10 L/min). Warm and humidified gases decrease airway inflammation and maintain mucociliary function to improve mucous clearance. They also decrease the work of breathing and oxygen demand in acute respiratory failure.
  - *Washout of nasopharyngeal dead space:* Upper airway dead space is washed out from the delivery of a large amount of oxygen to improve the efficiency of ventilation and enhance oxygen delivery. This improved washout with HFNC permits a higher fraction of minute ventilation to participate in alveolar gas exchange.
  - *Continuous positive airway pressure effect:* HFNC increases nasopharyngeal airway pressure that peaks at the end of expiration. This CPAP effect can decrease work of breathing and enhance oxygenation in the acute respiratory distress syndrome (ARDS). A better CPAP effect is achieved with the mouth closed. In general, every increase of 10 L/min of flow yields approximately 1 mm Hg of positive end-expiratory pressure (PEEP) with closed mouth breathing. The use of HFNC can also decrease preload by increasing intrathoracic pressure, commonly attributed to PEEP.
  - *High-flow rates:* High-flow rates cause alveolar recruitment and increased FRC as well as increased intrathoracic pressure likely due to added PEEP. High-flow rates result in minimal entrainment of room air, resulting in more accurate delivery of oxygen, especially when compared with conventional delivery systems. Patients in respiratory distress generate high inspiratory flow rates that exceed flow rates of standard oxygen equipment, resulting in entrainment of room air, and a reduction in FiO_2. The flow rate in HFNC generally exceeds that of the patient, entraining little room air and resulting in delivery of FiO_2. High-flow rates also improve the breathing pattern by decreasing inspiratory effort, increasing tidal volume, and decreasing respiratory rate.
- *Advantages:*
  - The work of breathing is reduced due to washout of dead space.
  - The ability to cough and clear secretions is preserved.

- Progress is better assessed due to improved communication with the patient.
- Excellent tolerance for extended periods as:
    - The HFNC cannula is lightweight, soft, and pliable, so extremely comfortable as compared to tight fitting CPAP or other face masks.
    - Patient can speak and eat while on HFNC.
    - Higher long-term compliance is seen with HFNC due to warm humidified gases.

  In a resource-constrained setting, HFNC for severe COVID-19 hypoxemic respiratory failure is feasible and nearly half of those who receive it can be successfully weaned without the need for mechanical ventilation.

- *Disadvantages:*
    - Positive end-expiratory pressure generated by HFNC is variable due to air leak, especially if the mouth is open.
    - Abdominal distension can lead to aspiration.
    - Rarely, barotrauma (e.g., pneumothorax) can occur

Noninvasive ventilation equipment:

Overview: NIV is the administration of ventilatory support via a patient-device interface without using invasive artificial airway. Thus, it eliminates the need for invasive airway in COVID-19 patients, thereby decreasing the ongoing damage to the lungs due to ventilator-induced lung injury. NIV provides almost similar physiological benefits as the conventional mechanical ventilation by improving gas exchange at alveolar level and reducing the work of breathing.[9]

Principle:[10] The working of NIV depends on developing a positive airway pressure within the lungs. This forces the air into the lungs, decreasing the respiratory efforts, and reducing the work of breathing. It also helps to keep lungs expanded by increasing the functional residual capacity after a normal tidal expiration, facilitating adequate gaseous exchange in the alveoli.

The two types of NIV are CPAP and BiPAP depending on either continuous or variable pressures of delivery of oxygen. The use of NIV in patients with COVID-19 and acute hypoxemic respiratory failure (AHRF) is favored by most organizations including the WHO, the English National Health Service, National Institutes of Health, the Society of Critical Care Medicine/European Society of Intensive Care Medicine Surviving Sepsis Campaign, and the Italian Respiratory Society.[9]

1. *Continuous positive airway pressure:*[10,11] CPAP is the most basic level of ventilatory support and provides continuous fixed positive pressure throughout inspiration and expiration. CPAP is beneficial in AHRF as it causes recruitment of collapsed alveoli and corrects ventilation-perfusion mismatch to improve oxygenation.

   Severe hypoxemia and well-preserved lung mechanics are characteristics of patients with COVID-19 pneumonia and ARDS; hence they benefit from CPAP therapy.

   Indications:
    - Management of hypoxemia in COVID-19 patients with ARDS who are unable to maintain adequate oxygen saturation on HFNC.
    - Type I respiratory failure
    - Obstructive sleep apnea (OSA)
    - Cardiogenic pulmonary edema and congestive heart failure

   Disadvantages: It is difficult to breathe against singular continuous pressure. Exhalation can be challenging at higher pressures.

2. *Bilevel positive airway pressure:* BiPAP provides differential airway pressure at inspiration and expiration. The inspiratory positive airway pressure (iPAP) is higher than the expiratory positive airway pressure (ePAP). Therefore, ventilation is provided mainly by iPAP, whereas ePAP recruits the collapsed alveoli for gas exchange. This facilitates the elimination of the exhaled gas, thus improving tidal volume and minute ventilation. BiPAP comes to rescue when the airway cannot be opened adequately with CPAP or when CPAP cannot be tolerated by the patient.

   BiPAP device therapy modes: Depending on the type of bilevel machine, it may have several modes of operation. A bilevel ST machine is the most advanced and acts like a ventilator.
    - *Continuous positive airway pressure:* CPAP maintains a constant level of pressure throughout the breathing cycle.
    - *Spontaneous (S) pressure support:* Breaths are patient-triggered and patient-cycled. The device triggers to iPAP in response to spontaneous inspiratory effort and cycles to ePAP during exhalation. The device also cycles a patient-triggered breath if no patient exhalation effort is detected for 3 seconds.
    - *Spontaneous/timed (S/T) pressure support:* Each breath is patient-triggered and patient-cycled or machine-triggered and machine-cycled. S/T mode is like S mode, except that the device also will enforce a set minimum breath rate by, if necessary, providing machine (time)-triggered breaths.
    - *Timed (T) pressure support:* Breaths are machine-triggered and machine-cycled. T mode provides mandatory pressure assist with bilevel pressures. The patient's breathing rate has no effect on the machine rate or pressure levels. The trigger to iPAP is determined by the breath rate setting, and the cycle time is determined by the inspiratory time setting.
    - *Pressure control (PC):* Each breath is patient or machine-triggered and machine-cycled. PC mode is similar to S/T mode, except that all breaths are machine-cycled. This is a pressure-limited,

machine- or patient-triggered, and time-cycled mode. The cycle time is determined by the inspiratory time setting.
- *Average volume-assured pressure support with auto-ePAP (AVAPS-AE):* It provides an automatically adjusting ePAP, pressure support, and back-up breath rate. The device monitors the patient's upper airway resistance and automatically adjusts the delivered ePAP required to maintain a patent airway.

Indications:
- COVID-19 positive patients with moderate ARDS (P/F ratio of 100–200) with hemodynamic stability and hypercapnia
- Type II respiratory failure
- Obstructive sleep apnea
- Acute exacerbation of chronic obstructive pulmonary disease (COPD)

Contraindications:
- Facial trauma and anatomical distortion
- Excessive secretions
- Increased risk of aspiration

Advantages:
- Positive end-expiratory pressure effect is better with BiPAP as compared to HFNC. The pressures are better controlled.
- With BiPAP machine, patients can breathe comfortably as the machine reduces the pressure level during exhalation, allowing the patient to exhale more easily.

Structure of CPAP/BiPAP machine:[11,12] Structure of CPAP/BiPAP machine is given in **Figures 4A and B**.

The CPAP/BiPAP machine includes:
- The flow generator/ventilator provides the pressurized airflow.
- The flexible tubing is a hose connecting the air outlet port on ventilator to the patient interface.
- The patient-device interfaces are varied and include:[13-15]
  - *Oral NIV interface* ***(Fig. 5):*** It is a mask covering only the mouth. Oral interface is used for patients needing long-term ventilation with severe chronic respiratory failure due to neuromuscular disease.
  - *Nasal mask* ***(Fig. 6):***[13,15] Nasal mask is the first choice for long-term ventilation but has also been used for acute respiratory failure cases.

    Advantages:
    - Less interference with speech and eating
    - Less likely to cause gastric distension
    - Better patient tolerance than nasal cannula

    Disadvantages:
    - Tidal volume monitoring is unreliable in the presence of an expiratory air leak.
    - It cannot be used in patients with soft palate defects.
  - *Oronasal/face mask*[13] ***(Fig. 7):*** Face masks are preferred for patients with acute respiratory failure because these patients generally breathe through the mouth to bypass nasal resistance. Many commercially available masks consist of two parts:
    1. Cushion of soft material (polyvinyl chloride, polypropylene, silicone elastomer, or hydrogel), which forms the seal against the patient's face.

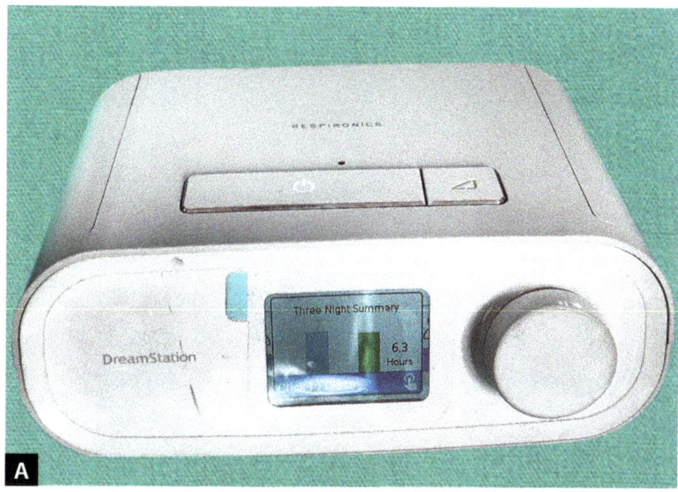

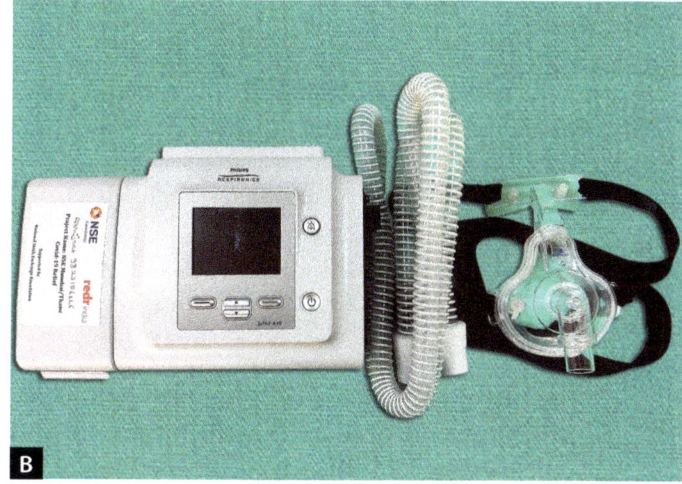

Figs. 4A and B: (A) CPAP machine; (B) BiPAP machine.

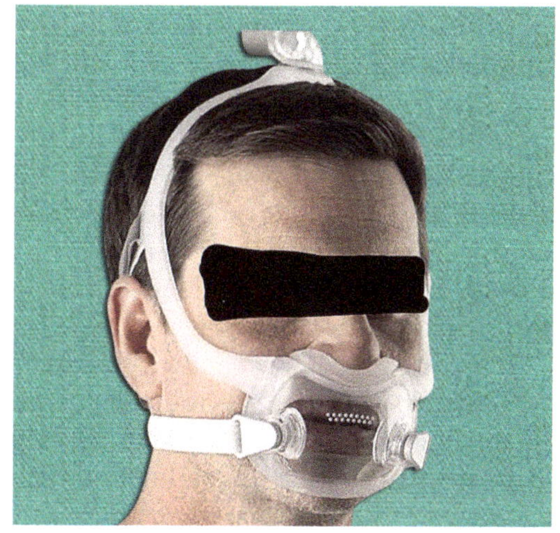

Fig. 5: Oral noninvasive ventilation (NIV) interface.

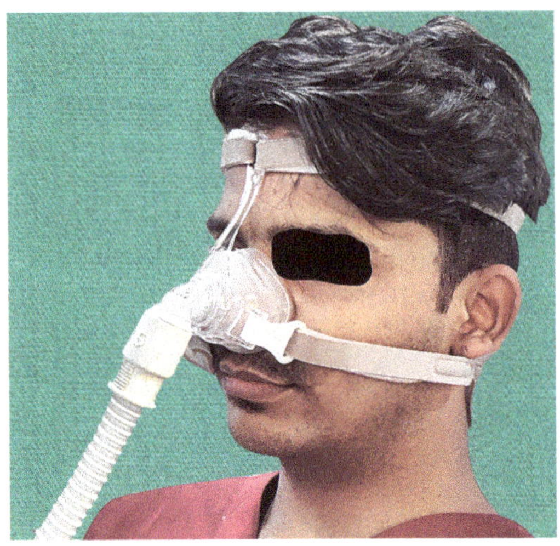

Fig. 6: Nasal noninvasive ventilation (NIV) interface.

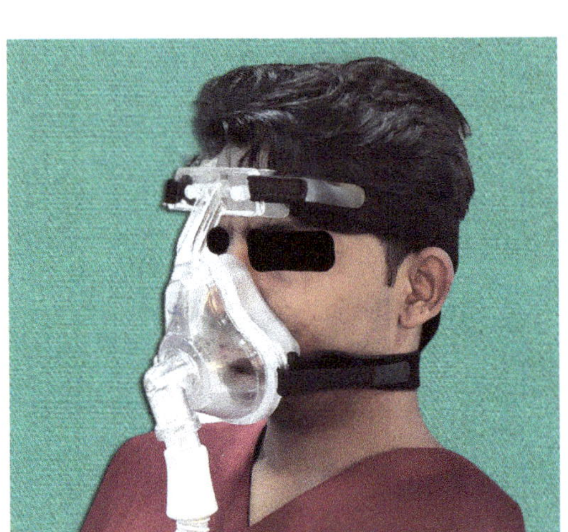

Fig. 7: Face noninvasive ventilation (NIV) mask.

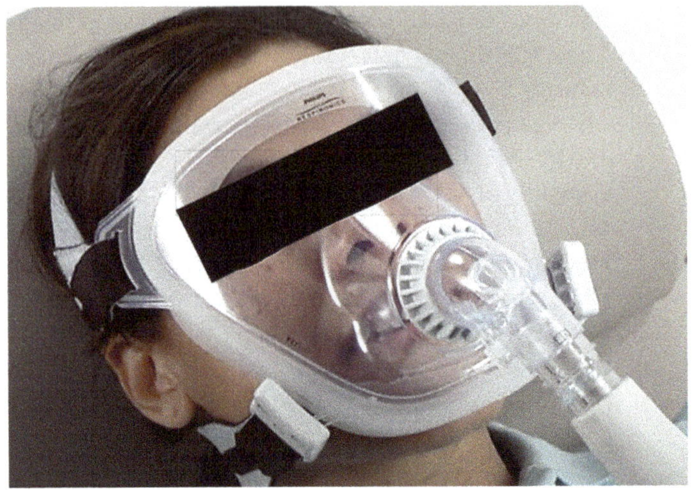

Fig. 8: Cephalic mask.

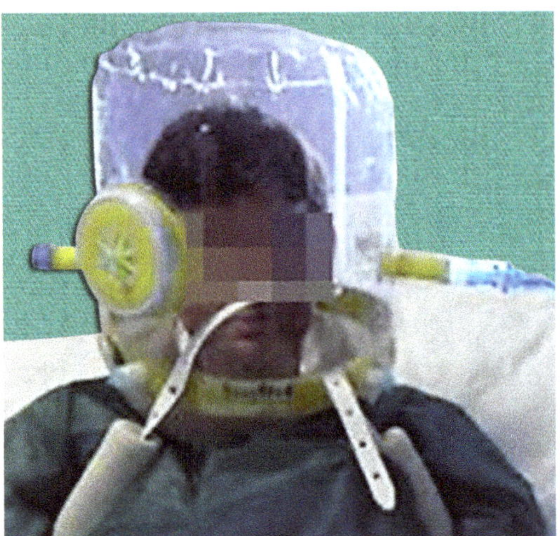

Fig. 9: Helmet noninvasive ventilation (NIV) interface.

2. Frame of stiff material (polyvinyl chloride, polycarbonate, or thermoplastic), which may be transparent.

The mask frame has several attachment points to fasten the headgear. More the number of attachment points, the better the chances of achieving the optimum seal. Some designs of CPAP face mask have a 22-mm female taper inlet such as anesthetic face masks. In this case, a "T"- or "Y"-shaped connector on the mask allows oxygen delivery to one limb with the CPAP valve situated on the other. Other designs have two taper inlets, one for oxygen delivery, and the second to accommodate the CPAP valve directly.

The masks are vented or nonvented. Vented masks allow exhaled gases to be vented to environment.

A total full face mask (cephalic mask) **(Fig. 8)** has a soft cuff that seals at the perimeter of the face to minimize pressure of oronasal mask contact areas. A cephalic mask covers the entire anterior surface of the face and hence, has a larger inner volume as compared with oronasal mask.

Conventional CPAP masks cannot be used for treating COVID-19 patients because the exhaled gases are vented to the room. To avoid contamination of the environment and for safety of clinicians, nonvented ventilation mask should be used. CPAP mask can cause claustrophobia.

- *Helmet interface*[13,15] ***(Fig. 9)****:* A helmet has a transparent hood and soft (polyvinyl chloride or silicone) collar that comes in contact with the body at the neck or shoulders. A helmet has at least two ports for entry and exit of the gases.

  Advantages:
  - It is superior in terms of safety for viral transmission as it is a closed system with viral filters in COVID-19 patients.
  - It reduces the risk of facial pressure sores.
  - It offers less interference with speech and cough
  - It offers less resistance to flow

Disadvantages: It may lead to swallowing of air, with resultant gastric distension and a risk of aspiration of gastric contents.

An ideal interface is one that gives the best combination of efficacy and comfort. The optimum interface differs in every patient, and trials of different interfaces are recommended for initial fitting and titration of the CPAP.

Contraindications to CPAP/BiPAP:[14]

- Impaired consciousness and raised ICP
- Hemodynamic instability
- Pneumothorax, lung abscess, and hemoptysis
- Facial fractures, trauma, and deformity
- Recent upper gastrointestinal (GI) surgery, hematemesis

Complications:

- *Aerosol generation:*[7] CPAP of 5–10 cmH_2O can cause aerosol generation up to 332 mm depending on different machines. In symptomatic patients, NIV generates aerosol of >10 μm diameter. BiPAP too can cause significant aerosol generation with increasing inspiratory pressures. At constant expiratory pressures of 4 cmH_2O, increasing inspiratory pressures from 10 to 18 cmH_2O increases aerosol spread from 0.65 to 0.85 m. A one-way valve, Whisper swivel adapter used to prevent rebreathing can increase aerosol spread beyond 1 m.
  Recommendations:
  - Noninvasive ventilation can be used in COVID-19 infection with all precautions related to the airborne spread.
  - Inspiratory pressures should be kept at a minimum level, preferably ≤10 cmH_2O.
  - Air leak should be minimized using snuggle-fitting masks or helmet.
  - Whisper swivel adapter and vented masks should be avoided.
  - Breathing circuits should be used with high-efficiency particulate air (HEPA) filters at the exhalation port.
- *Barotrauma:* Patients with less compliant lungs, as in COVID, are at risk of developing barotrauma. Pneumothorax must be recognized and assessed regularly with serial chest X-rays; if necessary, early intervention for the same should follow.
- *Facial pressure ulcers:* Grade I pressure ulcers can occur in many patients after a couple of hours and most patients after 48 hours of NIV therapy. These can be prevented by use of a nasal forehead spacer to reduce pressure on the bridge of the nose, use of forehead pads and by adequate skin, and mask hygiene.
- *Eye irritation:* Mask should be fitted correctly to prevent oxygen leaking upward to the eyes since this may cause eye irritation and conjunctivitis.
- *Retention of secretions:* The use of a full face mask and positive pressure created may affect the patient's ability to produce sufficient expiratory flow rates. This may hinder the ability to cough and impair the adequacy of mucociliary clearance.
- *Dry mouth:* Continuous positive pressure and high flows can cause severe drying and parching of the mouth. Patient needs to be well hydrated either with intravenous fluids or by water intake through Ryle's tube.

Ventilators (Refer Chapter 10): Invasive ventilation is used extremely late in COVID management, if patient deteriorates with NIV. Intubation and endotracheal suctioning are AGPs and demand highest level of personal protection in ICU. Proning helps in improving outcome. The mortality on invasive ventilation is quite high.

Extracorporeal membrane oxygenator ***(Fig. 10):*** ECMO is defined as the use of extracorporeal gas exchange and/or hemodynamic assistance to provide temporary life support in patients with reversible pulmonary or cardiac failure, alternatively known as extracorporeal carbon dioxide removal (ECCR), or extracorporeal life support (ECLS).

In COVID-19 patients who received ECMO, estimated mortality 90 days after ECMO was <40% compared to patients who did not receive ECMO.[16]

There are two types of ECMO:[17,18]

1. *Venovenous (VV)* ***(Fig. 11):***
   - In VV-ECMO, blood is removed from one or two large veins, circulated externally through the ECMO circuit (with membrane lung and pump), and then returned to the venous side of circulation.
   - It does not provide cardiac support to assist systemic circulation.
   - It requires only venous cannulation.
   - Higher perfusion rates may be required.

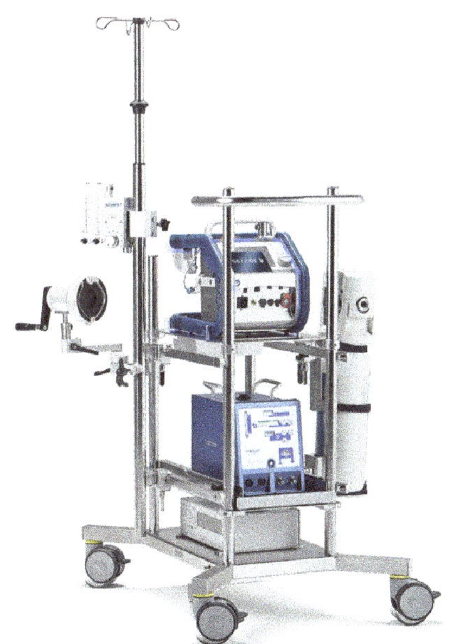

Fig. 10: Extracorporeal membrane oxygenator (ECMO) machine.

- It achieves lower arterial oxygen tension (PaO_2).
- ECMO circuit is in series to the heart and lungs.

2. *Venoarterial (VA)* ***(Fig. 12):***
   - In VA ECMO, blood is returned to the body into systemic arterial circulation. Both the patient's lungs and heart are bypassed, and cardiac output is supported by the ECMO pump.
   - It provides cardiac support to assist systemic circulation.
   - It requires arterial and venous cannulation.
   - Lower perfusion rates may be adequate.
   - It achieves higher PaO_2
   - Extracorporeal membrane oxygenator circuit is in parallel to the heart and lungs.

Components of ECMO ***(Fig. 13):*** A standard ECMO circuit consists of a mechanical blood pump, gas exchange device, and a heat exchanger. They are interconnected with circuit tubings.

- *Pump:* The ECMO pump provides flow appropriate for the patient within a safe range of pressures to avoid hemolysis. Pumps are of two types:
  1. *Roller pump:* Roller pumps have been in use since a long time. They generate direct suction on the venous catheter. There is a small transducer or collapsible bladder positioned at the lowest point of the venous line. It avoids excessive pressure by slowing or stopping the roller pump when a threshold suction is reached and vice versa. (i.e., restarts the

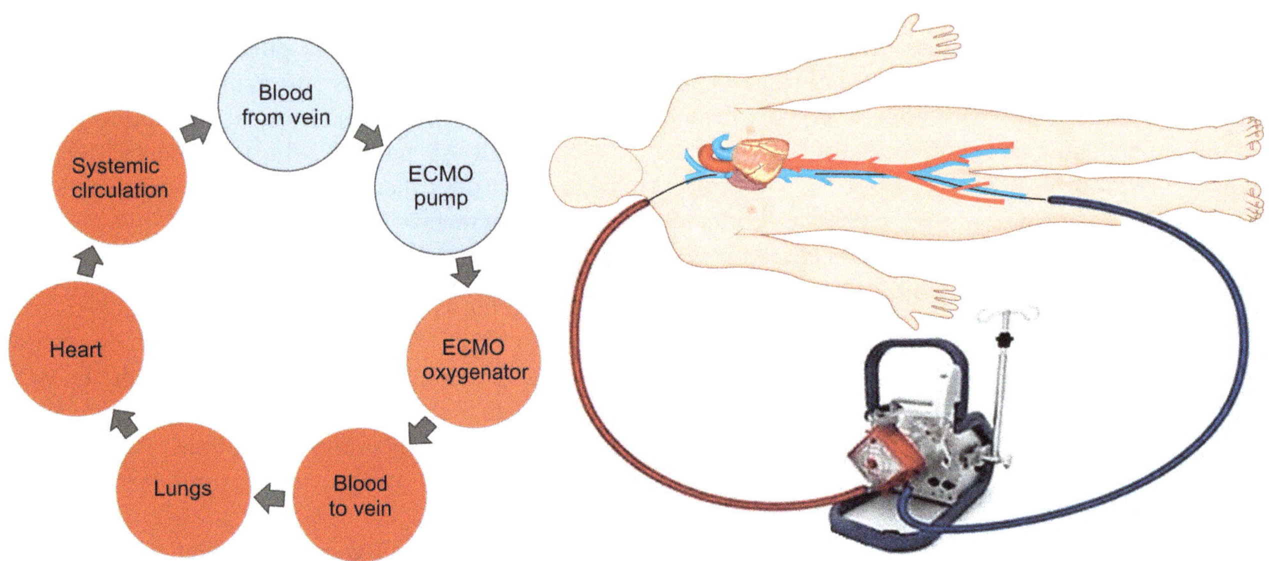

Fig. 11: Venovenous extracorporeal membrane oxygenator (VV-ECMO).

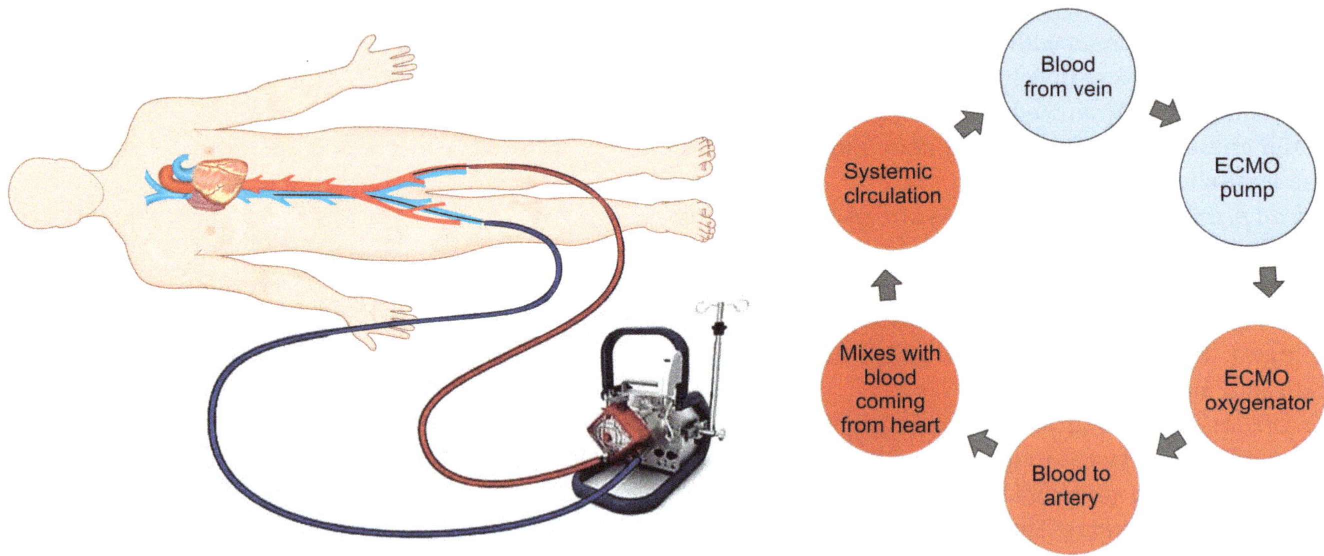

Fig. 12: Venoarterial extracorporeal membrane oxygenator (VA-ECMO).

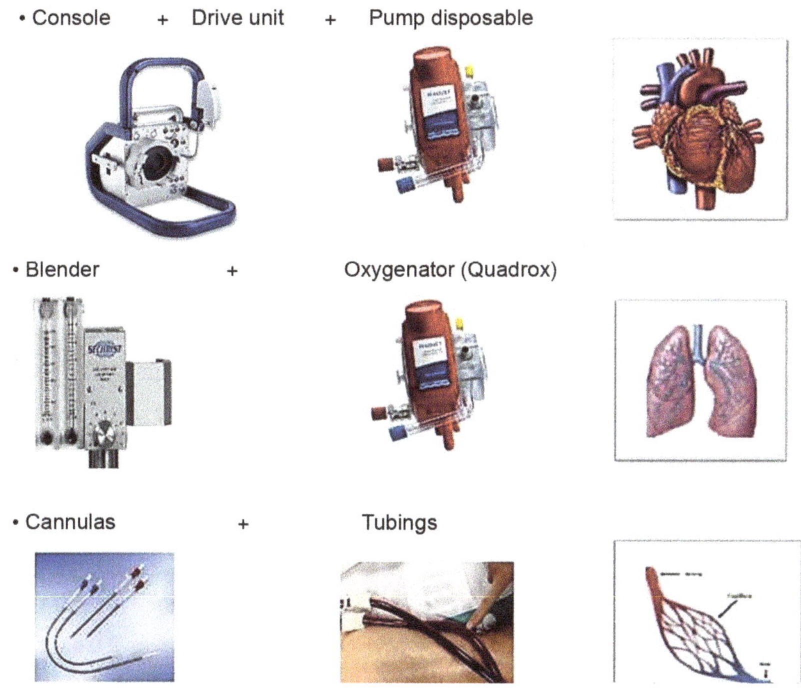

Fig. 13: Components of extracorporeal membrane oxygenator (ECMO).

pump when the venous drainage flow exceeds the pump flow). The disadvantages of roller pump are the need of heavy motor to run it and the rupture of tubing in the pump head with excessive infusion pressure.

2. *Centrifugal pump:* It is a newer pump in which a spinning rotor generates flow and pressure. It has longer pump head durability and can be used for prolonged extracorporeal circulation. Its motor is light and small, the components do not wear out, and the perfusion pressure is limited by the revolutions per minute (RPM), so circuit rupture is extremely rare. The potential problems of a centrifugal pump head include stagnation and heating in the pump head, leading to thrombus at low flows or when outlet line is occluded. Cavitation and hemolysis can occur when the inlet line is occluded. Maquet rotaflow pump (Maquet, Hirrlingen, Germany) is a new centrifugal pump which can reduce heat generation of the bearing and seal and lessen blood damage. Centrifugal pumps have a hole in the center of the rotor which prevents the stagnation, thrombosis, and heat problems.

- *Oxygenator:* Oxygenator is a gas exchange device with a semipermeable membrane. This membrane selectively permits diffusion of gas into and out of the blood. Deoxygenated blood is drained from a central vein via an external pump, passes through the oxygenator, and is returned to the patient through a reinfusion cannula. It is necessary to have a variety of sizes available to support patients of differing sizes.

Oxygenators are of two types:

1. *Silicone rubber membrane oxygenator:*
   - It is constructed of a flat reinforced sheet of silicone rubber membrane envelope wrapped around a wire mesh in a spiral coil. This membrane oxygenator is effective in gas exchange.
   - A separate heat exchanger is required for smaller silicone membrane lungs.
   - The silicone lung has a high resistance to flow which limits the maximum blood flow making it less suitable for use with centrifugal pumps.
   - Due to high resistance, a silicon oxygenator is much harder to de-air, so it takes longer to prime.
2. *Hollow fiber polymethylpentene (PMP) oxygenators:*
   - It has the hollow fibers bundled together with gas inside and blood outside the fibers within the oxygenator.
   - This design and the blood flow pattern through the device are all key factors in decreasing the priming volume, hence well suited for centrifugal blood pumps.
   - It is extremely efficient at gas exchange and demonstrates minimal plasma leakage.
   - This oxygenator is more compact with smaller surface area of the membrane and heat exchanger, thus reducing its potential for thrombus formation and inflammatory activation.
   - It also contains an integrated heat exchange device, thus controlling body temperature without the need for additional components.

- *Vascular cannula:*
  - *Single-lumen cannula:* It is used to provide venous and arterial access for patients receiving VA ECMO or multiple site venous access for patients receiving VV extracorporeal support. It is made up of biocompatible polyurethane, which may be coated with heparin or nonheparin polymers to prevent platelet activation and inflammatory response at the blood-cannula interface. Cannulae are available in different sizes ranging from 6F (2-mm diameter) to 51F (17-mm diameter). This cannula has wire-reinforced body to prevent luminal occlusion. Jugular and femoral cannulae have a long, multifenestrated flexible tip, whereas cannulae with a single end-hole or a short-fenestrated tip may be used for arterial or venous vascular access.
  - *Dual-lumen cannula:* It provides VV support via a single jugular venous access site. Blood is removed from the patient via one lumen and then returned to the patient via a smaller lumen. Proper positioning of the tip of the cannula near the inferior cavoatrial junction is necessary for optimal cannula performance. Echocardiographic or fluoroscopic imaging is necessary to confirm proper cannula placement. This cannula is available in sizes ranging from 13F to 31F, to be used to support neonates as well as adults.

Indications:
- Underlying disease process which is treatable and potentially reversible.
- Oxygenation index (PaO_2/FiO_2) < 200 mm Hg
- Air leak/barotrauma
- Hemodynamic or respiratory failure refractory to conventional therapy
- Arrhythmia refractory to conventional therapy

Contraindications:
- Multisystem organ failure of more than three organ systems
- Severe disseminated intravascular coagulation (DIC)
- Irreversible brain damage/irreversible lung disease/ irreversible cardiopulmonary failure
- Ongoing hemorrhagic condition/evidence of uncontrolled bleeding or coagulopathy
- Neonates with gestational age <34 weeks and or birth weight <1.6 kg

Failure of ECMO circuit (e.g., pump stops or power failure) is an emergency. One needs to call for help, perform CPR if necessary, support the patient with emergency drugs, and shift patient back to pre-ECMO ventilator settings.

Equipment Related to Intubation

Laryngoscope with Disposable Blade (Refer Chapter 12)

Conventional laryngoscopy poses great risk to healthcare personnel due to proximity with patient and higher aerosol generation during intubation. Disposable laryngoscope or disposable blades are preferred to prevent transmission of disease. Video laryngoscope is ideal for COVID intubation.

Video Laryngoscope (Refer Chapter 22)

Due to the COVID-19 pandemic, airway management guidelines in many countries have recommended video laryngoscopy for all patients requiring intubation.[19-23]

Advantages of video laryngoscope in COVID-19:[19,21]
- Use of a video laryngoscope increases the distance between the operator and the patient's airway, thereby decreasing risk of close patient contact in AGP.[22]
- Compared with conventional laryngoscopy, video laryngoscopy can enable better glottic view, thus reducing the number of attempts of intubation in patients with difficult airway.[22]
- Video laryngoscope facilitates intubation in patients with COVID-19 who may have a high incidence of laryngitis, periglottic edema, mucosal inflammation, and increased frailty or obesity, all factors that can make airway difficult.
- It also reduces the chances of requiring assistance in intubation, hence exposing fewer people to this AGP.
- Video laryngoscopy facilitates ability to use drapes or boxes over patient and also improves the visibility while wearing PPE.[19]

Heat and Moisture Exchanger (Refer Chapter 21) (Fig. 14)[24-27]

Passive humidifiers like the HME add heat and moisture to cool dry inspired gases and do not require external energy to function. They are also known as Swedish nose, thermal humidifying filter, and artificial nose. They are used in patients whose nasal passages (the body's own HME) are bypassed due to mechanical ventilation.

Principle: HME is a passive device that recovers and retains heat and moisture during expiration and then returns it

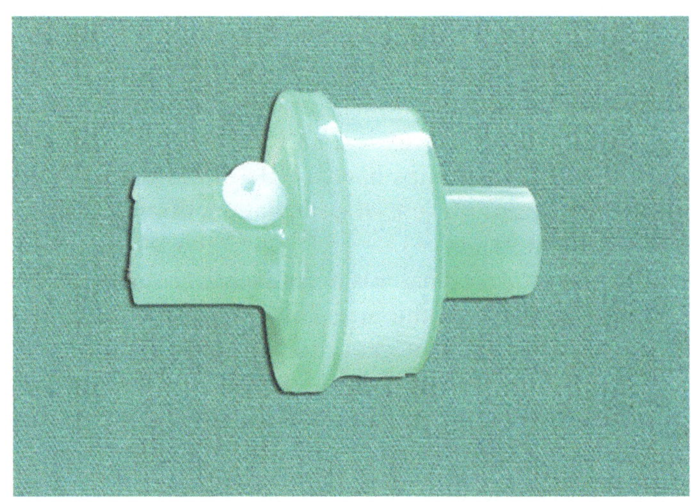

Fig. 14: Heat and moisture exchanger (HME).

to cool, dry gas that passes in the opposite direction during inspiration. Each HME has a 15-mm female connection port at the patient end and a 22-mm male port at the other end. There may be a port to attach the gas sampling line for a respiratory gas monitor. The internal volume of these devices can vary from approximately 12 to 100 mL, and resistance can be in the range of 0.7–3.8 $cmH_2O/L/s$.

An HME comprises a core of material within a plastic casing. HMEs can be classified into three groups, based on the nature and configuration of their core material:

1. *Hydrophobic (water repelling) HME:* These have an aluminum core. Hydrophobic devices are the simplest and cheapest, but the least efficient HME devices, producing modest moisture output of 10–14 mg H_2O/L at tidal volumes of 500–1,000 mL. In addition, these can suffer from problems caused by the pooling of condensed water.
2. *Hygroscopic (water retaining) HME:* A material with a low thermal conductivity such as paper or foam is saturated with hygroscopic salts such as calcium or lithium chloride. These adsorb water in expiration and release it in inspiration. These HME are more efficient and can produce higher humidity's of 22–34 mg H_2O/L at tidal volumes of 500–1,000 mL. There are higher chances of these getting saturated, resulting in increased resistance and reduced heat and moisture retention efficiency.
3. *Combined hygroscopic-hydrophobic HME:* Newer devices combine hygroscopic, hydrophobic, and electrostatic filters in varying configurations to produce even more efficient devices.

Heat and moisture exchangers are modified to prevent bidirectional passage of both airborne and water-borne pathogens with inclusion of a filter and are known as *heat and moisture exchanger filters* (HMEFs). HMEFs are designed to remove liquid or solid particles (aerosols) suspended in gas. This is achieved by reducing the pore size of the HME to <0.2 μm and/or coating it with a bacteriostatic or electrostatic substance.

Filter types:

- Pleated filters or mechanical filters carry high-density fiber hydrophobic membranes folded so that a large surface area is available in a smaller dimension.
- Electrostatic filters use low-density fiber, but the material has a high electrostatic charge, either fibrillated, or triboelectric charged.

Recommendations for COVID-19 patients:[24,28-30]

- It is recommended that one HMEF should be placed between tracheal tube and breathing circuit. The gas sampling line should be connected on the side of the filter away from the patient. A second HMEF is placed on the expiratory limb of the breathing circuit where it connects to the anesthesia machine. Thus, filtering is accomplished for the patient, the gas sampling line, and the breathing circuit. The patient inhales gas that is filtered once, and exhales gas that is filtered once before entering the gas analyzer sampling system and second time before entering the anesthesia machine. These HME filters can remove up to 99% of airborne particles 0.3 microns or greater and help in preventing contamination of OT atmosphere.
- In children <20 kg, one filter should be placed on the expiratory limb of the breathing circuit, but a filter with a smaller internal volume should be added at the patient end of the breathing circuit to avoid added dead space.
- It is recommended to change HMEF in every COVID-19 patient after every use in anesthesia setup. In an ICU, HMEF should be changed every 24 hours. It is for protection of breathing circuits and anesthesia machines and to prevent cross infection of patients.
- Proper management of HMEF involves continuous measurement of arterial SpO_2 using pulse oximetry and filter change after 24 hours. This is recommended to reduce the risk of filter obstruction by condensation.

Advantages:[24]

- It is simple and cost effective, no need for a power source.
- It enables 60–80% humidification of inspired gases and improves mucociliary function and sputum clearance.
- It is used to protect the patients from inhaled particles and viruses.

Disadvantages:[24]

- Increases the dead space of the breathing system and hence can cause rebreathing.
- Adding an HME to a breathing system increases the chances for disconnections and leaks.
- It can become occluded with secretions, blood or water and hence may increase the resistance of the breathing system, if used for prolonged period of ventilation.

High-efficiency particulate air filters:[31] HEPA filters are mechanical filters with a capacity for separating small particles at a much higher rate than other conventional filters. Apart from the HEPA filters, other filters available are the efficient particulate air (EPA) filters and the ultralow penetration air (ULPA) filters. These three types of filters are also known as "absolute filters."

The efficiency of HEPA filters specifically refers to the ability of capturing particles with maximum penetration particle size (MPPS) of diameter 0.3 μm. Bacterial and viral (B/V) filters are defined by their ability to filter particles with a diameter size of 3.0 μm and are used to reduce the risk of cross-contamination with pathogens.

High-efficiency particulate air filters have a hydrophobic membrane of coated glass fibers pleated which maximizes the total filter surface area. Due to the hydrophobicity, the HEPA filter cannot be passed by potentially contaminated fluids (e.g., blood, sputum, and condensate) under normal pressure conditions of mechanical ventilation (viral filtration efficiency: 99.97%).[31]

Uses of HEPA filter:

- The most critical particle size (MPPS) for each filter ranges from 0.12 to 0.25 µm. Coronaviruses are large viruses estimated to be between 0.12 and 0.16 µm. These viruses bind to respiratory droplets, which are the main mechanism of human-to-human transmission. These respiratory particles are more than 5 µm in size. Hence, HEPA filters can easily filter corona viruses.
- In addition to operation theaters, these filters are used in other sterilized clean rooms, inside vacuum cleaners, air conditioners, refrigerators, masks, and respirators.

Recommendations in COVID-19:[31]

- High-efficiency particulate air filters when attached at the helmet outlet in nonintubated patients on NIV can reduce the transmission of virus with great efficacy.
- When filters are placed on the expiratory limb of ventilator breathing circuit to preserve the reusable components, moisture may accumulate in the device which could increase exhalation resistance. Hence, the HEPA filter should be placed after the expiratory valve.
- If heat humidification system is not available, place a filter with both HEPA and HME capability between the Y-connection and the endotracheal tube. No other filter is required to prevent ICU air contamination on ventilator gas outlet.
- During manual ventilation, HEPA filter is between the manual resuscitator and endotracheal tube or face mask. During transport, HME + HEPA filter is placed between patient and ventilator circuit.
- Vertical laminar flow allowing the air through HEPA filter system is the most effective way to control viruses in the entire operating room.

Closed Suction Catheter System[32] (Fig. 15)

The closed suction catheter is enclosed within a flexible sterile plastic sleeve that allows a single catheter to be used multiple times, without having to break the ventilator circuit. There are different types available consisting of modular ports that allow for suctioning, bronchoscopic procedures, bronchoalveolar lavage, and drug therapy with a pressurized metered-dose inhaler (pMDI). Turbulent cleaning chamber creates cleansing action, resulting in a cleaner catheter and catheter tip.

Advantages:

- *For the patient:*
  - By avoiding disconnection during suctioning, risk of patient catching infection [ventilator-associated pneumonia (VAP)] from surrounding environment is minimal.
  - As the ventilation and oxygenation is maintained throughout suctioning, fall in lung volume is almost half of that when suctioning after disconnection from the ventilator.
  - It reduces colonization within the circuit.
  - It keeps the PEEP constant during the aspiration maneuver, reducing arterial desaturation and stabilizing vital parameters.
- *For the healthcare provider:*
  - It is possible to limit the contamination of the surrounding environment with patient's organisms, which is especially important while managing COVID patient on ventilator in ICU.
  - This technique facilitates any emergency maneuvers, which can be done simultaneously.

Personal Protective Equipment[33] (Fig. 16)

Personal protective equipment includes clothing and equipment that is worn or used to provide protection against hazardous substances or environments.

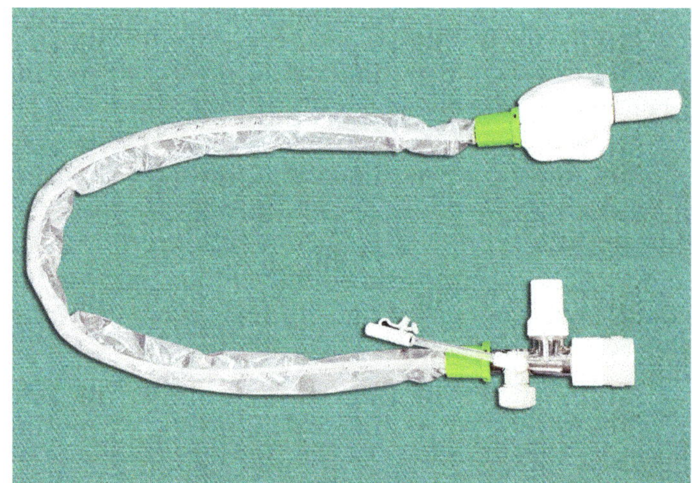

Fig. 15: Closed suction catheter system.

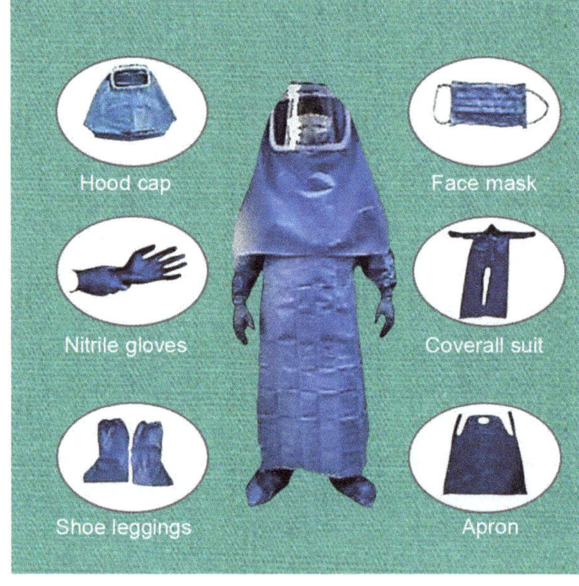

Fig. 16: Personal protective equipment kit.

The highest viral load is in sputum and upper airway secretions hence the virus is predominantly spread by droplet and contact routes. Larger respiratory particles, above 5 μm diameter are the source of droplet transmission. These do not travel more than 1 meter. Contact transmission occurs as virus remains on the surface for a period of hours or even days. This creates the risk that healthcare workers touching that surface will become contaminated and subsequently they, or others, will become infected.

Protection against exposure to SARS-CoV-2 virus includes both standard and transmission-based precautions. The PPE used to prevent exposure includes:

Gloves

Types of gloves are:

- *Latex:* These are closer fitting and provide a more effective barrier against microorganisms. These should be nonpowdered and have the lowest level of extractable protein available. If a healthcare worker has a suspected latex allergy, or the patient has latex allergy then latex gloves should not be used.
- *Nitrile (acrylonitrile):* These are comparable to natural rubber latex in terms of providing a biological barrier but are less elastic. Nitrile gloves are preferred to latex gloves.
- *Neoprene:* These have similar properties to natural rubber latex but are more expensive.
- *Polythene:* These gloves are thin and have tendency to tear, hence not preferred.
- *Vinyl:* These are less effective than latex gloves in terms of providing barrier against microorganisms. These are also loose-fitting.

Gown

- It is a fluid-resistant gown which covers the body from the neck to the mid-calf. There are shoe covers available which are of above ankle or knee length. There is a separate head cover for protection of head, hair, and neck.
- Coverall has a hood and shoe cover in it and is preferred when exposed to high viral load or during AGPs.
- Isolation gowns are made either of cotton or a spun synthetic material which are either disposable or reusable. If fluid penetration is likely, a fluid-resistant gown should be used.
- Gram per square meter (GSM) in fabric is the metric measurement of the weight of a fabric. This measurement helps one decide on the best weight to buy, considering the usage of the material at hand. The higher the GSM number, the denser the fabric will be. PPE suits of 70 GSM are preferred.

Face Masks (Figs. 17A to C)

There are different types of face masks available like cloth mask, surgical mask, N95 mask, and powered air-purifying respirator (PAPR). Depending on the COVID affected area to be visited and the procedure to be performed, selection of the mask should be done **(Table 1)**.

Face Shield (Fig. 18)

Face shield is made of clear plastic and provides good visibility to both the wearer and the patient. It has an adjustable band or elastic band to attach firmly around the head and fit snuggly against the forehead. It is fog resistant. It completely covers the sides and length of the face and extends below the chin. It may be reusable which can be cleaned and disinfected or disposable. It may be worn with an N95 respirator in place of goggles to provide eye and face protection.

Goggles

It provides barrier protection for the eyes and should fit snuggly over and around the eyes or prescriptive lenses.

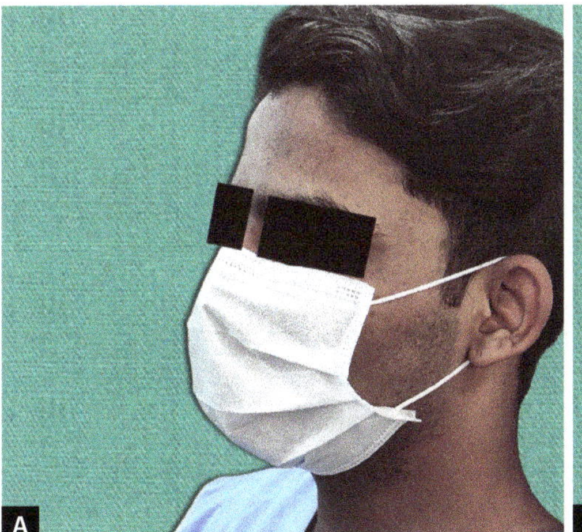

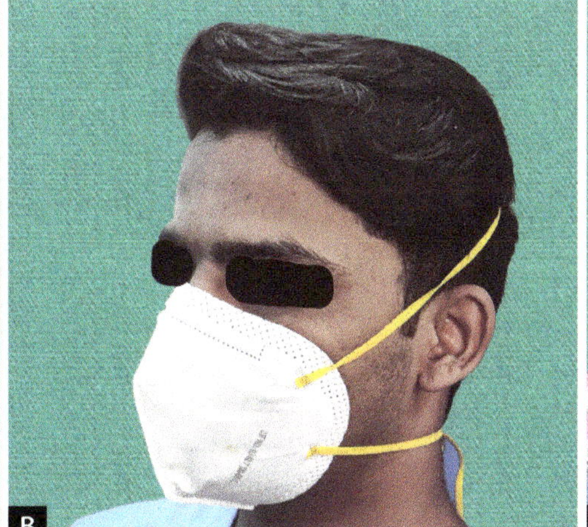

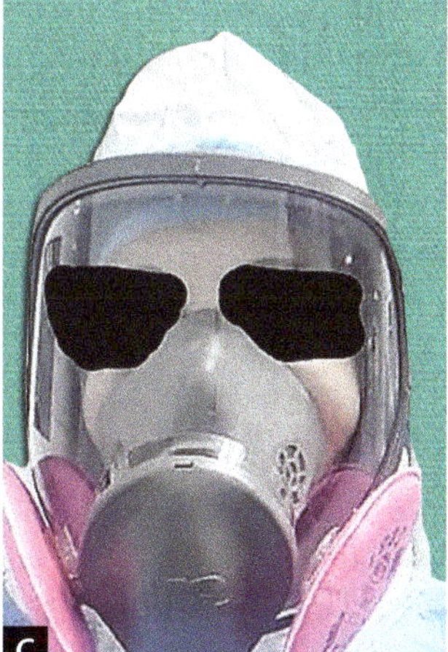

Figs. 17A to C: (A) Surgical mask; (B) N95 mask; and (C) Respirator.

TABLE 1: Comparison of different types of masks.

Type of mask	Cloth mask	Surgical mask	N95 mask	Respirator
Features	• Loose fitting made up of cotton or polyester • May have a layer of filter paper	• Loose fitting provides physical barrier • Used by healthcare workers	• Tight fitting, >95% filtration • To be used for AGPs	Loose head-top with battery powered blower to filter air
Benefits	Can be homemade, washed, and reused multiple times	• Cheaper, easily available • Disposable, single use	Greater protection against aerosols and droplets	• Greater protection as compared to N95 • More comfortable • No need of fit testing
Drawbacks	• Insufficient aerosol protection • Not useful in hospital	• No tight seal, so air leakage can occur • Cannot be used during AGP	• Requires regular fit-testing • Costly • Limited supply	• Expensive, limited availability • High cost • Difficult to maintain

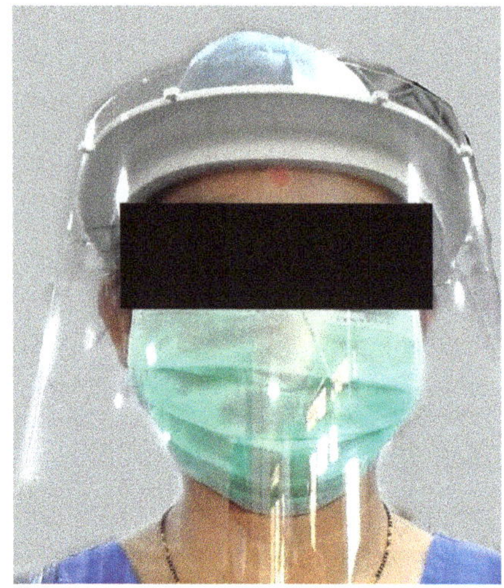

Fig. 18: Face shield.

TABLE 2: Steps of donning and doffing.

Donning	***Doffing***
Hand Wash	Outer gloves
↓	↓
Cap	Hood
↓	↓
Shoe cover	Coverall gown
↓	↓
Hand rub	Shoe cover
↓	↓
Inner gloves	Hand rub
↓	↓
Coverall gown	Goggles
↓	↓
N95 mask	Mask
↓	↓
Hood/visor	Cap
↓	↓
Outer gloves	Inner gloves

Biohazard Bag

It is a disposable autoclavable bag for biohazard waste. It is made up of high-density polyethylene (HDPE) or polypropylene (PP). It is red or yellow in color. It is puncture, tear, and leak resistant. It has leak proof flat bottom seal. It has a black imprint "Biohazard" with trisickle logo on one side. The capacity is approximately 20 L or 50 L.

Donning and Doffing of PPE (Table 2)

Before wearing PPE (donning), check all parts are available. Sufficiently hydrate and use washroom prior to donning. Wear surgical scrubs and remove all jewelry.

Removing PPE (doffing) is to be done very carefully and slowly in doffing area performing hand hygiene at all steps. Discard PPEs in appropriate bins.

When PPE is properly worn, removed, and discarded, it is effective in protecting both the wearer and those who meet the wearer.

CONCLUSION

COVID-19 pandemic has highlighted the role of the anesthetist in the ICU setting. The sudden spurt in the number of patients led to the establishment of new COVID facilities as well as the expansion of COVID wards and ICUs in established hospitals. There was a concurrent rise in the demand for anesthetists, many of whom were recruited on an urgent basis. A sizeable number were called upon to establish and manage new wards and ICUs with constraints of time and manpower. They innovated the ways to use an entire range of equipment for oxygen therapy right from an oxygen concentrator, BiPAP machine, HFNC, and conventional ventilator depending on the resources available at that location. They were also called upon to protect themselves as well as other healthcare workers especially during AGPs. Evolution of equipment for oxygen therapy and personal protection is ongoing; a pandemic such as the current one only serves to accelerate the process.

REFERENCES

1. Dorsch JA, Dorsch SE. Understanding Anesthesia Equipment, 5th edition. Philadelphia: Lippincott Williams & Wilkins; 2007.
2. Bland H, Borton C, Jafri S. The supply of anaesthetic and other medical gasses. In: Davey AJ, Diba A (Eds). Ward's Anaesthetic Equipment, 6th edition. Philadelphia: Elsevier Saunders; 2012.
3. Al Shaikh B, Stacey SG. Medical Gas Supply. In: Al Shaikh B, Stacey SG (Eds). Essentials of Equipment in Anaesthesia, Critical Care and Perioperative Medicine, 5th edition. Netherlands: Elsevier; 2019.
4. Aston D, Rivers A, Dharmadasa A. Medical gases. In: Aston D, Rivers A, Dharmadasa A (Eds). Equipment in Anaesthesia and Critical Care, A Complete Guide for the FRCA, 1st Edition. US: Scion; 2014.

5. WHO. (2020). Clinical management of COVID-19: interim guidance. [online] Available from https://www.who.int/publications/i/item/WHO-2019-nCoV-clinical-2021-1 [Last accessed April, 2021].
6. Whittle J, Pavlov I, Sacchetti A, et al. Respiratory support for adult patients with COVID-19. J Am Coll Emerg Physicians Open. 2020;1(2):95-101.
7. Roy A, Singh A, Khanna P. Oxygen delivery devices in COVID-19 patients: Review and recommendation. Bali J Anaesthesiol. 2020;4:3-7.
8. Gregory L, Calligaroa B, Lallac U, et al. The utility of high-flow nasal oxygen for severe COVID-19 pneumonia in a resource-constrained setting: A multicentre prospective observational study. eClinical Medicine. 2020;28:100570.
9. WHO. (2020). Clinical management of COVID-19: interim guidance. [online] Available from https://apps.who.int/iris/handle/10665/332196 [Last accessed April, 2021].
10. Lecavalier A, Goldberg P. Continuous positive airway pressure. In: Elliot M, Nava S, Schonfer B (Eds). Non-invasive Ventilation and Weaning Principles and Practice, 2nd edition. Florida: CRC press; 2019.
11. Al Shaikh B, Stacey SG. Additional equipment used in anaesthesia and intensive care. In: Al Shaikh B, Stacey SG (Eds). Essentials of Equipment in Anaesthesia, Critical Care and Perioperative Medicine, 5th edition. Netherlands: Elsevier; 2019.
12. Standley T, Wheeler DW. Equipment for the inhalation of oxygen and other gasses. In: Davey AJ, Diba A (Eds). Ward's Anaesthetic Equipment, 6th edition. Netherlands: Elsevier Saunders; 2005.
13. Gregoretti C, Russotto V, Chiumello D. Interfaces. In: Elliot M, Nava S, Schonfer B (Eds). Non-invasive ventilation and weaning Principles and Practice, 2nd Edition. Florida: CRC press; 2019.
14. Dobler CC, Murad MH, Wilson ME. Non-invasive Positive Pressure Ventilation in Patients With COVID-19. Mayo Clin Proc. 2020;95(12):2594-601.
15. Nava S, Navalesi P, Gregoretti C. Interfaces and humidification for noninvasive mechanical ventilation. Respir Care. 2009; 54(1):71-84.
16. Barbaro RP, MacLaren G, Boonstra PS, et al. Extracorporeal Life Support Organization. Extracorporeal membrane oxygenation support in COVID-19: an international cohort study of the Extracorporeal Life Support Organization registry. Lancet. 2020;396(10257):1071-8.
17. Lequier L, Horton SB, McMullan DM, et al. Extracorporeal membrane oxygenation circuitry. Pediatr Crit Care Med. 2013; 14(5 Suppl 1):S7-12.
18. Abrams D, Brodie D. Extracorporeal circulatory approaches to treat acute respiratory distress syndrome. Clin Chest Med. 2014;35(4):765-79.
19. Davies M, Hodzovic I. Video laryngoscopy post-COVID-19. Trends Anaesthesia Critical Care. 2021;36:49-51.
20. Maldini B, Hodžović I, Goranović T. Alternative Devices in Airway Visualization. Acta Clin Croat. 2016;55(Suppl 1):76-84.
21. Saito T, Taguchi A, Asai T. Video laryngoscopy for tracheal intubation in patients with COVID-19. Br J Anaesth. 2020; 125(3):e284-6.
22. Hamal PK, Chaurasia RB, Pokhrel N, et al. An affordable video laryngoscope for use during the COVID-19 pandemic. Lancet Glob Health. 2020;8(7):e893-4.
23. Kumar GP, Kulkarni AP, Govil D, et al. Airway Management and Related Procedures in Critically Ill COVID-19 Patients: Position Statement of the Indian Society of Critical Care Medicine. Indian J Crit Care Med. 2020;24(8):630-42.
24. Dorsch JA, Dorsch SE. Humidification equipment. In: Dorsch JA, Dorsch SE (Eds). Understanding Anaesthesia Equipment, 5th edition. Philadelphia: Lippincott Williams & Wilkins; 2007.
25. Aston D, Rivers A, Dharmadasa A. Filters and humidifiers. In: Aston D, Rivers A, Dharmadasa A (Eds). Equipment in Anaesthesia and Critical Care: A Complete Guide for the FRCA, 1st edition. US: Scion; 2014.
26. Shelly M, Spencer C. Humidification and Filtration. In: Ehrenwerth J, Eisenkraft JB, Berry JM (Eds). Anesthesia Equipment: Principles and Applications, 2nd edition. Philadelphia: Elsevier Saunders; 2014.
27. Wilkes AR. Breathing filters, humidifiers, and nebulizers. In: Davey AJ, Diba A (Eds). Ward's Anaesthetic Equipment, 6th edition. Philadelphia: Elsevier Saunders; 2012.
28. Malhotra N, Joshi M, Datta R, et al. Indian Society of Anaesthesiologists (ISA National) Advisory and Position Statement Regarding COVID-19. Indian J Anaesth. 2020;64:259-63.
29. De Seta D, Carta F, Puxeddu R. Management of tracheostomy during COVID-19 outbreak: Heat and moisture exchanger filter and closed suctioning system. Oral Oncol. 2020;106:104777.
30. Anesthesia Patient Safety Foundation. (2021). FAQ On Anesthesia Machine Use, Protection, And Decontamination During The COVID-19 Pandemic. [online] Available from https://www.apsf.org/faq-on-anesthesia-machine-use-protection-and-decontamination-during-the-covid-19-pandemic [Last accessed April, 2020].
31. Lucchini A, Giani M, Winterton D, et al. Procedures to minimize viral diffusion in the intensive care unit during the COVID-19 pandemic. Intensive Crit Care Nurs. 2020;60:102894.
32. Williams JP, Ari A, Shanmugam R, et al. The effect of different closed suction catheter designs and pMDI adapters on aerosol delivery in simulated adult mechanical ventilation with and without exhaled humidity. Respir Care. 2018;63(9):1154-61.
33. CDC. (2020). Using Personal Protective Equipment (PPE). [online] Available from https://www.cdc.gov/coronavirus/2019-ncov/hcp/using-ppe.html [Last accessed April, 2021].

Ventilation Strategies in COVID-19

Gunadhar Padhi, Balkrishna D Nimavat, Masood Ahmed

ABSTRACT

Coronavirus disease 2019 (COVID-19) pandemic is the burning issue of present time. High infective nature and predisposition for lung tissue are the real concern with severe acute respiratory syndrome coronavirus 2 (SARS-CoV-2). Early intubation in respiratory failure patient of COVID-19 is advocated to decrease viral transmission and aerosol spread. On other hand, noninvasive oxygen therapy is easy to apply and has less chances of ventilator associated lung injury or infection. There is emerging evidence of benefit of noninvasive ventilation (NIV) approach in particular subset of patients under close monitoring. The aim of this chapter is to emphasize that all the patients of respiratory failure cannot be put into one cart of invasive ventilation but should be individualized based on their need of oxygen support and risk benefit of invasive therapy. It is also important to identify the failure of noninvasive ventilatory strategies and timely recourse to invasive ventilation. We shall also discuss whether COVID-19-related acute respiratory distress syndrome (ARDS) ventilation should be managed same as classical ARDS or in different way.

Keywords: COVID-19, Noninvasive ventilation, Ventilation strategies.

INTRODUCTION

Coronavirus disease (COVID) is an infectious disease caused by newly discovered coronavirus, i.e., severe acute respiratory syndrome coronavirus 2 (SARS-CoV-2). COVID-19 can affect multiple organs and leads to multiorgan failure. But primarily, it targets the respiratory tract, causing widespread inflammation in the lungs. Around 14% of patients affected with COVID-19 develop respiratory failure and 5% become critically ill requiring critical care unit admission.[1] In other words, there is a subset of patients with COVID-19 who do not require intubation but are hypoxemic with increased work of breathing and not responding to simple oxygen supplementation and thus requiring noninvasive respiratory support.[2] So, in this chapter, we shall be discussing about types of noninvasive ventilation (NIV), their rationale to use, limitations, and advantages. We shall be also discussing about how to handle failure of NIV therapy and different invasive ventilatory strategies in COVID-19 patients.

PATHOPHYSIOLOGY OF LUNG INJURY IN COVID-19

There is significant gap in knowledge in understanding the complete pathophysiology of COVID-19-related lung injury. Current observations suggest that initial viral contact occurs at level of nasal mucosa through binding of the viral S (spike) protein to the ACE-2 (angiotensin-converting enzyme-2) receptor, followed by cleavage of S protein by TMPRSS2 (transmembrane serine protease 2). After entering, virus replicates within the nasal mucosa and travels to the conducting airways, where it triggers an immune and inflammatory response, manifesting as clinical signs and symptoms of COVID-19.[3] It is also seen that disease progression and worsening is not only related to virus but also due to consequences of dysregulated immune-mediated injury too. Other notable feature of severe COVID-19 is endothelialitis (inflammation of endothelial cell) leading to abnormal coagulation profile ranging from hypercoagulable state (elevated D-dimer and fibrinogen) to overt disseminated intravascular coagulation (DIC).[4] COVID-19 leads to impaired activity of NK cells and CD8+ T-cell subpopulation, leading to excessive cytokines production. Such phenomenon gives rise to cytokine storm like that seen in macrophage activation syndrome (MAS).[5] Giacomo Grasselli et al. showed that COVID-19-associated pulmonary injury with acute respiratory distress syndrome (ARDS) having decreased lung compliance with increased lung weight.[6]

STRATIFICATION OF DISEASE SEVERITY AND SELECTION OF MODALITIES

It is particularly important to monitor patient with subjective and objective parameters. Oxygen saturation with pulse oximetry is crucial to target oxygen saturation of >90% (target range 90–96%). It can be done by increase oxygen support through nasal cannula or Venturi mask. Along with oxygen saturation work of breathing is also crucial, as in patient having more work of breathing it is advisable to choose

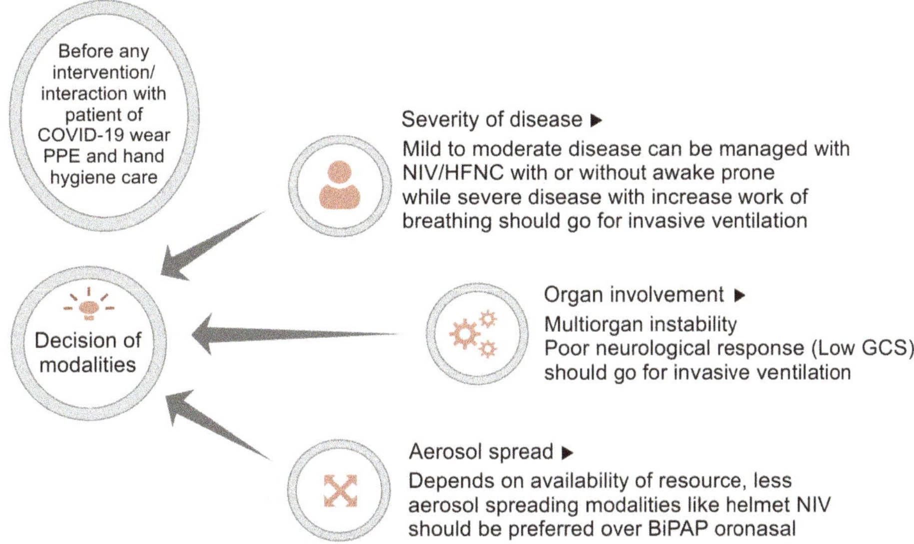

Fig. 1: Factors that help to make decision of ventilation strategies.
(GCS: Glasgow coma scale; NIV: noninvasive ventilation; HFNC: high-flow nasal cannula)

high-flow nasal therapy or NIV therapy. There are few key points that should be given importance while handling airway and initiating ventilation of COVID-19 patients:

- Selecting modalities with minimize aerosolizing spread or exposure
- Stratification of patients based on severity of disease and
- Reduce personnel exposure by wearing personal protective devices[7]

The risk of hasty intubation against the peril of sudden respiratory arrest with a cluttery emergency intubation which exposes to risk of infection must weighed carefully by the clinicians. Signs of impending respiratory arrest like increased efforts in breathing, hypoxemia that is refractory to supplemental oxygenation, multiple organ failure, hemodynamics instability, and encephalopathy, warrant for urgent endotracheal intubation (ETI) and mechanical ventilation **(Fig. 1)**.

Patient who having high work of breathing and hypoxemia but not requiring intubation should be treated with noninvasive positive pressure ventilation or with help of high-flow nasal cannula (HFNC) therapy. Noninvasive positive pressure ventilation use should be more beneficial particularly, if patient having cardiac component (pulmonary edema), obstructive sleep apnea, or having chronic obstructive lung disease. Noninvasive positive pressure ventilation is also helpful postextubation to decrease work of breathing and fatigue. When choosing noninvasive modalities, it is important to monitor patient clinical parameters and signs of deterioration. Early identification of failure of therapy and redirect to invasive ventilation is pivotal at that time **(Flowchart 1)**.[8]

Flowchart 1: How to approach hypoxemia COVID-19 patient.

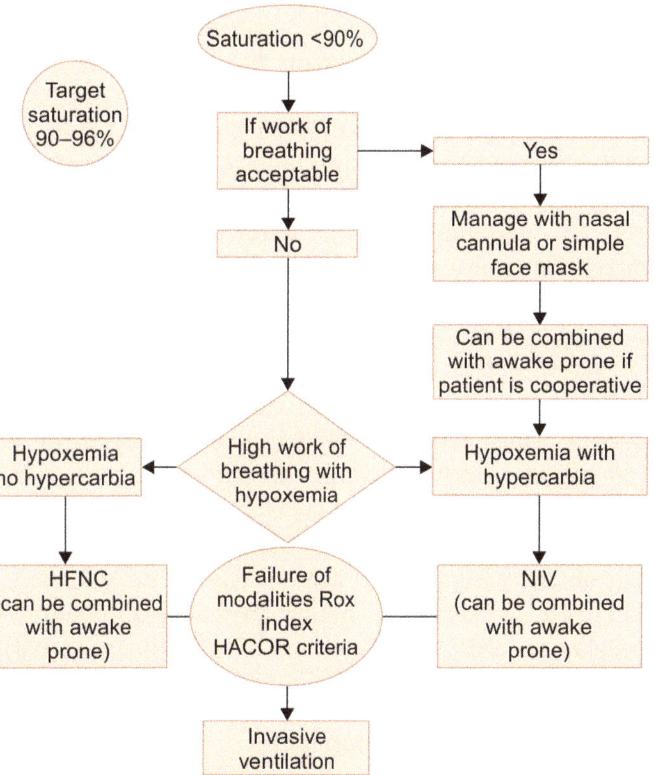

(COVID-19: coronavirus disease 2019; HFNC: high-flow nasal cannula; NIV: noninvasive ventilation)

STRATIFICATION OF SEVERITY OF DISEASE/ BERLIN DEFINITION FOR ARDS

Diagnostic criteria for acute lung injury stratification have changed to Berlin definition to define ARDS. Based on Berlin definition, ARDS stratified into mild, moderate, and severe according to partial pressure of oxygen/fraction of inspired oxygen (PAO_2/FiO_2) ratio (200–300, 200–100, and <100 mm Hg) with positive end-expiratory pressure/continuous positive airway pressure (PEEP/CPAP) of >5 cm of H_2O. ARDS classification helps to stratify both the severity of the disease and choice of treatment modalities.[9] If ratio is <150 mm Hg, it is advisable to choose ETI. Mild disease or ratio >150 mm Hg should be given attempt of HFNC or NIV trials under monitoring.[10]

Saturation/FiO_2 Ratio, Oxygen Saturation Index and Oxygen Index

The concept of oxygen saturation index (OSI) and oxygen index (OI) was given for pediatrics ARDS population. Later, it was studied in adult group too. OI is defined as $FiO_2/PaO_2 \times$ mean airway pressure × 100, is a marker of severity of ARDS. It is an independent risk factor for predicting mortality but requires invasive blood sampling. On other side, OSI is defined as mean airway pressure × 100 × FiO_2/SpO_2 is noninvasive bedside tool which correlates well with OI. OSI can be used as surrogate of OI for continuous monitoring and thus predicting mortality and ventilator free days in ARDS.[11,12] Patients with ARDS diagnosed by SF ratio have similar clinical characteristics and outcomes compared with patients diagnosed by PF ratio.[13]

NONINVASIVE VENTILATION APPROACH: BALANCING THE CART

On early COVID-19 era, people were dogmatic to practice early intubation in known or suspected COVID-19 with respiratory failure without giving them the option for less invasive treatments (like NIV or HFNC). But with further studies and data collected through them, WHO guidelines for the management of hypoxemia in COVID-19 advocate the use of NIV or HFNC, with proper use of proper personal protective equipment (PPE).[14] Early intubation in patient who is managing well with CPAP or NIV is not rational and in contrary it increases the risk of exposure to healthcare staffs and improper delivery of resource. A good interface fitting for CPAP or NIV systems will help to minimize widespread dispersion of exhaled air and thus reduce transmission of virus. During the severe acute respiratory syndrome epidemic, use of NIV with PPE in the intensive care unit (ICU) was not associated with an increased risk of transmission of the virus to healthcare workers, whereas ETI was associated with an increased risk of aerosolization and infection of healthcare workers. The notion that early intubation by passing use of NIV, to decrease risk of viral transmission with the use of PPE, is debatable.[14]

Noninvasive Ventilation Strategies

There are two types of NIV approach—(1) CPAP and (2) BiPAP (bilevel positive airway pressure). NIV (particularly BiPAP) is often selected in cases of short-term life-threatening respiratory conditions, such as pulmonary edema or when intubation carries a greater risk than other benefits, for example, patients with chronic type 2 respiratory failure from chronic obstructive pulmonary disease (COPD). HFNC differs in that it involves the use of nasal cannula to provide high flow of air to meet inspiratory efforts and thus decrease work of breathing.[15]

Bilevel Positive Airway Pressure

Bilevel positive airway pressure is beneficial modality for COPD exacerbation and cardiogenic pulmonary edema patient, but its role in other viral ARDS- or COVID-related ARDS is still controversial. For lung recruitment and to improve ventilation perfusion mismatch, the application of a PEEP is useful.

Evidence from Italy has shown NIV is not sufficient to manage type 1 respiratory failure in all patients presenting with severe COVID-19. For some patients, while NIV may temporarily improve oxygenation and work of breathing, it does not change natural disease progression and is not a replacement for intubation and invasive ventilation. But there are positive reports of role of NIV on postextubation phase. They have observed large number (around 50%) of extubated patients require reintubation because of fatigue, in this group where use of NIV to tide over the situation and prevent invasive ventilation.[16] As reported by several studies, in subset group of mild hypoxic respiratory failure in severe acute respiratory illness, the use of NIV has demonstrated that it can avoid intubation. Potential for aerosol generation and transmission of COVID-19 infection among healthcare professional is a setback for its use.

In contrary disadvantages of invasive ventilation are periprocedure aerosol exposure, ventilator-related lung injury, need of sedative-paralytic agent, and chances of pneumonia/secondary infections. So, it is advisable to select noninvasive method over invasive when patient having mild respiratory failure with younger age and no comorbidities.[17] Proper selection of mask size, fitting of mask (to minimize air leak), and monitoring of NIV for failure are crucial points when selecting NIV as modality. Undue continuation of NIV in worsening moderate to severe lung disease leads to increase mortality. An increase in ICU mortality was reported by a few studies on H1N1 who failed noninvasive positive pressure ventilation (NIPPV) trial compared to early invasive mechanical ventilation.

Noninvasive positive pressure ventilation failure was more common when applied to group of patients having higher Sequential Organ Failure Assessment (SOFA) scores and low P/F score (severe disease). In absence of randomized control trial or meta-analysis making statement on NIV role in COVID-19 is difficult, but once applied it should be done under close-controlled environment.[18] An NIPPV trial could be attempted for 2 hours, being aware that a prolonged NIPPV treatment can be harmful, delaying intubation, and provoking large tidal volumes increasing the risk of patient self-inflicted lung injury (P-SILI).

Concept of P-SILI and NIV Use

Any of acute respiratory failure (ARF) patient, those are nonintubated, spontaneously breathing having remarkably high air hunger and they breathe with high respiratory drive with generating high tidal volume. In such cases, large tidal volume generates more stress/strain to lung tissue. Such phenomenon leads to volutrauma and biotrauma even in nonintubated group of patients.

Not only alveolar level damage but due to high transmural pulmonary vascular pressure swings these patients develop vascular injuries too. Vascular leakage and worsening lung compliance seen particularly with group. This phenomenon is popularly known as patient self-inflicted lung injury.[19] Recent data suggest P-SILI as possible mechanism aggravating lung damage in patients using NIV.[20]

NIPPV/BiPAP Initial Setting

Inspiratory positive airway pressure (IPAP) should be set according to need of tidal volume and work of breathing. If patient having low tidal volume with more work of breathing, it can be supported by increasing IPAP. To achieve adequate tidal volumes, the IPAP can range from 12 to 20 cmH_2O. Expiratory positive airway pressure (EPAP) should be targeted based on oxygenation of patient. It works on the same principles as PEEP in invasive ventilator devices, preventing alveolar collapse on expiration which is maintained above atmospheric pressure. To overcome the difficulty of breathing on a ventilator (including valves) and increase in dead space from the ventilator tubing, it is achieved by pressure support (PS). PS is calculated by IPAP minus from EPAP (PS = IPAP – EPAP), and it is recommended that there should be a difference of at least 5 cmH_2O, with supplementary oxygen provided, if needed, to achieve oxygenation. Some BiPAP ventilators have additional setting of "ramp" and "rise time." It allows the pressure to be slowly increased over the first few minutes of ventilation until the required pressure is reached. Starting NIPPV with a PS of 5 cmH_2O and a PEEP between 5 and 10 cmH_2O, titrating the FiO_2 to reach the desired SpO_2 (mostly targeted as >89%). Trial of 2 hours should be given. During this trial, one should monitor clinical parameters like oxygenation, work of breathing, neurosensorium, and hemodynamics. ABG should be repeated after 30 minutes, if needed or after 2 hours. A reassessment is required after 30 minutes and repeated at the end of the trial. If desired SpO_2 and respiratory rate (RR) ≤ 25 breaths/min (bpm) with a low tidal volume of 6 mL/kg predicted body weight (PBW) is reached after the 60 minutes trial, then trial should consider as pass and NIPPV can be continued. In case of NIPPV failure, invasive ventilation should be performed without delay.[18]

Tool Used to Identify Failure of NIV Trial: HACOR Criteria

HACOR [heart rate (H), acidosis (A) pH, consciousness (C) GCS, oxygenation (O), and respiratory rate (R)] is a potentially useful bedside tool for the prediction of NIV failure. HACOR score accurately predicts NIV failure in patients with hypoxemic respiratory failure. A HACOR score >5 at 1 hour of NIV highlights patients with a >80% risk of NIV failure regardless of diagnosis, age, and disease severity. HACOR score should be used to detect failure of NIV thus facilitate early need of invasive ventilation and improve mortality.[21]

CONTINUOUS POSITIVE AIRWAY PRESSURE FOR COVID-19

Continuous positive airway pressure can solve the purpose as COVID-19 patient when they have hypoxemia without increase work of breathing. It will deliver PEEP that leads to alveolar recruitment improve oxygenation and avoid excessive negative pressure swings exerted by patient efforts. Due to its potential negative effects on hemodynamics and gastric distension, the lowest useful PEEP should be selected. CPAP modalities can be delivered by three different interfaces—(1) nasal CPAP (nCPAP), (2) face CPAP, and (3) helmet CPAP.

1. *Nasal CPAP (nCPAP):* nCPAP has advantage such as delivery of positive pressure, better patient tolerance, and adjustable and predicted oxygen delivery than nasal cannula. If patient presented with mild ARDS or respiratory failure and not maintaining with oxygen supplementation or having high work of breathing, one can initiate CPAP. A CPAP trial of 2 hours should be started. Initial setting will be start with PEEP/CPAP of 7.5 cmH_2O and a flow ≥60 L/min, titrating the FiO_2 to reach an $SpO_2 \geq 94\%$ and an RR ≤ 25 bpm. Vital monitoring every 30 minutes is necessary in this phase. If patient not achieved desired target in half hour then PEEP should be increased by 2.5 cmH_2O up to a maximum of 12.5 cmH_2O, while no modification of the setting is needed if target reached. If an $SpO_2 \geq 94\%$ and an RR ≤ 25 minutes is reached after the 120 minutes trial. In case of failure, early ETI should be considered. In patients who signed do not intubate (DNI) order, it is better to select noninvasive therapy like HFNC or CPAP.[18]
2. *Helmet CPAP:* The second method, a CPAP hood/helmet, requires the patient's head to be fully enclosed with a secure seal around the neck and the hood can be supported by straps. While such hoods reduce the risk of facial pressure sores, they can cause discomfort, pain and potentially with prolonged use, pressure sores. A potential complication is, it can lead to air being swallowed, which if not addressed will lead to gastric distention and vomiting, with a risk of aspiration of gastric contents. As with COVID-19 type diseases, patient with less compliant lungs, the risk of developing barotrauma and pneumothorax must be recognized and observations regularly taken and in the light of the rapid deterioration that occurs with COVID-19, early intervention is essential.

   Continuous positive airway pressure delivered by head helmet is as safe and effective as CPAP delivered by face mask and is tolerated better for prolonged ventilation periods. It is superior in terms of safety for viral transmission as it is a closed system and viral filters.

Continuous positive airway pressure delivers a constant flow of oxygen at a decided pressure, measured in cmH_2O, which remains constant during inspiration and expiration. CPAP is usually commenced at a higher level than normal intrinsic pressure around 5 cmH_2O. For most patients with type 1 respiratory failure, it is secondary to conditions which either collapse the alveoli or widen the gap between the alveoli and the blood vessels that surround them, thereby reducing gaseous exchange. The application of PEEP assists in maintaining the patient's airway pressure and prevents alveolar collapse, in turn increasing lung volumes and distends them to reduce the distance between the alveoli and the blood vessels to improve gaseous exchange. In severe COVID-19, initial CPAP settings have been suggested 10 cmH_2O and 60% oxygen. For CPAP to be effective, a sealed system is required, through application of a tight-fitting mask or a hood. Both methods for establishing a sealed system have benefits and disadvantages. With a face mask, the tight fit means patients may experience pressure damage to the nasal bridge. An ill-fitting mask leads to significant leaks, resulting in poor inflation of the lungs, with dry oxygen/air leaking round a mask likely to lead to irritation, abrasions, and edema of the cornea and conjunctiva.

3. *Helmet CPAP:* Evidence-COVID helmet trial shows that the use of helmet CPAP reduces the need for invasive mechanical ventilation compared to the use of HFNC without having a negative effect on survival.[22]

HFNC for Mild or Early Respiratory Failure

High-flow nasal cannula therapy gains its popularity in last couple of years in management of ARF. It is selected as alternative tool to NIV/CPAP. It is superior in terms of better compliance/tolerability by patients of ARF. By providing high flow, it satisfied the air hunger and work of breathing of ARF patients. With increasing flow, it develops low amount of PEEP too that helps to open alveoli and improve ventilation perfusion. It is simple to use, deliver humidified airflow, and allow patients to eat or talk while HFNC in place. It differs from nCPAP that it does not have valve. There are couple of limitations also there with HFNC like it is not advisable choice in cases of type 2 respiratory failure. Delivery of PEEP and oxygen is also variable as it depends on patient work of breathing and PEEP effect nullifies once patient open mouth or while talking.

A recent multicenter randomized controlled trial (RCT) showed benefits of HFNC in terms of mortality and need of intubation in patients with severe hypoxemic ARF.[23] In COVID-19, use of HFNC is little bit controversial as it is associated with aerosol dispersion. But it is advisable to consider use of HFNC over NIV for mild to moderate severity of COVID-19 patients as it is better tolerated and having less chances of P-SILI. There are data that show HFNC can reduce the incidence of intubation in patients with COVID-19, decrease the length of ICU stay, and complications related to mechanical ventilation. It also used for preoxygenation purpose like NIV while airway management. As it is aerosol generating device better to use in negative pressure room/single room with PPE use.[24]

High-flow Nasal Cannula

Evidence based on one multicenter prospective observational trial, for severe COVID-19 in a resource-constrained setting HFNC, is feasible and many who received it were successfully weaned without the need for mechanical ventilation.[25]

Tool to Identify HFNC Failure: ROX Index

Ratio of pulse oximetry (ROX/FiO_2 to RR) index helps in decision making when patient on HFNC. It should be monitor at 2, 6, and 12 hours. If value is <2.85, 3.47, and 3.85, it suggests HFNC failure and should go for intubation.[26]

HFNC versus nCPAP/NIV

Therapeutically, HFNC generates low PEEP, and this pressure is unstable, uncontrollable, and affected by multiple factors (such as work of breathing). Whereas, nCPAP can provide stable and adjustable airway pressure. Tolerance of oxygen therapy, as CPAP without interruption, seems important during AHRF, especially early ARDS. HFNC better tolerated than NIV/nCPAP and thus patient compliance is better with HFNC. In conclusion, there is lack of data on what to choose between HFNC and nCPAP treating mild AHRF due to COVID-19. Prospective RCTs are necessary to compare HFNC with nCPAP to provide more conclusive evidence on the use of different noninvasive respiratory support.[27]

Awake Proning

Role of proning in intubated severe ARDS patient is well documented but role of awake proning and particularly in COVID-19 patients is subject to debate. Recent guidance by the UK Intensive Care Society (ICS) advised awake prone positioning as standard of care for suspected or confirmed COVID-19, in whom $FiO_2 \geq 28\%$. The physiological rationale behind prone positioning in ARDS is to reduce ventilation/perfusion mismatching and shunting. This is believed to generate more homogenous lung aeration and strain distribution, thus enhancing recruitment of dorsal lung units. With improvements in ventilatory homogeneity and relatively constant perfusion patterns, a subsequent reduction in shunting is observed. Proning be used alone or in combination with HFNC or NIV. Proning tried cautiously in patients whose PaO_2/FiO_2 is <150/severe ARDS.

Presently, no published trials investigate the effectiveness of prone positioning in awake patients with typical ARDS. Evidence in awake prone positioning is limited to case series and small observational studies with heterogeneous approaches to noninvasive respiratory support.

These reports demonstrated short-term improvements in oxygen requirements (PaO_2) and demand (FiO_2) with no harm to patients.[28]

Evidence: Awake prone positioning demonstrated an improvement in oxygenation of the patients suffering from COVID-19-related respiratory disease. Need for intubation was observed in <30% of the patients. Thus, we recommend early and frequent proning in patients suffering from COVID-19-associated mild to moderate ARDS, however, RCTs are needed before any definite conclusions are drawn.[29]

Prone positioning plus HFNC/NIV: More recently, early prone positioning added to HFNC or NIV avoided the need for intubation in up to half of the patients with moderate to severe ARDS including those with viral pneumonia. No healthcare professional was infected during this study carried out in isolation negative pressure rooms. Randomized trial needed to get better insight on this topic.[30] Combination of both NIV and HFNC is also another alternative approach, when patient having long NIV course and when NIV break is needed, it can be supplemented with HFNC (e.g., while eating).[30]

COMPARISON OF AEROSOL SPREAD WITH DIFFERENT NONINVASIVE MODALITIES

Noninvasive support methods such as oxygen therapy, HFNC, and NIV can cause aerosol dispersion, especially in unprotected environments and pose risk for infection. Knowledge regarding the aerosol production distance of the various methods allows us to favor those with the lowest risk (e.g., helmet with an inflatable neck cushion) and to take the necessary precautions (e.g., correct placing of the HFNC).[31]

NONINVASIVE VENTILATION STRATEGIES CONCLUSION

The use of NIV and HFNC in severe COVID-19 disease remains contentious, with evidence for and against still being gathered, analyzed, and disseminated. In any pandemic where there is an incomplete knowledge of the disease trajectory and patient complications, all available respiratory support options must be considered and trialed. Noninvasive ventilatory methods cannot, and does not, replace invasive ventilation but it may, if used early, reduce deterioration to the point that invasive ventilation is not required **(Table 1)**.

Steps and Precaution while Intubation

Respirator masks such as N95 or FFP2 are made to block around 95–99% of aerosol particles. Surgical masks are designed to block large particles like droplets. Surgical masks are not the good choice for small particle aerosol (<5 μm) or for high-risk procedure. For all type of interaction with patient/procedure, it is advisable to wear full personal protective device (that includes gloves, gown, eye protection goggles, or face shield). Any high-risk aerosol generating procedure should be carried out in negative pressure room preferably.[32]

For patients those are of low risk of desaturation ambient pressure, preoxygenation with tight fitted face mask without mask ventilation is advisable. For high-risk patient (who having high risk of desaturation), manual bag assist positive pressure ventilation should be given with two people with two handed mask holding method to develop proper seal and reduce spread of aerosol.[7] Person who is expert/senior person must intubate the patient to decrease duration and attempt of procedure. Rapid sequence intubation is preferred in term of use of paralytic agent that eliminates coughing and achieves adequate relaxation. It is advisable to choose video laryngoscope compared to direct laryngoscopy. Less number of team members such as three to four should be allowed to stay inside cubicle.[32] High-efficiency particulate air (HEPA) filters should be placed in-line while positive pressure breath and at junction of tubing. Once tube is passed, the endotracheal tube (ETT) balloon should be inflated immediately and disconnection of tube

TABLE 1: Comparison of different oxygen and ventilation modalities used in COVID-19 patients.

Oxygen therapy with nasal cannula/Venturi mask	*Oxygen therapy with HFNC*		*NIV*		*Invasive ventilation*
Isolated hypoxemia patient	Isolated hypoxemia patient		Helps in type 1 respiratory failure		Definitive therapy
Does not help in work of breathing	Helps in work of breathing		Helps in reducing work of breathing		More invasive/chances of VAP (ventilation-associated pneumonia)/VILI (ventilator-induced lung injury)
Cannot be used in type 2 respiratory failure	Cannot be used in type 2 respiratory failure		Can be used in type 2 respiratory failure		Useful in both type of respiratory failure
Limitation of flow	High-flow satisfied flow hunger		Patient cooperation needed		High-risk aerosol generating procedure while intubation
Limitation of oxygen delivery	Deliver oxygen and limited amount of peep		More sustained oxygen delivery and PEEP		Least aerosol spread once secured
	HFNC	nCPAP	Oronasal	Helmet	
	No valve	Valve	Less tolerated/ air leak	Better tolerated/ less air leak	

(COVID-19: coronavirus disease 2019; HFNC: high-flow nasal cannula; nCPAP: nasal continuous positive airway pressure; NIV: noninvasive ventilation)

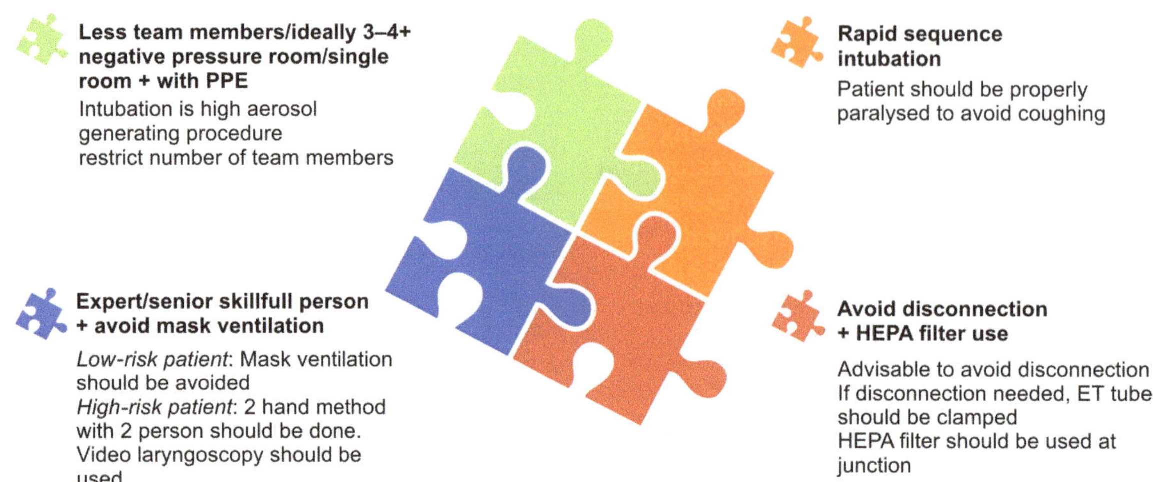

Fig. 2: Points to be considered while intubating COVID-19 patients.

should be avoided. In case of emergency or need, it should be disconnected with ETT clamped **(Fig. 2)**.[7]

CONCEPT OF DIFFERENT PHENOTYPES OF COVID-19-RELATED LUNG INJURY

In small series of intubated patient affected by COVID-19, Gattinoni et al. observed hypoxemia with relatively normal lung compliance. That was quite different than classical severe ARDS lung. In such group even low PEEP and normal lung volume 7–8 mL/kg of ideal body weight therapy with high FiO_2 suffice, rather than high PEEP and low tidal volume.

After above observation, they gave concept of different phenotype of COVID-19-associated lung injury. Where they mentioned two types of phenotypes—(1) type L and type H. Type L characterized by relatively normal lung compliance, normal lung weight. This lung will show least response to high PEEP and recruit ability. Type H in contrary is more of classical ARDS lung where it is characterized by low compliance, stiff lung shows response to high PEEP and recruit ability. They also mentioned that type L will turn into type H when etiology persists and sometime with iatrogenic issues, i.e., liberal fluid management and self-inflicted lung injury **(Fig. 3)**.[33,34.]

Is COVID-19 ARDS (CARDS) different than non-COVID ARDS or required different ventilatory strategies?

Normally, ARDS is characterized by noncardiogenic pulmonary edema, shunt-related hypoxemia, and reduced aerated lung size (popularly known as "baby lung"), responsible for poor lung compliance. In such scenario, prone or recruitment of lung by high PEEP strategy helps. Because high transpulmonary pressure induces stress across the lung, relatively low tidal volume, with permissive hypercapnia strategy, facilitates the goal of lung protective ventilation. It is important to understand that types L and H are the conceptual extremes of the COVID-19 ARDS spectrum, in clinical practice different proportional combination of these will be seen. Another peculiar feature of COVID-19 is variety of thromboinflammation complications and proinflammatory cascade-related organ injuries.

Ventilatory strategy of type L lung who having good lung compliance, requires larger tidal volumes (7–8 mL/kg ideal body weight), high FiO_2 to prevent hypoxemia-related pulmonary vasoconstriction and normal PEEP of 6–8 cmH_2O than high PEEP those classically prescribed for ARDS. Higher tidal volume (TV) could help avoid reabsorption atelectasis and hypercapnia. The clinician's first response, boosting FiO_2, may indeed prove effective early on.[35] In advanced state like H type, it is advisable to apply a more conventional lung-protective strategy in terms of higher PEEP (15 cmH_2O), lower tidal volume (6 mL/kg), and prone positioning while minimizing oxygen consumption **(Fig. 4)**.

PRONE VENTILATION FOR REFRACTORY HYPOXEMIA RATIONALE AND EVIDENCE

Patient who having severe ARDS, where conventional ventilatory strategies fail, it is advisable to go for prone ventilation. Prone decision should be beneficial, if done early such as within 36–48 hours. It should be selected for severe cases where P/F ration < 150. Early and extended prone (at least 16 hours) shows mortality in ARDS patients. Data of prone in COVID-19 patients are still emerging. But based on physiological rationale, it is recommended to go for early and extended prone with judicious use of neuromuscular blockade and low tidal volume strategies. Prone ventilation should be avoided in cases of cervical spine injuries, chest injuries (recent sternotomy) and brain injuries where there is high risk of increased intracranial pressure. Staff should be familiar with prone. Lines should be secured properly, and ETT connection should be watched for disconnection. Ryle's tube aspiration should be done prior to prone. Patient should be oxygenated with 100% pre- and postprone position. Sometime recruitment methods help to achieve oxygenation while proning. After prone watch for improvement in lung

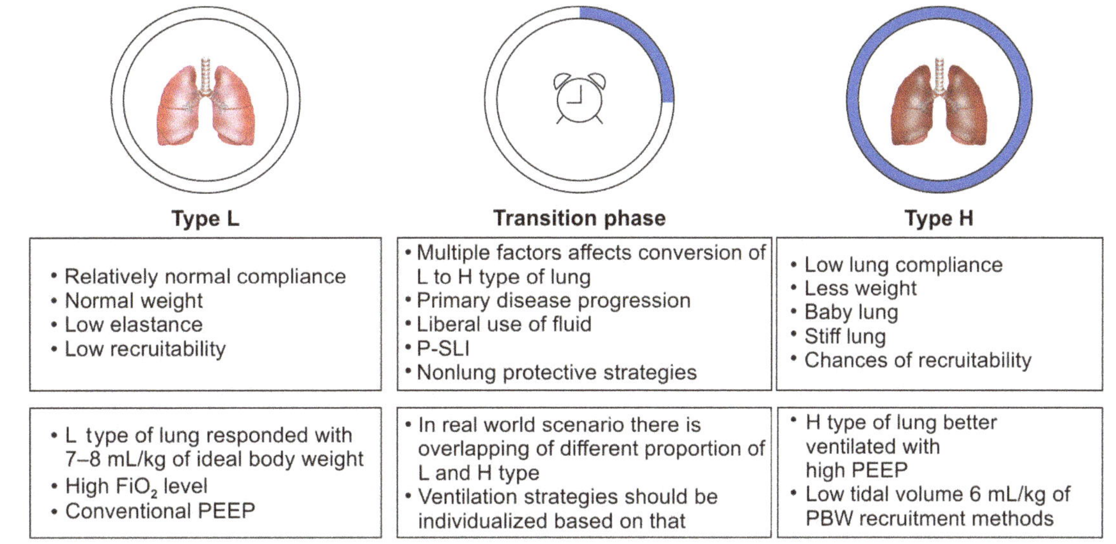

Fig. 3: Comparison of different phenotype and their transition. (FiO_2: fraction of inspired oxygen; PBW: predicted body weight; PEEP: positive end-expiratory pressure)

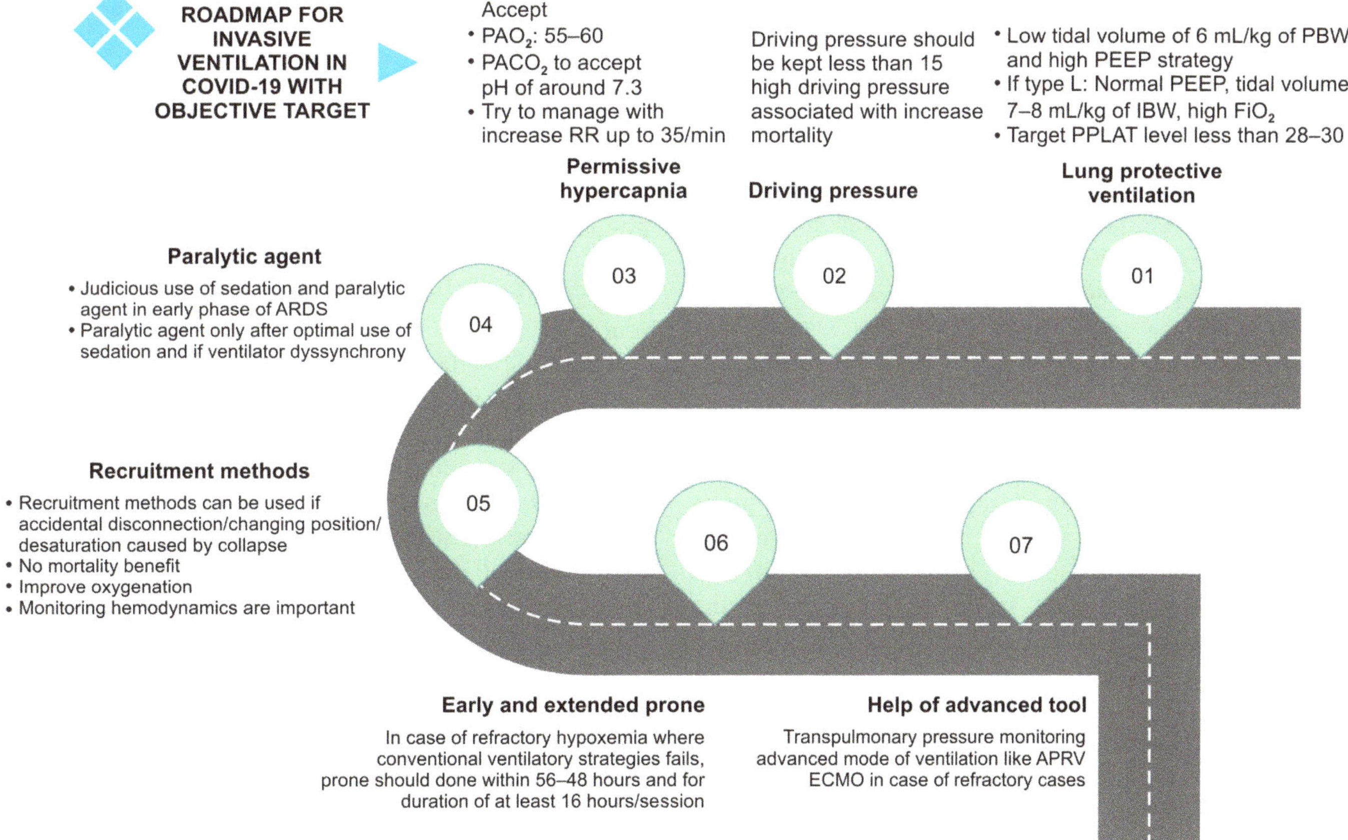

Fig. 4: Roadmap of invasive ventilation strategies in COVID-19 patients.

compliance and oxygenation, apply ECG leads on back and take care of pressure points by applying cushion. Eye should be taken care of. Corneal abrasion and pressure sore are quite common in prone cases.[36]

It is recommended to do early and frequent proning in patients suffering from COVID-19 associated ARDS, however, RCTs are needed before any definite conclusions are drawn.[29]

Open Lung Approach

Objective of ARDS lung ventilation is to achieve open and more homogenous ventilation. It is incredibly attractive concept and physiological right as it reduces shear stress and reduces atelectrauma. It can be done by low tidal volume high PEEP. Despite good biological plausibility, clinical evidence to support open lung concept is not that great. A meta-analysis comparing higher PEEP (13-15 cmH_2O)

and low PEEP ventilation strategies reported a reduction in mortality rate, but only in a subgroup analysis of patients with moderate to severe ARDS.[37]

Recruitment Methods: Different Methods

When low tidal volume strategies selected, it focusses on injury from alveolar overdistension. But it is also crucial to avoid injuries happen from repetitive opening-closing of alveoli and from atelectasis. Recruitment methods solve this problem by delivering sustain pressure to open collapsed alveoli and those newly opened alveoli should be kept open by postrecruitment increased PEEP. Role of recruitment methods is most controversial till date. It improves oxygenation in patients of ARDS but its role in reducing mortality is still lacking in existing literature.[38]

There are different methods of recruitment. Out of which, a sustained inflation is the recruitment maneuver that has probably been used most. It can be done by set the ventilator to CPAP mode and increases the pressure to 30–40 cmH_2O for 30–40 seconds. Prone ventilation also considers as recruitment method as it opens nonaerated alveoli, improve ventilation/perfusion mismatch leads to more homogenous oxygen delivery. There are other methods like sustained inflation followed by decremental PEEP, stepwise incremental PEEP, newer ventilation modes airway pressure release ventilation (APRV) and bilevel modes, sigh, and extended sigh.[39] It is pivotal to observe hemodynamics while recruitment methods, bradycardia, and hypotension are likely complications of such maneuvers. Overzealous methods will lead to barotrauma such as pneumothorax.

Optimizing PEEP: Methods to Use

Several methods have been suggested to set optimal PEEP in ARDS patients. They broadly classified into direct methods where lung recruit ability assesses based either on imaging (direct assessment) or indirect methods based on gas exchange/respiratory system mechanic variables during challenge tests (indirect methods). Direct methods rely on imaging like CT-scan, USG, and Electric impendence tomography (EIT). Indirect methods encompass P/F ratio PEEP table, incremental and decremental PEEP method with targeting lung compliance. Each of such methods having their own limitations/problems. Bed side portable CT scan is not available in all centers and shifting patients for CT scan is not always feasible and safe. The EIT is newer modalities that is quite promising as bed side tool, but it is semi-quantitative by nature. The ultrasound can only explore the portion/ 'shell' of the lung. All the tests do not take account the role of the hemodynamics and value of $PaCO_2$.[40]

Transpulmonary Pressure Monitoring to Optimize Ventilation

Transpulmonary pressure is defined as the pressure difference between the airway opening and the pleural surface. Esophageal manometry is most widely used method to measure pleural pressures now days. Conventional teaching has focused on airway Pplat pressure as measures of risk for barotrauma and lung injury. Values such as <28 or 30 have been cited as maximum safe limits during mechanical ventilation. The concept of transpulmonary pressure emphasizes that absolute airway pressures seen on mechanical ventilator are not the ultimate measure of lung stress. Instead, the transpulmonary pressure provides a more accurate measurement of lung stress and risk of injury. Such understanding will help in difficult to ventilate ARDS patient where lung compliance is high because of stiff chest wall or due to high abdominal pressure. In such cases to optimize PEEP, transpulmonary pressure monitoring is extremely helpful.[41] Despite strong physiological rationale, there is lack of evidence that it reduces mortality.

DRIVING PRESSURE CONCEPT AND EVIDENCE

Driving pressure (ΔP) can be derived from tidal volume divided by respiratory system compliance (CRS) (formula $\Delta P = TV/CRS$). High ΔP irrespective to tidal volume and Pplat pressure is associated with increased risk of mortality. Decreases in ΔP owing to changes in ventilator settings were strongly associated with increased survival (in non-COVID ARDS).[42] It is physiologically true for COVID-related lung too.

Role of Paralytic Agent and Evidence

Neuromuscular blocking agents (NMBAs) should be used after optimal sedation. Despite optimal sedation patient having cough, ventilator dyssynchrony, and desaturation, NMBAs should be used. It decreases risk of high tidal volume and transpulmonary swing that happens because of spontaneous air hunger breath. Thus, it reduces ventilation-related lung injury and improves lung conditions. There are two large RCTs done on role of paralytic agent in early ARDS patients. Those trials gave insight that if patient in supine position, it should be manage with isolated sedation preferably but in case of prone when despite sedation patient having high ventilation dyssynchrony and desaturation, it is advisable to use early paralytic agent that shows trends toward mortality benefit.[43]

Role of ECMO and Evidence

There are two large RCTs done on role of extracorporeal membrane oxygenation (ECMO) in severe ARDS. CESAR trial shows promising benefit with early ECMO in severe refractory cases of ARDS. While later EOLIA trial was negative trial and does not show any mortality benefit. Recently meta-analysis done on same topic including both trial and they came to conclusion that early ECMO leads to reduction in mortality and less treatment failure.[44] In COVID-19, data about role of ECMO are still limited. But one of the recent trials shows trends toward mortality benefit.[45]

REAL WORLD SCENARIO

Theoretically concept of L and H type of lung is extremely attractive. But in real world of COVID, it is exceedingly difficult to get such black and white picture, it is always overlap of L and H type of lung in different proportion (in shades of grey). It is very evident that ventilator strategies should be selected based on individual/personalized approach rather than practicing different phenotype strategies (author recommendation). Recently done multicenter trial shows that COVID-19 ARDS patients having nearly same clinical features, ventilatory management and outcome compared to non-COIVD-19 patients. They also mentioned that lung protective ventilation shows mortality benefit in COVID-19 group too.[46] So in view of lack of evidence, it is believed that ARDS patients with the same mechanical and clinical characteristics should be ventilated in the same way, without regard to whether they have COVID-19 ARDS or classical ARDS.[47]

Fluid Therapy in COVID-19

Positive fluid balance and low serum albumin concentration have been found to be independent risk factors for ARDS development. Moreover, an increased body weight related to cumulative fluid balance has been associated with a worse outcome. Fluid therapy in COVID-19 patients with ARDS should also be based on the timing of the disease. In the early phase, patients having low amount of lung edema, near normal elastance and low amount of atelectasis (phenotype L), whereas in the later phase, patients present with a higher amount of lung edema, atelectasis, and elastance (phenotype H).[48].

ROLE OF PHARMACOLOGICAL THERAPY

Remdesivir, along with three other repurposed antiviral drugs, was also studied in the WHO-SOLIDARITY trial, outcomes were hospital mortality, initiation of ventilation, and duration of hospitalization. None of the four drugs (hydroxychloroquine, lopinavir/ritonavir, remdesivir, or interferon-β1a) showed benefit amongst patients requiring mechanical ventilation. Convalescent plasma showed promise in early observational studies of COVID-19, but RCT data failed to show any benefit. Immunomodulatory therapies have so far failed to show convincing benefit. Tocilizumab, a monoclonal antibody that blocks the interleukin-6 receptor, appeared beneficial in early observational studies. But a recent RCT from Stone et al. did not show benefit with COVID-19 and lower respiratory tract involvement.[49] A higher risk of thrombosis has been described as a prominent feature of COVID-19. If patient did not have history of heparin-induced thrombocytopenia and no contraindication of venous thromboembolism (VTE) prophylaxis, ward patient should receive LMWH (low molecular weight heparin) 40 mg once daily (<120 kg weight) and 40 mg twice daily (if >120 kg weight). If CrCl (creatinine clearance) is <30 than unfractionated heparin should be given with dose of 5,000 U thrice daily. ICU patient should again stratify based on D-dimer level. If D-dimer level >3 μg/mL LMWH enoxaparin should be given with dose of 30 mg twice daily (for <120 kg) and 40 mg twice daily (for weight >120 kg).[50] The RECOVERY trial gave insight about role of steroid in COVID-19 patients, they conclude that dexamethasone (dose 6 mg once daily for 10 days) shows mortality benefit in patient who are on ventilator/respiratory support. They also pointed out that there is no benefit of steroid in patients who did not require oxygen.

PERSONALIZED MEDICINE VERSUS EVIDENCE-BASED MEDICINE

In conclusion, there is little evidence to support the use of one mode of ventilation over another in patients diagnosed with ARDS. The place of recruitment maneuvers is also debated. Individual trials evaluating the effects of higher versus lower levels of PEEP in patients with ARDS have largely been negative, although a meta-analysis demonstrated that higher PEEP was beneficial in patients with moderate or severe ARDS. Although theoretically appealing, PEEP titration based on esophageal pressure measurements has not resulted in better outcomes. The use of muscle relaxants should be individualized. It is also especially important for us to remember that COVID-19 is a disease, and ARDS is a syndrome. ARDS usually has an underlying identifiable cause, and the cause can often result in a specific therapy, such as antimicrobials/antiviral, anticoagulation, and corticosteroids.[51]

REFERENCES

1. Shang Y, Pan C, Yang X, et al. Management of critically ill patients with COVID-19 in ICU: statement from front-line intensive care experts in Wuhan, China: Springer; 2020.
2. Nicholson TW, Talbot NP, Nickol A, et al. Respiratory failure, and non-invasive respiratory support during the COVID-19 pandemic: an update for re-deployed hospital doctors and primary care physicians. BMJ. 2020;369:m2446.
3. Brosnahan SB, Jonkman AH, Kugler MC, et al. COVID-19 and respiratory system disorders current knowledge, future clinical and translational research questions. Arterioscler Thromb Vasc Biol. 2020;40(11):2586-97.
4. Cao W, Li T. COVID-19: towards understanding of pathogenesis. Cell Res. 2020;30(5):367-9.
5. Torres Acosta MA, Singer BD. Pathogenesis of COVID-19-induced ARDS: Implications for an ageing population. Eur Respir J. 2020;56(3):2002049.
6. Sacco F, Tonetti MT, Pizzilli G, et al. Pathophysiology of COVID-19-associated acute respiratory distress syndrome: a multicentre prospective observational study. Lancet Respir. 2020;8:1201-8.
7. Brown CA, Mosier JM, Carlson JN, et al. Pragmatic recommendations for intubating critically ill patients with suspected COVID-19. J Am Coll Emerg Physicians Open. 2020;1(2):80-4.
8. Berlin DA, Gulick RM, Martinez FJ. Severe COVID-19. N Engl J Med. 2020;383(25):2451-60.
9. Li X, Ma X. Acute respiratory failure in COVID-19: Is it "typical" ARDS? Crit Care. 2020;24(1):198.

10. Scala R, Pisani L. Noninvasive ventilation in acute respiratory failure: Which recipe for success? Eur Respir Rev. 2018; 27(149):180029.
11. Jakka S, Chandra S, Chaudhry D, et al. Oxygen saturation index as a surrogate to oxygenation index in predicting outcomes in ARDS. Euro Res J. 2020;3437.
12. DesPrez K, McNeil JB, Wang C, et al. Oxygenation Saturation Index Predicts Clinical Outcomes in ARDS. Chest. 2017;152(6):1151-8.
13. Chen W, Janz DR, Shaver CM, et al. Clinical characteristics and outcomes are similar in ARDS diagnosed by oxygen saturation/FiO_2 ratios compared with PaO_2/FiO_2 Ratio. Chest. 2015;148(6):1477-83.
14. Arulkumaran N, Brealey D, Howell D, et al. Use of non-invasive ventilation for patients with COVID-19: a cause for concern? Lancet Respir Med. 2020;8(6):e45.
15. Goligher EC, Slutsky AS. Not just oxygen? Mechanisms of benefit from high-flow nasal cannula in hypoxemic respiratory failure. Am J Respir Crit Care Med. 2017;195(9):1128-31.
16. Carter C, Aedy H, Notter J. COVID-19 disease: non-invasive ventilation and high frequency nasal oxygenation. Clin Integr Care. 2020;1:100006.
17. Singh A. Noninvasive versus invasive ventilation: one modality cannot fit all during COVID-19 outbreak. Korean J Anesthesiol. 2020;73(4):359-60.
18. Privitera D, Angaroni L, Capsoni N, et al. Flowchart for non-invasive ventilation support in COVID-19 patients from a northern Italy Emergency Department. Intern Emerg Med. 2020;15(5):767-71.
19. Brochard L, Slutsky A, Pesenti A. Mechanical ventilation to minimize progression of lung injury in acute respiratory failure. Am J Respir Crit Care Med. 2017;195(4):438-42.
20. Grieco DL, Menga LS, Eleuteri D, et al. Patient self-inflicted lung injury: Implications for acute hypoxemic respiratory failure and ARDS patients on non-invasive support. Minerva Anestesiol. 2019;85(9):1014-23.
21. Duan J, Han X, Bai L, et al. Assessment of heart rate, acidosis, consciousness, oxygenation, and respiratory rate to predict noninvasive ventilation failure in hypoxemic patients. Intensive Care Med. 2017;43(2):192-9.
22. Tverring J, Åkesson A, Nielsen N. Helmet continuous positive airway pressure versus high-flow nasal cannula in COVID-19: a pragmatic randomized clinical trial (COVID HELMET). Trials. 2020;21(1):994.
23. Frat JP, Coudroy R, Marjanovic N, et al. High-flow nasal oxygen therapy and noninvasive ventilation in the management of acute hypoxemic respiratory failure. Ann Transl Med. 2017;5(14):297.
24. Kaya AG, Öz M, Erol S, et al. High flow nasal cannula in COVID-19: a literature review. Tuberk Toraks. 2020;68(2):168-74.
25. Calligaro GL, Lalla U, Audley G, et al. (2020). The utility of high-flow nasal oxygen for severe COVID-19 pneumonia in a resource-constrained setting: A multi-centre prospective observational study. [online] Available from https://reader.elsevier.com/reader/sd/pii/S258953702030314X? token=7ED231DECF444F41F74E6726D715A778411922F65F0280DF98AA9C463193DA10A921A88F9E02349B 107437856C1E9E38 [Last accessed April, 2021].
26. Ricard JD, Roca O, Lemiale V, et al. Use of nasal high flow oxygen during acute respiratory failure. Intensive Care Med. 2020;46: 2238-47.
27. Guan L, Zhou L, Michael Le Grange J, et al. Non-invasive ventilation in the treatment of early hypoxemic respiratory failure caused by COVID-19: considering nasal CPAP as the first choice. Crit Care. 2020;24(1):333.
28. Koeckerling D, Barker J, Mudalige NL, et al. Awake prone positioning in COVID-19. Thorax. 2020;75(10):833-4.
29. Anand S, Baishya M, Singh A, et al. Effect of awake prone positioning in COVID-19 patients- A systematic review. Trends Anaesth Crit Care. 2021; 36:17-22.
30. Winck JC, Ambrosino N. COVID-19 pandemic and noninvasive respiratory management: Every Goliath needs a David. An evidence-based evaluation of problems. Pulmonology. 2020;26(4):213-20.
31. Ferioli M, Cisternino C, Leo V, et al. Protecting healthcare workers from sars-cov-2 infection: Practical indications. Eur Respir Rev. 2020;29(155):1-10.
32. Alhazzani W, Møller MH, Arabi YM, et al. Surviving Sepsis Campaign: guidelines on the management of critically ill adults with Coronavirus Disease 2019 (COVID-19). Intensive Care Med. 2020;46:854-87.
33. Fan E, Beitler JR, Brochard L, et al. Viewpoint COVID-19-associated acute respiratory distress syndrome: is a different approach to management warranted? Lancet Respir Med. 2020;8(8):816-21.
34. Gattinoni L, Chiumello D, Caironi P, et al. COVID-19 pneumonia: different respiratory treatments for different phenotypes? Intensive Care Med. 2020;46(6):1099-102.
35. Marini JJ, Gattinoni L. Management of COVID-19 Respiratory Distress. JAMA. 2020;323(22):2329-30.
36. Petrone P, Brathwaite CEM, Joseph DAK. Prone ventilation as treatment of acute respiratory distress syndrome related to COVID-19. Eur J Trauma Emerg Surg; 2020. pp. 1-6.
37. Van Der Zee P, Gommers D. Recruitment maneuvers and higher PEEP, the so-called open lung concept, in patients with ARDS. Crit Care. 2019;23(1):73.
38. Cui Y, Cao R, Wang Y, et al. Lung Recruitment Maneuvers for ARDS Patients: A Systematic Review and Meta-Analysis. Respiration. 2020;99(3):264-76
39. Hess DR. Recruitment maneuvers and PEEP titration. Respir Care. 2015;60(11):1688-704.
40. Gattinoni L, Collino F, Maiolo G, et al. Positive end-expiratory pressure: how to set it at the individual level. Ann Transl Med. 2017;5(14):288.
41. Williams EC, Motta-Ribeiro GC, Melo MFV. Driving pressure and transpulmonary pressure: how do we guide safe mechanical ventilation? Anesthesiology. 2019;131(1):155-63.
42. Amato MBP, Meade MO, Slutsky AS, et al. Driving pressure and survival in the acute respiratory distress syndrome. N Engl J Med. 2015;372(8):747-55.
43. Hraiech S, Yoshida T, Annane D, et al. Myorelaxants in ARDS patients. Intensive Care Med. 2020;46(12):2357-72.
44. Combes A, Peek GJ, Hajage D, et al. ECMO for severe ARDS: systematic review and individual patient data meta-analysis. Intensive Care Med. 2020;46(11):2048-57.
45. Barbaro RP, MacLaren G, Boonstra PS, et al. Extracorporeal membrane oxygenation support in COVID-19: an international cohort study of the Extracorporeal Life Support Organization registry. Lancet. 2020;396(10257):1071-8.
46. Ferrando C, Suarez-Sipmann F, Mellado-Artigas R, et al. Clinical features, ventilatory management, and outcome of ARDS caused by COVID-19 are similar to other causes of ARDS. Intensive Care Med. 2020;46(12):2200-11.
47. Goligher EC, Ranieri VM, Slutsky AS. Is severe COVID-19 pneumonia a typical or atypical form of ARDS? And does it matter? Intensive Care Med. 2021;47(1):83-5.
48. Vignon P, Evrard B, Asfar P, et al. Fluid administration and monitoring in ARDS: which management? Intensive Care Med. 2020;46(12):2252-64.
49. Tsang JLY, Binnie A, Fowler RA. Twenty articles that critical care clinicians should read about COVID-19. Intensive Care Med. 2021;47(3):337-41.
50. McBane RD, Torres Roldan VD, Niven AS, et al. Anticoagulation in COVID-19: A Systematic Review, Meta-analysis, and Rapid Guidance From Mayo Clinic. Mayo Clin Proc. 2020;95(11): 2467-86.
51. Vincent JL, Slutsky AS. We have never seen a patient with ARDS! Intensive Care Med. 2020;46(12):2133-5.

Infection Prevention and Control Guidelines and Recommendations for Healthcare Providers/Settings in the Times of COVID-19 Pandemic

Vaibhavi Baxi, Dwarkadas K Baheti

ABSTRACT

Healthcare-associated infections (HAIs) have a major impact on public health and a large percentage of them are preventable by effective infection prevention and control measures. Recommendations and guidelines help to formulate and implement effective prevention and control program which aims to reduce the transmission of HAIs, enhance safety of healthcare workers (HCWs), patients and their family members, and also enable the healthcare facilities to effectively respond to an outbreak. The strategies and practices that are recommended in this chapter are based on a broad consensus among international experts and institutions which form the core component of infection prevention to control the coronavirus disease 2019 (COVID-19) pandemic.

INTRODUCTION

Healthcare-associated infection is a major public health problem. An effective infection and prevention control (IPC) program in a healthcare facility reduces the transmission of HAI and enhances the safety of staff, patients, and visitors.

Additional practices have been recommended by Centers for Disease Control and Prevention (CDC) and World Health Organization (WHO) during coronavirus disease 2019 (COVID-19) pandemic, along with standard practices of infection prevention and control for all patients and not just those with suspected or confirmed SARS-CoV-2 (COVID-19) infection. These recommendations are made with the intention to guide healthcare providers and healthcare facilities to prevent healthcare-associated transmission of COVID-19 virus among healthcare workers (HCWs) and patients; while maintaining essential healthcare services. The major aspects of this include:

- Rapid identification of suspect cases
- Immediate isolation and referral for testing
- Safe clinical management
- Adherence to standard infection prevention and control precautions

These recommendations are based on the current available information about COVID-19. They are categorized as:

- Infection and prevention control practices for routine healthcare delivery during pandemic
- Infection and prevention control practices when caring for a patient with suspected or confirmed COVID-19 infection

RECOMMENDED ROUTINE IPC PRACTICES DURING COVID-19 PANDEMIC

Additional IPC practices are recommended during COVID-19 pandemic along with standard practices as a part of routine healthcare delivery to all patients.

- Using *telehealth technology* as a way to deliver acute, chronic, primary, and specialty care; helps maintaining high quality while reducing the risk of COVID-19 virus transmission in healthcare settings.
- Advise patients to wear their own cloth mask before they enter healthcare facility.
- *Screen and triage* everyone entering a healthcare facility for signs and symptoms of COVID-19. Postvisual alerts and posters at the entrance and strategic places.
- In the healthcare facility, provide supplies for respiratory hygiene/cough etiquette—alcohol (60–95%)-based hand sanitizer and tissues at multiple sites like at entrances, waiting rooms, etc.
- Reevaluate admitted patients for signs and symptoms of COVID-19.
- Healthcare worker should wear a well-fitting face mask; preferable over cloth mask as it gives both source control and protection for the wearer against exposure to spray and splash of infectious material.
- Face mask should be worn by HCW at all times that they are in healthcare facility including break-rooms where they may encounter coworkers.
- Patients and visitors should wear their own well-fitting cloth mask during their stay in the healthcare facility. However, masks should not be placed on children

below age of 2 years, anyone with breathing trouble, anyone who is unconscious, incapacitated, or otherwise is unable to remove mask without assistance.

- Educate patients, visitors, and HCW regarding significance of performing *hand hygiene* before and after any contact with mask and avoid the number of times they touch face to prevent self-contamination. Wash hands with soap and water for 40–60 seconds or rub hands with alcohol-based hand rub for 20–30 seconds.
- When possible *physical distancing* can be implemented for patients for example, limiting number of visitors along with patient, arranging seating 6 feet apart in waiting area, scheduling appointments to avoid overlap and crowding.
- *Use of personal protective equipment (PPE):*
  - *Healthcare workers working in areas with moderate to substantial community transmission* are more likely to encounter asymptomatic or presymptomatic patients with COVID-19 infection should apart from standard IPC practices also follow:
    - Wear eye protection in addition to face mask to protect eyes, nose, and mouth from respiratory secretions, e.g., face shield or goggles.
    - Wear N95 or equivalent respirator for aerosol generating procedures (AGPs) and surgical procedures that pose high risk of transmission, e.g., ear, nose, and throat (ENT) procedures, those generating potentially infectious aerosols.
  - *Healthcare workers working in areas with minimal to no community transmission* should continue standard IPC practices and may use eye protection, N95 mask, or other PPE depending on anticipated exposure or suspected/confirmed diagnosis.
- Healthcare facilities should consider implementing *preprocedure or preadmission diagnostic testing* with authorized nucleic acid or antigen detection assays for COVID-19 to identify those with asymptomatic or presymptomatic COVID-19 infection and further reduce the risk of exposure in healthcare settings. The results of testing may help decision of rescheduling elective procedures or for need of additional transmission-based precautions.
- *Balance the need to provide necessary services* to prevent potential harm to patient if care is deferred while minimizing risk of infection to patients and HCW when making decisions about providing elective procedures, surgeries and outpatient visits.
- *Optimized use of engineering controls to reduce exposure of HCW and other patients from infected individuals using:*
  - Physical barriers and dedicated pathways to guide symptomatic patients through triage
  - Remote triage facilities if possible
  - Vacuum shrouds for aerosol generating surgical procedures
  - Optimize air-handling systems (exchange rate, appropriate directionality, filtration, and updated maintenance)
  - Addition of portable solutions like high-efficiency particulate air (HEPA) filters to optimize air quality
- Healthcare facilities should notify the health department about suspected and confirmed COVID-19 cases in consultation with local health authorities in an established process so as to investigate, manage exposure, and allow contact tracing.

RECOMMENDED IPC PRACTICES WHEN CARING FOR A PATIENT WITH SUSPECTED OR CONFIRMED COVID-19 INFECTION

Following IPC practices are also recommended by CDC for patients who have met criteria for 14-day quarantine based on prolonged close contact with someone with COVID-19 infection. These patients should not be cohorted with patients' with COVID-19 infection (unless they test positive for COVID-19) though they should be isolated in a single person room and taken care by HCW using all personal protection equipment as recommended for a suspected or confirmed COVID-19 patient. This strategy is to reduce postquarantine transmission risks.

- *Reporting within and between healthcare facilities and to public health authorities:*
  - Implementing awareness for facility staff and frontline staff regarding policies of infection control, occupational health and facility plans for response.
  - Adequate training of HCW and monitoring of their compliance with standard precautions.
  - Specific persons in healthcare facility designated to communicate with public health officials and to provide necessary information to HCW.
- *Patient placement:*
  - Home care for patients with COVID-19 or other respiratory infections, if hospitalization is not medically essential.
  - Preferably a single room with closed door with dedicated bathroom. Natural ventilation with air flow of at least 160 L/s per patient or negative pressure room with at least 12 air changes per hour for a suspected or confirmed COVID-19 infected patient.
  - Airborne infection control room for AGPs
  - Larger designated units for higher number of suspected or confirmed COVID-19 patients with dedicated HCW
  - Minimize patient transfer outside the room and when possible perform procedures within his room/unit with portable equipment.
  - After COVID-19 infected patient's discharge, the vacated room should undergo sufficient air changes to remove potentially infectious particles and room should undergo appropriate cleaning and surface disinfection.

- *Personal protective equipment:* Healthcare worker entering the room/unit of suspected or confirmed COVID-19 patient's room should wear N95 mask or equivalent (or high level) respirator, isolation gown, one pair of sterile gloves, and eye protection such as goggles or face shield.
  - *Hand hygiene:* HCW should perform hand hygiene before and after contact with patient, infectious material, touching patient's surroundings, and before putting on and after removal of PPE (WHO's—my 5 moments for hand hygiene approach). For hand hygiene use alcohol-based hand solution (ABHS) with 60–95% alcohol or wash hands with soap and water for 20 seconds.
  - *Personal protective equipment training:* Appropriate PPE should be provided to HCW with training with respect to when to wear, how to don, use, and doff, and how to dispose PPE in a manner to prevent self-contamination.
  - *Respirator or face mask:* N95 respirator or equivalent or higher level respirator before entry into patient room or infected unit and during AGP. Other respirators are disposable filtering face-piece respirators, powered air purifying respirators, or elastomeric respirators.

    Reusable respirators should be removed out of the infected area and should be cleaned and disinfected as per manufacturer's instructions.

    While in use avoid touching the mask and when removing do not touch the front of mask but remove the lace from behind.
  - *Eye protection:* Goggles or face shield covering front and sides of face should be worn upon entering the infected area. They should be compatible with respirator so that the seal of respirator is not compromised.
  - *Gloves:* Clean, nonsterile gloves to be worn upon entry into infected area. Double gloving is not recommended. A change of gloves, if they get contaminated and on leaving the infected area followed by hand hygiene.
  - *Gown:* A clean isolation gown on entry to infected area with a change, if it gets soiled. Discard the gown in dedicated container on leaving. More than one gown at a time is not recommended.
- *Aerosol generating procedure:* Such procedures which generate infectious aerosols should be performed cautiously.
  - Healthcare worker should wear an N95 mask or equivalent or higher level respirator, eye protection, gloves, and an isolation gown.
  - Number of HCW in the room should be limited to minimum.
  - These procedures should be performed in airborne infection isolation room (AIIR) if possible.
  - Procedure room should be well ventilated with airflow of at least 160 L/s per patient or in negative pressure rooms with at least 12 air changes per hour and controlled direction of airflow.
  - Clean and disinfect the surfaces of procedure room promptly after the procedure.
- *Collection of diagnostic respiratory specimen (naso-pharyngeal/nasal swab):*
  - Healthcare worker should wear an N95 or equivalent or higher level respirator, eye protection, gloves, and a gown
  - Specimen collection to be done in a regular examination room with doors closed and transported in leak proof specimen bag with a separate sealable pocket for specimen.
  - During specimen collection, limit the number of people in the room to minimum essential for patient care.
  - Personnel collecting and transporting specimen should be trained in safe handling practices.
- *Visitor access:*
  - Alternative modes of patient visitor/relative interaction for example, video call on cell phones or tablets should be encouraged.
  - Visitation only if essential for patients physical or emotional care.
  - Visitors to enter only patients room and no other locations, to use hand hygiene PPE as per hospital facility.
  - Visitors not to be present during AGP.
- *Environmental infection control:*
  - Dedicated medical equipment for patients with suspected or confirmed COVID-19 infection, if possible
  - Environmental cleaning and disinfection of surfaces should be performed consistently and correctly using hospital disinfectants, e.g., 70% ethyl alcohol and sodium hypochlorite 0.5%.
  - Personal protective equipment to be worn by service personnel for cleaning and disinfection.
- *Biomedical waste management:* Biomedical waste to be managed as per the existing biomedical waste management rules and specific guidelines for COVID-19 include:
  - Dedicated trolleys and separate color-coded bins/bags/containers in COVID-19 isolation wards with proper segregation of waste
  - Double layered bags for waste collection to ensure strength and prevention of any leaks
  - COVID-19 waste bags to be labeled "COVID-19 waste" and to be stored separately till it is handed over to authorized staff of Common Biomedical Waste Treatment and Disposal Facility (CBWTF).

FREQUENTLY ASKED QUESTIONS WITH RESPECT TO INFECTION PREVENTION AND CONTROL FOR COVID-19

Q1: What are the options to reduce the quarantine for contacts of persons with COVID-19 infection?

Ans: CDC currently recommends a quarantine of 14 days. The following are, however, the acceptable alternatives:

- Quarantine ends after day 10 without testing, if no symptoms are reported during daily monitoring (transmission risk 1–10%).
- Quarantine ends on day 7, if diagnostic specimen tests negative with no symptoms reported during daily monitoring (transmission risk 5–12%).

Q2: Is a negative COVID test essential before discharge of a hospitalized patient?

Ans: No; decisions about discharge should be based on clinical status.

If a COVID positive patient has not met the criteria for discontinuation of transmission-based precautions, they can be transferred to a facility designated to take care of COVID-19-infected patients with adherence to IPC recommendations.

A non-COVID patient hospitalized for some other illness can be discharged without a test. To ensure that he was not exposed and acquired COVID infection, he may be placed in observation for 14 days with transmission-based precautions.

Q3: What are the special considerations for any surgery or planned procedure for patients during the COVID-19 pandemic?

Ans: The healthcare provider needs to assess the risk of exposure to infectious material during any surgery or planned procedures. When possible, nonoperative approach and techniques with minimal infectious aerosols should be chosen. Minimize the number of persons in the operating room. Use all recommended PPE. Where possible, use additional engineering controls for source control for example, smoke evacuation devices. Diagnostic testing for COVID-19 infection may be done to identify asymptomatic or presymptomatic to reduce risk of exposure.

Q4: Why is N95 disposable filtering face piece or equivalent/higher level respirator recommended for respiratory protection when caring for patients with suspected COVID-19?

Ans: Close range (and not long range) aerosol transmission by droplet and inhalation and contact followed by self-delivery to eye, nose, and mouth is a feature of COVID-19 infection. Potential routes for transmission in close range include splashes and sprays of infectious material on mucous membranes and inhalation of infectious microparticles exhaled by the infected person. The commonly used face mask during surgical procedures will provide barrier protection against splashes and sprays but an N95 mask or equivalent is designed to prevent inhalation of microparticles because of their tight-fit and filtration characteristics.

Q5: Which are the aerosol generating procedures in healthcare settings?

Ans: Certain medical procedures are more likely to generate higher concentrations of infectious aerosols such as:

- Open suction of airways
- Endotracheal intubation and extubation
- Tracheostomy
- Cardiopulmonary resuscitation
- Bronchoscopy
- Noninvasive ventilation, e.g., hand/manual ventilation, continuous positive airway pressure (CPAP), and bilevel positive airway pressure (BiPAP)

Q6: If an HCW has worked in healthcare setting while infected with COVID-19 infection and wore a mask at all times; are the patients he interacted with at risk COVID-19 infection?

Ans: Prolonged close contact, that is within 6 feet and for at least 15 minutes is considered to be potential exposure. If the infected HCW wore a face mask/respirator, face shield up to chin and adhered to other recommended IPC measures then the risk of transmission is less. Though, respirators with exhalation valves do not provide source control. Patients who did not wear a face mask, or who had a prolonged close contact or interaction with the infected HCW involving manipulation of patient's eyes, nose, or mouth, e.g., dental procedure are at a higher risk of transmission.

BIBLIOGRAPHY

1. CDC (2021). Clinical Questions about COVID-19: Questions and Answers. [online] Available from https://www.cdc.gov/coronavirus/2019-ncov/hcp/faq.html [Last accessed April, 2021].
2. CDC (2021). Interim Infection Prevention and Control Recommendations for Healthcare Personnel During the Coronavirus Disease 2019 (COVID-19) Pandemic. [online] Available from https://www.cdc.gov/coronavirus/2019-ncov/hcp/infection-control-recommendations.html [Last accessed April, 2021].
3. WHO (2020). World Health organization. Infection prevention and control during health care when COVID-19 is suspected: interim guidance. [online] Available from https://www.who.int/publications/i/item/10665-331495 [Last accessed April, 2021].
4. WHO (2021). Coronavirus disease (COVID-19) pandemic. [online] Available from https://www.who.int/emergencies/diseases/novel-coronavirus-2019 [Last accessed April, 2021].
5. WHO (2021). Country & Technical Guidance—Coronavirus disease (COVID-19). [online] Available from https://www.who.int/emergencies/diseases/novel-coronavirus-2019/technical-guidance/infection-prevention-and-control [Last accessed April, 2021].

Appendices

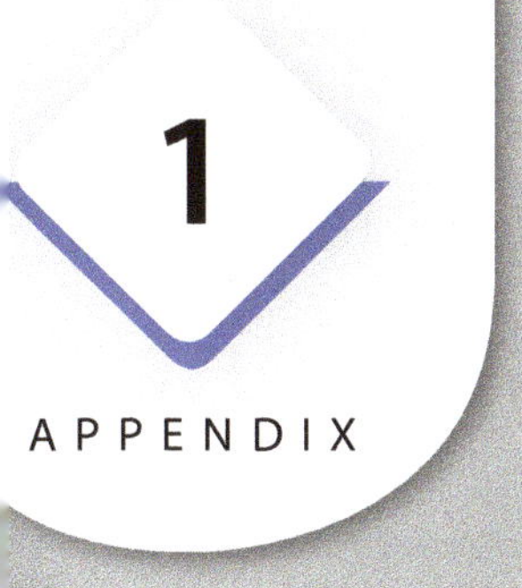

Safety Check of Anesthesia Machine

M Ravishankar

RECOMMENDED ESSENTIAL STEPS IN A "PREANESTHESIA CHECKOUT PROCEDURE 2008" PUBLISHED IN AMERICAN SOCIETY OF ANESTHESIOLOGISTS WEBSITE "TO BE COMPLETED DAILY, OR AFTER A MACHINE IS MOVED OR VAPORIZERS CHANGED"

Item to be completed		*Responsible party*
Item 1	Verify auxiliary O_2 cylinder and manual ventilation device (AMBU bag) are available and functioning	Provider and Tech
Item 2	Verify patient suction is adequate to clear the airway	Provider and Tech
Item 3	Turn on anesthesia delivery system and confirm that AC power is available	Provider or Tech
Item 4	Verify availability of required monitors, including alarms	Provider or Tech
Item 5	Verify that pressure is adequate on the spare O_2 cylinder mounted on the anesthesia machine	Provider and Tech
Item 6	Verify that the piped gas pressures are ≥50 psig	Provider and Tech
Item 7	Verify that vaporizers are adequately filled and, if applicable, that the filler ports are tightly closed	Provider or Tech
Item 8	Verify that there are no leaks in the gas supply lines between the flowmeters and the common gas outlet	Provider or Tech
Item 9	Test scavenging system function	Provider or Tech
Item 10	Calibrate, or verify calibration of the O_2 monitor and check the low O_2 alarm	Provider or Tech
Item 11	Verify CO_2 absorbent is fresh and not exhausted	Provider or Tech
Item 12	Perform breathing system pressure and leak testing	Provider and Tech
Item 13	Verify that gas flows properly through the breathing circuit during both inspiration and exhalation	Provider and Tech
Item 14	Document completion of checkout procedures	Provider and Tech
Item 15	Confirm ventilator settings and evaluate readiness to deliver anesthesia care (anesthesia time out)	Provider

RECOMMENDED ESSENTIAL STEPS IN A PREANESTHESIA CHECKOUT PROCEDURE, TO BE COMPLETED PRIOR TO EACH PROCEDURE

Subset of items in the daily checklist to be completed between cases		*Responsible party*
Item 2	Verify patient suction is adequate to clear the airway	Provider and Tech
Item 4	Verify availability of required monitors, including alarms	Provider or Tech
Item 7	Verify that vaporizers are adequately filled and if applicable that the filler ports are tightly closed	Provider
Item 11	Verify CO_2 absorbent is not exhausted	Provider or Tech
Item 12	Breathing system pressure and leak testing	Provider and Tech
Item 13	Verify that gas flows properly through the breathing circuit during both inspiration and exhalation	Provider and Tech
Item 14	Document completion of checkout procedures	Provider and Tech
Item 15	Confirm ventilator settings and evaluate readiness to deliver anesthesia care (anesthesia time out)	Provider

Source: Feldman JM, Olympio MA, Martin D, et al. (2008). New guidelines available for pre-anesthesia checkout. [online] Available from: http://www.apsf.org/newsletters/html/2008/spring/05_new_guidelines.htm [Last accessed February, 2014].

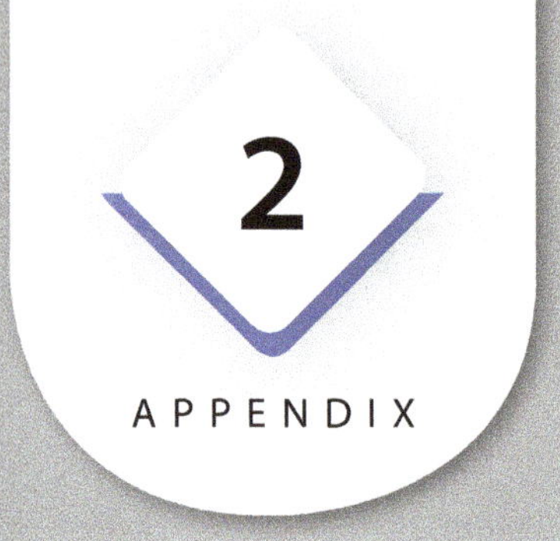

Protocol for Checking Anesthetic Equipment

M Ravishankar

MODERN ANESTHETIC WORKSTATIONS

The Association of Anaesthetists of Great Britain and Ireland (AAGBI) checklist for anesthetic equipment is applicable to all anesthetic workstations and should take only a few minutes to perform. It represents an important part of safe patient care. It is not intended to replace the manufacturer's preanesthetic checks, and should be used in conjunction with them. For example, some modern anesthetic workstations will enter a self-testing cycle when the machine is switched on, in which case those functions tested by the machine need not be retested by the user. The intention is to strike the right balance so that the AAGBI checklist for anesthetic equipment is not so superficial that its value is doubtful or so detailed that it is impractical to use. Manufacturers may also produce checklists specific to their device; these should be used in conjunction with the AAGBI checklist for anesthetic equipment.

The checking procedure described covers all aspects of the anesthetic delivery system from the gas supply pipelines, the machine and breathing systems, including filters, connectors, and airway devices. It includes an outline check for ventilators, suction, monitoring, and ancillary equipment.

PROCEDURES FOR CHECKING ANESTHETIC EQUIPMENT

The following checks should be carried out at the beginning of each operating theater session. In addition, specific checks should be carried out before each new patient during a session or when there is any alteration or addition to the breathing system, monitoring or ancillary equipment.

It is the responsibility of the anesthetist to make sure that these checks have been performed, and the anesthetist must be satisfied that they have been carried out correctly. In the event of a change of anesthetist during an operating session, the status of the anesthetic equipment must be confirmed, including that a formal check has been performed.

Before using any anesthetic equipment, ventilator, breathing system or monitor, it is essential to be fully familiar with it. Modern anesthetic workstations are complex devices. It is essential that anesthetists have full training and formal induction for any machines they may use. A quick "run-through" before the start of an operating session is not acceptable.

Careful note should be taken of any information or labeling on the anesthetic machine that might refer to its current status.

ALTERNATIVE MEANS OF VENTILATION

The early use of an alternative means of ventilation (a self-inflating bag that does not rely on a source of O_2 to function) may be lifesaving. A self-inflating bag must be immediately available in any location where anesthesia may be given. An alternative source of O_2 should be readily available.

Perform Manufacturer's Machine Check

Modern anesthesia workstations may perform many of the following checks automatically during start-up. Users must know which are included and ensure that the automated check has been performed.

Power Supply

Check that the anesthetic workstation and relevant ancillary equipment are connected to the mains electrical supply (where appropriate) and switched on. The anesthetic workstation should be connected directly to the mains electrical supply, and only correctly rated equipment connected to its electrical outlets. Multisocket extension leads must not be plugged into the anesthetic machine outlets or used to connect the anesthetic machine to the mains supply.

Hospitals should have backup generators, and many operating theaters will have their own backup system. Anesthetists should know what is available where they are working. Backup batteries for anesthetic machines and other equipment should be charged.

Switch on the gas supply master switch (if one is fitted). Check that the system clock (if fitted) is set correctly.

Gas Supplies and Suction

To check the correct function of the O_2 failure alarm involves disconnecting the O_2 pipeline on some machines, while on machines with a gas supply master switch, the alarm may be operated by turning the master switch off. As repeated disconnection of gas hoses may lead to premature failure of the Schrader socket and probe, these guidelines recommend that the regular presession check of equipment includes a "tug test" to confirm correct insertion of each pipeline into the appropriate socket.

It is, therefore, recommended that, in addition to these checks, the O_2 failure alarm must be checked on a weekly basis by disconnecting the O_2 hose whilst the O_2 flowmeter is turned on, and a written record kept. In addition to sounding an alarm, which must sound for at least 7 seconds, O_2 failure warning devices are also linked to a gas shutoff device. Anesthetists must be aware of both the tone of the alarm and also which gases will continue to flow on the particular model of anesthetic machine in use.

Medical Gas Supplies

Identify and take note of the gases that are being supplied by pipeline, confirming with a "tug test" that each pipeline is correctly inserted into the appropriate gas supply terminal. Note that excessive force during a "tug test" may damage the pipeline and/or gas supply terminal.

- Check that the anesthetic apparatus is connected to a supply of O_2 and that an adequate reserve supply of O_2 is available from a spare cylinder
- Check that adequate supplies of any other gases intended for use are available and connected as appropriate. All cylinders should be securely seated and turned off after checking their contents
- Carbon dioxide cylinders should not be present on the anesthetic machine. Where a blanking plug is supplied this should be fitted to any empty cylinder yoke
- Check that all pressure gauges for pipelines connected to the anesthetic machine indicate 400–500 kPa
- Check the operation of flowmeters, where these are present, ensuring that each control valve operates smoothly and that the bobbin moves freely throughout its range without sticking. If N_2O is to be used, the antihypoxia device should be tested by first turning on the N_2O flow and ensuring that at least 25% O_2 also flows. Then turn the O_2 flow off and check that the N_2O flow also stops. Turn on the O_2 flow and check that the O_2 analyzer display approaches 100%. Turn off all flow control valves (machines fitted with a gas supply master switch will continue to deliver a basal flow of O_2)
- Operate the emergency O_2 bypass control and ensure that flow occurs from the gas outlet without significant decrease in the pipeline supply pressure. Ensure that the emergency O_2 bypass control ceases to operate when released.

Suction

Check that the suction apparatus is functioning and all connections are secure; test for the rapid development of an adequate negative pressure.

Breathing System and Vaporizers

Whole breathing system: Check all breathing systems that are to be used and perform a "two-bag test" before use, as described further in this chapter. Breathing systems should be inspected visually and inspected for correct configuration and assembly. Check that all connections within the system and to the anesthetic machine are secured by "push and twist." Ensure that there are no leaks or obstructions in the reservoir bags or breathing system and that they are not obstructed by foreign material. Perform a pressure leak test (between 20 and 60 cmH_2O) on the breathing system by occluding the patient-end and compressing the reservoir bag.

Vaporizers: Manual leak testing of vaporizers was previously recommended routinely. It should only be performed on basic "Boyle's machines" and it may be harmful to many modern anesthetic workstations. Refer to the manufacturer's recommendation before performing a manual test.

Check that the vaporizer(s) for the required volatile agent(s) are fitted correctly to the anesthetic machine, that any locking mechanism is fully engaged and that the control knobs rotate fully through the full range(s). Ensure that the vaporizer is not tilted. Turn off the vaporizers.

Check that the vaporizer(s) are adequately filled but not overfilled, and that the filling port is tightly closed.

Manual leak test of vaporizer:

- Set a flow of O_2 at 5 L/min and with the vaporizer turned off, temporarily occlude the common gas outlet. There should be no leak from any part of the vaporizer and the flowmeter bobbin (if present) should dip.
- Where more than one vaporizer is present, turn each vaporizer on in turn and repeat this test. After this test, ensure that the vaporizers and flowmeters are turned off.

Changing and filling vaporizers during use: It may be necessary to change a vaporizer during use. Where possible, repeat the leak test; failure to do so is a common cause of critical incidents. Some anesthetic workstations will automatically test vaporizer integrity.

It is only necessary to remove a vaporizer from a machine to refill it if the manufacturer recommends this. Vaporizers must always be kept upright. Tilting a vaporizer can result in delivery of dangerously high concentrations of vapor.

Carbon Dioxide Absorber

Inspect the contents and connections and ensure there is adequate supply of CO_2 absorbent. Check the color of the absorbent.

Alternative Breathing Systems

For Bain-type and circle coaxial systems, perform an occlusion test on the inner tube and check that the APL valve, where fitted, can be fully opened and closed.

Correct Gas Outlet

Particular care must be exercised in machines with an auxiliary common gas outlet (ACGO). Incidents of patient harm have resulted from misconnection of a breathing system to an ACGO or misselection of the ACGO.

Whenever a breathing system is changed, either during a case or a list, its integrity and correct configuration must be confirmed. This is particularly important for pediatric lists when breathing systems may be changed frequently during a list.

Ventilator

- Check that the ventilator is configured correctly for its intended use
- Ensure that the ventilator tubing is securely attached
- Set the controls for use and ensure that adequate pressure is generated during the inspiratory phase
- Check that alarms are working and correctly configured
- Check that the pressure relief valve functions correctly at the set pressure.

Two-bag Test

A two-bag test should be performed after the breathing system, vaporizers and ventilator have been checked individually.

- Attach the patient-end of the breathing system (including angle piece and filter) to a test lung or bag
- Set the fresh gas flow to 5 L/min and ventilate manually. Check the whole breathing system is patent and the unidirectional valves are moving (if present)
- Check the function of the APL valve by squeezing both bags
- Turn on the ventilator to ventilate the test lung. Turn off the fresh gas flow or reduce to a minimum. Open and close each vaporizer in turn. There should be no loss of volume in the system.

Breathing systems should be protected with a test lung or bag when not in use to prevent intrusion of foreign bodies.

Scavenging

Check that the anesthetic gas scavenging system is switched on and functioning. Ensure that the tubing is attached to the appropriate exhaust port of the breathing system, ventilator, or anesthetic workstation.

Monitoring Equipment

Check that all monitoring devices, especially those referred to in the AAGBIs standards of monitoring during anesthesia and recovery guidelines, are functioning and that appropriate parameters and alarms have been set before using the anesthetic machine. This includes the cycling times, or frequency of recordings, of automatic noninvasive blood pressure monitors. Check that gas sampling lines are properly attached and free from obstruction or kinks. In particular, check that the O_2 analyzer, pulse oximeter, and capnograph are functioning correctly and that appropriate alarm limits for all monitors are set. Be aware of the "default" alarm settings if using these.

Gas monitoring lines are often the cause of a significant leak; check that they are properly attached and any sampling ports not in use have been blanked off. To eliminate the need to change the sampling line repeatedly, the gas monitoring line should be assembled as an integral part of the breathing circuit by attaching it proximal to the patient breathing filter.

Airway Equipment

These include bacterial filters, catheter mounts, connectors and tracheal tubes, laryngeal mask airways, etc., check that these are all available in the appropriate sizes, at the point of use, and that they have been checked for patency.

A new, single-use bacterial filter and angle piece/catheter mount must be used for each patient. It is important that these are checked for patency and flow, both visually and by ensuring gas flow through the whole assembly when connected to the breathing system.

Check that the appropriate laryngoscopes are available and function reliably. Equipment for the management of the anticipated or unexpected difficult airway must be available and checked regularly in accordance with departmental policies. A named consultant anesthetist must be responsible for difficult airway equipment and the location of this equipment should be known.

Source: Association of Anaesthetists of Great Britain and Ireland. (2012). Checking anaesthetic equipment 2012. [online] Available from http://www.aagbi.org/sites/default/files/checking_anaesthetic_equipment_2012.pdf [Last accessed February, 2014].

INDEX

Page numbers followed by *b* refer to box, *f* refer to figure, *fc* refer to flowchart, and *t* refer to table.

A

J

K

L

M

N

O

P

Q

R

S

EU GSPR Authorised Reprsentative
Logos Europe, 9 rue Nicolas Poussin
1700, La Rochelle, France
Phone: +33 (0) 6 67 93 73 78
E-mail: contact@logoseurope.eu

www.ingramcontent.com/pod-product-compliance
Ingram Content Group UK Ltd.
Pitfield, Milton Keynes, MK11 3LW, UK
UKHW061550190726
13845UKWH00030B/1097

* 9 7 8 9 3 5 4 6 5 0 0 6 2 *